Handbook of
Experimental Pharmacology

Continuation of Handbuch der experimentellen Pharmakologie

Vol. 55/I

Psychotropic Agents

Part I: Antipsychotics and Antidepressants

Contributors

M. Ackenheil · G. Bartholini · H. J. Bein · W.F.M. van Bever · S. Bhanji
M. H. Bickel · U. Breyer-Pfaff · T. B. Cooper · A. Delini-Stula · R. Fog
Y. Givant · G. Gogolák · R. Hempel · R. Hess · T. M. Itil · W. Janke
P.A.J. Janssen · I. Jurna · M. Karobath · B. Kjellberg · N.S. Kline
H. Kreiskott · R. Kretzschmar · M. H. Lader · G. Langer · E. Lehr
F. Leuschner · K. G. Lloyd · N. Matussek · P. L. Mobley · I. Møller Nielsen
B. Müller-Oerlinghausen · I. Munkvad · W. Neumann · C. W. Picard
A. Randrup · J. Roubicek · J. Scheel-Krüger · E. Schiørring · J. Schmutz
M. Schou · C. Soldatos · F. G. Sulman · F. Sulser · J. Teschendorf
P. Thomann · F. J. Zeelen

Editors

F. Hoffmeister · G. Stille

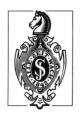

Springer-Verlag Berlin Heidelberg New York 1980

Professor Dr. F. HOFFMEISTER
Bayer AG, Institut für Pharmakologie, Aprather Weg 18 a, D-5600 Wuppertal 1

Professor Dr. G. STILLE
Institut für Arzneimittel des Bundesgesundheitsamtes,
Stauffenbergstraße 13, D-1000 Berlin 30

With 82 Figures

ISBN 3-540-09858-5 Springer-Verlag Berlin Heidelberg New York
ISBN 0-387-09858-5 Springer-Verlag New York Heidelberg Berlin

Library of Congress Cataloging in Publication Data. Main entry under title: Antipsychotics and antidepressants. (Handbook of experimental pharmacology; v. 55/I) (Psychotropic agents; pt. 1) Includes bibliographies and indexes. 1. Tranquilizing drugs – Physiological effect. 2. Antidepressants – Physiological effects. I. Ackenheil, M. II. Stille, Günther, 1923-. III. Hoffmeister, Friedrich. IV. Series. V. Series: Handbook of experimental pharmacology; v. 55/I. QP905.H3 vol. 55/I, pt. 1 [RM333] 615′.1s [615′.7882] 80-12230. 80-12210 (set)

Printed in Germany.

The use of registered names, trademarks, etc. in this publication does not imply, even in the absence of a specific statement, that such names are exempt from the relevant protective laws and regulations and therefore free for general use.

Typesetting, printing, and bookbinding: Brühlsche Universitätsdruckerei, Giessen. 2122/3130-543210

Preface

The volumes on „psychotropic substances" in the Handbook of Experimental Pharmacology series clearly show that the classical concept of this discipline has become too narrow in recent years.

For instance, what substances are psychotropic is determined not by the criteria of the animal trial, i.e. by experimental pharmacology, but by their action on the psyche, which in the final analysis is only accessible to us in man. Psychotropic substances force experimental pharmacology (and thus also this Handbook) outside its traditional limits, which have essentially depended on animal studies.

The antipsychotics and antidepressants were not discovered in animal experiments, but by chance (or more precisely, by clinical empiricism). Experienced psychiatrists trained in the observation of patients recognised the efficacy of drugs, the beneficial effect of which nobody had dreamed of before: DELAY and DENICKER in the case of chlorpormazine, KLINE in the case of the monoamine oxidase inhibitors and KUHN in the case of imipramine. It was only after these discoveries that the pharmacologists developed experimental models of the psychoses in animal experiments. However, even today we still do not know with certainty which of the effects shown in animals is relevant for the clinical effect despite the vast abundance of individual investigations. For many years, this uncertainty led to the testing of antipsychotics (e.g. of the neuroleptic type) in models which actually produced the undesired effects. For example, if one uses „catatonia" as selection criterion in animals, one will repeatedly develop antipsychotics with potentially strong extrapyramidal side effects.

Clozapine opened up a new dimension: this is an antipsychotic without significant extrapyramidal side effects. For other reasons, the hopes aroused by this preparation have unfortunately not been fulfilled.

Although an abundance of preparations is available for treatment of psychoses today, advances appear to be stagnating. The first volume of „psychotropic substances" reflects the present situation. The material gathered conveys an impression of the great activity in this field in recent years. However, it also shows that we have made hardly any real progress in fundamental knowledge in the last 20 years. Cooperation between different disciplines in the field of psychoactive agents is exemplary, as is also illustrated by the present volume. Research into the neuropharmacology, neurophysiology and neurochemistry of these preparations shows that they are not actually psychoactive agents, but in fact neuropharmacologically active agents. Their neuronal effects are reflected in psychic manifestations. The only real psychoactive drug is the placebo: it acts directly on the psyche.

As is legitimate for psychoactive agents, the clinicians, psychologists and behavioral researchers also have their say in this volume. It is clearly shown that to a greater extent than in other areas, in this field of drug research the observation of patients and test subjects constitutes the basis for new hypotheses which can only be tested secondarily in animals. The question may be asked as to why one needs the animal trial at all. However, it hardly likely to be disputed that brain function is more accessible both for the neurophysiologist and for the neurochemist in animals than in patients, in whom many investigations cannot be performed for ethical reasons. The path to knowledge is thus different from that in other groups of drugs.

With the large number of disciplines involved, overlapping standpoints cannot be avoided. Indeed, it is perhaps desirable to find a certain phenomenon interpreted by pharmacologists, and then by neurophysiologists, or even by behavioral researchers.

It is to be hoped that we have succeeded in reviewing research in the field of antipsychotics with an appropriate selection of authors and choice of topics. We also were concerned to do justice to the personal experience of the individual researchers. We hope that the volume will provide a bridge leading from the past into the future of psychosis pharmacotherapy.

Berlin, August 1980   G. STILLE

List of Contributors

Dr. M. Ackenheil, Nervenklinik der Universität München, Psychiatrische Klinik und Poliklinik, Nußbaumstraße 7, D-8000 München 2

Professor Dr. G. Bartholini, Research and Development Department, Synthélabo-L.E.R.S., 58 Rue de la Glacière, F-75013 Paris

Professor Dr. H.J. Bein, Meisenstraße 11, CH-4104 Oberwil

Dr. W.F.M. van Bever, Janssen Pharmaceutica Research Laboratories, B-2340 Beerse

Dr. S. Bhanji, Postgraduate Medical Institute, University of Exeter, Barrack Road, GB-Exeter, EX2 5 DW

Professor Dr. M.H. Bickel, Pharmakologisches Institut, Universität Bern, Friedbühlstraße 49, CH-3000 Bern

Professor Dr. Dr. U. Breyer-Pfaff, Institut für Toxikologie der Universität, Wilhelmstraße 56, D-7400 Tübingen

Dr. T.B. Cooper, Rockland Research Institute, Office of Mental Health, Orangeburg, NY 10962/USA

Dr. A. Delini-Stula, c/o Ciba-Geigy AG, Postfach, CH-4002 Basel

Dr. R. Fog, Centrallaboratoriet, Sct. Hans Mental Hospital, Dept. E, DK-4000 Roskilde

Dr. Y. Givant, The Hebrew University of Jerusalem, Department of Applied Pharmacology, Bioclimatology Unit, P.O.B. 12065, IL-Jerusalem 25432

Professor. Dr. G. Gogolák, Department of Neuropharmacology, Brain Research Institute, University of Vienna, Währinger Str. 13a, A-1090 Wien

R. Hempel, Laboratorium für Pharmakologie und Toxikologie, Francoper Str. 66b, D-2104 Hamburg 92

Professor Dr. R. Hess, Ciba-Geigy AG, Postfach, CH-4002 Basel

Professor Dr. T.M. Itil, HZI Research Center, 150 White Plains Road, Tarrytown, NY 10591/USA

Professor Dr. W. Janke, Psychologisches Institut der Universität Düsseldorf, Lehrstuhl für Psychologie II, Universitätsstraße 1, D-4000 Düsseldorf

Dr. P.A.J. Janssen, Janssen Pharmaceutica Research Laboratories, B-2340 Beerse

Professor Dr. I. JURNA, Institut für Pharmakologie und Toxikologie der Universität des Saarlandes, D-6650 Homburg

Doz. Dr. M. KAROBATH, Psychiatrische Universitätsklinik, Lazarettgasse 14, A-1097 Wien

Dr. B. KJELLBERG, Centrallaboratoriet, Sct. Hans Mental Hospital, Dept. E, DK-4000 Roskilde

Professor Dr. N.S. KLINE, Rockland Research Institute, Office of Mental Health, Orangeburg, NY 10962/USA

Dr. H. KREISKOTT, Knoll AG, BASF, Sparte Pharma, Biologische Forschung und Entwicklung, Postfach 210805, D-6700 Ludwigshafen

Professor Dr. R. KRETZSCHMAR, Biologische Forschung und Entwicklung, Sparte Pharma, BASF AG, D-6700 Ludwigshafen

Dr. M.H. LADER, Institute of Psychiatry, University of London, De Crespigny Park, Denmark Hill, GB-London SE5 8AF

Dr. G. LANGER, Psychiatrische Universitätsklinik, Lazarettgasse 14, A-1097 Wien

Priv. Doz. Dr. E. LEHR, Pharmakologisches Laboratorium D der Firma C.H. Boehringer Sohn, Postfach 200, D-6507 Ingelheim

Professor Dr. F. LEUSCHNER, Laboratorium für Pharmakologie und Toxikologie, Francoper Straße 66 b, D-2104 Hamburg 92

Dr. K.G. LLOYD, Synthélabo-L.E.R.S., 58 Rue de la Glacière, F-75013 Paris

Professor Dr. N. MATUSSEK, Psychiatrische Klinik und Poliklinik, Nußbaumstraße 7, D-8000 München 2

Dr. P.L. MOBLEY, Vanderbilt University School of Medicine, Tennessee Neuropsychiatric Institute, 5101 Murfreesboro Road, Nashville, TN 37217/USA

Dr. I. MØLLER NIELSEN, Himmelbjergvej 125, Laven, DK-8600 Silkeborg

Professor Dr. B. MÜLLER-OERLINGHAUSEN, Psychiatrische und Neurologische Klinik und Poliklinik, Nußbaumallee 36, D-1000 Berlin 19

Dr. I. MUNKVAD, Centrallaboratoriet, Sct. Hans Mental Hospital, Dept. E, DK-4000 Roskilde

W. NEUMANN, Laboratorium für Pharmakologie und Toxikologie, Francoper Str. 66 b, D-2104 Hamburg 92

Dr. C.W. PICARD, Wander Ltd., Forschungsinstitut, Postfach 2747, CH-3001 Bern

Dr. A. RANDRUP, Centrallaboratoriet, Sct. Hans Mental Hospital, Dept. E, DK-4000 Roskilde

Professor Dr. J. ROUBICEK, Hauptstraße 34, CH-4102 Binningen-Basal

Dr. J. SCHEEL-KRÜGER, Centrallaboratoriet, Sct. Hans Mental Hospital, Dept. E, DK-4000 Roskilde

Dr. E. SCHIØRRING, Centrallaboratoriet, Sct. Hans Mental Hospital, Dept. E, DK-4000 Roskilde

Dr. J. SCHMUTZ, Wander Ltd., Forschungsinstitut, Postfach 2747, CH-3001 Bern

Professor Dr. M. SCHOU, Psychopharmacology Research Unit, Aarhus University Institute of Psychiatry, DK-8240 Risskov

Professor Dr. C. SOLDATOS, New York Medical College, Department of Psychiatry, Division of Biological Psychiatry, 150 White Plains Road, Tarrytown, NY 10591/USA

Professor Dr. F.G. SULMAN, The Hebrew University of Jerusalem, Department of Applied Pharmacology, Bioclimatology Unit, P.O.B. 12065, IL-Jerusalem 25432

Professor Dr. F. SULSER, Vanderbilt University, School of Medicine, Tennessee Neuropsychiatric Institute, 1501 Murfreesboro Road, Nashville, TN 37217/USA

Dr. J. TESCHENDORF, Biologische Forschung und Entwicklung, Sparte Pharma, BASF AG, D-6700 Ludwigshafen

Dr. P. THOMANN, Ciba-Geigy Ltd., Postfach, CH-4002 Basel

Dr. F.J. ZEELEN, Organon Scientific Development Group, P.O. Box 20, NL-Oss

Contents

Antipsychotics: Chemistry (Structure and Effectiveness)

CHAPTER 4

Behavioral Pharmacology of Antipsychotics. H. KREISKOTT

CHAPTER 5

Testing Antipsychotic Drug Effects with Operant Behavioral Techniques.
E. LEHR

CHAPTER 6

Stereotyped Behavior and Its Relevance for Testing Neuroleptics.
A. RANDRUP, B. KJELLBERG, E. SCHIØRRING, J. SCHEEL-KRÜGER, R. FOG,
and I. MUNKVAD

CHAPTER 7

Neurophysiologic Properties of Neuroleptic Agents in Animals. I. JURNA.
With 14 Figures

CHAPTER 8

Antipsychotics: Neurophysiological Properties (in Man). J. ROUBICEK.
With 14 Figures

CHAPTER 12

Clinical Pharmacology (Pharmacokinetics). B. MÜLLER-OERLINGHAUSEN

CHAPTER 13

Metabolism and Kinetics. U. BREYER-PFAFF. With 6 Figures

CHAPTER 14

Psychometric and Psychophysiological Actions of Antipsychotics in Men. W. JANKE

CHAPTER 15

Endocrine Effects of Neuroleptics. F. G. SULMAN and Y. GIVANT. With 3 Figures

Antidepressants: Chemistry (Structure and Effectiveness)

CHAPTER 16

Chemistry (Structure and Activity). F. J. Zeelen

CHAPTER 17

Monoamine Oxidase Inhibitors as Antidepressants. N. S. KLINE and T. B. COOPER.
With 3 Figures

CHAPTER 18

Tricyclic Antidepressants: General Pharmacology. I. Møller Nielsen.
With 1 Figure

CHAPTER 19

Neurophysiological Properties (in Animals). G. Gogolák

CHAPTER 20

Clinical Neurophysiological Properties of Antidepressants. T. M. Itil and
C. Soldatos. With 20 Figures

CHAPTER 21 a

Biochemical Effects of Antidepressants in Animals. F. SULSER and P.L. MOBLEY.
With 3 Figures

CHAPTER 21 b

Biochemical Effects of Antidepressants in Man. G. LANGER and M. KAROBATH

CHAPTER 21 c

**Drug-Induced Alterations in Animal Behavior as a Tool for the Evaluation
of Antidepressants: Correlation with Biochemical Effects.** A. DELINI-STULA.
With 10 Figures

CHAPTER 22

Toxicology of Antidepressant Drugs. P. THOMANN and R. HESS. With 1 Figure

CHAPTER 23

Metabolism of Antidepressants. M. H. BICKEL

CHAPTER 24

Physiological and Psychological Effects of Antidepressants in Man.
M. LADER and S. BHANJI

CHAPTER 25

Pharmacology and Toxicology of Lithium. M. Schou

CHAPTER 26

Antipsychotics and Experimental Seizure Models. R. Kretzschmar and
H.J. Teschendorf

Antipsychotics
Chemistry (Structure and Effectiveness)

CHAPTER 1

Tricyclic Neuroleptics: Structure-Activity Relationships

J. SCHMUTZ and C. W. PICARD

A. Criteria for Neuroleptic Activity

In recent years, several excellent reviews dealing with the structure-activity relationships of the tricyclic neuroleptics have appeared (JANSSEN, 1973; ZIRKLE and KAISER, 1974; GSCHWEND, 1974; JANSSEN and VAN BEVER, 1975). In particular, the detailed review of ZIRKLE and KAISER (1974) will serve as a basis for our discussion. The latter authors have relied largely on the conditioned avoidance response (CAR) test in rats as a pharmacological measure of neuroleptic activity. Other authors have used central depressant activities, e.g. depression of locomotor activity in mice or the rotating rod test which is a measure of the degree of motor incoordination in mice.

In view of the continuing interest in the dopamine (DA) hypothesis of schizophrenia, however, we shall as far as possible base our structure-activity considerations upon in vivo and in vitro tests which are concerned with measuring DA receptor blocking action. The most important of such pharmacological tests are those measuring cataleptic effects and apomorphine- and amphetamine-antagonisms in the rat (JANSSEN et al., 1965, 1967, 1975), which have been shown to correlate well with the antipsychotic action in man. In recent years the results of biochemical studies on dopaminergic receptors (BURT et al., 1975, 1976; ENNA et al., 1976) and with DA-sensitive adenylate cyclase (MILLER et al., 1974; IVERSEN et al., 1976 a, b) have assumed increasing importance for structure-activity relationships. There is a close correlation between the clinical and pharmacological potencies of different types of neuroleptic agents on the one hand and their affinities for specific binding sites of [³H]haloperidol on the other (CREESE et al., 1976; SEEMAN et al., 1976), even though possible differences in absorption, distribution and metabolism cannot play a part in these in vitro tests. The correlations between the in vivo tests and the cyclic AMP assay, on the other hand, are generally less good. The inhibition of DA-sensitive adenylate cyclase of rat brain striatal homogenate does not appear to be a general and specific property of the neuroleptic agents. It has been found that tricyclic antidepressants also can be potent inhibitors (KAROBATH, 1975), whereas the clinically effective antipsychotic agent sulpiride fails to inhibit DA-stimulated adenylate cyclase (ROUFOGALIS et al., 1976) and the inhibitory effects of haloperidol and pimozide observed in vitro are much too weak in view of their high potencies in vivo (e.g. BURT et al., 1976; LADURON, 1976). However, within the group of the tricyclic neuroleptics, including the phenothiazines, thioxanthenes and dibenzo-epines, there is reasonable agreement between the in vivo tests and the cyclic AMP assay and also between the latter and the [³H]haloperidol binding assay (cf. Table 1). Today, [³H]spiperone tends to be preferred as ligand, because its receptor binding is more specific than that of [³H]haloperidol (LEYSEN et al., 1978).

As the effects of DA-blocking agents can be influenced by centrally active anticholinergic agents (SAYERS et al., 1976), Table 1 also includes the known anticholinergic effects of neuroleptics on muscarinic receptors of rat brain, as determined by the [³H] quinuclidine benzilate (QNB) assay (MILLER et al., 1974).

B. Chemical Classification of the Tricyclic Neuroleptics

A common characteristic of the tricyclic neuroleptics is a non-planar, more of less flexible ring system. The central ring may be six- or seven-membered and is linearly fused to two benzene rings, one of which may be replaced by an isosteric heterocyclic ring, e.g., thiophen[1]. One of the benzene rings must carry one substituent in a position that is equivalent for all classical tricyclic neuroleptics. The central ring carries a more or less flexible basic side chain, the tertiary amine function of which is separated from the tricyclic system by three atoms and is proximal to the substituted benzene ring. These structural requirements will be considered more fully in the succeeding sections.

The tricyclic neuroleptics are conveniently divided into two structural classes according to the size of the central ring: the 6-6-6 tricyclics (1), (2), and (3) and the 6-7-6 tricyclics, namely the dibenzo-epines (4) to (9) and the dibenzo[a,d]cycloheptenes (13) and (14). (For structures, see pp. 6–8.)

Two types of 6-7-6 neuroleptics do not, however, fit into the above general definition: clozapine (17 a) has a nuclear substituent in position 8 which is not equivalent to the substitution position of the other neuroleptics; and the benzocyclohepta-pyridoisoquinolines, dexclamol (15 b) and butaclamol (15 c), lack both the γ-aminopropyl side chain and a substituent in either of the aromatic rings.

Tricyclic neuroleptics in therapeutic use today are confined to the following structural types: the phenothiazines (1; X = S), aminopropylidene-thioxanthenes (3; X = S), dibenzo[b,f]thiepins (8; X = S), dibenzo[b,f][1,4]thiazepines and -oxazepines (7; X = O or S), and the dibenzo[b,e][1,4]diazepine (17 a).

C. Molecular Conformation

For biological activity, i.e. for interaction with the receptor, the molecular conformation is of great importance. However, the specific conformation in which a molecule is bound to the receptor is usually not known since most molecules possess more or less flexible structures capable of assuming different conformations which are in equilibrium with each other in solution. Only relatively few pharmacologically active agents have rigid molecular structures whose conformations can be determined in the crystal by X-ray diffraction methods or in solution by nuclear magnetic resonance (NMR) spectroscopy. Such molecules clearly exist in the perferred conformation for receptor binding.

Various attempts have been made in recent years to describe the topography of tricyclic neuroleptics by means of geometrical parameters and to determine their

---

1 Because of limited space these isosters will not be discussed here. In recent years such structures have figured mainly in the patent literature and none of them has so far proved of clinical importance. Some neuroleptically active thieno[1,4]benzothiazines, which are thieno-analogues of the phenothiazines, have been described by GROL and ROLLEMA (1975)

stereochemistry and conformational properties by various physical or physico-chemical methods (cf. WILHELM and KUHN, 1970; FENNER, 1970; SCHMUTZ, 1973, 1975; FOUCHÉ and COMBRISSON, 1973; MCDOWELL, 1974; KOCH, 1974; HORN et al., 1975; TOLLENAERE et al., 1977; REBOUL and CRISTAU, 1977 a, b, 1978; MOEREELS and TOLLENAERE, 1978; DE PAULIS et al., 1978 a, b). The determination of the three-dimensional structures in the crystalline state of different phenothiazines (1; X = S) and thioxanthenes (2; X = S), dibenzo[b,f]thiepins (8; X = S), dibenzo[b,e][1,4]diazepines and dibenz[b,f][1,4]oxazepines (7; X = NH and O respectively) has greatly contributed to a better understanding of the structure-activity relationships of these compounds (KOCH and EVRARD, 1974; PETCHER et al., 1975; ASCHWANDEN et al., 1976; PETCHER and WEBER, 1976; RODGERS et al., 1976; COSULICH and LOVELL, 1977; JAUNIN et al., 1977; REBOUL and CRISTAU, 1977 a; BÜRKI et al., 1978).

The phenothiazines (1) and thioxanthenes (3) are folded along an axis which passes through the two bridging atoms of the central ring. The dihedral angle formed by the planes of the two benzene rings is about 142° in the crystals of these compounds. The 9,10-dihydroanthracene derivative fluotracen (2e) possesses in the crystal a dihedral angle of approx 155° (CHU and CHUNG, 1976; cf. FOWLER et al., 1977b). A similar folding angle was also found in solution for the unsubstituted parent dihydroanthracene (ARONEY et al., 1971). Folding in solution was also demonstrated for acridan and xanthene, the unsubstituted parent compounds of (1; X = CH$_2$) and (2; X = O) respectively (AIZENSHTAT et al., 1972). The seven-membered ring in the 10,11-dihydrodibenzothiepins (8) folds along a line passing through the sulphur atom and the CH$_2$-group, the dihedral angle being approx. 113°. NMR studies of several dibenzo[a,d]cycloheptenes and their 10,11-dihydro-derivatives (9 and 8; X = CH$_2$) have shown that these molecules also are folded when in solution (FOUCHÉ and COMBRISSON, 1973). The dibenzoxazepines and dibenzodiazepines (7; X = O or NH) are folded about a line running through the bridging atom and the centre of the N = C double bond, the dihedral angle here being about 116°. Owing to the presence of the seven-membered central ring which is in the boat conformation, the 6-7-6 systems (4) to (9) are much more strongly bent than the 6-6-6 tricyclics (1) to (3). Although there appears to be no direct correlation between the dihedral angle and neuroleptic potency, a non-planar shape seems to be necessary for neuroleptic activity. Planar compounds with a five-membered central ring are inactive.

It should be noted, however, that most of the tricyclic systems are not fixed in one conformation but that their central rings are capable of inverting in solution. The degree of flexibility of the structures ranges from the very flexible 6-6-6 ring systems of the phenothiazines to the rigid 6-7-6 system of the dibenzo[a,d]cycloheptenes (14). The flexibility of the central ring depends on a number of factors, such as ring size, nature of the hetero-atom in the central ring and the type of linkage between the basic side chain and the central ring.

NMR studies of the 6-7-6 system (7) have shown that, in solution, molecules in which X = O or NH are the most flexible, those in which X = S or NCH$_3$ are the least flexible, with the morphanthridines (X = CH$_2$) occupying an intermediate position (HUNZIKER, unpublished results). Inversion may be inhibited or prevented altogether if the molecule contains conformation-stabilising elements. For example, in the case of the N,S-dioxide of clotiapine (7b) it was possible to isolate two conformers which in solution were in equilibrium (MICHAELIS and GAUCH, 1969).

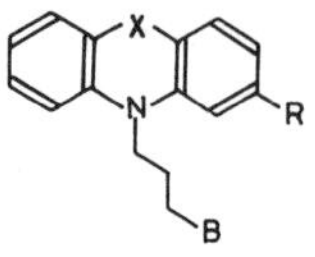

J. SCHMUTZ and C. W. PICARD

1

	X	R	B
(a)	S	H	NMe$_2$
(b)	S	Cl	NMe$_2$
(c)	S	Cl	N⌒N–CH$_2$CH$_2$OH
(d)	S	CF$_3$	NMe$_2$
(e)	S	CF$_3$	N⌒N–Me
(f)	S	CF$_3$	N⌒N–CH$_2$CH$_2$OH
(g)	S	COMe	N⌒N–CH$_2$CH$_2$OH
(h)	CMe$_2$	H	NMe$_2$

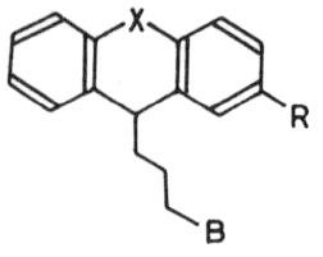

2

	X	R	B
(a)	S	CF$_3$	NMe$_2$
(b)	S	SO$_2$NMe$_2$	NMe$_2$
(c)	NH	Cl	NMe$_2$
(d)	CH$_2$	CF$_3$	NMe$_2$
(e)	CHMe	CF$_3$	NMe$_2$
(f)	CMe$_2$	H	NMe$_2$

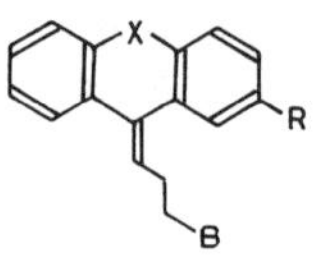

3

	X	R	B
(a)	S	Cl	NMe$_2$
(b)	S	Cl	N⌒N–CH$_2$CH$_2$OH
(c)	S	CF$_3$	N⌒N–CH$_2$CH$_2$OH
(d)	S	SO$_2$NMe$_2$	N⌒N–Me

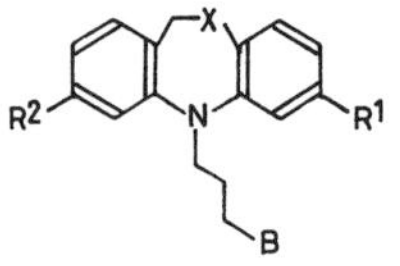

4

	X	R^1	R^2	B
(a)	O	CF$_3$	H	N⌒N–CH$_2$CH$_2$OH
(b)	O	H	Cl	N⌒N–CH$_2$CH$_2$OH

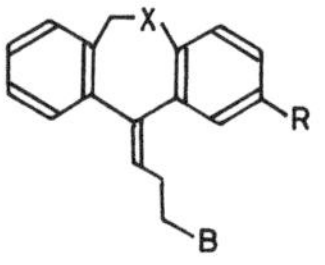

5

	X	R	B
(a)	O	Cl	N⌒N–CH$_2$CH$_2$OH
(b)	O	H	NMe$_2$

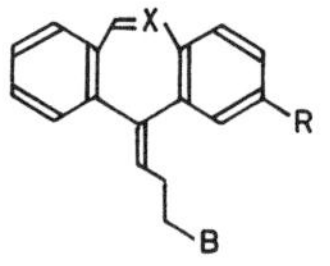

6

	X	R	B
(a)	N	Cl	NMe$_2$

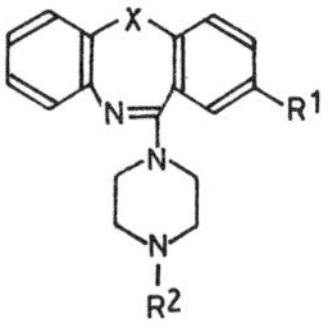

7

	X	R^1	R^2
(a)	S	Me	Me
(b)	S	Cl	Me
(c)	O	Cl	Me
(d)	NH	Cl	Me
(e)	CH$_2$	H	Me

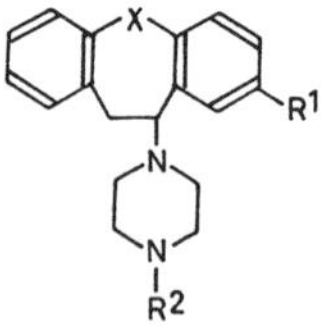

8

	X	R^1	R^2
(a)	S	Cl	Me
(b)	S	SMe	Me
(c)	S	H	Me

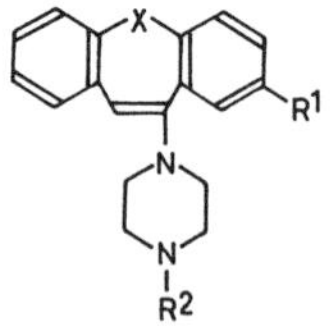

9

	X	R^1	R^2
(a)	O	Cl	Me
(b)	O	F	Me
(c)	O	OMe	Me

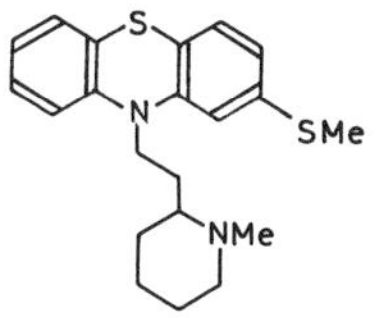

10

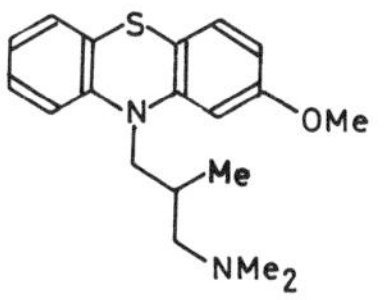

11

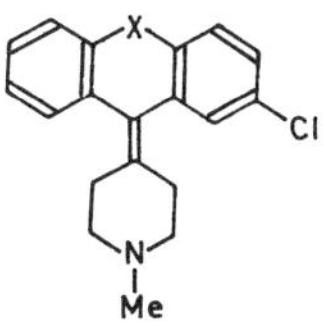

12

(a) X = S (b) X = NMe

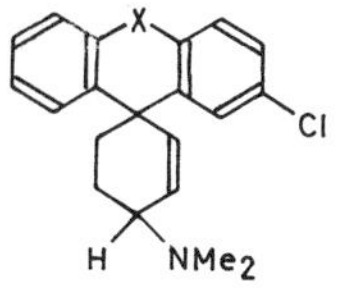

13

(a) X = -CH=CH-
(b) X = -CH₂CH₂-

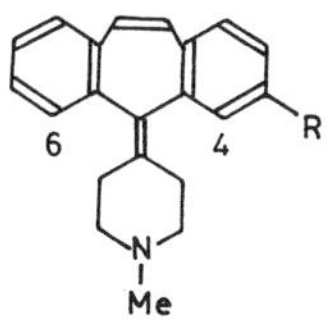

14

(a) R = Cl   (c) R = CN
(b) R = SCF₃ (d) R = H

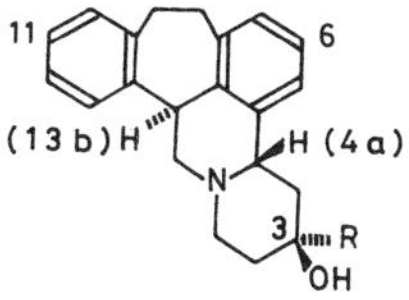

15

(a) R = Et
(b) R = CHMe₂ (c) R = CMe₃

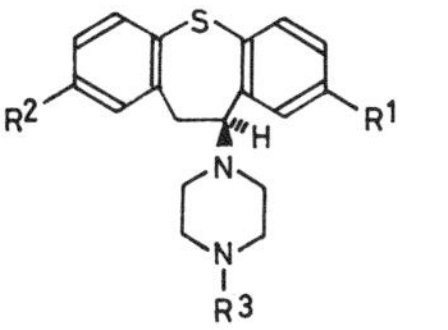

16

	R¹	R²	R³
(a)	Cl	H	Me
(b)	F	Me	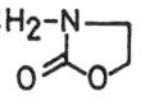 CH₂CH₂-N (morpholine)

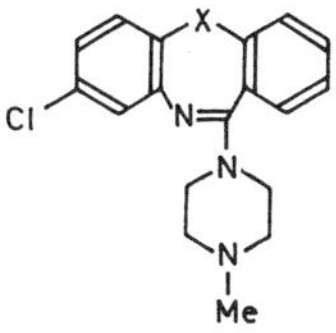

17

(a) X = NH   (c) X = O
(b) X = NMe (d) X = S
             (e) X = CH₂

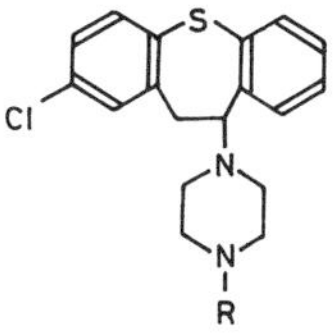

18

(a) R = Me
(b) R = CH₂CH₂OH

The dibenzo[a,d]cycloheptene system (9; X=CH₂) also is capable of rapidly inverting in solutions at 20 °C (FOUCHÉ and COMBRISSON, 1973). The system of (14) on the other hand is so rigid that no inversion can occur under normal conditions. This rigidity is due to the double bond in the central seven-membered ring and to steric hindrance produced by interaction between the protons in positions 4 and 6 of the aromatic rings and the allylic protons of the piperidine ring. Thus, it was possible to isolate the optically active isomers (atropisomers) of compounds (14a), (14b), and (14c) (EBNÖTHER et al., 1965; REMY et al., 1977; ROBINSON et al., 1977).

More significant for biological action may be the conformation of the basic side chain. In the aminopropyl-phenothiazines (1) the side chain is extended in the direction of the S-N axis and is intermediary between the pseudo-axial and pseudo-equatorial positions (COUBEILS and PULLMAN, 1972; FOUCHÉ and COMBRISSON, 1973; BARBE et al., 1973; BARBE and CHAUVET-MONGES, 1974). An analogous location of the side chain is encountered in the aminopropyl-thioxanthenes and -9,10-dihydroanthracenes (2; X=S or CH₂) (TERNAY and EVANS, 1974).

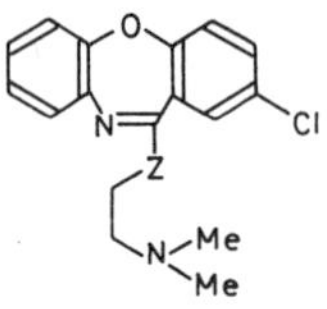

19

(a) Z = NMe

(b) Z = O   (c) Z = CH$_2$

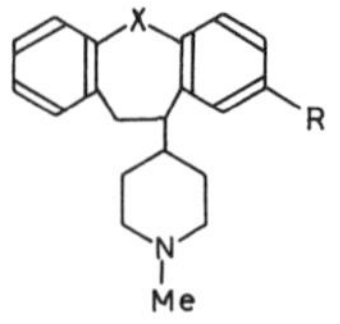

20

(a) X = S ; R = OMe

(b) X = CH$_2$; R = Cl

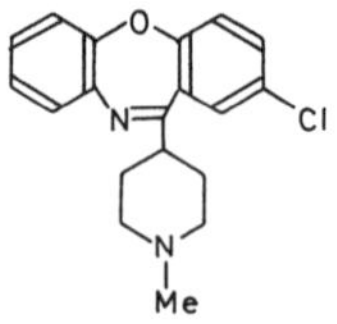

21

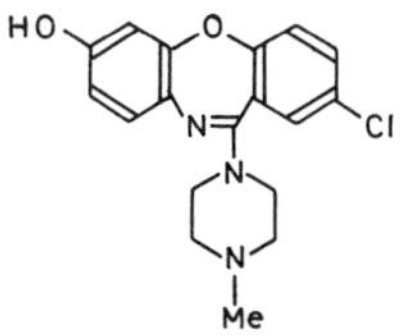

22

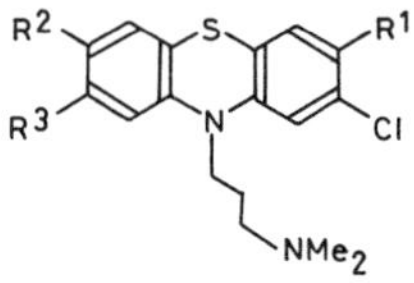

23

	R^1	R^2	R^3
(a)	OH	H	H
(b)	H	OH	H
(c)	H	H	OH
(d)	OH	OH	H
(e)	OH	H	OH
(f)	H	OH	OH
(g)	OH	OH	OH

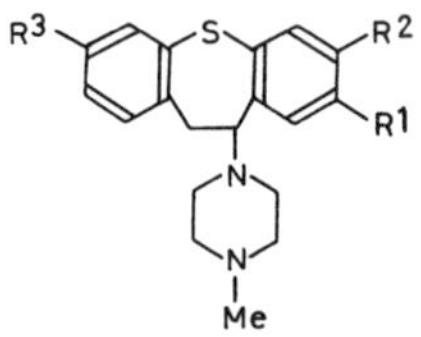

24

	R^1	R^2	R^3
(a)	Cl	H	OH
(b)	Cl	H	F
(c)	Cl	F	H
(d)	Cl	F	F
(e)	SMe	H	F

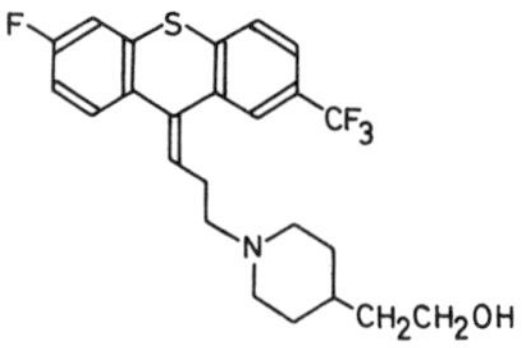

25

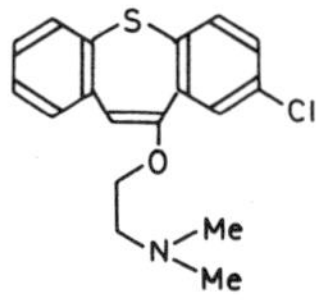

26

The conformational flexibility of the basic side chain is greatest in compounds having an aminopropyl chain which permits free rotation around all side-chain bonds (four degrees of freedom). Flexibility is progressively diminished as we pass through the aminopropylidene derivatives, having three degrees of freedom, to the dibenzo-epines (7) to (9) with essentially only one degree of freedom around the bond linking the basic moiety to the central ring. Rotation in the dibenzo-epines is hindered by the interaction between the α-protons of the piperazine ring and the proton in position 1 of the proximal benzene ring. Hindrance is particularly strong in the piperazinyldibenzo-epines (7), since the exocyclic C–N bond has a partial double-bond character. The tricyclic neuroleptics, including the most flexible systems, are capable of assuming asymmetric conformations very similar to that of the semi-rigid molecule of the highly active dibenzoxazepine derivative loxapine (7c), in which there is a more or less fixed geometrical relationship between the distal nitrogen and the two benzene rings. The mean plane of the piperazine ring of loxapine lies approximately parallel to the plane of the unsubstituted aromatic ring and is proximal to the substituted ring, the distance between the "outer" nitrogen atom of the piperazine moiety and the centre of the substituted aromatic ring being about 6 Å (PETCHER and WEBER, 1976; BÜRKI et al., 1978). In the most rigid compounds, e.g. the piperidylidene derivatives of thioxanthene and dibenzocycloheptene, (12a) and (14) respectively, and the spiroamines of the dibenzocycloheptenes (13), the distance between the basic nitrogen and either of the benzene rings is also about 6 Å. The neuroleptic potencies of these highly rigid compounds suggest that their structures fulfil the necessary requirements for interaction with the DA receptors.

D. Stereospecificity of Action

Most drug activities are stereospecific and involve, preferentially, one particular conformation of the drug molecule. This has obvious implications for the geometry of the receptor site, so that stereospecific agents are of considerable interest as research tools for elucidating mechanisms of drug action.

All neuroleptics capable of forming stereoisomers, i.e. diastereoisomers or enantiomers, exhibit stereospecific actions. Geometrical isomerism is exhibited by the γ-aminopropylidene-thioxanthenes (3) and the dibenzoxepin pinoxepin (5a), on account of their asymmetrically substituted exocyclic double bonds (KAISER et al., 1974 a, b). It is well-established that the neuroleptic properties are associated with the *cis* geometry[2], i.e. the configuration in which the side chain is oriented towards the substituted ring (PETERSEN et al., 1977). Of the thioxanthenes, flupenthixol (3c) has been studied in greatest detail. The *cis*-isomer (α-flupenthixol) is approximately equipotent pharmacologically with fluphenazine (lf), whereas the *trans*-isomer (β-flupenthixol) is practically inactive (MØLLER-NIELSEN et al., 1973). Similar conclusions were reached from biochemical studies. Thus, the *trans*-isomer is only $^1/_{50}$th as active as the *cis*-isomer in competing for the [³H]haloperidol binding with DA receptors in calf-brain membranes, and it is practically inactive in inhibiting DA-sensitive adenylate cyclase (cf. Table 1). Of particular interest are the findings of CROW and JOHNSTONE (1977) who tested the two isomeric flupenthixols in patients with acute schizophrenia. They showed that the antipsychotic activity was confined to the pharmacologically and biochemically active *cis*-isomer. Analogous results have been reported for clopenthixol (3b) (GRAVEM et al., 1978).

The spiroamines of the 3-chloro-dibenzocycloheptenes (13a and b) display geometrical as well as optical isomerism. In these molecules the cyclohexene ring is located perpendicularly to the tricyclic system and the amino group can occupy a position *cis* or *trans* to the substituted benzene ring. As the molecules contain two chiral centres, the *cis*- and *trans*-isomers can each be resolved into optically active enantiomers. Of the two racemates only the *cis*-isomers were pharmacologically and biochemically active, and the activities were confined entirely to the (−)-enantiomers (CARNMALM et al., 1976; ÖGREN et al., 1978). Again, in the active compounds the amino group is proximal to the substituted benzene ring.

---

2 The designation of the *cis-trans* isomers according to the sequential rule is Z for *cis* and E for *trans*

Table 1. Activities and chlorpromazine indices (C.I.) of some tricyclic neuroleptics in various pharmacological and biochemical tests (C.I.=activity of CPZ/activity of compound)

Generic	Formula	Catalepsy rat sc. ED$_{50}$[a] or ED 30 sec[b,c] μmol/kg	C.I.	Amphet. antag. rat sc., ED$_{50}$ μmol/kg	C.I.	Apomorph. antag. rat sc., ED$_{50}$ μmol/kg	C.I.	$[^3\mathrm{H}]$Haloperidol assay Ki(nM)	C.I.	Cyclic AMP assay Ki(nM)	C.I.	$[^3\mathrm{H}]$QNB assay ED$_{50}$(μM)	C.I.
Promazine	1a	143[a]	0.05	99.7[a]	0.02	>250[d]	<0.07	72[e]	0.14	2800[g]	0.02	0.65[i]	1.5
Chlorpromazine	1b	6.47[a]	1	1.69[a]	1	18.3[d]	1	10.2[e]	1	48[g]	1	1.0[i]	1
		10.7[c]	1			7.3[c]	1	17[k]	1			3.0[c]	
Perphenazine	1c	0.84[a]	7.7	0.14[a]	12	0.67[d]	27					11[i]	0.09
Triflupromazine	1d	4.37[a]	1.5	0.75[a]	2.3	4.63[d]	4	2.1[e]	4.9			1.0[i]	1
Trifluoperazine	1e	1.25[a]	5.2	0.17[a]	10	1.14[d]	16	2.1[e]	4.9	19[g]	2.5	13[i]	0.08
Fluphenazine	1f	0.33[a]	19	0.08[a]	22	0.26[d]	72	0.88[e]	12	4.3[g]	11	12[i]	0.08
Acetophenazine	1g	3.10[a]	2.1	0.34[a]	4.9	0.34[d]	54					10[i]	0.1
Thioridazine	10	34.4[a]	0.2	22.4[a]	0.08	>390[d]	<0.05	15[e]	0.7	130[g]	0.37	0.15[i]	6.7
								18[k]	0.9				
Chlorprothixene (cis, α)	3a	34.8[b]	0.31	4.26[a]	0.4	4.11[b]	1.8	4.4[e]	2.3	37[g]	1.3	—	—
				(19.3 ip)[m]									
trans (β)		12.7[m]	—	(>60 ip)[m]	—								
Clopenthixol (α, β)	3b	>60[m]	—										
cis (α)		2.35[b]	4.6	0.34[a]	5.0	1.61[b]	4.5	3.1[e]	3.3	16[g]	3	—	—
				(1.5 ip)[m]									
trans (β)		1.0[m]	—	(92.3 ip)[m]	—			88[e]	0.1	2800[g]	0.02		
Flupenthixol (α, β)	3c	244[m]	—										
cis (α)		1.29[b]	8.3	0.61[a]	2.8	0.37[b]	20	0.98[e]	10	3.5[g]	14	—	—
				0.17[l]		(0.66 ip)[l]							
trans (β)		0.32[m]	—	>370[l]	—	(>180 ip)[l]	—	48[e]	0.2	1.0[g]	48		
Thiothixene (cis, α)	3d	133[m]	—	0.46[a]	3.7	0.25[b]	29	1.5[e]	6.8	>5000[g]	0.01	—	—
trans (β)		5.86[b]	2					145[e]	0.1				

Table 1 (continued)

Generic	Formula	Catalepsy rat sc. ED$_{50}$[a] or ED 30 sec [b,c]		Amphet. antag. rat sc., ED$_{50}$		Apomorph. antag. rat sc., ED$_{50}$		[3H]Haloperidol assay		Cyclic AMP assay		[3H]QNB assay	
		μmol/kg	C.I.	μmol/kg	C.I.	μmol/kg	C.I.	Ki(nM)	C.I.	Ki(nM)	C.I.	ED$_{50}$(μM)	C.I.
Metiapine	7a	15.5[b]	0.7	—	—	6.18[b]	1.2	9[f]	1.9	—	—	—	1.5
Clotiapine	7b	2.09[c]	5.1	0.58[a]	2.9	0.79[c]	9.3	2.8[k]	6.1	25[h]	1.9	2[c]	1
Loxapine	7c	1.07[c]	10	0.37[a]	4.6	0.21[c]	35	11[k]	1.5	45[h]	1.1	3[c]	15
HF-2046	7d	10.7[c]	1	—	—	5.20[c]	1.4	20[f]	0.85	18[h]	2.7	0.2[c]	10
Clozapine	17a	0[c]	—	—	—	0[c]	—	120[e] 162[k]	0.09 0.1	170[h]	0.3	0.3[c]	
Clorotepine (Octoclothepin)	8a	4.06[b]	2.6	—	—	0.35[b]	21	2.0[f]	8.5	—	—	—	—
Metitepine (Methiothepin)	8b	4.66[b]	2.3	—	—	0.32[b]	23	1.4[e] 0.7[f]	7.3 24	—	—	—	—

[a] JANSSEN and VAN BEVER (1975)

[b] STILLE and SAYERS, unpublished data. For method and CPZ values, see (c)

[c] BÜRKI et al. (1977)

[d] JANSSEN et al. (1965)

[e] BURT et al. (1976). Inhibition of binding with DA-receptors in *calf*-brain striatal membranes

[f] BÜRKI, unpublished data. Inhibition of binding with DA-receptors in *rat*-brain striatal membranes; cf. method (k)

[g] IVERSEN et al. (1976a, b). Inhibition of DA-sensitive adenylate cyclase in rat striatal homogenates

[h] MILLER and HILEY (1976). Inhibition of DA-sensitive adenylate cyclase in rat striatal homogenates

[i] SNYDER et al. (1974). Inhibition of binding of [3H]quinuclidinyl benzilate with muscarinic receptors from rat brain homogenates

[k] BÜRKI (1978)

[l] MØLLER-NIELSEN et al. (1973)

[m] PETERSEN et al. (1977)

Introduction of a nuclear substituent into the 3-position of the rigid dibenzo-cycloheptene system, as in (14a), (14b), and (14c), gives rise to atropisomerism (Ebnö-ther et al., 1965). Of the optically active enantiomers of (14b) and (14c) only the (−)-isomers showed anti-avoidance and anti-apomorphine activities, while the central anticholinergic activity resided only in the (+)-isomers (Remy et al., 1977; Robin-son et al., 1977).

The stereospecific activities of the benzocyclohepta-pyridoisoquinolines (15a, b, and c) have been investigated fully. In this group the activity was found to be strongly dependent on the relative configuration of the three chiral centres at 3, 4a, and 13b. Thus, of the four possible racemic diastereoisomers of (15a) only the isomer having 4a,13b-*trans* and 3(OH),13b(H)-*trans* was pharmacologically active. Similarly, for dexclamol (15b) and butaclamol (15c) the same configuration is needed for high activities (Bruderlein et al., 1975). The structures of (15b) and (15c) were determined by X-ray crystallography (Bird et al., 1976). In both instances it was the (+)-enantiomer that exhibited the pharmacological and biochemical activities (Humber and Bruderlein, 1975; Voith and Cummings, 1976; Lippmann et al., 1975; Miller et al., 1975; Pugsley et al., 1976). Thus, (+)-butaclamol is over 1,000 times more potent than the (−)-enantiomer in inhibiting DA-sensitive adenylate cyclase (Iversen et al., 1976a, b) or [³H]haloperidol binding with DA receptors (Burt et al., 1976). For the (+)-enantiomer of dexclamol (15b) the absolute configuration 3S,4aS,13bS was established by X-ray crystallography, and the same configuration was assigned to (+)-butaclamol on the basis of a comparison of its molecular rotation with that of (+)-dexclamol (Bird et al., 1976). (+)-Dexclamol has recently been shown to possess an equally strong affinity for the [³H]haloperidol receptor as does (+)-butaclamol, whilst the (−−)-isomer is inactive (Pugsley and Lippmann, 1979).

The well-known neuroleptic levomepromazine (methotrimeprazine, 11) possesses a chiral centre in the side chain, the absolute configuration of which is as yet unknown. The pharmacologically active isomer is the (−)-enantiomer (Courvoisier et al., 1957; Julou et al., 1966).

The neuroleptic 10,11-dihydro-dibenzothiepins (8; X = S) have a chirality centre in the seven-membered ring. The pharmacological activities of clorotepine (8a) have been shown to be confined to the (+)-enantiomer (16a) which has the S configuration (Petcher et al., 1975; Metyšová and Protiva, 1975; Jaunin et al., 1977). Similarly, the activity of the oxazolidinone derivative (16b) was confined to the (+)-enantiomer, which again had the S configuration (Aschwanden et al., 1976). Both (+)-enantiomers (16a) and (16b) also have much higher affinities for [³H]haloperidol receptors of rat striatal membranes than their respective (−)-enantiomers (Bürki, unpublished results).

E. Nature of the Basic Side Chain

The basic nitrogen in the side chain must be tertiary and separated from the central ring by a three-carbon chain, as in the general structures (1) to (6), or by an N-C-C chain forming part of a piperazine ring, as in (7) to (9). Replacement of the γ-methylene group in the side chain of chlorpromazine (CPZ, 1b) by NH to form a terminal dimethylhydrazino group leads to an inactive compound (Corral et al., 1978). The three-carbon chain is most commonly a straight propylene as in CPZ (1b) itself, although it may be branched in β position with a methyl group as in levomepromazine (11) or be part of a piperidine ring as in thioridazine (10). However, if the side chain of CPZ is substituted in the β position by a phenyl, dimethylaminomethyl or hydroxyl group, practically inactive compounds are obtained (GORDON et al., 1963; CREESE et al., 1978). In the thioxanthene series, however, the aminopropyl derivatives (2) are as a rule comparatively weak neuroleptics, though there are exceptions like the 2-trifluoromethyl-thioxanthene (2a), which in the CAR test is equipotent with CPZ (KAISER et al., 1972), and the 2-dimethylsulphamoyl derivative (2b) which in the same test appears to be roughly ten times more potent than CPZ (MUREN and BLOOM, 1970). However, the introduction of an unsaturated aminopropylidene side chain generally results in much more potent neuroleptic compounds, the activity being concentrated in the *cis*-isomer as, for example, in chlorprothixene (3a) (cf. Table 1). For the aminopropylidene-morphanthridine (6a) antischizophrenic action in man has been reported (ANGRIST et al., 1976), but no pharmacological or stereochemical data have as yet been published.

The aminopropylidene chain may also be part of an N-methylpiperidylidene moiety, as in the dibenzocycloheptatrienes (14) already discussed or in the thioxanthenes and acridans described by KAISER et al. (1974a), the 2-trifluoromethyl analogues of (12a) and (12b) being a little more than half as active as trifluoperazine (1e) in producing ptosis in the rat.

The dimethylaminopropyl-acridans (2; X = NH), in contrast to the corresponding thioxanthenes, are potent neuroleptics, and recently the 2-chloro-derivative clomacran (2c) has received renewed attention. It has a similar pharmacological profile as CPZ, but is about twice as potent as CPZ in the apomorphine and cyclic AMP tests and about five times more potent in the amphetamine test (FOWLER et al., 1977a). Anthracenes carrying the saturated aminopropyl side chain also exhibit interesting CNS-activities. Thus, compound (2d) has potent neuroleptic effects, being about ten times more active than CPZ in the anti-apomorphine test, and in animal tests its 10-methyl analogue fluotracen (2e) displays a combination of the characteristic properties of antidepressants and antipsychotics (FOWLER et al., 1977b).

The nature of the terminal tertiary amino group in the side chain is a further factor determining neuroleptic potency. In the 2-substituted phenothiazines, the most important basic terminal groups increase neuroleptic potency generally in the following order:

$$-NMe_2 \sim -N\underset{\underline{\quad}}{\diagup} < -N\underset{\underline{\quad}}{\diagdown}NMe < -N\underset{\underline{\quad}}{\diagdown}NCH_2CH_2OH < -N\underset{\underline{\quad}}{\diagdown}NCH_2CH_2O\cdot COMe.$$

Other cycloalkylamino groups, e.g. 1-pyrrolidinyl or 1-morpholinyl, lead to compounds having much weaker neuroleptic potencies than the corresponding dimethylamino derivatives. Esterification of the 4-hydroxyethyl substituent of the piperazinyl- or piperidinyl-propyl side chain with a fatty acid produces compounds which, when given parenterally in an oily medium, exhibit prolonged neuroleptic activity extending over several weeks. The best-known of these long-acting neuroleptics are the enanthate and decanoate of fluphenazine (1f) and the decanoate of flupenthixol (3c). These esters probably do not act per se but diffuse from the oily depot where, by the action of esterases, they are hydrolysed to the parent compounds (YALE, 1978).

In the phenoxazines (1; X = O), thioxanthenes (2, 3; X = S) and dihydroanthracenes (2, 3; X = CH$_2$), the relative influences of the different basic groups on neuroleptic activity are very similar to those outlined above for the phenothiazines. In the acridans (1; $X = CH_2$), however, replacement of the dimethylamino moiety by N-methylpiperazinyl fails to increase neuroleptic potency, whereas activity in the di-benzo-epines (7–9) is practically confined to compounds having an N-alkylpiperazinyl group directly attached to the central ring. Replacement of the N-methyl group in the dibenzo-epines (7) by a hydroxyalkyl group decreases the activity, but in the dibenzo-thiepins (8, 9; $X = S$) hydroxyalkylation leads to an increase in activity.

For the dibenzo-epines, the importance of the N-methylpiperazinyl group for neuroleptic activity (Schmutz, 1975) has recently been further confirmed (Bürki et al., 1978). Compounds with an ethylenediamine side chain, as in (19a), and the di-methylaminoethoxy- and dimethylaminopropyl-derivatives (19b) and (19c) are inactive. Surprisingly, however, certain neuroleptic properties have been reported for the dibenzo[b,f]thiepin derivative zotepine (26) although it appears to be much weaker than clorotepine (8a) in the apomorphine test (Ueda et al., 1978). Of analogues carrying other heterocyclic groups, only N-methyl-4-piperidyl analogues have been reported as possessing some activity. Thus, the dibenzothiepin (20a) was more effective than CPZ in the rotating rod test in the mouse (Pelz et al., 1968), and for the diben-zocycloheptene (20b) biological activities comparable to those of its N-methyl-piperazinyl analogue have been reported (Fouché and Combrisson, 1973). Tranquil-lising properties have been claimed for the dibenzoxazepine (21) (Howell et al., 1970), though subsequently it has been shown that in the apomorphine test in the rat this compound possesses only about $1/_{250}$ th of the activity of its methylpiperazinyl analogue loxapine (7c); in vitro, in the [^{3}H]haloperidol binding assay, the compound is about one-half as active as loxapine (Bürki et al., 1978).

It has already been pointed out that the terminal amino group must be tertiary for optimal neuroleptic activity. Thus, N-desmethylation of chlorpromazine to the secondary and primary amines leads to a progressive loss of neuroleptic potency (Pos-NER et al., 1962; Brune et al., 1963; Creese et al., 1978). Secondary amines frequently display antidepressant activities, as for example the N-desmethyl analogue of triflu-promazine (ld) (Bickel and Brodie, 1964) or that of loxapine (7c), i.e. amoxapine (Schmutz et al., 1967; Gallant et al., 1971; Greenblatt et al., 1978). The quater-nary salts of the tertiary bases are ionised at physiological pH, and generally their pen-etration of the blood-brain barrier is poor. Thus, they have weak or no central activity as was shown in the case of the quaternary salt of CPZ (Watzman et al., 1968). CPZ-methiodide was found to be inactive in vitro in the [^{3}H]haloperidol assay using rat striatum homogenates (Schmutz and Bürki, unpublished results). It would appear that binding to the receptor site no longer occurs, either as a result of steric hindrance or because of the occupation of the lone electron pair of the nitrogen atom by the methyl group. The neuroleptic effects, manifested as amphetamine antagonism and catalepsy, that were seen after intrastriatal injection of quaternary salts of CPZ, flu-penthixol or perphenazine, were presumably due to some different mechanism (Fog et al., 1968). Quaternary haloperidol when given under identical conditions was inac-tive. The N-oxides of clotiapine (7b), loxapine (7c) and clozapine (17a) show neurolep-tic activity in the rat, varying from one-quarter to one-half of the activities of their respective parent drugs, but they all are inactive in vitro in the [^{3}H]haloperidol binding assay (Bürki et al., 1978). Chlorpromazine N-oxide is likewise inactive in vitro (Creese et al., 1978; Bürki et al., 1978). It is suggested that the N-oxides of all tricyclic neuroleptics probably exert their neuroleptic activity only after reduction to the parent drugs. These results emphasise the importance for receptor binding of the lone-pair electrons on the basic nitrogen atom of the side chain.

The nature of the basic side chain of the phenothiazines appears to be important also for the anticholinergic activities of these compounds. The piperazinyl derivatives (1c, e, f, and g) have only about one-tenth of the activity of CPZ in the [³H]QNB assay, whereas thioridazine (10) is about seven times more active than CPZ (cf. Table 1). Amongst the piperazinyl-dibenzo-epines tested, the dibenzodiazepines (7d and 17a) stand out as being 10–15 times more potent than CPZ in this in-vitro test (Table 1).

F. Aromatic Substitution

Substitution of one of the benzene rings is essential for strong neuroleptic activity. The unsubstituted parent compounds of any of the major tricyclic systems considered here are generally sedative with only weak neuroleptic activity, e.g. perlapine (7e); some have antidepressant properties, e.g. melitracen (2f), dimethacrine (1h) and doxepin (5b); and some have antihistamine and antiserotonin properties, e.g. promethazine (1a), cyproheptadine (14d) and perathiepine (8c) (METYŠ and METYŠOVÁ, 1966). The nuclear substituent must be in a position which is equivalent for all tricyclics and which is meta to the atom bearing the basic side chain. We shall refer to this as the "meta" position, because the numbering varies with different ring systems. The "meta" substituent as here defined is in the following positions:

Position:

2	in phenothiazines and -oxazines (1; X=S, 0)
2	in thioxanthenes and xanthenes (2 and 3; X=S, 0)
3	in acridans (1; X=C<), but
2	in acridans (2 and 3; X=NH)
2	in 9,10-dihydroanthracenes (2 and 3; X=C<)
3 or 7	in dibenz[b, e] [1,4]oxazepines and -thiazepines (4: X=0, S)
2	in dibenz[b, e]oxepins and -thiepins (5 and 6; X=0, S)
2	in dibenz[b, f] [1,4]oxazepines and -thiazepines (7; X=0, S)
2	in dibenzo[b, e] [1,4]diazepines (7; X=NH)
8	in dibenz[b, e] azepines (=morphanthridines) (7; X=CH₂)
8	in dibenz[b, f] oxepins and -thiepins (8 and 9; X=0, S)
3	in dibenzo[a, d] cycloheptene derivatives (8 and 9; X=CH₂).

Mono-substitution in other positions of the aromatic rings usually leads to compounds which are much less active or inactive neuroleptically. The special case of the 8-chloro-dibenzodiazepine clozapine (17a) will be considered later.

The benzocycloheptapyridoisoquinolines, dexclamol (15b) and butaclamol (15c), whose structures though derived from the tricyclic neuroleptics are different from them, do not fit into this concept. Here, the aromatic unsubstituted compounds are the most active, and chlorine substitution does not enhance the activity (HUMBER et al., 1978; VOITH et al., 1978; PUGSLEY and LIPPMANN, 1979).

There has been considerable discussion of the effect of the "meta" substituent on the activity of the tricyclic neuroleptics and of the mechanism whereby the substituent exerts its potency-enhancing effect. It does not seem to be due to any influence either on the conformation of the tricyclic nucleus or the side chain or on the lipophilicity of the compound (Schmutz, 1975; Tollenaere et al., 1976; Rodgers et al., 1976). It has been suggested that the most likely effect of the substituent in the phenothiazine series is one of direct interaction at the receptor site (Horn et al., 1975; Rodgers et al., 1976). There is much evidence that the effect is related to the electron-withdrawing properties of the substituent, in accord with the hypothesis that the psychotropic activity of the phenothiazines depends on a balance between the electron-donating power of the tricyclic nucleus and the electron-withdrawing effect of the 2-substituent (Mercier and Dupont, 1972). Feinberg and Snyder (1975), however, have argued on the basis of calculations of van der Waals' forces that, with changes of the substitution in position 2 of the phenothiazine nucleus and on the side-chain nitrogen, the force of attractive pull of the side chain in the direction of the ring substituent increases in the same way as the neuroleptic potency.

For the series of dibenz-oxazepines and -thiazepines (7; X = O, S), it has been shown (Schmutz, 1973, 1975) that the most strongly electron-withdrawing substituents confer the highest neuroleptic activity as measured by the apomorphine test in the rat, and the same general conclusion was reached in respect of the 10,11-dihydro-dibenzo[b,f]thiepins (8; X = S), the rotating rod test on mice being used as measure of neuroleptic potency of the latter (Tollenaere et al., 1976). In the phenothiazines, the relative effects of the different 2-substituents depend on the test model employed for measuring the biological activity. The data obtained with both the apomorphine and the amphetamine tests (Janssen et al., 1965) are in good general agreement with those reported for the dibenzo-epines. On the other hand, results based on the CAR test in the rat do not correlate so well with the electron-withdrawing powers of the substituents (Zirkle and Kaiser, 1974). Recent data for 2-substituted analogues of fluphenazine (lf) suggest that biological activity, at least as reflected by the catalepsy test in the rat, may not be solely related to the electron-withdrawing properties of the substituent (Bossle et al., 1976). For whereas the 2-nitro analogue of fluphenazine was about three times more potent in that test than fluphenazine itself, the 2-cyano analogue, possessing a substituent with electron-withdrawing properties intermediate between those of nitro and trifluoromethyl, was only about two-thirds as potent as fluphenazine.

The order in which "meta"-substituents in different tricyclic systems affect the neuroleptic potency as determined by different pharmacological tests is shown in Table 2.

The dibenz[b,e][1,4]oxazepines and -thiazepines (4; X = O or S) occupy a special position in that they possess two "meta" positions, i.e. 3 and 7, which are not equivalent on account of the asymmetrical nature of the 6-7-6 molecules. Indeed, it has been reported that a suitable substituent, e.g. Cl or CF$_3$, in either of the two "meta" positions produces compounds with marked CNS-depressant activities, provided that the side chain in the 5-position terminates in a 4-(N-hydroxyethyl)piperazinyl group as in compounds (4a) and (4b) (Yale et al., 1970).

Additional aromatic substitution generally leads to a marked reduction in neuroleptic potency, but there are important exceptions. In particular, the introduction of a fluorine atom in a position normally involved in the metabolisation of a compound can, by blocking metabolisation, result in increased potency and prolongation

Table 2. Influence of the "meta" substituent on neuroleptic activity in some tricyclic systems

System Structure Test	Phenothiazines (12)				Oxazepines/ Thiazepines (15)	Thiepins (17)
	Apo.[a]	Amphet.[b]	Catalep.[c]	CAR[d]	Apo.[e]	Rot. rod[f]
Decreasing potency →	SO_2NMe_2	SO_2NMe_2	NO_2	SO_2CF_3/CF_3	SO_2NMe_2	COMe
	CF_3	CF_3	CF_3	SO_2NMe_2	SO_2CF_3	CN
	Cl	Cl	CN	$Cl/Br/SCF_3$	NO_2	OMe
	COMe	COMe	SO_2NMe_2	$COMe/SO_2Me$	$Cl/CN/SO_2Me$	Cl
	OMe	OMe	OMe	$COOMe/CMe_3$	Br	CF_3
	H	H	Cl/COMe	Me	$F/OMe/SMe$	SMe
			H	$CHMe_2$	SCF_3/Me	F/Br
				CN	SOMe	Me
				OMe/H	NH_2	$CHMe_2$
				OH	H	H
						NH_2
						OH

[a] Apomorphine antagonismus, rat, sc. (JANSSEN et al., 1965)
[b] Amphetamine antagonism, rat, sc. (JANSSEN et al., 1965)
[c] Cataleptic effects, rat, sc. (JANSSEN et al., 1965), or im. (BOSSLE et al., (1976)
[d] Conditioned avoidance response, rat, ip. (ZIRKLE and KAISER, 1974)
[e] Apomorphine antagonism, rat, sc. (SCHMUTZ, 1975)
[f] Rotating rod test, mouse, iv. (TOLLENAERE et al., 1976)

of the neuroleptic effect. Such substitution might also enhance the affinity of the molecule for DA receptors. Thus, in the thioxanthene series, the 6-fluoro-derivative of chlorprothixene (3a) was found to have increased and protracted activity. It was two and a half times more potent than chlorprothixene both in the rotating rod test in mice and in the catalepsy test in rats (RAJŠNER et al., 1975).

More recently, high and prolonged neuroleptic activities have also been reported for piflutixol (25) (MØLLER-NIELSEN et al., 1977). This 2,6-disubstituted thioxanthene is four to ten times as potent as cis-flupenthixol (3c) in inhibiting stereotypies induced in rats by amphetamine and apomorphine respectively, and its cataleptogenic potency in rats is about three times as great as that of cis-flupenthixol. Piflutixol also exhibits very powerful sedative effects, being nearly 15 times more potent than cis-flupenthixol in inhibiting spontaneous motor activity in mice. In vitro, piflutixol is the most potent inhibitor of DA-sensitive adenyl cyclase described so far, being about four times as active as cis-flupenthixol.

It should be noted that piflutixol (25), in addition to having a second nuclear substituent, has a 4-hydroxyethylpiperidino group in the side chain in place of the 4-hydroxyethylpiperazino group present in flupenthixol (3c), and that the high activities reported for piflutixol appear to have been obtained with the cis-trans mixture.

In the dibenzo-epine series, some fluorinated derivatives of clorotepine (8a) and metitepine (8b) have shown enhanced neuroleptic activity as measured by the rotating rod test in mice. In this test, 3-fluoro-clorotepine (24b) was about three times as potent as clorotepine itself (RAJŠNER et al., 1975), whereas the 7-fluoro and 3,7-difluoro derivatives (24c) and (24d) were less active than clorotepine (Cervená et al., 1976; Šin-delář et al., 1977). Similarly, 3-fluoro-metitepine (24e) was about four times as potent as metitepine itself and the action was again protracted (Kopicová et al., 1975). In the dibenzodiazepines, however, introduction of a second halogen atom in the 8-position reduced neuroleptic activity as measured by the antiapomorphine test in the rat. The 8-chloro derivative of (7d) was about one-tenth and the 8-fluoro analogue one-fifth as potent as compound (7d) itself (Bürki et al., 1977).

Other examples of di- and tri-substituted tricyclics with significant neuroleptic activity are found among the metabolites of CPZ. Thus, 7-hydroxy-CPZ (23b), 3,7-di-hydroxy-CPZ (23d) and 7,8-dihydroxy-CPZ (23f) all retained significant activity in various behavioral tests in the rat (Barry et al., 1974). In vitro, the 7-hydroxy-metabolite (23b) was nearly as potent as CPZ itself in competing for [^{3}H]haloperidol binding, and the 3-hydroxy and 3,7-dihydroxy derivatives (23a) and (23d) were roughly twice as potent as CPZ in this assay. On the other hand, very weak or no affinity for these receptor sites was shown by the 8-hydroxy, 3,8- and 7,8-dihydroxy and the 3,7,8-trihydroxy derivatives (23c, e, f, and g) (Creese et al., 1978). In the dibenzo-epine series, 7-hydroxy-loxapine (22) showed significant in-vitro activity in the cyclic AMP assay (Coupet et al., 1976) and 3-hydroxy-clorotepine (24a) was nearly twice as potent as clorotepine (8a) in the rotating rod test in mice (Šindelář et al., 1974).

G. Nature of the Central Ring

The central ring of the tricyclic neuroleptics must be six- or seven-membered. Analogous compounds possessing a five- or eight-membered ring are neuroleptically inactive.

As will have been apparent from the discussion in Sect. E, the influence of different bridging atoms or groups (X) on the neuroleptic potency of compounds having the same substituent and the same basic side chain does not follow a uniform pattern. This is illustrated further by the following examples:

The phenothiazines (1; X=S) and the thioxanthenes (3; X=S) are more potent neuroleptics than the corresponding phenoxazines and xanthenes (1 and 3; X=O), respectively. Thioxanthenes of type (2), however, are generally less potent than their xanthene analogues (Zirkle and Kaiser, 1974).

The dibenz[b,e][1,4]oxazepines (4), the dibenz[b,e]oxepins (5) and the dibenz[b,f]-[1,4]oxazepines (7; X=O) are more potent than their respective thiazepine analogues, but the 10,11-dihydrodibenzo[b,f]thiepins (8; X=S) are more potent than the corresponding oxepins (8; X=O). Recently, however, several dibenz[b,f]oxepins (9; X=O) with potent neuroleptic properties have been reported (Coscia et al., 1975 a, b), in particular the derivatives (9a), (9b), and (9c) which are between 7 and 20 times more potent than CPZ in the amphetamine test and between six and ten times more cataleptogenic than CPZ.

Tricyclic neuroleptics with a sulphur atom in the central ring are metabolised to sulphoxides with some loss of activity. The sulphones are practically devoid of neuroleptic activity.

Replacement of the bridging atom by a methylene moiety increases neuroleptic potency in some series, e.g. the anthracenes (2; X=CH$_2$) are more potent than the corresponding thioxanthenes, and the morphanthridines (7; X=CH$_2$), though weaker than the corresponding dibenzoxazepines, are more potent than the dibenzo-thiazepines. However, in most of the other tricyclic systems (e.g. 1, 3, 4, 8) replacement of the sulphur atom by CH_2 results in reduced neuroleptic activity.

H. Non-Cataleptogenic Neuroleptics

Clozapine (17a), an antipsychotic drug which in clinical use has produced practically no extrapyramidal side-effects, is an agent which does not conform to the classical picture of a neuroleptic (STILLE et al., 1971; SCHMUTZ, 1975).

Pharmacologically, clozapine is strongly sedative and muscle-relaxant and, in relevant doses, produces neither cataleptic effects nor apomorphine antagonism. In vitro, its activity compared with that of CPZ is only about one-tenth in the [³H]haloperidol assay and one-third in the cyclic AMP assay, but in the [³H]QNB assay for anticholinergic activity it is ten times more potent than CPZ (Table 1). [³H]Clozapine binds specifically and with high affinity to rat-brain membranes. About two-thirds of reversibly bound [³H]clozapine are displaced by hyoscyamine in a stereospecific manner, suggesting interaction of clozapine with muscarinic cholinergic receptors. Most of the remaining [³H]clozapine binding is stereospecifically inhibited by butaclamol, but this binding component seems not to be related to dopamine receptors (HAUSER and CLOSSE, 1978).

Structurally, clozapine (17a) differs from the classical neuroleptics such as the 2-chloro-isomer (7d) or loxapine (7c) by having its nuclear substituent in position 8 of the tricyclic system. The clozapine molecule, though conformationally indistinguishable from the 2-substituted isomer (7d), has its piperazine ring not proximal but distal to the substituted benzene ring (SCHMUTZ, 1975; PETCHER and WEBER, 1976; BÜRKI et al., 1978).

In the absence of a specific screening test for neuroleptics of the clozapine type, it is difficult to make firm assertions concerning structure-activity relationships in this group of non-cataleptogenic, atypical neuroleptics. However, some conclusions may be drawn from their central depressant effects, as measured by their action on the locomotor activity in mice (SCHMUTZ et al., 1967; BÜRKI et al., 1977). In this model, clozapine is the most potent of the dibenzo-azepine analogues carrying an 8-chloro substituent, followed in order of decreasing potency by the dibenzoxazepine (17c), the morphanthridine (17e) and the dibenzothiazepine (17d). N-Methylation of clozapine in the 5-position (17b) reduces the central depressant activity. Of the 8-substituents tested, chlorine conferred the highest activity, followed in descending order of potency by methyl, hydrogen, trifluoromethyl, methylthio and methoxy. It will be noted that in this series there appears to be no relation between the electronic effects of the substituents and pharmacological potency, such as has been found for the classical neuroleptics discussed in Sect. F. However, replacement of the N-methyl group in the piperazine moiety by a hydroxyalkyl group or by hydrogen does reduce activity as it did in the "meta"-substituted dibenzo-epines of type (7).

Analogous substitution of the 10-piperazinyl-dibenzo[b,f]thiepins, as in (18), likewise led to non-cataleptogenic, clozapine-like, neuroleptics (ŠINDELÁŘ et al., 1975 a, b; JÍLEK et al., 1975). The 2-position in these compounds corresponds to the 8-position in the dibenzo[b,e][1,4]diazepines (17). The influence of the 2-substituent in (18) on the central depressing activity in the rotating rod test in mice was found to follow a similar structure-activity pattern as in the clozapine series. The most potent compounds (18a and b) are respectively three and five times more active than clozapine. In contrast to the clozapine series, the N-hydroxyethyl derivative (18b) is more potent than the N-methyl compound (18a). The 10,11-dehydro derivative of (18a) is about as strongly CNS-depressant as (18a) itself but, unlike the latter, antagonises apomorphine in the rat.

I. Conclusion

Our discussion of the structure-activity relationships of the different types of tricyclic neuroleptics has relied primarily on measurements of their DA-blocking activities. This approach is justified in the case of the "classical" neuroleptics by the fairly good correlation which exists between these activities and the antischizophrenic effects in man. The clozapine-type neuroleptics appear to have a different mechanism of action, and the structure-activity relationships observed for the classical neuroleptics do not apply to them. It is to be hoped that the intensive work on clozapine and other clozapine-like neuroleptics, which is continuing in many places, will throw fresh light on their mechanism of action and thus help to increase both our knowledge of the nature of schizophrenia itself and our chances of designing more effective and more specific antischizophrenic agents.

References

Aizenshtat, Z., Klein, E., Weiler-Feilchenfeld, H., Bergmann, E.D.: Conformational studies on xanthene, thioxanthene and acridan. Isr. J. Chem. *10*, 753–763 (1972)

Angrist, B., Rotrosen, J., Aronson, M., Gershon, S.: A morphanthridine derivative in schizophrenic patients. Lack of extrapyramidal symptoms. Curr. Therap. Res. *20*, 94–98 (1976)

Aroney, M.J., Cleaver, G., Le Fèvre, R.J.W., Pierens, R.K.: Molecular polarisability. The conformations as solutes of 9,10-dihydroanthracene, anthrone, and xanthone. J. Chem. Soc. (B) *1971*, 82–85

Aschwanden, W., Kyburz, E., Schönholzer, P.: Stereospezifität der neuroleptischen Wirkung und Chiralität von (+)-3-{2-[4-(8-Fluor-2-methyl-10,11-dihydrodibenzo[b,f]thiepin-10-yl)-1-piperazinyl]-äthyl}-2-oxazolidinon. Helv. Chim. Acta *59*, 1245–1252 (1976)

Barbe, J., Blanc, A., Hurwic, J.: Etude conformationnelle des phénothiazines N-substituées. Application aux relations structure-activités. C.R. Acad. Sci. (Paris) *277*, 1071–1074 (1973)

Barbe, J., Chauvet-Monges, A.-M.: Résonance magnétique nucléaire du proton à 250 MHz et conformations de la chaîne alkylamine de quelques phénothiazines-2,10 substituéees. C.R. Acad. Sci. (Paris) *279*, 935–938 (1974)

Barry, H.III., Steenberg, M.L., Manian, A.A., Buckley, J.P.: Effects of chlorpromazine and three metabolites on behavioral responses in rats. Psychopharmacologia *34*, 351–360 (1974)

Bickel, M.H., Brodie, B.B.: Structure and antidepressant activity of imipramine analogues. Int. J. Neuropharmacol. *3*, 611–621 (1964)

Bird, P.H., Bruderlein, F.T., Humber, L.G.: Crystallographic studies on neuroleptics of the benzocycloheptapyridoisoquinoline series. The crystal structure of butaclamol hydrobromide and the absolute configuration and crystal structure of dexclamol hydrobromide. Can. J. Chem. *54*, 2715–2722 (1976)

Bossle, P.C., Ferguson, C.P., Sultan, W.E., Lennox, W.J., Dudley, G.E., Rea, T.H., Miller, J.I.: Synthesis and biological activity of new 2-substituted analogs of fluphenazine. J. Med. Chem. *19*, 370–373 (1976)

Bruderlein, F.T., Humber, L.G., Voith, K.: Neuroleptic agents of the benzocycloheptapyridoisoquinoline series. I. Syntheses and stereochemical and structural requirements for activity of butaclamol and related compounds. J. Med. Chem. *18*, 185–188 (1975)

Brune, G.G., Kohl, H.H., Steiner, W.G., Himwich, H.E.: Relevance of the N,N-dimethyl configuration to the pharmacological action of chlorpromazine. Biochem. Pharmacol. *12*, 679–685 (1963)

Bürki, H.R.: Correlation between ^{3}H-haloperidol binding in the striatum and brain amine metabolism in the rat after treatment with neuroleptics. Life Sci. *23*, 437–442 (1978)

Bürki, H.R., Sayers, A.C., Ruch, W., Asper, H.: Effects of clozapine and other dibenzo-epines on central dopaminergic and cholinergic systems. Structure-activity relationships. Arzneim. Forsch. *27*, (II), 1561–1565 (1977)

Bürki, H.R., Fischer, R., Hunziker, F., Künzle, F., Petcher, T.J., Schmutz, J., Weber, H.P., White, T.G.: Dibenzo-epines: effect of the basic side-chain on neuroleptic activity. Eur. J. Med. Chem. *13*, 479–485 (1978)

Bürki, H.R., Fischer, R., Hunziker, F., Künzle, F., Petcher, T.J., Schmutz, J., Weber, H.P., White, T.G.: Dibenzo-epines: Effect of the basic side chain on neuroleptic activity. To be published

Burt, D.R., Enna, S.J., Creese, I., Snyder, S.H.: Dopamine receptor binding in the corpus striatum of mammalian brain. Proc. Natl. Acad. Sci. USA *72*, 4655–4659 (1975)

Burt, D.R., Creese, I., Snyder, S.H.: Properties of [^{3}H]haloperidol and [^{3}H]dopamine binding associated with dopamine receptors in calf brain membranes. Mol. Pharmacol. *12*, 800–812 (1976)

Carnmalm, B., Johansson, L., Rämsby, S., Stjernström, N.E., Ross, S.B., Ogren, S.-O.: Stereoselective effects of the potentially neuroleptic rigid spiro-amines. Nature *263*, 519–520 (1976)

Červená, I., Metyšová, J., Svátek, E., Kakáč, B., Holubek, J., Hrubantová, M., Protiva, M.: Potent neuroleptics with prolonged activity and diminished toxicity; 7,8-dihalogeno-10-piperazinodibenzo[b,f]thiepins. Coll. Czech. Chem. Commun. *41*, 881–905 (1976)

Chu, S.S.C., Chung, B.: The crystal structure of (+)-cis-9-(3-dimethylaminopropyl)-10-methyl-2-(trifluoromethyl)-9,10-dihydroanthracene hydrochloride monohydrate, SKFd-28175, acetone solvate. Acta Cryst. *B 32*, 836–842 (1976)

Corral, C., Lissavetzky, J., Madronero, R.: Analogues of antipsychotic phenothiazines. 10-(2-N′,N′-disubstituted hydrazinoethyl)phenothiazines. Eur. J. Med. Chem. *13*, 389–391 (1978)

Coscia, L., Causa, P., Giuliani, E.: New tricyclic enamine derivatives with CNS-depressant properties. Arzneim. Forsch. *25*, 1261–1265 (1975a)

Coscia, L., Causa, P., Giuliani, E., Nunziata, A.: Pharmacological properties of new neuroleptic compounds. Arzneim. Forsch. *25*, 1436–1442 (1975b)

Cosulich, D.B., Lovell, F.M.: The X-ray structure of loxapine {2-chloro-11-(4-methyl-1-piperazinyl)dibenz[b,f][1,4]oxazepine} and amoxapine {2-chloro-11-(1-piperazinyl)dibenz[b,f][1,4]oxazepine}. Acta Cryst. *B 33*, 1147–1154 (1977)

Coubeils, J.L., Pullman, B.: Molecular orbital study of the conformational properties of phenothiazines. Theor. Chim. Acta (Berl.) *24*, 35–41 (1972)

Coupet, J., Szucs, V.A., Greenblatt, E.N.: The effects of 2-chloro-11-(4-methyl-piperazinyl)-dibenz[b,f][1,4]oxazepine (loxapine) and its derivatives on the dopamine-sensitive adenylate cyclase of rat striatal homogenates. Brain Res. *116*, 177–180 (1976)

Courvoisier, S., Ducrot, R., Fournel, J., Julou, L.: Propriétés pharmacodynamiques générales de la lévomépromazine. C.R. Soc. Biol. (Paris) *151*, 1378–1382 (1957)

Creese, I., Burt, D.R., Snyder, S.H.: Dopamine receptor binding predicts clinical and pharmacological potencies of antischizophrenic drugs. Science *192*, 481–483 (1976)

Creese, I., Manian, A.A., Prosser, R.D., Snyder, S.H.: ^{3}H-Haloperidol binding to dopamine receptors in rat corpus striatum: influence of chlorpromazine metabolites and derivatives. Eur. J. Pharmacol. *47*, 291–296 (1978)

Crow, T.J., Johnstone, E.C.: Stereochemical specificity in the antipsychotic effects of flupenthixol in man. Br. J. Pharmacol. *59*, p. 466 (1977)

De Paulis, T., Kelder, D., Ross, S.B.: On the topology of the norepinephrine transport carrier in rat hypothalamus. The site of action of tricyclic uptake inhibitors. Mol. Pharmacol. *14*, 596–606 (1978a)

De Paulis, T., Liljefors, T.: Inhibition of amine uptake, conformations and inversion barriers of 5H-dibenzo[a,d]cycloheptene derivatives. A ¹H-DNMR study. Eur. J. Med. Chem. *13*, 327–335 (1978 b)

Ebnöther, A., Jucker, E., Stoll, A.: Atropisomerie in der Dibenzo[a,d]cyclohepten-Reihe. Helv. Chim. Acta *48*, 1237–1249 (1965)

Enna, S.J., Bennett, J.P., Burt, D.R., Creese, I., Snyder, S.H.: Stereospecificity of interaction of neuroleptic drugs with neurotransmitters and correlation with clinical potency. Nature *263*, 338–341 (1976)

Feinberg, A.P., Snyder, S.H.: Phenothiazine drugs: structure-activity explained by a conformation that mimics dopamine. Proc. Natl. Acad. Sci. USA *72*, 1899–1903 (1975)

Fenner, H.: Structure-activity relationship in the field of phenothiazine drugs. Pharmakopsych. Neuro-Psychopharmakol. *3*, 332–339 (1970)

Fog, R.L., Randrup, A., Pakkenberg, H.: Neuroleptic action of quaternary chlorpromazine and related drugs injected into various brain areas in rats. Psychopharmacologia *12*, 428–432 (1968)

Fouché, J., Combrisson, S.: Étude conformationnelle par RMN des composés neuroleptiques dérivés du dibenzo[a,d]cycloheptène. Comparaison avec les neuroleptiques dérivés de la phénothiazine et du thioxanthène. Bull. Soc. Chim. Fr. *1973*, 1693–1698

Fowler, P.J., Zirkle, C.L., Macko, E., Kaiser, C., Sarau, H., Tedeschi, D.H.: Pharmacological evaluation of clomacran, a new potent psychotropic agent. Arzneim. Forsch. *27* (I), 866–872 (1977 a)

Fowler, P.J., Zirkle, C.L., Macko, E., Setler, P.E., Sarau, H.M., Misher, A., Tedeschi, D.H.: Fluotracen: a tricyclic compound with the combined properties of antidepressants and antipsychotics in animals. Arzneim. Forsch. *27* (II), 1589–1595 (1977 b)

Gallant, D.M., Bishop, M.P., Guerrero-Figueroa, R.: CL-67,772: A preliminary evaluation of a potential antidepressant compound: animal and human correlations. Curr. Ther. Res. *13*, 364–368 (1971)

Gordon, M., Cook, L., Tedeschi, D.H., Tedeschi, R.E.: Some structure-activity relationships in the phenothiazines. Arzneim. Forsch. *13*, 318–320 (1963)

Gravem, A., Engstrand, E., Guleng, R.J.: Cis(Z)-clopenthixol and clopenthixol (Sordinol) in chronic psychotic patients. Acta Psychiatr. Scand. *58*, 384–388 (1978)

Greenblatt, E.N., Lippa, A.S., Osterberg, A.C.: The neuropharmacological actions of amoxapine. Arch. Int. Pharmacodyn. Ther. *233*, 107–135 (1978)

Grol, C.J., Rollema, H.: Synthesis and neuroleptic activity of isomeric thieno[1,4]benzothiazines. J. Med. Chem. *18*, 857–861 (1975)

Gschwend, H.W.: Chemical approaches to the development of neuroleptics. In: Industrial Pharmacology. Vol. I: Neuroleptics. Fielding, S., Lal, H. (eds.). Mount Kisco (N.Y.): Futura 1974, pp. 1–51

Hauser, D., Closse, A.: ³H-Clozapine binding to rat brain membranes. Life Sci. *23*, 557–562 (1978)

Horn, A.S., Post, M.L., Kennard, O.: Dopamine receptor blockade and the neuroleptics, a crystallographic study. J. Pharm. Pharmacol. *27*, 553–563 (1975)

Howell, C.F., Ramirez, P., Hardy, R.A.: Tranquilizing 11-(4-piperidyl)dibenz[b,f][1,4]-oxazepines and -thiazepines. U.S. Patent 3,501,483; Chem. Abs. *72*, 132813 (1970)

Humber, L.G., Bruderlein, F.T.: Neuroleptic agents of the benzocycloheptapyridoisoquinoline series. A hypothesis on their mode of interaction with the central dopamine receptor. Mol. Pharmacol. *11*, 833–840 (1975)

Humber, L.G., Sideridis, N., Asselin, A.A., Bruderlein, F.T.: Neuroleptics related to butaclamol. An investigation of the effects of chlorine substituents on the aromatic rings. J. Med. Chem. *21*, 1225–1231 (1978)

Iversen, L.L., Horn, A.S., Miller, R.J.: Structure-activity relationships for interactions of agonist and antagonist drugs with dopamine-stimulated adenylate cyclase of rat brain – a model for CNS dopamine receptors? In: Antipsychotic Drugs, Pharmacodynamics and Pharmacokinetics. Sedvall, G., Uvnäs, B., Zottermann, Y. (eds.). Oxford, New York: Pergamon 1976 a, pp. 285–303

Iversen, L.L., Rogawski, M.A., Miller, R.J.: Comparison of the effects of neuroleptic drugs on pre- and postsynaptic dopaminergic mechanisms in the rat striatum. Mol. Pharmacol. *12*, 251–262 (1976 b)

Janssen, P.A.J.: Structure-activity relationship (SAR) and drug design as illustrated with neuroleptic agents. In: International Encyclopedia of Pharmacology and Therapeutics. Peters, G. (ed.), Section 5: Structure Activity Relationship. Cavallito, C.J. (ed.). Oxford, New York: Pergamon 1973, pp. 37–73

Janssen, P.A.J., van Bever, W.F.M.: Advances in the research for improved neuroleptic drugs. In: Current Developments in Psychopharmacology. Essman, W.B., Valzelli, L. (eds.). New York: Spectrum 1975, Vol. 2, pp. 167–184

Janssen, P.A.J., Niemegeers, C.J.E., Schellekens, K.H.L.: Is it possible to predict the clinical effects of neuroleptic drugs from animal data? Part I: Neuroleptic activity spectra for rats. Arzneim. Forsch. *15*, 104–117 (1965)

Janssen, P.A.J., Niemegeers, C.J.E., Schellekens, K.H.L., Lenaerts, F.M.: An improved experimental design for measuring the inhibitory effects of neuroleptic drugs on amphetamine- or apomorphine-induced "chewing" and "agitation" in rats. Arzneim. Forsch. *17*, 841–854 (1967)

Jaunin, A., Petcher, T.J., Weber, H.P.: Conformations of some semi-rigid neuroleptic drugs. Part 2: Crystal structures of racemic and of (+)-(S)-octoclothepin{2-chloro-10,11-dihydro-11-(4-methylpiperazin-1-yl)dibenzo[b,f]thiepin} and the absolute configuration of the latter. J. Chem. Soc. [Perkin II] *1977*, 186–190

Jílek, J.O., Šindelář, K., Rajšner, M., Dlabač, A., Metyšová, J., Votava, Z., Pomykáček, J., Protiva, M.: Noncataleptic potential neuroleptics; 2-halogeno-10-piperazindibenzo[b,f]thiepins. Coll. Czech. Chem. Commun. *40*, 2887–2904 (1975)

Julou, L., Ducrot, R., Fouche, J.: Etude de quelques relations entre la structure chimique et l'activité neuroleptique. In: Convegno di Aggiornamento in Psicofarmacologia (Milano, 6–7 Nov. 1965). Atti Convegni Farmitalia. Torino: Edizione Minerva Medica 1966, pp. 20–54

Kaiser, C., Pavloff, A.M., Garvey, E., Fowler, P.J., Tedeschi, D.H., Zirkle, C.L.: Effects of structure upon neuropharmacological activity of some chlorpromazine analogs of the diphenylmethane type. J. Med. Chem. *15*, 665–673 (1972)

Kaiser, C., Fowler, P.J., Tedeschi, D.H., Lester, B.M., Garvey, E., Zirkle, C.L.: Synthesis and neuropharmacological activity of some piperidylidene derivatives of thioxanthenes, xanthenes, dibenzoxepines, and acridans. J. Med. Chem. *17*, 57–62 (1974a)

Kaiser, C., Warren, R.J., Zirkle, C.L.: Assignment of isomeric aminoalkylidene derivatives of xanthenes and thioxanthenes with neuropharmacological activity. J. Med. Chem. *17*, 131–133 (1974b)

Karobath, M.E.: Dopamin-Rezeptor-Blockade, ein möglicher Wirkungsmechanismus antipsychotisch wirksamer Pharmaka. Pharmakopsychatr. *8*, 151–161 (1975)

Koch, M.H.J.: The conformation of neuroleptic drugs. Mol. Pharmacol. *10*, 425–437 (1974)

Koch, M.H.J., Evrard, G.: 4-{2-(Methylthio)dibenzo[b,f]thiepin-11-yl}-1-piperazinylpropanol hemihydrate (oxyprothepine). Acta Cryst. *B 30*, 2925–2928 (1974)

Kopicová, Z., Metyšová, J., Protiva, M.: Neuroleptics with protracted action; 3-fluoro derivatives of methiothepin and oxyprothepin and their 2-fluoro analogues. Coll. Czech. Chem. Commun. *40*, 3519–3529 (1975)

Laduron, P.: Limiting factors in the antagonism of neuroleptics on dopamine-sensitive adenylate cyclase. J. Pharm. Pharmacol. *28*, 250–251 (1976)

Leysen, J.E., Gommeren, W., Laduron, P.M.: Spiperone: A ligand of choice for neuroleptic receptors. I. Kinetic and characteristics of in vitro binding. Biochem. Pharmacol. *27*, 307–316 (1978)

Lippmann, W., Pugsley, T., Merker, J.: Effect of butaclamol and its enantiomers upon striatal homovanillic acid and adenyl cyclase of olfactory tubercle in rats. Life Sci. *16*, 213–224 (1975)

McDowell, J.J.H.: The molecular structures of phenothiazine derivatives. Adv. Biochem. Psychopharmacol. *9*, 33–54 (1974)

Mercier, M.J., Dumont, P.A.: Influence of the electron-donating properties on the psychotropic activity of phenothiazine derivatives. J. Pharm. Pharmacol. *24*, 706–712 (1972)

Metyš, J., Metyšová, J.: Pharmacological properties of the potential neuroleptic drug perathiepine. II. Action on the autonomic nervous system and other pharmacological effects. Activ. Nerv. Sup. (Praha) *8*, 389–390 (1966)

Metyšová, J., Protiva, M.: Stereospecificity of neuroleptic effects in the 10-piperazino-10,11-dihydrodibenzo[b,f]thiepin series. Activitas nervosa superior (Praha) *17*, 218–219 (1975)

Michaelis, W., Gauch, R.: Intramolekulare Beweglichkeit eines Dibenzo[b,f]-1,4-thiazepin-5-oxids. Helv. Chim. Acta *52*, 2486–2491 (1969)

Miller, R.J., Horn, A.S., Iversen, L.L.: The action of neuroleptic drugs on dopamine-stimulated adenosine cyclic 3′,5′-monophosphate production in rat neostriatum and limbic forebrain. Mol. Pharmacol. *10*, 759–766 (1974)

Miller, R.J., Horn, A.S., Iversen, L.L.: Effect of butaclamol on dopamine-sensitive adenylate cyclase in the rat striatum. J. Pharm. Pharmacol. *27*, 212–213 (1975)

Miller, R.J., Hiley, C.R.: Anti-dopaminergic and anti-muscarinic effects of dibenzodiazepines. Naunyn-Schmiedebergs Arch. Pharmacol. *292*, 289–293 (1976)

Moereels, H., Tollenaere, J.P.: A comparison between the conformation of dexclamol and the tricyclic and butyrophenone type dopamine antagonists. Life Sci. *23*, 459–464 (1978)

Møller-Nielsen, I., Pedersen, V., Nymark, M., Frank, K.F., Boek, V., Fjalland, B., Christensen, A.V.: The comparative pharmacology of flupenthixol and some reference neuroleptics. Acta Pharmacol. Toxicol. *33*, 353–362 (1973)

Møller-Nielsen, I., Boek, V., Christensen, A.V., Danneskiold-Samsøe, P., Hyttel, J., Langeland, J., Pedersen, V., Svendsen, O.: The pharmacology of a new potent, long-acting neuroleptic, piflutixol. Acta Pharmacol. Toxicol. *41*, 369–383 (1977)

Muren, J.F., Bloom, B.M.: Thioxanthene psychopharmacological agents. I. 9-(3-Aminopropyl)-thioxanthene-2-sulfonamides. J. Med. Chem. *13*, 14–16 (1970)

Ögren, S.O., Hall, H., Köhler, C.: Studies on the stereoselective dopamine receptor blockade in the rat brain by rigid spiro amines. Life Sci. *23*, 1769–1774 (1978)

Pelz, K., Jirkovský, I., Adlerová, E., Metyšová, J., Protiva, M.: Über die in 8-Stellung durch die Methyl-, tert. Butyl-, Methoxy-, Methylthio- und Methansulfonylgruppe substituierten 10-(4-Methylpiperazino)-10,11-dihydrodibenzo[b,f]thiepin-Derivate. Coll. Czech. Chem. Commun. *33*, 1895–1910 (1968)

Petcher, T.J., Schmutz, J., Weber, H.P., White, T.G.: Chirality of (+)-octoclothepin, a stereospecific neuroleptic agent. Experientia *31*, 1389–1390 (1975)

Petcher, T.J., Weber, H.P.: Conformations of some semi-rigid neuroleptic drugs. Part 1: Crystal structures of loxapine, clozapine, and HUF-2046 monohydrate {2-chloro-11-(4-methylpiperazin-1-yl)dibenzo[b,f][1,4]oxazepine, 8-chloro-11-(4-methylpiperazin-1-yl)dibenzo-[b,e][1,4]diazepine, and 2-chloro-11-(4-methylpiperazin-1-yl)dibenzo[b,e][1,4]diazepine monohydrate}. J. Chem. Soc. [Perkin II] *1976*, 1415–1420

Petersen, P.V., Møller-Nielsen, I., Pedersen, V., Jørgensen, A., Lassen, N.: Thioxanthenes. In: Psychotherapeutic drugs, Part II. Usdin, E., Forrest, I.S. (eds.), pp. 827–867. New York, Basel: Dekker 1977

Posner, H.S., Hearst, E., Taylor, W.L., Cosmides, G.J.: Model metabolites of chlorpromazine and promazine: relative activities in some pharmacological and behavioral tests. J. Pharmacol. Exper. Therap. *137*, 84–90 (1962)

Pugsley, T.A., Lippmann, W.: Effects of chlorine substituents on the benzene rings of an analogue of the antipsychotic drug butaclamol on the interaction with dopamine and muscarinic receptors in rat brain. J. Pharm. Pharmacol. *31*, 47–49 (1979)

Pugsley, T.A., Merker, J., Lippmann, W.: Effect of structural analogs of butaclamol (a new antipsychotic drug) on striatal homovanillic acid and adenyl cyclase of olfactory tubercle in rats. Can. J. Physiol. Pharmacol. *54*, 510–515 (1976)

Rajšner, M., Metyšová, J., Svátek, E., Mikšík, F., Protiva, M.: 2- and 3-fluoro derivatives of clorotepin and related compounds; 6- and 7-fluoro derivatives of chlorprothixene. Coll. Czech. Chem. Commun. *40*, 719–737 (1975)

Reboul, J.-P., Cristau, B.: Analyse pharmacochimique des données fournies par la radiocristallographie des amines psychotropes polycycliques. I. Définition et calcul des paramètres conformationnels. Eur. J. Med. Chem. (Chim. Therap.) *12*, 71–75 (1977a)

Reboul, J.-P., Cristau, B.: Analyse pharmacochimique des données fournies par la radiocristallographie des amines psychotropes polycycliques. II. Confrontation des valeurs paramétriques. Eur. J. Med. Chem. (Chim. Therap.) *12*, 76–79 (1977b)

Reboul, J.P., Cristau, B.: Les amines psychotropes polycycliques «vues» par l'ordinateur. Annal. Pharm. Fr. *36*, 179–189 (1978)

Remy, D.C., Rittle, K.E., Hunt, C.A., Anderson, P.S., Arison, B.H., Engelhardt, E.L., Hirschmann, R., Clineschmidt, B.V., Lotti, V.J., Bunting, P.R., Ballentine, R.J., Papp, N.L., Flataker, L., Witoslawski, J.J., Stone, C.A.: Synthesis and stereospecific antipsychotic activity of (−)-1-cyclopropylmethyl-4-(3-trifluoromethylthio-5H-dibenzo[a,d]cyclohepten-5-ylidene)piperidine. J. Med. Chem. *20*, 1013–1019 (1977)

Robinson, S.E., Lotti, V.J., Sulser, F.: Cyanocyproheptadine: role of cholinolytic properties in modulating neuroleptic-induced elevation of striatal homovanillic acid (HVA). J. Pharm. Pharmacol. *29*, 564–566 (1977)

Rodgers, J.R., Horn, A.S., Kennard, O.: Antipsychotic phenothiazine drugs and the significance of the X-ray structure of promazine HCl. J. Pharm. Pharmacol. *28*, 246–247 (1976)

Roufogalis, B.D., Thornton, M., Wade, D.N.: Specificity of the dopamine-sensitive adenylate cyclase for antipsychotic antagonists. Life Sci. *19*, 927–934 (1976)

Sayers, A.C., Bürki, H.R., Ruch, W., Asper, H.: Anticholinergic properties of antipsychotic drugs and their relation to extrapyramidal side-effects. Psychopharmacol. *51*, 15–22 (1976)

Schmutz, J.: Absicht und Zufall in der Arzneimittelforschung, dargelegt am Beispiel der trizyklischen Psychopharmaka. Pharmacol. Acta Helv. *48*, 117–132 (1973)

Schmutz, J.: Neuroleptic piperazinyl-dibenzo-azepines. Chemistry and structure-activity relationships. Arzneim. Forsch. *25*, 712–720 (1975)

Schmutz, J., Hunziker, F., Stille, G., Lauener, H.: Constitution chimique et action pharmacologique d'un nouveau groupe de neuroleptiques tricycliques. Bull. Chim. Thérap. *1967*, 424–429

Seeman, P., Lee, T., Chau-Wong, M., Wong, K.: Antipsychotic drugs and neuroleptic/dopamine receptors. Nature *261*, 717–719 (1976)

Šindelář, K., Jílek, J.O., Metyšová, J., Pomykáček, J., Protiva, M.: 2- and 3-hydroxy derivatives of 8-chloro-10-(4-methylpiperazino)-10,11-dihydrodibenzo[b,f]thiepin and their methyl ethers. Coll. Czech. Chem. Commun. *39*, 3548–3559 (1974)

Šindelář, K., Dlabač, A., Kakáč, B., Svátek, E., Holubek, J., Šedivý, Z., Princová, E., Protiva, M.: Noncataleptic potential neuroleptics; 2-acetamido, 2-amino and 2-acetyl derivatives of 10-(4-methylpiperazino)-10,11-dihydrodibenzo[b,f]thiepin. Coll. Czech. Chem. Commun. *40*, 2649–2666 (1975a)

Šindelář, K., Dlabac, A., Metyšová, J., Kakáč, B., Holubek, J., Svátek, E., Šedivý, Z., Protiva, M.: Potential antipsychotics: 2-methoxy-, 2-methylthio-, 2-dimethylsulfamoyl- and 2-trifluoromethyl-10-piperazinodibenzo[b,f]thiepins. Coll. Czech. Chem. Commun. *40*, 1940–1959 (1975b)

Šindelář, K., Metyšová, J., Holubek, J., Šedivý, Z., Protiva, M.: Potential oral neuroleptics with protracted action; 8-chloro-3,7-difluoro-10-(4-methylpiperazino)-10,11-dihydrodibenzo[b,f]thiepin and further 3,7-substituted octoclothepin and dehydroclothepin derivatives. Coll. Czech. Chem. Commun. *42*, 1179–1199 (1977)

Snyder, S.H., Greenberg, D., Yamamura, H.I.: Antischizophrenic drugs and brain cholinergic receptors. Arch. Gen. Psychiatr. *31*, 58–61 (1974)

Stille, G., Lauener, H., Eichenberger, E.: The pharmacology of 8-chloro-11-(4-methyl-1-piperazinyl)-5H-dibenzo[b,e][1,4]diazepine (clozapine). Farmaco. [Prat.] *26*, 603–625 (1971)

Ternay, L.A., Evans, S.A.: Stereochemistry and conformational preferences of meso-alkylated thioxanthenes by proton magnetic resonance spectroscopy. J. Org. Chem. *39*, 2941–2946 (1974)

Tollenaere, J.P., Moereels, H., Protiva, M.: Quantitative structure activity relationship (QSAR) in a series of neuroleptic 10-piperazino-dibenzo[b,f]thiepins, ataxia in mice. Eur. J. Med. Chem. (Chim. Therap.) *11*, 293–298 (1976)

Tollenaere, J.P., Moereels, H., Koch, M.H.J.: On the conformation of neuroleptic drugs in the three aggregation states and their conformational resemblance to dopamine. Eur. J. Med. Chem. (Chim. Therap.) *12*, 199–211 (1977)

Ueda, I., Sato, Y., Maeno, S., Umio, S.: Synthesis and pharmacological properties of 8-chloro-10-(2-dimethylamino-ethoxy)dibenz[b,f]thiepin and related compounds. Neurotropic and psychotropic agents III. Chem. Pharm. Bull. (Tokyo) *26*, 3058–3070 (1978)

Voith, K., Cummings, J.R.: Behavioral studies on the enantiomers of butaclamol demonstrating absolute optical specificity for neuroleptic activity. Can. J. Physiol. Pharmacol. *54*, 551–560 (1976)

Voith, K., Bruderlein, F.T., Humber, L.G.: Neuroleptics related to butaclamol. Synthesis and some psychopharmacological effects of a series of 3-aryl analogues. J. Med. Chem. *21*, 694–698 (1978)

Watzman, N., Manian, A.A., Barry, H., Buckley, J.P.: Comparative effects of chlorpromazine hydrochloride and quaternary chlorpromazine hydrochloride on the central nervous systems of rats and mice. J. Pharm. Sci. *57*, 2089–2093 (1968)

Wilhelm, M., Kuhn, R.: Versuch einer stereochemisch-strukturellen Klassifizierung der Trizyklus-Psychopharmaka mit Einschluß der Dibenzobicyclooctadine. Pharmakopsychiatr. Neuropsychopharmakol. *3*, 317–332 (1970)

Yale, H.L.: The long-acting neuroleptics: A retrospective appraisal. Drug Metab. Rev. *8*, 251–262 (1978)

Yale, H.L., Beer, B., Pluscec, J., Spitzmiller, E.R.: Novel polycyclic heterocycles. Derivatives of 5,11-dihydrodibenz[b,e][1,4]oxazepine and 5,11-dihydrodibenzo[b,e][1,4]thiazepine. J. Med. Chem. *13*, 713–722 (1970)

Zirkle, C.L., Kaiser, C.: Antipsychotic agents (tricyclic). In: Psychopharmacological Agents. Gordon, M. (ed.). New York: Academic Press 1974, Vol. 3, pp. 39–128

CHAPTER 2

Butyrophenones and Diphenylbutylpiperidines

P.A.J. Janssen and W.F.M. van Bever

A. Introduction

The butyrophenones were discovered in 1957 as a result of a systematic investigation of structure–activity relationships of a series of propiophenones derived from norpethidine. At that time, our laboratory was using a simple screening procedure in mice, consisting of measurement of mydriatic activity (MD_{50}) (Jageneau and Janssen, 1956), the hot plate test for analgesic activity (AD_{50}) (Janssen and Eddy, 1960), and observation of gross behavioral effects. With this screening technique, morphine-like analgesics, characterized by MD_{50}/AD_{50} ratios not significantly different from unity, could easily be distinguished from chlorpromazine-like neuroleptics, characterized by MD_{50}/AD_{50} ratios considerably greater than unity.

The sequence of molecular modifications leading to the synthesis of haloperidol is summarized in Table 1. Ethyl 1-(3-oxo-3-phenylpropyl)-4-phenyl-4-piperidinecarboxylate (R 951), obtained by Mannich reaction from acetophenone and norpethidine, was found to be a morphine-like compound about 30 times more potent than pethidine. This interesting result encouraged further molecular manipulation, in-

Table 1. Sequence of molecular modifications leading to the development of the butyrophenones

$$A-\text{\textcircled{}}-CO-(CH_2)_n-N\text{\textless}\substack{B \\ C}$$

Serial number	Generic name	n	A	B	C	Morphine-like	Chlorpromazine-like	MD_{50}/AD_{50}[a]
R 951		2	H	COOEt	H	+ + +	0	1.7
R 1187		3	H	COOEt	H	+ +	+	5.7
R 1472		3	H	OH	H	0	+ +	>18
R 1589	Peridol	3	F	OH	H	0	+ + +	>35
R 1625	Haloperidol	3	F	OH	Cl	0	+ + + +	>71
	Morphine					+ +	0	1.3
	Chlorpromazine					0	+ +	>21

[a] Ratio of the median effective dose level "mydriatic activity" over the median effective dose level in the "hot plate test" in mice after sc administration

cluding lengthening of the side chain with one methylene unit. Surprisingly, the corresponding butyrophenone, R 1187, possessed mixed analgesic–neuroleptic activity. Furthermore, replacement of the 4-ethoxycarbonyl substituent of R 1187 by an hydroxyl group led to R 1472, which was completely devoid of morphine-like effects and almost indistinguishable from chlorpromazine in its pharmacologicl profile. Continued studies soon showed that introduction of appropriate aromatic substituents strikingly increased the neuroleptic potency of R 1472. Thus, introduction of a 4-fluoro substituent in the phenyl ring of the side chain gave rise to peridol (R 1589) and 4-chloro substitution of the phenyl ring attached to the piperidine ring of peridol led in 1958 to the synthesis of haloperidol (R 1625).

Subsequent pharmacologic (JANSSEN and NIEMEGEERS, 1959; JANSSEN et al., 1960 a, b) and clinical (DELAY et al., 1960; DIVRY et al., 1960 a) investigation of haloperidol, revealing it to be the most potent neuroleptic known at that time, has triggered major research efforts in many laboratories as reflected by numerous the patents which have been applied for and granted, and by a daily increasing number of publications dealing with known or newly synthesized butyrophenones. Reviews of the advances in the butyrophenones have been published regularly (JANSSEN, 1961, 1962, 1964, 1965, 1967 a, 1970 a, 1974; JANSSEN and VAN BEVER, 1977).

Five years after the synthesis of haloperidol, the diphenylbutylpiperidines were developed as a result of continued chemical modification of the keto function of the butyrophenone side chain. Pimozide (JANSSEN et al., 1968), the first representative of this series, is in fact a derivative of the butyrophenone, benperidol, in which the keto function is replaced by a 4-fluorophenylmethine moiety. As a group, the diphenylbutylpiperidines are characterized by their long duration of action, excellent oral activity, virtual absence of sedative and autonomic side effects, and a very low and transient incidence of neurological side effects when dosed appropriately. Owing to this particular activity profile, the diphenylbutylpiperidines are excellently suited for maintenance therapy. Today, four diphenylbutylpiperidines have been clinically investigated and three of them are currently used as drugs in human medicine. Advances in the diphenylbutylpiperidines have been reviewed regularly (JANSSEN, 1971, 1974; JANSSEN and VAN BEVER, 1977; VILLENEUVE and BORDELEAU, 1974).

For butyrophenones, diphenylbutylpiperidines, and structurally related compounds which are not explicitly mentioned in this chapter the reader is referred to other recent reviews (GSCHWEND, 1974; HOFFMANN and RUSHIG, 1972; JANSSEN, 1966, 1970 b, 1973; JANSSEN and VAN BEVER, 1975; PROTIVA, 1970; ZIRCLE and KAISER, 1970).

B. Structure-Activity Relationships

I. Chemistry

Owing to the large number of butyrophenones and diphenylbutylpiperidines that have been reported, particularly in patent literature, this discussion will be limited to the most relevant structural requirements as exemplified by 10 important butyrophenones and four diphenylbutylpiperidines. Their chemical structures are shown in Fig. 1 together with chlorpromazine as reference compound. The structures in Fig. 1 are drawn in a topographical fashion in order to demonstrate obvious structural simi-

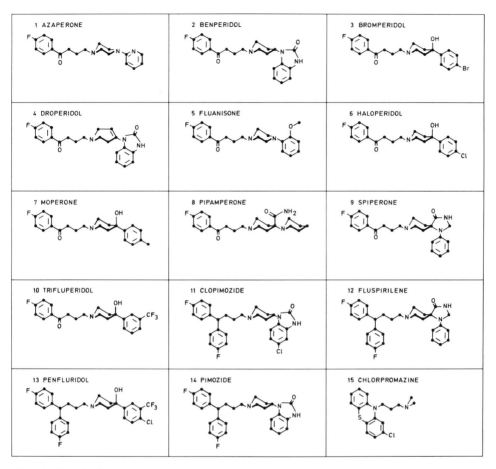

Fig. 1. Chemical structure of 10 butyrophenones, four diphenylbutylpiperidines and chlorpromazine

larities. All neuroleptics shown are tertiary amines. Butyrophenones have a 4-fluorobenzoyl moiety and diphenylbutylpiperidines have a bis-(4-fluorophenyl)methyl portion both linked by a straight unbranched propylene chain to the nitrogen atom of a 4-substituted piperidine ring or more exceptionally of a 4-substituted piperazine ring. The more potent butyrophenones are derived from 4-hydroxy-4-phenyl-piperidine or from 4-anilinopiperidine.

Structural formulas drawn topographically in Fig. 1 do not represent the preferred conformations shown in Fig. 2 for azaperone, benperidol, fluanisone, haloperidol, pipamperone, spiperone, clopimozide, and penfluridol in the solid state as derived from X-ray diffraction data. Conformational analysis of butyrophenones and diphenylbutylpiperidines has revealed their extremely flexible nature (KOCH, 1974; TOLLENAERE et al., 1977). As a direct consequence of the observed conformational flexibility it follows that conformation should be studied in several aggregation states since the actual shape of the molecule when bound to its receptor site is not necessarily re-

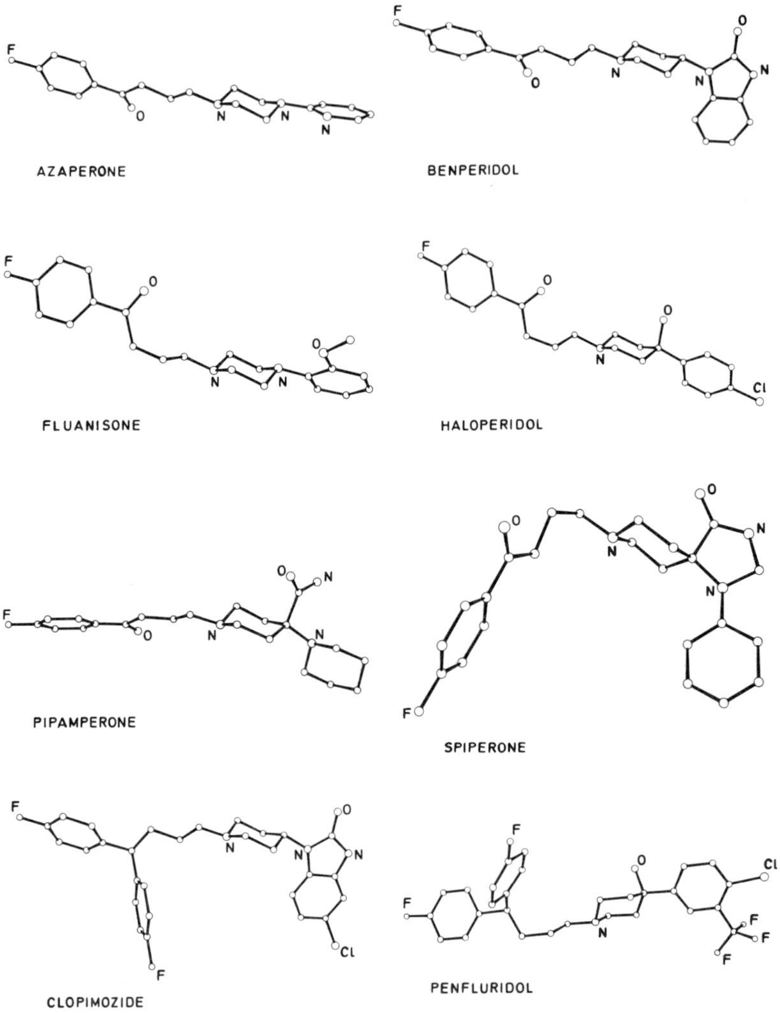

Fig. 2. Crystal structures of six butyrophenones and two diphenylbutylpiperidines

flected by one preferred conformation in one particular aggregation state nor even necessarily by any preferred conformation. However, within the limits of conformational flexibility, imposed by the molecular framework itself, the following general rules
can be stated: (1) All butyrophenones and diphenylbutylpiperidines are characterized
by a more or less fully extended side chain. (2) The more potent compounds possess
a planar aromatic ring attached to the 4-position of the piperidine (or piperazine) ring
and capable of orienting itself perpendicular to the mean plane of this piperidine (or
piperazine) ring. (3) The most potent compounds possess a hydrogen-bond-donating
moiety attached to the 4-position of the piperidine (or piperazine) ring oriented, with
respect to the mean plane of the piperidine (or piperazine) ring, toward the side opposite that of the lone pair of the basic nitrogen.

From a physicochemical point of view, all butyrophenones and diphenylbutyl-piperidines have a number of common properties: (1) They are all lipophilic compounds. Diphenylbutylpiperidines are significantly more lipophilic than the corresponding butyrophenones which probably explains their longer duration of action. (2) Their pK_a values and dipole moments range within the same order of magnitude. (3) All butyrophenones and diphenylbutylpiperidines are tensioactive compounds, capable of lowering surface tension in proportion to their neuroleptic potency (JANS-SEN, 1965).

II. Pharmacology

All butyrophenones and diphenylbutylpiperidines discussed in this section are very effective inhibitors of amphetamine- or apomorphine-induced stereotypies in rats and of apomorphine-induced emesis in dogs. At dose levels not significantly affecting gross behavior, they are specific inhibitors of conditioned operant behavior and of intracranial selfstimulation in most common laboratory animals. At more elevated dose levels they induce a typical state of catalepsy. At progressively higher doses, they induce palpebral ptosis, inhibit epinephrine – or norepinephrine – induced mortility, and finally prostration and other symptoms of CNS-depression.

It follows from the above that a discussion of "neuroleptic activity" cannot be adequately presented in terms of one experimental test procedure but should be defined in terms of a "neuroleptic activity profile" which allows meaningful predictions about such aspects of clinical efficacy as potency, onset and duration of action, oral versus parenteral efficacy, side effect liability etc. (JANSSEN et al., 1965a, b, 1966, 1967; NIE-MEGEERS, 1974). Although numerous experimental animal test models have been described for assaying the different aspects of neuroleptic activity, a few selected test systems are sufficient to define a major proportion (80–90%) of the neuroleptic activity profile as evidenced by principal component analysis and spectral mapping of existing pharmacologic and clinical data (LEWI, 1976a, b; LEWI et al., 1976). Such a set of comparative pharmacologic data in a few selected assays is summarized in Table 2 which lists ED_{50} values at the time of peak effect for amphetamine antagonism (AM), norepinephrine antagonism (NE), catalepsy (CA), and palpebral ptosis (PP) tests in rats and for apomorphine antagonism (AP) and jumpig box (JB) tests in dogs. General experimental procedures common to these tests (JANSSEN et al., 1963a, 1965a, b, 1966, 1967; NIEMEGEERS, 1974) and the detailed pharmacology of azaperone (NIEMEGEERS et al., 1974), benperidol (JANSSEN et al., 1965a, b), bromperidol (NIEMEGEERS and JANSSEN, 1974), droperidol (JANSSEN et al., 1963b), fluanisone (JANSSEN, 1961), haloperidol (JANSSEN, 1967b), moperone (JANSSEN, 1961), pipamperone (JANSSEN, 1961), spiperone (JANSSEN et al., 1965a, b), trifluperidol (JANSSEN, 1961), clopimozide (JANS-SEN et al., 1975), fluspirilene (JANSSEN et al., 1970a), penfluridol (JANSSEN et al., 1970b) and pimozide (JANSSEN et al., 1968) have been published earlier.

Visualization of the relative positioning of compounds (ratio concept) becomes difficult if one has to take into account more than two assays. A very useful aid to overcome this difficulty is the spectral mapping technique (LEWI, 1976a). This is illustrated in Fig. 3 for a combination of three assays (AM, NE, and PP). Characteristic of this technique is the separation of relative potencies from the activity spectra. The relative potencies are indicated by the magnitude of the circles identifying the respec-

Table 2

Generic name	Rat (sc) ED$_{50}$ [a]				Dog (sc) ED$_{50}$ [a]				Dog (po) ED$_{50}$ [a]			
	AM [b]	NE [c]	CA [d]	PP [e]	AP [f]	peak [g]	dura-tion [h]	JB [i]	AP [f]	peak [g]	dura-tion [h]	JB [i]
1. Azaperone	2.5	0.33	8.0	1.5	0.98	0.4	5.1	5.6	–	–	–	3.9
2. Benperidol	0.012	0.30	0.18	1.2	0.00052	2.4	8.4	0.0052	0.0014	2.8	8.2	0.0070
3. Bromperidol	0.053	7.2	0.12	1.7	0.018	0.6	20	0.040	0.033	6.4	31	0.080
4. Droperidol	0.023	0.10	0.38	0.38	0.0010	1	3.9	0.0090	0.0037	1.2	3.3	0.025
5. Fluanisone	0.20	0.10	2.0	0.65	0.070	0.3	2.3	0.31	1.2	0.5	6.7	1.3
6. Haloperidol	0.038	2.1	0.18	1.0	0.018	0.7	15	0.063	0.029	3.4	19	0.099
7. Moperone	0.030	1.5	0.80	2.3	0.020	0.7	6.3	0.040	0.25	1	6.2	0.29
8. Pipamperone	2.5	3.0	17	2.7	0.97	0.4	7.8	3.4	1.5	2.1	8.4	2.3
9. Spiperone	0.020	1.0	0.036	0.27	0.00024	4.4	12	0.0044	0.0014	4.2	9.2	0.015
10. Trifluperidol	0.025	0.30	0.13	0.34	0.053	1.3	6.8	0.058	0.066	1.8	9.1	0.16
11. Clopimozide	0.085 [j]	> 5 [j]	0.50 [j]	≧ 5 [j]	–	–	–	–	0.0049	31	144	0.19
12. Fluspirilene	0.31 [k]	>80 [k]	1.1 [k]	> 12 [k]	0.011 [k]	24 [k]	146 [k]	0.42 [k]	–	–	–	–
13. Penfluridol	0.45 [j]	6.2 [j]	0.95 [j]	36 [j]	–	–	–	–	0.023	24	165	0.17
14. Pimozide	0.10	40	0.18	4.5	0.011	4.2	22	0.091	0.017	4.2	21	0.18
15. Chlorpromazine	0.60	0.60	2.3	2.3	0.71	0.9	7.6	2.1	–	–	–	4.6

[a] In mg/kg, [b] Amphetamine antagonism, [c] Norepinephrine antagonism, [d] Catalepsy, [e] Palpebral ptosis, [f] Apomorphine antagonism, [g] Time of peak effect in hours, [h] Duration of action in hours of a dose corresponding to four times the lowest ED$_{50}$ value, [i] Jumping box, [j] Administration per os, [k] Intramuscular injection.

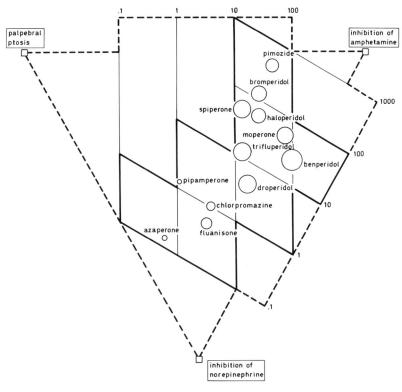

Fig. 3. Relative positioning of 10 butyrophenones, pimozide, and chlorpromazine by spectral mapping (LEWI, 1976a) for a combination of three assays (amphetamine antagonism, norepinephrine antagonism and palpebral ptosis) in rats. The relative potencies are reflected by the magnitude of the circles

tive compound. Thus, the most potent compound, benperidol, is indicated by the largest circle and is positioned according to the ratios NE/AM = 25, PP/AM = 100 and PP/NE = 4.

Without entering into detailed analysis of the data in Table 2, it can be briefly shown how these data allow predictions about clinical efficacy. One major difference between neuroleptics is potency and duration of action. The dose needed to produce a specific antipsychotic effect can vary tremendously. Although a specific animal test model of human psychosis does not exist, it has been observed that inhibition of amphetamine-induced stereotyped behavior correlates well with antipsychotic efficacy in humans. Neuroleptics that are very potent in the amphetamine antagonism test are also very potent antipsychotics in humans. Benperidol and spiperone, both very active in the amphetamine antagonism test are by far the most potent neuroleptics used in medical practice. The results in the amphetamine antagonism test correlate very well with those of the apomorphine antagonism test, inhibition of conditioned operant behavior (jumping box, Sidman avoidance, etc.), and inhibition of intracranial self-stimulation. Obviously, any of these tests can be used equally well to predict antipsychotic activity in humans.

Apomorphine-induced antagonism of emesis in dogs serves as a useful predictor for duration of action. For comparative purposes, the duration of action of a dose corresponding to four times the lowest ED_{50} value in the apomorphine antagonism test in dogs is given in Table 2. Long duration of action is a particular characteristic of the diphenylbutylpiperidines. Single oral doses of clopimozide and penfluridol or a single intramuscular dose of fluspirilene are active during one week.

Oral versus parenteral activity is another important factor to consider. Indeed, neuroleptics that are poorly absorbed in the gastro-intestinal tract are very likely to produce erratic clinical effects when given orally. Oral effectiveness ratios (OER) such as ED_{50} JBpo/ED_{50} JBsc or ED_{50} APpo/ED_{50} APsc can be used as a measure of gastro-intestinal absorption which is (1) excellent (OER ≤ 2) for azaperone, benperidol, bromperidol, haloperidol, pipamperone, clopimozide, penfluridol, and pimozide, (2) reasonable ($2 < OER \leq 4$) for droperidol, spiperone, trifluperidol, and chlorpromazine, and (3) poor (OER > 4) for fluanisone and moperone.

Side effect liability constitutes another difference among neuroleptics. Autonomic, sedative, and neurological effects are the three most commonly occuring side effects which can be a serious drawback for clinical use. Orthostatic hypotension, tachycardia, and other symptoms of autonomic blockade are unwanted side effects caused by the adrenolytic activity component of neuroleptics. The ratio of norepinephrine antagonism over amphetamine antagonism (NE/AM) can be used as an effective measure for the relative adrenolytic versus antipsychotic activity. Neuroleptics with low NE/AM possess a high potential for autonomic side effects, while compounds with a high NE/AM are relatively free of autonomic side effects. On the basis of the data in Table 1, autonomic side effects are predicted to be (1) a major problem (NE/AM ≤ 1) with azaperone, fluanisone, and chlorpromazine (2) a problem ($1 < $NE/AM ≤ 4) with pipamperone, (3) a minor problem ($4 < $NE/AM ≤ 16) with droperidol, trifluperidol and penfluridol, (4) a neglectable problem ($16 < $NE/AM ≤ 64) with benperidol, haloperidol, moperone, and spiperone, and (5) no problem at all (NE/AM > 64) with bromperidol, clopimozide, fluspirilene, and pimozide.

Oversedation, somnolence and hypokinesia are sometimes useful as they facilitate nursing, but more often a drawback as they impair intellectual and psychomotor skills. Sedative side effects can be effectively predicted with the ratio of palpebral ptosis over catalepsy (PP/CA). On the basis of the data in Table 2, it can be predicted that sedative side effects will occur (1) overwhelmingly (PP/CA < 1) with azaperone, fluanisone, and pipamperone, (2) frequently ($1 \leq $PP/CA < 2) with droperidol and chlorpromazine, (3) occasionally ($2 \leq $PP/CA < 4) with moperone and trifluperidol, (4) rarely ($4 \leq $PP/CA < 16) with benperidol, bromperidol, haloperidol, spiperone and clopimozide, and (5) virtually never (PP/CA ≥ 16) with fluspirilene, penfluridol and pimozide.

Extrapyramidal side effects such as akathisia, muscular rigidity, and tremor are more difficult to avoid. The ratio of the jumping box test over the apomorphine antagonism test (JB/AP), which can be used as an index for the relative neurological versus antipsychotic activity, varies between much narrower limits than the NE/AM and PP/CA ratios. Nevertheless, careful dosage control, taking into account JB/AP ratio and duration of activity (NIEMEGEERS, 1974), allows the choice of optimal daily dose regimens without producing neurological side effects.

III. Clinical Aspects

1. Butyrophenones

All butyrophenones discussed in this chapter, with the exception of bromperidol, presently undergoing extensive clinical investigation, are currently used in human and veterinary medicine. A few selected references are cited at the end of each paragraph.

a. Azaperone, exclusively used in veterinary practice, is a tranquillizer of choice in pigs and a variety of wild animals owing to its pronounced anti-aggresive effects (CALLEAR and VAN GESTEL, 1971; DEVLOO et al., 1972; SYMOENS and VAN DEN BRANDE, 1969).

b. Benperidol, a well-tolerated neuroleptic about eight times more potent than haloperidol, possesses pronounced antipsychotic effects in both acute and chronic psychotic patients. Owing the hypnotic and akinetic properties, it tends to improve sleep. An interesting indication is the inhibition of craving towards sexual behavior which the patient considers to be aberrant (BOBON, et al., 1962; FIELD, 1973; SCHWARZ, 1966; TENNENT et al., 1974).

c. Bromperidol is very similar to haloperidol *(vide infra)* but has a somewhat longer duration of action (AYD, 1975).

d. Droperidol is a potent, short-acting, well-tolerated neuroleptic drug with pronounced antishock and antiemetic properties. A single parenteral dose of 5–20 mg rapidly produces a state of tranquility without loss of consciousness; environment-induced anxiety disappears and the patient remains cooperative. In anesthesiology, droperidol is often used in combination with fentanyl. It is extremely effective against cardiac, traumatic, and hemorrhagic shock, both prophylactically and therapeutically. Other useful indications are its fast action in acutely agitated patients and its ability to almost immediately stop a typical attack of Menière's disease. In veterinary practice droperidol is effectively used as tranquillizer for monkeys and dogs (BOBON et al., 1968; NEFF et al., 1972; VAN LEEUWEN et al., 1977; WEISER, 1973).

e. Fluanisone resembles chlorpromazine and is characterized by a rapid onset but short duration of action. It is inferior to haloperidol against hallucinations and delirious episodes. Owing to its more sedative properties, it is often a useful adjunct to haloperidol therapy in oligophrenics. Particular indications are the treatment of senile agitation and mental retardation associated with impulsive and aggressive behavior both in children and adults. In veterinary practice, fluanisone is useful as a specific tranquillizer in poultry (DEBERDT, 1960; ISRAEL et al., 1967; PAQUAY et al., 1960; VILLA and PASINI, 1966).

f. Haloperidol is the most widely used butyrophenone. It is particularly useful in the treatment of psychomotor agitation, hallucinations, manic symptoms, paranoid ideation, aggresive and impulsive tendencies in psychopaths, choreic movements and tics, certain forms of anxiety and insomnia, nausea, vomiting, and hiccups. Besides its main use in psychiatry, haloperidol is also increasingly used in neurology, anesthesiology, radiotherapy, internal medicine, particularly in gastroenterology and obstetrics, as well as in veterinary practice. Recently haloperidol has been shown to be an effective inhibitor of drug craving and withdrawal symptoms in addicts. The most recent development is the use of high dose levels of haloperidol or so-called adequate individual dosage (AID) owing to a general tendency in psychiatry to abandon polypharmacy (drug cocktails) (AYD, 1972; GILLIS, 1977; PAQUAY et al.,1959; PLATH,1976).

g. Moperone is less potent than haloperidol and has a shorter duration of action. It is more effective against hallucinations than psychomotor agitation. When given on a *t.i.d.* schedule for maintenance therapy, it is surprisingly free of side effects and tends often to improve social contact in withdrawn and chronic underactive patients (Angst and Poldinger, 1963; Jones et al., 1970; Uytterschaut and Jacobs, 1962; Weiser, 1968).

h. Pipamperone is characterized by a peculiar pharmacologic profile and is also clinically different from known neuroleptics both in its effects and side effects. It has good hallucinolytic activity and remarkable resocializing effects in chronic delusions. It is inactive against mania and melancholia. Pipamperone normalizes mood and disturbed sleep patterns and has unexpected antianxiety effects in neurotics. It is particularly indicated in the treatment of psychopathic syndromes such as aggressive, destructive, explosive, and bellingerent behavior in both juvenile and adult delinquents (Ansoms et al., 1977; Auhagen and Breede, 1972; Bobon et al., 1961; Van Renynghe De Voxvrie and De Bie, 1976).

i. Spiperone is together with benperidol by far the most potent neuroleptic used in medical practice. Active daily maintenance doses range from 0.05 mg per adult upwards. Both benperidol and spiperone are beneficial in the treatment of alcoholic withdrawal. The therapeutic effectiveness of spiperone in many drug resistant chronic schizophrenics is quite striking (Bobon et al., 1963; Haase et al., 1964; Paquay et al., 1965).

j. Trifluperidol is about two to three times more potent than haloperidol to which it resembles in many respects. Withdrawn autistic schizophrenics generally derive more therapeutic benifit from trifluperidol than from haloperidol, whereas the latter drug is superior in the treatment of psychomotor agitation (Campbell et al., 1972; Divry et al., 1960b; Gross and Kaltenbäck, 1966; Sim et al., 1971).

2. Diphenylbutylpiperidines

Fluspirilene, penfluridol, and pimozide are currently used in human medicine. Clopimozide is presently undergoing clinical investigation. On June 1, 1977, three clinical investigations were published of clopimozide, 116 of fluspirilene, 133 of penfluridol, and 292 of pimozide. A few selected references are given at the end of each paragraph.

a. Clopimozide is qualitatively very similar to pimozide (vide infra) but has a considerably longer duration of action. A single oral dose is effective for one week. Clopimozide appears to possess unique reactivating properties (Bobon et al., 1976; Knapen et al., 1976).

b. Fluspirilene is an injectable neuroleptic with potent antihallucinatory, antidelusional and anti-autistic effects. A single intramuscular dose being effective for one week, it is mainly indicated for maintenance therapy, especially in ambutatory patients which are reluctant to continue or tempted to discontinue oral medication. Low dose levels of fluspirilene have a tranquillizing effect, providing mood-elevation, emotional stabilization and general reactivation (Cottrell and Magnus, 1973; Haase et al., 1968; Tanghe, 1976; Waniek and Pach, 1974).

c. Penfluridol is an orally effective neuroleptic particularly indicated for productive psychotic symptoms and autism. A single oral dose is effective for one week producing almost no sedative or autonomic side effects and only a few transient extrapyramidal side effects. Penfluridol is clearly indicated for maintenance therapy of hospitalized and ambulatory patients with schizophrenic and paranoid symptomatology, disturbed character and behavioral disorders (BOBON et al., 1970; CHOUINARD et al., 1977; GALLANT et al., 1974; MELLIEN, 1976).

d. Pimozide is a highly specific neuroleptic effective against productive psychotic symptoms such as hallucinations, delusions, bizarre mannierism, and autism. A single oral dose is effective for 24 h. Pimozide increases the patient's self-criticism and insight into his disease. As the other diphenylbutylpiperidines, pimozide is mostly used in maintenance therapy. It is also useful in the treatment of patients suffering from stress-related emotional lability (BRUGMANS, 1968; KLINE et al., 1977; WETZELS 1977 a, b; ZICK, 1969).

C. Conclusion

All potent butyrophenones and diphenylbutylpiperidines possess a strinkingly similar chemical structure, a similar conformation and similar physicochemical properties. From a pharmacologic and a clinical point of view, they share a great deal of common properties and differ only in potency, duration of action, and relative specificity of action. Clearly all these similarities suggest a common basic mechanism of action. An overwhelming amount of evidence supports the concept that neuroleptics exert their antipsychotic activity by dopamine receptor blockade in well-confined dopaminergic regions of the brain. Yet, the exact mechanism(s) remain(s) uncertain.

A clinical effective antipsychotic dose level of a highly potent and specific neuroleptic is characterized by specific distribution within the brain and high affinity specific binding to saturable receptor sites. Low dose levels of less specific neuroleptics or higher dose levels of specific neuroleptics show progressively more and more low affinity aspecific binding, at which point a variety of central and peripheral receptor sites are being occupied. A better understanding of the phenomena governing specific distribution and binding on the one hand and of the causes underlying schizophrenia on the other hand will undoubtedly lead to the development of yet more specific neuroleptic drugs and most likely to neuroleptics with profiles adapted to more particular aspects of the complex syndrome of schizophrenia.

References

Angst, J., Poldinger, W.: Clinical experiences with the butyrophenone derivative methylperidon (Lutraven) a comparative contribution to the methodology of pharmacopsychiatric investigations. Praxis *44*, 1348–1354 (1963)

Ansoms, G., De Backer-Dierick, G., Vereecken, J.L.T.M.: Sleep disorders in patients with severe mental depression: double-blind placebo-controlled evaluation of the value of pipamperone (Dipiperon). Acta Psychiatr. Scand. *55*, 116–122 (1977)

Auhagen, U., Breede, G.: Dipiperon bei kindlichen Verhaltensstörungen. Acta Psychiatr. Scand. *48*, 510–532 (1972)

Ayd, F.J.: Haloperidol: Fifteen years of clinical experience. Dis. Nerv. Syst. *33*, 459–469 (1972)

Ayd, F.J.: Bromperidol: a new potent, long acting neuroleptic. Int. Drug. Ther. Newsletter *10*, 25–28 (1975)

Bobon, J., Collard, J., Demaret, A.: Un nouveau neuroleptique à effect hypnogène différé: le dipipéron (R 3345); butyrophènone carbamidée. Acta Neurol. Belg. *61*, 611–630 (1961)

Bobon, J., Collard, J., Pinchard, A.: Un neuroleptique à effets hypnique et akinétique prépondérants: le benzpéridol (R 4584), 8° butyrophénone. Acta Neurol. Beleg. 62, 566–576 (1962)

Bobon, J., Collard, J., Delree, Ch., Gernay, J.M.: Spiroperidol. Acta Neurol. Belg. 63, 991–1003 (1963)

Bobon, J., Bobon, D.P., Breulet, M., Colinet, M., Devroye, A., Korn, M., Pinchard, A.: Un traitement d'urgence de l'agitation: le droperidol (R 4749). Acta Neurol. Belg. 68, 103–115 (1968)

Bobon, J., Melon, J., Mormont, C., Dufrasne, M., Pinchard, A.: Neuroleptiques à longue durée d'action. III. Etude pilote du penfluridol (R 16341). Acta Psychiatr. Belg. 70, 523–551 (1970)

Bobon, J., Parent, M., Toussaint, C., Pinchard, A.: Neuroleptiques à longue durée d'action. IV. Etude préliminaire du clopimozide (R 29764). Acta Psychiatr. Belg. 76, 138–148 (1976)

Brugmans, J.: A multicentric clinical evaluation of pimozide. Acta Neurol. Belg. 68, 875–887 (1968)

Callear, J.F.F., Van Gestel, J.F.E.: An analysis of the results of field experiments in pigs in the U.K. and Ireland with the sedative neuroleptic azaperone. Vet. Rec. 89, 453–458 (1971)

Campbell, M., Fish, E., Shapiro, T., Floyd, A.: Acute responses of schizophrenic children to a sedative and a "stimulating" neuroleptic: a pharmacologic yardstick. Curr. Ther. Res. 14, 759–766 (1972)

Chouinard, G., Annable, L., Kolivakis, T.N.L.: Penfluridol in the maintenance treatment of schizophrenic patients newly discharged from a brief therapy unit. J. Clin. Pharmacol. 162–167 (1977)

Cottrell, W.M., Magnus, R.V.: Fluspirilene in schizophrenia. J. Int. Med. Res. 1, 630–633 (1973)

Deberdt, R.: Expérimentation clinique et études „double blind" du R 2028 en psychiatrie. Acta Neurol. Belg. 60, 663–676 (1960)

Delay, J., Pichat, P., Lemperiere, T., Elisalde, B.: Halopéridol et chimiothérapie des psychoses. Presse Médicale 68, 1353–1355 (1960)

Devloo, S., Geerts, H., Symoens, J.: Einfluß von Azaperon auf Mortalität und Fleischqualität nach dem Transport von Schlachtschweinen. Tierärztl. Umschau, 302–318 (1972)

Divry, P., Bobon, J., Collard, J.: Rapport sur l'activité neuro-psychopharmacologique du halopéridol (R 1625). Acta Neurol. Belg. 60, 7–9 (1960a)

Divry, P., Bobon, J., Collard, J., Demaret, A.: Psychopharmacologie d'un troisième neuroleptique de la série des butyrophénones: le R 2498 ou tripéridol. Acta Neurol. Belg. 60, 465 (1960b)

Field, L.H.: Benperidol in the treatment of sexual offenders. Med. Sci. Law 13, 195–196 (1973)

Gallant, D.M., Mielke, D.H., Spirtes, M.A., Swanson, W.C., Bost, R.: Penfluridol: an efficacious long-acting oral antipsychotic compound. Am. J. Psychiatry 131, 699–702 (1974)

Gillis, J.S.: The effects of selected antipsychotic drugs on human judgment. Curr. Ther. Res. 21, 224–232 (1977)

Gross, H., Kaltenbäck, E.: Klinische Beurteilung eines Neuroleptikums aus der Butyrophenonreihe: Triperidol. Wien. Med. Wochenschr. 116, 998–1001 (1966)

Gschwend, H.W.: Chemical approaches to the development of neuroleptics. In: Industrial Pharmacology, Vol. 1. Fielding, S., Lal, H. (ed.). New York: Futura Publishing Company, Mount Kisko 1974, pp. 1–15

Haase, H.-J., Mattke, D., Schonbeck, M.: Klinisch-neuroleptische Prüfungen am Beispiel der Butyrophenonderivate Benzperidol und Spiroperidol. Psychopharmacologia 6, 435–452 (1964)

Haase, H.-J., Frank, Th., Knaack, M., Lehnardt, Ch., Richter-Peill, H.: Klinische Prüfung eines neuen Langzeitneuroleptikums (Fluspirilene) unter besonderer Berücksichtigung der neuroleptischen Schwelle. Nervenarzt 39, 275–279 (1968)

Hoffmann, I., Ruschig, H.: Neuroleptics. In: Arzneimittel, Vol. 1. Ehrhard, G., Ruschig, H. (eds.). Weinheim: Verlag Chemie 1972, pp. 218–234

Israel, MM.L., Depoutot, J.C., Wagner, J.: Etude EEG de l'action du 2028 MD (Haloanisone) dans l'agitation psychomotrice. Strasbourg Médical 1, 25–34 (1967)

Jageneau, A.H.M., Janssen, P.A.J.: The mydriatic activity of a series of atropine-like substances in mice. Arch. Int. Pharmacodyn. Thér. 106, 199–206 (1956)

Janssen, P.A.J.: Vergleichende pharmacologische Daten über sechs neue basische 4'-Fluorobu-tyrophenon-Derivate: Haloperidol, Haloanison, Triperidol, Methylperidid, Haloperidid und Dipiperon. Arzneim. Forsch. *11*, 819–827, 932–938 (1961)

Janssen, P.A.J.: The relationship between chemical structure and CNS-depressant activity of basic ketones related to haloperidol. Int. J. Neuropharmacol. *1*, 145 –148 (1962)

Janssen, P.A.J.: Recent advances in the butyrophenone series. In: Neuropsychopharmacology, Vol. 3, P.B. Bradley, F. Flügel, P. Hoch, (eds.). Amsterdam: Elsevier Publishing Company 1964, pp. 331–335

Janssen, P.A.J.: The evolution of the butyrophenones haloperidol and trifluperidol from me-peridine-like 4-phenylpiperidines. In: International Review of Neurobiology, Vol. 8. Pfeif-fer, C.C., Smythies, J.R. (eds.). New York: Academic Press 1965, pp. 221–263

Janssen, P.A.J.: The chemical anatomy of neuroleptic drugs. Särtryck ur Farmacevtisk Revy *65*, 272–295 (1966)

Janssen, P.A.J.: Haloperidol and related butyrophenones. In: Psychopharmacological Agents, Vol. 2. De Stevens, G. (ed.). New York: Academic Press 1967a, pp. 199–248

Janssen, P.A.J.: The pharmacology of haloperidol. Int. J. Neuropsychiatry *3*, Suppl. 1, 10–18 (1967b)

Janssen, P.A.J.: The butyrophenone story. In: Discoveries in Biological Psychiatry. Ayd, F.J., Blackwell, B. (eds.). Philadelphia: J.B. Lippincott Company 1970a, pp. 165–179

Janssen, P.A.J.: Chemical and pharmacological classification of neuroleptics. In: Modern Prob-lems in Pharmacopsychiatry. The Neuroleptics, Vol. 5, D.P. Bobon (ed.). Basel: J. Karger 1970b, pp. 33–44

Janssen, P.A.J.: A new series of neuroleptic drugs, the 4,4-diphenylbutylpiperidines and their relation with other neuroleptics. Clin. Trials J. *8*, Suppl. 11, 7–8 (1971)

Janssen, P.A.J.: Structureactivity relations (SAR) and drug design. In: International Encyclo-pedia of Pharmacology and Therapeutics, Vol. 1, G. Peters (ed.). Oxford: Pergamon Press 1973, pp. 37–73

Janssen, P.A.J.: Butyrophenones and diphenylbutylpiperidines. In: Psychopkarmacological Agents, Vol. 3, G. De Stevens (ed.). New York: Academic Press 1974, pp. 129–158

Janssen, P.A.J., Eddy, N.B.: Compounds related to pethidine. IV. Chemical methods of in-creasing the analgesic activity of pethidine. J. Med. Pharm. Chem. *2*, 31–45 (1960)

Janssen, P.A.J., Niemegeers, C.J.E.: Chemistry and pharmacology of compounds related to 4-(4-hydroxy-4-phenylpiperidino)-butyrophenone. Part II. Inhibition of apomorphine vomiting in dogs. Arzneim. Forsch. *9*, 765–767 (1959)

Janssen, P.A.J., Van Bever, W.F.M.: Advances in the search for improved neuroleptic drugs. In: Current Developments in Psychopharmacology, Vol. 2. W.B. Essman, L. Valzelli (ed.). New York: Spectrum Publications, Holliswood 1975, pp. 165–184

Janssen, P.A.J., Van Bever, W.F.M.: Butyrophenones and diphenylbutylamines. In: Psycho-therapeutic Drugs, Vol. 2, Part 2, E. Usdin, I.S. Forrest (eds.). New York: Marcel Dekker Inc. 1977, pp. 869–921

Janssen, P.A.J., Jageneau, A.H.M., Schellekens, K.H.L.: Chemistry and pharmacology of com-pounds related to 4-(4-hydroxy-4-phenylpiperidino)-butyrophenone. Psychopharma-cologia *1*, 389–392 (1960a)

Janssen, P.A.J., Niemegeers, C.J.E., Schellekens, K.H.L.: Chemistry and pharmacology of compounds related to 4-(4-hydroxy-4-phenylpiperidino)-butyrophenone. Arzneim. Forsch. *10*, 955 (1960b)

Janssen, P.A.J., Niemegeers, C.J.E., Dony, J.G.H.: A comparative study of the effects of sub-cutaneous and oral doses of haloperidol on avoidance-escape habits of rats and dogs in a "jumbing box" situation. Arzneim. Forsch. *13*, 401–403 (1963a)

Janssen, P.A.J., Niemegeers, C.J.E., Schellekens, K.H.L., Verbruggen, F.J., Van Nueten, J.M.: The pharmacology of dehydrobenzperidol a new potent and short acting neuroleptic agent chemically related to haloperidol. Arzneim. Forsch. *13*, 205–211 (1963b)

Janssen, P.A.J., Niemegeers, C.J.E., Schellekens, K.H.L.: Is it possible to predict the clinical effects of neuroleptic drugs from animal data? Arzneim. Forsch. *15* I, 104–117 (1965a)

Janssen, P.A.J., Niemegeers, C.J.E., Schellekens, K.H.L.: Is it possible to predict the clinical effects of neuroleptic drugs from animal data? Arzneim. Forsch. *15* II, 1196–1206 (1965b)

Janssen, P.A.J., Niemegeers, C.J.E., Schellekens, K.H.L.: Is it possible to predict the clinical effects of neuroleptic drugs from animal data? Arzneim. Forsch. *16* III, 339–346 (1966)

Janssen, P.A.J., Niemegeers, C.J.E., Schellekens, K.H.L.: Is it possible to predict the clinical effects of neuroleptic drugs from animal data? Part IV, Arzneim. Forsch. *17* IV, 841–854 (1967)

Janssen, P.A.J., Niemegeers, C.J.E., Schellekens, K.H.L., Dresse, A., Lenaerts, F.M., Schaper, W.K.A., Van Nueten, J.M., Verbruggen, F.J.: Pimozide a chemically novel highly potent and oral long-acting neuroleptic drug. Arzneim. Forsch. *18*, 261–287 (1968)

Janssen, P.A.J., Niemegeers, C.J.E., Schellekens, K.H.L., Lenaerts, F.M., Verbruggen, F.J., Van Nueten, J.M., Marsboom, R.H.M., Herin, V.V., Schaper, W.K.A.: The pharmacology of fluspirilene (R 6218) a potent long-acting and injectable neuroleptic drug. Arzneim. Forsch. *20*, 1689–1698 (1970a)

Janssen, P.A.J., Niemegeers, C.J.E., Schellekens, K.H.L., Verbruggen, F.J., Van Nueten, J.M., Schaper, W.K.A.: The pharmacology of penfluridol (R 16341) a new potent and orally long-acting neuroleptic drug. Eur. J. Pharmacol. *11*, 139–154 (1970b)

Janssen, P.A.J., Niemegeers, C.J.E., Schellekens, K.H.L., Lenaerts, F.M., Wauquier, A.: Clopimozide (R 29764) a new highly potent and orally long-acting drug of the diphenylbutylpiperidine series. Arzneim. Forsch. *25*, 1287–1294 (1975)

Jones, I.H., Davies, J.M., Buckle, R., Hanna, W.H., Pikler, N.: Comparison of methylperidol and trifluperazine in the treatment of chronic, underactive schizophrenic patients. Aust. N.Z.J. Psychiatry *4*, 143–147 (1970)

Kline, F., Burgoyne, R.W., Yamamoto, J.: Comparison of pimozide and trifluperazine as once-daily therapy in chronic schizophrenic outpatients. Curr. Ther. Res. *21*, 768–778 (1977)

Knapen, J., Bollen, J., Brugmans, J., Rombaut, N.: Traitement des psychoses chroniques par le clopimozide oral. Acta Psychiatr. Belg. *76*, 644–657 (1976)

Koch, M.H.J.: The conformation of neuroleptic drugs. Mol. Pharmacol. *10*, 425–427 (1974)

Lewi, P.J.: Spectral mapping, a technique for classifying biological activity. Arzneim. Forsch. *26*, 1295–1300 (1976a)

Lewi, P.J.: Clinical and pharmacological spectral maps of the neuroleptics. Int. Pharmacopsychiatry *11*, 181–189 (1976b)

Lewi, P.J., Van Bever, W.F.M., Janssen, P.A.J.: Classification and discrimination for data analysis in pharmacology. Eur. J. Pharmacol. *35*, 403–407 (1976)

Mellien, G.: Semap, ein neues orales Langzeitneuroleptikum. Therapiewiche *26*, 5588–5592 (1976)

Neff, K.E., Denney, D., Blachly, P.H.: Control of severe agitation with droperidol. Dis. Nerv. Sys. *33*, 594–597 (1972)

Niemegeers, C.J.E.: Prediction of side-effects. In: Industrial Pharmacology, Neuroleptics, Vol. 1, S. Fielding, H. Lal (eds.). New York: Futura Publishing Company, Mount Kiska 1974, pp. 98–129

Niemegeers, C.J.E., Janssen, P.A.J.: Bromoperidol a new potent neuroleptic of the butyrophenone series. Arzneim. Forsch. *24*, 45–52 (1974)

Niemegeers, C.J.E., Van Nueten, J.M., Janssen, P.A.J.: Azaperone a sedative neuroleptic of the butyrophenone series with pronounced anti-aggressive and anti-shock activity in animals. Arzneim. Forsch. *24*, 1798–1806 (1974)

Paquay, J., Arnould, F., Burton, P.: Etude clinique de l'action du R 1625 à doses modérées en psychiatrie. Acta Neurol. Belg. *59*, 882–891 (1959)

Paquay, J., Arnould, F., Burton, P.: Etude clinique du R 2028 en psychiatrie. Acta Neurol. Belg. *60*, 677–682 (1960)

Paquay, J., Arnould, F., Burton, P.: Le spiropéridol (R 5147) en milieu psychiatrique. Acta Neurol. Belg. *65*, 720–726 (1965)

Plath, P.: Die medikamentöse Behandlung des Stotterns. Therapiewoche *26*, 5705–5708 (1976)

Protiva, M.: Neurotrope und psychotrope Pharmaka. Pharmaceutische Industrie *32*, 923–933 (1970)

Schwarz, H.: Zur klinisch psychiatrischen Behandlung mit Benperidol. Med. Welt *17*, 2642–2643 (1966)

Sim, M., Armitage, G.H., Davies, M.H., Gordon, E.B.: A controlled trial of trifluperidol (triperidol) with trifluperazine. Clin. Trials J. *8*, 34–40 (1971)

Symoens, J., Van Den Brande, M.: Prevention and cure of aggressiveness in pigs using the sedative azaperone. Vet. Rec. *85*, 64–67 (1969)

Tanghe, A.: A retrospective evaluation of long-term fluspirilene (IMAP) treatment. Acta Psychiatr. Belg. *76*, 480–490 (1976)

Tennent, G., Bancroft, J., Cass, J.: The control of deviant sexual behavior by drugs: A double-blind controlled study of benperidol, chlorpromazine, and placebo. Arch. Sex. Behav. *3*, 261–271 (1974)

Tollenaere, J.P., Moereels, H., Koch, M.H.J.: On the conformation of neuroleptic drugs in the three aggregation states and their conformational resemblance to dopamine. Eur. J. Med. Chem. *12*, 199–211 (1977)

Uytterschaut, P., Jacobs, R.: Etude clinique de l'activité neuropsychopharmacologique du méthylpéridol (R 1658). Acta Neurol. Belg. *62*, 677–701 (1962)

Van Leeuwen, A.M.H., Molders, J., Sterkmans, P., Mielants, P., Martens, C., Toussaint, C., Hovent, A.M., Desseilles, M.F., Koch, H., Devroye, A., Parent, M.: Droperidol in acutely agitated patients, N. Nerv. Ment. Dis. *164*, 280–283 (1977)

Van Renynghe de Voxvrie, G., De Bie, M.: Character neuroses and behavioural disorders in children: their treatment with pipamperone (Dipiperon). Acta Psychiatr. Belg. *76*, 688–695 (1976)

Villa, J.-L., Pasini, W.: Une année d'expérimentation avec l'haloanisone 2028 MD en gérontopsychiatrie. Praxis *55*, 46–49 (1966)

Villeneuve, A., Bordeleau, J.M.: The diphenylbutylpiperidines. Québec: Les Presses de l'Université Laval 1973

Waniek, W., Pach, J.: Vegetativ-emotionale Syndrome in der Praxis: Therapieerfahrungen mit einem Langzeitpharmakon. Münch. Med. Wochenschr. *116*, 1339–1344 (1974)

Weiser, G.: Erfahrungen mit dem Butyrophenonpräparat Luvatren in der Behandlung der Schizophrenie. Wien Med. Wochenschr. *118*, 444–446 (1968)

Weiser, G.: Initialbehandlung der Schizophrene mit Droperidol. Wien Z. Nervenheilkd. *31*, 176–188 (1973)

Wetzels, M.H.: The stress-related emotional lability syndrome. I. Definition, psychophysiological mechanisms and a pilot experience with Orap. Acta Psychiatr. Belg. *77*, 267–276 (1977a)

Wetzels, M.H.: The stress-related emotional lability syndrome. II. A multicentre evaluation of Orap. Acta Psychiatr. Belg. *77*, 277–283 (1977b)

Zick, W.H.: Klinischer Bericht über ein hochpotentes Neuroleptikum mit sicherer substanzeigener Vierundzwanzigstundenwirkung nach oraler Verabreichung. Med. Welt *20*, 1659–1661 (1969)

Zircle, C.I., Kaiser, C.: Antipsychotic agents. In: Medicinal Chemistry, Vol. 2, A. Burger (ed.) Wiley-Interscience New York: 1970, pp. 1410–1469

CHAPTER 3

Centrally Acting Rauwolfia Alkaloids*

H.J. Bein

A. Introduction and History

Rauwolfia (a genus of the family *Apocynaceae*) is one of the most abundant single sources of alkaloids in the entire vegetable realm. Biologically active compounds have been isolated from the root, the stem, the branches, and the leaves (Bein, 1956; Schlittler and Bein, 1967). With the exception of thebaine and papaverine, all the Rauwolfia alkaloids are indole bases. The principal active constituent, reserpine, was isolated in 1952 by Mueller et al. Reserpine, together with chlorpromazine, ushered in the era of modern antipsychotic drug therapy (Deniker, 1975). By now, several thousand papers have been published on the pharmacology and the use of reserpine; for the purposes of the present review, judicious selection had to be made. The early literature will not be reviewed in detail; interested readers will find it covered in previous articles by Bein (1956), Carlsson (1965), and Rand and Jurevics (1977). The present review will not discuss every central action of reserpine, but only some central effects of special importance to its use in psychiatry. Moreover, no reference will be made to the results of studies with tetrabenazine. Although the mechanisms of action of tetrabenazine and reserpine are generally considered identical, several lines of evidence suggest that there are subtle differences between them (Kuczenski, 1977).

The Rauwolfia plant was so named by the French botanist Plumier in honour of the 16th century German botanist Leonhard Rauwolf. It seems unlikely that Rauwolf himself was actually acquainted with Rauwolfia (Rieppel, 1956). Although Rauwolfia has been used for centuries in India, in the Ayurvedic and other indigenous systems of medicine, it was chiefly administered as a febrifuge, in painful conditions of the intestine, and as an antidote against insect stings and snake bite. The earliest reference to Rauwolfia in western literature appeared in a Portuguese work published in 1563 (Rieppel, 1956), which was likewise chiefly concerned with the antivenomous action of the drug. Its author, Garcia Da Orta, who practised as a physician in India for 36 years, does not mention its use as a hypnotic (Markham, 1913). In ancient Indian medicicine, it does not appear to have been used in the treatment of mental disorders (Chopra, 1933). Nevertheless, although not borne out by the historic sources, the assumption that Rauwolfia had been employed for centuries to calm agitated psychotics seems to have been so attractive that it pervades the entire western literature on the plant. In this connection, one must also remember that in other cultures the attitude to mental illnesses is, as a rule, completely different from that of the present-day, western world. This does not exclude the possibility that the hypnotic effect of Rauwolfia may have been known in contemporary folk medicine. Rauwolfia vomitoria was em-

---

* Review of literature published up to the autumn of 1977

ployed by Africans to treat insomnia and agitation (RAYMOND-HAMET, 1939; PRINCE, 1960). Their familiarity with the calming effects of Rauwolfia vomitoria was presumably empirical, for Rauwolfia vomitoria and Rauwolfia serpentina are so unlike each other in appearance – the former is a large tree and the latter a shrub not quite as tall as a man – as to make it improbable that hearsay knowledge of the properties of non-African species of Rauwolfia would lead them to credit Rauwolfia vomitoria with the same powers. One striking fact, however is that in all the regions to which Rauwolfia is indigenous (India, Africa, and South America), it is associated with the snake in various ways extending beyond its use as a simple antidote (BEIN, 1956). In view of the profound mythologic symbolism investing the snake throughout the various cultures, it seems not unlikely that the association of the Rauwolfia plant with the snake is simply a reflection of the effects it is capable of exerting upon the human organism.

Although it recently proved necessary to review the history of chlorpromazine owing to the fictions, confusions and distortion coming into currency (DENIKER, 1975), there can be no doubt that Indian authors first described the beneficial effects of Rauwolfia in hypertension and mania and also recognized other effects characteristic of Rauwolfia or reserpine, viz. "flushing of the face, running of the nose, congestion of the eyes, diarrhoea," bradycardia ("occurring with very small doses") and finally extrapyramidal symptoms (SEN and BOSE, 1931; DE 1944/1945). DE reported typical cases of Parkinsonism, reversible after withdrawal of Rauwolfia and susceptible to tincture of Belladonna. This was the first published account of drug-induced extrapyramidal symptoms.

Besides reserpine, other naturally occuring Rauwolfia alkaloids with reserpine-like properties have been isolated, e.g., (in descending order of potency) deserpidine, rescinnamine, raunescine, and pseudoreserpine (SCHLITTLER and BEIN, 1967). Reserpine, however, proved to be by far the most widely investigated compound, so that this review will be concentrated on it. Reserpine is a colorless, crystalline, readily liposoluble substance which is almost insoluble in water at neutral pH but soluble in solutions of organic acids, such as acetic, ascorbic, or citric acid.

B. Biologic Fate and Mechanisms of Action of Reserpine

The finding that reserpine depletes brain tissue of 5-hydroxytryptamine (5-HT) (PLETSCHER et al., 1955), of noradrenaline (NA) (HOLZBAUER and VOGT, 1956), and of dopamine (DA) (CARLSSON et al., 1958) afforded a completely new insight into the function of the nervous system. Because of its liposolubility, reserpine shows a characteristic pattern of distribution in the body. STITZEL (1976) has recently summarized the data on the biologic fate of reserpine:

Reserpine is rapidly absorbed after p.o., s.c., or i.p. administration. It is also rapidly eliminated from the blood, as a result of both tissue uptake and metabolism. During the process of absorption from the gastrointestinal tract, a portion of the drug is hydrolyzed by the intestinal mucosa. Further biotransformation occurs through the action of serum exterases and in the liver where probably both microsomal oxidative and hydrolytic enzymes contribute to the degradation of reserpine.

Reserpine is excreted in the urine and faeces even after i.v. administration. It crosses the placenta.

Its high lipid solubility probably facilitates the passage of reserpine across lipid cell membranes, and the accumulation of the drug within tissues is primarily the result of rapid permeation through these membranes. The reserpine found within the tissues probably consists initially of both reversibly and irreversibly bound drug. The irreversibly bound reserpine is assumed to be associated with the lipid sites of the granular membranes of amine-containing nerves (WAGNER, 1975); the degree of its binding correlates with the effect of the drug (NORN and SHORE, 1971 a, b). In blood platelets it is also associated with the phospholipids of the membrane of vesicles containing 5-HT (ENNA et al., 1974).

The most likely mode of action of reserpine is that it inhibits the Mg^{2+}-ATP-dependent pump in the vesicle membrane, which maintains a high concentration of amine inside the vesicle, and thus prevents any amine that diffuses out of the vesicle from being pumped back in again. In the case of NA, the free amine is rapidly degraded by monoamine oxidase (MAO) largely within the neurone. During the early phase of the action of reserpine, leakage into the extracellular space may be of sufficient magnitude to cause activation of receptors but under most experimental conditions a direct releasing action is weak (CARLSSON, 1965). Reserpine does not impair the movement of amine across the neuronal membrane (LINDMAR and MUSCHOLL, 1964) and may even increase membrane permeability of adrenergic neurones to the outward movements of amines (FIBIGER and McGEER, 1973). Vesicular amine uptake is mediated by a carrier system whose activity is correlated to the activity of a membrane-bound ATPase activity. Reserpine, however, has only little effect on ATPase activity (TAUGNER and HASSELBACH, 1966; FERRIS et al., 1970). SLOTKIN (1973) therefore suggested the existence of separate sites of action for reserpine and ATPase and discussed separate processes for uptake and storage; in this case reserpine would block the transport of amines by inhibiting their attachment to the carrier.

There is also a mechanism, insensitive to reserpine and independent of ATP and Mg^{2+}, by means of which noradrenaline is taken up into amine-storing vesicles from the hypothalamus (PHILIPPU et al., 1969).

The decrease in tissue amine levels following reserpine administration is thought to be due to blockade of re-uptake into the storage granules. Depletion of catecholamines by reserpine is not uniform in its rate of onset and intensity throughout the whole brain, but varies in different areas; this variation might reflect differences in rates of release (CARLSSON, 1965). The pharmacologic actions of reserpine appear to be more closely correlated to the storage function than to the amine content of the stores. In addition, small, functionally critical pools of biogenic amines must be considered, a concept suggested by HÄGGENDAL and LINDQUIST (1964 a, b). Such a functionally critical pool may consist mainly of newly synthesized amine and may be extremely small (ANTONACCIO and SMITH, 1974).

After chronic administration of reserpine there is a feedback-regulated increase in the activity or synthesis of tyrosine hydroxylase (MUELLER et al., 1969; SEGAL et al., 1971; ZIGMOND et al., 1974) and of tryptophan hydroxylase (GAL et al., 1968; ZIVKOVIC et al., 1973), so that synthesis of NA, DA, and 5-HT would be expected to be gradually increased during long-term administration of reserpine (COSTA and MEEK, 1974). The axoplasmic transport of amines may be accelerated (FIBIGER and McGEER, 1973) and the striatal turnover of dopamine is increased (SANER and PLETSCHER, 1977).

MAO activity was found to increase after repeated administration of reserpine (BI-DARD and CRONENBERGER, 1974; RAND and JUREVICS, 1977).

Various investigators have suggested that the effects of reserpine are due to its action on NA, DA, or 5-HT in the brain. The following sections show that it is not possible to explain the various effects of reserpine in terms of a single biochemical point of attack. This is especially evident when complex central processes are involved. Moreover, besides NA, DA, and 5-HT, other endogenous substances have to be considered. Numerous investigators have tried to modify the action of reserpine by administration of precursors of the neurotransmitters. In view of evidence that exogenously administered 5-HT may be taken up unspecifically (CHASE and MURPHY, 1973) and that L-Dopa causes an accumulation of DA not only in dopaminergic but also in 5-hydroxytryptaminergic neurones (BARTHOLINI et al., 1968), any results of experiments with both reserpine and Dopa or reserpine and 5-HT should be interpreted with caution. In addition to the concentrations of NA, DA, and 5-HT, reserpine reduces the concentrations of p-tyramine and m-tyramine in the rat brain (BOULTON et al., 1977). Moreover, it reduces the concentration of histamine in the brain of the cat (ADAM and HYE, 1966; WHITE, 1966) and the mouse (ATACK, 1971) and modifies histamine metabolism in the rat brain (POLLARD et al., 1973). The reserpine-induced release of histamine in vitro is different from that evoked by potassium depolarization (TAYLOR and SNYDER, 1973).

In view of the increased interest in the cholinergic system in psychiatric patients, it is noteworthy that reserpine increases the amount of acetylcholine in the brain (MALPICA et al., 1970; HRDINA and LING, 1973) and stimulates the activity of choline acetyltransferase (MANDELL and KNAPP, 1971).

Reserpine stimulates the turnover of glutamate and associated amino acids in various brain areas (SANTINI and BERL, 1972), stimulates glutamate decarboxylase activity (ITOH et al., 1976) and lowers homocarnosine levels (MARSHALL, 1973). Only large doses decrease the concentration of γ-aminobutyric acid (BERL and FRIGYESI, 1969; POPOV and MATHIES, 1967). Reserpine inhibits prostaglandin biosynthesis (KUNZE et al., 1975).

C. Central Actions of Reserpine

I. Effect of Reserpine on Behavior

Reserpine evokes a calming effect in all the animals species in which it has been tested and in man. Not even very large doses of reserpine produce genuine anesthesia; experimental animals can still be roused by external stimuli. This peculiar sedative effect led at the time of its first pharmacologic characterization to the coining of the term "tranquillizer" by F.F. YONKMAN.

The studies of the effects of reserpine in the monkey carried out by PLUMMER et al. (1954) provided the first demonstration of the taming action of a tranquillizer in frightened and aggressive animals. The sham-rage response induced in decerebrate cats was found to be suppressed by reserpine (SCHNEIDER et al., 1955). In the monkey, chronic administration diminishes locomotor activity and visual exploration, increases "self-huddling" and posturing and induces tremor (McKINNEY et al., 1971).

It is highly characteristic that the quieting effect of reserpine only occurs after a certain latency period, which can be somewhat shortened by increasing the dose, but not altogether eliminated, and that single doses have a long duration of effect. Repeated administration can therefore lead to accumulation of the drug in the body.

Under certain experimental conditions, individual effects of reserpine may become attenuated despite continued treatment, and even paradoxical reactions may occur. Gross behavior in rabbits (HÄGGENDAL and LINDQUIST, 1964b) and spontaneous locomotor activity in rats (PIRCH and RECH, 1968; PIRCH, 1969) revert to normal in the course of chronic reserpine treatment. In rats, a subsequent phase of hyperactivity may occur, which is, however, only transient and can only be observed within a certain dosage range (PIRCH, 1969). GLUCKMAN (1964) reported stimulation in mice and increased irritability in rats was noted by MORPURGO and THEOBALD (1966). Mice treated with reserpine had no spontaneous seizures but showed convulsions on handling (GOLDSTEIN, 1973). Bursts of coordinated, stereotyped activity seen in otherwise sedated rats after high doses of reserpine have been compared with the stereotyped behavior produced by small doses of amphetamine (SCHIORRING and RANDRUP, 1968); this stereotyped behavior in reserpinized rats is inhibited by centrally acting anticholinergics (KRÜGER and RANDRUP, 1968). SEGAL et al. (1971), however, assume that hyperactivity after reserpine may be associated with an increase in tyrosine hydroxylase activity in the midbrain (and in the caudate). Reserpine-induced weight loss is not in itself sufficient to produce the hyperactivity and increased enzymatic activities (SEGAL et al., 1971).

The suppression of locomotor activity in the rodent is reversed by large doses of Dopa (CARLSSON et al., 1957; BLASCHKO and CHRUSCIEL, 1960; STRÖMBOM, 1975), but not by 5-HT (CARLSSON et al., 1957; SMITH and DEWS, 1962; AHLENIUS et al., 1973) or by a combination of 5-HT and of a low dose of Dopa (AHLENIUS et al., 1973). The intraventricular infusion of relatively low doses of NA reverses reserpine-induced sedation (GEYER and SEGAL, 1973). Many years ago BLASCHKO and CHRUSCIEL (1960) raised the question whether the reversal by Dopa of reserpine akinesia was due only to the restoration of brain DA or whether NA formation was also important. ANDÉN et al. (1973), MARSDEN et al. (1975) and STRÖMBOM (1975) concluded that activation of postsynaptic dopamine receptors is a prerequisite for locomotion in reserpinized rodents, but that the involvement of NA release cannot be excluded, even though it may only be subservient to that of dopamine.

Various effects of reserpine differ in their duration, possibly because they are mediated by different neurochemical pathways in the brain. The recovery of the depressed conditioned avoidance response is especially slow, compared with that of spontaneous locomotor activity, for instance (FAITH et al., 1968; LEVISON and FREEDMAN, 1967; PIRCH et al., 1967).

Reserpine depresses well-established performance patterns in the rhesus monkey, e.g., pressing a bar to avoid shock or to obtain food (WEISKRANTZ and WILSON, 1955); it probably diminishes learning capacity, as well as performance (WEISKRANTZ and WILSON, 1956; CARLSON et al., 1965).

The administration of a single large dose of Dopa to reserpine-pretreated animals can partially and temporarily reverse reserpine-induced suppression of the conditioned avoidance response: this effect has been observed in mice and rats (SEIDEN and CARLSSON, 1964; SEIDEN and PETERSON, 1968a) and in cats (SEIDEN and HANSON, 1964). The dosages of both reserpine and Dopa are important in this respect (AHLENIUS, 1974). Experiments performed by SEIDEN and PETERSON (1968b), AHLENIUS and ENGEL (1971) and ENGEL (1971) indicate that stimulation of DA receptors as well as NA receptors is essential to the maintenance of a conditioned avoidance response in reserpine-treated mice (see also SEIDEN et al., 1975). Although it is generally thought that a reduction of catecholamines and not of 5-HT in the brain is responsible for the suppressive effects of reserpine on conditioned behavior, the possibility that the depletion of 5-HT by reserpine is also of some importance cannot be excluded (BUTCHER et al., 1972; AHLENIUS, 1974).

Reserpine has also been reported to produce time-dependent retention impairments; depending on the task, the effect of reserpine could be counteracted either by Dopa (DISMUKES and RAKE, 1972) or by 5-HTP (ALLEN et al., 1974). The effect of reserpine on retention of a single passive avoidance trial in mice could, however, not be blocked by Dopa or 5-HTP given alone, but only a combination of both substances (PALFAI et al., 1977).

Rats with lesions in the medial forebrain bundle have decreased brain concentrations of 5-HT and NA without showing signs of sedation, but their sensitivity to reserpine, measured in terms of the reduction in the frequency of lever pressing for a reward of water, is increased (GRABARITS and HARVEY, 1966). Lesions of the medial forebrain bundle, however, not only affect the brain concentration of catecholamines and of 5-HT but also produce a fall in forebrain histidine decarboxylase which is exclusively stored in histamine neurones (SCHWARTZ et al., 1974).

A monoamine-depleting action of reserpine seems, however, not to be involved in its effect on the grooming behavior of mice, which was found to be suppressed by reserpine. ROHTE and MÜNTZING (1973) found no relation between this effect of reserpine and the reduction of the transmitter content of central and peripheral serotonergic and adrenergic neurones.

Reserpine depresses the rate of self-stimulation in rats with electrodes implanted in the hypothalamus (STEIN, 1964; HALEY et al., 1968; STINUS et al., 1976), in the midbrain tegmentum (STEIN, 1964; STINUS et al., 1976), or in the medial forebrain bundle (BARRETT and LEITH, 1976). In the experiments conducted by HALEY et al. (1968), there did not appear to be any correlation between the rate of self-stimulation and brain-stem concentration of 5-HT; it seems that dopaminergic neurones, or dopaminergic and noradrenergic neurones, are involved (STINUS et al., 1976).

Mice treated with reserpine showed a decrease in shock-elicited aggression and mobility, but slightly elevated shock thresholds (BUTCHER and DIETRICH, 1973). RAY (1965) assumes that reserpine diminishes the effectiveness of an external conditioned stimulus in eliciting anxiety responses.

The effect of reserpine on an alleged analog of anxiety in the animal, the conditioned emotional response (CER), has been found to be inconsistent. MILLENSON and LESLIE (1974) have critically reviewed the results obtained with reserpine and other central depressants: reserpine generally proved to be effective when administered chronically, but was either ineffective or augmented anxiety when administered acutely. In contrast to reserpine, the benzodiazepines yield uniformly positive results only when administered acutely.

II. Effect of Reserpine on the Motor System

The use of Dopa in the treatment of Parkinson patients is a direct consequence of the research on reserpine and its influence on amine metabolism, stemming on the one hand from the finding of CARLSSON et al. (1958) that reserpine lowers the dopamine content of the brain and on the other from the observations of EHRINGER and HOR-NYKIEWICZ (1960) that the dopamine concentration in the corpus striatum of Parkinsonian patients is markedly reduced.

A cataleptic effect of high doses of reserpine in experimental animals (BEIN et al., 1953) and a Parkinson-like picture in man (WEBER, 1954) were described in the very first publications on the drug, and have since been confirmed by numerous investigators. STEG (1964) proposed the extrapyramidal syndrome induced by reserpine as a model for the investigation of Parkinsonian neurophysiology. In rats, reserpine produces tremor, rigidity of supraspinal origin and a dose-dependent increase in the electromyogram activity. It reduces γ- and increases α-motoneurone responses (STEG, 1964; MORRISON and WEBSTER, 1973 a). In spinal rats, the numbers of α- and γ-reflex discharges are not changed significantly by reserpine (GROSSMANN et al., 1975). Decortication did not diminish the rigidity (ARVIDSSON et al., 1967), which was abolished after section of the spinal cord (ARVIDSSON et al., 1966). In rats with chronic (DIVAC, 1972) as well as acute (ARVIDSSON et al., 1967) neostriatal lesions, reserpine did not produce rigidity. Reserpine-induced catatonia in the rat, as well as certain alterations in the EEG, was suppressed by the injection of 25% KCl into the striatum (STILLE, 1971). Catalepsy and sedation induced by reserpine in rats were accelerated in their onset and intensified in their severity by prior application of acute or chronic electroconvulsive shocks (PAPESCHI et al., 1974); the catatonia-like state was potentiated by the simultaneous administration of histamine (CESARE et al., 1967). In the decerebrate cat, reserpine prevented not only the development of rigidity, but also of the so-called Schiff-Sherrington phenomenon (HERMAN and BARNES, 1967) and suppressed the activity of tonic γ fibres (BALTZER and BEIN, 1973).

In decerebrated rabbits, reserpine blocked the excitation of fusimotor neurones by cord stimulation (ELLAWAY and PASCOE, 1968).

In the dog, muscle tremors and a Parkinson-like syndrome appeared to increase as the duration of reserpine administration was lengthened (ADAMS et al., 1971).

In monkeys with certain brain lesions, reserpine gave rise to postural tremor, which was abolished by Dopa and apomorphine, but not by amphetamine; reserpine-induced catatonia in these monkeys was reversed by Dopa, apomorphine, amphetamine and, to a lesser degree, by benztropine (LAROCHELLE et al., 1971).

Reserpine-induced rigidity in the rat was abolished by MAO inhibitors, but was unaffected by Dopa or 5-HTP in dosages of 20 mg/kg, i.p. On the basis of these results, MORRISON and WEBSTER (1973 b) speculated that the reserpine rigidity might be due to dopamine depletion in the brain or to an increase in deaminated metabolites, or both. The doses of Dopa used by these authors were probably inadequate. The i.v. injection of larger amounts of Dopa causes a reversible disappearance of the rigidity, reappearance of the fusimotor activity, and a reduction of the exaggerated monosynaptic reflexes; a similar effect was seen after the injection of 5-HTP (ROOS and STEG, 1964). Reserpine-induced rigidity as well as the increased α- and γ-activity were furthermore antagonized by metamphetamine, phenytoin (JURNA and LANZER, 1969), amantadine (JURNA et al., 1972), and antimuscarinic agents (JURNA and LANZER, 1969; MORRISON and WEBSTER, 1973 a).

The mechanisms of action of reserpine on various spinal responses depend on the pathway studied, the experimental conditions, the dosages of reserpine used, and the animal species involved: SCHNEIDER et al. (1955) reported a facilitation of the monosynaptic responses in spinal and decerebrate cats and inconstant facilitation of a poly-

synaptic reflex in decerebrate cats, while KRIVOY (1957) observed a predominant inhibition of monosynaptic transmission in the spinal cord of anesthetized and decerebrate cats. BEIN (1957) found no significant alterations of the patellar-tendon reflex
in the anesthetized rabbit and in the anesthetized cat. Inconstant effects on the patellar
reflex and the crossed-extension reflex in anesthetized rabbits and cats were noted by
SILVESTRINI and MAFFII (1959).

In chronic spinal dogs, the flexor reflex was intensified by acute treatment and decreased after chronic treatment with reserpine (MARTIN and EADES, 1967).

According to ANDÉN et al. (1964), reserpine by itself produced little effect in the
acute spinal cat, but when given after the administration of a MAO inhibitor, it blocked the transmission from the flexor reflex afferants to primary afferents and motoneurones. This effect was possibly due to the release of both NA and 5-HT (ANDÉN
et al., 1964; ENGBERG et al., 1968). In the chronic spinal cat, however, reserpine had
no effect on the flexor reflex afferents (ENGBERG et al., 1968). In the decerebrate cat,
reserpine blocked the reticulospinal excitation of motoneurones produced by stimulation of the caudal medulla (ANDÉN et al., 1964).

In the intact rat, reserpine increased monosynaptic and depressed polysynaptic
mass reflexes, effects suggested to be due to a change in the interaction of dopaminergic transmission in the nigrostriatal system (GROSSMANN et al., 1973). In spinal rats,
reserpine (and Dopa) increased ventral and dorsal root responses evoked by stimulation of dorsal roots and of afferent nerves. GROSSMANN et al. (1975) therefore concluded that reserpine exerted this effect via a spinal site of action and by releasing NA
from the terminals of descending noradrenergic pathways. In the rabbit and the rat
all the 5-HT is assumed to be associated with descending fibres, whereas in the cat
5-HT might also be associated with some segmental interneurons (ANDERSON, 1972).
With regard to the spinal mechanisms of reserpine, it should be recognized that there
are possibly other indole amines present in the spinal cord besides 5-HT. BJÖRKLUND
et al. (1970) have shown the presence of an amine in the rat spinal cord that is depleted
by reserpine, but has a fluorescent spectrum slightly different from that of serotonin.

III. Effects of Reserpine on Bioelectric Signals

Early work with reserpine on bioelectric signals has been reviewed in detail by DOMINO
(1962).

On the EEG, reserpine causes a biphasic response, consisting of an initial arousal
phase, followed by slow-wave activity (PIRCH et al., 1967; TABUSHI and HIMWICH,
1969). Slow waves of high amplitude (EEG-synchronization) were observed in rats at
a time when the animals showed motor impairment; the EEG-synchronization was,
however, of shorter duration than the behavioral depression (PIRCH et al., 1967). In
cats, EEG-synchronization after reserpine coincided with a decrease in the homoval-
linic acid concentration in the cerebrospinal fluid (BUCKINGHAM and RADULOVACKI,
1976). The initial period of synchronization in the rabbit was assumed to be due to
a release of physiologically active 5-HT (GAILLARD et al., 1974).

Slow-wave sleep was restored in the reserpinized cat with 5-HTP and REM-sleep
with Dopa (MATSUMOTO and JOUVET, 1964); this reversal by Dopa was, however, not
observed by STERN and MORGANE (1973). In the cat, reserpine shortened both stages
of sleep (HOFFMAN and DOMINO, 1969). Similar REM-suppressing effects of reser-

pine have also been observed in the rabbit (TABUSHI and HIMWICH, 1969) and rat (GOTTESMANN, 1969). Reserpine, however, has an opposite action in the monkey (REITE et al., 1969) and in man (HARTMANN, 1966; HOFFMAN and DOMINO, 1969). After acute (COULTER et al., 1971) and chronic (HARTMANN and CRAVENS, 1973) administration of reserpine there is an increase in the number of REM-sleep episodes but not in their duration, which, in fact, is diminished. The amount of slow-wave sleep is decreased. Subjective aspects of sleep were not greatly changed (HARTMANN and CRAVENS, 1973).

An increase in REM-sleep can also be produced in the cat by intraventricular injection of reserpine (STERN and MORGANE, 1973), although in this connection the localization of the injection proved to be important (BROOKS et al., 1972). The decrease in REM-wave activity in the cat after the systemic administration of reserpine appears to be due to a disorganization of REM, because the activity in the forebrain is not decreased and the pontogeniculo-occipital (PGO) spikes, which are considered to be the most important phasic characteristics of REM-sleep in the cat, are actually increased by reserpine. Moreover, reserpine induces PGO-waves in animals that remain awake. (DELORME et al., 1965; JEANNEROD and KIYONO, 1969; MUNSON and GRAHAM, 1971; BROOKS and GERSHON, 1971, 1972; BROOKS et al., 1972; SATOH, 1972; STERN and MORGAN, 1973). The PGO-spikes occurring after the administration of reserpine in rats can be recorded from a somewhat larger area than in untreated animals (MUSON and GRAHAM, 1973). The reserpine-induced increase of PGO-activity is depressed by 5-HTP (DELORME et al., 1965). The lateral geniculate body is also the area where the retinopalpebral reflex in the cat is facilitated under reserpine (FEGER et al., 1972).

In studies of the acoustic input to the basal ganglia in rats, it has been observed that the effects of L-Dopa and reserpine on the caudate nucleus, globus pallidus and substantia nigra may be synergistic or antagonistic, depending on the experimental conditions and on the anatomical localization of the electrodes (DAFNY and GILMAN, 1973, 1974; DAFNY, 1975).

D. Comparison with Other Neuroleptics

I. General Clinical Effects

The first clinical publications on reserpine already pointed out its close similarity to chlorpromazine: it was only later that decisive differences between the two classes of substances were noted.

On the one hand, the onset of action of clorpromazine is, as a rule, more rapid than that of reserpine; this is probably one of the reason why chlorpromazine gained preference in clinical use. On the other hand, reserpine exerts effects that could warrant a reappraisal of its activity, e.g., in connection with the syndrome referred to as "tardive dyskinesia," which has developed into a serious therapeutic problem in the course of the last few years. It is assumed that the prolonged administration of neuroleptics increases the sensitivity of the dopaminergic receptors. Reserpine, however, not only lowers the concentrations of DA, but also it does not block the DA receptors so that it does not contribute to the pathogenesis of tardive dyskinesia; in established cases of dyskinesia it has beneficial effects (SATO et al., 1971; KLAWANS and RUBOVITS, 1975; KOBAYASHI, 1977).

II. Alleged Depression-Inducing Effect of Neuroleptics

At an early stage in its history, it was pointed out that reserpine could induce depressions. An effect of this nature is pathogenetically extremely complex and multifaceted and there is no common denominator applicable to all cases (HELMCHEN and HIPPIUS, 1969; SIMPSON and WAAL-MANNING, 1971). It certainly cannot be equated with depression in every case; and often it is indistinguishable from psychomotor inhibition; it is largely dose-related. In this context, it is especially interesting to note that the original psychiatric publications reported that not only reserpine, but also chlorpromazine could lead to depressive reactions, similar in intensity and frequency (AYD, 1956; FELDMAN, 1957). It is nowadays an accepted fact in psychiatry that all neuroleptics can give rise to such reactions (DENIKER and GINESTET, 1975); their incidence is reckoned as being 10–30% of all cases treated (HELMCHEN and HIPPIUS, 1969). The frequent experimental use of reserpine in evaluating so-called antidepressive activity in animals is, therefore, not based on any specific clinical effect of the substance; what is demonstrated is not antidepressive efficacy as such, but a possible pharmacologic antagonism, which in the case of the known antidepressive agents is mediated by a catecholaminergic and perhaps also serotoninergic mechanism.

References

Adam, H.M., Hye, H.K.A.: Concentration of histamine in different parts of brain and hypophysis of cat and its modification by drugs. Br. J. Pharmacol. 28, 137–152 (1966)

Adams, H.R., Smookler, H.H., Clarke, D.E., Jandhyala, B.S., Dixit, B.N., Ertel, R.J., Buckley, J.P.: Clinicopathologic effects of chronic reserpine administration in mongrel dogs. J. Pharm. Sci. 60, 1134–1138 (1971)

Ahlenius, S.: Effects of L-Dopa on conditioned avoidance responding after behavioral suppression by α-methyltyrosine or reserpine in mice. Neuropharmacology 13, 729–739 (1974)

Ahlenius, S., Engel, J.: Behavioral and biochemical effects of L-Dopa after inhibition of dopamine-β-hydroxylase in reserpine pretreated rats. Naunyn Schmiedebergs Arch. Pharmacol. 270, 349–360 (1971)

Ahlenius, S., Andén, N.E., Engel, J.: Restoration of locomotor activity in mice by low L-Dopa doses after suppression by α-methyltyrosine but not by reserpine. Brain Res. 62, 189–199 (1973)

Allen, C., Allen, B.S., Rake, A.V.: Pharmacological distinctions between "active" and "passive" avoidance memory formation as shown by manipulation of biogenic amine active compounds. Psychopharmacologia 34, 1–10 (1974)

Andén, N.E., Jukes, M.G.M., Lundberg, A.: Spinal reflexes and monoamine liberation. Nature 202, 1222–1223 (1964)

Andén, N.E., Strömbom, U., Svensson, T.H. : Dopamine and noradrenaline receptor stimulation: Reversal of reserpine-induced suppression of motor activity. Psychopharmacologia 29, 289–298 (1973)

Anderson, E.G.: Bulbospinal serotonin-containing neurons and motor control. Fed. Proc. 31, 107–112 (1972)

Antonaccio, M.J., Smith, C.B.: Effects of chronic pretreatment with small doses of reserpine upon adrenergic nerve function. J. Pharmacol. Exp. Ther. 188, 654–667 (1974)

Arvidsson, I., Jurna, I., Steg, G.: Descending pathways mediating reserpine rigidity. Acta Physiol. Scand. 68, [Suppl. 277] 16 (1966)

Arvidsson, I., Jurna, I., Steg, G.: Striatal and spinal lesions eliminating reserpine and physostigmine rigidity. Life Sci. 6, 2017–2020 (1967)

Atack, C.: Reduction of histamine in mouse brain by N 1-(DL-seryl)-N 2-(2,3,4-trihydroxybenzyl) hydrazine and reserpine. J. Pharm. Pharmacol. 23, 992–993 (1971)

Ayd, F.J.: New pharmacotherapeutic drugs for psychic disturbances. Curr. Med. Digest. *23*, 59–64 (1956)

Baltzer, V., Bein, H.J.: Pharmacological investigations with benzoctamine (Tacitin), a new psycho-active agent. Arch. Int. Pharmacodyn. Ther. *201*, 25–41 (1973)

Barrett, R.J., Leith, N.J.: Gradual depression of self stimulation behavior produced by chronic administration of d-amphetamine or reserpine. Pharmacologist *18*, (No. 471) (1976)

Bartholini, G., Da Prada, M., Pletscher, A.: Decrease of cerebral 5-hydroxytryptamine by 3,4-dihydroxyphenylalanine after inhibition of extracerebral decarboxylase. J. Pharm. Pharmacol. *20*, 228–229 (1968)

Bein, H.J.: The pharmacology of Rauwolfia. Pharmacol. Rev. *8*, 435–483 (1956)

Bein, H.J.: Effects of reserpine on the functional strata of the nervous system. In: Psychotropic Drugs. Garattini, S., Ghetti, V. (eds.). Amsterdam: Elsevier 1957, pp. 325–331

Bein, H.J., Gross, F., Tripod, J., Meier, R.: Experimentelle Untersuchungen über „Serpasil" (Reserpin), ein neues, sehr wirksames Rauwolfiaalkaloid mit neuartiger zentraler Wirkung. Schweiz. Med. Wochenschr. *82*, 1007–1012 (1953)

Berl, S., Frigyesi, T.L.: Effect of reserpine on the turnover of glutamate, glutamine, aspartate and GABA labeled with (1-14C) acetate in caudate nucleus, thalamus and sensorimotor cortex (cat). Brain Res. *14*, 683–695 (1969)

Bidard, J.N., Cronenberger, L.: Effets du nialamide et de la réserpine sur les activités enzymatiques monoamine oxydase (M.A.O.) et catéchol-o-methyltransferase (C.O.M.T.) chez le rat in vivo. J. Pharmacol. (Paris) *5*, 479–494 (1974)

Björklund, A., Falck, B., Stenevi, U.: On the possible existence of a new intraneuronal monoamine in the spinal cord of the rat. J. Pharmacol. Exp. Ther. *175*, 525–532 (1970)

Blaschko, H., Chrusciel, T.L.: The decarboxylation of amino acids related to tyrosine and their awakening action in reserpine-treated mice. J. Physiol. *151*, 272–284 (1960)

Boulton, A.A., Juorio, A.V., Philips, S.R., Wu, P.H.: The effects of reserpine and 6-hydroxydopamine on the concentrations of some arylalkylamines in rat brain. Br. J. Pharmacol. *59*, 209–214 (1977)

Brooks, D.C., Gershon, M.D.: Eye movement potentials in the oculomotor and visual systems of the cat. A comparison of reserpine induced waves with those present during wakefulness and rapid eye movement sleep. Brain Res. *27*, 223–239 (1971)

Brooks, D.C., Gershon, M.D.: An analysis of the effect of reserpine upon ponto-geniculo-occipital wave activity in the cat. Neuropharmacology *11*, 499–510 (1972)

Brooks, D.C., Gershon, M.D., Simon, R.P.: Brain stem serotonin depletion and ponto-geniculo-occipital wave activity in the cat treated with reserpine. Neuropharmacology *11*, 511–520 (1972)

Buckingham, R.L., Radulovacki, M.: The effects of reserpine, L-Dopa and 5-hydroxytryptophan on 5-hydroxyindoleacetic and homovanillic acids in cerebrospinal fluid, behavior and EEG in cats. Neuropharmacology *15*, 389–392 (1976)

Butcher, L.L., Rhodes, D.L., Yuwiler, A.: Behavior and biochemical effects of preferentially protecting monoamines in the brain against the action of reserpine. Eur. J. Pharmacol. *18*, 204–212 (1972)

Butcher, L.L., Dietrich, A.P.: Effects on shock-elicited aggression in mice of preferentially protecting brain monoamines against the depleting action of reserpine. Naunyn Schmiedebergs Arch. Pharmacol. *277*, 61–70 (1973)

Carlson, N.J., Doyle, G.A., Bidder, T.G.: The effects of dl-amphetamine and reserpine on runway performance. Psychopharmacologia *8*, 157–173 (1965)

Carlsson, A.: Drugs which block the storage of 5-hydroxytryptamine and related amines. In: Handb. Exp. Pharmakol. Erg. Werk, Vol. XIX (Erspamer, V. (ed.). Berlin, Heidelberg, New York: Springer 1965, pp. 529–592

Carlsson, A., Lindquist, M., Magnusson, T.: 3,4-Dihydroxyphenyl-alanine and 5-hydroxytryptophan as reserpine antagonists. Nature *180*, 1200 (1957)

Carlsson, A., Lindquist, M., Magnusson, T., Waldeck, B.: On the presence of 3-hydroxytyramine in brain. Science *127*, 471 (1958)

Cesare, L.C., Carlini, G.R., Carlini, E.A.: Influence of histamine on the catatonia induced in mice by tetrabenazine and reserpine. Arch. Int. Pharmacodyn. Ther. *169*, 26–34 (1967)

Chase, T.N., Murphy, D.L.: Serotonin and central nervous system function. Ann. Rev. Pharmacol. *13*, 181–197 (1973)

Chopra, R.N.: Indigenous drugs of India. Their Medical and Economic Aspects. Calcutta: Art Press 1933

Costa, E., Meek, J.L.: Regulation of biosynthesis of catecholamines and serotonin in the CNS. Ann. Rev. Pharmacol. *14*, 491–511 (1974)

Coulter, J.D., Lester, B.K., Williams, H.L.: Reserpine and sleep. Psychopharmacologia *19*, 134–147 (1971)

Dafny, N.: Effects of reserpine and L-Dopa in the globus pallidus of freely behaving rats. Arch. Int. Pharmacodyn. Ther. *215*, 31–39 (1975)

Dafny, N., Gilman, S.: L-Dopa and reserpine: effects on evoked potentials in basal ganglia of freely moving rats. Brain Res. *50*, 187–191 (1973)

Dafny, N., Gilman, S.: Alteration of evoked potentials in caudate nucleus of freely moving rats by L-Dopa, reserpine, and pentobarbital. Exp. Neurol. *42*, 51–64 (1974)

De, N.: Neurological and mental symptoms produced by therapeutic dose of Rauwolfia serpentina and mepacrine hydrochloride. Trans. Med. Coll. Reun. (Calcutta) *7*, 27–29 (1944/1945)

Delorme, F., Jeannerod, M., Jouvet, M.: Effets remarquables de la réserpine sur l'activité EEG phasique ponto-géniculo-occipitale. C.R.Soc. Biol. (Paris) *159*, 900–903 (1965)

Deniker, P.: Qui a inventé les neuroleptiques? Confront. Psychiatr. *13*, 7–17 (1975)

Deniker, P., Ginestet, D.: Les effets psychiques des neuroleptiques. Confront. Psychiatr. *13*, 135–153 (1975)

Dismukes, R.K., Rake, A.V.: Involvement of biogenic amines in memory formation. Psychopharmacologia *23*, 17–25 (1972)

Divac, I.: Drug-induced syndromes in rats with large, chronic lesions in the corpus striatum. Psychopharmacologia *27*, 171–178 (1972)

Domino, E.F.: Sites of action of some central nervous system depressants. Ann. Rev. Pharmacol. *2*, 215–250 (1962)

Ehringer, H., Hornykiewicz, O.: Verteilung von Noradrenalin und Dopamin (3-hydroxytyramin) im Gehirn des Menschen und ihr Verhalten bei Erkrankungen des extrapyramidalen Systems. Klin. Wochenschr. *38*, 1236–1239 (1960)

Ellaway, P.H., Pascoe, J.E.: Noradrenaline as a transmitter in the spinal cord. J. Physiol. *197*, 8P–9P (1968)

Engberg, I.: Lundberg, A., Ryall, R.W.: The effect of reserpine on transmission in the spinal cord. Acta Physiol. Scand. *72*, 115–122 (1968)

Engel, J.: Metatyrosine-induced reversal of the suppression of the conditioned avoidance response in reserpine-treated rats. Acta Pharmacol. Toxicol. *30*, 278–288 (1971)

Enna, S.J., Da Prada, M., Pletscher, A.: Subcellular distribution of reserpine in blood platelets: evidence for multiple pools. J. Pharmacol. Exp. Therap. *191*, 164–171 (1974)

Faithe, M.E., Young, L.D., Grabarits, F., Harvey, J.A.: Differences in the duration of reserpine action in the rat depending on the measure employed. Int. J. Neuropharmacol. *7*, 575–585 (1968)

Feger, J., Boulu, R., Rossignol, P.: Le réflexe de clignement à la lumière: étude de son trajet et de sa facilitation par la réserpine. Electroenceph. Clin. Neurophysiol. *32*, 247–258 (1972)

Feldman, P.E.: A comparative study of ataractic drugs. Am. J. Psychiatry *113*, 589–594 (1957)

Ferris, R.M., Viveros, O.H., Kirschner, N.: Effects of various agents on the Mg^{++}-ATP stimulated incorporation and release of catecholamines by isolated bovine adrenomedullary storage vesicles and on secretion from the adrenal medulla. Bioch. Pharmacol. *19*, 505–514 (1970)

Fibiger, H.C., McGeer, E.G.: Increased axoplasmic transport of H3-dopamine in nigro-neostriatal neurons after reserpine. Life Sci. *13*, 1565–1571 (1973)

Gaillard, J.M., Herkert, B., Tissot, R.: Reversal of the reserpine electro encephalographic synchronization in the rabbit by parachlorophenylalanine. Neuropharmacology *13*, 789–793 (1974)

Gál, E.M., Heater, R.D., Millard, S.A.: Studies on the metabolism of 5-hydroxytryptamine (serotonin) VI. Hydroxylation and amines in cold-stressed reserpinized rats. Proc. Soc. Exp. Biol. Med. *128*, 412–415 (1968)

Geyer, M.A., Segal, D.S.: Differential effects of reserpine and α-methyl-p-tyrosine on norepinephrine and dopamine induced behavioral activity. Psychopharmacologia *29*, 131–140 (1973)

Gluckman, M.I.: Reserpin stimulation in mice. Fed. Proc. *23*, 197 (1964)

Goldstein, D.B.: Convulsions elicited by handling: a sensitive method of measuring CNS excitation in mice treated with reserpine or convulsant drugs. Psychopharmacologia *32*, 27–32 (1973)

Gottesmann, C.: Réserpine et vigilance chez le rat. C.R. Soc. Biol. (Paris) *160*, 2056–2061 (1966)

Grabarits, F., Harvey, J.A.: The effects of reserpine on behavior and on brain concentrations of serotonin and norepinephrine in control rats and rats with hypothalamic lesions. J. Pharmacol. Exp. Ther. *153*, 401–411 (1966)

Grossmann, W., Jurna, I., Nell, T., Theres, C.: The dependence of the antinociceptive effect of morphine and other analgetic agents on spinal motor activity after central monoamine depletion. Eur. J. Pharmacol. *24*, 67–77 (1973)

Grossmann, W., Jurna, I., Nell, T.: The effect of reserpine and Dopa on reflex activity in the rat spinal cord. Exp. Brain Res. *22*, 351–361 (1975)

Häggendal, J., Lindquist, M.: Disclosure of labile monoamine fractions in brain and their correlation to behaviour. Acta Physiol. Scand. *60*, 351–357 (1964a)

Häggendal, J., Lindquist, M.: Brain monoamine levels and behavior during long-term administration of reserpine. Int. J. Neuropharmacol. *3*, 59–64 (1964b)

Haley, T.J., Flesher, A.M., Komesu, N.: Influence of reserpine, tetrabenazine and iproniazid on self-stimulation by rats. Arch. Int. Pharmacodyn. Ther. *171*, 198–205 (1968)

Hartmann, E.: Reserpine: its effect on the sleep-dream cycle in man. Psychopharmacologia *9*, 242–247 (1966)

Hartmann, E., Cravens, J.: The effects of long-term administration of psychotropic drugs on human sleep. II. The effects of reserpine. Psychopharmacologia *33*, 169–184 (1973)

Helmchen, H., Hippius, H.: Pharmakogene Depressionen. In: Das depressive Syndrom. Hippius, H., Selbach, H. (eds.). München: Urban und Schwarzenberg 1969, pp. 443–448

Herman, E.H., Barnes, C.D.: Drug modification of the Schiff-Sherrington phenomenon. J. Pharmacol. Exp. Ther. *156*, 48–54 (1967)

Hoffman, J.S., Domino, E.F.: Comparative effects of reserpine on the sleep cycle of man and cat. J. Pharmacol. Exp. Ther. *170*, 190–198 (1969)

Holzbauer, M., Vogt, M.: Depression by reserpine of the noradrenaline concentration in the hypothalamus of the cat. J. Neurochem. *1*, 8–11 (1956)

Hrdina, P.D., Ling, G.M.: Effects of desipramine and reserpine on "free" and "bound" acetylcholine in rat brain. J. Pharm. Pharmacol. *25*, 504–507 (1973)

Itoh, M., Uchimura, H., Hirano, M., Saito, M., Nakahara, T.: Effects of reserpine and pargyline on glutamate decarboxylase activity in rat hypothalamic nuclei. Brain Res. *115*, 529–534 (1976)

Jeannerod, M., Kiyono, S.: Décharge unitaire de la formation réticulée pontique et activité phasique ponto-géniculo-occipitale chez le chat sous réserpine. Brain Res. *12*, 112–128 (1969)

Jurna, I., Lanzer, G.: Inhibition of the effect of reserpine on motor control by drugs which influence reserpine rigidity. Arch. Pharmakol. Exp. Pathol. *262*, 309–324 (1969)

Jurna, I., Grossmann, W., Nell, T.: Depression by amantadine of drug-induced rigidity in the rat. Neuropharmacology *11*, 559–564 (1972)

Klawans, H.L., Rubovits, R.: The pharmacology of tardive dyskinesia and some animal models. In: Neuropsychopharmacology. Boissier, J.R., Hippius, H., Pichot, P. (eds.). Amsterdam: Excerpta Med. 1975, pp. 355–364

Kobayashi, R.M.: Drug therapy of tardive dyskinesia. New Engl. J. Med. *296*, 257–260 (1977)

Krivoy, W.A.: Actions of chlorpromazine and of reserpine on spinal reflex activity in the cat. Proc. Soc. Exp. Biol. Med. *96*, 18–20 (1957)

Krüger, J.S., Randrup, A.: Pharmacological evidence for a cholinergic mechanism in brain involved in a special stereotyped behaviour of reserpinized rats. Br. J. Pharmacol. *34*, 217P–218P (1968)

Kuczenski, R.: Differential effects of reserpine and tetrabenazine on rat striatal synaptosomal dopamine biosynthesis and synaptosomal dopamine pools. J. Pharmacol. Exp. Ther. *201*, 357–367 (1977)

Kunze, H., Bohn, E., Bahrke, G.: Effects of psychotropic drugs on prostaglandin biosynthesis in vitro. J. Pharm. Pharmacol. *27*, 880–881 (1975)

Larochelle, L., Bedard, P., Poirier, L.J., Sourkes, T.L.: Correlative neuroanatomical and neuropharmacological study of tremor and catatonia in the monkey. Neuropharmacology *10*, 273–288 (1971)

Levison, P.K., Freedman, D.X.: Recovery of a discriminated leverpress avoidance performance from the effects of reserpine, chlorpromazine and tetrabenazine. Arch. Int. Pharmacodyn. Ther. *170*, 31–38 (1967)

Lindmar, R., Muscholl, E.: Die Wirkung von Pharmaka auf die Elimination von Noradrenalin aus der Perfusionsflüssigkeit und die Noradrenalinaufnahme in das isolierte Herz. Naunyn Schmiedebergs Arch. Pharmacol. *247*, 469–492 (1964)

Markham, C.(Translator): Garcia da Orta: Colloquies on the simples and drugs of India. London: H. Sotheran 1913

Malpica, J.F., Jurupe, H., Campos, H.A.: Actions of reserpine and tyramine on the acetylcholine content of brain stem, heart and blood of the rat. Arch. Int. Pharmacodyn. Ther. *185*, 13–19 (1970)

Mandell, A.J., Knapp, S.: The effects of chronic administration of some cholinergic and adrenergic drugs on the activity of choline acetyltransferase in the optic lobes of the chick brain. Neuropharmacology *10*, 513–516 (1971)

Marsden, C.D., Duvoisin, R.C., Jenner, P., Parkes, J.D., Pycock, C., Tarsy, D.: Relationship between animal models and clinical parkinsonism. Adv. Neurol. *9*, 165–175 (1975)

Marshall, F.D. (Jr.): The effect of reserpine, chlorpromazine and nembutal on levels of dipeptides in rat brain and muscle. Life Sci. *13*, 135–140 (1973)

Martin, W.R., Eades, C.G.: Pharmacological studies of spinal cord adrenergic and cholinergic mechanisms and their relation to physical dependence on morphine. Psychopharmacologia *11*, 195–223 (1967)

Matsumoto, J., Jouvet, M.: Effets de réserpine, Dopa et 5HTP sur les deux états de sommeil. C.R.Soc. Biol. (Paris) *158*, 2137–2140 (1964)

McKinney, W.T. (Jr.), Eising, R.G., Moran, E.C., Suomi, S.J., Harlow, H.F.: Effects of reserpine on the social behavior of rhesus monkeys. Dis. Nerv. Syst. *32*, 735–741 (1971)

Millenson, J.R., Leslie, J.: The conditioned emotional response (CER) as a baseline for the study of anti-anxiety drugs. Neuropharmacology *13*, 1–9 (1974)

Morpurgo, C., Theobald, W.: Behavioral reactions to amphetamine in reserpinized rats. Int. J. Neuropharmacol. *5*, 375–377 (1966)

Morrison, A.B., Webster, R.A.: Drug induced experimental parkinsonism. Neuropharmacology *12*, 715–724 (1973 a)

Morrison, A.B., Webster, R.A.: Reserpine rigidity and adrenergic neurones. Neuropharmacology *12*, 725–733 (1973 b)

Mueller, J.M., Schlittler, E., Bein, H.J.: Reserpin, der sedative Wirkstoff aus Rauwolfia Serpentina Benth. Experientia 8, 338 (1952)

Mueller, R.A., Thoenen, H., Axelrod, J.: Increase in tyrosine hydroxylase activity after reserpine administration. J. Pharmacol. Exp. Ther. *169*, 74–79 (1969)

Munson, J.B., Graham, R.B.: Lateral geniculate spikes in sleeping, awake, and reserpine-treated cats: correlated excitability changes in superior colliculus and related structures. Exp. Neurol. *31*, 326–336 (1971)

Munson, J.B., Graham, R.B.: Localization of lateral geniculate spikes in alert, sleeping and reserpine-treated cats. Electroencephalogr. Clin. Neurophysiol. *35*, 323–326 (1973)

Norn, S., Shore, P.A.: Further studies on the nature of persistent reserpine binding: evidence for reversible and irreversible binding. Biochem. Pharmacol. *20*, 1291–1295 (1971 a)

Norn, S., Shore, P.A.: Failure to affect tissue reserpine concentrations by alteration of adrenergic nerve activity. Bioch. Pharmacol. *20*, 2133–2135 (1971 b)

Palfai, T., Walsh, T.J., Albala, B.J., Brown, O.M.: Effects of 1-Dihydroxyphenylalanine (L-Dopa) and d, 1, 5-Hydroxytryptophan (d, 1, 5-HTP) on reserpine-induced amnesia. Psychopharmacology *53*, 269–276 (1977)

Papeschi, R., Randrup, A., Lai, S.: Effect of ECT on dopaminergic and noradrenergic mechanisms. I. Effect on the behavioural changes induced by reserpine, alpha-methyl-p-tyrosine or amphetamine. Psychopharmacologia *35*, 149–158 (1974)

Philippu, A., Becke, H., Burger, A.: Effect of drugs on the uptake of noradrenaline by isolated hypothalamic vesicles. Eur. J. Pharmacol. *6*, 96–101 (1969)

Pirch, J.H.: Behavior "recovery" during chronic reserpine treatment: effect of dose of reserpine. Psychopharmacologia *16*, 253–260 (1969)

Pirch, J.H., Rech, R.H.: Behavioral recovery in rats during chronic reserpine treatment. Psychopharmacologia *12*, 115–122 (1968)

Pirch, J.H., Rech, R.H., Moore, K.E.: Depression and recovery of the electrocorticogram, behavior, and brain amines in rats treated with reserpine. Int. J. Neuropharmacol. *6*, 375–385 (1967)

Pletscher, A., Shore, P.A., Brodie, B.B.: Serotonin release as a possible mechanism of reserpine action. Science *122*, 374–375 (1955)

Plummer, A.J., Earl, A., Schneider, J.A., Trapold, J., Barrett, W.: Pharmacology of Rauwolfia alkaloids, including reserpine. Ann. N.Y. Acad. Sci. *59*, 8–21 (1954)

Pollard, H., Bischoff, S., Schwartz, J.C.: Increased synthesis and release of 3H-histamine in rat brain by reserpine. Eur. J. Pharmacol. *24*, 399–401 (1973)

Popov, N., Matthies, H.J.: Die Wirkung von Monoaminoxydase-Hemmstoffen und Reserpin auf den γ-Amino-Buttersäure-Gehalt des Rattenhirns. Acta Biol. Med. Ger. *18*, 91–98 (1967)

Prince, R.: The use of Rauwolfia for the treatment of psychosis by Nigerian native doctors. Am. J. Psychiatry *117*, 147–149 (1960)

Rand, M.J., Jurevics, H.: The pharmacology of Rauwolfia alkaloids. In: Hdb. Exp. Pharmacology. Gross, F. (ed.). New Series XXXIX. Berlin, Heidelberg, New York: Springer 1977, pp. 77–159

Ray, O.S.: Tranquilizer effects as a function of experimental anxiety procedures. Arch. Int. Pharmacodyn. Ther. *153*, 49–68 (1965)

Raymond-Hamet, M.: Le „Rauwolfia vomitoria" Afzelius possède-t-il réellement les vertus thérapeutiques que lui attribuent les guérisseurs indigènes? Bull. Acad. Méd. *122*, 30–38 (1939)

Reite, M., Pegram, G.V., Stephens, L.M., Bixler, E.C., Lewis, O.L.: The effect of reserpine and monoamine oxidase inhibitors on paradoxical sleep in the monkey. Psychopharmacologia *14*, 12–17 (1969)

Rieppel, F.W.: Zur Frühgeschichte der Rauwolfia. Sudhoffs Arch. *40*, 231–239 (1956)

Rohte, O., Müntzing, J.: Effects of reserpine, 6-hydroxydopamine, p-chlorophenylalanine and a combination of these substances on the grooming behaviour of mice. Psychopharmacologia *31*, 333–342 (1973)

Roos, B.E., Steg, G.: The effect of L-3, 4-dihydroxyphenylalanine and DL-5-hydroxytryptophan on rigidity and tremor induced by reserpine, chlorpromazine and phenoxybenzamine. Life Sci. *3*, 351–360 (1964)

Saner, A., Pletscher, A.: Increase of striatal dopamine turnover by drugs: interference with granular storage or receptor blockade? Eur. J. Pharmacol. *42*, 155–160 (1977)

Santini, M., Berl, S.: Effects of reserpine and monoamine oxidase inhibition on the levels of amino acids in sensory ganglia, sympathetic ganglia and spinal cord. Brain Res. *47*, 167–176 (1972)

Sato, S., Daly, R., Peters, H.: Reserpine therapy of phenothiazine induced dyskinesia. Dis. Nerv. Syst. *32*, 680–685 (1971)

Satoh, T.: Cortical responsiveness during reserpine-induced PGO-spike in the cat. Int. J. Neurosci. *3*, 201–204 (1972)

Schiorring, E., Randrup, A.: "Paradoxical" stereotyped activity of reserpinized rats. Int. J. Neuropharmacol *7*, 71–73 (1968)

Schlittler, E., Bein, H.J.: Rauwolfia alkaloids in "Antihypertensive Agents." New York: Academic Press 1967 pp. 191–221

Schneider, J.A., Plummer, A.J., Earl, A.E., Gaunt, R.: Neuropharmacological aspects of reserpine. Ann. N.Y. Acad. Sci. *61*, 17–26 (1955)

Schwartz, J.C., Julien, C., Feger, J., Garbarg, M.: Histaminergic pathway in rat brain evidenced by hypothalamic lesions. Fed. Proc. *33*, 285 (1974)

Segal, D.S., Sullivan, J.L., Kuczenski, R.T., Mandell, A.J.: Effects of long-term reserpine treatment on brain tyrosine hydroxylase and behavioral activity. Science *173*, 847–849 (1971)

Seiden, L.S., Carlsson, A.: Brain and heart catecholamine levels after L-Dopa administration in reserpine treated mice: correlations with a conditioned avoidance response. Psychopharmacologia *5*, 178–181 (1964)

Seiden, L.S., Hanson, L.C.F.: Reversal of the reserpine-induced suppression of the conditioned avoidance response in the cat by L-Dopa. Psychopharmacologia 6, 239–244 (1964)

Seiden, L.S., Peterson, D.D.: Reversal of the reserpine-induced suppression of the conditioned avoidance response by L-Dopa: correlation of behavioral and biochemical differences in two strains of mice. J. Pharmacol. Exp. Ther. 159, 422–428 (1968a)

Seiden, L.S., Peterson, D.D.: Blockade of L-Dopa reversal of reserpine-induced conditioned avoidance response suppression by disulfiram. J. Pharmacol. Exp. Ther. 163, 84–90 (1968b)

Seiden, L.S., MacPhail, R.C., Oglesby, M.W.: Catecholamines and drug-behavior interactions. Fed. Proc. 34, 1823–1831 (1975)

Sen, G., Bose, K.C.: Rauwolfia serpentina, a new Indian drug for insanity and high blood pressure. Indian Med. World 2, 194–201 (1931)

Silvestrini, B., Maffii, G.: Effects of chlorpromazine, promazine, diethazine, reserpine, hydroxyzine and morphine upon some mono- and polysynaptic motor reflexes. J. Pharm. Pharmacol. 11, 224–233 (1959)

Simpson, F.O., Waal-Manning, H.J.: Hypertension and depression, interrelated problems in therapy. J. R. Coll. Physicians Lond. 6, 14–24 (1971)

Slotkin, Th.A.: Hypothetical model of catecholamine uptake into adrenal medullary storage vesicles. Life Sci. 13, 675–683 (1973)

Smith, C.B., Dews, P.B.: Antagonismus of locomotor suppressant effects of reserpine in mice. Psychopharmacologia 3, 55–59 (1962)

Steg, G.: Efferent muscle innervation and rigidity. Acta Physiol. Scand. 61, Suppl. 225 (1964)

Stein, L.: Self-stimulation of the brain and the central stimulant action of amphetamine. Fed. Proc. 23, 836–850 (1964)

Stern, W.C., Morgane, P.J.: Effects of reserpine on sleep and brain biogenic amine levels in the cat. Psychopharmacologia 28, 275–286 (1973)

Stille, G.: Zur Pharmakologie katatonigener Stoffe. 2. Mitteilung: Ausschaltung des N. caudatus und die katatonigene Wirkung der Neuroleptika. Arzneimittel-Forsch. 21, 386–390 (1971)

Stinus, L., Thierry, A.M., Cardo, B.: Effects of various inhibitors of tyrosine hydroxylase and dopamine β hydroxylase on rat self stimulation after reserpine treatment. Psychopharmacologia 45, 287–294 (1976)

Stitzel, R.E.: The biological fate of reserpine. Pharm. Rev. 28, 179–205 (1976)

Strömbom, U.: On the functional role of pre- and postsynaptic catecholamine receptors in brain. Acta Physiol. Scand. [Suppl.] 431, 1–43 (1975)

Tabushi, K., Himwich, B.E.: The acute effects of reserpine on the sleep-wakefulness cycle in rabbits. Psychopharmacologia 16, 240–252 (1969)

Taugner, G., Hasselbach, W.: Über den Mechanismus der Catecholamin-Speicherung in den „chromaffinen Granula" des Nebennierenmarks. Naunyn Schmiedebergs Arch. Pharmacol. 255, 266–286 (1966)

Taylor, K.M., Snyder, S.H.: The release of histamine from tissue slices of rat hypothalamus. J. Neurochem. 21, 1215–1223 (1973)

Wagner, L.A.: Minireview. Subcellular storage of biogenic amines. Life Sci. 17, 1755–1762 (1975)

Weber, E.: Ein Rauwolfia-Alkaloid in der Psychiatrie: Seine Wirkungsähnlichkeit mit Chlorpromazin. Schweiz. Med. Wochenschr. 84, 968–970 (1954)

Weiskrantz, L., Wilson, W.A. (Jr.): The effects of reserpine on emotional behavior of normal and brain-operated monkeys. Ann. N.Y. Acad. Sci. 61, 36–55 (1955)

Weiskrantz, L., Wilson, W.A. (Jr.): Effect of reserpine on learning and performance, Science 123, 1117–1118 (1956)

White, T.: Histamine and methylhistamine in cat brain and other tissues. Br. J. Pharmacol. 26, 494–501 (1966)

Zigmond, R.E., Schon, F., Iversen, L.L.: Increased tyrosine hydroxylase activity in the locus coeruleus of rat brain stem after reserpine treatment and cold stress. Brain Res. 70, 547–552 (1974)

Zivkovic, B., Guidotti, A., Costa, E.: Increase of tryptophan hydroxylase activity elicited by reserpine. Brain Res. 57, 522–526 (1973)

CHAPTER 4

Behavioral Pharmacology of Antipsychotics

H. KREISKOTT

A. Introduction

It is the task of behavioral pharmacology to find and to differentiate substance actions in animals and in man by observation or instrumental analysis of spontaneous individual and social behavior, of the antagonistic and/or synergistic influence on stimulus and/or drug-induced behavioral changes as well as of effects on learning and memorizing capacity.

The term antipsychotic specifies substances of various chemical compounds which are able to prevent, to suppress or to abolish processes of extreme excitation in man which may be accompanied by pathological experiences such as illusions, hallucinations and delusional conditions. Stereotyped thinking and behavior are characteristic for schizophrenias. Stereotyped movements are described particularly for catatonic types as "rhythmic turning" of the head to one side, mimicking gestures, frowning, lifting the upper lip, shaking the arms (MUNKVAD, 1970).

The terms neuroleptic and major tranquillizer are used in the literature synonymously with antipsychotic. The term antipsychotic is mainly applied in connection with the inhibition of extreme excitation conditions and stereotyped processes in motor activity and thinking (MUNKVAD, 1970); neuroleptic has a similar meaning but is more often used with emphasis on accompanying effects such as in neuroleptic threshold (HAASE, 1966, 1977). Major tranquillizers describe substances with sedating, tranquillizing characters which cause only slight or no extrapyramidal side-effects in the doses used. The antipsychotics introduced in clinical practice belong to the groups of phenothiazines, thioxanthenes, butyrophenones and of reserpine; substances with other structures, e.g. oxypertine and sulpiride, are more recent additions.

B. Basic Aspects and Considerations in Regard to Investigations

The behavior of both man and animal is composed of observable activities including the expressive movements. The transition from normal to pathologic reactions such as excessive aggression and iterations is gradual and depends on the excitation pattern of the organism. A lack of excitation may lead to stupor, strong excitation to hypermotility and even convulsions but also to immobility, to catalepsy. Extreme physiological conditions such as coma, or paralysis caused by neuromuscular block or anaesthesia do not fall within our subject.

KRAEPELIN and BLEULER realized that schizophrenia is not a uniform pathologic picture with only a single cause. In more modern psychiatry a multifactor aetiology of the various types of schizophrenia is therefore assumed (ACKENHEIL et al., 1978).

Nosological diagnostic findings are assessed by considering the syndrome, if possible even on a symptomatic level (HIPPIUS and MATUSSEK, 1978). Symptoms may be assessed more precisely because of the introduction of rating-scales and the AMP[1]-system and have become comparable in spite of different investigators (ANGST et al., 1969). Pharmacotherapy of psychoses is a restitution of behavioral patterns and condition of the patient. But antipsychotics exert their action not only on disturbed behavior but also on normal processes which form the basis for disturbed reactions. This enables us to investigate the action of psychotropic substances in healthy test persons. Symptoms, syndromes and psycho-physiological reaction abilities indicate gradual transitions from healthy to afflicted individuals (DEBUS, 1977). This is one of the bases for the investigation of neurotropic drugs in intact experimental animals.

Animal experiments are imperative in order to find new drugs, to characterize them pharmacologically and to select them in view of their clinical use. Disregarding verbal expression, which is specific to man, the changes of behavior after application of antipsychotics in animals and in man are closely related. All living creatures show a restricted number of drives and reactions. Reflexes, movements, gestures, signals and ceremonies as a whole are characteristic for individual species but nevertheless comparable since they developed like the anatomical substrate, phylogenically. Psycho-pathological types of expression as well may to a large extent be attributed to motor reactions and parts of specific drives common to all mammals (PLOOG, 1964; HEINRICH, 1965; ITIL[2]; KREISKOTT, 1979). The comparison of different behavioral processes is epistemologically based on the same principles which have led to the natural system of animals, to comparative anatomy and to phylogenesis as not only cells, organs and organic systems but also behavioral patterns and parts thereof have an evolutionary history. They are hereditary structures and may therefore be homologized. The criteria were formulated and discussed by REMANE (1952) and WICKLER (1961). Not only organs and organic systems but also the functions based on them are homologous. The homology of processes is more secure the more they conform in regard to differentiated characteristics, the more similar they are and the more frequently they occur in related species. Drives secure the basic functions of organism, which are necessary for the survival of the individual and the species. They are particularly conservative as their loss or significant changes due to mutation would imperil the individual and thus the species. This presents a further basis in scientific theory for the investigation of psychotropic substances in animals to make predictions to their effects in man.

Essential suggestions for pharmacological investigations will always be clinical results. The importance of animal experiments in finding new antipsychotics and in differentiating between their qualities arises from the history of modern psychopharmacology.

With promethazine at the onset LABORIT and HUGENARD developed the potentiated anaesthesia, and they controlled hypothermia with chlorpromazine (due to its sedative-hypnotic, anaesthesia-potentiating and hypothermic components) (reviews: LABORIT, 1954; WEESE, 1954). In 1952 DELAY et al. recognized the antipsychotic action of chlorpromazine, and almost at the same time COURVOISIER et al. (1953), in a large-

---

1 Arbeitsgemeinschaft für Methodik und Dokumentation in der Psychiatrie (Working group for methodology and documentation in psychiatry)
2 Year of publication unknown

scale animal experiment, proved not only the properties used in anaesthesia and the adrenolytic and anticholinergic components but also the essential effects on behavior: muscle relaxation, antiemetic action and inhibition of conditioned avoidance. In 1957 the same working group made a supplementary contribution to behavioral pharmacology by observing catalepsy in rats, dogs and rhesus monkeys. WIRTH et al. (1958) introduced the inhibition of the spontaneous motor impulse of the mouse as well as the fright reaction and posture reflexes of the Syrian golden hamster as further differentiating behavioral tests. BEIN (1953) postulated a central action of reserpine based on cardiovascular studies. He and his colleagues observed impaired spontaneous motility, indifference towards external stimuli, somnolence, reduced food intake, ptosis, catalepsy and hypothermia, in various species as sedative-neuroleptic properties (TRIPOD et al., 1954). With animal experiments, carried out in 1958, JANSSEN et al. succeeded in finding neuroleptics of varying strength among the butyrophenones which gained great importance in the treatment of psychoses (HAASE, 1966, 1977). The screening methods proved that there are simple behavioral criteria which are more expressive than highly complicated non-transparent models and allow predictions of clinical effects (STILLE, 1974).

It is a rare occurrence in the history of pharmacology for the recognition of new clinical signs, due to the introduction of psychotropic substances, to result in such an explosive development of new animal experimental methods. One experimental idea is to look for equivalents in the behavior of animals which correspond to effects and side-effects of antipsychotics in man. Sedative-hypnotic, antiemetic and muscle-relaxing effects, for example, are thus determined. The parkinsonoid syndrome in man including tremor, catalepsy, glosso-pharyngeal dyskinesia and akathisia corresponds, in animals, to cataleptic immobilization with lack of impulses, passiveness and tolerance of bizarre positions. The other experimental idea also involves studying innate and learned animal behavior, whereby behavioral patterns which have no direct relation to pathological pictures in man such as prey catching and maternal behavior are also included. Pharmacologists use influences on specific impulses of various species to obtain a pharmacological profile of action. Physiologists and ethologists disturb the behavioral pattern by drugs (among them antipsychotics) to investigate the behavior, because a disturbed biological process is often more informative for the exact assessment, description and analysis of the basic normal process than is the rule.

Both ideas resulted in important results and allow the pharmacological characterization not only of the individual antipsychotics but also of the antipsychotics as a group. KREISKOTT (1965a, 1974a) and recently FIELDING and LAL (1978) have presented summaries under this aspect. The latter, using numerous experimental designs, gives data of up to 40 neuroleptics which were made available to the authors JANSSEN, VAN BEVER and NIEMEGEERS. This compilation of data is highly informative, due to uniform acquisition and treatment and shall be repeatedly referred to. The following section is intended to give a selection of important ideas for characterization of chemical substances, and trends in investigating the action of antipsychotics on behavior.

C. Action of Antipsychotics on Spontaneous Behavior

The action of antipsychotics on spontaneous behavior is best categorized according to drives or parts thereof, giving examples of different methods and species, but also of different actions of individual neuroleptics.

I. Pattern of Action on Behavior

The consideration that drugs exert the same or similar actions in animals and in man caused IRWIN (1957, 1964) and IRWIN et al. (1971) to investigate the total behavior in the animal as a model for effects in man. As clinical investigations are preceded by the pharmacological selection of substances the assessment of numerous parameters of action in an experimental design using the same species may result in better, faster and more economical investigations. The methods were developed in mice and cats but may easily be applied to any other mammal which is to be kept under laboratory conditions. The parameters are body posture and limb position, convulsions, tremor and motor activity, furthermore aggression, rigidity, irritability, palpebral aperture, pupil size and body temperature. This procedure proved to be so highly efficient that IRWIN and KONOHI (1971) applied it to the clinical investigation of substances in man as well. NORTON (1957) assessed 25 behavioral patterns including social behavior, in each cats, golden hamsters and rhesus monkeys, and the changes occurring after drug administration, including chlorpromazine. The 25 patterns were summarized in 5 groups: sociability, contentment, excitement, defensive hostility and aggressive hostility. A "scoring-system" allows a classification (this was also done by IRWIN).

To determine the quantitative action of antipsychotics, individual behavioral parameters are mostly assessed and demonstrated in a dose-dependent manner and as a time function.

II. Locomotion

In healthy test persons antipsychotics cause sedation and drowsiness of various degree depending on chemical structure and doses, in agitated schizophrenic patients suffering from insomnia they reduce motor activity and exert soporific effects (HAASE, 1966; GREENBLATT and SHADER, 1977). A variability of methods to assess locomotor activity has been described on which a review was given by KINNARD and WATZMAN (1966) and a critique by ROBBINS (1977).

The following five principles of assessment are predominantly used in animal experiments:
1) Open field;
2) jiggle cages recording the movements of a small spring suspended box into which the animal is placed;
3) light barrier cages recording horizontal or vertical movements of the animal(s);
4) inductive and capacitive frequency shift methods;
5) running wheels which mostly allow moving in one direction only whereby the movements are recorded.

Open field describes a test situation in which the locomotor activity of the test animal is observed when placed in a larger area than its usual home cage. The floor is devided into squares allowing the recording of changes either by observation or by means of an apparatus (ROBBINS, 1977; VOITH and HERR, 1975). JANSSEN et al. (1960b, 1965) investigated numerous antipsychotics in rats applying this method which also proved to be applicable to other experimental animals. HUGHES et al. (1977) differentiated the actions of azaperone and acetylpromazine using sheep as experimental animals. This and numerous other papers demonstrate that not only locomotor activity

– walking, running, jumping, rearing and motionless posturing – but also a number of other parameters are frequently used for the further characterization of antipsychotics, e.g. preening, sniffing, food intake, urination, defaecation and vocalization. LJUNGBERG and UNGERSTEDT (1978) using automatic equipment recorded eight parameters of this type simultaneously. Mere observation and these methods are well-suited for the assessment of exploration but also of the continuous activity of the animals.

Exploratory behavior of rodents may also be recorded applying separate experimental designs. The animals orientate themselves in a new environment by sniffing and feeling movements of the vibrissae and turning movements of the head, running is increased. There is naturally a particular tendency to dip the head into holes and to crawl into tunnels.

BOISSIER and SIMON (1964) used an open field fitted with holes in which the mice could dip and draw back their heads. KRNJEVIC and VIDEK (1967), using rats, placed a cage underneath a one-hole plate. To measure the activity they assess the period between dipping of the nose and disappearing of the tail base. Chlorpromazine, acetyl-promazine, thioridazine and reserpine significantly slow down the downward movement.

A particular of locomotor activity is the tendency of rodents to run upwards on sloping surfaces. The usual compulsion to move is additionally stimulated by the activation of the posture reflexes. WIRTH et al. (1958) took advantage of this fact. A board, covered with coarse canvas, is placed at a slope of 75°. Mice put onto the lower edge of the board feel compelled to run up the board. Sedating substances more or less reduce the activity of the animals. Tone and strength of the muscles and posture reflexes are stressed. Remaining at the lower edge may be regarded as sedation but cataleptic effects cannot be excluded. KNEIP (1960) did not put the mice directly onto the sloping surface but employed their exploratory behavior to make them climb up. A group of mice was placed in a cage with transparent walls, they climbed a sloping ladder of wire net within 10 min. Neuroleptics inhibit this reaction in some of the animals depending on the doses given (SANDBERG, 1959).

Running wheels were developed to assess perseverance and performance; the running activity at the inner side of the drum is measured by the number of revolutions. OBERST and CROOK (1967) subjected dogs to a sustained physical exercise test. The animals were trained to run in a treadmill for 15 min and, after a 2 min break, continued up to 1 h. The test was interrupted and the time recorded when the dog stopped running after i.v. treatment with antipsychotics. Pulse rate and body temperature were additionally measured before and after the test.

The reduced activity may also be easily investigated in fish. (CHARI-BITRON and CHARI-BITRON, 1970). Minnows *(Gambusia affinis)* tend to rise to the surface of the test vessel. Vibration stimuli caused the control animals to sink, they remained at the bottom of the vessel and then resumed an evenly distributed pattern. Minnows treated with 0.2 and 0.3 µg/ml of chlorpromazine, contained in the water, show only a slight tendency to sink and quickly resume their position at the surface. The animals receiving 0.4 and 0.5 µg/ml remained at the surface, also when applying external stimuli.

Clinical experience and the results of the experiments described uniformly demonstrate that locomotion is inhibited by the administration of neuroleptics and may result in immobility when giving neuroleptics in higher dose ranges.

III. Immobilization

Neuroleptic-induced inhibition of locomotion is of particular significance as it stands in contrast to the inquisitive behavior of animals; this gave rise to numerous experimental investigations. Antipsychotics, administered in doses higher than those necessary to reduce mobility, cause a lack of motor impulses, passiveness towards external stimuli, hunchback posture, abnormal cataleptic postures and rigidity (COURVOISIER et al., 1957). The most simple experimental design to be applied to rodents, insectivores, carnivores and primates is to place the animals at a block (WIRTH et al., 1958; KREISKOTT, 1965a) recording mobility of the animals, intensity of the reaction and duration of motionless posturing. MENGE and BRAND (1978) tried to analyse the reactions of rats to different cataleptogenic substances by employing various trigger mechanisms. Besides static tests (placing the animals in upright position, spreading of the extremities, back position, tolerance of a wooden rod sticking in the mouth) they applied dynamic methods: the animals are turned in a horizontal and vertical wire-net tube as well as use of a treadmill. In static tests the abnormal position is maintained in spite of different trigger mechanisms such as constant and variable muscle relaxation, changes of position, provocation of movement and trigeminal stimulation whereas the animal is unable to do this in dynamic tests. Intrinsic reflexes are maintained, extrinsic reflexes increased. Escape and defence reactions are inhibited. According to COSTALL and NAYLOR (1973) antipsychotics of the phenothiazine and butyrophenone group, reserpine and oxypertine as well as loxapine and clothiapine induce marked catalepsy, clozapine, however, exerts only a slight cataleptogenic action in spite of its pronounced clinical antipsychotic effect. With the exception of loxapine and clothiapine the cataleptic action of the substances mentioned, e.g. including clozapine, is increased when combining them with cholinergic agents. KOSTOWSKI and CZLONKOWSKI (1973) and ZETLER (1975) studied the cataleptic effect of antipsychotics in rats and mice, respectively, which had been socially isolated for 3 and 4 weeks. Rats, which seemed indolent and "socially indifferent" (VALZELLI and GARATTINI, 1972) after longer-term isolation react less sensitively to chlorpromazine and haloperidol than other animals in the group. Mice, however, which become more aggressive by isolation (YEN et al., 1958; VALZELLI et al., 1967) were more sensitive to the cataleptogenic action of haloperidol. ZETLER (1975) concludes from these findings and from antidote trials that catalepsy is not due to central depression, but is much rather caused by stimulation of certain cerebral structures. This conclusion is supported by many studies carried out by STILLE (1971) in rats and rabbits from which he concludes that antipsychotic-induced catalepsy is a reaction of active inhibition. Strong cataleptogenic substances such as loxapine, fluphenazine, perphenazine and haloperidol cause an increased functional readiness of limbic structures in contrast to the reduced vigilance in the cortex. A clear correlation is existent between cataleptogenic and antipsychotic action in the sence of the influence on paranoid–hallucinotic patterns. The cortical arousal reaction in the EEG of rabbits is most intensely inhibited by neuroleptics with slight cataleptogenic properties, e.g. perlapine, chlorprothixene, clozapine and thioridazine. Strong neuroleptics are lacking this component in animal experiments and in the clinical equivalent, i.e. the depressing, sleep-inducing action.

Neuroleptic catatonia is also connected with increased electrical irritability of the neostriatum which may be concluded from the fact that a functional failure of the caudate nucleus is followed by a reduction of neuroleptic-induced rigidity and catalepsy (STILLE, 1971). The striatal aetiology of cataleptic conditions in mammals gives rise to the question as to the action of cataleptogenics on other animal species.

Octopus shows centralization of the nervous system, cephalization, localizable functions in the brain and a hierarchy of the centres but no striatum and no extra-pyramidal-motor system in the sense of mammalian anatomy. Still, the octopus given 1 mg/litre of chlorpromazine, administered via the water pumped through the respiratory cavity, reacts with slight catalepsy which is indicated by bizarre positions, a lack of impulses and marked muscle relaxation. Butyrylperazine, in doses of 0.1–2 mg/litre, causes complete immobilization after 30–60 min (KREISKOTT, 1963b, 1965b). MERCIER and DESSAIGNE (1970) investigated chlorpromazine and reserpine in the scorpion *(Androctonus australis)*. Chlorpromazine, after dorsal administration of 50–100 µg/g into the front region of the abdomen, reduced muscle tone and inhibited defensive reflexes but did not influence motor activity. As compared to that, reserpine did not influence the muscle tone but induced a catalepsy-like condition.

The site of action of antipsychotics is also at the nerve structures in groups with entirely different systems. Even details of cataleptic conditions such as tense and relaxed catalepsy become evident. The equidirection of the influence on the motor system is remarkable, but should not be overrated as compared to other systems as our senses present an especially pronounced ability to recognize movements and their changes.

IV. Muscle Relaxation and Ptosis

The flexible relaxed form of catalepsy in invertebrates and vertebrates can be explained by the reduced muscle tone due to phenothiazines of the chlorpromazine type. KINNARD and CARR (1957) recorded the muscle relaxation after chlorpromazine in mice using a rotarod in which the animals must prove their ability to hold on to the rotating rod. This method is well-suited for screening purposes but also for the differentiation of new antipsychotic substances, as has been shown by COSCIA et al. (1975) who used several methylpiperazines. The tube test, performed in the golden hamster, is very useful for a more precise assessment of muscle relaxation in the intact animal (KREISKOTT, 1963c). The animals are placed in a plexiglass tube kept in a horizontal position. Normal animals and also those with suppressed effect hold fast when the tube is gradually brought into a vertical position. Hamsters with muscle relaxation, prestages of anaesthesia or toxic damages, however, slip through after a more or less short period.

In connection with the muscle relaxing action of antipsychotics ptosis of the eyelids, i.e. the passive closing of the palpebral aperture which is removable for a short period by external stimuli, must be mentioned. TEDESCHI (1967) points out that the reduction of sympathetic outflow is paralleled by sedation. Ptosis is induced by activation of branches of the facial nerve and a central depression of the upper part of the sympathicus in the cervical region. The palpebral width is reduced after reserpine, and a third independent mechanism of action is the retraction of the eyeballs into the orbit (TEDESCHI, 1967). Further possibilities for the investigation of motor reactions using operant conditioning methods are discussed by LEHR in another chapter of this handbook.

According to LOEW (1970) the inhibition of locomotion allows the prediction of sedating actions in clinical practice: the same holds for catalepsy in regard to the affinity to the extrapyramidal-motor system, i.e. in regard to neuroleptic qualities and dyskinesias. FIELDING and LAL (1978) discussed the correlation of locomotor inhibition and cataleptic action as another possibility. This becomes evident by comparing the ED_{50}-values of both parameters in 40 antipsychotics as described by JANSSEN and VAN BEVER (1978). Deviations in the ratio might, for example, be due to differences in muscle relaxation.

V. Excitation Conditions

Excitation is the response of the organism to one or more stimuli exceeding a threshold value. Conditions of unrest due to hyperexcitation become evident, besides increased locomotion, in repetitive reactions, rhythmic movement sequences which are stereotyped, of compulsive character and clearly different from normal behavior. They are characteristic for all amniotes, birds and mammals, including man. Very strong stimuli induce defence reactions of the organism. The most pronounced reaction is fright. All ergotropic mechanisms are suddenly mobilized by a vigorous stimulus, according to LEYHAUSEN (1967) the only case in which vigilance and tone come near to "general excitation."

An easily arousable and reproducible effect reaction in the mammal is a characteristic fright reaction of the golden hamster *(Mesocricetus auratus)*. It rolls over and stretches its extremities, defaecation is often observed, also sharpening of the teeth and preening at the end of the reaction.

In an ethogram of the golden hamster set up by NORTON (1957) the most frequently occurring reaction of spontaneous social behavior out of 25 reactions observed is rolling over. The reaction can be experimentally induced by a vigorous, measured air blast on the neck. Antipsychotics influence the intensity of the reaction (WIRTH et al., 1958; KREISKOTT and VATER, 1959; THER et al., 1959; KREISKOTT, 1963c; Table 1). Reserpine, administered orally, reached its maximal effect, similar to clinical results, only after approx. 24 h. 0.1 mg/kg resulted in a 50%, 0.25 mg/kg in an 80% inhibition of defensive behavior (KREISKOTT, 1963c).

Table 1. Inhibition of the fright reaction of the golden hamster after oral administration of the test substances (KREISKOTT, unpublished data)

Substance	ED_{50} mg/kg p.o.[a] (95% confidence interval)	t_{max}
Fluphenazine	1.8 (0.24/ 4.0)	5 h
Haloperidol	3.5 (1.72/ 7.5)	2 h
Chlorpromazine	5.4 (1.36/13.1)	3 h
Melperone	15.6 (2.9 /40)	4 h
Clozapine	15.7 (2.6 /97)	5 h

[a] The ED_{50} values are listed at the time of the maximal effect of the substance (t_{max})

The cotton rat *(Sigmidon hispidus)* shows a hereditary escape reaction at a low stimulation threshold which may be triggered off by sounds or air jets, and its inhibition can be used to assess centrally depressing substances. As described for the golden hamster the hereditary impulse is suppressed by antipsychotics in doses far lower than those required to cause coordination disorders (VOGEL and THER, 1960). Fear and tension in conditioned escape reactions but also in fright reactions cause vegetative signs, among others defaecation. The inhibition of emotional defaecation of the rat was used by HUNT (1956) and TAESCHLER and CERLETTI (1960) to investigate antipsychotics. The latter found predominantly an inhibition of motor reaction in the case of perphenazine and thiopropazate whereas thioridazine mainly suppressed emotional defaecation; chlorpromazine and prochlorperazine influence both functions to an equal extent.

Socially isolated animals which are kept in a small area tend to repetitive reactions. Caged canaries exhibit route tracing and spot picking. 30 mg/kg of chlorpromazine p.o. inhibits both parameters after 60 min without influencing posture reflexes and inquisitive behavior (KEIPER, 1969). Nociceptive stimuli induce increased locomotion up to escape behavior, motionless posturing and, in the presence of conspecifics, behavior directed towards the other animal. A particularly well-suited design for behavioral pharmacological analysis is the aggressive–defensive behavior of the mouse aroused by electrical foot shocks in pairs of mice, (TEDESCHI et al., 1959b; HOFFMEISTER and WUTTKE, 1969). Two male mice are placed onto a metal grid floor and foot shocked with certain intensity and frequency. These stimuli induce behavior regarded as aggression. The animals make attempts to escape, they vocalize and then stand upright opposite one another. The behavior is initially aggressive, the animals may wound one another by biting, and then becomes defensive or even submissive. The frequency of contacts between the animals is taken to measure the intensity of the reaction. The inhibitory action of amphetamine demonstrates that defensive behavior is an essential part (LAL et al., 1968), the animals exhibit rigidity due to over-excitation. Antipsychotics, chlorpromazine, prochlorpromazine and trifluperazine exert significant actions on aggressive–defensive behavior in approx. those doses which also inhibit spontaneous motor activity (TEDESCHI et al., 1969). HOFFMEISTER and WUTTKE (1969) proved the effect of chlorpromazine on hand of the attack and aggressive–defensive behavior of the cat, EMLEY and HUTCHINSON (1971) used the defensive biting reaction of the squirrel monkey. SACKETT (1968) regards disturbing influences on young animals, e.g. isolation from conspecifics, as an essential cause of abnormal behavior later in life. MCKINNEY et al. (1973) isolated rhesus monkeys from their mothers for 11 months, isolation beginning directly after birth. They developed abnormal behavior such as mutilation by self-biting, scratching and stereotypies. The animals were then treated with 7.5 mg/kg of chlorpromazine/day by nasogastric intubation for 12 weeks. In three of four monkeys the self-disturbance activity was significantly reduced.

VI. Aggression

Aggressive behavior among members of the same species may occur as sexual rival fights or rank order fights but also as territorial fighting. It depends on external and internal factors and is connected with other drives (WELCH and WELCH, 1969).

So-called aggressive behavior accompanying maternal behavior and prey cateching is dealt with when discussing these drives. The Siamese fighting fish *(Betta splendens)* was used in investigations by ABRAMSON and EVANS (1954), WALASZEK and ABOOD (1956), WIRTH et al. (1958) and THOMPSON (1969). Male fighting fish responded to one another by display, colour intensification and attack. The midline fins and opercula are erect, exposing the branchiostegal membrane. The fight is initially of ritual type but escalates later and culminates in vigorous biting into fins and flanks. The defeated tries to escape. Antipsychchotics reduce the tendency to fight, the animals become pale, the gill covers remain closed, the membranes unexposed. Inhibitory effects on circulation, colour hormones and activity as a whole are furthermore likely to occur. THOMPSON (1969) presented an analysis on the physiology of behavior. The method was used to differentiate neuroleptics qualitatively and quantitatively (WIRTH et al., 1958).

Isolated mice are very aggressive towards conspecifics. YEN et al. (1958) placed an "unisolated" mouse with an "isolated" animal. In the resulting attacks the intruder exhibits defensive behavior. Aggression increases the longer the duration of isolation (LAL et al., 1972) and decreases the larger the group (WELCH and WELCH, 1970). Antipsychotics inhibit isolation-induced aggression (JANSSEN et al., 1960a; VALZELLI et al., 1967) only in high doses, however (LAL et al., 1975). Aggressive behavior of the cat towards conspecifics occurs as two types (LEYHAUSEN, 1973), one is the purely aggressive behavior in the rival fight, the animals stand upright opposite one another, the hairs of back and tail are erected, the ears stand upright. Both animals whine and thrash their tails. After this initial phase the fight starts and culminates in biting in the neck. The other type is a defence–fear behavior overlapped by aggression: crouching body posture, the head slightly bent forward, the ears lie backwards to the side, the animals strike with their paws (see Sect. C. V.). Antipsychotics exert an inhibitory action on both behavioral patterns. 2.5 mg/kg of chlorpromazine p.o. exerts a slightly inhibitory action, the attack behavior is strongly reduced at 8 mg/kg p.o. and the defence–fear behavior at 10 mg/kg p.o. (HOFFMEISTER and WUTTKE, 1969).

Rank orders must also be considered in animals exhibiting this feature. This applies particularly to primates. GIONO-BARBER et al. (1970) investigated this parameter in the dominant food behavior of cynocephalic monkeys *(Papio papio)*. 1 mg/kg of methotrimepromazine, 0.05–0.2 mg/kg of haloperidol and 0.1–0.5 mg/kg of reserpine, administered intramuscularly, reduced aggression towards the inferior animal; the effect was paralleled by drowsiness and staggering. BERRY et al. (1972) investigated drugs by taking advantage of the fights for the rank order. The intruder was not represented by a potentially superior monkey but by the investigator himself, he was accepted as a partner. The younger group members immediately acknowledged his dominance. The group leader initially showed aggressive fear behavior, hanging at the railings and, if junior animals attempted to eat and came near to the intruder, cries, anxiety, restlessness and frequent changes of position. Within 30 min to 2 h after administration of 0.25 mg/kg of oxypertine p.o. the leader climbed down and started eating, drinking and preening. Slight side-effects in the form of sedation occur only at doses of 8 mg/kg and more.

A basis for natural experiments on aggression is given by modern pig production and transport. For economic reasons the animals are kept in a very small space. Excitation conditions increase the innate aggressiveness of pigs. Fighting results in loss of weight, wounding and strain on the heart; the mortality rate is high. The animals are subjected to even greater stress during transport. Azaperone of the butyrophenone group gives almost complete protection within the dose range of 1.5–2.9 mg/kg, administered intramuscularly (SYMOENS, 1970).

The treatment of aggression and excitation in man is more complicated, arousal more variable than in animals. According to SHEARD (1977) there are two types of aggression, either external stimulus or pain induced aggression or anxious, defensive aggression. Depressive conditions of exogenous and endogenous origin and drug influences may furthermore play a part. Antipsychotics with a strong inhibitory action on motor activity exert depressant effects also in this case; phenothiazine and butyrophenone act almost selectively even on aggression within psychotic syndromes.

VII. Reproduction

TAGLIAMONTE et al. (1974) increased the rate of mounts, intromission and ejaculation in sexually sluggish male rats either by apomorphine or by combining L-Dopa with a peripherally acting decarboxylase inhibitor. Haloperidol completely inhibits conditioned and spontaneous activities. ELIASSON and MEYERSON (1976) induced lordosis responses in ovariectomized rats by the combined treatment with oestrogen and progesterone. LSD and apomorphine inhibited the frequency, pimozide (0.1, 0.5 mg/kg) blocked the apomorphine (0.2 mg/kg)-induced decrease of lordosis response, while only a certain abbreviation of the LSD (0.10 mg/kg) inhibition was achieved by pimozide (0.5 mg/kg). Chlorpromazine (0.5 mg/kg) in a dose without effects on lordosis of its own had an action similar to pimozide on the LSD effect.

VIII. Maternal Behavior

The maternal behavior of rats was investigated on days 4, 5, 6, 8, and 10 after the birth of the young by removing the mother or the young from the cage. The parameters used were latency up to the first contact, nest building, exploration, grooming and immobility. 3 mg/kg of chlorpromazine s.c. markedly reduced the duration of the contact with the newborn, reduced the other parameters and increased immobility (FRANKOVA, 1977). BLÖSCH (1972) investigated the action of several phenothiazines on the maternal behavior of free-living herring gulls. Chlorpromazine (12–75 mg/kg), given in the bait, caused increasing motor excitement, the animals stopped brooding and moved aimlessly within their brooding territory. Nevertheless they kept returning to their nest in hunched posture to sit down for a while. After 25–50 mg/kg of methotrimepromazine the gulls left their nest only for a short time and, after performing some retching movements, continued with their normal brooding. 4 mg/kg of fluphenazine and 2.5–7.5 mg/kg of butyrylperazine did not induce any behavioral changes.

IX. Feeding Behavior

Search, selection and intake of food are physiological basic functions which are controlled centrally (HOEBEL, 1971). The pharmacological disturbance of these functions comes to mind and there are numerous experimental designs to assess food and water intake and weight development (SPENGLER and WASER, 1959; OPITZ, 1967). JANSSEN'S method (1961), the conditional food intake in rats (Δ-W-test), has been used to investigate numerous antipsychotics (JANSSEN et al., 1965; FIELDING and LAL, 1978). Rats are trained to cover their total daily requirements of food within 2 h. There is no food available otherwise, water is ad libitum. The substances are administered subcutaneously 30 min before the test period. The amount of food and water ingested, but also body weight differences, are simple criteria for the substance effects. Most potent antipsychotics reduce food intake in the rat, but the doses required are higher than those needed to inhibit avoidance behavior and amphetamine stereotypies, they are equally high or in most cases lower than those required to inhibit locomotion and to induce catalepsy (Tables in FIELDING and LAL, 1978).

X. Prey Catching

Prey catching biologically belongs to food selection and intake but must be separated from them as it is an instinctive act. The behavior of the rat is similar to that of carnivores and was described as "killing-response" by KARLI (1956) and KARLI et al. (1969). The specific instinctive action is a general prey catching reaction of the rat towards small mammals (KREISKOTT, 1963a, 1969). The total process consists of perception – visual, olfactory and tactile – chasing, seizing, orientation by hair line, holding, striking, biting and eating. Only a small percentage of laboratory rats, depending on the strain, show this reaction. Antipsychotics of the phenothiazine type inhibit the final act markedly only at a catalepsy-inducing dose range (KARLI, 1958; KREISKOTT, 1963a; SOFIA, 1969).

The influence on earlier phases cannot be precisely assessed in the rat, the ferret *(Putoris putoris)* is better suited here. Its prey catching consists of individual instinctive actions which follow a certain hierarchy and which are performed in regard to their specific releasers and in a stereotyped way. Haloperidol (0.14 mg/kg i. m.) shortened the total period for capture and killing of prey, improved orientation reactions and produced a better placement of bites. Haloperidol had no influence on the use of paws and rolling to the side. Chlorpromazine (4 mg/kg i. m.) also increased the total period for capture and decreased the number of bites in several cases, the paw movements were unaffected. Clozapine (10 mg/kg i. m.) increased the total period for capture and in some cases a delay or lack of interest in the prey was observed. There was a greater number of bites on captured prey observed with clozapine than with haloperidol. The sedative action is especially evident in the case of clozapine. The orientation reaction is more pointed than in normal behavior and may be due to the protective action of neuroleptics towards additional stimuli (SCHMIDT and APFELBACH, 1977).

XI. Memory and Learning

Memory functions may be experimentally assessed in man and in various animal species by conditioned reactions (training and arousal). This subject is discussed in a separate chapter of this handbook by LEHR (Chapter 5).

D. Actions of Antipsychotics on Induced Behavioral Patterns

The first part of this review was concerned with actions of antipsychotics on spontaneous behavior. The drives or parts thereof may also be stimulated by systemic drug application, topical chemical and electrical stimuli or surgery at the brain. These complete or even excessive reactions may be influenced by antipsychotics, the extent of the influence may be carried over to clinical practice and vice versa.

I. Stimulant-Induced Excitation Patterns

Amphetamine and chemically related compounds which are mostly used in therapy as appetite depressants cause hyperconscious conditions with anxiety and increased motor activity which may culminate in exogenous psychoses (ELLINWOOD et al., 1973). Various animal species show similar motor symptoms with stereotypies. These behavioral patterns predominantly belong to locomotion, licking and compulsive gnawing to preening behavior (KREISKOTT, 1979). ASHCROFT and co-workers (1965) observed stereotyped grinding movements of the jaws and licking in amphetamine addicts. RANDRUP et al. (see Chapter 6) discuss "stereotypies and their relevance for testing neuroleptics" in greater detail elsewhere in this handbook. ED_{50} values of various neuroleptics acting on amphetamine-induced stereotypies of rats are given by FIELDING and LAL (1978). Agitation is paralleled by the O_2 consumption after amphetamine as has been demonstrated by NIEMEGEERS and JANSSEN (1975). This parameter is also a means for assessing the inhibitory action of antipsychotics.

LAL et al. (1976) increased the action of amphetamine by additionally giving L-Dopa, a high rate of upward jumping was observed in the mice when placed individually. Haloperidol, pimozide, chlorpromazine, thioridazine and clozapine antagonized mouse jumping in a dose-dependent manner; promethazine was inactive. The amplitude of the acoustic startle-response of rats can be reduced by pimozide (2.5 mg/kg i. p.). Potentiation of the startle-response by amphetamine isomers is completely blocked by the same dose of pimozide (KEHNE and SORENSON, 1978).

The amphetamine-induced increase of locomotion inhibits the activity of other drives. High doses of amphetamine inhibit the preening behavior of rats. KJELLBERG and RANDRUP (1974) partially restored the preening behavior by spiramide. Complete restoration seems impossible as the normal comfort behavior is impaired by neuroleptics. The results of the anti-amphetamine effects of neuroleptics seem to have a good correlation with the antipsychotic action of the substances in clinical practice. ELLINWOOD and KILBEY (1977), by comparing symptoms in various species, demonstrated the extent to which chronic intoxication with stimulants may even be a model for psychoses. Comparing man, rhesus monkeys, cats and rats, the symptoms observed in man and in cats correspond particularly well. A similar excitation pattern after the daily administration of 10 mg/kg of cocaine i. m. to cats is therefore described in the same paper. The following symptoms occurred in part of the collective as of the third week of treatment: Hyper-reactivity, increase in startle-response, sudden reaction to apparently non-existent stimuli, e. g. sudden recoil or fly-catching behavior involving tongue, specific increase in head and paw shake, fearful crouching; dysjunctive behavior, lack of proper relationship among postures or movements, often isolated remnant or abortive behaviors (e. g. grooming), dystonia, awkward movement or posture, twitches and dyskinesias, e. g. torsion of tongue, blepharospasm, facial twitches, obstinate progression, akathisia, ataxia. The excitation pattern of four strongly reacting cats was abolished in three animals by 2.5 mg/kg of clozapine i. m., in all animals by 5 mg/kg. 0.8 mg/kg of pimozide i. m. was inactive but had an effect in two of four animals at 2 mg/kg.

Apomorphine causes motor excitement, vomiting and repetitive reactions in mammals and birds (KREISKOTT, 1979). Licking and compulsive gnawing are regarded as phases of head preening. Sharpening of the teeth, differing from the gnawing in its frequency, has cleaning functions but also occurs as displacement activity and as a threat. RANDRUP et al., in a separate section (Chapter 6) of this handbook, discuss stereotypies with relation to neuroleptic effects, the other impulse drives stimulated by apomorphine and antagonized by neuroleptics shall be mentioned here.

Apomorphine (5 mg/kg s. c.) increases the total activity and locomotion in the rat, the legs are flexed, hunchback formation and erected tail are observed and, at the same time, sniffing, repetitive movements of head and forepaws and compulsive gnawing.

Table 2. Antagonistic actions of neuroleptics on apomorphine-induced behavioral parameters in the rat[a]

Neuroleptics	ED_{50} mg/kg i. p.		
	Activity	Locomotion	Gnawing
Metoclopramide	17	15	2.5
Haloperidol	0.5	0.5	0.14
Chlorpromazine	28	6	9
Thioridazine	10	1	20
Clozapine	13	3	32
Sulpiride	50	50	>200

[a] Substances, i.p. 30 min before apomorphine [ED_{50} values determined graphically (LJUNGBERG and UNGERSTEDT, 1978)]

Apomorphine-induced activities are influenced by antipsychotics in different ways, most intensely locomotion. NYMARK (1972) investigated motor stereotypies after i. v. administration of apomorphine during investigations of antiemetics: 0.1 mg/kg which is four times the vomit-inducing dose, does not cause running, 0.4 mg/kg induce motor stereotypies persisting for approx. 1 h; 0.8 mg/kg has a maximum effect. The pharmacological influence on both parameters was investigated in dogs receiving 1.6 mg/kg of apomorphine i. v. Fluphenazine, flupentixol and haloperidol were highly effective apomorphine antagonists. Metoclopramide did not influence motor activity in vomit-preventing doses (NYMARK, 1972). After direct activation of cerebral dopamine receptors rats in a social situation show interactions between the animals. The rat runs around in its cage and, when it meets a partner rat, the animals confront each other in upright position with their noses in close contact. They make rhythmic movements with their front legs and produce vocalizations. This bizarre reaction is triggered off for example by 0.84 mg/kg of apomorphine i. p. and blocked by 0.12 mg/kg of haloperidol (VAN ROSSUM, 1970). Attacks occur as of 1 mg/kg of apomorphine i. v. (SENAULT, 1970). Wounding and bleeding are observed in the highest dose range of 20 mg/kg of apomorphine i. p. which is used to investigate antipsychotics. LAL and GIANUTSOS (quoted in FIELDING and LAL, 1978) could inhibit the parameters attacks, rearing and vocalization in a dose-dependent manner with 0.63, 1.25, and 2.5 mg/kg of haloperidol i. p.

Birds, solidungulates, ruminants and rodents show stereotypies and locomotor excitation, carnivores and primates vomiting and increased locomotion as apomorphine-induced reactions (KREISKOTT, 1979). Apomorphine-induced vomiting in the dog is frequently used to investigate antipsychotics (WANG, 1958; BHARGAVA and CHANDRA, 1963; JANSSEN et al., 1963; NYMARK, 1972). The most frequently used dose is 0.31 mg/kg of apomorphine s. c. The parameters used are: Onset of licking and vomiting, duration of emesis, time of maximum effect (JANSSEN and VAN BEVER, 1978).

Many other stimulants, e. g. LSD, mescaline and tetrahydrocannabinol have been used in the most different animal species to investigate neuroleptics. The phenylethylamine-induced stereotypy after chronic administration to the rat has recently been described as being particularly selective for antipsychotics (BORISON et al., 1977).

The experimental models with excitation patterns after stimulants are manifold and have been described in greater detail as the action of antipsychotics can be assessed in different ways depending on animal species and parameters used. One of many examples is clozapine. Whereas BÜRKI et al. (1975) explicitly characterize the substance as being inactive on apomorphine stereotypies of the rat, LJUNGBERG and UNGERSTEDT (1978) could observe pronounced effects on locomotor activity and slight effects on compulsive gnawing, also using rats (Table 2).

II. Tryptamine-Induced Convulsion

The convulsion-inducing action of TRYPTAMINE was used by TEDESCHI et al. (1959a) to characterize monoamine oxidase inhibitors in the rat. JANSSEN (1961), also using rats, investigated the inhibitory action of neuroleptics on the "bilateral clonic-convulsive movements of the forepaws" due to tryptamine. Excitation is followed by a long-lasting phase of intensive central depression which is regarded as catatonic syndrome by ERNST et al. (1961). Analysis of tryptamine-induced convulsions in rats (KREISKOTT, 1979) resulted in pronounced up and down movements of the forepaws interrupted only occasionally by movements of the hindpaws. Appearance and frequency of this reaction indicate scratching as the basic mechanism. The up and down movements of the forepaws push the convulsing animal backwards resulting in characteristic retropulsion (KREISKOTT, 1979). JANSSEN (1961) administered the neuroleptics subcutaneously 5 h before giving 40 mg/kg of tryptamine i. v. and observed the forepaw movements. In our laboratories 16 mg/kg of tryptamine are given intravenously after administration of the test substances i. p. 30 min or p. o. 1 h previously whereby four parameters are assessed: movements of forepaws, hunchback formation, retropulsion and stereotyped gnawing. The test is suitable particularly to investigate potent antipsychotics.

III. Withdrawal Syndrome

Withdrawal symptoms must be regarded as a special type of excitation as they are induced by discontinuing the administration of a substance. Substances with centrally depressing qualities of the morphine and barbiturate-alcohol type cause habituation and physical dependence. The withdrawal symptoms may be induced by sudden withdrawal of the substance or, in the case of substances similar to morphine, also by morphine antagonists. The action of antipsychotics on withdrawal symptoms of the rhesus monkey was investigated (KREISKOTT, 1963c). The excitation pattern in morphine-addicted animals can be reliably aroused by morphine antagonists whereby the withdrawal symptoms are accumulated in time. The symptoms observed are: compulsive gnawing, tremor, rigidity, erected hairs, intestinal spasms, extreme restlessness alternating with bizarre body postures, loss of appetite, vomiting, erections and masturbation, bellicosity, cries, lateral position, convulsions. The symptoms were induced by levallorphan 0.3 mg/kg s.c., the antipsychotics were administered also s.c. 1 h previously. The withdrawal symptoms were reduced in a dose-dependent manner, 1.0, 5.0, and 7.5 mg/kg of chlorpromazine resulted in slight up to strong inhibition, 5 and 7.5 mg/kg of butyrylperazine induced slight up to marked inhibition and 0.3–0.5 mg/kg of haloperidol s.c. slight to moderate inhibition, higher doses could not be investigated in this case due to severe catalepsy and impaired respiration.

LAL and NUMAN (1976) and LAL and HYNES (1977) could reduce the withdrawal wet shakes in morphine-addicted rats by haloperidol and benperidol. The addicted rats become hypersensitive towards external stimuli during the withdrawal period and show attack behavior after 3 days at the latest (BOSHKA et al., 1966; LAL et al., 1975). Neuroleptics act very effectively on this withdrawal symptom too (FIELDING and LAL, 1978).

WILSON and SCHUSTER (1972) studied the D-amphetamine i.v. self-administration in the rhesus monkey. Following stabilization of total drug intake within 14 days the monkeys were treated with at least four doses of chlorpromazine. Dosages of 0.25 and 0.5 mg/kg i.m. increased D-amphetamine intake, 1.0 mg/kg severely depressed self-administration. HOFFMEISTER (1975) also employing self-administration demonstrated that neuroleptics are strongly aversive, have intensive effects in addicted rhesus monkeys. Similar effects as to dose and action could also be obtained with haloperidol in 400 addicted patients (LAL and HYNES, 1977).

IV. Topical Brain Stimulation

Various methods have been developed for the *topical stimulation of the brain*. Four examples are given in the following: BANERJEE et al. (1968) injected reserpine into the lateral ventricle of the conscious rabbit via permanently implanted cannulae; 0.5 mg induced a rise in temperature, central depression and defaecation; 0.25 mg were inactive. Cats showed the same symptoms but the reduction of temperature was followed by a rise. COSTALL et al. (1972) induced stereotypies in rats by intrastriatal and/or intrapallidal administration of 50–400 μg of apomorphine; these, like stereotypies, induced by systemic administration of 5 mg/kg of apomorphine, were inhibited by intrastriatal, intrapallidal and intranigral administration of 50 μg of haloperidol.

BERGMANN et al. (1974) implanted apomorphine pellets of 100 μg into various brain regions of the rat. In 25–30% of cases compulsive gnawing was triggered off by the globus pallidus and the putamen. Initiated by the nucleus ventralis thalami a period of intensive compulsive gnawing was observed following general excitation. These effects were inhibited by chlorpromazine (2 mg/kg i. p.), haloperidol (2–10 mg/kg p. o.) and pimozide (4 mg/kg i. p.).

KOSHELEVA (1975) stimulated the nucleus caudatus of cats by implanted electrodes. The motion inhibition occurring was assessed on an estimation scale. 0.1 mg/kg of reserpine i. p. reduced even motility, induced drowsiness and increased the skeletal muscle tone. The stimulation threshold for motion inhibition was increased reaching its maximum after 3 h; an action was no longer detectable after 24 h. Reserpine (0.3 mg/kg) exerted stronger actions on all parameters. Normalization was reached only 10–12 days after injection.

V. Self-Stimulation

Self-stimulation via electrodes in various mesencephalic and prosencephalic regions which is reinforcing and "pleasurable" can be performed in mice, rats, gerbils, cats, guinea-pigs, dogs, monkeys and in man (FIELDING and LAL, 1978; FRANCIS et al., 1978). This subject will be discussed by LEHR (Chapter 5).

VI. Rotational Model

Unilateral striatal dopaminergic stimulation causes contralateral rotation in rodents. ANDÉN et al. (1966 a) removed the nucleus caudatus by suction and used dopamine antagonists, the indirectly acting agent amphetamine and apomorphine acting as direct receptor stimulant; rotation was abolished by haloperidol (ANDÉN et al., 1967). UNGERSTEDT (1968) differentiated this method by the topical administration of 6-hydroxydopamine into the striatum or the zona compacta of the substantia nigra. In unilateral 6-hydroxydopamine-induced lesions of the nigrostriatal bundle apomorphine stimulates the intact, due to the lesion probably hypersensitive, dopamine receptors of the striatum so intensely that contralateral rotation results, whereas amphetamine as an agonist acting indirectly by the release of dopamine causes rotation towards the lesioned side (STAWARZ et al., 1975). Table 3 gives the ratio between the inhibitory effects of various antipsychotics on rotational behavior and extrapyramidal-motor disorders in man.

Table 3. Effect of antipsychotic drugs in rats with unilateral lesions of the substantia nigra[a]

Antipsychotic drug	Rotational antagonism[b] ED_{50} mg/kg, i.p. 95% c.i.	Extrapyramidal side-effects in man
Haloperidol	0.05 (0.02– 0.15)	+++
Pimozide	0.08 (0.06– 0.10)	+++
Chlorpromazine	2.0 (1.1 – 4.6)	++
Thioridazine	13.6 (6.5 –31.9)	+
Clozapine	25.4 (15.0 –55.2)	(±)

[a] 2 mg/kg D-amphetamine i.p. (STAWARZ et al., 1975)
[b] ED_{50} mg/kg, i.p. (95% c.i.)

Various authors investigated the action of neuroleptics on amphetamine, metamphetamine or apomorphine induced rotational behavior of the rat. The ED_{50} values comply to a surprising extent even at varying doses and different application and observation times. Haloperidol is the strongest acting, closely followed by pimozide. The chlorpromazine dose is approx. 100 times higher but still within a range of clinical relevance. Clozapine and thioridazine have only very slight inhibitory actions (summary by Echols and Ursillo, 1977). Similar effects can be obtained in the mouse with this lesion technique (Von Voigtländer and Moore, 1973). Echols and Ursillo (1977) investigated the same antipsychotics after injection of 6-hydroxydopamine into the nucleus caudatus and apomorphine-stimulated rotation (0.2 mg/kg s. c.). Contrary to the investigations in rats chlorpromazine, thioridazine and clozapine exert almost equal actions, haloperidol, as compared to these, is only three to four times stronger. This refined method shows behavioral influences which may be directly correlated with changes of transmission systems (Stawarz et al., 1975; Bartholini, 1976). The obvious differences of actions depending on the species again demonstrate the necessity of comparative pharmacological methods.

VII. Brain Lesions

Brady and Nauta (1953, 1955) described that bilateral lesions in the septal region of the forebrain of the rat cause emotional hyperactivity which becomes evident in attacks after neutral stimuli. Various authors, Hunt (1957), Raitt et al. (1961) and Malick et al. (1969) reported on an inhibition of excitation due to chlorpromazine observed in acute trials, Cytawa and Kutulas (1972) confirmed this effect also for chronic administration. Sofia (1969) compared the mean doses of various antipsychotics obtained by using this model with those used in the rotarod test (rat and mouse), and those applied in isolation-induced aggression (mouse) and aggressive-defensive behavior induced by electrical foot shock (rat). The doses required proved to be so high, already showing neurological effects, that none of the substances could specifically inhibit the septal lesions aggression.

Akinesia, rigidity and flexibilitas cerea in rats may be induced by larger lesions in the transitory zone between mesencephalic and diencephalic region (Andén et al., 1966b). Slighter lesions do not arouse any symptoms on part of the animals; by administering antipsychotics such as chlorpromazine, perphenazine and haloperidol in doses inducing only slight or no cataleptogenic actions in normal animals, Delini-Stula (1972) observed states of marked immobilization in the rats. Due to the fact that catalepsy cannot be induced by cataleptogenics of the cholinergic type in rats with brain lesions the method allows not only a more sensitive but also a more differentiated assessment of antipsychotics.

E. Side-Effects Following Acute
and Chronic Administration and Tolerance Phenomena

Antipsychotics administered to man exert not only the desired therapeutic action but also cause side-effects. Engelmeier (1964) pointed out that considerations under these aspects are of little value to gain knowledge. It is more reasonable to present spectra of action to demonstrate pharmacological effects in animals and in man. Soon after the introduction of neuroleptics into therapy, parkinsonoid symptoms (FLÜGEL, 1955) such as dyskinesias of the upper extremities with abnormal postures, buccolingual dyskinesias and akathisia became evident after more or less long treatment periods. Other extrapyramidal disturbances are tremor, akinesia and involuntary movements of the mouth (munching) (SOVNER and DI MASCIO, 1978). Equivalents in animal experiments are catalepsy, oral automatism and tremor. Some species show extrapyramidal-motor irritations after acute administration of antipsychotics; DOMINO et al. (1968) described increased aggression with biting and hypersexuality in dogs after perphenazine and chlorpromazine. JANSSEN and VAN BEVER (1978) recorded the relative neurological side-effects by quotients from the jumping box test and apomorphine-induced vomiting in the dog thus providing further information for therapy. The equivalent of sedative effects in clinical practice which occur particularly in less potent antipsychotics accompanied by slight tendency to extrapyramidal-motor disorders is the inhibition of motility in animal experiments. JANSSEN and VAN BEVER (1978) suggest here the quotient ptosis/catalepsy in the rat.

The paroxysmal extrapyramidal early dyskinesias in man, occurring occasionally even within the first week of treatment, with potent antipsychotics may be cut short within a few minutes by 1 or 2 injections of 2.5–5 mg of biperiden i. v. or i. m. (HUBER, 1977).

To obtain the desired therapeutic effects antipsychotics must be administered to in- and out-patients over a longer period of time. Longer-term treatment causes not only the desired effects but also pronounced side-effects. The neuroleptic parkinsonoid syndrome of the patients occurs after 1–2 weeks at the earliest, not considering early dyskinesias described in the previous section. Only long-term administration and high doses of neuroleptics will lead to persisting extrapyramidal hyperkinesias (HUBER, 1977; BALDESSARINI and TARSY, 1978). These tardive dyskinesias affect distal extremities as well as oral and facial muscles (BERCHTOLD et al., 1974). The involuntary, compulsive stereotyped movements of lips, tongue, jaws and extremities are related to comfort reactions and displacement activity (KREISKOTT, 1979).

Pharmacological actions in the animal are predominantly determined in acute, i. e. short-term trials. Only long-term pharmacological investigations allow the comparison with clinical results and a prediction to therapy. The profile of action of a substance is represented as longitudinal profile after longer-term administration whereby the total effects should, if possible, be assessed as a function of time. The first attempts to establish a relation between pharmacological investigations and clinical results of antipsychotics were made by BOYD (1960) as well as LIM and co-workers (1961). They both were concerned with the question of a modified action on the test animal after repeated administration over a longer period. BOYD injected chlorpromazine intramuscularly to rats for a period of 40 weeks. He concluded that habituation and dependence will develop after continuous administration of chlorpromazine. LIM and co-workers compared the toxicity and part of the pharmacological profile of action of various substances after acute and subchronic administration (20–28 days). These authors observed habituation in the case of prochlorperazine and chlorpromazine; reserpine is reported to accumulate. Papers on the investigation of actions after continuous administration using particular experimental designs also belong to this category: after chlorpromazine, perphenazine (IRWIN, 1961, 1962) and reserpine (ASTON et al., 1962) using conditioned reactions of the rat, after chlorpromazine using aggressive behavior of isolated mice (DAVANZO, 1969) and after various phenothiazines on hand of the EEG-arousal reaction of the rabbit (DOYLE et al., 1968).

THEOBALD and co-workers (1968) observed decreasing actions on the one hand, constant effects on the other hand after the administration of chlorpromazine, thioproperazine and thioridazine for 4–5 days assessing various test parameters. The administration period is too short, however. Already by 1961, IRWIN had succeeded in differentiating the profile of action of chlorpromazine by comparing various experimental designs. Habituation was not observed in regard to holding on at the rotating wheel after 26 days of substance application, tolerance at varying degrees depending on the period of time was found, however, in regard to a conditioned reaction. MØLLER-NIELSEN et al. (1974) investigated antipsychotics after repeated administration to mice, rats and dogs for up to 14 days; tolerance was observed in all experimental designs in regard to stereotypies but could not be detected in regard to catalepsy and inhibition of conditioned reactions. The development of tolerance was dependent on doses and duration of treatment. EZRIN-WATERS and SEEMAN (1977) investigated haloperidol-induced catalepsy alone in rats. The animals received an acute injection of haloperidol (0.5–2.0 mg/kg i. p. or 1.0–4.0 mg/kg p. o.) and catalepsy was scored. Haloperidol (0.75 and 1.5 mg/kg p. o.) was administered to the rats daily for a period of 16 days. After 16 days on haloperidol, all animals became tolerant to the drug, exhibiting decreased cataleptic response to haloperidol; after 16 days of abstinence from the drug the degree of catalepsy was the same as on the 1st day. In addition, a group of animals treated and tested daily for catalepsy demonstrated that the time course of the development of tolerance to haloperidol was biphasic, with a rapid phase of 2.5 days and a slower phase of 5.5 days. VOTAVA (1972) administered increasing doses of 10–20 mg/kg of perphenazine p. o. to rabbits on 7 subsequent days; he observed habituation and, after abrupt discontinuation, withdrawal symptoms which became manifest in behavior and EEG.

A further approach to this problem became possible by pharmacokinetic methods. DREYFUSS and his colleagues (1972) could establish a correlation between the half-life for the elimination of ^{14}C-fluphenazine and its metabolites, and the duration of extrapyramidal-motor disorders. They investigated 2.5 and 5 mg/kg of fluphenazine, administered via the food, in baboons *(papio papio)* for a period of 14 days. Between the 2nd and the 8th day all animals showed rest tremor or intentional tremor, masklike faces and rigidity. All symptoms disappeared only 12–13 days after discontinuation.

MØLLER-NIELSEN et al. (1974) investigated the behavior of several species in regard to tolerance and cross-tolerance of various neuroleptics using excitation patterns induced by amphetamine and apomorphine. They found that habituation was most pronounced 3 days after termination of a 12-day treatment period. Tolerance was observed up to 3–4 weeks after discontinuation of treatment and occurred most readily with fluphenazine, haloperidol, pimozide and flupenthixole. Cross-tolerance was found between haloperidol and flupenthixole, habituation did not develop in regard to the catatonigenic action of flupenthixole.

SCHELKUNOV (1967) investigated the adrenergic tone after chronic administration of neuroleptics (haloperidol, perchlorperazine, trifluperazine and chlorpromazine) for a period of 6 weeks in amphetamine- and apomorphine-induced stereotypies of rats which, as excitation patterns, clearly differ from normal behavior. Single administration of these neuroleptics either prevented the occurrence of stereotypies or reduced their duration, whereas chronic administration prolonged the time of stereotyped behavior. SCHELKUNOV interpreted this as a compensatory rise of the central adrenergic tone and discussed its connection with the increase of homovanillic acid at unchanged dopamine content in the corpus striatum of the cat and various rodents. It seems of particular interest to assess the behavior simultaneously with electrophysiological and biochemical parameters. STILLE and LAUENER (1971) and ASPER et al. (1973) investigated the development of habituation in the rat after haloperidol, fluphenazine and loxapine administered in daily doses of 2 mg/kg p. o. for a period of up to 4 weeks. The protective action against apomorphine-induced stereotypies and the neuroleptic-induced rise of homovanillic acid in the corpus striatum was impaired after one week. The development of cataleptic conditions was pronounced to varying degrees depending on the individual substances. Tolerance was also observed with regard to the characteristic EEG-changes after neuroleptics.

Longitudinal profiles of the actions of psychopharmacological drugs, whereby time is represented by the longitudinal axis, are of importance not only for repeated administration over a longer period, but also for single administration of substances with long-term effect. Penfluridol, fluspirilene, fluphenazine enanthate and decanoate act for a period of 1–3 weeks, pipotiazine palmitate even for 4 weeks, following intramuscular administration (SIMPSON and LEE, 1978). The papers mentioned demonstrate that the degrees of habituation differ in regard to the individual qualities of action. Thus, complying with clinical experience in man, the initially pronounced inhibition of activity and muscle relaxation due to substances belonging to the group of neuroleptics is reduced after several days of treatment. Many questions remain unanswered: Is the reduction of initial sedation in man the only parallel to tolerance phenomena in animal experiments? Are therapy-resistent forms and relapses occurring when administering neuroleptics possibly connected with tolerance phenomena? What is the basis for careful gradual dosing of neuroleptics whereby the neuroleptic threshold dose may be exceeded without great complications? (HAASE, 1966, 1977). And how as compared to that, can it be explained that a high initial neuroleptic dose markedly above the neuroleptic threshold induces sedation and increased tendency to fall asleep in addition to the antipsychotic effect, but only rarely coarse tremor, named "surprise effect" of the extrapyramidal-motor system by HAASE (1966, 1977)?

SCHELKUNOV's experience (1967) that treatment with antipsychotics causes an increase of substance-induced stereotypies and increased sensitivity towards dopamine agonists has been proved by numerous investigators and in various animal species. It cannot be clarified, as yet, how far the persistence of the symptoms is due to neurotoxic or degenerative actions of antipsychotics (BALDESSARINI and TARSY, 1978). As a biochemical correlate BURT et al. (1977) found a 20–30% increase of the dopamine receptors in the striatum of rats after daily administration of haloperidol, fluphenazine and reserpine for a period of 1–3 weeks.

GUNNE and BÁRÁNY (1976) induced tardive dyskinesia in cebus monkeys using haloperidol. In three cebus *(C. apella)* monkeys chronic daily administration of haloperidol (0.5 mg/kg/day p. o.) induced sedation and parkinsonism during the first 5–7 weeks. Subsequently the animals developed signs of acute dystonia which were dose-dependent and, in extreme cases, included tonic and clonic seizures. After 3 and 12 months, respectively, two of the monkeys showed grimacing and protrusion of the tongue; the symptoms of tardive dyskinesia were reduced in a dose-dependent manner after each haloperidol administration, being most pronounced in the morning before haloperidol application. Biperiden (70 mg/kg i. m.) reduced acute dystonia but brought back signs of tardive dyskinesia which had been abolished by haloperidol.

WEISS and SANTELLI (1978) were able to provoke tardive dyskinesias by administration of haloperidol only once per week. In two cebus *(Cebus albifrons)* monkeys given 0.25 mg/kg of haloperidol p. o. the tenth weekly dose induced movement disorders 1–8 h after drug administration. These disorders included tongue and mouth movements, peculiar postures and stretching. Further treatment induced sedation; increased doses exacerbated dyskinesias.

Another cebus monkey which did not respond to haloperidol (0.25 mg/kg, 5 days/ wk, p. o.) administered for a period of 1 year, received haloperidol (0.5 mg/kg/wk p. o.). Haloperidol produced abnormal mouth movements when given in a higher dose (0.5 mg/kg p. o.) only once per week. After 8 weeks haloperidol induced sedation. Similar effects were observed in a squirrel monkey treated with 0.5 mg/kg p. o. only once per week.

F. Conclusions

Experiences on the use of antipsychotics in man confirm results of animal experiments representing equivalents to clinical practice. This holds for methods to assess sedative-hypnotic, antiemetic and muscle-relaxing effects and parkinsonoid-inducing qualities. The conformity between man and animal is particularly high in regard to the action of antipsychotics on extreme anxiety conditions which may be of endogenous or exogenous origin. But also, behavioral patterns of other drives may be influenced which cannot be homologized with reactions in man, such as prey catching and maternal behavior in mammals or locomotion in invertebrates. These findings can be used to characterize antipsychotics as there is a homogenous influence on the transmitters (FISCHER, 1971). Within the past few years great progress has been made in the biochemical analysis of schizophrenic processes and mechanisms of action of antipsychotics. It was found that antipsychotic effectiveness, extrapyramidal-motor excitation conditions (SULSER and ROBINSON, 1978) and the development of tolerance phenomena (MOORE and KELLY, 1978) are due to the blockade of dopamine and noradrenaline receptors. Tardive dyskinesias are explained by the hypersensitivity of dopamine receptors at continuous administration (BALDESSARINI and TARSY, 1978). Influences on the metabolism of serotonin, γ-aminobutyric acid, histamine and peptides have furthermore been proved. Disorders in one system will disturb other systems. Hypothetical explanations are complicated by the multifactor aetiology of schizophrenia and that is why a reproducible model on biochemical basis of schizophrenic symptoms does not yet exist (ACKENHEIL et al., 1978). Even though there has been essential progress on the part of biochemistry we must still rely on behavioral studies. Simple criteria of the behavior of normal animals and test animals influenced by pharmacological or physiological methods make it possible to assess the profile of action of antipsychotics and to make predictions to clinical effects (STILLE, 1974).

Further progress is possible in regard to man and animal by the differentiated assessment of symptomatology. HEINRICH (1977) demonstrated that only the early recognition of schizophrenic psychoses and their therapy thus rendered possible will have the greatest prospects of success. Early symptoms of the disease within the affective and motor range can even be diagnosed by the patient himself, his relatives and his physician. The animal, too, offers simple methods to study antipsychotics based on pointed questioning, subtle recording and exact assessment; some examples are the fright reaction of the golden hamster, excitation patterns of the cat, withdrawal symptoms in rats after centrally acting stimulants, or rhesus monkeys and the induction of tardive dyskinesias by repeated drug application to various species.

References

Abramson, H.A., Evans, L.T.: Lysergic acid diethylamide (LSD 25): II. Psychobiological effects on the Siamese fighting fish. Science *120*, 990–991 (1954)

Ackenheil, M., Hippius, H., Matussek, N.: Ergebnisse der biochemischen Forschung auf dem Schizophrenie-Gebiet. Nervenarzt *49*, 634–649 (1978)

Andén, N.-E., Dahlström, A., Fuxe, K., Larsson, K.: Functional role of the nigro-neostriatal dopamine neurons. Acta Pharmacol. Toxicol. (Kbh.) *24*, 263–274 (1966a)

Andén, N.-E., Fuxe, K., Larsson, K.: Effect of large mesencephalic-diencephalic lesions on the noradrenalin, dopamine and 5-hydroxytryptamine neurons of the central nervous system. Experientia *22*, 842–843 (1966b)

Andén, N.-E., Rubenson, A., Fuxe, K., Hökfelt, T.: Evidence for dopamine receptor stimulation by apomorphine. J. Pharm. Pharmacol. *19*, 627–629 (1967)

Angst, J., Battegay, R., Bente, D., Berner, P., Broeren, W., Cornu, F., Dick, P., Engelmeier, M.-P., Heimann, H., Heinrich, K., Helmchen, H., Hippius, H., Pöldinger, W., Schmidlin, P., Schmitt, W., Weis, P.: Das Dokumentations-System der Arbeitsgemeinschaft für Methodik und Dokumentation in der Psychiatrie (AMP). Arzneim. Forsch. *19*, 399–405 (1969)

Ashcroft, G.W., Eccleston, D., Waddell, J.L.: Recognition of amphetamine addicts. Br. Med. J. *1*, 57 (1965)

Asper, H., Baggiolini, M., Bürki, H.R., Lauener, H., Ruch, W., Stille, G.: Tolerance phenomena with neuroleptics catalepsy, apomorphine stereotypies and striatal dopamine metabolism in the rat after single and repeated administration of loxapine and haloperidol. Eur. J. Pharmacol. *22*, 287–294 (1973)

Aston, R., Sekino, E., Greifenstein, F.E.: Quantitation of drug effects upon conditioned avoidance behavior in the rat. Toxicol. Appl. Pharmacol. *4*, 393–401 (1962)

Baldessarini, R.J., Tarsy, D.: Tardive dyskinesia. In: Psychopharmacology. A generation of progress. Lipton, M.A., Di Mascio, A., Killam, K.F. (eds.), pp. 993–1004. New York: Raven Press 1978

Banerjee, U., Burks, T.F., Feldberg, W., Goodrich, C.A.: Temperature effects of reserpine injected into the cerebral ventricles of rabbits and cats. J. Physiol. *197*, 221–231 (1968)

Bartholini, G.: Differential effect of neuroleptic drugs on dopamine turnover in the extrapyramidal and limbic system. J. Pharm. Pharmacol. *28*, 429–433 (1976)

Bein, H.J.: Zur Pharmakologie des Reserpin, eines neuen Alkaloids aus Rauwolfia serpentina Benth. Experientia *9*, 107–110 (1953)

Berchtold, P., Hinssen, M., Irmscher, K.: Tardive Dyskinesie, ein wenig bekanntes extrapyramidales Syndrom als Folge der Therapie mit Neuroleptika. Dtsch. Med. Wochenschr.*99*, 420–421 (1974)

Bergmann, F., Chaimovitz, M., Pasternak, V., Ramu, A.: Compulsive gnawing in rats after implantation of drugs into the ventral thalamus. A contribution to the mechanism of morphine action. Br. J. Pharmacol. *51*, 197–205 (1974)

Berry, P.A., Lister, R.E., Beattie, I.A.: Oxypertine and primate behaviour. Postgrad. Med. J. *48*, Suppl. 4, 11–14 (1972)

Bhargava, K.P., Chandra, O.: Anti-emetic activity of phenothiazines in relation to their chemical structure. Br. J. Pharmacol. *21*, 436–440 (1963)

Blösch, M.: Über die Wirkung einiger Phenothiacine auf das Verhalten von freilebenden Silbermöven (Larus a. argentatus Pontopp). Psychopharmacologia *25*, 380–387 (1972)

Boissier, J.R., Simon, P.: Dissociation de deux composantes dans le comportement d'investigation de la souris. Arch. Int. Pharmacodyn. Thér. *147*, 372–387 (1964)

Borison, R.L., Havdala, H.S., Diamond, B.I.: Chronic phenylethylamine stereotypy in rats: A new animal model for schizophrenia. Life Sci. *21*, 117–122 (1977)

Boshka, S.E., Weissman, M.C., Thor, D.H.: A technique for inducing aggression in rats utilizing morphine withdrawal. Psychol. Rec. *16*, 541–543 (1966)

Boyd, E.M.: Chlorpromazine tolerance and physical dependence. J. Pharmacol. *128*, 75–78 (1960)

Brady, J.V., Nauta, W.J.H.: Subcortical mechanism in emotional behavior: affective changes following septal and habenular lesions in the albino rat. J. Comp. Physiol. Psychol. *46*, 339–346 (1953)

Brady, J.V., Nauta, W.J.H.: Subcortical mechanism in emotional behavior: the duration or affective changes following septal and habenular lesions in the albino rat. J. Comp. Physiol. Psychol. *48*, 412–420 (1955)

Bürki, H.R., Eichenberger, E., Sayers, A.C., White, T.C.: Clozapine and the dopamine hypothesis of schizophrenia, a critical appraisal. Pharmakopsychiatr. Neuropsychopharmacol. *8*, 115–121 (1975)

Burt, D.R., Creese, I., Snyder, S.H.: Antischizophrenic drugs: chronic treatment elevates dopamine receptor binding in brain. Science *196*, 326–328 (1977)

Chari-Bitron, A.A., Chari-Bitron, A.: Estimation of low chlorpromazine concentrations by surfacing and sinking reaction of minnows (Gambusia affinis). Psychopharmacologia *18*, 407–411 (1970)

Coscia, L., Causa, P., Giuliani, E., Nunziata, A.: Pharmacological properties of new neuroleptic compounds. Arzneim. Forsch. *25*, 1436–1442 (1975)

Costall, B., Naylor, R.J.: Neuroleptic and non-neuroleptic catalepsy. Arzneim. Forsch. *23*, 674–683 (1973)

Costall, B., Naylor, R.J., Olley, J.E.: Stereotypic and anticataleptic activities of amphetamine after intracerebral injections. Eur. J. Pharmacol. *18*, 83–94 (1972)

Courvoisier, S., Fournel, J., Ducrot, R., Kolsky, M., Koetschet, P.: Propriétés pharmacologiques du chlorhydrate de chloro-3-(diméthylamino-3′-propyl)-10-phénothiazine (4.560 R.P.). Arch. Int. Pharmacodyn. Thér. *92*, 305–361 (1953)

Courvoisier, S., Ducrot, R., Julou, L.: Nouveaux aspects expérimentaux de l'activité centrale des dérivés de la phénothiazine. In: Psychotropic drugs. Garattini, S., Ghetti, V. (eds.), pp. 373–391. Amsterdam: Elsevier 1957

Cytawa, J., Kutulas, G.: Influence of chlorpromazine on emotional hyperreactivity resulting from septal forebrain injury. Psychopharmacologia *27*, 389–392 (1972)

Davanzo, J.P.: Observations related to drug-induced alterrations in aggressive behaviour. In: Aggressive behaviour. Garattini, S., Sigg, E.B. (eds.), pp. 263–272. Amsterdam: Excerpta Medica 1969

Debus, G.: Wirkung von Psychopharmaka und zugrundeliegende theoretische Vorstellungen. Pharmakopsychiatr. Neuropsychopharmacol. *10*, 109–118 (1977)

Delay, J., Deniker, T., Harl, J.M.: Utilisation en que psychiatrique d'une phénothiazine d'action centrale sélective. Ann. Med. Psychol. Fr. *110*, 112–117 (1952)

Delini-Stula, A.: Increased sensitivity to neuroleptics in rats with lesions of the central nervous system. Psychopharmacologia *26*, 84–90 (1972)

Domino, E.F., Hudson, R.D., Zografi, G.: Substituted phenothiazines: Pharmacology and chemical structure. In: Drugs affecting the central nervous system. Burger, A. (ed.), pp. 327–397. New York: Marcel Dekker 1968

Doyle, C., Shimizu, A., Himwich, H.E.: Effects of chronic administration of some psychoactive drugs on EEG arousal on rabbit. Int. J. Neuropharmacol. *7*, 87–95 (1968)

Dreyfuss, J., Beer, B., Devine, D.D., Roberts, B.F., Schreiber, E.C.: Fluphenazine-induced parkinsonism in the baboon: Pharmacological and metabolic studies. Neuropharmacology *11*, 223–230 (1972)

Echols, S.D., Ursillo, R.C.: Significance of species differences: Rotational models. In: Animal models in psychiatry and neurology. Hanin, I., Usdin, E. (eds.), pp. 27–34. Oxford: Pergamon Press 1977

Eliasson, M., Meyerson, B.J.: Comparison of the action of lysergic acid diethylamide and apomorphine on the copulatory response in the female rat. Psychopharmacology 49, 301–306 (1976)

Ellinwood, E.H., Kilbey, M.M.: Chronic stimulant intoxication models of psychosis. In: Animal models in psychiatry and neurology. Hanin, I., Usdin, E. (eds.), pp. 61–74. Oxford: Pergamon Press 1977

Ellinwood, E.H., Sudilovsky, A., Nelson, L.M.: Evolving behavior in the clinical and experimental amphetamine (model) psychosis. Am. J. Psychiatry 130, 1088–1093 (1973)

Emley, G.S., Hutchinson, R.R.: Similar and selective actions of chlorpromazine, chlordiazepoxide, and nicotine on shock-produced aggressive and anticipatory motor responses in the squirrel monkey. Proceedings, 79th Annual Convention, APA, pp. 759–760 (1971)

Engelmeier, M.-P.: Das Gesamtwirkungsspektrum enzephalotroper Medikamente und seine Bedeutung für die psychiatrische Pharmakotherapie. In: Begleitwirkungen und Mißerfolge der psychiatrischen Pharmakotherapie. Kranz, H., Heinrich, K. (eds.), pp. 4–12. Stuttgart: Thieme 1964

Ernst, A.M., van Andel, H., Charbon, G.A.: Beruht die experimentelle Katatonie durch Tryptamin auf einer Verdrängung des 5-Hydroxytryptamin? Psychopharmacologia 2, 425–435 (1961)

Ezrin-Waters, C., Seeman, P.: Tolerance to haloperidol catalepsy. Eur. J. Pharmacol. 41, 321–327 (1977)

Fielding, S., Lal, H.: Behavioral actions of neuroleptics. In: Neuroleptics and schizophrenia. Handbook of Psychopharmacology. Iversen, L.L., Iversen, S.D., Snyder, S.H. (eds.), Vol. 10,, 91–128. New York: Plenum Press 1978

Fischer, H.: Vergleichende Pharmakologie von Überträgersubstanzen in tiersystematischer Darstellung. In: Handbuch der experimentellen Pharmakologie, Vol. XXVI. Berlin, Heidelberg, New York: Springer 1971

Flügel, F.: Über medikamentös erzeugte parkinsonähnliche Zustandsbilder. Med. Klin. 50, 634–635 (1955)

Francis, N., Marley, E., Stephenson, J.D.: Effects of spiperone on self-stimulation and other activities of the mongolian gerbil. Br. J. Pharmacol. 63, 43–49 (1978)

Fraňková, S.: Drug-induced changes in the maternal behavior of rats. Psychopharmacology 53, 83–87 (1977)

Giono-Barber, H., Giono-Barber, P., Bertuletti, G.: Methode d'essai des substances psychotropes sur le comportement de domination du Singe Cynocephale (Papio papio). Compt. Rend. Soc. Biol. 164, 199–203 (1970)

Greenblatt, D.J., Shader, R.I.: Rational use of psychotropic drugs. In: Drug therapy reviews. Miller, R.R., Greenblatt, D.J. (eds.), Vol. 1, pp. 59–72. New York: Masson 1977

Gunne, L.M., Bárány, S.: Haloperidol-induced tardive dyskinesia in monkeys. Psychopharmacology 50, 237–240 (1976)

Haase, H.J.: Therapie mit Psychopharmaka und anderen psychotropen Medikamenten. Düsseldorf: Janssen 1966

Haase, H.J.: Therapie mit Psychopharmaka und anderen seelisches Befinden beeinflussenden Medikamenten. Stuttgart: Schattauer 1977

Heinrich, K.: Zur Bedeutung der Stammesgeschichte des menschlichen Erlebens und Verhaltens für Neurologie und Psychopathologie. Homo 16, 65–77 (1965)

Heinrich, K.: Die psychiatrische Frühklinik bei psychotischen Störungen. Therapiewoche 27, 6450–6459 (1977)

Hippius, H., Matussek, N.: Bemerkungen zur Biologischen Psychiatrie. Nervenarzt 49, 650–653 (1978)

Hoebel, B.G.: Feeding: Neural control of intake. Am. Rev. Physiol. 33, 533–568 (1971)

Hoffmeister, F.: Negative reinforcing properties of some psychotropic drugs in drug-naive rhesus monkeys. J. Pharmacol. Exp. Ther. 192, 468–477 (1975)

Hoffmeister, F., Wuttke, W.: On the actions of psychotropic drugs on the attack- and aggressive-defensive behaviour of mice and cats. In: Aggressive behaviour. Garattini, S., Sigg, E.B. (eds.), pp. 273–280. Amsterdam: Excerpta Medica 1969

Huber, G.: Langzeittherapie der Schizophrenie in der Praxis. Med. Welt 28, 213–217 (1977)

Hughes, R.N., Syme, L.A., Syme, G.J.: Open-field behaviour in sheep following treatment with the neuroleptics azaperone and acetylpromazine. Psychopharmacology 52, 107–109 (1977)

Hunt, H.F.: Some effects of drugs on classical (Type S) conditioning. Ann. N.Y. Acad. Sci. *65,* 258–267 (1956)

Hunt, H.F.: Some effects of meprobamate on conditioned fear and emotional behavior. Ann. N.Y. Acad. Sci. *67,* 712–723 (1957)

Irwin, S.: The value of animal experimentation. In: Psychopharmacology frontiers. Kline, N.S. (ed.). Boston: 1957

Irwin, S.: Differential tolerance development to the avoidance and locomotor suppressant actions of perphenazine and chlorpromazine. Pharmacologist *3,* 75 (1961)

Irwin, S.: Influence of experimental variables on the rate of tolerance development to chlorpromazine and perphenazine. Fed. Proc. *21,* 419 (1962)

Irwin, S.: Drug screening and evaluation of new compounds in animals. In: Animal and clinical pharmacologic techniques in drug evaluation. Nodine, J.H., Siegler, P.E. (eds.), Vol. 1, pp. 36–54. Chicago: Year Book Medical 1964

Irwin, S., Konohi, R.G.: Single and repeat dose effects of imipramine and chlorpromazine in man. Psychopharmacol. Bull. *7,* 23–24 (1971)

Irwin, S., Kinohi, R., Van Sloten, M., Workman, M.P.: Drug effects on distress-evoked behavior in mice: methodology and drug class comparisons. Psychopharmacologia *20,* 172–185 (1971)

Itil, T.M.: Quantitative analysis of "motor pattern" in schizophrenia. In: Schizophrenia current concepts and research. Siva Sankar, D.V. (ed.), Hicksville, N.Y.: PJD Publications Ltd. (year of publication unknown)

Janssen, P.A.J.: Vergleichende pharmakologische Daten über sechs neue basische 4'-Fluorobutyrophenon-Derivate. Arzneim. Forsch. *11,* 932–938 (1961)

Janssen, P.A.J., van Bever, W.F.M.: Structure-activity relationships of the butyrophenones and diphenylbutylpiperidines. In: Neuroleptics and schizophrenia. Handbook of Psychopharmacology, Iversen, C.L., Iversen, S.D., Snyder, S.H. (eds.), Vol. 10, pp. 1–35. New York: Plenum Press 1978

Janssen, P.A.J., Jageneau, A.H., van Proosdij-Hartzema, E.G., De Jongh, D.K.: The pharmacology of a new potent analgesic R 951 2-[N(4-carbethoxy-4-phenyl)-piperidino] propiophenone HCl. Acta Physiol. Pharmacol. Neerl. *7,* 373–402 (1958)

Janssen, P.A.J., Jageneau, A.H., Niemegeers, C.J.E.: Effects of various drugs on isolation-induced fighting behavior of male mice. J. Pharmacol. Exp. Ther. *129,* 471–475 (1960a)

Janssen, P.A.J., Niemegeers, C.J.E., Schellekens, K.H.L.: Is it possible to predict the clinical effects of neuroleptic drugs (major tranquillizers) from animal data. Arzneim. Forsch. *15,* 104–117 (1965)

Karli, P.: The norway rat's killing response to the white mouse: an experimental analysis. Behaviour *10,* 81–103 (1956)

Karli, P.: Action de l'amphétamine et de la chlorpromazin sur l'agressivité interspécifique rat-souris. Compt. Rend. Soc. Biol. *152,* 1796–1798 (1958)

Karli, P., Vergnes, M., Didiergeorges, F.: Rat-mouse interspecific aggressive behaviour and its manipulation by brain ablation and by brain stimulation. In: Aggressive behaviour. Garattini, S., Sigg, E.B. (eds.), pp. 47–55. Amsterdam: Excerpta Medica 1969

Kehne, J.H., Sorenson, C.A.: The effects of pimozide and phenoxybenzamine pretreatments on amphetamine and apomorphine potentiation of the acoustic startle response in rats. Psychopharmacology *58,* 137–144 (1978)

Janssen, P.A.J., Jageneau, A.H.M., Schellekens, K.H.L.: Chemistry and pharmacology of compounds related to 4-(4-hydroxy-4-phenyl-piperidino)-butyrophenone. Psychopharmacologia *1,* 389–392 (1960b)

Janssen, P.A.J., Niemegeers, C.J.E., Schellekens, K.H.L., Verbruggen, F.J., Van Nueten, J.M.: The pharmacology of Dehydrobenzperidol, a new potent and short acting neuroleptic agent chemically related to Haloperidol. Arzneim. Forsch. *13,* 205–211 (1963)

Keiper, R.R.: Drug effects on canary stereotypies. Psychopharmacologia *16,* 16–24 (1969)

Kinnard, W.J., Carr, C.J.: A preliminary procedure for the evaluation of central nervous system depressants. J. Pharmacol. Exp. Ther. *121,* 354–361 (1957)

Kinnard, W.J., jr., Watzman, N.: Techniques utilized in the evaluation of psychotropic drugs on animal activity, J. Pharm. Sci. *55,* 995–1012 (1966)

Kjellberg, B., Randrup, A.: Partial restoration by a neuroleptic (spiramide) of items of grooming behaviour suppressed by Amphetamine. Arch. Int. Pharmacodyn. Thér. *210*, 61–66 (1974)

Kneip, P.: Kletter-Trieb und Kletter-Test. Arch. Int. Pharmacodyn. Thér. *126*, 238–245 (1960)

Kosheleva, O.V.: Reserpine action on the arrest reaction following stimulation of the caudate nucleus in cats. Farmakol. Toksikol. *38*, 650–652 (1975)

Kostowski, W., Czlonkowski, A.: The activity of some neuroleptic drugs and amphetamine in normal and isolated rats. Pharmacology *10*, 82–87 (1973)

Kreiskott, H.: Einfluß von Pharmaka auf das Beutefangverhalten der Ratte. Arch. Exp. Path. Pharmak. *245*, 54 (1963 a)

Kreiskott, H.: Die experimentelle Erzeugung von Starrezuständen an Octopus vulgaris durch Kataleptica (Bulbocapnin und Phenothiazine). Arch. Exp. Path. Pharmak. *246*, 24 (1963 b)

Kreiskott, H.: Zur Verhaltensforschung im Rahmen der Psychopharmakologie. Medizin und Chemie *7*, 57–78 (1963 c)

Kreiskott, H.: Verhaltensänderungen an Tieren unter dem Einfluß von antipsychotischen Drogen. Diskussion. In: Bente, D., Bradley, P.B. (eds.), Neuropsychopharmacology *4*, 115–117. Amsterdam: Elsevier 1965 a

Kreiskott, H.: Kataleptische Zustände von Octopus vulgaris nach Butyrylperazin und Bulbocapnin. In: Bente, D., Bradley, P.B. (eds.), Neuropsychopharmacology *4*, 172. Amsterdam: Elsevier 1965 b

Kreiskott, H.: Some comments on the killing response behavior of the rat. In: Aggressive behaviour. Garattini, S., Sigg, E.B. (eds.). Amsterdam: Excerpta Medica 56–58, 1969

Kreiskott, H.: Verhaltensänderungen durch psychotrope Substanzen bei Versuchstieren. Arzneim. Forsch. *24*, 1294–1297 (1974 a)

Kreiskott, H.: Einführung zum Thema Längsschnittprofile von Psychopharmakawirkungen. Arzneim. Forsch. *24*, 974–976 (1974 b)

Kreiskott, H.: Erregungszustände von Tier und Mensch. Stuttgart: Fischer 1979

Kreiskott, H., Vater, W.: Verhaltensstudien am Goldhamster unter dem Einfluß zentral wirksamer Substanzen. Arch. Exp. Path. Pharmakol. *236*, 100 (1959)

Krnjević, H., Videk, M.: A new method of testing CNS-active compounds (hole test). Psychopharmacologia *10*, 308–315 (1967)

Laborit, H.: Potenzierte Narkose und künstlicher Winterschlaf. Arch. Exp. Pathol. Pharmakol. *222*, 41–58 (1954)

Lal, H., Numan, R.: Blockade of morphine- withdrawal body shakes by haloperidol. Life Sci. *18*, 163–168 (1976)

Lal, H., Hynes, M.D.: Effectiveness of butyrophenones and related drugs in narcotic withdrawal. In: Proceedings Collegium International Neuro-Psychopharmacology. Deniker, P., Radouco-Thomas, G., Villeneuve, A. (eds.), Vol. 1, pp. 289–295. New York: Pergamon Press 1978

Lal, H., Defeo, J.J., Thut, P.: Effect of amphetamine on pain induced aggression. Comm. Behav. Biol. *1*, 333–336 (1968)

Lal, H., Defeo, J.J., Pittermann, A., Patel, G., Baumel, I.: Effects of prolonged social deprivation or enrichment on neuronal sensitivity for CNS depressants and stimulant. In: Drug addiction. Singh, J.M., Miller, L.H., Lal, H. (eds.), Vol. 1, pp. 255–266. New York: Futura 1972

Lal, H., Gianutsos, G., Puri, S.K.: Comparison of narcotic analgesics with neuroleptics on behavior measures of dopaminergic act. Life Sci. *17*, 29–34 (1975)

Lal, H., Marky, M., Fielding, S.: Effect of neuroleptic drugs on mouse jumping induced by l-dopa in amphetamine treated mice. Neuropharmacology *15*, 669–671 (1976)

Leyhausen, P.: Zur Naturgeschichte der Angst. Politische Psychologie *6*, (1967). In: Antriebe tierischen und menschlichen Verhaltens. Lorenz, K., Leyhausen, P. (eds.). München: Pieper 1968

Leyhausen, P.: Verhaltensstudien an Katzen 3 rd ed. Berlin, Hamburg: Parey 1973

Lim, R.K.S., Rink, K.G., Glass, H.G., Soaje-Echague, E.: A method for the evaluation of cumulation and tolerance by the determination of acute and subchronic median effective doses. Arch. Int. Pharmacodyn. Thér. *130*, 336–353 (1961)

Ljungberg, T., Ungerstedt, U.: Classification of neuroleptic drugs according to their ability to inhibit apomorphine-induced locomotion and gnawing: evidence for two different mechanism of action. Psychopharmacology *56*, 239–247 (1978)

Loew, D.M.: The prediction of sedative potency of neuroleptics. In: The neuroleptics. Bobon, D.P., Janssen, P.A.J., Bobon, J. (eds.), pp. 47–50. Basel: Karger 1970

Malick, J.B., Sofia, R.D., Goldberg, M.E.: A comparative study of the effects of selected psychoactive agents upon three lesion-induced models of aggression in the rat. Arch. Int. Pharmacodyn. Thér. *181*, 459–465 (1969)

McKinney, W.T., Young, L.D., Suomi, S.J., Davis, J.M.: Chlorpromazine treatment of disturbed monkeys. Arch. Gen. Psychiatry *29*, 490–494 (1973)

Menge, H.G., Brand, U.: Zur Differenzierung der Wirkung kataleptogener Stoffe. Arzneim. Forsch. *28*, 1506–1507 (1978)

Mercier, J., Dessaigne, S.: Influence exercée par quelques drogues psycholeptiques sur le comportement du scorpion (Adroctonus australis Hector). Compt. Rend. Soc. Biol. *164*, 341–344 (1970)

Møller Nielsen, I., Fjalland, B., Pedersen, V., Nymark, M.: Pharmacology of neuroleptics upon repeated administration. Psychopharmacologia *34*, 95–104 (1974)

Moore, K.E., Kelly, P.H.: Biochemical pharmacology of mesolimbic and mesocortical dopaminergic neurons. In: Psychopharmacology. A generation of progress. Lipton, M.A., DiMascio, A., Killam, K.F. (eds.), pp. 221–234. New York: Raven Press 1978

Munkvad, I.: Neuroleptics in the treatment of schizophrenia. In: The neuroleptics. Bobon, D.P., Janssen, P.A.J., Bobon, J. (eds.), pp. 44–47. Basel: Karger 1970

Niemegeers, C.J.E., Janssen, P.A.J.: Differential antagonism to amphetamine-induced oxygen consumption and agitation by psychoactive drugs. In: Antidepressants. Fielding, S., Lal, H. (eds.), pp. 125–141. New York: Futura 1975

Norton, S.: Behavioral patterns as a technique for studying psychotropic drugs. In: Psychotropic drugs. 73–82. Garattini, S., Ghetti, V. (eds.). Amsterdam: Elsevier 1957

Nymark, M.: Apomorphine provoked stereotypy in the dog. Psychopharmacologia *26*, 361–368 (1972)

Oberst, F.W., Crook, J.W.: Behavioral, physical, and pharmacodynamic effects of haloperidol in dogs and monkeys. Arch. Int. Pharmacodyn. Thér. *167*, 450–464 (1967)

Opitz, K.: Anorexigene Phenylalkylamine und Serotoninstoffwechsel. Arch. Pharmakol. exp. Pathol. *259*, 56–65 (1967)

Ploog, D.: Verhaltensforschung und Psychiatrie. In: Forschung und Praxis. Gruhle, H.W., Jung, R., Mayer-Gross, W., Müller, M. (eds.), Psychiatrie der Gegenwart, Vol. I/1B, pp. 291–443. Verlin, Göttingen, Heidelberg, New York: 1964

Raitt, J.R., Nelson, J.W., Tye, A.: Effect of chlorpromazine on septal hyperactivity in the rat. Br. J. Pharmacol. *17*, 473–478 (1961)

Remane, A.: Die Grundlagen des natürlichen Systems, der vergleichenden Anatomie und der Phylogenetik. Leipzig: Geest & Portwig 1952

Robbins, T.W.: A critique of the methods available for the measurement of spontaneous motor activity. In: Principles of behavioral pharmacology. Iversen, L.L., Iversen, S.D., Snyder, S.H. (eds.), Vol. 7, pp. 37–82. New York: Plenum Press 1977

Sackett, G.P.: Abnormal behavior in laboratory-reared rhesus monkeys. In: Abnormal behavior in animals. Fox, M.W. (ed.), pp. 293–331. Philadelphia: Saunders 1968

Sandberg, F.: A comparative quantitative study of the central depressant effect of seven clinically used phenothiazine derivatives. Arzneim. Forsch. *9*, 203–206 (1959)

Schelkunov, E.L.: Adrenergic effect of chronic administration of neuroleptics. Nature *214*, 1210–1212 (1967)

Schmidt, W., Apfelbach, R.: Psychopharmakologische Beeinflußung des Beutefangverhaltens beim Frettchen (Putorius furo L.). Psychopharmacology *51*, 147–152 (1977)

Senault, B.: Comportement d'agressivité intraspécifique induit par l'apomorphine chez le rat. Psychopharmacologia *18*, 271–287 (1970)

Sheard, M.H.: The role of drugs in precipitating or inhibiting human aggression. Psychopharmacology *13*, 23–25 (1977)

Simpson, G.M., Lee, J.H.: A ten-year review of antipsychotics. In: Psychopharmacology. A generation of progress. Lipton, M.A., DiMascio, A., Killam, K.F. (eds.), pp. 1131–1137. New York: Raven Press 1978

Sofia, R.D.: Effects of centrally active drugs on four models experimentally-induced aggression in rodents. Life Sci. *8*, 705–716 (1969)

Sovner, R., DiMascio, A.: Extrapyramidal syndromes and other neurological side effects of psychotropic drugs. In: Psychopharmacology. A generation of progress. Lipton, M.A., DiMascio, A., Killam, K.F. (eds.), pp. 1021–1032. New York: Raven Press 1978

Spengler, J., Waser, P.: Der Einfluß verschiedener Pharmaka auf den Futterkonsum von Albino-Ratten im akuten Versuch. Arch. Exp. Pathol. Pharmakol. *237*, 171–185 (1959)

Stawarz, R.J., Hill, H., Robinson, S.E., Setler, P., Dingell, J.V., Sulser, F.: On the significance of the increase in homovanillic acid (HVA) caused by antipsychotic drugs in corpus striatum and limbic forebrain. Psychopharmacologia *43*, 125–130 (1975)

Stille, G.: Zur Pharmakologie katatonigener Stoffe. Aulendorf: Editio Cantor 1971

Stille, G.: Entwicklung von Psychopharmaka. Dtsch. Ärztebl. *45*, 3249–3251 (1974)

Stille, G., Lauener, H.: Die Wirkung von Neuroleptika im chronischen pharmakologischen Experiment. Vortrag 2. Zentraleur. Symposion, Neuropsychopharmacol. and Pharmacopsychiatr. Split 1971

Sulser, F., Robinson, S.E.: Clinical implications of pharmacological differences among antipsychotic drugs (with particular emphasis on biochemical central synaptic adrenergic mechanism). In: Psychopharmacology. A generation of progress. Lipton, M.A., DiMascio, A., Killiam, K.F. (eds.), pp. 943–954. New York: Raven Press 1978

Symoens, J.: Vorbeugen und Heilung von Aggressivität und Streß bei Schweinen durch das Neuroleptikum Azaperone. Dtsch. Tierärztl. Wochenschr. *77*, 144–148 (1970)

Taeschler, M., Cerletti, A.: Zur Pharmakologie psychoaktiver Wirkstoffe. Münch. Med. Wochenschr. *102*, 1000–1005 (1960)

Tagliamonte, A., Fratta, W., Gessa, , G.L.: Aphrodisiac effect of L-Dopa and Apomorphine in male sexually sluggish rats. Experientia *30*, 381–382 (1974)

Tedeschi, D.H.: Techniques for evaluating neuroleptics: comments on their mechanism of action. In: Animal and clinical pharmacologic techniques in drug evaluation. Siegler, P.E., Moyer, J.H. (eds.), Vol. 2, pp. 297–304. Chicago: Year Book Medical 1967

Tedeschi, D.H., Tedeschi, R.E., Fellows, E.J.: The effects of tryptamine on the central nervous system, including a pharmacological procedure for the evaluation of iproniazid-like drugs. J. Pharmacol. Exp. Ther. *126*, 223–232 (1959a)

Tedeschi, R.E., Tedeschi, D.H., Mucha, A., Cock, L., Mattis, P.A., Fellows, E.J.: Effects of various centrally acting drugs on fighting behavior of mice. J. Pharmacol. Exp. Ther. *125*, 28–34 (1959b)

Tedeschi, D.H., Fowler, P.J., Miller, R.B., Macko, E.: Pharmacological analysis of footshock-induced fighting behavior. In: Aggressive behaviour. Garattini, S., Sigg, E.B. (eds.), pp. 245–252. Amsterdam: Excerpta Medica 1969

Theobald, W., Büch, O., Delina-Stula, A., Eigenmann, R., Levin, P.: Pharmakologische Untersuchungen zur Wirkung von Neuroleptica am Tier nach einmaliger und wiederholter Applikation. Arzneim. Forsch. *18*, 1491–1495 (1968)

Ther, L., Vogel, G., Werner, P.: Zur pharmakologischen Differenzierung und Bewertung der Neuroleptika. Arzneim. Forsch. *9*, 351–354 (1959)

Thompson, T.: Aggressive behavior of siamese fighting fish. In: Aggressive behavior. Garattini, S., Sigg, E.B. (eds.), pp. 15–31. Amsterdam: Excerpta Medica 1969

Tripod, J., Bein, H.J., Meier, R.: Characterization of central effects of serpasil (reserpin, a new alkaloid of rauwolfia serpentina B.) and their antagonistic reactions. Arch. Int. Pharmacodyn. Thér. *96*, 406–425 (1954)

Ungerstedt, U.: 6-Hydroxy-dopamine induced degeneration of central monoamine neurons. Eur. J. Pharmacol. *5*, 107–110 (1968)

Valzelli, L., Garattini, S.: Biochemical and behavioral changes induced by isolation in rats. Neuropharmacology *11*, 17–22 (1972)

Valzelli, L., Giacalone, E., Garattini, S.: Pharmacological control of aggressive behavior in mice. Eur. J. Pharmacol. *2*, 144–146 (1967)

Van Rossum, J.M.: Antagonism by neuroleptics of abnormal behavior induced by activation of brain dopamine receptors. In: The neuroleptics. Bobon, D.P., Janssen, P.A.J., Bobon, J. (eds.), pp. 65–67. Basel: Karger 1970

Vogel, G., Ther, L.: Das Verhalten der Baumwollratte zur Beurteilung der neuroleptischen Breite zentral-depressiver Stoffe. Arzneim. Forsch. *10*, 806–808 (1960)

Voith, K., Herr, F.: The behavioral pharmacology of butaclamol hydrochloride (Ay-23,028), a new potent neuroleptic drug. Psychopharmacologia *42*, 11–20 (1975)

Von Voigtländer, P.F., Moore, K.E.: Turning behavior of mice with unilateral 6-hydroxydopamine lesions in the striatum. Neuropharmacology *12*, 451–463 (1973)

Votava, Z.: Habituation and withdrawal symptoms after one week administration of perphenazine in rabbits. Psychopharmacologia *26*, Suppl. 100, (1972)

Walaszek, E.J., Abood, L.G.: Effect of tranquilizing drugs on fighting response of siamese fighting fish. Science *124*, 440–441 (1956)

Wang, S.C.: Perphenazine, a potent and effective antiemetic. J. Pharmacol. Exp. Ther. *123*, 306–310 (1958)

Weese, H.: „Potenzierte Narkose" und „Hibernation durch Phenothiazine". Arch. Exp. Pathol. Pharmakol. *222*, 15–20 (1954)

Weiss, B., Santelli, S.: Dyskinesias evoked in monkeys by weekly administration of haloperidol. Science *200*, 799–801 (1978)

Welch, B.L., Welch, A.S.: Aggression and the biogenic amine neurohumors. In: Aggressive Behavior. Garattini, S., Sigg, E.B. (eds.), pp. 188–202. Amsterdam: Excerpta Medica 1969

Welch, B.L., Welch, A.S.: Some aspects of brain biochemistry correlated with general nervous reactivity and aggressiveness. In: Animal aggression: Selected readings. Southwick, C.H. (ed.), pp. 187–200. New York: Van Nostrand-Reinhold 1970

Wickler, W.: Ökologie und Stammesgeschichte von Verhaltensweisen. Fortschr. Zool. *13*, 303–365 (1961)

Wilson, M.C., Schuster, C.R.: The effects of chlorpromazine on psychomotor stimulant self-administration in the rhesus monkey. Psychopharmacologia *26*, 115–126 (1972)

Wirth, W., Gösswald, R., Hörlein, U., Risse, K.-H., Kreiskott, H.: Zur Pharmakologie acylierter Phenothiazin-Derivate. Arch. Int. Pharmacodyn. Thér. *115*, 1–31 (1958)

Yen, H.D.Y., Stanger, R.L., Millman, N.: Isolation-induced aggressive behavior in ataractic tests. J. Pharmacol. Exp. Ther. *122*, 85 A (1958)

Zetler, G.: Haloperidol catalepsy in grouped and isolated mice. Pharmacology *13*, 526–532 (1975)

CHAPTER 5

Testing Antipsychotic Drug Effects with Operant Behavioral Techniques

E. LEHR

A. General Advantages of Operant Procedures for the Demonstration of Behavioral Drug Effects

Operant techniques offer one of the best possible controls of behavior. Depending on the pattern of reinforcement the animals produce characteristic patterns of responding (FERSTER and SKINNER, 1957). As these patterns have been found highly reproducible in different species (even in man), schedule controlled behavior is a phenomenon of great generality; and it is on these patterns that the critical behavioral effects of drugs depend upon (KELLEHER and MORSE, 1968, 1969). That is why especially operant procedures can uniquely provide very stable and reproducible baselines for drug studies, and it also explains the broad use of these techniques in drug testing, even if they require a lot of time and effort (COOK and SEPINWALL, 1976a; DEWS, 1978). The specifity of behavioral changes and the sensitivity to drugs is a further advantage of operant procedures (COOK and KELLEHER, 1963), as is the possibility of testing drug effects on the behavior of an intact living system (COOK and SEPINWALL, 1976b).

B. Operant Procedures for Evaluating Antipsychotic Drug Actions

I. Active Avoidance Tests

Operant active avoidance procedures are the behavioral techniques most commonly used to study antipsychotics (COOK and SEPINWALL, 1976a). In these tests animals are trained to prevent punishment, usually electric shock, by an operant behavior, e.g. by climbing a pole (COOK and WEIDLEY, 1957) or pressing a lever (DOBRIN and RHYNE, 1969). And antipsychotics generally block this active avoidance in a dose-dependent manner. There are two main variations of the active avoidance techniques being used: in the so-called discriminated active avoidance tasks the animals receive stimuli that discriminate the preshock time in which the trained activity leads to avoidance of the electric shock; the so-called Sidman avoidance or continuous avoidance does not present any discriminative stimulus, but uses the contingency to postpone the electric shock by every operant action, to a defined degree (SIDMAN, 1953). Both variations have their advantages. The continuous procedures seem to be a little more sensitive to the blocking effects of antipsychotics (DOBRIN and RHYNE, 1969). NIEMEGEERS et al. (1974) demonstrated the sensitivity of such a test: always being similar and correlated to that of antiamphetamine tests that are considered to be the most sensitive ones for antipsychotics. Discrete procedures allow one to compare drug effects on avoidance behavior (actions that prevent the punishment) and escape behavior (reactions after received punishment that prevent further punishments). And it is typical for anti-psychotic drugs to suppress avoidance responses at lower doses than those that suppress escape responses (COOK and WEIDLEY, 1957; COOK and CATANIA, 1964; OKA and SHIMIZU, 1975). This so-called selective avoidance blocking is not shared by other CNS depressant agents like meprobamate or barbiturates (FELLOWS and COOK, 1957; VERHAVE et al., 1958; COOK and KELLEHER, 1962, 1963; COOK and SEPINWALL, 1976b), but may be produced by serotonin and morphine (FELLOWS and COOK, 1957; COOK and KELLEHER, 1962). Operant avoidance techniques also proved their sensitivity by demonstrating tolerance effects after long-term application of antipsychotics to the trained animals (DANNESKIOLD-SAMSOE and PEDERSEN, 1976).

There exist many variations in the described active avoidance procedures. It has been demonstrated that similar results are obtained testing different species, e. g., mice (OKA and SHIMIZU, 1975) or dogs (FIELDING and AL, 1974), besides the commonly used rat. Even when the technique was applied to human test persons chlorpromazine caused a selective avoidance block (FISCHMAN et al., 1976), as in animal tests.

An important reason for many of the variations is to get the best possible sensitivity for drug testing. The sort of stimuli used in discriminated avoidance procedures can influence this sensitivity (COOK and CATANIA, 1964). DEWS and MORSE (1961) described that chlorpromazine blocked discriminated active avoidance more if the discriminated stimuli were reduced in the strengths they exerted over the avoidance responses. By testing the trained rats under extinction conditions the avoidance blocking of antipsychotics in a Sidman avoidance procedure could be further increased, and this blocking drug effect was less predominant in the times close to the shock delivery than in the other fractions before.

Other variations improve the active avoidance techniques by reducing the experimental effort. KURIBARA et al. (1975) reported that training of rats for Sidman avoidance could be optimized by giving not more than one training session a day, but delivering a high number of shocks during that session. The careful selection of proper responses in a given animal is important to achieve rapid learning. A rat, e. g., usually learns more easily to run in a shuttle box or to jump at a pole for avoidance of electric shocks (applied via the bottom grid) than how to prevent those shocks by pressing a lever. The one-way shuttle task (start always in the same compartment and escape to the other side of the box for avoiding the shock) was found to give remarkably better results than the usual two-way shuttle task when OKA and SHIMIZU (1975) successfully trained mice for active avoidance in less than 50 successive trials. DAVIDSON and WEIDLEY (1976), using a swinging lever that prevented holding, demonstrated the blocking of avoidance by antipsychotics in rats even during the first training session. It has, however, not proved advantageous to use too short test sessions for testing antipsychotic activities. After testing a lot of different antipsychotics, NIEMEGEERS et al. (1974) stated that even 3 h often appeared to be not enough time for a testing session. Even if many variations like, for example, changing the sort of aversive stimuli used, do not seem to influence avoidance behavior too much (MCMILLAN, 1975), with any new modification it has to be considered that variables in techniques may change the effects of antipsychotics on responding. Already changes in the rate of responding caused by using different sorts of responses can lead to changes in drug effects (KELLEHER and MORSE, 1969).

II. Other Operant Procedures

MIGLER (1975) trained squirrel monkeys by using an analogous procedure of conditioned avoidance that consisted of signalized food approach. Chlorpromazine had a selective suppressing effect on the behavior controlled by the food indicating signal without reducing the reward controlled behavior itself, quite similar to its action in discriminated active avoidance tests.

As drug effects depend more on the pattern of schedule controlled behavior than on any other experimental influences (KELLEHER and MORSE, 1968), antipsychotics proved characteristic changes in special schedules of operant behavior. For example, CANON and LIPPA (1977) demonstrated in rats that fixed ratio schedule responding (reward after a ratio of 20 responses = FR 20) was reduced by chlorpromazine and clozapine. In rats performing a fixed interval responding (the first response following a fixed interval of 2 min after the last reward is reinforced = FI 2 min), behavior was also suppressed, but mostly during the end of the time interval where under control conditions responding regularly increases to a high rate. By training animals to perform multiple schedules of operant behavior several different kinds of response patterns can be sampled from individuals within a short time period and many other variables that may change the performance of an individual over time are controlled (KELLEHER and MORSE, 1968, 1969). In the often used multiple FR/FI program the schedule is alternating from FR to FI, the different schedules being indicated to the test animals by discriminative stimuli. In general antipsychotics reduce responding a bit more and at lower doses in FI components than in FR components. This effect is dose-dependent and not shared by other drug classes, as, for example, minor tranquilizers tend to increase in special doses FI rates like amphetamine (COOK and KELLEHER, 1962; COOK, 1964; KELLEHER and MORSE, 1968). It must be taken into account, however, that in contrast to their actions in many mammals antipsychotics tend to stimulate rather than to reduce FR/FI responding if given to pigeons (DEWS, 1958).

Responding can be reinforced by using electric stimulation of special brain sites (mostly the median fore brain bundle in hypothalamic levels) as a reinforcer instead of, for example, food. Antipsychotics of different chemical classes inhibit this electric self-stimulation of the brain in a dose-related manner (KAMEI et al., 1974; WAUQUIER and NIEMEGEERS, 1976) and this inhibition is probably not due to motoric deficits (WAUQUIER, 1976). These procedures are as sensitive to antipsychotics as are the above described avoidance tests (KAMEI et al., 1975), the relative potency of these drugs in suppressing electric brain self-stimulation parallels their antipsychotic effectivity in man (FIELDING and AL, 1974). The observed behavioral changes are typical for neuroleptics, they are not shared by antidepressants or minor tranquilizers though barbiturates may cause similar effects by motoric deficits (KAMEI et al., 1974; FIELDING et al., 1974). The effects of antipsychotics on intracranial self-stimulation do, however, not differ principally from the effects these drugs have on other forms of operant behavior (WAUQUIER, 1976). This was also demonstrated when FIBIGER et al. (1976) trained rats to similar rates of responding using either food or electric brain stimulation for reinforcement and found that haloperidol reduced this responding identically in both cases. Once more the rule was proved that it is mainly the rate of responding that the drug effects depend on (KELLEHER and MORSE, 1968).

Operant techniques may also help to find out the stimulus qualities of drugs. Hoffmeister (1975) proved negative reinforcing qualities for chlorpromazine when rhesus
monkeys avoided chlorpromazine self-applications in a similar manner to the way in
which they avoided electric shocks, but tolerated the injections if pentobarbital was
applied instead. Besides being used as reinforcing stimuli, drugs can also serve as discriminative stimuli. Colpaert et al. (1975) varied this context, using apomorphine vs
saline injections to signal to their rats whether to press one or the other lever. Additional haloperidol reduced this discriminability in a dose-related manner.

C. Value of Operant Techniques
for Detecting Antipsychotic Drug Effects

One critical question about the practical value of techniques for drug development is
whether the results are specific to a certain class of drugs, or whether drugs with different clinical actions produce similar experimental effects. The described operant
procedures not only differentiate between such opposite types of drugs as stimulants
or depressants; being much more specific, they also allow distinctions between antipsychotics and minor tranquilizers or barbiturates, as pointed out for active avoidance tests (Verhave et al., 1958; Cook and Kelleher, 1962, 1963; Cook and Sepinwall, 1976b), for actions on schedules of behavior (Cook and Kelleher, 1962;
Cook, 1964; Kelleher and Morse, 1968; Canon and Lippa, 1977), and intracranial
electric self-stimulation (Kamei et al., 1974; Fielding and Al, 1974). It should be mentioned that there exist also specific operant procedures that give typical results for
non-antipsychotics, as do the so-called conflict techniques for minor tranquilizers that
selectively counteract the inactivity in avoidance–approach conflicts, whereas antipsychotics are ineffective there, even in pigeons that are stimulated in other behaviors by
these drugs (Morse, 1964). Appropriate operant techniques may help to further increase the differentiating value. McKearney (1975), e. g., clearly demonstrated that
morphine and chlorpromazine had opposite effects in animals trained to respond for
electric shock. The specifity of results is of course increased if the findings of different
experiments are combined. Comparing different operant techniques when calculating
the ratio of the effects on electric brain self-stimulation to conditioned avoidance responses Kamei et al. (1975) found differences among antipsychotics that allowed the
behavioral classification into phenothiazine derivates, butyrophenone derivates, and
dibenzoheteropine derivates. And it is evident that the information about antipsychotic drug values will be increased if all data of other pharmacologic and biochemical
techniques besides operant procedures are included.

   Another important question about the value of test procedures is the predictive
information for clinical efficiency. As none of the described operant procedures reflects a model situation for human psychotic disorders, but uses healthy test animals,
there is no possibility to directly compare the effects to clinical drug actions. But correlation analyses clearly showed that antipsychotics have the same order of potency
in operant animal tests like active avoidance procedures (Cook and Kelleher, 1962;
Cook and Catania, 1964; Cook and Sepinwall, 1976a; Davidson and Weidley,
1976), or intracranial electric self-stimulation (Fielding and Al, 1974). The objection
that such correlations could be misleading, since the animal experiments migh reflect

side effects like extrapyramidal disturbances rather than antipsychotic properties, can be partly counteracted. For clozapine and thioridazine have acted in such operant procedures despite their lack of extrapyramidal side effects (KAMEI et al., 1975; COOK and SEPINWALL, 1976a; CANON and LIPPA, 1977).

Attempts to interpret the effects of antipsychotics on operant behavior follow two different routes. In one case an attempt is made to find some indications about the physiologic mechanism of action, in particular it has been demonstrated that the results are compatible with the biochemical hypothesis about the influencing of transmitter functions by antipsychotics (DAVIS, 1965; WAUQUIER and NIEMEGEERS, 1976). It must be realized, however, that all these attempts remain indirect evidence as long as they are based on behavioral data only.

In the other case, attempts are made to interpret the behavioral animal data in comparison to human psychological function. DOBRIN and RHYNE (1969), e. g., suggested that the inhibition of active avoidance could reflect anxiolytic actions. Many experts of operant techniques prefer, however, to be very cautious with such interpretations. The fact that the nature of the reinforcer has not much influence on drug actions compared to the pattern of responding is not easily compatible with interpretations that try to include "motivation" (KELLEHER and MORSE, 1968). As COOK and CATANIA (1964) have pointed out the use of interpretative anthropomorphic terms can be misleading. As operant procedures proved to give reproducible, specific, and predictive results for clinical potency their main value is not dependent on such interpretative attempts.

D. Summary

Selective blocking of active avoidance behavior, reduction of FR/FI responding, and inhibition of intracranial electric self-stimulation have proved to be specific and reproducible actions of antipsychotics on sensitive operant procedures. There exist strong correlations between effectiveness in those operant procedures and antipsychotic potency in man. Antipsychotics also proved that there are special stimulus qualities in operant responding. Interpretations of the behavioral results in terms of physiologic mechanisms of drug action, or direct comparison with human behavior, may be misleading and they are not basically needed to prove the value of operant procedures for finding antipsychotic drug properties.

References

Canon, J.G., Lippa, A.S.: Effects of clozapine, chlorpromazine and diazepam upon adjunctive and schedule controlled behaviors. Pharmacol. Biochem. Behav. 6, 581–587 (1977)

Colpaert, F.C., Niemegeers, C.J.E., Kuyps, J.J.M.D., Janssen, P.A.J.: Apomorphine as a discriminative stimulus, and its antagonism by haloperidol. Eur. J. Pharmacol. 32, 383–386 (1975)

Cook, L.: Effects of drugs on operant conditioning. In: Ciba foundation symposium jointly with the co-ordinating committee for symposia on drug action on animal behavior and drug action. London: Churchill 1964

Cook, L., Catania, A.C.: Effects of drugs on avoidance and escape behavior. Fed. Proc. 23, 818–835 (1964)

Cook, L., Kelleher, R.T.: Drug effects on the behavior of animals. Ann. N.Y. Acad. Sci. *96*, 315–335 (1962)

Cook, L., Kelleher, R.T.: Effects of drugs on behavior. Annu. Rev. Pharmacol. *3*, 205–222 (1963)

Cook, L., Sepinwall, J.: Reinforcement schedules and extrapolations to humans from animals in behavioral pharmacology. In: Behavioral pharmacology: The current status. Weiss, B., Laties, V.G. (eds.), pp. 265–282. New York: Plenum 1976a

Cook, L., Sepinwall, J.: Animal psychopharmacological procedures: Predictive value for drug effects in mental and emotional disorders. In: Proceedings of the sixth international congress of pharmacology, Vol. 3: Central nervous system and behavioral pharmacology. Oxford: Pergamon 1976b

Cook, L., Weidley, E.: Behavioral effects of some psychopharmacological agents. Ann. N.Y. Acad. Sci. *66*, 740–752 (1957)

Danneskiold-Samsoe, P., Pedersen, V.: Inhibition of conditional avoidance response by neuroleptics upon repeated administration. Psychopharmacology *51*, 9–14 (1976)

Davidson, A.B., Weidley, E.: Differential effects of neuroleptic and other psychotropic agents on acquisition of avoidance in rats. Life Sci. *18*, 1279–1284 (1976)

Davis, J.L.: Antagonism of a behavioral effect of d-amphetamine by chlorpromazine in the pigeon. J. Exp. Anal. Behav. *8*, 325–327 (1965)

Dews, P.B.: Effects of chlorpromazine and promazine on performance on a mixed schedule of reinforcement. J. Exp. Anal. Behav. *1*, 73–82 (1958)

Dews, P.B.: Origins and future of behavioral pharmacology. Life Sci. *22*, 1115–1122 (1978)

Dews, P.B., Morse, W.H.: Behavioral pharmacology. Annu. Rev. Pharmacol. *1*, 145–174 (1961)

Dobrin, P.B., Rhyne, R.L.: Effects of chlorpromazine on two types of conditioned avoidance behavior. Arch. Int. Pharmacodyn. Ther. *178*, 351–356 (1969)

Fellows, E.J., Cook, L.: The comparative pharmacology of a number of phenothiazine derivatives. In: Psychotropic drugs. Garattini, S., Ghetti, V. (eds.), pp. 397–404. Amsterdam: Elsevier 1957

Ferster, C.B., Skinner, B.F.: Schedules of reinforcement. New York: Appleton-Century-Crofts 1957

Fibiger, H.C., Carter, D.A., Phillips, A.G.: Decreased intracranial self-stimulation after neuroleptics or 6-hydroxydopamine: Evidence for mediation by motor deficits rather than by reduced reward. Psychopharmacology *47*, 21–27 (1976)

Fielding, S., Lal, H.: Screening tests using higher animals. In: Neuroleptics. Fielding, S., Lal, H. (eds.), pp. 64–75. New York: Futura 1974

Fischman, M.W., Smith, R.C., Schuster, C.R.: Effects of chlorpromazine on avoidance and escape responding in humans. Pharmacol. Biochem. Behav. *4*, 111–114 (1976)

Hoffmeister, F.: Negative reinforcing properties of some psychotropic drugs in drug-naive rhesus monkeys. J. Pharmacol. Exp. Ther. *192*, 468–477 (1975)

Kamei, C., Masuda, Y., Shimizu, M.: Effects of psychotropic drugs on hypothalamic self-stimulation behavior in rats. Jpn. J. Pharmacol. *24*, 613–619 (1974)

Kamei, C., Fujitani, Y., Oka, M., Shimizu, M.: Comparison of the effects of neuroleptics on self-stimulation and conditioned avoidance responses in rats. Jpn. J. Pharmacol. [Suppl.] *25*, 50P–51P (1975)

Kelleher, R.T., Morse, W.H.: Determinants of the specifity of behavioral effects of drugs. Ergeb. Physiol. *60*, 1–56 (1968)

Kelleher, R.T., Morse, W.H.: Determinants of the behavioral effects of drugs. In: Importance of fundamental principles in drug evaluation. Tedeschi, D.H., Tedeschi, R.E. (eds.), pp. 383–405. New York: Raven Press 1969

Kuribara, H., Okuizumi, K., Tadokoro, S.: Analytical study of acquisition on free-operant avoidance response for evaluation of psychotropic drugs in rats. Jpn. J. Pharmacol. *25*, 541–548 (1975)

McKearney, J.W.: Drug effects on behavior maintained by aversive events. Psychopharmacol. Bull. *11*, 52–53 (1975)

McMillan, D.E.: Determinants of drug effects on punished responding. Fed. Proc. *34*, 1870–1879 (1975)

Migler, B.: Conditioned approach: An analogue of conditioned avoidance; effects of chlorpromazine and diazepam. Pharmacol. Biochem. Behav. *3*, 961–965 (1975)

Morse, W.H.: Effect of amobarbital and chlorpromazine on punished behavior in the pigeon. Psychopharmacologia *6*, 286–294 (1964)

Niemegeers, C.J.E., Verbruggen, F.J., Janssen, P.A.J.: The influence of various neuroleptic drugs on shock avoidance responding in rats. In: Neuroleptics. Fielding, S., Lal, H. (eds.), pp. 76–97. New York: Futura 1974

Oka, M., Shimizu, M.: A simple avoidance procedure for testing psychotropic drugs in mice. Jpn. J. Pharmacol. *25*, 121–127 (1975)

Sidman, M.: Avoidance conditioning with brief shock and no exteroceptive warning signal. Science *118*, 157–158 (1953)

Verhave, T., Owen, J.E. Jr., Robbins, E.B.: Effects of chlorpromazine and secobarbital on avoidance and escape behavior. Arch. Int. Pharmacodyn. Ther. *116*, 45–53 (1958)

Wauquier, A.: The influence of psychoactive drugs on brain self-stimulation in rats: A review. In: Brain-stimulation reward. Wauquier, A., Rolls, E.T. (eds.), pp. 158–160. Amsterdam, Oxford: North-Holland; New York: American Elsevier 1976

Wauquier, A., Niemegeers, C.J.E.: Restoration of self-stimulation inhibited by neuroleptics. Eur. J. Pharmacol. *40*, 191–194 (1976)

CHAPTER 6

Stereotyped Behavior and Its Relevance for Testing Neuroleptics

A. RANDRUP, B. KJELLBERG, E. SCHIØRRING, J. SCHELL-KRÜGER, R. FOG, and I. MUNKVAD

During the early Sixties it became clear that the characteristic clinical effects of neuroleptics (antimanic, antischizophrenic, neurologic) correlated with their ability to antagonize stereotypies elicited in animals by amphetamine or apomorphine (JANSSEN et al., 1965;RANDRUP and MUNKVAD, 1965). Most studies were made with rats, a species whose most extreme stereotyped behavior is continuous sniffing, licking, or biting; later, stereotyped behavior was also observed in other animal species, e. g., continuous looking from side to side or sniffing in cats, repetitive head and hand movements or locomotor repertoires in monkeys, pecking in pigeons (RANDRUP and MUNKVAD, 1967, 1968, 1974; ELLINWOOD and DUARTE-ESCALANTE, 1972; ANDERSEN et al., 1975).

Almost concurrently it was found that the dopamine in brain mediated both the production of stereotyped behavior by amphetamines and its antagonism by neuroleptics (RANDRUP et al., 1963; RANDRUP and SCHEEL-KRÜGER, 1966; MUNKVAD et al., 1968 with references).

Other types of stereotyped behavior, e. g., cholinergic and GABA-ergic forms were found later (SCHEEL-KRÜGER and RANDRUP, 1968, 1969; FOG and PAKKENBERG, 1971; RANDRUP et al., 1975 a; SCHEEL-KRÜGER et al., 1977) but only the dopaminergic type has been used for testing neuroleptic drugs. In recent years much has been learnt about this dopaminergic stereotypy and its usefulness and limitations for neuroleptic testing. In the following we shall discuss some of these newer developments.

A. Similarities and Differences Between Endogenous Psychoses and States Induced by Amphetamines in Man or Animals

I. Amphetamine Psychosis and Endogenous Psychoses

The literature about the effects of amphetamines in man is very comprehensive. Here we shall consider only amphetamine *psychosis* and its comparison with endogenous psychoses.

In his 1958 monograph on amphetamine psychosis, CONNELL stated that the symptomatology was very similar to that of schizophrenia, and that many patients were initially diagnosed as schizophrenics. At about the same time Japanese authors, drawing on a larger patient base, described a schizophrenic-like state among the effects of methamphetamine addiction (TATETSU et al., 1956; SANO and NAGASAKA, 1956; TATETSU, 1960). Since then, these results have been tested and generally confirmed during extensive experience with amphetamine abusers and in more controlled experimental settings (BEAMISH and KILOH, 1960; KELLNER, 1960; BELL, 1965, 1973; VAN

Table 1. Some literal examples from interviews of amphetamine addicts concerning stereotypies (punding) and social withdrawal. (From SCHIØRRING, 1977)

"'Punding' is an autistic state."

"You are in a special world – a world of your own."

"You do not listen to anybody, when 'punding'."

"Some are 'punding' in the way that they are staring at others. They are not interested in the others, only a constant gazing."

"A heavily 'punding' human is 'insnoead' (hung up) ('snowed up'). Does not answer, when talked to. Totally autistic."

"When you are hung up (insnoea), you are not in contact with anybody."

"They are sitting like insane people, talking with themselves."

"I have so many ideas myself when high, I find it difficult to follow the world of ideas of others."

"A girl I know can tidy up her handbag in a mechanical way for many hours (even a whole day). She takes the things out and puts them back. She had done this for 6–7 years now."

"The higher the dose, the more isolated I feel."

"At the final examination I was really high on Preludin. I wrote my name a hundred times on the paper, and thought that I had solved the problem."

"It is almost impossible for me to get contact, and if I get it – I withdraw."

"He's snowed up (hung up) – give up talking to him."

"– it was just rough fucking, a complete desexualized process, could go on for hours – but it was false feelings. Chemical love."

"Several people can be 'punding' in the same room, without any contact with each other."

Wife of addict (anamnestic record):

... initially she was fond of his increasing talkativeness and sexual interest, but at the same time, she had had a feeling as if there were a glass wall between them.

PRAAG, 1968; ANGRIST and GERSHON, 1969, 1972; TATETSU, 1972; ELLINWOOD and SUDILOVSKY, 1973; KALANT, 1973, 1974; DAVIS, 1974; ANGRIST et al., 1974b; DAVISON, 1976; JANOWSKI and DAVIS, 1976; BRON et al., 1976; JANOWSKI et al., 1977; VAN KAMMEN et al., 1977; ANGRIST and SUDILOVSKY, 1978). In addition, certain more specific issues have become progressively clarified during the later years.

In early 1966, one of us (A. R.) searched the literature for reports of stereotyped behavior in amphetamine psychosis, but found only some descriptions of abnormal behavior, indicating that stereotypy did occur (RANDRUP and MUNKVAD, 1967). Later in the same year, however, RYLANDER (1966) published a special study of stereotypy ("punding") in amphetamine addicts and mentioned that patients seldom report this symptom spontaneously. Subsequently, comprehensive evidence has confirmed the frequent occurrence of stereotypies in man as well as in animals after larger doses of amphetamine; in humans the many types of stereotyped activities include: continuous but aimless mechanical work, washing, grooming, searching, sorting of things (Table 1; RYLANDER, 1972; KRAMER, 1972; ELLINWOOD et al., 1973; ANGRIST and SUDILOVSKY, 1978; see also KELLNER, 1960; which was not found by our literature search in 1966).

Work by RYLANDER (RYLANDER, 1972; SCHIØRRING, 1977) and by one of us (Table 1; SCHIØRRING, 1977; see also RANDRUP et al., 1975a, pp. 94 and 98) demonstrates the pronounced autistic social withdrawal of amphetamine addicts performing stereotyped behavior (punding). SCHIØRRING states that withdrawal is less pronounced in patients who are "high" without punding, and this observation may help to reconcile the results with earlier reports which state that autistic lack of contact is relatively infrequent in amphetamine psychosis (SANO and NAGASAKA, 1956). Differences between observations may also be due to different degrees of chronicity of the amphetamine intake (MACHIYAMA et al., 1970, 1974; ELLINWOOD et al., 1973; RANJE and UNGERSTEDT, 1974; ELLISON et al., 1978, see also discussion by KELLNER, 1960, p. 529). ELLINWOOD (1972) writes that amphetamine psychotics often retain a relatively appropriate affect, while ANGRIST et al., (1974b) report that, in their experience with addicts and experimentally induced cases, affectual flattening was encountered frequently but by no means in all subjects. Incongruous affect was also reported (ANGRIST and GERSHON, 1969, 1972).

There has been some ambiguity in the literature with respect to the occurrence of thought disorder. BELL (1973) describes amphetamine psychosis as a "schizophrenic-like state … without thought disorder," while ÄNGGARD et al. (1970) found that "disorganization of thought" was one of the most consistent symptoms. In 1974, ANGRIST et al. concluded "that large doses of amphetamine can indeed cause disruption of thinking of various types, some quite severe, but that, on the other hand, amphetamine psychosis is not necessarily accompanied by the degree of disorganization generally seen in schizophrenia" (see also ANGRIST and SUDILOVSKY, 1978). Thought disorder, including thought blocking, was also reported by SANO and NAGASAKA (1956), TATETSU (1960, and McCONNELL (1963).

In an experiment by ANGRIST et al (1974a), the psychotic symptoms elicited by amphetamine were antagonized by haloperidol just as those of endogenous psychoses. ANGRIST observed that antipsychotic effect "within an hour after the administration of haloperidol;" this links the acute effects of neuroleptics tested on amphetaminized animals (see Sect. B) and the slowly developing antipsychotic effect frequently seen in the clinic.

In his 1958 monograph, CONNELL also noted that visual hallucinations were experienced by many patients. This observation has been corroborated by several later authors (BELL, 1965; ANGRIST and GERSHON, 1972; KALANT, 1973) and may constitute a difference between schizophrenia and amphetamine psychosis. It should be considered, however, that CONNELL (1958) noted that the visual hallucinations were of minor importance and far less disturbing than their auditory accompaniments (similar observation by DAUBE, 1942), and that TATESU (1960) found visual hallucinations infrequent; see also discussion by SNYDER (1973).

The most important difference, however, between "amphetamine schizophrenia" and endogenous schizophrenia, may be amphetamine itself, since there is no evidence of amphetamine in schizophrenic patients. The related substance, phenylethylamine, has been found in the human organism and its involvement in endogenous psychoses suggested; this issue is, however, unsettled (MOSNAIM and WOLF, 1978; BRÆSTRUP and RANDRUP, 1978; ANDERSEN and BRÆSTRUP, 1977).

Finally, not all amphetamine addicts develop psychosis, and not all psychotic cases are schizophrenic-like. Several authors report cases similar to manic-depressive psychosis, hypomania, agitated depression, or mixed manic-depressive and schizophrenic states (HARDER, 1947; O'FLANAGAN and TAYLOR, 1950; SANO and NAGASAKA, 1956; TATETSU, 1960, 1972; KELLNER, 1960; VAN PRAAG, 1968; ANGRIST et al., 1969; SCHILDKRAUT et al., 1971; RYLANDER, 1972; ELLINWOOD, 1972; BRON et al., 1976).

It may, therefore, be most relevant to compare amphetamine psychosis with "endogenous psychoses" rather than with "schizophrenia." This issue is of course related to the more general problem of classification of psychoses (OLLERENSHAW, 1973; JAROSZYNSKI, 1975; SHEPHERD, 1976). There seems to be a continuum, rather than a distinct categorization, which ranges from the classical schizophrenias over the schizoaffective schizophrenics, mixed psychoses, and Urstein psychoses to the classical manic-depressive psychoses; dopamine appears to be involved in all (RANDRUP and MUNKVAD, 1966, 1968; MUNKVAD and RANDRUP, 1970; RANDRUP et al., 1975 b).

II. Comparison of Animal and Human Data

Stereotypy is a very conspicuous feature of the behavior of amphetaminized animals (mammals, birds, less prominent in reptiles: KIRKBY et al., 1972; ELLINWOOD and DUARTE-ESCALANTE, 1972; RANDRUP and MUNKVAD, 1974, 1975; ANDERSEN et al., 1975; SCHIØRRING, 1977) and in humans it is a conspicuous symptom in endogenous psychoses (references in RANDRUP et al., 1975 a, p. 98, and 1975, p. 218; RANDRUP and MUNKVAD, 1975) as well as in amphetamine psychoses. Stereotypy, therefore, forms an important link between human and animal studies (see also Sect. B about testing neuroleptic drugs).

In recent years, other features of the behavior of amphetaminized animals have also been investigated and related to human data. We found that amphetamine strongly affects social behavior and usually results in social isolation (SCHIØRRING and RANDRUP, 1971; KJELLBERG and RANDRUP, 1973; SCHIØRRING, 1977; SCHIØRRING and HECHT, 1979). Our observations were made in acute experiments with rats and monkeys, but similar results have been found in other laboratories after acute, subchronic, or chronic administration of amphetamines (MACHIYAMA et al., 1970; GARVER et al., 1975; GAMBILL and KORNETSKY, 1976). Abnormal forms of social behavior, including social stereotypies and excessive or inappropriate aggression, have also been seen (MACHIYAMA et al., 1970; VAN ROSSUM, 1972; RANDRUP et al., 1973; RANDRUP and MUNKVAD, 1973; KJELLBERG and RANDRUP, 1973; ROLINSKI, 1974; GARVER et al., 1975; SCHIØRRING, 1977; ELLISON et al., 1978).

Direct parallels to human thought disorder (as observed in the speech and writings of psychotic patients) cannot be studied in animals. However, GARVER et al. (1975) suggest that the fragmentation of sequential patterns of behavior, seen in amphetaminized animals, could be a related phenomenon. The study of behavioral patterns is difficult, but some beginnings have been made, e. g., in our laboratory (SCHIØRRING, 1971, 1977, and in press; NORTON, 1973) and it seems to be a very promising line of research.

With respect to delusions, ELLINWOOD (1969 and 1972) describes an interesting parallel between stereotyped delusions of parasitosis with accompanying rubbing, scratching, etc., in humans and similar repetitive but abortive grooming in cats, monkeys, and chimpanzees. Sores and scars from the repetitive grooming, self-picking, and digging of parasites were observed in both humans and animals (see also KJELLBERG and RANDRUP, 1972, i.a. "Drawing out hair" in Table 3 a).

In rats and more prominently in monkeys, there are some individual differences in the response to amphetamines (RANDRUP et al., 1963; LYON and RANDRUP, 1972; KJELLBERG and RANDRUP, 1972), but we have so far not seen anything that could be regarded as a parallel to the difference between the schizophrenic and the manic responses in humans.

In humans, amphetamine also induces neurologic effects, such as mouth and tongue movements (VAN PRAAG, 1968; RYLANDER, 1972; ELLINWOOD and DUARTE-ESCALANTE, 1972; SCHIØRRING, 1977; further references in KJELLBERG and RANDRUP, 1972). Similar phenomena have been observed in monkeys (KJELLBERG and RANDRUP, 1972; ELLINWOOD and DUARTE-ESCALANTE, 1972), but in rats no neurologic effects have been observed which are clearly distinguishable from behavioral effects.

Since amphetamine itself seems to be the most important flaw in the model, nonpharmacologic models may be of interest, i. e., models produced without drugs, but, for example, by genetic selection and specific changes in the animals' environment. Such models, preferably in monkeys, might be closer to the psychotic patient and also helpful in the study of the pathogenesis of psychoses. The detailed knowledge now available about amphetamine behavior and its relations to psychotic behavior aids development of such nonpharmacologic models (RANDRUP et al., 1976).

B. Relevance of Stereotypies in Testing Antipsychotic Drugs

The drugs used around 1965 showed a very high correlation between clinical neuroleptic effects (antimanic, antischizophrenic, "extrapyramidal") and antagonism of amphetamine- and apomorphine-stereotypies in rats. Reserpine, however, one of the best known neuroleptics, was not able to antagonize the stereotypies and thus appeared as a "false negative" in the test. Later it was found that reserpine is active in various stereotypy tests modified by the use of amphetamine derivatives or by using cats instead of rats (SCHEEL-KRÜGER, 1971; PEDERSEN and CHRISTENSEN, 1972; WALLACH and GERSHON, 1972; BRÆSTRUP, 1977).

In recent years other "false negatives" have been found and studied, notably clozapine, sulpiride, and thioridazine. These drugs are also active in various modified amphetamine tests using smaller or chronic doses of amphetamines, intracerebral application of the test drugs, animals made supersensitive to dopamine, special behavioral observations, etc. (KELLY et al., 1974; NIEMEGEERS, 1974; see Fig. 5; FOG, 1975; COSTALL and NAYLOR, 1975, 1976; SAYERS et al., 1975; COSTENTIN et al., 1976; BUUS LASSEN, 1976, 1977; BOISSIER et al., 1977; BORISON et al., 1977; ELLIOTT et al., 1977; UNGERSTEDT and LJUNGBERG, 1977; LJUNGBERG and UNGERSTEDT, 1978).

With all the false negatives it seems to be true that their peculiarities in the stereotypy tests are associated with special ways of interfering with brain dopamine (RANDRUP and JONAS, 1967; SCHEEL-KRÜGER, 1971; BUNNEY et al., 1975; DAY and BLOWER, 1975; BÜRKI et al., 1975 and 1977; WILK et al., 1975; COSTALL and NAYLOR, 1976; WALDMEIER and MAITRE, 1976 a, b; SAYERS et al., 1976; PERINGER et al., 1976; SEDVALL et al., 1976; SEEMAN et al., 1976; HYTTEL, 1976; SQUIRES, 1976; v. STRALENDORFF et al., 1976; SMITH and DAVIS, 1976; RÜTHER, 1976; KOOB et al., 1977; BRÆSTRUP, 1977; BOISSIER et al., 1977; BUUS LASSEN, 1977; CLOW et al., 1977; ELLITOTT et al., 1977; WESTERINK et al., 1977; SCATTON et al., 1977; STANLEY and WILK, 1977; VAN PRAAG, 1977; UNGERSTEDT and LJUNGBERG, 1977; LJUNGBERG and UNGERSTEDT, 1978; COOLS, in press). The nondopaminergic (i. e., noradrenergic, cholinergic, serotonergic) effects of these drugs, as well as of other neuroleptics, probably also contribute to the net behavioral effects. The exact nature of these contributions has not yet been clarified (see GORDON, 1964, 1967; JANSSEN et al., 1965; MARCO et al., 1976; BÜRKI et al., 1975, 1977; WESTERINK et al., 1977; PEROUTKA et al., 1977; COOLS, in press; LJUNGBERG and UNGERSTEDT, 1978).

Table 2. Suppression of social behavior of pairs of monkeys (♂ and ♀) by amphetamine and partial prevention by neuroleptics. Each experiment comprised three or four (always same number within one horizontal line) 30 min observation periods distributed between $1/_2$ and $3^1/_2$ h after the s.c. injection of 0.37 mg amphetamine (A) per kg. The neuroleptics (N), haloperidol and chlorpromazine, were injected $1/_2$ h, and pimozide 3 h before amphetamine. A placebo (P) experiment was performed on the day before each drug experiment.

The social behaviors comprise: grooming of the other monkey, stretching to be groomed, touching the other monkey with the hand, ♀ presents rear to ♂, mounting, fighting, and biting. The number of social behaviors were counted in each experiment and the averages are shown in the Table. Total number of times of occurence of social behaviors and total time spent with these behaviors were also evaluated and show the same trend as the figures in the Table; these evaluations were dominated by one of the behaviors, mutual grooming (compare Table 3). [From Kjellberg (in preparation), details about the technique in Kjellberg & Randrup (1972, 1973)]

Monkey pairs	Neuroleptic	Dose[a] (mg/kg s.c.)	No. of different items of social behavior			No. of experiments		
			P	A	N+A	P	A	N+A
A+B	Pimozide	0.03 –0.06	9.5	0	0.7	6	3	3
J+Si	Pimozide	0.03 –0.06	6.7	0.3	4.0	6	3	3
O+So	Pimozide	0.03 –0.06	4.9	1.7	2.2	9	3	6
Jo+Ju	Haloper.	0.015–0.04	5.8	0.3	2.0	13	4	9
G+V	Haloper.	0.015–0.04	6.1	0.7	1.3	9	3	6
A+B	Haloper.	0.015–0.04	6.4	1.0	0.7	5	2	3
Au+Aua	Haloper.	0.015–0.04	6.0	0	0.7	7	4	3
O+So	Chlorprom.	0.2 –0.6	6.4	1.5	4.6	12	4	8
A+B	Chlorprom.	0.2 –0.6	7.5	0	0.3	8	2	6
G+V	Chlorprom.	0.2 –0.6[b]	7.2	0	2.3	9	2	7

[a] Doses were regulated so that amphetamine-stereotypies were just inhibited and no "extrapyramidal" effects of the neuroleptics appeared; amphetamine gives a surmountable protection against the latter (compare Table 3)
[b] Monkey V was given up to 1.5 mg clorpormazine/kg

At the moment, then, the classical amphetamine and apomorphine tests seem to predict classical neuroleptic clinical effects which lie within the range of variation described, e.g., by Bobon and colleagues (Bobon et al., 1972; Bobon and Gottfries, 1974).

It has been suggested that these tests should predict "extrapyramidal" side effects better than antipsychotic effects. However, reserpine would again be a false negative and the clinically important combinations of neuroleptics with antiparkinson drugs would be false positives (Setler et al., 1976). These side effects are probably better predicted from tests with monkeys (Weissman, 1968; Crane and Gardner, 1969; Gunne and Bárány, 1976; own observations: Kjellberg unpublished, see Table 3).

If a new drug is negative in the classical tests, but positive in some of the abovementioned modified tests, an unusual but perhaps desirable antipsychotic effect might be possible.

Finally, since effects on brain dopamine seem to be so important, it may prove profitable to look into series of drugs acting on brain dopamine and to investigate further some of the members with unusual effects. This might lead to drugs with new types of antischizophrenic effects, to antidepressives (Angst and Gram , 1976; Ran-

Table 3. Reduction by neuroleptics of only one social activity (mutual grooming) in three couples of monkeys.
The dose range covers that in Table 2 for each drug. The monkeys were observed for 6×30 min during a period of $5^1/_2$ h, starting $^1/_2$ h after injection except in experiments with pimozide[b]. One experiment was performed with each dose of the neuroleptics and a placebo experiment on the day before each experiment with neuroleptics. "Extrapyramidal" symptoms were also recorded; these comprise: backwards walking, sudden stop of movement, unusual postures, unusual (compulsive) movements, and tremor. (From KJELLBERG (in preparation), see also Table 2)

Drug	Dose (mg/kg s.c.)	Mutual grooming minutes			"Extrapyramidal" symptoms. Average total number of times observed	
		O+S	G+V	A+Aa	♂	♀
Placebo[a]		29.5±10.3	11.5±6.1	9.8±7.6	0	0
	0.01	38.7	2.5	25.4	0	0
Haloperidol	0.02	0.7	0	0	13	19
	0.04	0	0	0	11	27
Chlorpromazine	0.4	2.7	0	5.2	0	3
	0.8	10.5	0.3	0	5	7
	1.6	0	0	3.5	2	22
Pimozide[b]	0.03	0	0.4	0	3	0
	0.06	2.2	0	0	9	20
	0.12	0	0	0	10	14
Placebo for pimozide[b]		26.4± 6.0	10.3±8.2	8.0±9.7	0	0

[a] Average ± standard error
[b] Observation 4×30 min during a period of 3 h 50 min starting 2 h 10 min after injection

DRUP and BRÆSTRUP, 1977), or to milder, nonaddictive sedative, stimulant, or analgetic drugs (HAASE, 1972; COLLARD, 1976; ZAPLETALEK et al., 1977).

Theoretically, nondopaminergic antipsychotic drugs are possible but no conclusive clinical evidence for them exists. Search for such drugs could be based on knowledge about interactions and connections between dopaminergic and certain nondopaminergic (e.g., cholinergic, GABA-ergic) systems in the brain (see VAN KAMMEN, 1977).

New developments in the therapy of schizophrenia emphasizing personal contact and resocialization (e.g., JØRSTAD and UGELSTAD, 1976; ALANEN et al., 1977; MOSHER and MENN, 1977; LEHRER and LANOIL, 1977) call for drugs with a more subtle or "mild" antipsychotic effect, which would not only mitigate psychotic symptoms, but also restore normal, including social, *activity*.

The known neuroleptics only partially restore normal activities in amphetaminized animals and in schizophrenic patients (Table 2; NIEMEGEERS et al., 1970; KJELLBERG and RANDRUP, 1974; AHLENIUS and ENGEL, 1976; RANDRUP et al., 1976; SPOHN et al., 1977). To this extent the various amphetamine models parallel the disease, but it is unclear whether the models also parallel the disease with respect to differences between individual neuroleptics (DEL RIO and FUENTES, 1969) and to what extent the models are able to select new drugs which may restore normal activities. The amphetamine or apomorphine models using smaller or chronic doses of amphetamines may be preferable here and non-pharmacologic models, as conjectured in the previous section, could hopefully also become useful in due time.

The fact that neuroleptics do not completely restore normal activities can be partly due to their own action on behavior, which in the doses needed also suppress normal activities, i.a., social activities (Table 3; RIFKIN et al., 1977).

As neuroleptics and amphetamine (or schizophrenia) here act in the same direction, the effects of new potentially antipsychotic drugs on normal animals are crucial (see BUUS LASSEN, 1976, 1977). The ideal antipsychotic drug would be one that antagonized psychotic behavior but not normal behavior.

References

Ahlenius, S., Engel, J.: Normalization by antipsychotic drugs of biochemically induced abnormal behavior in rats. Psychopharmacology 49, 63–68 (1976)

Alanen, Y.O., Eberhard, G., Gerle, B.O., Hansson, B., Rosman, C., Sedvall, G.: Behandling av schizofreni. Svenska Läkartidningen 74, 2195–2202 (1977)

Andersen, H., Bræstrup, C.: Mass fragmentographic demonstration of low amounts of β-phenylethylamine in human urine. Scand. J. Clin. Lab. Invest. 37, 33–37 (1977)

Andersen, H., Bræstrup, C., Randrup, A.: Apomorphine-induced stereotyped biting in the tortoise in relation to dopaminergic mechanisms. Brain Behav. Evol. 11, 365–373 (1975)

Änggard, E., Gunne, L.-M., Jönsson, L.-E., Niklasson, F.: Pharmacokinetic and clinical studies on amphetamine dependent subjects. Eur. J. Clin. Pharmacol. 3, 3–11 (1970)

Angrist, B., Gershon, S.: Some recent studies on amphetamine psychosis – Unresolved issues. In: Current Concepts on Amphetamine Abuse. Ellinwood, E.H., Cohen, S. (eds.). Washington: U.S. Government Printing Office, DHEW Publication No. (HSM) 72-9085 1972, pp. 193–204

Angrist, B., Lee, H.K., Gershon, S.: The antagonism of amphetamine-induced symptomatology by a neuroleptic. Am. J. Psychiatr. 131, 817–819 (1974a)

Angrist, B., Sathananthan, G., Wilk, S., Gershon, S.: Amphetamine psychosis: Behavioral and biochemical aspects. J. Psychiatr. Res. 11, 13–23 (1974b)

Angrist, B., Sudilovsky, A.: Central nervous system stimulants, historical aspects and clinical effects. In: Handbook of Psychopharmacology. Iversen, L., Iversen, S., Snyder, S. (eds.). N.Y., London, Washington DC – Boston: Plenum Vol. XI, pp. 99–165 (1978)

Angrist, B.M., Gershon, S.: Amphetamine induced schizophreniform psychosis. In: Schizophrenia Current Concepts and Research. Siva Sankar, D.V. (ed.), Hickville, N.A.: PJD 1969, pp. 508–524

Angrist, B.M., Schweitzer, J., Friedhoff, A.J., Gershon, S., Hekimian, L.J., Floyd, A.: The clinical symptomatology of amphetamine psychosis and its relationship to amphetamine levels in urine. Int. Pharmacopsychiatry 2, 125–139 (1969)

Angst, J., Gram, L.F.: New trends in the treatment of depressive states. In: Collegium Internationale Neuro-Psychopharmacologicum (C.I.N.P.). Baronet-Lacroix, D. (ed.). Abstracts. 10th Congress Quebec 1976, pp. 162–165

Beamish, P., Kiloh, L.G.: Psychoses due to amphetamine consumption. J. Ment. Sci. 106, 337–343 (1960)

Bell, D.S.: Comparison of amphetamine psychosis and schizophrenia. Br. J. Psychiatr. 111, 701–707 (1965)

Bell, D.S.: The experimental reproduction of amphetamine psychosis. Arch. Gen. Psychiatry 29, 35–40 (1973)

Bobon, J., Bobon, D.P., Pinchard, A., Collard, J., Ban, T.A., De Buck, R., Hippius, H., Lambert, P.-A., Vinar, O.: A new comparative physiognomy of neuroleptics: a collaborative clinical report. Acta Psychiatr. Belg., 72, 542–554 (1972)

Bobon, D.P., Gottfries, C.G.: Clinical physiognomy of thioxanthenes. Acta Psychiatr. Belg. 74, 442–568 (1974)

Boissier, J.R., Puech, A.J., Simon, P.: Action of classic and unusual neuroleptics on various behavioral apomorphine-induced effects. In: Advances in Biochemical Psychopharmacology. Costa, E., Gessa, G.L. (eds.). New York: Raven Press 1977, pp. 631–634

Borison, R.L., Havdala, H.S., Diamond, B.I.: Chronic phenylethylamine stereotypy in rats: A new animal model for schizophrenia? Life Sci. *21*, 117–122 (1977)

Bræstrup, C.: Biochemical differentiation of amphetamine vs methylphenidate and nomifensine in rats. J. Pharm. Pharmacol. *29*, 463–470 (1977)

Bræstrup, C., Randrup, A.: Stereotyped behavior in rats induced by phenylethylamine, dependence on dopamine and noradrenaline and possible relation to psychoses? In: Noncatecholic Phenylethylamines. Part I. Mosnaim, A.D., Wolf, M. (eds.). New York: Marcel Dekker, pp. 245–269 (1978)

Bron, B., Fröscher, W., Gehlen, W.: Differentialdiagnostische und syndromgenetische Probleme und Aspekte drogeninduzierter Psychosen bei Jugendlichen. Fortschr. Neurol. Psychiatr. *44*, 673–682 (1976) and *45*, 53–75 (1977)

Bunney, B.S., Roth, R.H., Aghajanian, G.K.: Effects of molindone on central dopaminergic neuronal activity and metabolism: Similarity to other neuroleptics. Psychopharmacol. Commun. *1*, 349–358 (1975)

Buus Lassen, J.: Inhibition and potentiation of apomorphine-induced hypermotility in rats by neuroleptics. Eur. J. Pharmacol. *36*, 385–393 (1976)

Buus Lassen, J.: Inhibition of apomorphine-induced hypermotility in rats by chlorpromazine, perphenazine, thioridazine and melperone. Acta Pharmacol. Toxicol. (Kbh.) *40*, 418–429 (1977)

Bürki, H.R., Ruch, W., Asper, H.: Effects of clozapine, thioridazine, perlapine and haloperidol on the metabolism of the biogenic amines in the brain of the rat. Psychopharmacologia *41*, 27–33 (1975)

Bürki, H.R., Sayers, A.C., Ruch, W., Asper, H.: Effects of clozapine and other dibenzo-epines on central dopaminergic and cholinergic systems. Arzneim. Forsch./Drug Res. *27*, 1561–1565 (1977)

Clow, A., Elliott, P.N.C., Jenner, P., Marsden, C.D., Pycock, C.: Interactions of substituted benzamide drugs with cerebral dopamine pathways. Br. J. Pharmacol. *60*, 268P–269 (1977)

Collard, J.: Long-term clinical trial of pimozide (R 6239) in the treatment of "social maladjustments" in patients with personality disorders. In: Collegium Internationale Neuro-Psychopharmacologicum (C.I.N.P.). Baronet-Lacroix, D. (ed.). 10th Congress. Québec: 1976, p. 181

Connell, P.H.: Amphetamine Psychosis. Maudsley Monograph no. 5. London: The Institute of Psychiatry, Chapman & Hall 1958

Cools, A.R.: The influence of neuroleptics on central dopaminergic systems. To be published in: Neurotransmission and Disturbed Behavior. Van Praag, H.M. (ed.). Amsterdam: De Erven Bohn BV. (in press)

Costall, B., Naylor, R.J.: Detection of the neuroleptic properties of clozapine, sulpiride and thioridazine. Psychopharmacologia *43*, 69–74 (1975)

Costall, B., Naylor, R.J.: A comparison of the abilities of typical neuroleptic agents and of thioridazine, clozapine, sulpiride and metochlopramide to antagonise the hyperactivity induced by dopamine applied intracerebrally to areas of the extrapyramidal and mesolimbic systems. Eur. J. Pharmacol. *40*, 9–19 (1976)

Costentin, J., Protais, P., Marcais, H., Schwartz, J.-C.: The climbing behavior, a sensitive test to study the activity of antipsychotics and the modulations in sensitivity of dopamine receptors in mouse striatum. In: Collegium Internationale Neuro-Psycopharmacologicum (C.I.N.P.). Baronet-Lacroix, D. (ed.). 10th Congress Abstracts. Québec: 1976, p. 159

Crane, G.E., Gardner, R.: Psychotropic drugs and dysfunctions of the basal ganglia. A multidisciplinary Workshop. In: Public Health Service Publication no. 1938. Washington: U.S. Government Printing Office 1969

Daube, H.: Pervitinpsychosen. Nervenarzt *15*, 20–25 (1942)

Davis, J.M.: A two factor theory of schizophrenia. J. Psychiatr. Res. *11*, 25–29 (1974)

Davison, K.: Drug-induced psychoses and their relationship to schizophrenia. In: Schizophrenia Today. Kemali, D., Bartholini, G., Richter, D. (eds.). Oxford, New York, Toronto, Sidney, Paris, Frankfurt: Pergamon Press 1976, pp. 105–133

Day, M., Blower, P.: Cardiovascular dopamine receptor stimulation antagonized by metoclo-pramide. J. Pharm. Pharmacol. 27, 276–278 (1975)

Del Rio, J., Fuentes, J.A.: Further studies on the antagonism of stereotyped behavior induced by amphetamine. Eur. J. Pharmacol. 8, 73–78 (1969)

Ellinwood, E.H.: Amphetamine psychosis: A multi-dimensional process. Semin. Psychiatry 1, 208–226 (1969)

Ellinwood, E.H.: Amphetamine psychosis: Individuals, settings, and sequences. In: Current Concepts on Amphetamine Abuse. Ellinwood, E.H., Cohen, S. (eds.). Washington: U.S. Government Printing Office DHEW Publication no. (HSM) 72-9085 1972, pp. 143–157

Ellinwood, E.H., Duarte-Escalante, O.: Chronic methamphetamine intoxication in three species of experimental animals. In: Current Concepts on Amphetamine Abuse. Ellinwood, E.H., Cohen, S. (eds.). Washington: U.S. Government Printing Office. DHEW Publication no. (HSM) 72-9085 1972, pp. 59–68

Ellinwood, E.H., Sudilovksy, A.: The relationship of the amphetamine model psychosis to schizophrenia. In: Psychopharmacology, Sexual Disorders and Drug Abuse. Ban, T.A. et al. (eds.). Amsterdam, London: North-Holland, Prague: Avicenum, Czechoslovak Medical Press 1973, pp. 189–203

Ellinwood, E.H., Sudilovsky, A., Nelson, L.: Evolving behavior in the clinical and experimental amphetamine (model) psychosis. Am. J. Psychiatry 130, 1088–1093 (1973)

Elliott, P.N., Jenner, P., Huizing, G., Marsden, C.D., Miller, R.: Substituted benzamides as cerebral dopamine antagonists in rodents. Neuropharmacology 16, 333–342 (1977)

Ellison, G., Eison, M.S., Huberman, H.S.: Stages of constant amphetamine intoxication: Delayed appearance of paranoid-like behaviors in rat colonies. Psychopharmacology 56, 293–299 (1978)

Fog, R.: Neuroleptic action of clozapine injected into various brain areas in rats. Int. Pharmacopsychiatry 10, 89–93 (1975)

Fog, R., Pakkenberg, H.: Intracerebral lesions causing stereotyped behavior in rats. Acta Neurol. Scand. 47, 475–484 (1971)

Gambill, J.D., Kornetsky, C.: Effects of chronic d-amphetamine on social behavior of the rat: Implications for an animal model of paranoid schizophrenia. Psychopharmacology 50, 215–223 (1976)

Garver, D.L., Schlemmer, F., Maas, J.W., Davis, J.M.: A schizophreniform behavioral psychosis mediated by dopamine. Am. J. Psychiatry 132, 33–38 (1975)

Gordon, M.: Psychopharmacological Agents. New York, London: Academic Press 1964, Vol. I

Gordon, M.: Psychopharmacological Agents. New York, London: Academic Press 1967, Vol. II

Gunne, L.-M., Bárány, S.: Haloperidol-induced tardive dyskinesia in monkeys. Psychopharmacology 50, 237–240 (1976)

Haase, H.-J.: Therapie mit Psychopharmaka und anderen psychotropen Medikamenten. Stuttgart, New York: F. K. Schattauer Verlag 1972

Harder, A.: Über Weckamin-Psychosen. Schweiz. Med. Wochenschr. 37/38, 982–985 (1947)

Hyttel, J.: Effects of a single administration of clozapine on mouse brain catecholamines. Acta Pharmacol. Toxicol. (Kbh.) 38, 358–365 (1976)

Janowsky, D.S., Davis, J.M.: Methylphenidate, dextroamphetamine, and levamfetamine. Arch. Gen. Psychiatry 33, 304–308 (1976)

Janowsky, D.S., Huey, L., Storms, L.: Psychologic test responses and methylphenidate. In: Cocaine and Other Stimulants. Ellinwood, E.H., Kilbey, M.M. (eds.). New York, London: Plenum Press 1977, pp. 675–682

Janssen, P.A.J., Niemegeers, C.J.E., Schellekens, K.H.L.: Is it possible to predict the clinical effects of neuroleptic drugs (major tranquillizers) from animal data? Drug Res. (Arzneim. Forsch.) 15, 104–117 (1965)

Jaroszynski, J., Rzewuska-Szatkowska, M., Skowronska, J., Tarczynska, K.: The course of treatment in schizophrenia in relation to the presence of affective disturbances. Pol. Med. Sci. Hist. Bull. 15, 479–485 (1975)

Jørstad, J., Ugelstad, E. (eds.): Schizophrenia 75. Psychotherapy. Family Studies, Research. Oslo, Norway: Universitetsforlaget 1976

Kalant, O.J.: The Amphetamines. Toxicity and Addiction. University of Toronto Press: Brookside Monograph of the Addiction Research Foundation No. 5, 1973

Kalant, O.J., Kalant, H.: Amphetamines and Related Drugs. Clinical Toxicity and Dependence. Addiction Research Foundation, Canada 1974

Kammen, D., van: γ-Aminobutyric acid (GABA) and the dopamine hypothesis of schizophrenia. Am. J. Psychiatry *134*, 138–143 (1977)

Kammen, D., van, Bunney, W.E., Docherty, J.P., Jimerson, D.C., Post, R.M., Siris, S., Ebert, M., Gillin, J.C.: Amphetamine-induced catecholamine activation in schizophrenia and depression: Behavioral and physiological effects. In: Advances in Biochemical Pyschopharmacology. Costa, E., Gessa, G.L. (eds.). New York: Raven Press 1977, Vol. XVI, pp. 655–659

Kellner, E.: Preludinsucht und Preludinpsychose. Ther. Ggw. *99*, 524–530 (1960)

Kelly, P., Miller, R.J., Sahakian, B.: Interaction of neuroleptic and cholinergic drugs with central dopaminergic mechanisms. Br. J. Pharmacol. *52*, 430P–431P (1974)

Kirkby, R.J., Bell, D.S., Preston, A.C.: The effects of methylamphetamine on stereotyped behavior, activity, startle, and orienting responses. Psychopharmacology *25*, 41–48 (1972)

Kjellberg, B., Randrup, A.: Stereotypy with selective stimulation of certain items of behavior observed in amphetamine treated monkeys (Cercopithecus). Pharmakopsychiatrie. Neuropharmakologie *5*, 1–12 (1972)

Kjellberg, B., Randrup, A.: Disruption of social behavior of vervet monkeys (Cercopithecus) by low doses of amphetamines. Pharmakopsychiatry *6*, 287–293 (1973)

Kjellberg, B., Randrup, A.: Partial restoration by neuroleptic (spiramide) of items of grooming behavior suppressed by amphetamine. Arch. Int. Pharmacodyn. *210*, 61–66 (1974)

Koob, G.F., Del Fiacco, M., Iversen, S.D.: Dissociable properties of dopamine neurons in the nigrostriatal and mesolimbic dopamine systems. In: Advances in Biochemical Psychopharmacology. Costa, E., Gessa, G.L. (eds.). New York: Raven Press 1977, Vol. XVI, pp. 589–595

Kramer, J.C.: Introduction of amphetamine abuse. In: Current Concepts on Amphetamine Abuse. Ellinwood, E.H., Cohen, S. (eds.). Washington: U.S. Government Printing Office DHW Publication No. (HSM) 72-9085 1972, pp. 177–184

Lehrer, P., Lanoil, J.: Natural reinforcement in a psychiatric rehabilitation program. Schizophrenia Bull. *3*, 297–302 (1977)

Ljungberg, T., Ungerstedt, U.: Classification of neuroleptic drugs according to their ability to inhibit apomorphine induced locomotion and gnawing. Evidence for two different mechanisms of action. Psychopharmacology *56*, 239–247 (1978)

Lyon, M., Randrup, A.: The dose-response effect of amphetamine upon avoidance behavior in the rat seen as a function of increasing stereotypy. Psychopharmacologia *23*, 334–347 (1972)

Machiyama, Y., Utena, H., Kikuchi, M.: Behavioral disorders in Japanese monkeys produced by the long-term administration of methamphetamine. Proc. Jap. Acad. *46*, 738–743 (1970)

Machiyama, Y., Hsu, S.C., Utena, H., Katagiri, M., Hirata, A.: Aberrant social behavior induced in monkeys by the chronic methamphetamine administration as a model for schizophrenia. In: Biological Mechanisms of Schizophrenia and Schizophrenia-Like Psychoses. Mitsuda, H., Fikuda, I. (eds.). Tokyo: Igaku Shoin 1974, pp. 97–105

Marco, E., Mao, C.C., Cheney, D.L., Revuelta, A., Costa, E.: The effects of antipsychotics on the turnover rate of GABA and acetylcholine in rat brain nuclei. Nature *264*, 363–365 (1976)

McConnell, W.B.: Amphetamine substances in mental illnesses in Northern Ireland. Br. J. Psychiatry *109*, 218–224 (1963)

Mosher, L.R., Menn, A.Z.: Soteria House: One-year outcome data. Psychopharmacol. Bull. *13*, 46–47 (1977)

Mosnaim, A.D., Wolf, M. (eds.): Noncatecholic Phenylethylamines. New York: Marcel Dekker 1978

Munkvad, I., Randrup, A.: Evidence indicating the role of brain dopamine in the psychopharmacology of schizophrenic psychoses. Psihofarmakologija (Yugoslavia) *2*, 45–47 (1970)

Munkvad, I., Pakkeberg, H., Randrup, A.: Aminergic systems in basal ganglia associated with stereotyped hyperactive behavior and catalepsy. Brain Behav. Evol. *1*, 89–100 (1968)

Niemegeers, C.: Predictions of side effects. In: Neuroleptics. Fielding, S., Lal, H. (eds.). USA: Futura 1974, pp. 98–129

Niemegeers, C.J.E., Verbruggen, F.J., Janssen, P.A.J.: The influence of various neuroleptic drugs on shock avoidance responding in rats. III. Amphetamine antagonism in the discriminated sidman avoidance procedure. Psychopharmacologia 17, 151–159 (1970)

Norton, S.: Amphetamine as a model for hyperactivity in the rat. Physiol. Behav. 11, 181–186 (1973)

O'Flanagan, P., Taylor, R.: A case of recurrent psychosis associated with amphetamine addiction. N. Ment. Sci. 96, 1033–1036 (1950)

Ollerenshaw, D.P.: The classification of the functional psychoses. Br. J. Psychiatry 122, 517–530 (1973)

Pedersen, V., Christensen, A.V.: Antagonism of methylphenidate-induced stereotyped gnawing in mice. Acta Pharmacol. Toxicol. (Kbh.) 31, 488–496 (1972)

Peringer, E., Jenner, P., Donaldson, I.M., Marsden, C.D., Miller, R.: Metoclopramide and dopamine receptor blockade. Neuropharmacology 15, 463–469 (1976)

Peroutka, S.J., U'Prichard, D.C., Greenberg, D.A., Snyder, S.H.: Neuroleptic drug interactions with norepinephrine alpha receptor binding sites in rat brain. Neuropharmacology 16, 549–556 (1977)

Praag, H.M., van: Abuse of, dependence on and psychoses from anorexigenic drugs. In: Drug-Induced Diseases. Meyer, L., Peck, H.M. (eds.). Amsterdam, New York, London, Paris, Milan, Tokyo, Buenos Aires: Excerpta Medica Foundation 1968, Vol. III, pp. 281–294

Praag, H.M., van: The significance of dopamine for the mode of action of neuroleptics and the pathogenesis of schizophrenia. Br. J. Psychiatry 130, 463–474 (1977)

Randrup, A., Bræstrup, C.: Uptake inhibition of biogenic amines by newer antidepressant drugs, relevance to the dopamine hypothesis of depression. Psychopharmacology 53, 309–314 (1977)

Randrup, A., Jonas, W.: Brain dopamine and the amphetamine-reserpine interaction. J. Pharm. Pharmacol. 19, 483–484 (1967)

Randrup, A., Munkvad, I.: Special antagonism of amphetamine-induced abnormal behavior. Psychopharmacologia 7, 416–422 (1965)

Randrup, A., Munkvad, I.: Dopa and other naturally occurring substances as causes of stereotypy and rage in rats. Acta Psychiatr. Scand. [Suppl.] 191 (ad vol. 42), 193–199 (1966)

Randrup, A., Munkvad, I.: Stereotyped activities produced by amphetamine in several animal species and man. Psychopharmacologia 11, 300–310 (1967)

Randrup, A., Munkvad, I.: Behavioral stereotypies induced by pharmacological agents. Pharmakopsychiatr. Neuropsychopharmakol. 1, 18–26 (1968)

Randrup, A., Munkvad, I.: Roles of brain noradrenaline and dopamine in pharmacologically induced aggressive behavior. In: Symposium on Pharmacological Agents and Biogenic Amines in the Central Nervous System. Knoll, J., Magyar, K. (eds.). Budapest: Akadémiai Kiadó 1973, Vol. I, pp. 131–139

Randrup, A., Munkvad, I.: Pharmacology and Physiology of stereotyped behavior. In: Neuropathology of Schizophrenia. Kety, S., Mathysse, S. (eds.). J. Psychiatr. Res. 11, 1–10 (1974)

Randrup, A., Munkvad, I.: Stereotyped behavior. Pharmacol. Ther. [B.] 1, 757–768 (1975)

Randrup, A., Scheel-Krüger, J.: Diethyldithiocarbamate and amphetamine stereotyped behavior. J. Pharm. Pharmacol. 18, 752 (1966)

Randrup, A., Munkvad, I., Udsen, P.: Adrenergic mechanisms and amphetamine induced abnormal behaviour. Acta Pharmacol. Toxicol. (Kbh.) 20, 145–157 (1963)

Randrup, A., Munkvad, I., Scheel-Krüger, J.: Mechanisms by which amphetamines produce stereotypy, aggression and other behavioral effects. Psychopharmacologia 26, 37 suppl. (1972)

Randrup, A., Munkvad, I., Scheel-Krüger, J.: Mechanisms by which amphetamines produce stereotypy, aggression and other behavioral effects. In: Psychopharmacology, Sexual Disorders and Drug Abuse. Ban, T., Boissier, J., Gessa, G., Heimann, H., Hollister, L., Lehmann, H., Munkvad, I., Steinberg, H., Sulser, F., Sundwall, A. & Vinar, O. (eds.). VIII Congr. of the Collegium Internationale Neuro-Psychopharmacologicum, Copenhagen, 1972. North-Holland Publishing Company, Amsterdam, London and Avicenum, Czechoslovak Medical Press, Prague 1973, pp. 659–673

Randrup, A., Munkvad, I., Fog, R., Ayhan, I.H.: Catecholamines in activation, stereotypy, and level of mood. In: Catecholamines and Behavior. Friedhoff, A.J. (ed.). New York: Plenum Press 1975 a, Vol. I, pp. 89–107

Randrup, A., Munkvad, I., Fog, R., Gerlach, J., Molander, L., Kjellberg, B., Scheel-Krüger, J.: Mania, depression and brain dopamine. In: Current Developments in Psychopharmacology. Essman, W.B., Valzelli, L. (eds.). New York: Spectrum 1975 b, Vol. II, pp. 205–248

Randrup, A., Munkvad, I., Fog, R., Kjellberg, B., Lyon, M., Nielsen, E., Svennild, I., Schiørring, E.: Behavioral correlates to antipsychotic efficacy of neuroleptic drugs. In: International Symposium on "Antipsychotic Drugs, Pharmacodynamics and Pharmacokinetics." Sedvall, G., Uvnäs, B., Zotterman, Y. (eds.). Oxford: Wenner-Gren Center Internat. Symp. Ser. Pergamon Press 1976, pp. 331–341

Ranje, C., Ungerstedt, U.: Chronic amphetamine treatment: vast individual differences in performing a learned response. Eur. J. Pharmacol. 29, 307–311 (1974)

Rifkin, A., Quitkin, F., Kane, J., Klein, D.F.: Fluphenazine decanoate, oral fluphenazine, and placebo in the treatment of remitted schizophrenics. II. Rating Scale Data. Psychopharmacol. Bull. 13, 49–50 (April, 1977)

Rolinski, Z.: Analysis of the aggressiveness-stereotypy complex induced in mice by amphetamine or D,L-dopa. Pol. J. Pharmacol. Pharm. 26, 369–378 (1974)

Rossum, J.M., van: Psychopharmacology of amphetamines. Psychiatr. Neurol. Neurochir. (Amst.) 75, 165–178 (1972)

Rüther, E.: Interaction of neuroleptics: haloperidol and clozapine. In: Collegium Internationale Neuro-Psychopharmacologicum (C.I.N.P.). Baronet-Lacroix, D. (ed.). Abstracts. 10th Congress Quebec, Canada 1976, p. 54

Rylander, G.: Preludin-narkomaner fran klinisk och medicins-kkriminologisk synpunkt. Svenska Läkartidningen 63, 4973–4980 (1966)

Rylander, G.: Psychoses and the punding and choreiform syndromes in addiction to central stimulant drugs. Psychiatr. Neurol. Neurochir. (Amst.) 75, 203–212 (1972)

Sano, I., Nagasaka: Über chronische Weckaminsucht in Japan. Fortschr. Neurol. Psychiatr. 24, 391–394 (1956)

Sayers, A.C., Bürki, H.R., Ruch, W., Asper, H.: Neuroleptic-induced hypersensitivity of striatal dopamine receptors in the rat as a model of tardive dyskinesia. Effects of clozapine, haloperidol, loxapine and chlorpromazine. Psychopharmacologia 41, 97–104 (1975)

Sayers, A.C., Bürki, H.R., Ruch, W., Asper, H.: Anticholinergic properties of antipsychotic drugs and their relation to extrapyramidal side-effects. Psychopharmacology 51, 15–22 (1976)

Scatton, B., Bischoff, S., Dedek, J., Korf, J.: Regional effects of neuroleptics on dopamine metabolism and dopamine-sensitive adenylate cyclase activity. Eur. J. Pharmacol. 44, 287–292 (1977)

Scheel-Krüger, J.: Comparative studies of various amphetamine analogues demonstrating different interactions with the metabolism of the catecholamines. Eur. J. Pharmacol. 14, 47–59 (1971)

Scheel-Krüger, J., Randrup, A.: Pharmacological evidence for a cholinergic mechanism in brain involved in a special stereotyped behavior of reserpinized rats. Br. J. Pharmacol. 34, 217P (1968)

Scheel-Krüger, J., Randrup, A.: Evidence for a cholinergic mechanism in brain involved in the tetrabenazine reversal by thymoleptic drugs. J. Pharm. Pharmacol. 21, 403–406 (1969)

Scheel-Krüger, J., Arnt, J., Magelund, G.: Behavioural stimulation induced by muscimol and other GABA agonists injected into the substantia nigra. Neuroscience Letters 4, 351–356 (1977)

Schildkraut, J.J., Watson, R., Draskoczy, P.R., Hartmann, E.: Amphetamine withdrawal: depression and M.H.P.G. excretion. Lancet August 28 1971 II, 485–486

Schiørring, E.: Amphetamine induced selective stimulation of certain behavior items with concurrent inhibition of others in an open-field test with rats. Behavior 39, 1–17 (1971)

Schiørring, E.: Changes in individual and social behavior induced by amphetamine and related compounds in monkeys and man. In: Advances in Behavioral Biology. Ellinwood, E.H., Kilbey, M.M. (eds.). New York, London: Plenum Press 1977, Vol. XXI, pp. 373–407

Schiørring, E.: An open-field study on spontaneous locomotion with amphetamine treated rats. Psychopharmacology (in press).

Schiørring, E., Hecht, A.: Behavioral effects of low, acute doses of d-amphetamine on the dyadic interaction between mother and infant vervet monkeys (Cercopithecus aethiops) during the first six postnatal months. Psychopharmacology 64, 219–224 (1979).

Schiørring, E., Randrup, A.: Social isolation and changes in the formation of groups induced by amphetamine in an open-field test with rats. Pharmakopsychiatr. Neuropsychopharmakol. 4, 1–11 (1971)

Sedvall, G., Uvnas, B., Zotterman, Y. (eds.): Antipsychotic Drugs: Pharmacodynamics and Pharmacokinetics. Oxford, New York, Toronto, Sydney, Paris, Frankfurt: Pergamon Press 1976

Seeman, P., Lee, T., Chau-Wong, M., Wong, K.: Antipsychotic drug doses and neuroleptic/dopamine receptors. Nature 261, 717–718 (1976)

Setler, P., Sarau, H., McKenzie, G.: Differential attenuation of some effects of haloperidol in rats given scopolamine. Eur. J. Pharmacol. 39, 117–126 (1976)

Shepherd, M.: Definition, classification and nomenclature: A clinical overview. In: Schizophrenia Today. Kemali, D., Bartholini, G., Richter, E. (eds.). Oxford, New York, Toronto, Sydney, Paris, Frankfurt: Pergamon Press 1976, pp. 3–12

Smith, R.C., Davis, J.M.: Behavioral evidence for supersensitivity after chronic administration of haloperidol, clozapine, and thioridazine. Life Sci. 19, 725–732 (1976)

Snyder, S.H.: Amphetamine psychosis: A "model" schizophrenia mediated by catecholamines. Am. J. Psychiatry 130, 61–67 (1973)

Spohn, H.E., Lacoursiere, R.B., Thompson, K., Coyne, L.: Phenothiazine effects on psychological and psychophysiological dysfunction in chronic schizophrenics. Arch. Gen. Psychiatry 34, 633–644 (1977)

Squires, R.F.: Some in vitro properties of striatal tyrosine hydroxylase (TH) activated in vivo by neuroleptics. In: Acta Physiologica Scandinavica. Suppl. 40. Abstract. 1976, p. 135

Stanley, M., Wilk, S.: The effect of antipsychotic drugs and their clinically inactive analogs on dopamine metabolism. Eur. J. Pharmacol. 44, 293–302 (1977)

Stralendorff, B., von, Ackenheil, M., Zimmermann, J.: Akute und chronische Wirkung von Carpipramin, Clozapin, Haloperidol und Sulpirid auf den Stoffwechsel biogener Amine im Rattengehirn. Arzneim. Forsch. 26, 1096–1098 (1976)

Tatetsu, S.: Pervitin-Psychosen. Folia Psychiatr. Neurol. Jap. suppl. 6, 25–33 (1960)

Tatetsu, S.: Methamphetamine Psychosis. In: Current Concepts on Amphetamine Abuse. Ellinwood, E.H., Cohen, S. (eds.). Washington: U.S. Government Printing Office, DHEW Publ. No. (HSM) 72-9085 1972, pp. 159–161

Tatetsu, S., Goto, A., Fujiwara, T.: The methamphetamine-psychosis (Kakuseizai chudoku). Igaku Shoin, Tokyo 1956 (in Japanese).

Ungerstedt, U., Ljungberg, T.: Behavioral patterns related to dopamine neurotransmission: Effect of acute and chronic antipsychotic drugs. In: Advances in Biochemical Psychopharmacology. Costa, E., Gessa, G.L. (eds.). New York: Raven Press 1977, Vol. XVI, pp. 193–199

Waldmeier, P.C., Maitre, L.: On the relevance of preferential increases of mesolimbic versus striatal dopamine turnover for the prediction of antipsychotic activity of psychotropic drugs. J. Neurochem. 27, 589–597 (1976 a)

Waldmeier, P.W., Maitre, L.: Clozapine: Reduction of the initial dopamine turnover increase by repeated treatment. Eur. J. Pharmacol. 38, 197–203 (1976 b)

Wallach, M., Gershon, S.: The induction and antagonism of central nervous system stimulant-induced stereotyped behavior in the cat. Eur. J. Pharmacol. 18, 22–26 (1972)

Weissman, A.: Psychopharmacological effects of thiothixene and related compounds. Psychopharmacologia 12, 142–157 (1968)

Westerink, B.H.C., Lejeune, B., Korf, J., Praag, H.M., van: On the significance of regional dopamine metabolism in the rat brain for the classification of centrally acting drugs. Eur. J. Pharmacol. 42, 179–190 (1977)

Wilk, S., Watson, E., Stanley, M.: Differential sensitivity of two dopaminergic structures in rat brain to haloperidol and to clozapine. J. Pharmacol. Exp. Ther. 195, 265–270 (1975)

Zapletalek, M., Hübsch, T., Zbytovsky, Polackova, J., Kindernayova, H.: Klinische und experimentelle Erfahrungen mit Maprotilin, Clomipramin, Sydnocarb und Mefexamid bei psychisch kranken und gesunden Personen. Schweiz. Arch. Neurol., Neurochir. Psychiatr. 120, 323–334 (1977)

CHAPTER 7

Neurophysiological Properties of Neuroleptic Agents in Animals

I. Jurna

A. Pre- and Postsynaptic Action of Antipsychotic Drugs

When one tries to give an account of the action of neuroleptic agents on neurons in the central nervous system, it seems reasonable to start from the principle that drugs such as reserpine or CPZ impair impulse transmission at synapses where monoamines act as transmitter substances. Reserpine depletes NA from sympathetically innervated tissues (for literature see Carlsson et al., 1957b; Carlsson, 1966), and diminishes or abolishes the effect of electrical or chemical stimulation of adrenergic nerves due to lack of the transmitter (Bertler et al., 1956; Bertler et al., 1958; Muscholl and Vogt, 1957, 1958, Trendelenburg and Gravenstein, 1958). There is better time correlation between the depression of adrenergic impulse transmission and a reduced tissue uptake of NA than between the disturbed nerve function and the reduced NA levels in the tissues (Andén et al., 1964f). Similarly, reserpine decreases the content of NA, DA, and 5HT in the brain and spinal cord (Shore and Brodie, 1957; Shore et al., 1957; Carlsson, 1959, 1965; Andén et al., 1967b) and inhibits the accumulation of NA in the brain when the amine is administered into the lateral ventricles (Glowinski and Axelrod, 1965, 1966). It is now generally accepted that changes in central nervous functions produced by reserpine are due to lack of the monoamines as transmitters (Carlsson, 1964), i.e., reserpine acts presynaptically in inhibiting monoaminergic impulse transmission. However, there is considerable disagreement when an attempt is made to correlate central effects in terms of changes in animal behavior with the impairment of the function of a particular monoaminergic transmitter. Sedation produced by reserpine has been ascribed to depletion of 5HT in the brain (Brodie et al., 1961; Costa et al., 1962). This view was advocated because treatment with αMT re-

---

Abbreviations

A	= adrenaline	5 HTP	= 5-hydroxytryptophan
ACh	= acetylcholine	IPSP	= inhibitory postsynaptic potential
ATP	= adenosine triphosphate	α MT	= α-methyl-*p*-tyrosine
cAMP	= cyclic adenosine monophosphate (adenosine-3',5'-cyclic mono-phosphate)	NA	= noradrenaline
		6-OH-DA	= 6-hydroxydopamine
		TTX	= tetrodotoxin
CPZ	= chlorpromazine	low spinalization	
DA	= dopamine (3,4-dihydroxyphenyl-ethylamine)		= transection of the spinal cord at the lower thoracic or upper lumbar region
Dopa	= L-Dopa ((−)-3,4-dihydroxy-phenylalanine)	high spinalization	
EPSP	= excitatory postsynaptic potential		= transection of the spinal cord at the upper cervical region (C 1)
GABA	= γ-aminobutyric acid		
5 HT	= 5-hydroxytryptamine		

duced the content of brain catecholamines but not of 5HT without producing sedation. On the other hand, it had been shown by GADDUM and VOGT (1956) that an intraventricular injection of 5HT did not antagonize the sedative effect of reserpine. Moreover, p-chlorphenylalanine did not produce sedation, although it selectively depleted the stores of 5HT in the brain (KOE and WEISSMAN, 1966).

Chronic treatment with reserpine enhanced DA-receptor binding in the rat striatum (UNGERSTEDT et al., 1975) and increased the number of adrenergic receptors of the α- and β-type in the rat cortex (U'PRICHARD and SNYDER, 1978). This effect of reserpine resembles the result produced by 6-OH-DA-induced degeneration of the nigrostriatal DA-containing path, i.e., supersensitivity of the DA receptors in the striatum developed (UNGERSTEDT, 1971 b; UNGERSTEDT and PYCOCK, 1974; SCHULTZ and UNGERSTEDT, 1978) and the binding of labeled apomorphine or spiroperidol in the striatum was increased (CREESE and SNYDER, 1979). Supersensitivity of DA receptors also followed from chronic treatment with neuroleptic agents such as CPZ, haloperidol, or clozapine (KLAWANS and RUBOVITS, 1972; TARSY and BALDESSARINI, 1973; SAYERS et al., 1975; DUNSTAN and JACKSON, 1976).

As compared with reserpine, the action of CPZ is considerably more complex. CPZ may inhibit the effects of 5HT in the periphery (GYERMEK, 1955; COSTA, 1956) and in the central nervous system. It exerted a blocking effect on adrenergic α-receptors (POCIDALO et al., 1952; HUIDOBRO, 1954; MELVILLE, 1954; GOKHALE et al., 1964; WEBSTER, 1965), but also prolonged or potentiated the pressor effect of NA (MARTIN et al., 1960; GOKHALE et al., 1964). The result produced by CPZ probably depended on the dosages used and on the experimental condition. Since CPZ partially blocked the uptake of NA into adrenergic nerves (AXELROD et al., 1961; DENGLER et al., 1961; HERTTING et al., 1961; AXELROD et al., 1962; MALMFORS, 1963; CARLSSON and WALDECK, 1965; IVERSEN, 1965), the concentration of NA at the receptor sites could have increased so that the blockade was eventually overcome. For adrenergic α-receptor affinity of neuroleptic drugs in the brain see PEROUTKA et al. (1977). In the brain, CPZ was found to block NA and DA receptors equally well; perphenazine, clothiapine, haloperidol, and particularly spiroperidol were more effective on DA and NA receptors, while pimozide and fluspirilene blocked only DA receptors (ANDÉN et al., 1970a). The uptake mechanism for DA apparently differs from that for NA since it was hardly inhibited by CPZ, while that for NA was blocked as in the periphery (HÄGGENDAL and HAMBERGER, 1967). Because of conformation similarities between the molecules of DA and those of CPZ and related neuroleptic agents, it has been assumed that these drugs act on DA receptors (HORN and SNYDER, 1971). Labeled haloperidol and DA showed a high affinity for the same membrane binding sites indicating an association with postsynaptic DA receptors, and this was also true for apomorphine (BURT et al., 1976) which is considered to be a DA-receptor agonist (ANDÉN et al., 1967c; ERNST, 1967). DA was more potent inhibitor than NA or GABA at the crayfish stretch receptor, and its effect was abolished by CPZ, but also by the adrenergic α-receptor blocking agent phenoxybenzamine (McGEER et al., 1961). In the snail, *Helix aspersa,* one group of neurons was excited, another inhibited by DA (STRUYKER BOUDIER et al., 1974). Neurons excited by DA were also activated by apomorphine, and the excitation produced by DA or apomorphine was abolished by haloperidol (Fig. 1) or droperidol. Neither apomorphine nor haloperidol were effective on neurons inhibited by DA. Indirect evidence has been presented that two functionally

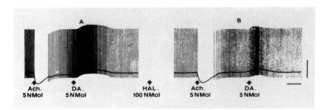

Fig. 1 A and B. Antagonism by haloperidol (HAL) of DA-induced excitation of cell 7 in the snail *Helix aspersa*. Horizontal calibration: 30 s; vertical calibration: 25 mV. (From STRUYKER et al., 1974)

different types of DA-sensitive neuron also exist in the cat caudate nucleus, and that only the type excited by either DA or apomorphine was influenced by haloperidol (COOLS et al., 1976; see also SCHWARCZ et al., 1978). It has been assumed that neuroleptic agents acting postsynaptically block DA receptors by forming monolayers at the surface of the sensitive membrane thus reducing membrane permeability (SEEMAN and BIALY, 1963; JANSSEN, 1967; JANSSEN and ALLEWIJN, 1969; JANSSEN et al., 1968 b).

On account of physico-chemical data SEEMAN (SEEMAN et al., 1974; SEEMAN and LEE, 1975) concluded that neuroleptic drugs must not necessarily act according to the "receptor-blockade hypothesis," but that their effects might as well be explained by the "coupling-blockade hypothesis." This hypothesis implies that neuroleptic drugs act either as local or as general anesthetic agents (RITCHIE and GREENGARD, 1961; QUASTEL et al., 1972; SEEMAN et al., 1974) and block the release of DA coupled with the impulse generation in presynaptic terminals (Fig. 2).

Results from binding studies suggest that there are at least two classes of DA receptors (NAGY et al., 1978; SEEMAN et al., 1978; TITELER and SEEMAN, 1978). One receptor possesses low affinity for DA, micromol concentrations are required to inhibit binding of neuroleptic agents, and this receptor is possibly located postsynaptically. The other receptor exhibits high affinity for DA or apomorphine (which bind in the nanomolar range), a low affinity for neuroleptic agents (which bind in the micromolar range) and is possibly located presynaptically. Reviews are given, for example, by COOLS and VAN ROSSUM (1976), HYTTEL (1978), and KEBABIAN (1978). The characteristics of the two classes of DA receptors have been summarized by IVERSEN (1978a) in Table 1.

To assess the effect of the neuroleptic drugs as inhibitors of monoaminergic impulse transmission in a particular area of the central nervous system, the minimum condition to be fulfilled is that the system under study contains neurons which on activation release a known monoamine as transmitter substance. Although neurons containing NA, DA, and 5 HT together with their synthesizing and metabolizing enzymes have been localized in various parts of the central nervous system, the effect of each monoamine on the neuron at which it is released is often all but clear. This is due to numerous reasons, the principal one being that monoaminergic neurons cannot be isolated together with their target cells in the brain or spinal cord as in the periphery. Changes observed in the activity of more or less complex neuronal systems after either depleting monoamines or enhancing their synthesis may lead to false conclusions because more than one type of monoaminergic neuron could be involved; different types

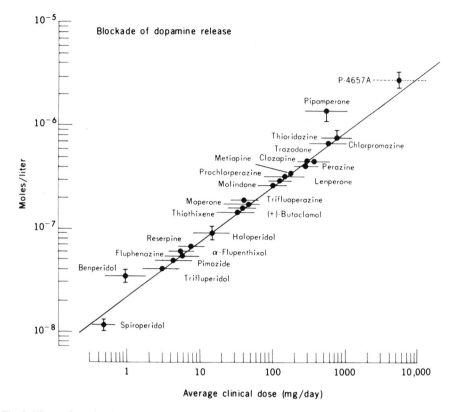

Fig. 2. The antipsychotic IC$_{50}$ values (the antipsychotic concentrations which inhibited the stimulated release of DA by 50%) correlate with the average clinical doses (mg/day) for controlling schizophrenia. The horizontal bars show the 20% variation of the IC$_{50}$ values. (From SEEMAN and LEE, 1975)

of such neurons possibly even exert opposite effects. When an attempt is made to restore activity impaired by depletion of a monoamine, or to enhance a particular monoaminergic activity by administration of the respective precursor, it is possible that a false transmitter is formed. Dopa may be transformed into DA not only in dopaminergic neurons but also in neurons normally synthesizing 5 HT (VOGT, 1965; NG et al., 1970; WUERTHELE and MOORE, 1977; but see also HILLARP et al., 1966), and decarboxylation of 5 HTP can occur in adrenergic tissues (CARLSSON, 1960). Considerable progress in the determination of central transmitter action has been made since the introduction of the technique of recording activity from single neurons with a micropipette in combination with microionophoretic administration of drugs. However, certain rules have to be obeyed to obtain reliable and relevant results (BLOOM, 1974). It seems to be of particular importance whether the experiments have been carried out under anesthesia (SALMOIRAGHI and STEFANIS, 1965) and which type of anesthetic agent was used. In cats anesthetized with a barbiturate, microionophoretic administration of NA to spinal or thalamic neurons was ineffective, while in unanesthetized animals it produced inhibition (CURTIS et al., 1961; ENGBERG and RYALL, 1965, 1966; PHILLIS and TE-

Table 1. DA receptor types (after IVERSEN, 1978a)

Denomination by		
COOLS and VAN ROSSUM (1976)	DA$_e$	DA$_i$
KEBABIAN (1978)	Alpha	Beta
KEBABIAN and CALNE (1979)	D-2	D-1
cAMP	Not linked	Linked
Most potent antagonists	Spiperone Benperidol Haloperidol	α-Flupenthixol Pifluthixol Fluphenazine
Selective antagonists	Metoclopramide Sulpiride Domperidone Oxiperomide Molindone	None known
Selective agonists	Bromocriptine and other ergolines Piribedil	None known – ergolines may act as antagonists
Apomorphine	Potent agonist	Partial agonist or antagonist
Labeled ligands	^{3}H-haloperidol ^{3}H-spiperone ^{3}H-domperidone ^{3}H-dihydroergocriptine	[^{3}H]DA [^{3}H] apomorphine [^{3}H]α-flupenthixol
Model	Inhibition of prolactin secretion from anterior pituitary gland	Bovine parathyroid

BĒCIS, 1967a). Tryptamine excited spinal neurons in unanesthetized spinal cats or in cats anesthetized with chloralose, but it had no effect when barbiturate anesthesia was employed (CURTIS, 1962; MARLEY and VANE, 1963).

B. Spinal Neurons and Descending Pathways

The presence of NA and 5HT in pathways descending from the brain stem and making extensive contact with neurons in distinct regions of the spinal cord has been demonstrated in various species using histochemistry and fluorescence microscopy methods (CARLSSON et al., 1962, 1963; MAGNUSSON and ROSENGREN, 1963; ANDÉN et al., 1964c; CARLSSON et al., 1964; DAHLSTRÖM and FUXE, 1965a; ANDERSON and HOLGERSON, 1966). On electrical stimulation of these tracts, NA and 5 HT were released from the endings (ANDÉN et al., 1964b, 1965; DAHLSTRÖM et al.,1965). The presence of DA in the spinal cord (MCGEER and MCGEER, 1962; MCGEER et al., 1963) has been disputed (ANTON and SAYRE, 1964) but was later confirmed for the rat (ANDÉN et al., 1967a; MAGNUSSON,1973; COMMISSIONG et al.,1979) and man (COMMISSIONG and SEDGWICK, 1975).

An intravenous injection of large doses of A produced an initial increase in the patellar reflex which coincided with the period of rise in blood pressure; this increase in reflex activity was followed by a long lasting reflex depression, which was also present in low spinal cats (SCHWEITZER and WRIGHT, 1937; SIGG et al., 1955; TEN CATE et al., 1959). Reflex facilitation by A depended on the level of anesthesia and could disappear in deep anesthesia (SIGG et al, 1955). McLENNAN (1961) observed that A, NA, and DA injected to anesthetized cats depressed the patellar reflex, A exerting the strongest effect and DA nearly none. The depression was abolished by CPZ and phenoxybenzamine. When the catecholamines were topically applied to the surface of the spinal cord, DA was more potent than A or NA in depressing the patellar reflex, and the reflex inhibition produced by the amines could not be blocked by CPZ or phenoxybenzamine, but was antagonized by dichlorisoprenaline or strychnine. In high spinal cats intravenously administered A increased monosynaptic extensor reflexes and either depressed monosynaptic flexor reflexes or left them unchanged; these effects were independent of changes in blood pressure (BERNHARD et al., 1952). Close intra-arterial injection or local administration of A or NA to the spinal cord equally increased the monosynaptic extensor reflex, while mono- and polysynaptic flexor reflexes were depressed (BERNHARD et al., 1947; BERNHARD and SKOGLUND, 1953; WILSON, 1956). The significance of the results obtained with systemically administered A or NA has been seriously questioned by LUNDBERG (1965) because of the improbability that the amines penetrated into the spinal cord (HAMBERGER, 1967; SCHILDKRAUT and KETY, 1967).

Dopa and 5 HTP – precursors in the synthesis of the catecholamines and 5 HT, respectively – have been reported to pass the blood-brain barrier in appreciable amounts (UDENFRIEND et al., 1957 a, b; CARLSSON et al., 1957; CARLSSON et al., 1958; SOURKES, 1961; WEBER and HORITA, 1965). The observation that Dopa and 5 HTP injected to acutely spinalized rabbits produced a powerful enhancement of flexor reflexes in the hind limbs (CARLSSON et al., 1963) prompted LUNDBERG and co-workers to analyze the changes induced by Dopa in the activity of spinal reflex pathways in low spinal cats. It was found that Dopa inhibited the impulse transmission from flexor reflex afferents to motoneurons, primary afferents and ascending pathways. At the same time when the short latency dorsal root potential and flexor reflexes evoked by single stimuli were depressed, a long latency dorsal root potential and a vigorous late flexor reflex discharge was evoked by repetitive stimulation of flexor reflex afferents (ANDÉN et al.,1963; ANDÉN et al., 1964e, 1966e, f). The changes in flexor reflex activity were probably due to an overflow of NA from the terminals of a descending pathway (JURNA and LUNDBERG, 1968) which produced inhibition of the short latency flexor reflex pathway and a simultaneous release of a normally inhibited long latency flexor reflex pathway. An injection of 5 HTP produced effects similar to those following the administration of Dopa with additional spontaneous motor discharges (ANDÉN et al, 1964d). Depression of dorsal root potentials and flexor reflexes with a concomitant increase in monosynaptic reflex activity was observed by BAKER and ANDERSON (1965, 1970a) after the injection of moderate doses of Dopa to high spinal cats. On account of the catecholamine levels determined in the spinal cord these authors concluded that DA was involved in the effects of Dopa. In fact, apomorphine injected to high spinal cats depressed polysynaptic reflexes, the dorsal root reflex and the impulse transmission to ascending pathways; however, it did not increase but inhibited monosynaptic reflexes (SCHLOSSER et al., 1972). The depressant effects of apomorphine were blocked by haloperidol but not by CPZ, phenoxybenzamine or propranolol. On the

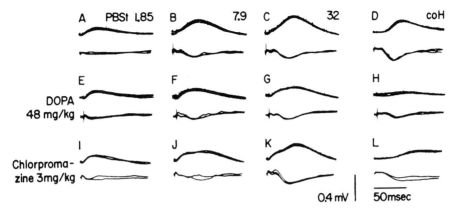

Fig. 3 A–L. Partial reversal of the inhibitory effect of Dopa on the dorsal root potentials by CPZ. Upper traces of each pair of records are the dorsal root potentials evoked by electric stimulation of the posterior biceps-semitendinosus (PBSt) or contralateral hamstring (coH) nerves at the strengths indicated (multiples of threshold). The lower traces are the potentials recorded from the dorsal root entry zone. The control records **A–D** were obtained and then Dopa (48 mg/kg) was intravenously injected and records **E–H** taken, showing the depression of the dorsal root potentials evoked from high threshold muscle afferents. Later CPZ (3 mg/kg) was intravenously injected and there was an immediate, but only partial, reversal of the effect of Dopa, shown in records **I–L**. Same time and voltage calibrations for all records. Low spinal cat. (From ANDÉN et al., 1966d)

other hand, the facilitation of flexor reflex activity produced by clonidine, a NA receptor-stimulating agent, was blocked by CPZ and phenoxybenzamine (ANDÉN et al., 1970b). Likewise, the effects of Dopa were inhibited by the adrenergic α-receptor blocking agents CPZ and phenoxybenzamine, but not by the β-receptor blocker, pronethalol (BAKER and ANDERSON, 1970b).

It is conceivable that part of the effects observed after the administration of Dopa or 5 HTP were due to an excessive formation of false transmitter substances in cells containing decarboxylase. This might explain why a specific NA-releasing agent (4,α-dimethyl-m-tyramine, H 77/77) depressed short latency impulse transmission from flexor reflex afferents, but failed to evoke the late long lasting reflex discharge (FEDINA et al., 1971). The effects of Dopa were prevented by reserpine or decarboxylase inhibition, and those of the NA liberator by pretreatment with reserpine and a tyrosine hydroxylase inhibitor. CPZ (Figs. 3 and 4) and phenoxybenzamine reduced or abolished the effects of both Dopa and the NA liberator (ANDÉN et al., 1964e, 1966d; FEDINA et al., 1971). Microionophoretic administration of DA, NA, and 5 HT enhanced the field potentials of motoneurons in rats kept under halothane anesthesia (BARASI and ROBERTS, 1977). Flupenthixol antagonized the effect of DA, left that of 5 HT uninfluenced and potentiated the effect of NA. In the spinal cat, reserpine by itself was ineffective on the reflexes tested (ESPLIN and HEATON, 1955; ANDÉN et al., 1964d). However, in the spinal rat both reserpine and Dopa increased monosynaptic as well as short latency flexor reflexes and the dorsal root potentials, and evoked a late long lasting flexor reflex; both substances antagonized the effects of each other (GROSSMANN et al., 1975). The increase in primary afferent depolarization giving rise to the dorsal root potential indicated that the organization of the pathways involved

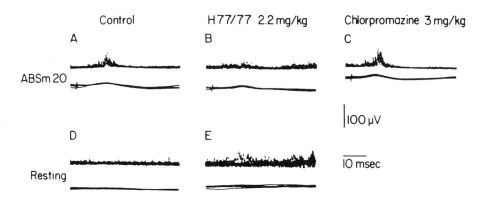

Fig. 4 A–E. The effect of the NA liberator H 77/77 on ventral root discharges evoked from high threshold muscle afferents (flexor reflex afferents) in a spinal cat. Transection of the cord at Th 11. The upper traces are from the ventral root S 1 and the lower from the dorsal root entry zone L 7. **A** was recorded immediately before, **B** 8 min after, H 77/77 (2.2 mg/kg), and **C** 18 min after CPZ (3 mg/kg). **D** represents resting ventral root discharges before, and **E** 4 min after, H 77/77. All records consist of 3–4 superimposed traces. (From FEDINA et al., 1971)

in the action of Dopa and reserpine are different in cats and rats. The increase in the (late) flexor reflex activity produced by Dopa in the rat has been ascribed to a NA receptor activation either by newly formed NA or DA, or by NA released from storage sites by DA (ANDÉN et al., 1972 b).

The changes induced by Dopa in the activity of spinal reflex pathways facilitated reciprocal interneuron innervation from which reciprocal activation of extensor and flexor motoneurons resulted; this was the basis for stepping movements (JANKOWSKA et al., 1965, 1967 a, b; FU et al., 1975). Stepping movements were initiated in spinal animals not only by Dopa but also by the NA receptor-stimulating agent clonidine (FORSSBERG and GRILLNER, 1973; GRILLNER, 1973).

The involvement of NA in motor control at the spinal level is also suggested by the following observations. In the acute spinal cat tonic stretch reflexes cannot be elicited because of the inactivity of the γ-motoneurons innervating the muscle spindles in the extensor muscles. After an injection of Dopa, however, the γ-motoneurons showed tonic activity as in the intercollicularly decerebrate preparation, and a stretch reflex could easily be evoked (GRILLNER, 1969). Likewise, extensor fusimotor activity followed repetitive electrical stimulation of descending pathways below the site of spinal cord transection (ELLAWAY and PASCOE, 1966, 1968). Since only the descending facilitation was blocked by CPZ or phenoxybenzamine (fusimotor activity facilitated by peripheral nerve stimulation remained unchanged), it appeared to be mediated by NA. A short period of potentiated facilitation could precede the inhibition, possibly because CPZ and phenoxybenzamine reduced the uptake of NA into the presynaptic terminals (ELLAWAY and PASCOE, 1968). COMMISSIONG and SEDGWICK (1974) observed that Dopa injected to intercollicularly decerebrate cats made it possible to elicit a tonic stretch reflex when no rigidity was present, or to first enhance and then depress the stretch reflex in preparations with rigidity; dihydroxyphenylserine (DOPS), which is transformed directly into NA, produced only inhibition of the reflex. From these results it has been concluded that Dopa enhanced the stretch reflex via DA, and inhibited the reflex via NA. Pretreatment with reserpine prevented the development of rigidity after intercollicular transection, but it enhanced the effect of Dopa on the stretch reflex. Furthermore, systemically administered 5 HTP also facilitated the tonic reflex activity in low spinal cats, either because of an increased impulse discharge from extensor γ-motoneurons (AHLMAN et al., 1971; ELLAWAY and TROTT, 1975) or independent of fusimotor activity (WAND, 1976). In this connection it is worth noting that intercollicular decerebration not only sets up a rigidity resulting from hyperactivity of the γ-motor system, but also produced changes in spinal reflex activity similar to those following the administration of Dopa or 5 HTP (ENGBERG et al., 1968) and which have been ascribed to a release of tonic activity in descending monoaminergic pathways. The rigidity due to hyperactivity of the γ-motor system was abolished by CPZ (HENATSCH and INGVAR, 1956). CPZ depressed tonic activity of the γ-motoneurons as well as it inhibited the activation of the γ-motor system produced either by pinna (see also WITKIN et al., 1959) or by electrical stimulation in the reticular formation or of skin nerves. Since it did not influence the rigidity caused by anemic decerebration, which is due to hyperactivity of the α-motoneurons, it had been suggested that CPZ specifically depressed the γ-motor system by an action on the mesencephalic reticular formation (see also CHIN and SMITH, 1962). Although CPZ did not markedly influence the post-tetanic potentiation of monosynaptic mass reflexes evoked by electrical stimulation of primary afferents, it abolished the post-tetanic potentiation of single α motoneurons evoked by repeated muscle stretch (HENATSCH and INGVAR, 1956) and the activation of α motoneurons by chemical stimulation of extensor muscle spindles with suxamethonium in spinal cats (SCHULTE and HENATSCH, 1958). It also depressed the monosynaptic reflex based on the rigidity resulting from spinal ischemia (SMITH and MURAYAMA, 1964).

CPZ depressed the facilitation or inhibition of the patellar reflex evoked in high spinal cats by electrical stimulation of descending pathways (HUDSON, 1966). CPZ, as well as the phenothiazine derivative pecazine, and phenoxybenzamine abolished the inhibition of the reflex evoked by stimulation of the bulbar reticular formation (CRANMER et al., 1959; KRUGLOV and SINITSYN, 1959). Likewise, reserpine blocked the reticulospinal excitation of motoneurons obtained in decerebrate cats by stimulation of the caudate medulla (ANDÉN et al., 1964d). The motor effects elicited by electrical stimulation of the cerebral and cerebellar cortex and of the cerebellar nuclei were depressed by CPZ (DASGUPTA and WERNER, 1955; KREINDLER et al., 1958; KRUGLOV and SINITSYN, 1959). The effect of the drug on the patellar reflex facilitated or inhibited by stimulation of various brain stem areas varied with the structures activated (VALDMAN, 1962). Facilitation of spinal monosynaptic reflexes evoked by electrical stimulation of the substantia nigra was markedly reduced by CPZ (Fig. 5). In intact animals reserpine, CPZ and various other phenothiazine derivatives decreased or abolished mono- or polysynaptic reflex activity (SILVESTRINI and MAFFII, 1959; WITKIN et al., 1960; HUDSON and DOMINO, 1963, 1964). CPZ influenced not only descending but also ascending activity in the spinal cord, as followed from the depression by the drug of the Schiff-Sherrington phenomenon (HENATSCH and INGVAR, 1956; HERMAN and BARNES, 1964), i.e., the increase in the rigidity of the forelimbs after spinalization at the lower thoracic level of intercollicularly decerebrate animals.

When NA was administered by microionophoresis to cat spinal motoneurons and interneurons including Renshaw cells and was found to exert an effect. This effect was

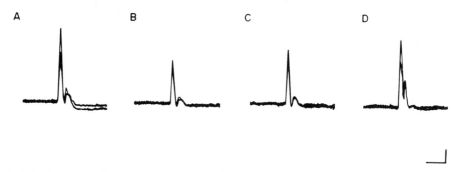

Fig. 5 A–D. Averaged records (16 sweeps) of nigral-potentiated monosynaptic reflex (MSR) superimposed on the control MSR obtained by stimulation of the dorsal root L 6 and recording from the ventral root of the same segment. **A** Control, nigral-induced potentiation (stimulation of the substantia nigra 0.05 mA, 0.1 ms, pulse train 200 Hz–20 ms. Stimulation dorsal root 35 ms after substantia nigra). **B** 3 min after intravenous injection of CPZ (1 mg/kg) showing marked reduction in nigral effect. **C** 22 min later a partial recovery was apparent. **D** 55 min after CPZ almost complete recovery. Calibration 0.5 mV, 2 ms (From YORK, 1973 b)

mostly a depression of the neuron activity which could not be abolished by intravenous or microionophoretic administration of phenoxybenzamine, phentolamine or propranolol (ENGBERG and RYALL, 1965, 1966; BISCOE et al., 1966), nor by picrotoxin or strychnine (BISCOE and CURTIS, 1966; PHILLIS et al., 1968), although strychnine antagonized the depressant effect of NA on cortical neurons (PHILLIS and YORK, 1967). NA hyperpolarized the membrane of the motoneurons and, in contrast to inhibitory amino acids such as GABA, increased the membrane resistance and reduced the membrane conductance (PHILLIS et al., 1968; ENGBERG and MARSHALL, 1971, 1973; ENGBERG and THALLER, 1970). Similar observations have been made in cerebellar Purkinje cells (Fig. 14). The membrane hyperpolarization produced by NA was proportional to the membrane potential immediately before the ejection of the amine and reversed to depolarization at a membrane potential of about − 20 mV, indicating an essential difference in the mode of action betwen NA and other central inhibitory transmitter substances (ENGBERG and MARSHALL, 1971, 1973; SIGGINS et al., 1971b; ENGBERG and THALLER, 1970; ENGBERG et al., 1974). 5 HT as well as DA produced effects identical with those of NA. The apparent lack of specificity of the amines might be ascribed to a liberation of NA from presynaptic terminals (ENGBERG et al., 1974). In some cases, the effects were antagonized by adrenergic α- and β-receptor blocking agents and by CPZ and haloperidol. Difficulties were encountered when it was tried to assess the antagonistic effects, because also the blocking agents hyperpolarized the neuronal membrane (ENGBERG et al., 1974). Some investigators observed not only inhibition but also excitation of interneurons, especially of Renshaw cells, during microionophoretic administration of NA (KOLMODIN and SKOGLUND, 1954; WEIGHT and SALMOIRAGHI, 1965, 1966 a, b, 1967).

C. Presence of Monoamines in the Brain Stem

The brain stem is relatively rich in NA and 5 HT (VOGT, 1954; BOGDANSKI et al., 1957; BERTLER and ROSENGREN, 1959; SANO et al., 1959; CARLSON et al., 1962; McGEER et al., 1963; GLOWINSKI and IVERSEN, 1966; HILLARP et al., 1966). Part of the NA and 5 HT is present in cell bodies whose axons either descend to spinal cord neurons or ascend to other brain areas, such as the tuberculum olfactorium, nucleus accumbens, limbic forebrain, neocortex and hypothalamus (ANDÉN et al., 1965 b, c; DAHLSTRÖM and FUXE, 1965 b; ANDÉN et al., 1966 b, c; UNGERSTEDT, 1971 a). The role of 5 HT-containing neurons in the brain stem, particularly in the raphé nuclei, and the spinal cord in nociception has been reviewed by MAYER and PRICE (1976) and MESSING and LYTLE (1977). For distribution of DA neurons see Chap. D, E and F.

I. Arousal

Systemic administration of catecholamines activated or inhibited neurons in the reticular formation (BONVALLET et al., 1956; BRADLEY and MOLLICA 1958) and produced a pattern of arousal in the electrocorticogram (BONVALLET et al., 1954; BRADLEY, 1960; DELL, 1961) which was abolished by destroying the mesencephalic reticular formation (BONVALLET et al., 1954; ROTHBALLER, 1956). It has been questioned whether the effects produced by A or NA were due to a direct action on the reticular neurons, because arousal following from an injection into the cerebral circulation was not observed until the amines had recirculated and increased the blood pressure (LONGO and SILVESTRINI, 1957; CAPON, 1960; MANTEGAZZINI et al., 1959). On the other hand, microinjections of NA (CORDEAU et al., 1963) and amphetamine (BRADLEY and ELKES, 1957) into the brain stem of unrestrained animals produced an arousal. A similar result was obtained by YAMAGUCHI et al. (1964) with A, but not with amphetamine. In a recent investigation (KEY, 1975) NA and A administered with a push-pull cannula to the pontine and mesencephalic reticular formation were found to produce desynchronization in the electrocorticogram of the *encéphale isolé* preparation; high concentrations of catecholamines elicited a secondary "sedative" effect.

NA administered by microionophoresis to brain stem neurons of unanesthetized decerebrate cats produced excitation or inhibition; A and DA exerted an effect less frequently, but when they did, it was in the same direction as after NA (BRADLEY and WOLSTENCROFT, 1962, 1965; BRADLEY et al., 1966). The effects of NA could not be blocked by microionophoretic administration of dibenamine or dihydroergotamine (BRADLEY and WOLSTENCROFT, 1965). Systemic administration of CPZ inhibited single brain stem neurons exhibiting convergence of activation by peripheral stimuli (Fig. 6), and inhibition was also produced by local application of CPZ with the "microtap" technique (AVANZINO et al., 1966). When CPZ was administered by microionophoresis, it produced inhibition of neurons inhibited by NA and antagonized the excitation caused by NA and 5 HT (BRADLEY et al., 1966).

The tranquillization produced in animals by reserpine (BEIN, 1953; SCHNEIDER, 1954 a, 1955; SCHNEIDER and EARL, 1954) and CPZ (DASGUPTA et al., 1954; BRADLEY and HANCE, 1957) has been ascribed rather to an inhibition of the activation of the brain stem reticular formation by afferent impulse than to a direct depressant effect exerted on the reticular neurons. CPZ as well as other phenothiazine derivatives, inhibited the arousal response in the electrocorticogram. They diminished the spontaneous activity in the reticular formation of the brain stem and its sensitivity to sensory and nociceptive inputs, and blocked its activation by A, the major effect being exerted on the rostral, ascending diffuse projecting system (HIEBEL et al., 1954; LONGO

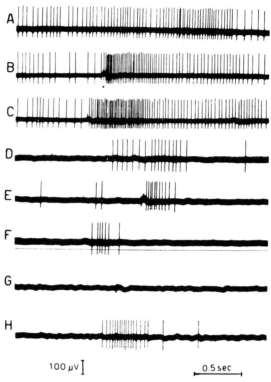

Fig. 6 A–H. The effect of CPZ on the activity of a unit in the mesencephalic reticular formation.
A Normal spontaneous discharge. **B** Response to tapping the right anterior leg. **C** Response
to trigeminal stimulation (rubbing the nose). **D** Spontaneous activity after CPZ (2 mg/kg) had
been injected. **E** Tapping of the right anterior leg. **F** Trigeminal stimulation. **G** Following the
injection of thiopental (5 mg/kg) showing complete inhibition of the activity of the unit. **H** Recovery 30 min later. (From BRADLEY, 1957)

et al., 1954; KILLAM et al., 1957; BRADLEY and KEY, 1958; MARTIN et al., 1958). The
thresholds of electrocortical arousal in the neocortex to electrical stimulation of the
reticular formation or peripheral nerves was raised less by CPZ than those for the
arousal in the limbic cortex (KILLAM and KILLAM, 1956). The arousing effect of DL-amphetamine in unrestrained rabbits was abolished by CPZ and phenoxybenzamine,
partially inhibited by dibenamine, and not changed by phentolamine, azapetine and
dihydroergotamine; dichlorisoprenaline had itself a stimulant effect which was blocked
by phenoxybenzamine and which potentiated the arousing effect of DL-amphetamine
(MUNOZ and GOLDSTEIN, 1960). Reserpine, however, was ineffective on the arousal
response evoked from the brain stem reticular formation (KILLAM and KILLAM, 1956;
KILLAM et al., 1957). It depressed spontaneous and evoked activity in thalamic nuclei
and the sensorimotor cortex (GANGLOFF and MONNIER, 1955) and elicited seizure activity in the hippocampus and amygdala (GANGLOFF and MONNIER, 1955; KILLAM and
KILLAM, 1956; KILLAM et al., 1957). PRESTON (1956 a, b) did not observe an effect of
CPZ on cortical arousal evoked by stimulation of the brain stem reticular formation
but found that it produced seizure activity in the amygdala. This seizure activity might

result from a block of monoamine receptors at neurons in the limbic system, because NA, DA and 5HT applied by microionophoresis to hippocampal cells and relay nuclei neurones depressed spontaneous, amino acid-induced and synaptical activity (STEFANIS, 1964; HERZ and GOGOLÁK, 1965; HERZ and NACIMIENTO, 1965; BISCOE and STRAUGHAN, 1966).

A or NA injected into the carotid arteries, under the dura or into the brain, intracisternally or into the ventricles produced sleep, analgesia, and general anesthesia (BASS 1914; IVY et al., 1944; LEIMDORFER, 1948, 1950; LEIMDORFER and METZNER, 1949; FELDBERG and SHERWOOD, 1954). These observations are obviously contrary to the finding that NA administered locally by cannulae placed stereotaxically into the mesencephalic reticular formation elicited alertness (HERNÁNDEZ-PEÓN, 1963), or that amphetamine or metamphetamine exert an analeptic action. Moreover, they are not easily to be reconciled with the findings that CPZ injected intraventricularly also causes general anesthesia (CATHALA and POCIDALO, 1952) and that CPZ and reserpine potentiate the effects of analgesic agents, barbiturates, and ethanol (LABORIT and HUGUENARD, 1951; COURVOISIER et al., 1953; BRODIE et al., 1955; SHORE et al., 1955). Very likely, the potentiation is due to a depression of the neuronal activity in the systems which are involved in the arousal produced by peripheral stimuli and/or facilitate the perception of these stimuli.

II. Analgesia and Nociceptive Reflexes

Starting from the observation that pretreatment with reserpine diminished or abolished the antinociceptive effect of morphine (SCHNEIDER, 1954b; SCHAUMANN, 1958; SIGG et al., 1958), numerous attempts have been made to correlate the content of monoamines in the brain with analgesia and with the effect of analgesic agents (for a survey of the literature see CLOUET, 1971; KOSTERLITZ et al., 1972; PEPEU, 1976). Recently, it has been found that the DA agonists apomorphine and amantadine or Dopa reduce the antinociceptive effect of morphine, and that DA antagonists such as perphenazine, spiroperidol, pimozide, or haloperidol enhance it (VAN DER WENDE and SPOERLEIN, 1973; MCGILLIARD and TAKEMORI, 1979). This agrees with the original observation of a potentiating effect of antipsychotic drugs on morphine analgesia (LABORIT and HUGUENARD, 1951; COURVOISIER et al., 1953; BRODIE et al., 1955; SHORE et al., 1955). Obviously, the effect of morphine and related agents on spinal reflexes including nociceptive reflexes depends on central monoamines, since spinal reflex activity is regulated by central monoaminergic activities (GROSSMAN et al., 1973). There seems also to be little doubt that monoamines, particularly 5HT, are involved in pain processing (for literature see NATHAN, 1977).

Nociceptive reflex activity such as that manifesting itself in the tail-flick response to noxious heat is depressed by morphine at the spinal level without the participation of monoamines (IRWIN et al., 1951; JURNA, 1972; GROSSMANN et al., 1973; YAKSH and RUDY, 1976, 1977). This spinal antinociceptive effect of morphine may be ascribed to a depression of repetitive activation of motoneurons (JURNA et al., 1973; ZIEGLGÄNSBERGER and SATOH, 1975; ZIEGLGÄNSBERGER and BAYERL, 1976) and is subject to monoaminergic and nonmonoaminergic control from supraspinal centers. It is hazardous, however, to deduce a change in the analgesic effect of morphine in its proper sense from a change in the effect of morphine on a nociceptive reflex. In rats with prenigral decerebration, in which morphine failed to exert an antinociceptive effect on the tail-flick response (JURNA et al., 1978), morphine depressed the activity in ascending axons of the spinal cord evoked by stimulation of nociceptive afferent C fibers (JURNA, unpublished results); this ascending activity would certainly have been perceived as painful by man, and its depression is therefore a true analgesic effect. Moreover, it must be borne in mind that an antinociceptive effect, i.e., depression of nociceptive reflex activity, may easily be mistaken for an analgesic one. Reserpine inhibited nociceptive reflex activity in intact rats as did morphine (GROSSMANN et al., 1973; HEINZ and JURNA, 1979) but it increased rather than reduced the sensation of pain in patients suffering from chronic pain (STERNBACH et al., 1976). Likewise, clonidine was found to increase the thresholds of vocalization to noxious stimulation in rats, and this effect was enhanced by reserpine, CPZ, or phenoxybenzamine (PAALZOW and PAALZOW, 1976), but reports on an analgesic effect of clonidine determined in man are still missing.

Neuroleptic agents very much resemble morphine and opioid analgesic agents in depressing nociceptive reflex activity from the nigrostriatal system. The caudate nucleus of the rat is particularly rich in opiate receptors (PERT and SNYDER, 1973; LEE et al., 1975; PERT et al., 1975; ATWEH and KUHAR, 1977) and contains a considerable number of encephalinergic neurons (HONG et al., 1977). Opiate receptors and neuroleptic receptors were found enriched in the microsomal fraction prepared from the rat striatum (LEYSEN and LADURON, 1972). Bilateral microinjections of morphine or haloperidol into the caudate nucleus depressed nociceptive reflex activity; this antinociceptive effect was reduced by systemic administration of naloxone or apomorphine (JURNA and HEINZ, 1979). Systemic administration of morphine or haloperidol increased the spontaneous activity of nigral neurons, whilst Dopa or apomorphine decreased the spontaneous activity of nigral neurons and reduced the effects of morphine and haloperidol (IWATSUBO and CLOUET, 1977). LEE et al. (1977) also found an increase in spontaneous activity of nigral neurons after systemic administration of morphine and, at the same time, predominantly a depression of caudate neuron activity (see also DAFNY et al., 1979) which could be prevented by haloperidol or pimozide. Increasing the activity of nigral neurons by electrical stimulation depressed the tail-flick response to noxious heat (JURNA et al., 1978). The effect of morphine on the nigroneostriatal system may be attributed to either an interference of morphine with dopaminergic impulse transmission in the striatum (KUSCHINSKY and HORNYKIEWICZ, 1972) or stimulation of nigral neurons (LEE et al., 1977). Microinjection of morphine into the substantia nigra, which is rich in opiate receptors (POLLARD et al., 1978), blocked the haloperidol-induced activation of striatal tyrosine hydroxylase (GALE et al., 1979, see also Chapter 8 Sect. B). The activity of DA-sensitive adenylate cyclase, which is closely related to the DA receptor (see Chap. 11), was increased by morphine as well as by haloperidol (IWATSUBO and CLOUET, 1975). Since DA-stimulated activity of the adenylate cyclase was inhibited by haloperidol but not by morphine (IWATSUBO and Clouet, 1975), it is assumed that morphine does not act on the DA receptor, as do the neuroleptic agents, but blocks DA-mediated impulse transmission in some other way. This would explain why CPZ but not morphine blocked apomorphine-induced stereotyped behavior in rats (MCKENZIE and SADOF, 1974). It is also worth noting in this context that naloxone abolished locomotor activity and circling behavior evoked by D-amphetamine (DETTMAR et al., 1978). By contrast, it was postulated that morphine and β-endorphine facilitate DA-containing neurons in the substantia nigra, as they produce circling to the opposite side following unilateral intranigral injection, and sniffing and gnawing after bilateral injection which were antagonized by naloxone (IWAMOTO and WAY, 1977). It would fit into the picture that morphine inhibited in a dose-dependent way spontaneous and evoked release of ACh in the caudate nucleus (YAKSH and YAMAMURA, 1977). Opiate receptors, endogenous opioids, and opiates in the nigroneostriatal system are obviously involved in motor behavior and the control of spinal motor activity including nociceptive reflexes. Very probably they also play a role in normal and disturbed psychic functions. It is doubtful, however, that they participate in the process of pain perception.

III. Seizure Activity

The intensity of convulsions resulting from the administration of nikethamide or nicotine is reduced by CPZ (COURVOISIER et al., 1953) and the incidence of insulin-induced seizures reduced (RYALL, 1956). Convulsions evoked by tryptamine and 5 HTP were depressed by CPZ, prochlorperazine, and trifluoperazine (TEDESCHI et al., 1959). Audiogenic seizures in mice and rats appeared to depend on monoaminergic activity in the brain; reserpine increased the incidence and severity of the seizures, whilst Dopa D-amphetamine and apomorphine reduced them (LEHMAN, 1964, 1967; BOGGAN and SEIDEN, 1971; ANLEZARK and MELDRUM, 1975). Pretreatment with haloperidol blocked the effect against seizure activity of apomorphine and ergot alkaloids considered to act as DA agonists (ANLEZARK et al., 1976). Reserpine lowered the threshold of seizures induced by electrical stimulation and by an injection of penetrazol or caffeine (CHEN and ENSOR, 1954; CHEN et al., 1954; JENNEY, 1954; DE SCHAPDRYVER et al., 1962) and, like CPZ, promoted grand mal seizures in man (KINROSS-WRIGHT, 1955). Electroseizures increased the turnover of NA in the brain and spinal cord (KETY et al., 1967). The facilitation by reserpine of seizure activity was abolished by metamphetamine (KOBINGER, 1958; DE SCHAPDRYVER et al., 1962), by Dopa and by antiparkinsonism drugs with cholinolytic properties (JURNA and REGÉLHY, 1968). The findings pointed to a disturbance by reserpine of an interaction between monoaminergic and cholinergic impulse transmission in the brain similar to that made responsible for the motor syndrome in Parkinson's disease (BARBEAU, 1962). However, inhibition by αMT of tyrosine hydroxylase had no effect on the electroseizure threshold, whilst inhibition by diethyldithiocarbamate (DTC) of DA-β-hydroxylase elevated the seizure threshold and antagonized the effect of Dopa, which also was an increase in the threshold (JURNA and REGÉLHY, 1968); moreover, metamphetamine, atropine, and biperiden in doses antagonizing the effect of reserpine lowered the threshold when given alone, and metamphetamine lost its effect either on repeated administration or after pretreatment with αMT. It is conceivable that the facilitation by reserpine of seizure activity was due to an effect on more than one monoaminergic system in the brain. Reserpine induced seizure activity in parts of the limbic system (GANGLOFF and MONNIER, 1955; KILLAM and KILLAM, 1956; KILLAM et al., 1957). Electrical stimulation within the amygdala produce "sham rage" in unrestrained cats (HILTON and ZBROŻYNA, 1963) and a marked depletion of catecholamines in terminals of the forebrain, a less pronounced depletion in the lower brain stem, and no change in the terminals of the mesencephalon (FUXE and GUNNE, 1964). Recently, it has been observed that lowering by 6-OH-DA of the NA levels in the spinal cord facilitated and enhanced spinal convulsions; this was attributed to a reduction by NA depletion of descending tonic noradrenergic inhibition in the spinal cord (JOBE et al., 1978).

IV. Vomiting, Swallowing

Stimulation of the chemoreceptor trigger zone for vomiting in the area postrema of the medulla oblongata by apomorphine, morphine, ergot alkaloids, and cardiac glycosides evokes vomiting (BORISON, 1952, 1974; WANG and BORISON, 1952; BORISON and WANG, 1953; WANG and GLAVIANO, 1954; GAITONDÉ et al., 1965). Lesioning of the chemoreceptor trigger zone abolished apomorphine-induced vomiting (WANG and BORISON, 1952; SHARE et al., 1965) but did not preclude vomiting evoked by stimulation of the gastric mucosa by oral administration of copper sulfate (WANG and BORISON, 1952). Vomiting due to gastric stimulation evoked by oral copper sulfate did not occur after lesioning of the nucleus of the solitary tract, whose stimulation elicited vomiting (WANG, 1965). Apomorphine enhanced the activity of neurons in this nucleus not only on systemic but also on local administration to the area postrema, and the stimulant effect of apomorphine was blocked by CPZ or metoclopramide (TAKAORI et al., 1968, 1970). It appears that apomorphine acts on receptors in the chemoreceptor trigger zone which, in turn, activates a neuron population in the nucleus of the solitary tract constituting the emetic center. Connections exist between the chemoreceptor trigger zone and the emetic center (BORISON and BRIZZEE, 1951; MOREST, 1960, 1966).

There is an important difference in the emetic response of animals treated with CPZ and animals with their chemoreceptor trigger zone lesioned: systemic administration of cardiac glycosides or copper sulfate produced vomiting in animals treated with CPZ but not in the animals with lesioning of the trigger zone. Thus, the cardiac glycosides and copper sulfate must act on the emetic centers whilst apomorphine, morphine, and ergot alkaloids provoke vomiting by acting on DA receptors which can be blocked by CPZ (BRAND et al., 1954; GLAVIANO and WANG, 1955; FELLOWS and COOK, 1957). Also DA may produce vomiting when it is administered systemically (WANG, 1965), probably because it is able to penetrate, as do other drugs (WILSON and BRODIE, 1961; WILSON et al., 1962), the blood-brain barrier in the area postrema.

Reserpine, CPZ, a great number of butyrophenone derivatives including haloperidol, droperidol, and spiroperidol, and pimozide are protected against the vomiting induced by apomorphine, morphine, Dopa, and ergot alkaloids (BOYD et al., 1953; CASSELL and BOYD, 1953; COURVOISIER et al., 1953; MALHOTRA and SIDHU, 1956; JANSSEN, 1967; JANSSEN et al., 1965a, b; JANSSEN et al., 1968; LEE et al., 1979). The antiemetic effect of promazine was weaker, and that of prochlorperazine was stronger than the effect of CPZ, whilst promethazine was devoid of any antiemetic effect (BRAND et al., 1954; FELLOWS and COOK, 1957).

Phenothiazine derivatives have been divided by COURVOISIER et al. (1957) into two groups; one group comprises drugs with antiemetic and cataleptogenic effects and is used in the treatment of psychoses, the other is formed by derivatives with a sedative effect and is used in the treatment of neuroses. The cataleptogenic effect is paralleled by the protection against apomorphine-induced vomiting (JANSSEN et al., 1965a, b), which is considered an equivalent to the Parkinson syndrome in man. A mechanism of selective retention of haloperidol and pimozide was found in the chemoreceptor trigger zone, the caudate nucleus, the floor of the third ventricle and in the ventral part of the mesencephalon (JANSSEN et al., 1968).

It has recently been shown that spontaneous swallowing as well as swallowing evoked by reflex activation in the rat was enhanced by Dopa, DA, Apomorphine, and D-amphetamine (BIEGLER et al., 1977). This is paralleled by the observation made by UNGERSTEDT (1971c) in rats that lesioning of the nigrostriatal DA system produced adipsia and aphagia along with hypoactivity and loss of exploratory behavior; adipsia was also produced by pimozide, a DA-receptor blocker (ANDÉN et al., 1970a), but followed from apomorphine, too.

D. Nigrostriatal System

I. DA as a Transmitter

The striatum (caudatum and putamen) contains DA in large amounts but very little NA (CARLSSON et al., 1958; BERTLER and ROSENGREN, 1959; CARLSSON, 1959; SANO et al., 1959). DA is present in nerve terminals which belong to cell bodies localized in the substantia nigra (mainly the zona compacta) and send their axons ipsilaterally to the striatum via the crus cerebri and the internal capsule (CARLSSON et al., 1962; ANDÉN et al., 1964a, 1965b, c; POIRIER and SOURKES, 1965; HILLARP et al., 1966; GOLDSTEIN et al., 1967; MOORE et al., 1971; MALER et al., 1973).

When perfusion was performed of the lateral ventricles labeled DA was released into the prefusion medium by adding D-amphetamine, amantadine, tyramine, or potassium ions to it (BESSON et al., 1971; VON VOIGTLANDER and MOORE, 1973a), and by electrical stimulation of the caudate nucleus (VON VOIGTLANDER and MOORE, 1971) or the substantia nigra (CHIUEH and MOORE, 1973). The release by D-amphetamine or amantadine of labeled DA was reduced not only after chronic but also after acute lesioning of the nigrostriatal pathway, which suggested that the releasing effect of the two drugs depended on an intact impulse flow in the pathway (VON VOIGTLANDER and MOORE, 1973a). Inhibition of the formation of labeled DA from [^{3}H]tyrosine by αMT abolished the releasing effect of amphetamine (CHIUEH and MOORE, 1974). When [^{3}H]tyrosine was administered to the substantia nigra with a push-pull cannula, labeled DA appeared in the perfusates of the substantia nigra and the caudate nucleus (NIEOULLON et al., 1977a). When the DA containing neurons in the substantia nigra were activated, DA was released not only from their terminals in the neostriatum but also from their cell bodies and dendrites (GROVES et al., 1975a, b; GEFFEN et al., 1976; KORF et al., 1976). This release of DA at the dendrites and cell bodies was interpreted in terms of a *self-* or *auto-inhibition* of the DA-containing neurons since microionophoretic administration of DA, apomorphine, and amphetamine to these neurons inhibited their activity (BUNNEY and AGHAJANIAN, 1973) and systemically administered CPZ and haloperidol blocked the inhibition (AGHAJANIAN and BUNNEY, 1973). The concept of self-inhibition offers an alternative to the nigrostriatal feedback system (Fig. 10) in the regulation of the activity of the nigral dopaminergic neurons (CARLSSON et al., 1972; AGHAJANIAN and BUNNEY, 1973; GROVES et al., 1975b; GEFFEN et al., 1976).

Blocking the sodium channels with TTX administered by a push-pull cannula to the caudate nucleus decreased the release of labeled DA, probably because the DA-containing terminals were made inactive. Similar administration of TTX to the substantia nigra resulted in a decreased release of DA collected from the substantia nigra (NIEOULLON et al., 1977a).

The dopaminergic pathway from the substantia nigra to the striatum appears to end at least in part on neurons containing ACh (LYNCH et al., 1972; BUTCHER and BUTCHER, 1974; McGEER et al., 1975). Dopa, D-amphetamine, metamphetamine, amantadine, and piribedil increased the ACh content in the rat striatum, while reserpine, CPZ, haloperidol, clozapine, or pimozide reduced it (SETHY and VAN WOERT, 1973, 1974a; McGEER et al., 1974b; GUYENET et al., 1975; LADINSKI et al., 1975) as well as 6-OH-DA-induced degeneration of the nigrostriatal DA pathway (AGID et al., 1975). Systemic administration of DA, apomorphine, and D-amphetamine increased the concentration of ACh in the striatum; reserpine, CPZ, haloperidol, pimozide, or clozapine reduced striatal ACh levels, and pretreatment with Dopa inhibited reserpine or CPZ to reduce the striatal concentration of ACh (SETHY and VAN WOERT, 1974a, b; GUYENET et al., 1975). Apomorphine or piribedil failed to increase the ACh content after treatment with pimozide (LADINSKY et al., 1975). As haloperidol and CPZ increased the synthesis of ACh in the rat striatum (TRABUCCHI et al., 1974), it must be assumed that DA-receptor blocking agents increase the turnover of ACh. When CPZ was administered with a push-pull cannula to caudate neurons, the amount of ACh released was increased, and this effect could be inhibited by apomorphine (STADLER et al., 1973). The turnover rate of labeled ACh in the striatum was decreased after the administration of Dopa, D-amphethamine, and apomorphine (TRABUCCHI et al., 1975). These results strongly support the view that dopaminergic neurons make synaptic contact with ACh-containing neurons, and that DA acts as an inhibitory transmitter on the cholinergic neurons. Systemic administration of physostigmine inhibited the circling movements evoked by unilateral 6-OH-DA-induced lesioning of the nigrostriatal DA path, whereas scopolamine enhanced it (MARSDEN et al., 1975). Since physostigmine reduced the contrariwise circling resulting from low doses of apomorphine but not that produced by high doses of apomorphine, and as scopolamine-induced circling was abolished by haloperidol or αMT, it has been suggested that scopolamine acted only on the side with an intact nigrostriatal pathway.

In early investigations performed with the microelectrode technique in unanesthetized cats, microionophoretic administration of DA to neurons in the caudate nucleus was found to depress the spontaneous activity as well as the activity evoked by microionophoretically administered excitant amino acids (e.g., glutamic acid) or by electrical stimulation of thalamic nuclei in most of the neurons tested (BLOOM et al., 1965; HERZ and ZIEGLGÄNSBERGER, 1966, 1968). The depression by DA of spontaneous activity or of the excitation produced by amino acids or stimulation of the substantia nigra could be prevented by previous microionophoretic administration of phenoxybenzamine and not by dichlorisoprenaline; the excitation evoked by nigral stimulation was not influenced by phenoxybenzamine (McLENNAN and YORK, 1967). A good correlation existed between the inhibition of caudate neurons produced by DA and that exerted by electrical stimulation of the substantia nigra in the anesthetized rat (GONZALEZ-VEGAS, 1974). However, results obtained with substances administered microionophoretically to caudate neurons in anesthetized animals must be judged carefully, because the responses appear to depend considerably on the stage of anesthesia (BLOOM et al., 1964).

Stimulation of the substantia nigra produced not only inhibition but also excitation of caudate neurons. In the experiments of CONNOR (1968, 1970) performed on unanesthetized cats, a greater number of caudate neurons was inhibited than facilitated, and neurons inhibited by nigral stimulation were also inhibited by microionophoretic administration of DA. YORK (1970) recorded from an about equal number of neurons excited or inhibited by nigral stimulation or microionophoretically administered DA; the excitatory effects were blocked by CPZ, phenoxybenzamine, and phentolamine. In lightly anesthetized monkeys, DA excited about half as many neurons as were inhibited by it; CPZ administered by microionophoresis exerted an initial weak local anesthetic effect which was followed by a block of both the excitatory and inhibitory effects of DA (YORK, 1972a). Obviously, there are two types of caudate neurons exhibiting opposite reactions to stimulation of the substantia nigra: spontaneously active neurons were mostly depressed by the stimulation, the other type was silent and could be found only when excited by stimulation of the substantia nigra (FELTZ and ALBE-FESSARD, 1972). In anesthetized and unanesthetized cats, electrical stimulation of the substantia nigra and microionophoretic administration of DA depressed the spontaneous activity and the activity evoked by administration of excitant amino acids; however, even large amounts of DA, NA, or ACh released from the micropipettes had no effect on those caudate neurons which were excited by stimulation of the substantia nigra (FELTZ, 1969, 1970). In an identified population of caudate neurons excited monosynaptically from the substantia nigra (FELTZ and MACKENZIE, 1969; see also FRIGYESI and PURPURA, 1967, and KITAI et al., 1975), this synaptic activation was not influenced by microionophoretic administration of DA, NA, or 5HT, but the stimulant effect of amino acids on the neurons was depressed by the monoamines (FELTZ, 1971a). On microionophoretic administration to caudate neurons not affected by DA, haloperidol produced a longlasting blocking action which was explained by a local anesthetic effect of haloperidol (FELTZ, 1971b). When DA containing terminals in the cat caudate nucleus were selectively damaged by an injection of 6-OH-DA into the lateral ventricles, caudate neurons could still be activated monosynaptically by stimulation of the substantia nigra (FELTZ and DE CHAMPLAIN, 1972a). In cats having been treated with an injection of 6-OH-DA into the lateral ventricles, DA inhibited the effect of nigral stimulation in a small number of neurons only; it always blocked the activation of the neurons by amino acids in this preparation, while in cats not pretreated with 6-OH-DA the number of neurons in which the excitatory effect of amino acids was reduced or abolished was much higher (FELTZ and DE CHAMPLAIN, 1972b). Similar results as after pretreatment with 6-OH-DA were obtained after monoamine depletion caused by reserpine and αMT. Intracellular recordings made from caudate neurons of unanesthetized cats revealed that electrical stimulation of the substantia nigra produced excitation often followed by inhibition (HULL et al., 1970). On account of experiments with temporal and spatial combinations of stimuli, and taking into consideration anatomic data, it had been concluded that all input fibers to caudate neurons, including those from the substantia nigra, are excitatory, and that the caudate nucleus consists primarily of inhibitory interneurons which, when activated from

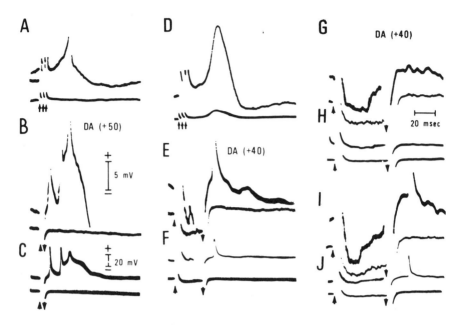

Fig. 7. A EPSP and an action potential triggered in a caudate neuron by substantia nigra stimulation (3 pulses, 400 Hz). **B** Depolarization and spikes produced by microionophoretic administration of DA with a current of 50 nA. Up-going and down-going arrows indicate the onset and offset of DA currents, respetively. **C** Comparable DC records. **D** Substantia nigra stimulation evoked EPSP and action potentials in another caudate neuron. Bottom trace: comparable DC record. **E** Depolarization and spike potential evoked by administration of DA with a current of 40 nA. **F** Comparable DC records. **G–I** Effects of DA on the same neuron with a longer duration of electrophoretic current. The traces of **I** and **J** were recorded 6 s after those of **G** and **H** during which some DA was ejected with the same current pulse every 2 s. **H** and **J** are comparable DC records. Calibrations: 5 mV for upper AC records, 20 mV for DC records; 20 ms. Upper traces: intracellular recordings. Bottom trace in **A–J** except **D**, extracellular controls. Cat, pentobarbital anesthesia. (From Kitai et al., 1976)

outside the nucleus, will inhibit neighboring neurons in the nucleus (Buchwald et al., 1973; Hull et al., 1973). Convincing evidence has recently been presented showing that microionophoretic administration of DA (Fig. 7) mimics the monosynaptic EPSPs evoked in caudate neurons by electrical stimulation of the substantia nigra or the dopaminergic pathway to the caudate nucleus (Kitai et al., 1976). The excitation is blocked by CPZ (Fig. 8). IPSPs built up in caudate neurons are secondary to activation of other caudate neurons. An excitatory effect of DA on caudate neurons has also been postulated by Cools (1971, 1973) on account of the changes in motor behavior produced in cats by microinjections of DA, procaine, and haloperidol into, and by electrical stimulation of the caudate nucleus. However, it seems that even though the DA-containing nigrostriatal pathway is excitatory the eventual result of its activation is inhibition of caudate (cholinergic) neurons, and an impairment of dopaminergic transmission by reserpine or DA receptor blocking agents will release these neurons. Discrepancies in results may also find a solution in the existence of two classes of DA receptors (see Chap. A).

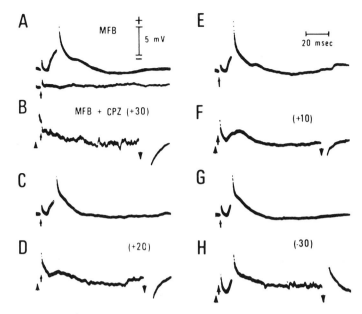

Fig. 8 A–H. Effect of CPZ on intracellularly recorded EPSPs and action potentials evoked in a caudate neuron by electric stimulation of the median forebrain bundle. **A** Control records; bottom trace, extracellular record. CPZ was administered with currents of 30 nA in **B,** 20 nA in **D** and 10 nA in **F. C, E,** and **G** control records in absence of CPZ. **H** CPZ ejection current was reversed to negative 30 nA. Calibrations: 5 mV and 20 ms. Cat, pentobarbital anesthesia. (From Kitai et al., 1976)

II. The Neuronal Feedback Loop and Self-Inhibition

Impairment of catecholamine-mediated impulse transmission by CPZ, haloperidol, or reserpine is associated with an increase in the amount of catecholamine metabolites in the brain (Carlsson and Lindqvist, 1963; Andén et al., 1964g). This is explained by a compensatory activation of monoaminergic neurons leading to an increased release of the transmitters from their terminals and consequently to an enhanced formation of metabolites. Since antipsychotic drugs also inhibit the reuptake of the transmitter into the presynaptic terminals, it is fully exposed to metabolization by catecholamine-O-methyltransferase, COMT (Janssen, 1967). Conversely, increased activation of the receptor should reduce transmitter synthesis. The results have since been confirmed, and the observations were extended to a greater number of neuroleptic agents (Gey and Pletscher, 1964; Juorio et al., 1966; Laverty and Sharman, 1965; da Prada and Pletscher, 1966 a, b; Sharman, 1966; O'Keeffe et al., 1970; Besson et al., 1971). Phenothiazine derivatives without a neuroleptic property (prothipendyl, promazine) were significantly less potent in stimulating catecholamine metabolism in the neostratium than the derivatives with a pronounced neuroleptic action (Roos, 1965). Reserpine inhibited the storage as well as the synthesis of DA in the striatum (Besson et al., 1971), and D-amphetamine decreased the latter (Laverty and Sharman, 1965; Besson et al., 1971). Inhibition of monoamine synthesis entailed loss of catecholamines and 5 HT in the brain and spinal cord, and this loss was reduced by clonidine; the effect of clonidine was abolished by phenoxybenzamine and haloperidol (ANDÉN et al., 1970b). CPZ, haloperidol, pimozide, and fluspirilen accelerated the disappearance of NA from the brain after inhibition of its synthesis; the loss in DA was accelerated by haloperidol and only slightly affected by CPZ (ANDÉN et al., 1972a; see also O'KEEFFE et al., 1970). On the other hand, CPZ increased the formation of DA but not of NA from labeled tyrosine (NYBÄCK et al., 1967, 1968; NY-BÄCK and SEDVALL, 1968). Contrary to this result, CORRODI et al. (1967) reported that an acute administration of CPZ and haloperidol accelerated exclusively the disappearance from the brain of NA; DA neurons were depleted but after repeated administration of both drugs.

In the absence of nervous impulse flow, i.e., after acute interruption of the dopaminergic nigrostriatal pathway, neuroleptic drugs such as CPZ, haloperidol, spiroperidol, and pimozide did not accelerate the DA depletion in the striatum (ANDÉN et al., 1971; NYBÄCK and SEDVALL, 1971). However, since apomorphine inhibited the accumulation of Dopa, and haloperidol counteracted the inhibition produced by apomorphine after interruption of the nigrostriatal pathway, it seemed that the stimulation of DA synthesis did not require an intact impulse flow but depended rather on a feedback between the postsynaptic receptors and the tyrosine hydroxylase in the presynaptic terminals (KEHR et al., 1972). This feedback is very likely operated via a presynaptic receptor (WALTERS and ROTH, 1974).

Reserpine, CPZ and haloperidol markedly enhanced, whereas clozapine only slightly increased tyrosine hydroxylase activity; apomorphine decreased the activity of the enzyme and piribedil, a DA agonist, was ineffective (LEONARD, 1977). Morphine as well as haloperidol enhanced tyrosine hydroxylase activity in the striatum as determined by the accumulation of DOPA, and naloxone abolished the effect of morphine (PERSSON, 1979). The decrease in the content of DA and NA in the brain after tyrosine hydroxylase inhibition is accelerated by haloperidol; pretreatment with anticholinergic drugs, such as atropine, hyoscine, or the antiparkinsonism agent trihexyphenidyl, markedly reduced the effect of haloperidol on the disappearance of DA but not of NA (ANDÉN and BÉDARD, 1971). This observation suggested that the anticholinergic drugs acted on a neuronal feedback loop consisting of at least two types of neuron, a dopaminergic and a cholinergic one. The finding that oxotremorine, a cholinergic agent, increased the metabolism of catecholamines in the brain (LAVERTY and SHARMAN, 1965) supports this view. However, the possibility of a feedback loop consisting of two neurons only, a nigroneostriatal and a strionigral one, has been excluded by results obtained when the interconnections between caudate and nigral neurons were studied. They clearly showed that there is no direct reciprocal relationship. Evidence exists (see below) that GABA containing neurons form part of the feedback loop and that GABA inhibits dopaminergic neurons in the nigra. Intranigral microinjections of GABA increased the DA concentration in the regions of dopaminergic terminals, i.e., in the striatum and in the olfactory tubercle, possibly because of a reduced activity of the dopaminergic neurons (KELLY and MOORE, 1978).

Direct evidence for the existence of a neuronal feedback system derives from electrophysiologic studies. Electrical stimulation of the substantia nigra produced antidromic activation of caudate neurons which indicated that there is a direct uninterrupted strionigral pathway (FRIGYESI and PURPURA, 1967; KITAI et al., 1975; see also SZABO, 1970, 1972). Electrical stimulation of various parts of the caudate nucleus evoked short and long latency EPSPs, long latency IPSPs, and delayed

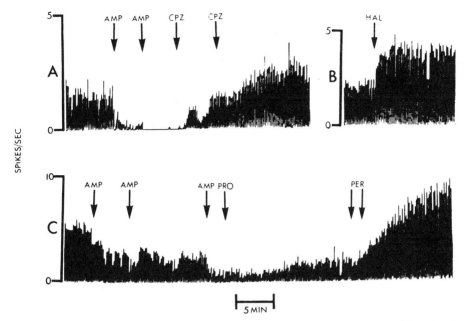

Fig. 9. A Antagonism by CPZ of D-amphetamine (AMP)-induced slowing of activity of a dopaminergic neuron in the substantia nigra of a nonanesthetized rat. D-Amphetamine given intravenously in an initial dose (0.25 mg/kg) significantly decreased firing rate. An additional 0.5 mg D-amphetamine/kg stopped the cell completely. After CPZ was administered intravenously (0.25 mg/kg initially followed by 0.5 mg/kg), cell firing resumed and increased to above basal rate. **B** Effect of haloperidol (HAL) on a dopaminergic cell in the nonanesthetized animal. Intravenous injection of haloperidol (0.04 mg/kg) increased basal activity 100%. **C** Effect of promethazine (PRO) on cell firing rate subsequent to D-amphetamine depression in an anesthetized animal. D-Amphetamine in these doses (0.25, 0.50, 0.50 mg/kg) markedly decreased unit activity. Promethazine (10 mg/kg intraperitoneally) failed to elicit the usual increase in rate induced by antipsychotic phenothiazines. The slow moderate increase in rate following promethazine was no greater than the spontaneous recovery from amphetamine seen with these cells. Perphenazine (PER; 0.2 mg/kg, total dose) produced a rapid increase in rate to above baseline levels. (From BUNNEY et al., 1973b)

EPSP-IPSP sequences (FRIGYESI and PURPURA, 1967, which suggested a complex pattern of innervation of the nigral neurons projecting to the caudate nucleus. From electronmicroscopic essays it appeared that there are at least four different types of synaptic bouton on the dendrites and somata of nigral neurons (GULLEY and SMITHBERG, 1971). Spontaneously active nigral neurons were inhibited by electrical stimulation in the caudate nucleus (YOSHIDA and PRECHT, 1971; McNAIR et al., 1972) and by microionophoretic application of GABA (OLPE and KOELLA, 1979). The inhibition is due to membrane hyperpolarization by true IPSPs which, despite their relatively long latency, were considered to be monosynaptic (YOSHIDA and PRECHT, 1971). Picrotoxin, a putative GABA antagonist, reduced the inhibition (PRECHT and YOSHIDA, 1971). Dopa, apomorphine, D-amphetamine, and piribedil depressed the activity of DA-containing neurons in the substantia nigra, haloperidol, and phenothiazine derivatives with a neuroleptic property (CPZ, thioridazine, perphenazine, fluphenazine, trifluperazine) increased it or blocked the depressant effect (Fig. 9; BUNNEY et al., 1973a,b; WALTERS et al., 1975). Lesions

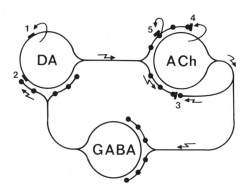

Fig. 10. Schematic presentation of different mechanisms by which the activity of DA containing neurons in the nigro-neostriatal feedback system may be inhibited. The hypothetical receptors are indicated by small bars. Direction of impulse propagation is indicated by flashes, and diffusion paths by arrows. *1* DA released from cell body acts on receptor on cell body and mediates self-inhibition. *2* GABA released from terminals of strio-nigral axon acts on receptor on cell body and produces inhibition (neuronal negative feedback). *3* ACh-containing neuron acts on terminals of DA-containing neuron via axo-axonal synapses. *4* ACh-containing neuron acts on terminals of DA-containing neuron by diffusion of a chemical compound across the synaptic cleft. *5* DA released from terminals acts on receptors on DA-containing terminals. (Modified from Andén, 1974)

placed in the nigrostriatal pathway markedly attenuated the depressant effect of δ-amphetamine (Bunney and Aghajanian, 1976). From these results it might be inferred that the dopaminergic nigrostriatal neurons from part of a negative feedback loop: enhanced dopaminergic activity increases the inhibition of the DA-containing neurons, and diminished inhibition of the DA-containing neurons will result from decreased dopaminergic activity. The composition of the feedback loop is still far from being fully understood, but there is much evidence that GABA-containing neurons form part of the strionigral pathway (Kim et al., 1971; McGeer et al, 1973; Okada and Hassler, 1973; McGeer et al., 1974a, b; Fonnum et al., 1974). Direct evidence for the role of GABA-containing neurons in the feedback loop has been provided by the observation that electrical stimulation of the caudate nucleus as well as microionophoretic administration of GABA depressed the activity of nigral neurons, and that picrotoxin could antagonize the inhibitory effects (Crossman et al., 1973, 1974; Feltz, 1971 c). Thus, the minimum number of neurons forming the feedback loop would be three (Fig. 10): the *nigrostriatal DA-containing neuron*, acting on the *intracaudate ACh-containing neuron*, which acts on the *strionigral GABA-containing neuron*, acting on the nigrostriatal DA-containing neuron).

Most probably, the feedback loop does not operate on such a simple circuitry. Otherwise it would be difficult to explain why drugs enhancing DA-mediated impulse transmission to ACh-containing neurons reduced the ACh content in, and enhanced the release of ACh from the striatum (see Chap. D Sect. I.). An interesting alternative or complement of the negative feedback loop is the self-inhibition of the nigral DA-containing neurons (Fig. 10). The observation that haloperiodol accelerated the release of GABA in the substantia nigra (Kim and Hassler, 1975) is not compatible with the hypothesis of a negative feedback: under the influence of haloperidol an excitation from DA-containing neurons of ACh-containing neurons should be reduced. The ACh-containing neurons should, therefore, produce less excitation of the GABA-containing neurons which, in turn, released less GABA. However, if it is assumed that the DA-containing neurons limit their firing rate by DA released from their cell bodies and dendrites and acting on receptors located on the cell bodies and dendrites (GROVES et al., 1975; GEFFEN et al., 1976), the effect of haloperidol should be as if the drug acted on a positive feedback system: haloperidol, by abolishing the DA-induced self-inhibition, would render the dopaminergic neurons more active, and more GABA would finally be released. The receptors acted upon by DA and DA agonists (e.g., apomorphine) and blocked by neuroleptic drugs have recently been termed dopamine "autoreceptors" by AGHAJANIAN and BUNNEY (1977); they are clearly distinct from the classical adrenergic α- and β-receptors, because neither clonidine and isoprenaline, nor adrenergic α- and β-receptor blocking agents were found to influence the activity of the neurons on microionophoretic administration.

There is also convincing evidence for ACh being a transmitter in the substantia nigra, as ACh occurs in the substantia nigra (JACOBOWITZ and GOLDBERG, 1971) together with choline acetylase (FONNUM et al., 1974) and ACh-esterase (BUTCHER et al., 1975). Blockade of ACh receptors in the substantia nigra increased, and stimulation of the receptors reduced the release of DA in the ipsilateral striatum (BARTHOLINI and PLETSCHER, 1971; JAVOY et al., 1974). Unilateral microinjection of hemicholinium (which lowers the concentration of ACh in cholinergic neurons) into the substantia nigra reduced the DA concentration and increased the homovanillic acid concentration in the ipsilateral striatum; unilateral intranigral carbachol injection produced opposite effects, the increase in the concentration of DA and the decrease in the concentration of homovanillic acid being abolished by simultaneous administration of α-flupenthixol (JAMES and MASSEY, 1978). These results were explained by an inhibition of activity in the nigrostriatal path, ACh exerting its effect probably by way of an inhibitory (dopaminergic) interneuron.

Moreover, there is evidence that GABA is involved in the regulation of the activity of caudate neurons. Microionophoretically applied GABA depressed the firing of caudate neurons (HERZ and VON FREYTAG-LORINGHOVEN, 1968), and the spontaneous release of DA collected from the caudate nucleus with the push-pull technique was enhanced by the GABA antagonists picrotoxin or bicuculline (BARTHOLINI and STADLER, 1977).

Recent studies which also involved neuroleptic agents revealed that the two nigrostriatal paths can be made to operate in a reciprocal fashion (NIEOULLON et al., 1977 b, c; NIEOULLON et al., 1979).

III. Spinal Motor Activity

The nigrostriatal feedback loop controls motor behavior. Bilateral impairment of dopaminergic as well as enhancement of cholinergic impulse transmission in the nigrostriatal system produced by microinjection of drugs into parts of the system results in catalepsy (COSTALL and OLLEY, 1971 a, b; COSTALL et al., 1972). Unilateral change in dopaminergic impulse transmission produced circling movements of the animals, the animals circled to the side of reduced transmission (UNGERSTEDT et al., 1973; UN-

Gerstedt and Pycock, 1974). After intrastriatal microinjection of 6-OH-DA or CPZ to rats the animals turned to the side of injection, whereas an injection of DA or apomorphine made the animals turn to the opposite side (Ungerstedt, 1968; Ungerstedt et al., 1969; von Voigtlander and Moore, 1973 b; for "paradoxical" rotation see Ungerstedt et al., 1973). However, it is unclear why after unilateral intranigral microinjection of GABA, which is assumed to act on the DA containing neurons as an inhibitory transmitter released from stroinigral neurons (see Chap. D, Sect. II) rats circled away from the side of injection (Kelly and Moore, 1978). When the dopaminergic nigrostriatal path had been interrupted, systemic administration of reserpine, CPZ, or haloperidol produced circling of the animals to the unoperated side (Andén et al., 1966a), i.e., the animals behaved as if not operated on and as if the drugs had been injected into the neostriatum of one (the intact) side.

Circling evoked in mice with unilateral 6-OH-DA-induced nigrostriatal lesions by systemic administration of apomorphine or D-amphetamine was inhibited in a dose-dependent manner by haloperidol, pimozide, CPZ, metoclopramide, and clozapine (listed in descending rank of potency), but not by phenoxybenzamine (Pycock et al., 1975). Likewise, the circling produced by D-amphetamine was inhibited by α-flupenthixol and α-clopenthixol, but not by their β-isomers; CPZ and pimozide also inhibited the circling, but not thioridazine or clozapine (Kelly and Miller, 1975).

In rats with unilateral lesion of the DA-containing nigrostriatal pathway, systemic administration of ergocornine and bromocriptine produced circling movements of longer duration than those resulting from apomorphine; the circling was blocked by pimozide (Corrodi et al., 1973). In a detailed analysis, the activity of bromocriptine was compared with that of apomorphine, D-amphetamine, and Dopa (Johnson et al., 1976): bromocriptine induced stereotypies (licking and sniffing); it made rats rotate to the side contralateral to the lesioning of the nigrostriatal DA pathway; it abolished reserpine-induced catalepsy; it stimulated locomotor activity after initially having depressed it; it was inhibited in its effects by pretreatment with pimozide, reserpine, or αMT. Because of its DA-receptor stimulant effect, bromcriptine has rather successfully ben employed in the Parkinson model of the monkey and in patients with parkinsonism (Calne, 1976; Goldstein et al., 1978)

Ipsilateral circling movements were evoked not only by unilateral injection of haloperidol into the striatum, but also by unilateral injections made into the globus pallidus or the substantia nigra (Costall et al., 1972). Atropine or the DA agonists, apomorphine, δ- or λ-amphetamine, amantadine, and relatively large amounts of DA made the animals turn to the side opposite to the microinjection in the neostriatum or globus pallidus; pretreatment with haloperidol enhanced the sensitivity of caudate tissue to DA, and lesioning of the substantia nigra abolished the effect of DA (Costall et al., 1972; Costall and Naylor, 1974 a). Microinjection of DA, NA, apomorphine, or 3-methoxytyramine into one caudate nucleus of the cat evoked a pattern of motor responses which was similar to the one produced by electrical stimulation of the area into which the drugs were injected; the effects were inhibited by locally administered haloperidol or procaine (Cools, 1971, 1973). Since DA and procaine exerted opposite effects when injected into the same part of the caudate nucleus, it has been proposed that DA produced excitation (Cools, 1971). DA-induced contralateral head-turning was selectively mimicked by apomorphine and inhibited by haloperidol; DA-induced ipsilateral head-turning was mimicked by 3,4-dihydroxyphenylamino-2-

imidazoline and inhibited by ergometrine, piribedil, and NA (COOLS et al., 1976). In principle, the results agreed with those obtained in DA-sensitive neurons of the snail, *Helix aspersa,* (STRUYKER BOUDIER et al., 1974): the first type of response was ascribed to an action on DA receptors mediating excitation, the second type to an action on DA receptors mediating inhibition.

Unilateral microinjection of hemicholinium into the substantia nigra of rats produced circling to the side opposite of the injection, and this circling was abolished by haloperidol; an identical injection of carbachol produced ipsilateral circling which was abolished by α-flupenthixol but not by β-flupenthixol, showing that the antagonism was stereospecific (JAMES and MASSEY, 1978). These results were explained by an indirect inhibitory effect exerted by ACh in the substantia nigra via dopaminergic neurones acting on the nigrostriatal path (JAMES and MASSEY, 1978).

Soon after the initiation of reserpine and phenothiazine derivatives into antipsychotic therapy, reports appeared dealing with a Parkinsonlike syndrome caused by these drugs (WEBER, 1954; FLACH, 1955; KINROSS-WRIGHT, 1955; KLINE and STANLEY, 1955; LAUNAY and DESPATURE, 1956; SIGWALD et al., 1959). In animals, these drugs produced catalepsy which has been characterized by loss of motor initiative and fixation combined with an active maintenance of abnormal attitudes (BARUK et al., 1957; BEAULNES and VIENS, 1961). This catalepsy was considered as an equivalent in animals of the Parkinson syndrome in man and suitable to test drugs on their prospective effectiveness in Parkinson's disease (MORPURGO, 1962). However, rigidity, tremor, and akinesia appeared also in animals after the administration of reserpine or CPZ (WINDLE et al., 1956; KAELBER and JOYNT, 1956; WINDLE and CAMMERMEYER, 1958; GLOW, 1959; STEG, 1964).

The rigidity produced in rats by either depleting central monoamines with reserpine, tetrabenazine, or αMT or by blocking central catecholamine receptors with CPZ, haloperidol, or phenoxybenzamine is due to tonic hyperactivity of the α motoneurons supplying the skeletal muscle fibers, while the activity of the γ motoneurons controlling the tone of the intrafusal muscle fibers and thus the sensitivity of the muscle spindles is simultaneously depressed (Fig. 11; STEG, 1964; ROOS and STEG, 1964; ARVIDSSON et al., 1966; JURNA et al., 1969, 1972b). The motor disturbance following administration of drugs inhibiting central monoaminergic impulse transmission must result from an action of the drugs on the nigrostriatal system, because identical changes in spinal motor activity were obtained by lesioning the substantia nigra by electrocoagulation or microinjection of 6-OH-DA (JURNA et al., 1972b). Since the rigidity produced by neuroleptic agents was always present when the γ-motor activity was depressed and persisted as well as the α-motor hyperactivity after deafferentation, i.e., cutting the dorsal roots, it has been classified as an α type of rigidity (STEG, 1966). It differs thus from the rigidity induced by intercollicular decerebration which is due to hyperactivity of the γ-motor system and is abolished by deafferentation (GRANIT, 1955). Moreover, rigidity based on hyperactivity of the α-motoneurons was evoked by drugs which enhance cholinergic impulse transmission, such as physostigmine and oxotremorine (ARVIDSSON et al., 1966; JURNA et al., 1970; JURNA, 1976b). This indicated that, as in the Parkinson syndrome (BARBEAU, 1962), Parkinsonlike motor symptoms produced in animals resulted from an imbalance between dopaminergic and cholinergic impulse transmission in the nigrostriatal system. These symptoms are due either to a reduced dopaminergic or to an increased cholin-

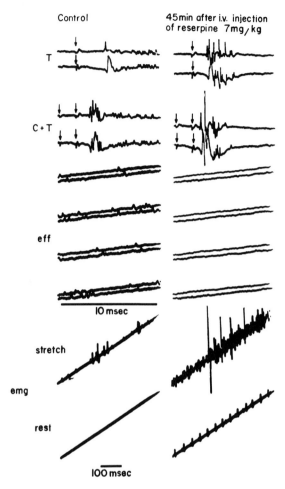

Fig. 11. The reflex and spontaneous activity of α- and γ-efferents recorded before and after injection of reserpine to a rat. The discharges of α- and γ-motoneurons were recorded from a filament isolated from a ventral root with two pairs of recording electrodes 9 mm apart, amplified and displayed on the upper and lower beam of a dual beam oscilloscope (upper and lower tracing in each pair of recordings). The action potentials are distinguished into α- and γ-fiber potentials by the difference in conduction velocity and spike amplitude. The reflex response shown in *T* (test stimulus) and *C + T* (conditioning and test stimulus) were evoked by electric stimulation of the corresponding dorsal root with single pulses supramaximal for α reflex discharges. Conditioning stimulation of the dorsal root to which the test stimulus was delivered facilitated the α-reflex discharge. Spontaneous activity *(eff)* shows only γ-discharges and the electromyogram *(emg)* recorded from the calf muscle phasis activity during quick stretch of the muscle. After reserpine, α reflex activity is markedly increased and γ-activity reduced, and tonic activity is present in the electromyogram during sustained muscle stretch and in the muscle at rest. (From STEG, 1964)

ergic activity, as was first proposed by STEG and co-workers (ARVIDSSON et al., 1966, 1967) and later supported by KLAWANS (1968) and other authors. Accordingly, drugs which enhance dopaminergic impulse transmission (i.e., Dopa, apomorphine, metamphetamine, and amantadine) or inhibit cholinergic transmission (i.e., atropine, biperiden, and trihexyphenidyl) abolished the motor disturbance following from cholinergic predominance in the nigroneostriatal system (STEG, 1964; ARVIDSSON et al., 1966; JURNA and LANZER, 1969; JURNA et al., 1969a, 1972b; JURNA, 1976a). Similarly, increased α and reduced γ-reflex activity following systemic administration of reserpine or bilateral intranigral microinjections of 6-OH-DA were abolished by bilateral intracaudate injection of DA or apomorphine (JURNA et al., 1978a).

In the untreated rat, the α-motoneurons discharge impulses to reflex activation with a long latency, that is polysynaptic activation prevails; after the administration of drugs producing rigidity, the reflex latency is shifted towards values corresponding with a monosynaptic activation (JURNA and LANZER, 1969; JURNA et al., 1969). An increase in the amplitude of monosynaptic mass reflexes was produced by CPZ or electrical stimulation of the globus pallidus in cats (STERN and WARD, 1962). Likewise, reserpine or lesioning of the substantia nigra increased monosynaptic reflex activity and simultaneously depressed polysynaptic reflexes in the rat (GROSSMANN et al., 1973).

Reserpine or physostigmine rigidity was abolished by bilateral ablation of the striata or by transecting the dorsolateral funiculi (ARVIDSSON et al., 1967); it remained unchanged after decortication, ablation of the cerebellum, destruction of the vestibular and red nuclei, and after pyramidectomy or cutting the dorsal funiculi which, in the rat, contain the pyramidal tract (KING, 1910; RANSON, 1913, 1914; LINOWIECKI, 1914). It seems that impairment of dopaminergic impulse transmission in the nigrostriatal feedback system set up an increased impulse barrage which reached the spinal motoneurons via the dorsolateral funiculi; because of the sustained descending facilitation, the α-motoneurons exhibited tonic impulse activity producing tonic contractions of the skeletal muscles and a monosynaptic response to reflex activation (JURNA and THERES, 1969). It has not yet been clarified whether the depression of the γ-motor activity is also due to the changes induced by neuroleptic drugs in the nigrostriatal system, or to the depressant action on the brain stem reticular formation responsible for the elimination of hyperactivity in the γ-motor system in intercollicularly decerebrate cats (HENATSCH and INGVAR, 1956). Mapping out the neuronal connections from the nigrostriatal system to the spinal motoneurons is required to directly correlate the biochemical and electrophysiologic data obtained with antipsychotic drugs within the feedback loop with the changes in motor activity and behavior induced by these substances. An outlet from the feedback loop might be formed by neurons in the substantia nigra which facilitated monosynaptic reflexes when electrically stimulated (YORK, 1972b). Moreover, unilateral electrical stimulation of the substantia nigra performed in unrestrained cats produced an "arrest" reaction with subsequent head-turning and circling movements to the side contralateral to the stimulation (YORK, 1973a). However, both the enhancement of monosynaptic reflex activity and the effects in motor behavior elicited by nigral stimulation were abolished by CPZ or haloperidol (YORK, 1973a, b). Moreover, bilateral microinjections of GABA, which is an inhibitory transmitter acting on nigral dopaminergic neurons (see Chap. D, Sect. II), or procaine produced an increase in α-reflex discharges but did not depress

γ-reflex discharges (JURNA et al., 1978a). This showed that the α- and the γ-motor system are not influenced by the nigroneostriatal system in a strictly reciprocal way. The blockade by procaine of nigral neurons and axons passing through the substantia nigra indicated also that there are outlets from the nigroneostriatal system to the spinal cord other than the substantia nigra.

Despite the obvious similarity of the biochemical causes of the rigidity in Parkinson's disease and drug-induced parkinsonism on one hand (cf. BARBEAU and SOURKES, 1961; HORNYKIEWICZ, 1966) and in animals treated with neuroleptic drugs on the other, it should be noted that it is still an open question whether Parkinson rigidity in man is maintained by the α- or the γ-motor system. The importance of an undisturbed balance between dopaminergic and cholinergic impulse transmission in the nigroneostriatal system for normal motor performance would sufficiently explain why the incidence of Parkinsonlike motor symptoms is much higher with neuroleptic drugs of little or no aticholinergic property (e.g., fluphenazine, flupenthixol, or spiroperidol) than with those exhibiting relatively strong anticholinergic activity (thioridazine, clozapine). Strong neuroleptic potency and marked extrapyramidal effects must not necessarily be combined in a drug. Clozapine is a potent neuroleptic agent with little risk to evoke extrapyramidal motor disturbance (BERZEWSKI et al., 1969; GROSS and LANGNER, 1966; DE MAIO, 1972), nor does it produce catalepsy in animals (STILLE and HIPPIUS, 1971; STILLE et al., 1971). The increase in α reflex activity and the depression in γ-reflex activity produced by reserpine 10 mg/kg in rats were abolished by systemic administration of clozapine 30 mg/kg (JURNA, unpublished results). Clozapine enhanced the DA turnover in the mesolimbic system (see Chap. E) but not in the striatum, whilst haloperidol increased the turnover of DA in both systems to the same extent (ANDÉN and STOCK, 1973). In combination with the anticholinergic effect of clozapine (STILLE et al., 1971) this difference in the effect of the drug on the two DA-containing systems may account for the peculiarity that clozapine is a potent but not a "typical" (i.e., catalepsy-inducing) neuroleptic agent. Further studies with neuroleptic agents revealed that CPZ and haloperidol increased the turnover of DA in the striatum and mesolimbic system (nucleus accumbens) to nearly the same extent, while clozapine was more effective on mesolimbic than on striatal DA turnover (ZIVKOVIC et al., 1975); from these results it was concluded that neuroleptic drugs with a high incidence of extrapyramidal side effects exert a strong effect on the nigrostriatal dopaminergic pathway. Similarly, it was found with the help of a concurrent semiautomatic fluorometric assay technique that "typical" or "traditional" neuroleptic agents like haloperidol, pimozide, and thioridazine produced practically identical changes in the DA turnover in the striatum and the accumbens, while clozapine and sulpiride may be considered as "atypical" neuroleptic agents as they enhance like morphine or oxotremorine preferentially the DA turnover in the accumbens (WESTERINK and KORF, 1976). It is still a matter of debate whether a predilective increase of the DA turnover in the mesolimbic system (see Chap. E) warrants a better ratio of neuroleptic potency versus extrapyramidal side effects (WALDMEIER and MAITRE, 1976; WESTERINK et al., 1977).

Apparently, the therapeutic effect exerted by neuroleptic agents in schizophrenia cannot be due to an action of these drugs on the nigrostriatal system, whose paramount task seems to be the control of motor performance. As VOGT (1973) has put it, "the neurons involved in the antipsychotic effect are not those of the nigrostriatal pathway, the destruction of which in parkinsonism neither protects from, nor predisposes to, schizophrenia; if we assume that the therapeutic effect is mediated by dopaminergic neurons, they must lie outside the nigrostriatal pathway".

Promising candidates for this role would be the dopaminergic ascending neurons of the mesolimbic system. However, interest has lately been directed to the nigrostriatal system as a stage for the development of particular symptoms in schizophrenia (CROW, 1979).

E. Mesolimbic System

Apart from the nigroneostriatal pathway another dopaminergic ascending system exists in the forebrain, the so-called mesolimbic DA system (UNGERSTEDT, 1971a). Axons with their cell bodies in the ventral mesencephalic tegmentum follow a route medial to the nigrostriatal pathway and end in the nucleus accumbens, the tuberculum olfactorium, the nucleus striae terminalis, and the amygdala; moreover, axons containing DA have recently been traced till the cerebral cortex (FUXE et al., 1974; LINDVALL and BJÖRKLUND, 1974; LINDVALL et al., 1974). This system has been shown to be important in the locomotor behavior produced by DA-receptor stimulants such as DA and ergometrine injected into the nucleus accumbens (PIJNENBURG and VAN ROSSUM, 1973; PIJNENBURG et al., 1975, 1976); the effect of these substances was antagonized by the neuroleptic agents haloperidol and pimozide. Although bromocriptine and ergocornine have been shown to produce circling in rats with unilateral lesioning of the dopaminergic nigrostriatal path (CORRODI et al., 1973), bromocriptine failed to produce circling movements when injected into the nucleus accumbens (PIJNENBURG et al., 1976). After bilateral microinjection of ergometrine into the nucleus accumbens of the rat, there was first a period of ptosis and sedation; this was followed by strong and longlasting locomotor stimulation (PIJNENBURG et al., 1973) which was abolished by low doses of systemic haloperidol and pimozide.

The nuclei of the mesolimbic system seem to play a differential role in the development of catalepsy induced by haloperidol, fluphenazine, clothiapine, or clozapine, and in the antagonism of the drugs against amphetamine-induced stereotypic behavior (COSTALL and NAYLOR, 1974b). Clozapine, haloperidol, thioridazine, morphine, and sulpiride increased the DA turnover in the mesolimbic system (nucleus accumbens and olfactory tubercle) and the striatum of rats (WESTERINK and KORF, 1976). As in the nigrostriatal system, a disturbed interaction between cholinergic and dopaminergic impulse transmission appears to be an important factor in the mesolimbic system for the development of catalepsy (COSTALL and NAYLOR, 1974c); acutely placed lesions interrupting the pathways from the ventral tegmentum to the mesolimbic nuclei initially potentiated and then reduced the cataleptogenic effect of neuroleptic drugs and potentiated the cholinergic (arecoline-induced) catalepsy.

Neurons in the nucleus accumbens were inhibited by microionophoretically applied DA, ergometrine, and dibutyryl cAMP, as were neurons in the caudate nucleus (WOODRUFF et al., 1976); ACh caused excitation of accumbens neurons that were antagonized by atropine. Intravenously administered D-amphetamine reduced the activity of single DA-containing neurons in the ventral tegmentum of rats, and this inhibition was abolished by CPZ (BUNNEY and AGHAJANIAN, 1974). Bilateral microinjection of dibutyryl cAMP into the nucleus accumbens increased coordinated locomotor activity as did DA; pretreatment with haloperidol had no effect on the responses to dibutyryl cAMP but abolished those of DA, whilst administration of haloperidol after dibutyryl cAMP blocked the effect of the nucleotide (HEAL et al., 1978). After unilateral injection of GABA or baclofen into the olfactory tubercle, rats circled away from the side of drug injection (KELLY and MOORE, 1978). Lesioning of DA neurons in the nucleus accumbens by the administration of 6-OH-DA blocked amphetamine-induced rotation to the side of a 6-OH-DA-induced lesion of the dopaminergic nigrostriatal path, and enhanced the contralateral rotation produced by apomorphine (KELLY and MOORE, 1976). From these results it was concluded that the mesolimbic system modulates the control exerted by the nigrostriatal system on motor behavior.

At present, the DA receptors in the nuclei of the mesolimbic system seem to be the most likely site of the therapeutic action of neuroleptic drugs (MATTHYSSE, 1973; STEVENS, 1973; VOGT, 1973; TORREY and PETERSEN, 1974; BARTHOLINI, 1976). Schizophrenia is most faithfully mimicked by an amphetamine-induced psychosis which depends as well as the amphetamine-induced stereotyped behavior in animals, on the integrity of DA stores in the brain (RANDRUP and MUNKVAD, 1967; GRIFFITH et al., 1972; ANGRIST et al., 1974). The symptoms produced by amphetamine are abolished by DA-receptor-blocking neuroleptic agents (ANGRIST et al., 1974; BERGER, 1978; JOHNSTONE et al., 1978). Experiments performed with lesioning of the two main DA-containing paths arising in the mesencephalon (the nigrostriatal and the mesolimbic; UNGERSTEDT, 1971 a; UNGERSTEDT and PYCOCK, 1974) suggest that these systems subserve motivation and orientation towards external and internal stimuli. There is as yet no positive evidence of an increased release or turnover of DA in schizophrenia (IVERSEN, 1978 b). However, the density of DA receptors has been demonstrated to be increased in post mortem brains of schizophrenic patients (OWEN et al., 1978; LEE et al., 1978). A good correlation exists between the clinical potency of neuroleptic drugs and their displacing of labeled haloperidol from DA receptors in vitro (CREESE et al., 1976; SEEMAN et al., 1976). The therapeutic effect of the neuroleptic agents could thus be explained by a binding to surplus receptors. It is an open question, however, why it takes so long a time for the neuroleptic drugs to depress the symptoms of schizophrenia. Moreover, supersensitivity of the DA receptors should be expected to develop during chronic treatment with neuroleptic agents (LEE et al., 1978).

F. Locus Coeruleus and Other Brain Stem Nuclei: Ascending Pathways

Large amounts of catecholamines have been detected in the cells of the locus coeruleus (DAHLSTRÖM and FUXE, 1975b; GERARDY et al., 1969; LOIZOU, 1969). Pathways were traced by autoradiographic analysis after microinjections of [³H]proline made into the nucleus from their origin to their terminals in the limbic cortex, hippocampus, neocortex, and, brain stem nuclei (SEGAL et al., 1973), which form the dorsal noradrenergic bundle (UNGERSTEDT, 1971 a). Moreover, NA-containing fibers were found to reach the cerebellar cortex (UNGERSTEDT, 1971 a). Since the spontaneous activity of NA-containing neurons in the locus coeruleus was depressed by an intravenous injection of small doses of D-amphetamine (GRAHAM and AGHAJANIAN, 1971), it was proposed that these neurons are inhibited via a neuronal feedback after presynaptic release by D-amphetamine of catecholamines from the terminals: CPZ reduced the effect of

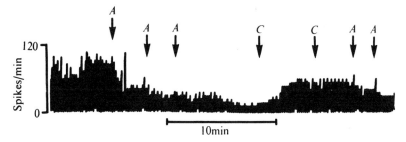

Fig. 12. Typical response of a locus coeruleus unit to amphetamine *(A)* and CPZ *(C)*. Spontaneous rate was 90 spikes/min. The record consists of the number of spikes counted over consecutive 10 s intervals. Within 30 s after the intravenous injection of amphetamine (0.2 mg/kg), a marked decrease in rate was observed. Two subsequent doses of amphetamine (0.4, 1.0) produced additional slowing (to 12 spikes/min). A recovery rate to two thirds of the original was observed with 1 min of intravenous injection of CPZ (1 mg/kg). Additional CPZ (1.0) had no additional effect. Subsequent doses of amphetamine (0.5, 1.0) were less effective in decreasing the rate than in the untreated animal. Rat, anesthetized (chloral hydrate). (From GRAHAM and AGHAJANIAN, 1971)

D-amphetamine in part of the neurons (Fig. 12). On the other hand, spontaneous firing of NA-containing neurons in the locus coeruleus was inhibited by intravenously administered clonidine and by microoonophoretically applied NA and clonidine (SVENSSON et al., 1975), while the spontaneous activity of DA-containing neurons in the substantia nigra was not influenced by clonidine (see also SATOH et al., 1976). The effect of clonidine and NA on the locus coeruleus neurons was interpreted in terms of self-inhibition of these neurons. The dorsal noradrenergic bundle has been proposed as being involved in the extinction of conditioned behavior (MASON and IVERSEN, 1975, 1977) or the control of attentional processes (MASON and IVERSEN, 1978).

In *encéphale isolé* preparations of the cat, CPZ decreased the rate of impulses discharged from single neurons in the nucleus vestibularis lateralis (TAKAORI et al., 1970). CPZ did not affect the spontaneous activity of single neurons in the nucleus tractus solitarii, but blocked the activity accelerated by an intravenous injection or local administration of apomorphine to the area postrema (see Chap. IV).

Ascending catecholamine-containing neurons were found to send their axons from the brain stem to thalamic nuclei (ANDÉN et al., 1966 c). Microionophoretically administered A and NA depressed or excited thalamic neurons, or exerted no effect on the spontaneous impulse discharges; DA produced depression in nearly all neurons recorded from with extracellular microelectrodes (PHILLIS and TEBĒCIS 1967 b). Excitation by catecholamines was mostly observed in neurons which were also excited by ACh. Electrical stimulation within the reticular formation of the brain stem excited some neurons and depressed others. The inhibition produced by microionophoretic administration of the catecholamines and by electrical stimulation in the brain stem could be blocked by picrotoxin and strychnine. It has therefore been suggested that NA might be an inhibitory transmitter in the thalamus. After repeated administration of NA to neurons exhibiting excitation, some of the neurons developed tachyphylaxis, and some of the neurons thus desensitized to the excitatory effect of NA responded to NA with inhibition of spontaneous activity. CPZ, phentolamine and phenoxybenzamine as well as adrenergic β-receptor antagonists had either a pronounced depressant effect on some neurons or excited neurons that were also excited by the catecholamines. Only a rather coarse differentiation of the neurons with regard to their depth in the thalamus had been attempted in this study. To obtain information about specific effects of antipsychotic drugs on the impulse transmission in the thalamus it will be necessary to investigate the influence of these drugs with respect to the different function of the thalamic nuclei in the processing of sensory information and in the regulation of motor activity.

NA-containing neurons have been found to ascend from their origin in the pons and the medulla oblongata via the medial forebrain bundle to the neocortex (ANDÉN et al., 1965b, 1966b, c). Moreover, there seem to exist DA-containing terminals in the rat cerebral cortex (THIERRY et al., 1973). In anesthetized cats or *cerveau isolé* preparations, catecholamines administered by microionophoresis to cortical neurons depressed the spontaneous impulse discharges and the activity evoked by synaptic excitation or by administration of excitant amino acids (KRNJEVIĆ and PHILLIS, 1963; LEGGE et al., 1966; PHILLIS and YORK, 1967; JORDAN et al., 1972). DA was found to be particularly potent (KRNJEVIĆ and PHILLIS, 1963; LEGGE et al., 1966), while 5 HT was reported to produce depression or excitation (ROBERTS and STRAUGHAN, 1966). CPZ was ineffective on neuronal activity (KRNJEVIĆ and PHILLIS, 1963) and the depression induced by NA could not be antagonized by adrenergic α- or β-receptor blocking agents (LEGGE et al., 1966) but was antagonized by strychnine (PHILLIS and YORK, 1967).

The effects of microionophoretically administered catecholamines have been studied in many neurons in various other parts of the central nervous system, and from the results obtained a transmitter role for NA has been suggested at the Purkinje cells in the cerebellar cortex and neurons in the medial and lateral geniculate nucleus, in the olfactory bulb and in the hypothalamus, but data concerning an effect of neuroleptic drugs on these neurons are lacking.

The hypophysial portal blood contains significant amounts of DA (BEN-JONATHAN et al., 1977), which is known to inhibit prolactin secretion (KAMBERI et al., 1970; LU et al., 1970; MACLEOD, 1976). DA receptors have been detected in the anterior pituitary by employing labeled DA agonists and neuroleptic agents and were found to belong to two different types; one type of receptor exhibits low affinity for classical DA agonists (concentrations in the micromolar range are effective) (CREESE et al., 1977) and is linked to adenylate cyclase (AHN et al., 1979), the other receptor type has a high affinity for DA agonists (these are effective in nanomolar concentrations) and controls prolactin release (CARON et al., 1978; KEBABIAN and CALNE, 1979; SIBLEY and CREESE, 1979). The prolactin secretion increased by sulpiride (an "atypical" neuroleptic agent which does not evoke extrapyramidal side effects) is depressed by the DA agonist bromocriptine (HOFMANN et al., 1979). Bromocriptine and ergocornine as DA receptor stimulants inhibit prolactin secretion (FLÜCKIGER and WAGNER, 1968). DA, NA, A, and apomorphine inhibited the release of prolactin in vitro (BIRGE et al., 1970; MACLEOD et al., 1970; SHAAR et al., 1973; SMALSTIG et al., 1974) and in vivo (DE WIED, 1967; FRANTZ, 1973; KLEINBERG et al., 1971), and neuroleptic agents antagonized this inhibition.

Reserpine produced inhibition of the firing of 5 HT-containing neurons in the dorsal raphé nuclei which was prevented by intraventricular injection of 6-OH-DA but not be pretreatment with parachlorphenylalanine; the inhibition was abolished by systemic administration of amphetamine or clonidine and by microionophoretic application of NA (BARABAN et al., 1978). It was suggested that the 5 HT-containing neurons are subject to inhibition from GABAergic neurons, which, in turn, are inhibited by noradrenergic neurons.

Spontaneous discharges in sympathetic nerves and the activity evoked in these nerves by hypothalamic stimulation were depressed by CPZ and haloperidol, while trifluoperazine produced facilitation (CLUBLEY and ELLIOTT, 1977).

G. Cyclic-AMP

Since KEBABIAN et al. (1972) demonstrated that DA activated adenylate cyclase in the brain, evidence has accumulated which strongly suggests that this enzyme may act as a receptor for the central transmitters NA or DA, or is closely associated with the receptors. Detailed accounts of the role of adenylate cyclase in central monoaminergic impulse transmission were given by BLOOM (1975) and SCHWARTZ et al. (1978). Adenylate cyclase and phosphodiesterase were found to be associated to a considerable extent with the synaptosomal fraction of brain homogenates (DE ROBERTIS et al., 1967). By employing a specific immunofluorescence method to detect cAMP, it has been shown that local treatment with NA or electrical stimulation of the NA-containing pathway from the locus coeruleus to the cerebellar cortex strikingly increased the number of Purkinje cells exhibiting an intense cAMP reactivity (SIGGINS et al., 1973). Also in the human striatum DA stimulated selectively the formation of cAMP, and this effect was inhibited by haloperidol; no difference existed in the basal activity and the DA-stimulated activity of the striatal adenylate cyclase between control subjects and schizophrenic patients (CARENZI et al., 1975). DA and apomorphine are similarly potent in stimulating the formation of cAMP in the rat caudate nucleus (KEBABIAN et al., 1972). The stimulating effect of DA on striatal and mesolimbic tissue could be blocked by low concentrations of CPZ, haloperidol, and other neuroleptic drugs (KE-BABIAN et al., 1972; MILLER et al., 1974; MILLER and IVERSEN, 1974). The antagonism seems to be a specific one, because several compounds structurally closely related to the antipsychotic drugs but lacking their antipsychotic property as well as the capacity to produce extrapyramidal symptoms exhibited a low inhibitor potency (CLEMENT-CORMIER et al., 1974; KAROBATH and LEITICH, 1974; MILLER et al., 1974). Moreover, α-flupenthixol inhibited the DA-induced formation of cAMP, whilst β-flupenthixol did not (Table 2). On the other hand, CPZ increased the concentration of cAMP in the cerebral cortex instead of reducing it (PALMER et al., 1975, 1977). This has been explained by the observation that CPZ blocks not only DA-induced stimulation of cAMP formation but also the activation of phosphodiesterase, a process involving competition with the endogenous protein activator of the cAMP metabolizing enzyme (LEVIN and WEISS, 1976); thus, CPZ might cause a drop in the concentration of cAMP in a brain area relatively rich in catecholamine-sensitive adenylate cyclase, and a rise in areas containing large amounts of activable phosphodiesterase, as in the cerebral cortex. After intraventricular administration of 6-OH-DA the formation of cAMP in the rat cortex, brain stem and hypothalamus was stimulated by NA and isoprenaline to a greater extent than in nonpretreated brains (PALMER, 1972; HUANG et al., 1973; KALISKER et al., 1973). In the acute experiment performed under both in vitro and in vivo conditions, CPZ and haloperidol inhibited NA-induced activation of adenylate

Table 2. Drug concentrations causing 50% inhibition of stimulation of cAMP production (IC_{50}) in striatal homogenates by 100 μM dopamine, and calculated K_i values[a]

K_i values were calculated from the relationship $IC_{50} = K_i(I + S/K_m)$, where S is the concentration of dopamine (100 μM) and K_m is the concentration of dopamine required for half-maximal stimulation of adenylate cyclase activity (5 μM). Competitive inhibition has been assumed for all compounds tested

Drug	IC_{50}	K_i
	M	M
1. α-Flupenthixol	2.2×10^{-8}	1.0×10^{-9}
2. (α,β)-Flupenthixol	7.5×10^{-8}	3.5×10^{-9}
3. Fluphenazine	9.2×10^{-8}	4.3×10^{-9}
4. Trifluoperazine	4.0×10^{-7}	1.9×10^{-8}
5. α-Clopenthixol	3.3×10^{-7}	1.6×10^{-8}
6. α-Chlorprothixene	7.8×10^{-7}	3.7×10^{-8}
7. Chlorpromazine	1.0×10^{-6}	4.8×10^{-8}
8. Prochlorperazine	2.2×10^{-6}	1.0×10^{-7}
9. Spiroperidol	2.0×10^{-6}	9.5×10^{-8}
10. Thioridazine	2.8×10^{-6}	1.3×10^{-7}
11. Clozapine	3.5×10^{-6}	1.7×10^{-7}
12. Pimozide	3.0×10^{-6}	1.4×10^{-7}
13. Chlorimipramine	9.0×10^{-6}	4.2×10^{-7}
14. Promazine	6.0×10^{-5}	2.8×10^{-6}
15. Morphine	1.0×10^{-4}	4.8×10^{-6}
16. β-Chlorprothixene	2.0×10^{-5}	9.5×10^{-7}
17. β-Clopenthixol	6×10^{-5}	2.8×10^{-6}
18. β-Flupenthixol	$>10^{-4}$	$>5 \times 10^{-6}$
19. Promethazine	$>10^{-4}$	$>5 \times 10^{-6}$
20. Benztropine	$>10^{-4}$	$>5 \times 10^{-6}$

[a] From Miller et al. (1974)

cyclase, while during subchronic administration of the neuroleptic agents, other factors (enhanced receptor sensitivity and/or inhibition of phosphodiesterase) seem to come into play (Palmer et al., 1978).

Intraventricular injection of dibutyryl cAMP evoked circling movements in rats to the side opposite of intranigral 6-OH-DA injection, as did DA, NA, apomorphine, or theophylline, while clonidine was ineffective (Satoh et al., 1976). Theophylline potentiated the effect of apomorphine on rotational behavior and on the formation of cAMP, while haloperidol blocked the stimulation by apomorphine (and DA or NA) of adenylate cyclase activity.

Classification of adenylate cyclase in the brain in terms of the classical α- or β-adrenergic receptors is a matter of controversy. In the rat cerebral cortex the accumulation of cAMP induced by NA was reduced to about one-half by either phentolamine or propranolol, and completely blocked by the combination of both sympatholytic agents (Perkins and Moore, 1973). A, NA, and isoprenaline enhanced the formation of cAMP in the rat cerebral cortex to nearly the same extent, whereas in the mouse cerebral cortex the stimulation seemed to be mediated predominantly by adrenergic

β-receptors (SCHULTZ and DALY, 1973). Both DA and NA increased the rate of the formation of cAMP in the rat striatum, DA being more potent in stimulating the synthesis; in the cerebral cortex, however, only NA enhanced the formation of cAMP (WALKER and WALKER, 1973); the effect of DA was blocked by haloperidol and slightly reduced by phenoxybenzamine. Propranolol abolished the stimulation by NA of the synthesis of cAMP in the cortex. It has, therefore, been suggested that two independent receptors for the activation of cAMP formation exist in the striatum, one being sensitive to DA and the other to NA. Recently, a highly specific inhibition by phenoxybenzamine of DA-stimulated adenylate cyclase has been reported, and a direct interaction between phenoxybenzamine and the DA-binding component of the enzyme has been suggested (WALTON et al., 1978). HARRIS (1976), however, reported that the formation of cAMP in the rat striatum depended on a mechanism bearing the characteristics of an adrenergic β-receptor. DA and apomorphine produced a relatively weak stimulation, and adrenergic β-receptor blockers effectively inhibited the stimulated formation of cAMP, while the adrenergic α-receptor blocker phentolamine as well as CPZ and trifluperazine had nearly no effect. HARRIS (1976), therefore, proposed that the DA-induced accumulation of cAMP is not associated with specific DA receptor-coupled adenylate cyclase but might involve an adrenergic β-receptor-linked cyclase weakly responsive to non-β-hydroxylated catecholamines. When reviewing the information concerning the role of adenylate cyclase as a catecholamine receptor in the central nervous system, IVERSEN (1975) concluded that the inhibitory effects of NA may be mediated by a NA-sensitive enzyme with adrenergic β-receptor properties; the DA-sensitive adenylate cyclase has properties distinguishing it clearly from either of the traditional α- or β-receptor classes and is extremely sensitive to the stimulant effect of apomorphine and the blocking action of antipsychotic drugs. In the zona reticulata of the substantia nigra, which contains dendrites of the dopaminergic nigrostriatal neurons in the zona compacta, a DA-sensitive adenylate cyclase has been demonstrated to show characteristics similar to those of the enzyme in the striatum; DA was more potent than NA in stimulating its activity and was competitively inhibited by CPZ (KEBABIAN and SAAVEDRA, 1976).

Biochemical data suggest that the formation of cAMP may be involved in the synthesis of DA and NA in the central nervous system. Electrical stimulation of the dopaminergic nigroneostriatal and mesolimbic pathways increased the activity of tyrosine hydroxylase in the neostriatum and olfactory tubercles, respectively, and cAMP produced changes in the enzyme kinetics similar to those evoked by electrical stimulation of the dopaminergic pathways (MURRIN et al., 1976). In slices and synaptosomes prepared from the rat cerebral cortex and striatum, cAMP and its derivatives such as dibutyryl cAMP stimulated the activity of tyrosine hydroxylase (GOLDSTEIN et al., 1973; HARRIS et al., 1974a, b; ROBERGE et al., 1974). The activation of the synthesis was stereospecific for the L-isomer of tyrosine and could be inhibited by low concentrations of DA (HARRIS et al., 1974b) and apomorphine (GOLDSTEIN et al., 1973). The stimulation in striatal synaptosomes of tyrosine hydroxylase by dibutyryl cAMP, which is a poor substrate for the phosphodiesterase, appeared to be independent of the concentration of potassium ions in the suspension medium; therefore, it has been assumed that cAMP-stimulated synthesis of the transmitter and the potassium-induced transmitter release are not mediated by one and the same mechanism but that the formation of cAMP may reduce the inhibition of

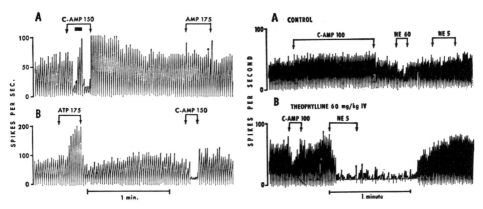

Fig. 13 A and B. (left). Effects of microionophoretic administration of adenine nucleotides on spontaneous Purkinje cell discharge. A and B illustrate continuous record from the same cell. Duration of drug administration is indicated by arrows. The numbers after each drug indicate ejection current in nA. The solid bar in **A** represents application of a cathodal current through the micropipette. The restauration of spontaneous discharge by cathodal current indicates that the slowing seen with cAMP is not secondary to local anesthetic action or hyperdepolarization (cathodal block). (right) Potentiation of microionophoretically administered NA and cAMP by parenteral injection of theophylline. **A** Control. **B** The same cell after intravenous injection of theophylline (60 mg/kg). Duration of drug administration indicated by arrows. Numbers after each drug indicate ejection current in nanoamperes. The residual discharge after 5 nA or NA in **B** consisted almost entirely of climbing fiber bursts. All records obtained from rats anesthetized with chloral hydrate. (From SIGGINS et al., 1969)

tyrosine hydroxylase activity resulting from the accumulation of the end-product DA (ROBERGE et al., 1974).

Microionophoretical administration of cAMP and NA to cerebellar Purkinje cells of the rat reduced the frequency of impulses discharged spontaneously. The effect of cAMP was faster in onset and termination than that of NA, as should be the case if the effect of NA was mediated by the formation of cAMP, and the depression exerted by both NA and cAMP was potentiated by drugs inhibiting phosphodiesterase activity, that is by intravenous injection of theophylline (Fig. 13) or locally administered aminophylline (HOFFER et al., 1969; SIGGINS et al., 1969, 1971a). The prostaglandins E_1 and E_2, which have been reported to reduce the level of cAMP in peripheral neuroeffector systems, antagonized the depressant effect of NA but not of cAMP on the Purkinje cell activity (HOFFER et al., 1969; SIGGINS et al., 1971a). In contrast to cAMP, ATP, and 5'-AMP accelerated the activity of these neurons (SIGGINS et al., 1969). A particularly convincing argument for the mediation by cAMP of the depressant effect of NA derived from the observation that, although GABA as well as NA and cAMP hyperpolarized the membrane of the Purkinje cells, the mechanism by which these agents produce hyperpolarization and thereby inhibit the impulse discharge must be entirely different: GABA decreased the transmembrane resistance as do other amino acids possibly acting as inhibitory transmitters in the central nervous system, whereas cAMP mimicked NA (Fig. 14) in its unique effect of elevating the membrane resistance (SIGGINS et al., 1969, 1971b). In the cat medulla oblongata, microionophoretic administration of cAMP depressed the activity in the majority of

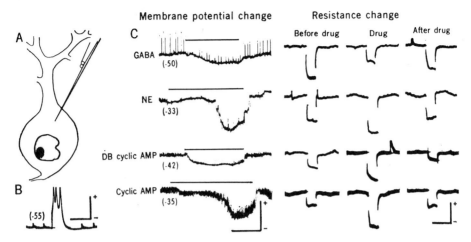

Fig. 14 A–C. Intracellular recordings from rat cerebellar Purkinje cells. **A** Schematic representation of a three-barrel micropipette with a Purkinje cell. The intracellular electrode protrudes beyond the orifices of the two extracellular microionophoresis barrels. **B** Multispiked spontaneous climbing fiber discharge obtained during intracellular recording from a Purkinje cell. Number in parentheses is resting potential in mV; calibration bars are 20 ms and 25 mV. **C** Changes in membrane potential and membrane resistance of four different Purkinje cells in response to GABA, NA, dibutyryl cAMP (DB cyclic AMP) and cAMP. All specimens in each horizontal row of records are from the same cell. Solid bar above each record indicates the extracellular ionophoresis of the indicated drug (100–150 nA). Number in parentheses below each recording is resting potential in mV; calibration bar under membrane potential records is 10 s and 20 mV for NA, DB cyclic AMP, and cAMP, and is 5 s and 10 mV for GABA. The effective input resistance was judged by the size of pulses resulting from the passage across the membrane of a brief constant current (1 nA) pulse before, during, and after ionophoresis of the respective drugs (1 mV = 1 MΩ). Discontinuities in the fast transients of the pulses result from the loss of high frequencies (> 10 kHz) and from the chopped nature of the frequency-modulated magnetic tape recording used. All "pulse" records were graphically normalized to the same baseline level. Calibration bar on right indicates 80 ms and 15 mV for all pulse records. (From SIGGINS et al., 1971 b)

the neurons tested; excitation never occurred after the administration of cAMP, and neurons inhibited by microionophoresis of NA were also inhibited by cAMP, whereas neurons excited by NA were not affected by cAMP (ANDERSSON et al., 1973). Spontaneous and amino acid-induced activity of rat caudate neurons was depressed not only by DA and apomorphine but also by cAMP (SIGGINS et al., 1974). Phosphodiesterase inhibition produced by xanthine derivatives potentiated the effect of DA, and CPZ antagonized the depression produced by DA but not that following from cAMP.

According to the view advocated by GREENGARD and collaborators the sequence of events triggered by NA or DA released from presynaptic terminals would be the following: the catecholamines bind to their postsynaptic receptors activating adenylate cyclase to convert ATP into cAMP. The cAMP acts as a second messenger by phosphorylating a protein kinase which changes the ion permeability of the neuronal membrane (KEBABIAN and GREENGARD, 1971; KEBABIAN et al., 1972; MCAFEE and GREENGARD, 1972; UEDA et al., 1973). Thus, microionophoretic administration of catecholamines and cAMP must result in the same changes of the membrane characteristics, and antipsychotic drugs will block the effect of DA or NA but not that evoked by cAMP. However, for the cerebellar Purkinje cells and the neurons in the sensory cortex a mediation of the effect of NA by cAMP has seriously been questioned, because microionophoretically administered cAMP or dibutyryl cAMP were not found to mimic the strong inhibitory effect of NA on these neurons in various species (JORDAN et al., 1972; LAKE et al., 1972, 1973; LAKE and JORDAN, 1974). Inhibition by aminophylline or papaverine of phosphodiesterase enhanced the depressant effect of NA, but also depressed the activity of neurons not inhibited by NA, and prostaglandins did not consistently block the depression following from the administration of NA.

Discrepancies observed in studies performed on DA-receptor binding and DA-sensitive adenylate cyclase suggest that two different DA-receptor populations exist (LEYSEN and LADURON, 1972; MINNEMAN et al., 1978; SCHWARCZ et al., 1978; QUIK and IVERSEN, 1979 see also Chap. A).

H. Concluding Remarks

Neuroleptic drugs may antagonize the transmitter effects of DA and NA in particular central neuron systems. Apparently, DA-mediated impulse transmission is more sensitive to the blocking effect of these drugs than is NA-mediated transmission. As for the target neurons of the antipsychotic action of the drugs, interest has lately been focused on the mesolimbic system. Parkinsonlike motor symptoms induced by antipsychotic drugs derive from an impairment of dopaminergic impulse transmission in the nigrostriatal system. In the two systems containing dopaminergic pathways, the nigrostriatal and the mesolimbic, the activity of the DA-containing neurons is regulated by way of a neuronal feedback as well as by auto- or self-inhibition of these neurons. Both mechanisms are influenced by neuroleptic drugs.

The manuscript for this article had been finished at the end of September 1977. Due to delay in the process of editing, a revision became indispensable but had to be restricted to parts of the manuscript. The author apologizes if some relevant, recently published papers are not included.

Acknowledgements. The author wishes to thank Mrs. FLORENTINE ECKER and Mrs. BIRGIT KILTHAU for valuable technical assistance in preparing the manuscript.

References

Aghajanian, G.K., Bunney, B.S.: Central dopaminergic neurons: neurophysiological identification and responses to drugs. In: Frontiers in Catecholamine Research, Snyder, S.H., Usdin, E., Eds., pp. 643–648, Pergamon Press, New York (1973)
Aghajanian, G.K., Bunney, B.S.: Dopamine "autoreceptors": pharmacological characterization by microionotophoretic single cell recording studies. Naunyn Schmiedebergs Arch. Pharmacol. *297*, 1–7 (1977)
Agid, Y., Guyenet, P., Glowinski, J., Beaujouan, J.C., Javoy, F.: Inhibitory influence of the nigrostriatal dopamine system on the striatal cholinergic neurons in the rat. Brain Res. *86*, 488–492 (1975)
Ahlman, H., Grillner, S., Udo, M.: The effect of 5-HTP on the static fusimotor activity and the tonic stretch reflex of an extensor muscle. Brain Res. *27*, 393–396 (1971)
Ahn, H.S., Gardner, E., Makman, M.H.: Anterior pituitary adenylate cyclase: stimulation by dopamine and other monoamines. Eur. J. Pharmacol. *53*, 313–317 (1979)

Andén, N.-E.: Antipsychotic drugs and catecholamine synapses. J. Psychiatr. Res. *11*, 97–104 (1974)

Andén, N.-E., Bédard, P.: Influences of cholinergic mechanisms on the function and turnover of brain dopamine. J. Pharm. Pharmacol. *23*, 460–462 (1971)

Andén, N.-E., Stock, G.: Effect of clozapine on the turnover of dopamine in the corpus striatum and in the limbic system. J. Pharm. Pharmacol. *25*, 346–348 (1973)

Andén, N.-E., Lundberg, A., Rosengren, E., Vyklický, L.: The effect of DOPA on spinal reflexes from the FRA (flexor reflex afferents). Experientia *19*, 654–655 (1963)

Andén, N.-E., Carlsson, A., Dahlström, A., Fuxe, K., Hillarp, N.-Å., Larsson, K.: Demonstration and mapping out of nigro-neostriatal dopamine neurons. Life Sci. *3*, 523–530 (1964a)

Andén, N.-E., Carlsson, A., Hillarp, N.-Å., Magnusson, T.: 5-Hydroxytryptamine release by nerve stimulation of the spinal cord. Life Sci. *3*, 473–478 (1964b)

Andén, N.-E., Häggendal, J., Magnusson, T., Rosengren, E.: The time course of the disappearance of noradrenaline and 5-hydroxytryptamine in the spinal cord after transection. Acta Physiol. Scand. *62*, 115–118 (1964c)

Andén, N.-E., Jukes, M.G.M., Lundberg, A.: Spinal reflexes and monoamine liberation. Nature *202*, 1222–1223 (1964d)

Andén, N.-E., Jukes, M.G.M., Lundberg, A., Vyklický, L.: A new spinal flexor reflex. Nature *202*, 1344–1345 (1964e)

Andén, N.-E., Magnusson, T., Waldeck, B.: Correlation between noradrenaline uptake and adrenergic nerve function after reserpine treatment. Life Sci. *3*, 19–25 (1964f)

Andén, N.-E., Roos, B.-E., Werdenius, B.: Effects of chlorpromazine, haloperidol and reserpine on the levels of phenolic acids in rabbit corpus striatum. Life Sci. *3*, 149–158 (1964g)

Andén, N.-E., Carlsson, A., Hillarp, N.-Å., Magnusson, T.: Noradrenaline release by nerve stimulation of the spinal cord. Life Sci. *4* 129–132 (1965a)

Andén, N.-E., Dahlström, A., Fuxe, K., Larsson, K.: Mapping out of catecholamine and 5-hydroxytryptamine neurons innervating the telencephalon and diencephalon. Life Sci. *4*, 1275–1279 (1965b)

Andén, N.-E., Dahlström, A., Fuxe, K., Larsson, K.: Further evidence for the presence of nigro-neostriatal dopamine neurons in the rat. Am. J. Anat. *116*, 329–334 (1965c)

Andén, N.-E., Dahlström, A., Fuxe, K., Larsson, K.: Functional role of the nigro-neostriatal dopamine neurons. Acta Pharmacol. Toxicol. *24*, 263–274 (1966a)

Andén, N.-E., Dahlström, A., Fuxe, K., Olson, L., Ungerstedt, U.: Ascending noradrenaline neurons from the pons and the medulla oblongata. Experientia *22*, 44–45 (1966b)

Andén, N.-E., Dahlström, A., Fuxe, K., Olson, L., Ungerstedt, U.: Ascending monoamine neurons to the telecephalon and diencephalon. Acta Physiol. Scand. *67*, 313–326 (1966c)

Andén, N.-E., Jukes, M.G.M., Lundberg, A.: The effect of DOPA on the spinal cord. 2. A pharmacological analysis. Acta Physiol. Scand. *67*, 387–397 (1966d)

Andén, N.-E., Jukes, M.G.M., Lundberg, A., Vyklický, L.: The effect of DOPA on the spinal cord. 1. Influence on transmission from primary afferents. Acta Physiol. Scand. *67*, 373–386 (1966e)

Andén, N.-E., Jukes, M.G.M., Lundberg, A., Vyklický, L.: The effect of DOPA on the spinal cord. 3. Depolarization evoked in the central terminals of ipsilateral Ia afferents by volleys in the flexor reflex afferents. Acta Physiol. Scand. *68*, 322–336 (1966f)

Andén, N.-E., Corrodi, H., Fuxe, K., Hökfelt, T.: Increased impulse flow in bulbospinal noradrenaline neurons produced by catecholamine receptor blocking agents. Eur. J. Pharmacol. *2*, 59–64 (1967a)

Andén, N.-E., Fuxe, K., Hökfelt, T.: Effect of some drugs on central monamine nerve terminals lacking nerve impulse flow. Eur. J. Pharmacol. *1*, 226–232 (1967b)

Andén, N.-E., Rubenson, A., Fuxe, K., Hökfelt, T.: Evidence for dopamine receptor stimulation by apomorphine. J. Pharm. Pharmacol. *19*, 627–629 (1967c)

Andén, N.-E., Butcher, S.G., Corrodi, H., Fuxe, K., Ungerstedt, U.: Receptor activity and turnover of dopamine and noradrenaline after neuroleptics. Eur. J. Pharmacol. *11*, 303–314 (1970a)

Andén, N.-E., Corrodi, H., Fuxe, K., Hökfelt, B., Hökfelt, T., Rydin, C., Svensson, T.: Evidence for a central noradrenaline receptor stimulation by clonidine. Life Sci. *9*, 513–523 (1970b)

Andén, N.-E., Corrodi, H., Fuxe, K., Ungerstedt, U.: Importance of nervous impulse flow for the neuroleptic induced increase in amine turnover in central dopamine neurons. Eur. J. Pharmacol. *15*, 193–199 (1971)

Andén, N.-E., Corrodi, H., Fuxe, K.: Effect of neuroleptic drugs on central catecholamine turnover assessed using tyrosine- and dopamine-β-hydroxylase inhibitors. J. Pharm. Pharmacol. *24*, 177–182 (1972 a)

Andén, N.-E., Engel, J., Rubenson, A.: Mode of action of L-Dopa on central noradrenaline mechanisms. Naunyn Schmiedebergs Arch. Pharmacol. *273*, 1–10 (1972 b)

Anderson, E.G., Holgerson, L.O.: Distribution of 5-hydroxytryptamine and norepinephrine in cat spinal cord. J. Neurochem. *13*, 479–485 (1966)

Anderson, E.G., Haas, H., Hösli, L.: Comparison of effects of noradrenaline and histamine with cyclic AMP on brain stem neurons. Brain Res. *49*, 471–475 (1973)

Angrist, B., Sathanathan, G., Wilk, S., Gershon, S.: Amphetamine psychosis: behavioral and biochemical aspects. J. Psychiatr. Res. *11*, 13–23 (1974)

Anlezark, G.M., Meldrum, B.S.: Effects of apomorphine, ergocornine and piribedil on audiogenic seizures in DBA/2 mice. Br. J. Pharmacol. *53*, 419–421 (1975)

Anlezark, G., Pycock, C., Meldrum, B.: Ergot alkaloids as dopamine agonists: comparison in two rodent models. Eur. J. Pharmacol. *37*, 295–302 (1976)

Anton, A.H., Sayre, D.F.: The distribution of dopamine and dopa in various animals and a method for their determination in diverse biological material. J. Pharmacol. Exp. Ther. *145*, 326–336 (1964)

Arvidsson, J., Roos, B.-E., Steg, G.: Reciprocal effects on α- and γ-motoneurones of drugs influencing monoaminergic and cholinergic transmission. Acta Physiol. Scand. *67*, 398–404 (1966)

Arvidsson, J., Jurna, I., Steg, G.: Striatal and spinal lesions eliminating reserpine and physostigmine rigidity. Life Sci. *6*, 2017–2020 (1967)

Atweh, S., Kuhar, M.J.: Autoradiographic localization of opiate receptors in rat brain. III. The telencephalon. Brain Res. *134*, 393–405 (1977)

Avanzino, G.L., Bradley, P.B., Comis, S.D., Wolstencroft, J.H.: A comparison of the actions of ergothioneine and chlorpromazine applied to single neurons by two different methods. Neuropharmacology *5*, 331–332 (1966)

Axelrod, J., Whitby, L.G., Hertting, G.: Effect of psychotropic drugs on the uptake of H^3-norepinephrine by tissues. Science *133*, 383–384 (1961)

Axelrod, J., Hertting, G., Potter, L.: Effect of drugs on the uptake and release of ^3H-norepinephrine in the rat heart. Nature *194*, 297 (1962)

Baker, R.G., Anderson, E.G.: The effect of L-3,4, dihydroxyphenylalanine on spinal activity. Pharmacologist *7*, 142 (1965)

Baker, R.G., Anderson, E.G.: The effects of L-3,4-dihydroxyphenylalanine on spinal activity. J. Pharmacol. Exp. Ther. *173*, 212–223 (1970 a)

Baker, R.G., Anderson, E.G.: The antagonism of the effects of L-3,4-dihydroxyphenylalanine on spinal reflexes by adrenergic blocking agents. J. Pharmacol. Exp. Ther. *173*, 224–231 (1970 b)

Baraban, J.M., Wang, R.Y., Aghajanian, G.K.: Reserpine suppression of dorsal raphe neuronal firing: mediation by adrenergic system. Eur. J. Pharmacol. *52*, 27–36 (1978)

Barasi, S., Roberts, M.H.T.: Responses of motoneurones to electrophoretically applied dopamine. Br. J. Pharmacol. *60*, 29–34 (1977)

Barbeau, A.: The pathogenesis of Parkinson's disease: a new hypothesis. Can. Med. Assc. J. *87*, 802–807 (1962)

Barbeau, A., Sourkes, T.L.: Some biochemical aspects of extrapyramidal diseases. Rev. Can. Biol. *20*, 197–203 (1961)

Bartholini, G.: Differential effect of neuroleptic drugs on dopamine turnover in the extrapyramidal and limbic system. J. Pharm. Pharmacol. *28*, 429–433 (1976)

Bartholini, G., Pletscher, A.: Atropine-induced changes of cerebral dopamine turnover. Experientia *27*, 1302–1303 (1971)

Bartholini, G., Stadler, H.: Evidence for an intrastriatal GABA-ergic influence on dopamine neurones of the cat. Neuropharmacology *16*, 343–347 (1977)

Baruk, H., Launay, J., Berges, J.: Action des drogues psychotropes sur le comportement psychomoteur animal. In: Psychotropic Drugs. S. Garattini and V. Ghetti, Eds., pp. 160–168, Elsevier Publishing Company, Amsterdam (1957)

Bass, A.: Über eine Wirkung des Adrenalins auf das Gehirn. Z. ges. Neurol. Psychiat. 26, 600–601 (1914)

Beaulnes, A., Viens, G.: Catatonie et catalepsie. Rev. Can. Biol. 20, 215–220 (1961)

Bein, H.J.: Zur Pharmakologie des Reserpin, eines neuen Alkaloides, aus Rauwolfia serpentina Benth. Experientia 9, 107–110 (1953)

Ben-Jonathan, N., Oliver, C., Weiner, H.J., Mical, R.S., Porter, J.C.: Dopamine in hypophysial portal plasma of the rat during the estrous cycle and throughout pregnancy. Endocrinology (Phil.) 100, 452–458 (1977)

Berger, P.A.: Medical treatment of mental illness. Science 200, 974–981 (1978)

Bernhard, C.G., Skoglund, C.R.: Potential changes in spinal cord following intra-arterial administration of adrenaline and noradrenaline as compared with acetylcholine effects. Acta Physiol. Scand. 29, suppl. 106, 435–454 (1953)

Bernhard, C.G., Skoglund, C.R., Therman, P.O.: Studies on the potential level in the ventral root under varying condition. Acta Physiol. Scand. 14, suppl. 47. pp. 1–10 (1947)

Bernhard, C.G., Gray, J.A.B., Widén, L.: The difference in response of monosynaptic extensor and monosynaptic flexor reflexes to d-tubocurarine and adrenaline. Acta Physiol. Scand. 29, suppl. 106, 73–78 (1952)

Bertler, Å, Rosengren, E.: Occurence and distribution of dopamine in brain and other tissues. Experientia 15, 10–11 (1959)

Bertler, Å, Carlsson, A., Rosengren, E.: Release by reserpine of catecholamines from rabbit's hearts. Naturwissenschaften 43, 521 (1956)

Bertler, Å, Carlsson, A., Lindqvist, M., Magnusson, T.: On the catecholamine levels in blood plasma after stimulation of the sympathoadrenal system. Experientia 14, 184–185 (1958)

Berzewski, H., Helmchen, H., Hippius, H., Hoffmann, H., Kanowski, S.: Das klinische Wirkungsspektrum eines neuen Dibenzodiazepin-Derivates. Arzneim. Forsch. 19, 495–498 (1969)

Besson, M.J., Chéramy, A., Feltz, P., Glowinski, J.: Dopamine: spontaneous and drug-induced release from the caudate nucleus in the cat. Brain Res. 32, 407–424 (1971)

Besson, M.J., Chéramy, Glowinski, J.: Effects of some psychotropic drugs on dopamine synthesis in the rat striatum. J. Pharmacol. Exp. Ther. 177, 196–205 (1971)

Biegler, D., Giles, S.A., Hockman, C.H.: Dopaminergic influences on swallowing. Neuropharmacology. 16, 245–252 (1977)

Birge, C.A., Jacobs, L.S., Hammer, C.T., Daughaday, W.H.: Catecholamine inhibition of prolactin secretion by isolated rat adenohypophyses. Endocrinology 86, 120–130 (1970)

Biscoe, T.J., Curtis, D.R.: Noradrenaline and inhibition of Renshaw cells. Science 151, 1230–1231 (1966)

Biscoe, T.J., Straughan, D.W.: Micro-electrophoretic studies of neurones in the cat hippocampus. J. Physiol. (Lond.) 183, 341–359 (1966)

Biscoe, T.J., Curtis, D.R., Ryall, R.W.: An investigation of catecholamine receptors of spinal interneurones. Neuropharmacology 5, 429–434 (1966)

Bloom, F.E.: Minireview. To spritz or not to spritz: the doubtful value of aimless iontophoresis. Life Sci. 14, 1819–1834 (1974)

Bloom, F.E.: The role of cyclic nucleotides in central synaptic functions. Rev. Physiol. Biochem. Pharmacol. 74, 1–103 (1975)

Bloom, F.E., Costa, E., Oliver, A.P., Salmoiraghi, G.C.: Caudate nucleus neurons: their responsiveness to iontophoretically administered amines and the effects of anesthetic agents. Fed. Proc. 23, 249 (1964)

Bloom, F.E., Costa, E., Salmoiraghi, G.C.: Anesthesia and the responsiveness of individual neurons of the caudate nucleus of the cat to acetylcholine, norepinephrine and dopamine administered by microelectrophoresis. J. Pharmacol. Exp. Ther. 150, 244–252 (1965)

Bogdanksi, D.F., Weissbach, H., Udenfriend, S.: The distribution of serotonin, 5-hydroxytryptamine decarboxylase and monoamine oxidase in brain. J. Neurochem. 1, 272–278 (1957)

Boggan, W.O., Seiden, L.S.: Dopa reversal of reserpine enhancement of audiogenic seizure susceptibility in mice. Physiol. Behav. 6, 215–217 (1971)

Bonvallet, M., Dell, P., Hiebel, G.: Tonus sympathique et activité électrique corticale. Electroencephalogr. Clin. Neurophysiol. *6*, 119–144 (1954)

Bonvallet, M., Hugelin, A., Dell, P.: Milieu intérieur et activité automatique des cellules réticulaires mésencéphaliques. J. Physiol. (Paris) *48*, 403–406 (1956)

Borison, H.L.: Role of gastrointestinal innervation in digitalis emesis. J. Pharmacol. Exp. Ther. *104*, 396–403 (1952)

Borison, H.L.: Area postrema: chemoreceptor trigger zone for vomiting – is that all? Life Sci. *14*, 1807–1817 (1974)

Borison, H.L., Brizzee, K.R.: Morphology of emetic chemoreceptor trigger zone in cat medulla oblongata. Proc. Soc. Exp. Biol. Med. *77*, 38–42 (1951)

Borison, H.L., Wang, S.C.: Physiology and pharmacology of vomiting. Pharmacol. Rev. *5*, 193 (1953)

Boyd, E.M., Cassell, W.A., Boyd, C.E.: Prevention of apomorphine-induced vomiting by (dimethylamino-1-n-propyl-3)-N-(2-chloro)-phenothiazine hydrochloride. Fed. Proc. *12*, 303 (1953)

Bradley, P.B.: Microelectrode approach to the neuropharmacology of the reticular formation. In: Psychotropic Drugs. S. Garattini and V. Ghetti, Eds., pp. 207–216. Elsevier Publishing Company, Amsterdam (1957)

Bradley, P.B.: Electrophysiological evidence relating to the role of adrenaline in the central nervous system. Ciba Foundation Symposium on "Adrenergic Mechanisms", pp. 410–420. Churchill Ltd., London (1960)

Bradley, P.B., Elkes, J.: The effects of some drugs on the electrical activity of the brain. Brain *80*, 77–117 (1957)

Bradley, P.B., Hance, A.J.: The effect of chlorpromazine and methopromazine on the electrical activity of the brain in the cat. Electroencephalogr. Clin. Neurophysiol. *9*, 191–215 (1957)

Bradley, P.B., Key, B.J.: The effect of drugs on arousal responses produced by electrical stimulation of the reticular formation of the brain. Electroencephalogr. Clin. Neurophysiol. *10*, 97–110 (1958)

Bradley, P.B., Mollica, A.: The effect of adrenaline and acetylcholine on single unit activity in the reticular formation of the decerebrate cat. Arch. Ital. Biol. *96*, 168–186 (1958)

Bradley, P.B., Wolstencroft, J.H.: Excitation and inhibition of brain stem neurons by noradrenaline and acetylcholine. Nature *196*, 840 and 873 (1962)

Bradley, P.B., Wolstencroft, J.H.: Actions of drugs on single neurones in the brain stem. Br. Med. Bull. *21*, 15–18 (1965)

Bradley, P.B., Wolstencroft, J.H., Hösli, L., Avanzino, G.L.: Neuronal basis for the central action of chlorpromazine. Nature *212*, 1425–1427 (1966)

Brand, E.D., Harris, T.D., Borison, H.L., Goodman, L.S.: The anti-emetic activity of 10-(γ-dimethylamino propyl)-2-chlorophenothiazine (chlorpromazine) in dog and cat. J. Pharmacol. Exp. Ther. *110*, 86–92 (1954)

Brodie, B.B., Shore, P.A., Silver, S.L., Pulver, R.: Potentiating action of chlorpromazine and reserpine. Nature *175*, 1133–1134 (1955)

Brodie, B.B., Sulser, F., Costa, E.: Theories on mechanism of action of psychotherapeutic drugs. Rev. Can. Biol. *20*, 279–285 (1961)

Buchwald, N.A., Price, D.D., Vernon, L., Hull, C.D.: Caudate intracellular response to thalamic and cortical inputs. Exp. Neurol. *38*, 311–323 (1973)

Bunney, B.S., Aghajanian, G.K.: Electrophysiological effects of amphetamine on dopaminergic neurons. In: Frontiers in Catecholamine Research, S.H. Snyder, E. Usdin, Eds., pp. 957–962, Pergamon Press, Oxford (1973)

Bunney, B.S., Aghajanian, G.K.: A comparison of the effects of chlorpromazine, 7-hydroxychlorpromazine and chlorpromazine sulfoxide on the activity of central dopaminergic neurons. Life Sci. *15*, 309–318 (1974)

Bunney, B.S., Aghajanian, G.K.: d-Amphetamine-induced inhibition of central dopaminergic neurons: mediation by a striato-nigral feedback pathway. Science *192*, 391–393 (1976)

Bunney, B.S., Aghajanian, G.K., Roth, R.H.: Comparison of effect of L-DOPA, amphetamine and apomorphine on firing rate of rat dopaminergic neurones. Nature New Biol. *245*, 123–125 (1973a)

Bunney, B.S., Walters, J.R., Roth, R.H., Aghajanian, G.K.: Dopaminergic neurones: effect of antipsychotic drugs and amphetamine on single cell activity. J. Pharmacol. Exp. Ther. *185*, 560–571 (1973b)

Burt, D.R., Creese, I., Snyder, S.H.: Properties of [³H]haloperidol and [³H]dopamine binding associated with dopamine receptors in calf brain membranes. Mol. Pharmacol. *12*, 800–812 (1976)

Butcher, S.G., Butcher, L.L.: Origin and modulation of acetylcholine activity in the neostriatum. Brain Res. *71*, 167–171 (1974)

Butcher, L.L., Talbot, K., Bilizikjian, L.: Acetylcholinesterase neurones in dopamine-containing regions of the brain. J. Neural. Transm. *37*, 127–153 (1975)

Calne, D.B.: Developments in the treatment of Parkinsonism. New Engl. J. Med. *295*, 1433–1434 (1976)

Capon, A.: Analyse de l'effect d'éveil exercé par l'adrénaline et la noradrénaline et d'autres amines sympathomimétiques sur l'électrocorticogramme du lapin non narcotisé. Arch. Int. Pharmacodyn. Ther. *127*, 141–162 (1960)

Carenzi, A., Gillin, J.C., Guidotti, A., Schwartz, M.A., Trabucchi, M., Wyatt, R.J.: Dopamine-sensitive adenyl cyclase in human caudate nucleus. A study in control subjects and schizophrenic patients. Arch. Gen. Psychiatry *32*, 1056–1059 (1975)

Carlsson, A.: The occurrence, distribution and physiological role of catecholamines in the nervous system. Pharmacol. Rev. *11*, 490–493 (1959)

Carlsson, A.: Discussion. In: Ciba Foundation Symposium on "Adrenergic Mechanisms", p. 551, J.R. Vane, W. Wolstenholme, M. O'Connor Eds., Little, Brown & Co., Boston (1960)

Carlsson, A.: Evidence for a role of dopamine in extrapyramidal functions. Acta Neuroveget. *26*, 484–493 (1964)

Carlsson, A.: Drugs which block the storage of 5-hydroxytryptamine and related amines. In: Handbook of Experimental Pharmacology. Vol. 19: 5-Hydroxytryptamine and Related Indolealkylamines, O. Eichler and A. Farah, Eds., pp. 529–592, Springer-Verlag, Berlin (1965)

Carlsson, A.: Pharmacological depletion of catecholamine stores. Pharmacol. Rev. *18*, 541–549 (1966)

Carlsson, A., Lindqvist, M.: Effect of chlorpromazine and haloperidol on the formation of 3-methoxytyramine and normetanephrine in mouse brain. Acta Pharmacol. Toxicol. (Kbh.) *20*, 140–144 (1963)

Carlsson, A., Waldeck, B.: Inhibition of ³H-metaraminol uptake by antidepressive and related agents. J. Pharm. Pharmacol. *17*, 243–244 (1965)

Carlsson, A., Lindqvist, M., Magnusson, T.: 3,4-Dihydroxyphenylalanine and 5-hydroxytryptophan as reserpine antagonists. Nature *180*, 1200 (1957a)

Carlsson, A., Rosengren, E., Bertler, Å, Nilsson, J.: Effect of reserpine on the metabolism of catechol amines. In: Psychotropic Drugs. S. Garattini, V. Ghetti, Eds., pp. 363–372, Elsevier Publishing Company, Amsterdam (1957b)

Carlsson, A., Lindqvist, M., Magnusson, T., Waldeck, B.: On the presence of 3-hydroxytyramine in brain. Science *127*, 471 (1958)

Carlsson, A., Falck, B., Hillarp, N.-Å.: Cellular localization of brain monoamines. Acta Physiol. Scand. *56*, suppl. 196: 1–28 (1962)

Carlsson, A., Magnusson, T., Rosengren, E.: 5-Hydroxytryptamine of the spinal cord normally and after transection. Experientia *19*, 359 (1963)

Carlsson, A., Falck, B., Fuxe, K., Hillarp, N.-Å.: Cellular localization of monoamines in the spinal cord. Acta Physiol. Scand. *60*, 112–119 (1964)

Carlsson, A., Kehr, W., Lindqvist, M., Magnusson, T., Atack, C.V.: Regulation of monoamine metabolism in the central nervous system. Pharmacol. Rev. *24*, 371–384 (1972)

Caron, M.G., Raymond, V., Lefkowitz, R.J., Labrie, F.: Dopaminergic receptors in the anterior pituitary gland, correlation of [³H]-dihydroergocryptine binding with the dopaminergic control of prolactin release. J. Biol. Chem. *253*, 2244–2253 (1978)

Cassell, W.A., Boyd, C.E.: Prevention of apomorphine-induced vomiting by (dimethylamino-1-n-propyl-3)-N-(2-chloro)-phenothiazine hydrochloride. Fed. Proc. *12*, 303 (1953)

Cathala, H.P., Pocidalo, J.J.: Sur les effets de l'injection dans les ventricules cérébraux du chien du chlorhydrate de diméthylaminopropyl-N-chloro-phénothiazine (4560 RP). Action centrale de ce produit. C. R. Soc. Biol. (Paris) *146*, 1709–1711 (1952)

Chen, G., Ensor, C.R.: Antagonism studies on reserpine and certain CNS depressants. Proc. Soc. Exp. Biol. Med. *87*, 602–608 (1954)

Chen, G., Ensor, C.R., Bohner, B.: A facilitation action of reserpine on the central nervous system. Proc. Soc. Exp. Biol. Med. *86*, 507–510 (1954)

Chin, J.H., Smith, C.M.: Effects of some central nervous system depressants on the phasic and tonic stretch reflex. J. Pharmacol. Exp. Ther. *136*, 276–283 (1962)

Chiueh, C.C., Moore, K.E.: Release of endogenously synthesized catechols from the caudate nucleus by stimulation of the nigro-striatal pathway and by the administration of d-amphetamine. Brain Res. *50*, 221–225 (1973)

Chiueh, C.C., Moore, K.E.: Effects of α-methyltyrosine on d-amphetamine-induced release of endogenously synthesized and exogenously administered catecholamines from the cat brain in vivo. J. Pharmacol. Exp. Ther. *190*, 100–108 (1974)

Clement-Cormier, Y.C., Kebabian, J.W., Petzold, G.L., Greengard, P.: Dopamine-sensitive adenylate cyclase in mammalian brain: a possible site of action of antipsychotic drugs. Proc. Natl. Acad. Sci. USA *71*, 1113–1117 (1974)

Clouet, D.H.: Narcotic Drugs: Biochemical Pharmacology. Plenum Press, New York (1971)

Clubley, M., Elliott, R.C.: Centrally active drugs and the sympathetic nervous system of rabbits and cats. Neuropharmacology *16*, 609–616 (1977)

Commissiong, J.W., Sedgwick, E.M.: A pharmacological study of the adrenergic mechanisms involved in the stretch reflex of the decerebrate rat. Br. J. Pharmacol. *50*, 365–374 (1974)

Commissiong, J.W., Sedgwick, E.M.: Dopamine and noradrenaline in human spinal cord. Lancet I 347 (1975)

Commissiong, J.W., Gentleman, S., Neff, N.H.: Spinal cord dopaminergic neurons: evidence for an uncrossed nigrospinal pathway. Neuropharmacology *18*, 565–568 (1979)

Connor, J.D.: Caudate unit responses to nigral stimuli: evidence for a possible nigro-neostriatal pathway. Science *160*, 899–900 (1968)

Connor, J.D.: Caudate nucleus neurones: correlation of the effects of substantia nigra stimulation with iontophoretic dopamine. J. Physiol. (Lond.) *208*, 691–703 (1970)

Cools, A.R.: The function of dopamine and its antagonism in the caudate nucleus of cats in relation to the stereotyped behaviour. Arch. Int. Pharmacodyn. Ther. *194*, 259–269 (1971)

Cools, A.R.: Chemical and electrical stimulation of the caudate nucleus in freely moving cats: the role of dopamine. Brain Res. *58*, 437–451 (1973)

Cools, A., Van Rossum, J.M.: Excitation-mediating and inhibition-mediating dopamine-receptors: a new concept towards a better understanding of electrophysiological, biochemical, pharmacological, functional and clinical data. Psychopharmacology (Berlin) *45*, 243–254 (1976)

Cools, A.R., Struyker Boudier, H.A.J., Van Rossum, J.M.: Dopamine receptors: relective agonists and antagonists of functionally distinct types within the feline brain. Eur. J. Pharmacol. *37*, 283–293 (1976)

Cordeau, J.P., Moreau, A., Beaulnes, A., Laurin, C.: EEG and behavioural changes following microinjection of acetylcholine in the brain stem of cats. Arch. Ital. Biol. *101*, 30–47 (1963)

Corrodi, H., Fuxe, K., Hökfelt, T.: The effect of neuroleptics on the activity of central catecholamine neurones. Life Sci. *6*, 767–774 (1967)

Corrodi, H., Fuxe, K., Hökfelt, T., Lidbrink, P., Ungerstedt, U.: Effect of ergot drugs on central catecholamine neurons: evidence for a stimulation of central dopamine neurons. J. Pharm. Pharmacol. *25*, 409–412 (1973)

Costa, E.: Effects of hallucinogenic and tranquilizing drugs on serotonin evoked uterine contractions. Proc. Soc. Exp. Biol. Med. *91*, 39–41 (1956)

Costa, E., Gessa, G.L., Hirsch, C., Kuntzman, R., Brodie, B.B.: On current status of serotonin as a brain neurohormone and on action of reserpine-like drugs. Ann. N. Y. Acad. Sci. *96*, 118–130 (1962)

Costall, B., Naylor, R.J.: Specific asymmetric behaviour induced by the direct chemical stimulation of neostriatal dopaminergic mechanisms. Naunyn Schmiedebergs Arch. Pharmacol. *285*, 83–98 (1974a)

Costall, B., Naylor, R.J.: Mesolimbic involvement with behavioural effects indicating antipsychotic activity. Eur. J. Pharmacol. *27*, 46–58 (1974b)

Costall, B., Naylor, R.J.: The importance of the ascending dopaminergic systems to the extrapyramidal and mesolimbic brain areas for the cataleptic action of the neuroleptic and cholinergic agents. Neuropharmacology *13*, 353–364 (1974c)

Costall, B., Olley, J.E.: Cholinergic- and neuroleptic-induced catalepsy: Modification by lesions in the caudate-putamen. Neuropharmacology *10*, 297–306 (1971a)

Costall, B., Olley, J.E.: Cholinergic and neuroleptic induced catalepsy: modification by lesions in the globus pallidus and substantia nigra. Neuropharmacology *10*, 581–594 (1971b)

Costall, B., Naylor, R.J., Olley, J.E.: Catalepsy and circling behavior after intracerebral injections of neuroleptic, cholinergic and anticholinergic agents into the caudate-putamen, globus pallidus and substantia nigra of rat brain. Neuropharmacology *11*, 645–663 (1972)

Courvoisier, S., Fournel, J., Ducrot, R., Kolsky, M., Koetschet, P.: Propriétés pharmacodynamiques du chlorhydrate de chloro-3 (diméthylamino-3'-propyl)-10 phénothiazine (4.560 R.P.). Etude expérimentale d'un nouveau corps utilisé dans l'anesthésie potentialisé et dans l'hibernation artificielle. Arch. Int. Pharmacodyn. Ther. *92*, 305–361 (1953)

Courvoisier, S., Ducrot, R., Julou, L.: Nouveaux aspects expérimentaux de l'activité centrale des dérivés de la phénothiazine. In: Psychotropic Drugs. S. Garattini, V. Ghetti, Eds., pp. 373–391, Elsevier Publishing Company, Amsterdam (1957)

Cranmer, J.I., Brann, A.W., Bach, L.M.N.: An adrenergic basis for bulbar inhibition. Am. J. Physiol. *197*, 835–838 (1959)

Creese, I., Snyder, S.H.: Nigrostriatal lesions enhance striated ^{3}H-apomorphine and ^{3}H-spiroperidol binding. Eur. J. Pharmacol. *56*, 277–281 (1979)

Creese, I.N.R., Burt, D.R., Snyder, S.H.: Dopamine receptor binding predicts clinical and pharmacological potencies of antischizophrenic drugs. Science *129*, 481–483 (1976)

Creese, I., Schneider, R., Snyder, S.H.: ^{3}H-spiroperidol labels dopamine receptors in pituitary and brain. Eur. J. Pharmacol. *46*, 377–381 (1977)

Crossman, A.R., Walker, R.J., Woodruff, G.N.: Picrotoxin antagonism of γ-aminobutyric acid inhibitory responses and synaptic inhibition in the rat substantia nigra. Br. J. Pharmacol. *49*, 696–698 (1973)

Crossman, A.R., Walker, R.J., Woodruff, G.N.: Problems associated with iontophoretic studies in the caudate nucleus and substantia nigra. Neuropharmacology *13*, 547–552 (1974)

Crow, T.J.: What is wrong with dopaminergic transmission in schizophrenia? Trends Neurosci. *2*, 52–55 (1979)

Curtis, D.R.: The action of 3-hydroxytyramine and some tryptamine derivatives upon spinal neurones. Nature *194*, 292 (1962)

Curtis, D.R., Phillis, J.W., Watkins, J.C.: Cholinergic and non-cholinergic transmission in the mammalian spinal cord. J. Physiol. (Lond.) *158*, 296–323 (1961)

Dafny, N., Brown, M., Burks, T.F., Rigor, B.M.: Morphine tolerance and dependence: sensitivity of caudate nucleus neurons. Brain Res. *162*, 363–368 (1979)

Dahlström, A., Fuxe, K.: Experimentally induced changes in the intraneuronal amine levels of bulbospinal neurone systems. Acta Physiol. Scand. *64*, suppl. 247: 1–36 (1965a)

Dahlström, A., Fuxe, K.: Evidence for the existence of monoamine-containing neurons in the central nervous system. Acta Physiol. Scand. *62*, suppl. 232 (1965b)

Dahlström, A., Fuxe, K., Kernell, D., Sedvall, G.: Reduction of the monoamine stores in the terminals of bulbospinal neurones following stimulation in the medulla oblongata. Life Sci. *4*, 1207–1212 (1965)

Da Prada, M., Pletscher, A.: On the mechanism of chlorpromazine-induced changes of cerebral homovanillic acid levels. J. Pharm. Pharmacol. *18*, 628–630 (1966a)

Da Prada, M., Pletscher, A.: Acceleration of the cerebral dopamine turnover by chlorpromazine. Experientia *22*, 465–466 (1966b)

Dasgupta, S.R., Werner, G.: Inhibitory action of chlorpromazine on motor activity. Arch. Int. Pharmacodyn. Ther. *100*, 409–417 (1955)

Dasgupta, S.R., Mukherjee, K.L., Werner, G.: The activity of some central depressant drugs in acute decorticate and diencephalic preparations. Arch. Int. Pharmacodyn. Ther. *97*, 149–156 (1954)

Dell, P.: Intervention of an adrenergic mechanism during brain stem reticular activation. In: Ciba Foundation Symposium (General Series) on "Adrenergic Mechanisms", pp. 393–409, G.E.W. Wolstenholme, Maeve O'Connor., Eds., Churchill, London (1961)

De Maio, D.: Clozapine, a novel major tranquilizer. Arzneim. Forsch. *22*, 919–923 (1972)

Dengler, H.J., Spiegel, H.E., Titus, E.O.: Effects of drugs on uptake of isotopic norepinephrine by cat tissues. Nature *191*, 816–817 (1961)

De Robertis, E., Arnaiz, G., Alberici, M., Butcher, R., Sutherland, E.: Subcellular distribution of adenyl cyclase and cyclic phosphodiesterase in rat brain cortex. J. Biol. Chem. *242*, 3487–3493 (1967)

De Schaepdryver, A.F., Piette, Y., De Launois, A.L.: Brain amines and electroshock threshold. Arch. Int. Pharmacodyn. Ther. *140*, 358–367 (1962)

Dettmar, P.W., Cowan, A., Walter, D.S.: Naloxone antagonizes behavioural effects of d-amphetamine in mice and rats. Neuropharmacology *17*, 1041–1044 (1978)

De Wied, D.: Chlorpromazine and endocrine function. Pharmacol. Rev. *19*, 251–288 (1967)

Dunstan, R., Jackson, D.M.: The demonstration of a change in adrenergic receptor sensitivity in the central nervous system of mice after withdrawal from long term treatment with haloperidol. Psychopharmacology (Berlin) *48*, 105–114 (1976)

Ellaway, P.H., Pascoe, J.E.: Blockage of a spinal pathway by chlorpromazine. J. Physiol. (Lond.) *183*, 46–47 P (1966)

Ellaway, P.H., Pascoe, J.E.: Noradrenaline as a transmitter in the spinal cord. J. Physiol. (Lond.) *197*, 8–10 P (1968)

Ellaway, P.H., Trott, J.R.: The mode of action of 5-hydroxytryptophan in facilitating a stretch reflex in the spinal cat. Exp. Brain Res. *22*, 145–162 (1975)

Engberg, I., Marshall, K.C.: Mechanism of noradrenaline hyperpolarization in spinal cord motoneurones of the cat. Acta Physiol. Scand. *83*, 142–144 (1971)

Engberg, I., Marshall, K.C.: Reversal potential for noradrenaline-induced hyperpolarization of spinal motoneurones of cats. J. Gen. Physiol. *61*, 261 (1973)

Engberg, I., Ryall, R.W.: The action of mono-amines upon spinal neurones. Life Sci. *4*, 2223–2227 (1965)

Engberg, I., Ryall, R.W.: The inhibitory action of noradrenaline and other monoamines on spinal neurones. J. Physiol. (Lond.) *185*, 298–322 (1966)

Engberg, I., Thaller, A.: Hyperpolarizing actions of noradrenaline in spinal motoneurones. Acta Physiol. Scand. *80*, 34A–35A (1970)

Engberg, I., Lundberg, A., Ryall, R.W.: Is the tonic decerebrate inhibition of reflex paths mediated by monoaminergic pathways? Acta Physiol. Scand. *72*, 123–133 (1968)

Engberg, I., Flatman, J.A., Kadzielawa, K.: The hyperpolarization of motoneurones by electrophoretically applied amines and other agents. Acta Physiol. Scand. *91*, 3A–4A (1974)

Ernst, A.M.: Relation between the action of dopamine and apomorphine and their O-methylated derivatives upon the CNS. Psychopharmacologia *7*, 391–399 (1967)

Esplin, D.W., Heaton, D.G.: Effects of reserpine on spinal cord synaptic transmission. J. Pharmacol. Exp. Ther. *121*, 267–271 (1955)

Fedina, L., Lundberg, A., Vyklický, L.: The effect of a noradrenaline liberator (4,alpha-dimethyl-meta-tyramine) on reflex transmission in spinal cats. Acta Physiol. Scand. *83*, 495–504 (1971)

Feldberg, W., Sherwood, S.L.: Injections of drugs into the lateral ventricle of the cat. J. Physiol. (Lond.) *123*, 148–167 (1954)

Fellows, E.J., Cook, L.: The comparative pharmacology of a number of phenothiazine derivatives. In: Psychotropic Drugs. S. Garattini, V. Ghetti, Eds., pp. 397–404, Elsevier Publishing Company, Amsterdam (1957)

Feltz, P.: Dopamine, aminoacids and caudate unitary responses to nigral stimulation. J. Physiol. (Lond.) *205*, 8–9 P (1969)

Feltz, P.: Relation nigro-striatale: essai de differentiation des excitations et inhibitions par micro-iontophorèse de dopamine. J. Physiol. (Paris) *62*, 151 (1970)

Feltz, P.: Monoamines and the excitatory nigro-striatal linkage. Experientia *27*, 1111–1112 (1971 a)

Feltz, P.: Sensitivity to haloperidol of caudate neurones excited by nigral stimulation. Eur. J. Pharmacol. *14*, 360–364 (1971 b)

Feltz, P.: γ-Aminobutyric acid and a caudato-nigral inhibition. Can. J. Physiol. Pharmacol. *49*, 1113–1115 (1971 c)

Feltz, P., Albe-Fessard, D.: A study of an ascending nigrocaudate pathway. Electroencephalogr. Clin. Neurophysiol. *33*, 179–193 (1972)

Feltz, P., De Champlain, J.: Persistence of caudate unitary responses to nigral stimulation after destruction and functional impairment of the striatal dopaminergic terminals. Brain Res. *43*, 595–600 (1972a)

Feltz, P., De Champlain, J.: Enhanced sensitivity of caudate neurons to microiontophoretic injections of dopamine in 6-hydroxydopamine treated rats. Brain Res. *43*, 601–605 (1972b)

Feltz, P., Mackenzie, J.S.: Properties of caudate unitary responses to repetitive nigral stimulation. Brain Res. *13*, 612–616 (1969)

Flach, F.: Clinical effectiveness of reserpine. Ann. N. Y. Acad. Sci. *61*, 161–166 (1955)

Flückiger, E., Wagner, H.R.: 2-Br-α-Ergokryptin: Beeinflussung von Fertilität und Laktation bei der Ratte. Experientia *24*, 1130–1131 (1968)

Fonnum, F., Grofová, I, Rinvik, E., Storm-Mathisen, J., Walberg, F.: Origin and distribution of glutamine decarboxylase in the substantia nigra of the cat. Brain Res. *71*, 77–92 (1974)

Forssberg, H., Grillner, S.: The locomotion of the acute spinal cat injected with clonidine i.v. Brain Res. *50*, 184–186 (1973)

Frantz, A.G.: Catecholamines and the control of prolactin secretion in humans. Prog. Brain Res. *39*, 311–322 (1973)

Frigyesi, T.L., Purpura, D.P.: Electro-physiological analysis of reciprocal caudato-nigral relations. Brain Res. *6*, 440–456 (1967)

Fu, T.-C., Jankowska, E., Lundberg, A.: Reciprocal Ia inhibition during the late reflexes evoked from the flexor reflex afferents after DOPA. Brain Res. *85*, 99–102 (1975)

Fuxe, K., Gunne, L.-M.: Depletion of the amine stores in brain catecholamine terminals on amygdaloid stimulation. Acta Physiol. Scand. *62*, 493–494 (1964)

Fuxe, K., Hökfelt, T., Johansson, O., Jonsson, G., Lidbrink, P., Ljungdahl, Å: The origin of the dopamine nerve terminals in limbic and frontal cortex. Evidence for meso-cortico dopamine neurons. Brain Res. *82*, 349–355 (1974)

Gaddum, J.H., Vogt, M.: Some central actions of 5-hydroxytryptamine and various antagonists. Br. J. Pharmacol. *11*, 175–179 (1956)

Gaitondé, B.B., McCarthy, L.E., Borison, H.L.: Central emetic action and toxic effects of digitalis in cats. J. Pharmacol. Exp. Ther. *147*, 409–415 (1965)

Gale, K., Moroni, F., Kumakura, K., Guidotti, A.: Opiate-receptors in substantia nigra: role in the regulation of striatal tyrosine hydroxylase activity. Neuropharmacology *18*, 427–430 (1979)

Gangloff, H., Monnier, M.: Topische Bestimmung des zerebralen Angriffs von Reserpin (Serpasil). Experientia *11*, 404–407 (1955)

Geffen, L.B., Jessell, T.M., Cuello, A.C., Iversen, L.L.: Release of dopamine from dendrites in rat substantia nigra. Nature *260*, 258–260 (1976)

Gérardy, J., Quinaux, N., Maeda, T., Dresse, A.: Analyse des monoamines du locus coeruleus et d'autres structures cérébrales par chromatographie sur couche mince. Arch. Int. Pharmacodyn. Ther. *177*, 492–496 (1969)

Gey, K.F., Pletscher, A.: Effects of chlorpromazine on the metabolism of dl-2-C^{14}-Dopa in the rat. J. Pharmacol. Exp. Ther. *145*, 337–343 (1964)

Glaviano, V.V., Wang, S.C.: Dual mechanism of anti-emetic action of 10 (γ-dimethylaminopropyl)-2-chlorphenothiazine hydrochloride (chlorpromazine) in dogs. J. Pharmacol. Exp. Ther. *114*, 358–366 (1955)

Glow, P.: Some aspects of the effects of acute reserpine treatment on behaviour. J. Neurol. Neurosurg. Psychiatry *22*, 11–32 (1959)

Glowinski, J., Axelrod, J.: Effect of drugs on the uptake, release, and metabolism of H^3-norepinephrine in the rat brain. J. Pharmacol. Exp. Ther. *149*, 43–49 (1965)

Glowinski, J., Axelrod, J.: Effects of drugs on the disposition of ^{3}H-norepinephrine in the rat brain. Pharmacol. Rev. *18*, 775–785 (1966)

Glowinski, J., Iversen, L.L.: Regional studies of catecholamines in the rat brain. I. The disposition of [^{3}H] norepinephrine, [^{3}H] dopamine and [^{3}H] dopa in various regions of the brain. J. Neurochem. *13*, 655–669 (1966)

Gokhale, S.D., Gulati, O.D., Parikh, H.M.: An investigation of the adrenergic blocking action of chlorpromazine. Br. J. Pharmacol. *23*, 508–520 (1964)

Goldstein, M., Anagnoste, B., Owen, W.S., Battista, A.F.: The effects of ventromedial segmental lesions on the disposition of dopamine in the caudate nucleus of the monkey. Brain Res. *4*, 298–300 (1967)

Goldstein, M., Anagnoste, B., Shirron, C.: The effect of trivastal, haloperidol and dibutyryl cyclic AMP on [¹⁴C] dopamine synthesis in rat striatum. J. Pharm. Pharmacol. *25*, 348–351 (1973)

Goldstein, M., Lieberman, A., Battista, A.F., Lew, J.Y., Matsumoto, Y.: Experimental and clinical studies on bromocriptine in the Parkinsonism syndrome. Acta Endocrinol. (Copenh.) *88*, suppl. *216*, 57–66 (1978)

Gonzalez-Vegas, J.A.: Antagonism of dopamine-mediated inhibition in the nigro-striatal pathway: a mode of action of some catatonia-inducing drugs. Brain Res. *80*, 219–228 (1974)

Graham, A.W., Aghajanian, G.K.: Effects of amphetamine on single cell activity in a catecholamine nucleus, the locus coeruleus. Nature *234*, 100–102 (1971)

Granit, R.: Receptors and Sensory Perception. Yale University Press, New Haven (1955)

Griffith, J.D., Cavanaugh, J., Held, J., Oates, J.A.: Dextroamphetamine, evaluation of psychomimetic properties in man. Arch. Gen. Psychiatry *26*, 97–100 (1972)

Grillner, S.: The influence of DOPA on the static and the dynamic fusimotor activity to the triceps surae of the spinal cat. Acta Physiol. Scand. *77*, 490–509 (1969)

Grillner, S.: Locomotion in the spinal cat. In: Control of Posture and Locomotion. R.B. Stein, K.B. Pearson, R.S. Smith, and J.B. Redford, Eds., pp. 515–535, Plenum Press, New York (1973)

Gross, H., Langner, E.: Das Wirkungsprofil eines chemisch neuartigen Breitbandneuroleptikums der Dibenzodiazepingruppe. Wien. Med. Wochenschr. *116*, 814–816 (1966)

Grossmann, W., Jurna, I., Nell, T.: The effect of reserpine and DOPA on reflex activity in the rat spinal cord. Exp. Brain Res. *22*, 351–361 (1975)

Grossmann, W., Jurna, I., Nell, T., Theres, C.: The dependence of the anti-nociceptive effect of morphine and other analgesic agents on spinal motor activity after central monoamine depletion. Eur. J. Pharmacol. *24*, 67–77 (1973)

Groves, P.M., Rebec, G.V., Harvey, J.A.: Alteration of the effects of (+)-amphetamine on neuronal activity in the striatum following lesions of the nigrostriatal bundle. Neuropharmacology *14*, 369–376 (1975a)

Groves, P.M., Wilson, C.J., Young, S.J., Rebec, G.V.: Self-inhibition by dopaminergic neurons. An alternative to the "neuronal feedback loop" hypothesis for the mode of action of certain psychotropic drugs. Science *190*, 522–529 (1975b)

Gulley, R.L., Smithberg, M.: Synapses in the rat substantia nigra. Tissue Cell *3*, 691–700 (1971)

Guyenet, P.G., Agid, Y., Javoy, F., Beaujouan, J.C., Rossier, J., Glowinsky, J.: Effects of dopaminergic receptor agonists and antagonists on the activity of the neo-striatal cholinergic system. Brain Res. *84*, 227–244 (1975a)

Guyenet, P.G., Javoy, F., Agid, Y., Beaujouan, J.C., Glowinski, J.: Dopamine receptors and cholinergic neurons in the rat neostriatum. Adv. Neurol. *9* 43–51 (1975b)

Gyermek, L.: Chlorpromazine: a serotonin antagonist? Lancet II: 724 (1955)

Häggendal, J., Hamberger, B.: Quantitative in vitro studies on noradrenaline uptake and its inhibition by amphetamine, desipramine and chlorpromazine. Acta Physiol. Scand. *70*, 277–280 (1967)

Hamberger, B.: Reserpine-resistant uptake of catecholamines in isolated tissues of the rat. Acta Physiol. Scand. *71*, 1–56 (1967)

Harris, J.E.: Beta adrenergic receptor-mediated adenosine cyclic 3′,5′-monophosphate accumulation in the rat corpus striatum. Mol. Pharmacol. *12*, 546–558 (1976)

Harris, J.E., Baldessarini, R., Wheeler, S.: Stimulation of tyrosine hydroxylation in striatal synaptosomes by derivatives of adenosine 3′,5′-cyclic phosphate. Fed. Proc. *33*, 521 (1974a)

Harris, J.E., Morgenroth III, V.H., Roth, R.H., Baldessarini, R.J.: Regulation of catecholamine synthesis in the rat brain in vitro by cyclic AMP. Nature *252*, 156–158 (1974b)

Heal, D.J., Phillips, A.G., Green, A.R.: Studies on the locomotor activity produced by injection of dibutyryl cyclic 3′5′AMP into the nucleus accumbens of rats. Neuropharmacology *17*, 265–270 (1978)

Heinz, G., Jurna, I.: The anti-nociceptive effect of reserpine and haloperidol mediated by the nigro-striatal system: antagonism by naloxone. Naunyn Schmiedebergs Arch. Pharmacol. *306*, 97–100 (1979)

Henatsch, H.D., Ingvar, D.H.: Chlorpromazin und Spastizität: Eine experimentelle elektrophysiologische Untersuchung. Arch. Psychiatr. Z. Neurol. *195*, 77–93 (1956)

Herman, E.H., Barnes, C.D.: Evidence for an action of chlorpromazine on the spinal cord. Fed. Proc. *23*, 456 (1964)

Hernández-Peón, R.: Central neuro-humoral transmission in sleep and wakefulness. In: Sleep Mechanisms. Progress in Brain Research, Vol. 18, pp. 96–117. Akert, K., Bally, C., Schadé, J.P., Eds., Elsevier Publishing Company, Amsterdam (1963)

Hertting, G., Axelrod, J., Whitby, L.G.: Effect of drugs on the uptake and metabolism of H^3-norepinephrine. J. Pharmacol. Exp. Ther. *134*, 146–153 (1961)

Herz, A., Gogolák, G.: Mikroelektrophoretische Untersuchungen am Septum des Kaninchens. Pflügers Arch. *285*, 317–330 (1965)

Herz, A., Nacimiento, A.: Über die Wirkung von Pharmaka auf Neurone des Hippocampus nach mikroelektrophoretischer Verabfolgung. Naunyn Schmiedebergs Arch. Pharmacol. *251*, 295–314 (1965)

Herz, A., Von Freytag-Loringhoven, H.: Über die synaptische Erregung im Corpus striatum und deren antagonistische Beeinflussung durch mikroelektrophoretisch verabfolgte Glutaminsäure und Gamma-Aminobuttersäure. Pflügers Arch. Ges. Physiol. *229*, 167–184 (1968)

Herz, A., Zieglgänsberger, W.: Synaptic excitation in the corpus striatum inhibited by microelectrophoretically administered dopamine. Experientia *22*, 839–840 (1966)

Herz, A., Zieglgänsberger, W.: The influence of microelectrophoretically applied biogenic amines, cholinomimetics and procaine on synaptic excitation in the corpus striatum. Neuropharmacology *7*, 221–230 (1968)

Hiebel, G., Bonvallet, M., Dell, P.: Action de la chlorpromazine ("Largactil", 4560 RP) au niveau du système nerveux central. Hop. Paris *30*, 2346–2353 (1954)

Hillarp, N.-Å., Fuxe, K., Dahlström, A.: Demonstration and mapping of central neurons containing dopamine, noradrenaline, and 5-hydroxytryptamine and their reactions to psychopharmaca. Pharmacol. Rev. *18*, 727–741 (1966)

Hilton, S.M., Zbrożyna, A.W.: Amygdaloid region for defence reactions and its efferent pathway to the brain stem. J. Physiol. (Lond.) *165*, 160–173 (1963)

Hoffer, B.J., Siggins, G.R., Bloom, F.E.: Cyclic 3′,5′-adenosine monophosphate (c-AMP) mediation of the response of rat cerebellar Purkinje cells to norepinephrine (NE): Blockade with prostaglandins. Pharmacologist *11*, 238 (1969)

Hofmann, M., Battaini, F., Tonon, G., Trabucchi, M. Spano, P.: Interaction of sulpiride and ergot derivatives on rat brain DOPAC concentration and prolactin secretion in vivo. Eur. J. Pharmacol. *56*, 15–20 (1979)

Hong, J.S., Yang, H.-Y.T., Costa, E.: On the location of methionine enkephalin neurons in rat striatum. Neuropharmacology *16*, 451–453 (1977)

Horn, A.S., Snyder, S.H.: Chlorpromazine and dopamine: conformational similarities that correlate with the antischizophrenic activity of phenothiazine drugs. Proc. Natl. Acad. Sci. USA *68*, 2325–2328 (1971)

Hornykiewicz, O.: Dopamine (3-hydroxytyramine) and brain function. Pharmacol. Rev. *18*, 925–964 (1966)

Huang, M., Ho, A.K.S., Daly, J.W.: Accumulation of adenosine cyclic 3′,5′-monophosphate in rat cerebral cortical slices. Stimulatory effect of alpha and beta adrenergic agents after treatment with 6-hydroxydopamine, 2,3,5-trihydroxyphenethylamine and dihydroxytryptamines. Mol. Pharmacol. *9*, 711–717 (1973)

Hudson, R.D.: Effects of chlorpromazine on spinal cord reflex mechanisms. Neuropharmacology *5*, 43–58 (1966)

Hudson, R.D., Domino, E.F.: Effects of chlorpromazine on some motor reflexes. Neuropharmacology *2*, 143–162 (1963)

Hudson, R.D., Domino, E.F.: Comparative effects of three substituted phenothiazines on the patellar reflex and mean arterial blood pressure of the rabbit. Arch. Int. Pharmacodyn. Ther. *147*, 36–42 (1964)

Huidobro, F.: Some pharmacological properties of chloro-3(dimethylamine-3′propyl)10-phenothiazine or 4.560 R. P. Arch. Int. Pharmacodyn. Ther. *98*, 308–319 (1954)

Hull, C.D., Bernardi, G., Buchwald, N.A.: Intracellular responses of caudate neurons to brain stem stimulation. Brain Res. *22*, 163–179 (1970)

Hull, C.D., Bernardi, G., Price, D.D., Buchwald, N.A.: Intracellular responses of caudate neurons to temporaly and spatially combined stimuli. Exp. Neurol. *38*, 324–336 (1973)

Hyttel, J.: Effects of neuroleptics on ³H-haloperidol and ³H-cis(Z)-flupenthixol binding and on adenylate cyclase activity in vitro. Life Sci. *23*, 551–556 (1978)

Irwin, S., Houde, R.W., Bennet, D.R., Hendershot, L.C., Seevers, M.H.: The effects of morphine, methadone and meperidine on some reflex responses in spinal animals to nociceptive stimulation. J. Pharmacol. Exp. Ther. *101*, 132–143 (1951)

Iversen, L.L.: The inhibition of noradrenaline uptake by drugs. In: Advances in Drug Research. Harper, N.J., Simmonds, A.B., Eds., *2*, 1–46, Academic Press, London (1965)

Iversen, L.L.: Dopamine receptors in the brain (A dopamine-sensitive adenylate cyclase models synaptic receptors, illuminating antipsychotic drug action). Science *188*, 1084–1089 (1975)

Iversen, L.L.: More than one type of dopamine receptor in brain? Trends Neuro Sci. *1*, V–VI (1978 a)

Iversen, L.L.: Biochemical and pharmacological studies: the dopamine hypothesis. In: Schizophrenia: Towards a New Synthesis. J.K. Wing, Ed., Academic Press, London, pp. 89–116 (1978 b)

Ivy, A.C., Goetzel, F.R., Harris, S.C., Burril, D.Y.: The analgesic effect of intracarotid and intravenous injection of epinephrine in dogs and of subcutaneous injection in man. Quart. Bull. Northwestern University Med. School *18*, 298–306 (1944)

Iwamoto, E., Way, L.: Circling behaviour and stereotypy induced by intranigral opiate microinjections. J. Pharmacol. Exp. Ther. *203*, 347–359 (1977)

Iwatsubo, K., Clouet, D.H.: Dopamine-sensitive adenylate cyclase of the caudate nucleus of rats treated with morphine or haloperidol. Biochem. Pharmacol. *24*, 1499–1503 (1975)

Iwatsubo, K., Clouet, D.H.: Effects of morphine and haloperidol on the electrical activity of rat nigrostriatal neurons. J. Pharmacol. Exp. Ther. *202*, 429–436 (1977)

Jacobowitz, D.M., Goldberg, A.M.: Determination of acetylcholine in discrete regions of the rat brain. Brain Res. *122*, 575–577 (1971)

James, T.A., Massey, S.: Evidence for a possible dopaminergic link in the action of acetylcholine in the rat substantia nigra. Neuropharmacology *17*, 687–690 (1978)

Jankowska, E., Jukes, M.G.M., Lund, S., Lundberg, A.: Reciprocal innervation through interneuronal inhibition. Nature *206*, 198–199 (1965)

Jankowska, E., Jukes, M.G.M., Lund, S., Lundberg, A.: The effect of dopa on the spinal cord. 5. Reciprocal organization of pathways transmitting excitatory action to alpha-motoneurones of flexors and extensors. Acta Physiol. Scand. *70*, 369–388 (1967 a)

Jankowska, E., Jukes, M.G.M., Lund, S., Lundberg, A.: The effect of DOPA on the spinal cord. 6. Halfcentre organization of interneurones transmitting effects from the flexor reflex afferents. Acta Physiol. Scand. *70*, 389–402 (1967 b)

Janssen, P.A.J.: The pharmacology of haloperidol. Int. J. Neuropsychiatr. *3*, suppl. 1, S 10–S 18 (1967)

Janssen, P.A.J., Allewijn, F.T.N.: The distribution of the butyrophenones haloperidol, trifluperidol, moperone, and clofluperidol in rats, and its relationship with their neuroleptic activity. Arzneim. Forsch. *19*, 199–208 (1969)

Janssen, P.A.J., Niemegeers, C.J.E., Schellekens, K.H.L.: Is it possible to predict the clinical effects of neuroleptic drugs (major tranquillizers) from animal data? Part I: "Neuroleptic activity spectra" for rats. Arzneim. Forsch. *15*, 104–117 (1965 a)

Janssen, P.A.J., Niemegeers, C.J.E., Schellekens, K.H.L.: Is it possible to predict the clinical effects of neuroleptic drugs (major tranquillizers) from animal data? Part II: "Neuroleptic activity spectra" for dogs. Arzneim. Forsch. *15*, 1196–1206 (1965 b)

Janssen, P.A.J., Niemegeers, C.J.E., Schellekens, K.H.L., Dresse, A., Lenaerts, F.M., Pinchard, A., Schaper, W.K.A., Van Nueten, J.M., Verbruggen, F.J.: Pimozide, a chemically novel, highly potent and orally long-acting neuroleptic drug. Part I: The comparative pharmacology of pimozide, haloperidol, and chlorpromazine. Arzneim. Forsch. *18*, 261–279 (1968 a)

Janssen, P.A.J., Soudijn, W., Van Wijngaarden, I., Dresse, A.: Pimozide, a chemically novel, highly potent and orally long-acting neuroleptic drug. Part III: Regional distribution of pimozide and haloperidol in the dog brain. Arzneim. Forsch. *18*, 282–287 (1968 b)

Javoy, P., Agid, Y., Bouvet, D., Glowinski, J.: Changes in neostriatal DA metabolism after carbachol or atropine microinjections into the substantia nigra. Brain Res. *68*, 253–260 (1974)

Jenney, E.H.: Changes in convulsant thresholds after Rauwolfia serpentina, reserpine and veriloid. Fed. Proc. *13*, 370–371 (1954)

Jobe, P.C., Geiger, P.F., Ray, T.B., Woods, T.W., Mims, M.E.: The relative significance of spinal cord norepinephrine and 5-hydroxytryptamine in electrically induced seizure in the rat. Neuropharmacology *17*, 185–190 (1978)

Johnson, A.M., Loew, D.M., Vigouret, J.M.: Stimulant properties of bromocriptine on central dopamine receptors in comparison to apomorphine, (+)-amphetamine and L-DOPA. Br. J. Pharmacol. *56*, 59–68 (1976)

Johnstone, E.C., Crow, T.J., Frith, C.D., Carney, M.W.P., Price, J.S.: Mechanism of the antipsychotic effect in the treatment of acute schizophrenia. Lancet I: 848–851 (1978)

Jordan, L.M., Lake, N., Phillis, J.W.: Mechanism of noradrenaline depression of cortical neurones: a species comparison. Eur. J. Pharmacol. *20*, 381–384 (1972)

Juorio, A.V., Sharman, D.F., Trajkov, T.: The effect of drugs on the homovanillic acid content of the corpus striatum of some rodents. Br. J. Pharmacol. *26*, 385–392 (1966)

Jurna, I.: Dämpfung repetivier Aktivierungsvorgänge an der spinalen Motorik durch Morphin. In: Schmerz (Pain). R. Janzen, W.D. Keidel, A. Herz, C. Steichele, J.P. Payne and R.A.P. Burt, Eds., pp. 267–269. Stuttgart: Thieme 1972

Jurna, I.: Striatal monoamines and reserpine and chlorpromazine rigidity. Pharmacol. Ther. [B] *2*, 113–128 (1976a)

Jurna, I.: The cholinergic rigidity. Pharmacol. Ther. [B] *2*, 413–421 (1976b)

Jurna, I., Heinz, G.: Anti-nociceptive effect of morphine, opioid analgesics and haloperidol injected into the caudate nucleus of the rat. Naunyn Schmiedebergs Arch. Pharmacol. *309*, 145–151 (1979)

Jurna, I., Lanzer, G.: Inhibition of the effect of reserpine on motor control by drugs which influence reserpine rigidity. Naunyn Schmiedebergs Arch. Pharmacol. *262*, 309–324 (1969)

Jurna, I., Lundberg, A.: The influence of an inhibitor of dopamine-beta-hydroxylase on the effect of DOPA on transmission in the spinal cord. In: Structure and Functions of Inhibitory Neuronal Mechanisms, pp. 215–219, C. von Euler, S. Skoglund, U. Söderberg, Eds., Pergamon Press, Oxford, New York (1968)

Jurna, I., Regélhy, B.: The antagonism between reserpine some antiparkinson drugs in electroseizure. Naunyn Schmiedebergs Arch. Pharmacol. *259*, 442–459 (1968)

Jurna, I., Theres, C.: The effect of phenytoin and metamphetamine on spinal motor activity. Naunyn Schmiedebergs Arch. Pharmacol. *265*, 244–259 (1969)

Jurna, I., Theres, C., Bachmann, T.: The effect of physostigmine and tetrabenazine on spinal motor control and its inhibition by drugs which influence reserpine rigidity. Naunyn Schmiedebergs Arch. Pharmacol. *263*, 427–438 (1969)

Jurna, I., Nell, T., Schreyer, I.: Motor disturbance induced by tremorine and oxotremorine. Naunyn Schmiedebergs Arch. Pharmacol. *267*, 80–98 (1970)

Jurna, I., Grossmann, W., Nell, T.: Depression by amantadine of drug-induced rigidity in the rat. Neuropharmacology *11*, 559–564 (1972a)

Jurna, I., Ruždić, N., Nell, T., Grossmann, W.: The effect of α-methyl-p-tyrosine and substantia nigra lesions on spinal motor activity in the rat. Eur. J. Pharmacol. *20*, 341–350 (1972b)

Jurna, I., Grossmann, W., Theres, C.: Inhibition by morphine of repetitive activation of cat spinal motoneurons. Neuropharmacology *12*, 983–993 (1973)

Jurna, I., Brenner, M., Drum, P.: Abolition of spinal motor disturbance by injections of dopamine receptor agonists, atropine and GABA into the caudate nucleus. Neuropharmacology *17*, 35–44 (1978a)

Jurna, I., Heinz, G., Blinn, G., Nell, T.: The effect of substantia nigra stimulation and morphine on α-motoneurones and the tail-flick response. Eur. J. Pharmacol. *51*, 239–250 (1978b)

Kaelber, W.W., Joynt, R.J.: Tremor production in cats given chlorpromazine. Proc. Soc. Exp. Biol. Med. *92*, 399–402 (1956)

Kalisker, A., Rutledge, C.O., Perkins, J.P.: Effect of nerve degeneration by 6-hydroxydopamine on chatecholamine-stimulated adenosine 3′,5′-monophosphate formation in rat cerebral cortex. Mol. Pharmacol. *9*, 619–629 (1973)

Kamberi, I.A., Mical, L.S., Porter, J.C.: Effect of anterior pituitary perfusion and intraventricular injection of catecholamines and indolamines in LH release. Endocrinology *87*, 1–12 (1970)

Karobath, M., Leitich, H.: Antipsychotic drugs and dopamine-stimulated adenylate cyclase prepared from corpus striatum of rat brain. Proc. Natl. Acad. Sci. USA *71*, 2915–2918 (1974)

Kebabian, J.W.: Multiple classes of dopamine receptors in mammalian central nervous system: the involvement of dopamine-sensitive adenyl cyclase. Life Sci. *23*, 479–484 (1978)

Kebabian, J.W., Calne, D.B.: Multiple receptors for dopamine. Nature *277*, 93–96 (1979)

Kebabian, J.W., Greengard, P.: Dopamine-sensitive adenyl cyclase: possible role in synaptic transmission. Science *174*, 1346–1349 (1971)

Kebabian, J.W., Saavedra, J.M.: Dopamine-sensitive adenylate cyclase occurs in a region of substantia nigra containing dopaminergic dendrites. Science *193*, 683–685 (1976)

Kebabian, J.W., Petzold, G.L., Greengard, P.: Dopamine-sensitive adenylate cyclase in caudate nucleus of rat brain, and its similarity to the dopamine receptor. Proc. Natl. Acad. Sci. USA *69*, 2145–2149 (1972)

Kehr, W., Carlsson, A., Lindqvist, M., Magnusson, T., Atack, C.: Evidence for a receptor-mediated feedback control of striatal tyrosine hydroxylase activity. J. Pharm. Pharmacol. *24*, 744–747 (1972)

Kelly, P.H., Miller, R.J.: The interaction of neuroleptic and muscarinic agents with central dopaminergic system. Br. J. Pharmacol. *54*, 115–121 (1975)

Kelly, P.H., Moore, K.E.: Mesolimbic dopaminergic neurones in the rotational model of nigrostriatal function. Nature *263*, 695–696 (1976)

Kelly, P.H., Moore, K.E.: Dopamine concentrations in the rat brain following injections into the substantia nigra of baclofen, γ-aminobutyric acid, γ-hydroxybutyric acid, apomorphine and amphetamine. Neuropharmacology *17*, 169–174 (1978)

Kety, S.S., Javoy, F., Thierry, A.-M., Julou, L., Glowinski, J.: A sustained effect of electroconvulsive shock on the turnover of norepinephrine in the central nervous system of the rat. Proc. Natl. Acad. Sci. USA *58*, 1249–1254 (1967)

Key, B.J.: Electrocortical changes induced by perfusion of catecholamines into the brainstem reticular formation. Neuropharmacology *14*, 41–51 (1975)

Killam, E.K., Killam, K.F.: A comparison of the effects of reserpine and chlorpromazine to those of barbiturates on central afferent systems in the cat. J. Pharmacol. Exp. Ther. *116*, 35 (1956)

Killam, E.K., Killam, K.F., Shaw, T.: The effects of psychotherapeutic compounds on central afferent and limbic pathways. Ann. N. Y. Acad. Sci. *66*, 784–805 (1957)

Kim, J.-S., Hassler, R.: Effects of acute haloperidol on the gamma-aminobutyric acid system in rat striatum and substantia nigra. Brain Res. *88*, 150–153 (1975)

Kim, J.S., Bak, I.J., Hassler, R., Okada, Y.: Role of γ-aminobutyric acid (GABA) in the extrapyramidal motor system. 2. Some evidence for the existence of a type of GABA-rich strionigral neurons. Brain Res. *14*, 95–104 (1971)

King, J.L.: The cortico-spinal tract of the rat. Anat. Rec. *4*, 245–252 (1910)

Kinross-Wright, V.: Chlorpromazine and reserpine in the treatment of psychoses. Ann. N.Y. Acad. Sci. *61*, 174–182 (1955)

Kitai, S.T., Wagner, A., Precht, W., Ohno, T.: Nigro-caudate and caudato-nigral relationship: an electrophysiological study. Brain Res. *85*, 44–48 (1975)

Kitai, S.T., Sugimori, M., Kocsis, J.D.: Excitatory nature of dopamine in the nigro-caudate pathway. Exp. Brain Res. *24*, 351–363 (1976)

Klawans, H.L.: The pharmacology of Parkinsonism (a review). Dis. Nerv. Syst. *29*, 805–817 (1968)

Klawans, H.L., Rubovits, R.: An experimental model of tardive dykinesia. J. Neural. Transm. *33*, 235–246 (1972)

Kleinberg, D.L., Noel, G.L., Frantz, A.G.: Chlorpromazine stimulation and L-DOPA suppression of plasma prolactin in man. J. Clin. Endocrinol. Metab. *33*, 873–876 (1971)

Kline, N.S., Stanley, A.M.: Use of reserpine in a neuropsychiatric hospital. Ann. N. Y. Acad. Sci. *61*, 85–91 (1955)

Kobinger, W.: Reversibility of a facilitatory action of reserpine on the central nervous system, by methylamphetamine. Experientia *14*, 337–338 (1958)

Koe, B.K., Weissman, A.: p-chlorophenylalanine: a specific depletor of brain serotonin. J. Pharmacol. Exp. Ther. *154*, 499–516 (1966)

Kolmodin, G.M., Skoglund, C.R.: Properties and functional differentiation of interneurons in the ventral horn of the cat's lumbar cord as revealed by intracellular recording. Experientia *10*, 505–506 (1954)

Korf, J., Zieleman, M., Westerink, B.H.C.: Dopamine release in substantia nigra. Nature 260, 257–258 (1976)

Kosterlitz, H.W., Collier, H.O.J., Villareal, J.E.: Agonist and Antagonist Actions of Narcotic Analgesic Drugs. Macmillan, London (1972)

Kreindler, A., Steriade, M., Zuckermann, E., Chimon, D.: The influence of chlorpromazine upon cerebello-cortical and cerebello-spinal circuits. Electroencephalogr. Clin. Neurophysiol. 10, 515–520 (1958)

Krnjević, K., Phillis, J.W.: Actions of certain amines on cerebral cortical neurones. Br. J. Pharmacol. 20, 471–490 (1963)

Kruglov, N.A., Sinitsyn, L.N.: The effect of aminozine and mepazine on the cerebellar and bulbar inhibitory mechanisms. Farmak. Toksikol. 22, 97–101 (1959)

Kuschinsky, K., Hornykiewicz, O.: Morphine catalepsy in the rat: relation to striatal dopamine metabolism. Eur. J. Pharmacol. 19, 119–122 (1972)

Laborit, H., Huguenard, P.: L'hibernation artificielle par moyens pharmacodynamiques et physiques. Presse Med. 59, 1329 (1951)

Ladinsky, H., Consolo, S., Bianchi, S., Samanin, R., Ghezzi, D.: Cholinergic-dopaminergic interaction in the striatum: the effect of 6-hydroxydopamine or pimozide treatment on the increased striatal acetylcholine levels induced by apomorphine, piribedil and d-amphetamine. Brain Res. 84, 221–226 (1975)

Lake, N., Jordan, L.M.: Failure to confirm cyclic AMP as second messenger for norepinephrine in rat cerebellum. Science 183, 663–664 (1974)

Lake, N., Jordan, L.M., Phillis, J.W.: Mechanisms of noradrenaline action in cat cerebral cortex. Nature New Biol. 240, 249–250 (1972)

Lake, N., Jordan, L.M., Phillis, J.W.: Evidence against cyclic adenosine 3′,5′-monophosphate (cAMP) mediation of noradrenaline depression of cerebral cortical neurones. Brain Res. 60, 411–421 (1973)

Launay, J. Despature, M.: Syndromes psycho-moteurs et syndromes extra-pyramidaux au cours de traitements prolongés par la chlorpromazine. Ann. Med. Psychol. (Paris) 114, 340–344 (1956)

Laverty, R., Sharman, D.F.: Modification by drugs of the metabolism of 3,4-dihydroxyphenylethylamine, noradrenaline and 5-hydroxytryptamine in the brain. Br. J. Pharmacol. 24, 759–772 (1965)

Legge, K.F., Randić, M., Straughan, D.W.: The pharmacology of neurones in the pyriform cortex. Br. J. Pharmacol. 26, 87–107 (1966)

Lee, C.-Y., Akera, T., Stolman, S., Brody, T.M.: Saturable binding of dihydromorphine and naloxon to rat brain tissue in vitro. J. Pharmacol. Exp. Ther. 194, 583–592 (1975)

Lee, C.M., Wong, P.C.L., Chan, S.H.H.: The involvement of dopaminergic neurotransmission in the inhibitory effect of morphine on caudate neurone activities. Neuropharmacology 16, 571–576 (1977)

Lee, T., Seeman, P., Tourtelotte, W.W., Farley, I.J., Hornykiewicz, O.: Binding of ^{3}H-neuroleptics and ^{3}H-apomorphine in schizophrenic brains. Nature 274, 897–900 (1978)

Lee, H.K., Chai, C.Y., Chung, P.M., Wang, S.C.: Central antiemetic actions of pimozide and haloperidol in the dog. Neuropharmacology 18, 341–346 (1979)

Lehmann, A.: Contribution à l'étude psycho-physiologique et neuropharmacologique de l'épilepsie acoustique de la souris et du rat. II. Etude expérimentale. Agressologie 5, 311–351 (1964)

Lehmann, A.: Audiogenic seizures data in mice supporting new theories of biogenic amines mechanisms in the central nervous system. Life Sci. 6, 1423–1431 (1967)

Leimdorfer, A.: Über zentrale Wirkungen von Adrenalin. Wien. Klin. Wochenschr. 60, 382–385 (1948)

Leimdorfer, A.: The action of sympathomimetic amines on the central nervous system and the blood sugar. Mechanism of action. J. Pharmacol. Exp. Ther. 98, 62–71 (1950)

Leimdorfer, A., Metzner, W.R.T.: Analgesia and anaesthesia induced by epinephrine. Am. J. Physiol. 157, 116–121 (1949)

Leonard, B.E.: Drug-induced changes in brain tyrosine hydroxylase activity in vivo. Neuropharmacology 16, 47–52 (1977)

Levin, R.M., Weiss, B.: Mechanism by which psychotropic drugs inhibit adenosine cyclic 3′,5′-monophosphate phosphodiesterase of brain. Mol. Pharmacol. 12, 581–589 (1976)

Leysen, J., Laduron, P.: Differential distribution of opiate and neuroleptic receptors and the dopamine sensitive adenylate cyclase in rat brain. Life Sci. *20*, 281–288 (1972)

Lindvall, O., Björklund, A.: The organization of the ascending catecholamine neurone system in the rat brain as revealed by glyoxylic acid fluorescence method. Acta Physiol. Scand. [Suppl.] *412*, 1–48 (1974)

Lindvall, O., Björklund, A., Moore, R.Y., Stenevi, U.: Mesencephalic dopamine neurons projecting to neocortex. Brain Res. *81*, 325–331 (1974)

Linowiecki, A.J.: The comparative anatomy of the pyramidal tract. J. Comp. Neurol. *24*, 509–530 (1914)

Loizou, L.A.: Projections of the nucleus coeruleus in the albino rat. Brain Res. *15*, 563–560 (1969)

Longo, V.G., Silvestrini, B.: Effect of adrenergic and cholinergic drugs injected by intracarotid route on electrical activity of brain. Proc. Soc. Exp. Biol. Med. *95*, 43–47 (1957)

Longo, V.G., von Berger, G.P., Bovet, D.: Action of nicotine and of the "ganglioplégiques centraux" on the electrical activity of the brain. J. Pharmacol. Exp. Ther. *111*, 349–359 (1954)

Lu, K.-H., Amenomori, Y., Chen, C.-L., Meites, J.: Effects of central acting drugs on serum and pituitary prolactin levels in rats. Endocrinology (Philadelphia) *87*, 667–672 (1970)

Lundberg, A.: Monoamines and spinal reflexes. In: Studies in Physiology. D.R. Curtis and A.K. McIntyre, Eds., pp. 186–190, Springer-Verlag, Berlin (1965)

Lynch, G.S., Lucas, PA., Deadwyler, S.A.: The demonstration of acetylcholinesterase-containing neurones within the caudate nucleus of the rat. Brain Res. *45*, 617–621 (1972)

MacLeod, R.M.: Regulation of prolactin secretion. In: Frontiers in Neuroendocrinology, Vol. 4. L. Martini, W.F. Ganong, Eds., New York, Raven Press, pp. 169–194 (1976)

MacLeod, R.M., Fontham, E.H., Lehmeyer, J.E.: Prolactin and growth hormone production as influenced by catecholamines. Neuroendocrinology *6*, 283–294 (1970)

Magnusson, T.: Effect of chronic transection on dopamine, noradrenaline and 5-hydroxytryptamine in the rat spinal cord. Naunyn Schmiedebergs Arch. Pharmacol. *278*, 13–22 (1973)

Magnusson, T., Rosengren, E.: Catecholamines of the spinal cord normally and after transection. Experientia *19*, 229–230 (1963)

Maler, L., Fibiger, H.C., McGeer, P.L.: Demonstration of the nigro striatal projection by silver staining after nigral injection of 6-hydroxydopamine. Exp. Neurol. *40*, 505–515 (1973)

Malhotra, C.L., Sidhu, R.K.: The anti-emetic activity of alkaloids of Rauwolfia serpentina. J. Pharmacol. Exp. Ther. *116*, 123–129 (1956)

Malmfors, T.: Studies on adrenergic nerves. The use of rat and mouse iris for direct observations on their physiology and pharmacology at cellular and subcellular levels. Acta Physiol. Scand. *64*, Suppl. 248, 1–93 (1963)

Mantegazzini, P., Poeck, K., Santibañez, H.G.: The action of adrenaline and noradrenaline on the cortical electrical activity of the "encéphale isolé" cat. Arch. Ital. Biol. *97*, 222–242 (1959)

Marley, E., Vane, J.R.: Tryptamine receptors in the central nervous system. Nature *198*, 441–444 (1963)

Marsden, C.D., Milson, J., Parkes, J.D., Pycock, C., Tarsy, D.: The effect of cholinergic and anticholinergic drugs on rotational behavior in mice with destruction of one nigrostriatal pathway. J. Physiol. (Lond.) *249*, 64p–65p (1975)

Martin, W.R., Demaar, E.W.J., Unna, K.R.: Chlorpromazine: I. The action of chlorpromazine and related phenothiazines on the EEG and its activation. J. Pharmacol. Exp. Ther. *122*, 343–358 (1958)

Martin, W.R., Riehl, J.L., Unna, K.R.: Chlorpromazine. III. The effects of chlorpromazine and chlorpromazine sulfoxide on vascular responses to l-epinephrine and levarterenol. J. Pharmacol. Exp. Ther. *130*, 37–45 (1960)

Mason, S.T., Iversen, S.D.: Learning in the absence of forebrain noradrenaline. Nature *258*, 422–424 (1975)

Mason, S.T., Iversen, S.D.: Effects of selective forebrain noradrenaline loss on behavioural inhibition in the rat. J. Comp. Physiol. Psychol. *91*, 165–173 (1977)

Mason, S.T., Iversen, S.D.: Reward, attention and the dorsal noradrenergic bundle. Brain Res. *150*, 135–148 (1978)

Matthysse, S.: Antipsychotic drug actions: A clue to the neuropathology of schizophrenia? Fed. Proc. *32*, 200–205 (1973)

Mayer, D.J., Price, D.D.: Central nervous system mechanisms of analgesia. Pain *2*, 379–404 (1976)

McAfee, D.A., Greengard, P.: Adenosine 3′,5′-monophosphate: electrophysiological evidence for a role in synaptic transmission. Science *178*, 310–312 (1972)

McGeer, E.G., McGeer, P.L.: Catecholamine content of spinal cord. Can. J. Biochem. Physiol. *40*, 1141–1151 (1962)

McGeer, E.G., McGeer, P.L., McLennan, H.: The inhibitory action of 3-hydroxytyramine, gamma-aminobutyric acid (GABA) and some other compounds towards the crayfish stretchreceptor neuron. J. Neurochem. *8*, 36–49 (1961)

McGeer, E.G., Fibiger, H.C., McGeer, P.L., Brooke, S.: Temporal changes in amine synthesizing enzymes of rat extrapyramidal structures after hemitransection or 6-hydroxydopamine administration. Brain Res. *52*, 289–300 (1973)

McGeer, P.L., Fibiger, H.C., Hattori, T., Singh, V.K., McGeer, E.G., Maler, L.: Biochemical neuroanatomy of the basal ganglia. In: Neurohumoral Coding and Brain Function, Advances in Behaviour and Biology *10*, 27–48, R.D. Myers, R.R.Drucker-Colin, Eds. (1974a)

McGeer, P.L., Grewaal, D.S., McGeer, E.G.: Influence of noncholinergic drugs on rat striatal acetylcholine levels. Brain Res. *80*, 211–217 (1974b)

McGeer, E.G., McGeer, P.L., Grewaal, D.S., Singh, V.K.: Striatal cholinergic interneurons and their relation to dopaminergic nerve endings. J. Pharmacol. (Paris) *6*, 143–152 (1975)

McGeer, P.L., McGeer, E.G., Wada, J.A.: Central aromatic amine levels and behavior. II. Serotonin and catecholamine levels in various cat brain areas following administration of psycho-active drugs on amine precursors. Arch. Neurol. *9*, 81–89 (1963)

McGillard, K.L., Takemori; A.E.: The effect of dopaminergic modifiers on morphine-induced analgesia and respiratory depression, Eur. J. Pharmacol. *54*, 61–68 (1979)

McKenzie, G.M., Sadof, M.: Effects of morphine and chlorpromazine on apomorphine-induced stereotyped behaviour. J. Pharm. Pharmacol. *26*, 280–282 (1974)

McLennan, H.: The effect of some catecholamines upon a monosynaptic reflex pathway in the spinal cord. J. Physiol. (Lond.) *158*, 411–425 (1961)

McLennan, H., York, D.H.: The action of dopamine on neurons of the caudate nucleus. J. Physiol. (Lond.) *189*, 393–402 (1967)

McNair, J.L., Sutin, J., Tsubokawa, T.: Suppression of cell firing in the substantia nigra by caudate nucleus stimulation. Exp. Neurol. *37*, 395–411 (1972)

Melville, K.I.: Observations on the adrenergic-blocking and antifibrillatory actions of chlorpromazine. Fed. Proc. *13*, 386–387 (1954)

Messing, R.B., Lytle, L.D.: Serotonin-containing neurons: their possible role in pain and analgesia. Pain *4*, 1–21 (1977)

Miller, R.J., Iversen, L.L.: Effect of chlorpromazine and some of its metabolites on the dopamine-sensitive adenylate cyclase of rat brain striatum. J. Pharm. Pharmacol. *26*, 142–144 (1974)

Miller, R.J., Horn, A.S., Iversen, L.L.: The action of neuroleptic drugs on dopamine-stimulated adenosine cyclic 3′,5′-monophosphate production in rat neostriatum and limbic forebrain. Mol. Pharmacol. *10*, 759–766 (1974)

Minneman, K.P., Quik, M., Emson, P.C.: Receptor linked cyclic AMP systems in rat neostriatum: differential localization revaled by kainic acid injection. Brain Res. *151*, 507–521 (1978)

Moore, R.Y., Bhatnagar, R.K., Heller, A.: Anatomical and chemical studies of a nigro-neostriatal projection in the cat. Brain Res. *30*, 119–135 (1971)

Morest, D.K.: A study of the structure of the area postrema with Golgi methods. Am. J. Anat. *107*, 291–303 (1960)

Morest, D.K.: Experimental study of the projections of the nucleus of the tractus solatarius and the area postrema in the cat. J. Comp. Neurol. *130*, 277–300 (1966)

Morpurgo, C.: Effects of anti-Parkinson drugs on a phenothiazine induced catatonic reaction. Arch. Int. Pharmacodyn. Ther. *137*, 84–90 (1962)

Munoz, C., Goldstein, L.: Quantitative EEG studies on the action of adrenergic blocking drugs upon the analeptic effects of DL amphetamine in rabbits. Pharmacologist *2*, 80 (1960)

Murrin, L.C., Morgenroth, V.H., Roth, R.H.: Dopaminergic neurons: effects of electrical stimulation on tyrosine hydroxylase. Mol. Pharmacol. *12*, 1070–1081 (1976)

Muscholl, E., Vogt, M.: The action of reserpine on sympathetic ganglia. J. Physiol. (Lond.) *136*, 7 P (1957)

Muscholl, E., Vogt, M.: The action of reserpine on the peripheral sympathetic system. J. Physiol. (Lond.) *141*, 132–155 (1958)

Nagy, J.I., Lee, T., Seeman, P., Fibiger, H.C.: Direct evidence for presynaptic and postsynaptic dopamine receptors in brain. Nature *274*, 278–281 (1978)

Nathan, P.W.: Pain. Brit. med. Bull. *33*, 149–156 (1977)

Ng, K.Y., Chase, T.N., Colburn, R.W., Kopin, I.J.: L-Dopa induced release of cerebral monoamines. Science *170*, 76–77 (1970)

Nieoullon, A., Chéramy, A., Glowinski, J.: Release of dopamine in vivo from cat substantia nigra. Nature *266*, 375–377 (1977 a)

Nieoullon, A., Cheramy, A., Glowinski, J.: Nigral and striatal dopamine release under sensory stimuli. Nature *269*, 340–342 (1977 b)

Nieoullon, A., Cheramy, A., Glowinski, J.: Interdependence of the nigrostriatal dopaminergic systems on the two sides of the brain in the cat. Science *198*, 416–418 (1977 c)

Nieoullon, A., Cheramy, A., Leviel, V., Glowinski, J.: Effects of the unilateral nigral application of dopaminergic drugs on the in vivo release of dopamine in the two caudate nuclei of the cat. Euro. J. Pharmacol. *53*, 289–296 (1979)

Nybäck, H., Sedvall, G.: Effect of chlorpromazine on accumulation and disappearance of catecholamines formed from tyrosine-C^{14} in brain. J. Pharmacol. Exp. Ther. *162*, 294–301 (1968)

Nybäck, H., Sedvall, G.: Effect of nigral lesion on chlorpromazine-induced acceleration of dopamine synthesis from [^{14}C]tyrosine. J. Pharm. Pharmacol. *23*, 322–326 (1971)

Nybäck, H., Sedvall, G., Kopin, I.J.: Accelerated synthesis of dopamine-C^{14} from tyrosine-C^{14} in rat brain after chlorpromazine. Life Sci. *6*, 2307–2312 (1967)

Nybäck, H., Borzecki, Z., Sedvall, G.: Accumulation and disappearance of catecholamines formed from tyrosine-^{14}C in mouse brain; effect of some psychotropic drugs. Eur. J. Pharmacol. *4*, 395–403 (1968)

Okada, Y., Hassler, R.: Uptake and release of γ-aminobutyric acid (GABA) in slices of substantia nigra of rat. Brain Res. *49*, 214–217 (1973)

O'Keeffe, R., Sharman, D.F., Vogt, M.: Effect of drugs used in psychoses on cerebral dopamine metabolism. Br. J. Pharmacol. *38*, 287–304 (1970)

Olpe, H.-R., Koella, W.P.: Inhibition of nigral and neocortical cells by γ-hydroxy butyrate: a microiontophoretic investigation. Eur. J. Pharmacol. *53*, 359–364 (1979)

Owen, F., Cross, A.J., Crow, T.J., Longen, A., Poulter, M., Riley, G.J.: Increased dopamine-receptor sensitivity in schizophrenia. Lancet II: 223–226 (1978)

Paalzow, G., Paalzow, L.: Clonidine antinociceptive activity: effects of drugs influencing central monoaminergic and cholinergic mechanisms in the rat. Naunyn Schmiedebergs Arch. Pharmacol. *292*, 119–126 (1976)

Palmer, G.C.: Increased cyclic AMP response to norepinephrine in the rat brain following 6-hydroxydopamine. Neuropharmacology *11*, 145–149 (1972)

Palmer, G.C., Jones, D.J., Medina, M.A., Stavinoha, W.B.: Action of psychoactive drugs on cyclic AMP levels in mouse cerebral cortex and lung following microwave irradiation. Pharmacologist *17*, 233 (1975)

Palmer, G.C., Jones, D.J., Medina, M.A., Stavinoha, W.B.: Influence of injected psychoactive drugs on cyclic AMP levels in mouse brain and lung following microwave irradiation. Neuropharmacology *16*, 435–443 (1977)

Palmer, G.C., Jones, D.J., Medina, M.A., Palmer, S.J., Stavinoha, W.B.: Actions in vitro and in vivo of chlorpromazine and haloperidol on cyclic nucleotide systems in mouse cerebral cortex and cerebellum. Neuropharmacology *17*, 491–498 (1978)

Pepeu, G.: Involvement of central transmitters in narcotic analgesia. In: Advances in Pain Research and Therapy. J.J. Bonica, D. Albe-Fessard, Eds., Vol. 1: 595–600, Raven Press, New York (1976)

Perkins, J.P., Moore, M.M.: Characterization of the adrenergic receptors mediating a rise in cyclic 3′,5′-adenosine monophosphate in rat cerebral cortex. J. Pharmacol. Exp. Ther. *185*, 371–378 (1973)

Peroutka, S.J., U'Prichard, D.C., Greenberg, D.A., Snyder, S.H.: Neuroleptic drug interactions with norepinephrine alpha receptor binding sites in rat brain. Neuropharmacology *16*, 549–556 (1977)

Persson, S.-Å.: Effect of morphine on the accumulation of DOPA after decarboxylase inhibition in the rat. Eur. J. Pharmacol. *55*, 121–128 (1979)

Pert, C.B., Snyder, S.H.: Opiate receptor: demonstration in nervous tissue. Science *179*, 1011–1014 (1973)

Pert, C.B., Kuhar, M.J., Snyder, S.H.: Autoradiographic localization of the opiate receptor in rat brain. Life Sci. *16*, 1849–1854 (1975)

Phillis, J.W., Tebēcis, A.K.: The effects of pentobarbitone sodium on acetylcholine excitation and noradrenaline inhibition of thalamic neurones. Life Sci. *6*, 1621–1625 (1967a)

Phillis, J.W., Tebēcis, A.K.: The responses of thalamic neurones to iontophoretically applied monoamines. J. Physiol. (Lond.) *192*, 715–745 (1967b)

Phillis, J.W., York, D.H.: Strychnine block of neural and drug induced inhibition in the cerebral cortex. Nature *216*, 922–923 (1967)

Phillis, J.W., Tebēcis, A.K., York, D.H.: Depression of spinal motoneurones by noradrenaline, 5-hydroxytryptamine and histamine. Eur. J. Pharmacol. *4*, 471–475 (1968)

Pijnenburg, A.J.J., Van Rossum, J.M.: Stimulation of locomotor activity following injection of dopamine into the nucleus accumbens. J. Pharm. Pharmacol. *25*, 1003–1005 (1973)

Pijnenburg, A.J.J., Woodruff, G.N., Van Rossum, J.M.: Ergometrine induced locomotor activity following intracerebral injection into the nucleus accumbens. Brain Res. *59*, 289–302 (1973)

Pijnenburg, A.J.J., Honig. W.M.M., Van Rossum, J.M.: Effects of antagonists upon locomotor stimulation induced by injection of dopamine and noradrenaline into the nucleus accumbens of nialamide-pretreated rats. Psychopharmacology (Berlin) *41*, 175–180 (1975)

Pijnenburg, A.J.J., Honig, W.M.M., Struyker Boudier, H.A.J., Cools, A.R., Van der Heyden, J.A.M., Van Rossum, J.M.: Further investigations on the effects of ergometrine and other ergot derivatives following injection into the nucleus accumbens of the rat. Arch. Int. Pharmacodyn. Ther. *222*, 103–115 (1976)

Pocidalo, J.J., Cathala, H.P., Himbert, J.: Action sur l'excitabilité sympathique du chlorhydrate de diméthylaminopropyl-N-chlorophénothiazine (4560 R. P.). C. R. Soc. Biol. (Paris) *146*, 368–370 (1952)

Poirier, L.J., Sourkes, I.L.: Influence of the substantia nigra on the catecholamine content of the striatum. Brain *88*, 181–192 (1965)

Pollard, H., Llorens, C., Schwartz, J.C., Cross, C., Dray, F.: Localization of opiate receptors and enkephalins in the rat striatum in relationship with the nigro striatal dopaminergic system. Brain. Res. *151*, 392–398 (1978)

Precht, W., Yoshida, M.: Blockage of caudate-evoked inhibition of neurons in the substantia nigra by picrotoxin. Brain Res. *32*, 229–233 (1971)

Preston, J.B.: Chlorpromazine: a possible mechanism of action. Fed. Proc. *15*, 468–469 (1956a)

Preston, J.B.: Effects of chlorpromazine on the central nervous system of the cat: A possible neural basis for action. J. Pharmacol. Exp. Ther. *118*, 100–115 (1956b)

Pycock, C., Tarsy, D., Marsden, C.D.: Inhibition of circling behavior by neuroleptic drugs in mice with unilateral 6-hydroxydopamine lesions of the striatum. Psychopharmacology (Berlin) *45*, 211–219 (1975)

Quastel, D.M.J., Hackett, J.T., Okamoto, K.: Presynaptic action of central depressant drugs: inhibition of depolarization-secretion coupling. Can. J. Physiol. Pharmacol. *50*, 279 (1972)

Quik, M., Iversen, L.L.: Regional study of ^{3}H-spiperone binding and the dopamine-sensitive adenylate cyclase in rat brain. Eur. J. Pharmacol. *56*, 323–330 (1979)

Quik, M., Iversen, L.L., Larder, A., Mackay, A.U.P.: Use of ADTN to define specific ^{3}H-spiperone binding to receptors in brain. Nature *274*, 513–514 (1978)

Randrup, A., Munkvad, I.: Stereotyped activities produced by amphetamine in several animal species and man. Psychopharmacology (Berlin) *11*, 300–310 (1967)

Ranson, S.W.: The fasciculus cerebro-spinalis in the albino rat. Am. J. Anat. *14*, 411–424 (1913)

Ranson, S.W.: A note on the degeneration of the fasciculus cerebro-spinalis in the albino rat. J. Comp. Neurol. *24*, 503–507 (1914)

Ritchie, J.M., Greengard, P.: On the active structure of local anesthetics. J. Pharmacol. Exp. Ther. *133*, 241–245 (1961)

Roberge, C., Ebstein, B., Goldstein, M.: Stimulation of tyrosine hydroxylase (T.H.) activity by dibutyryl cyclic AMP (dB-cAMP) in synaptosomal preparations (S.P.). Fed. Proc. *33*, 521 (1974)

Roberts, M.H.T., Straughan, D.W.: An excitatory effect of 5-hydroxytryptamine on single cerebral cortical neurones. J. Physiol. (Lond.) *188*, 27–28 P (1966)

Roos, B.-E.: Effects of certain tranquillisers on the level of homovanillic acid in the corpus striatum. J. Pharm. Pharmacol. *17*, 820–821 (1965)

Roos, B.-E., Steg, G.: The effect of L-3,4-dihydroxyphenylalanine and DL-5-hydroxytryptophan on rigidity and tremor induced by reserpine, chlorpromazine and phenoxybenzamine. Life Sci. *3*, 351–360 (1964)

Rothballer, A.B.: Studies on the adrenaline-sensitive component of the reticular activating system. Electroencephalogr. Clin. Neurophysiol. *8*, 603–621 (1956)

Ryall, R.W.: Some actions of chlorpromazine. Br. J. Pharmacol. *11*, 339–345 (1956)

Salmoiraghi, G.C., Stefanis, C.N.: Patterns of central neurons responses to suspected transmitters. Arch. Ital. Biol. *103*, 705–724 (1965)

Sano, I., Gamo, T., Kakimoto, Y., Taniguchi, K., Takasada, M., Nishinuma, K.: Distribution of catechol compounds in human brain. Biochim. Biophys. Acta *32*, 586–587 (1959)

Satoh, H., Satoh, Y., Notsu, Y., Honda, F.: Adenosine 3′,5′-cyclic monophosphate as a possible mediator of rotational behaviour induced by dopaminergic receptor stimulation in rats lesioned unilaterally in the substantia nigra. Eur. J. Pharmacol. *39*, 365–377 (1976)

Sayers, A.C., Burki, H.R., Ruch, W., Asper, H.: Neuroleptic-induced hypersensitivity of striatal dopamine receptors in the rat as a model of tardive dyskinesias. Effects of clozapine, haloperidol, loxapine and chlorpromazine. Psychopharmacology (Berlin) *41*, 97–104 (1975)

Schaumann, W.: Beeinflussung der analgetischen Wirkung des Morphins durch Reserpin. Naunyn Schmiedebergs Arch. Pharmacol. *235*, 1–9 (1958)

Schildkraut, J.J., Kety, S.S.: Biogenic amines and emotion. Science *156*, 21–30 (1967)

Schlosser, W., Horst, W.D., Spiegel, H.E., Sigg, E.B.: Apomorphine and its effects on the spinal cord. Neuropharmacology *11*, 417–426 (1972)

Schneider, J.A.: Further studies on the central action of reserpine (Serpasil). Am. J. Physiol. *179*, 670–671 (1954a)

Schneider, J.A.: Reserpine antagonism of morphine analgesia in mice. Proc. Soc. Exp. Biol. Med. *87*, 614–615 (1954b)

Schneider, J.A.: Further characterization of central effects of reserpine (Serpasil). Am. J. Physiol. *181*, 64–68 (1955)

Schneider, J.A., Earl, A.E.: Effects of Serpasil on behavior and autonomic regulating mechanisms. Neurology *4*, 657–667 (1954)

Schulte, F.J., Henatsch, H.D.: Unterdrückung tonischer Eigenschaften von Alpha- und Gamma-Motoneuronen durch Phenothiazinkörper. Pflügers Arch. Ges. Physiol. *268*, 65–66 (1958)

Schultz, J., Daly, J.W.: Accumulation of cyclic adenosine 3′,5′-monophosphate in cerebral cortical slices from rat and mouse: stimulatory effect of α- and β-adrenergic agents and adenosine. J. Neurochem. *21*, 1319–1326 (1973)

Schultz, W., Ungerstedt, U.: Striatal cell supersensitivity to apomorphine in dopamine-lesioned rats correlated to behaviour. Neuropharmacology *17*, 349–353 (1978)

Schwarcz, R., Creese, I., Coyle, J.T., Snyder, S.H.: Dopamine receptors localized on cerebral cortical afferents to rat corpus striatum. Nature *271*, 766–768 (1978)

Schwartz, J.C., Costentin, I., Martes, M.P., Protais, P., Baudry, M.: Review: modulation of receptor mechanisms in the CNS: hyper- and hyposensitivity to catecholamines. Neuropharmacology *17*, 665–685 (1978)

Schweitzer, A., Wright, S.: The action of adrenaline on the knee jerk. J. Physiol. (Lond.) *88*, 476–491 (1937)

Seeman, P.M., Bialy, H.S.: The surface activity of tranquilizers. Biochem. Pharmacol. *12*, 1181–1191 (1963)

Seeman, P., Lee, T.: Antipsychotic drugs: direct correlation between clinical potency and pre-synaptic action on dopamine neurons. Science *188*, 1217–1219 (1975)

Seeman, P., Lee, T., Chau-Wong, M., Wong, K.: Antipsychotic drug doses and neuroleptic/ dopamine receptors. Nature *261*, 717–719 (1976)

Seeman, P., Staiman, A., Chau-Wong, M.: The nerve impulse-blocking actions of tranquilizers and the binding of neuroleptics to synaptosome membranes. J. Pharmacol. Exp. Ther. *190*, 123–130 (1974)

Seeman, P., Tedesco, J., Titeler, M., Hartley, E.J.: Antischizophrenic drugs: membrane sites of action. Advan. Pharmacol. Therap. Vol. 5. Neuropsychopharmacol. C. Dumont (Ed.), Oxford: Pergamon Press, pp. 3–20 (1978)

Segal, M., Pickel, V., Bloom, F.: The projections of the nucleus locus coerulus: an autoradiographic study. Life Sci. *13*, 817–821 (1973)

Sethy, V.H., Van Woert, M.H.: Effect of L-DOPA on brain acetylcholine and choline in rats. Neuropharmacology *12*, 27–31 (1973)

Sethy, V.H., Van Woert, M.H.: Regulation of striatal acetylcholine concentration by dopamine receptors. Nature *251*, 529–530 (1974a)

Sethy, V.H., Van Woert, M.H.: Modification of striatal acetylcholine concentration by dopamine receptor agonists and antagonists. Res. Commun. Chem. Path. Pharmacol. *8*, 13–28 (1974b)

Shaar, C.J., Smalstig, E.B., Clemens, J.A.: The effect of catecholamines, apomorphine, and monoamine oxidase on rat anterior pituitary prolactin release in vitro. Pharmacologist *15*, 256 (1973)

Share, N.N., Chai, C.Y., Wang, S.C.: Emesis induced by intra-cerebroventricular injections of apomorphine and deslanoside in normal and chemoreceptive trigger zone ablated dogs. J. Pharmacol. Exp. Ther. *147*, 416–421 (1965)

Sharman, D.F.: Changes in the metabolism of 3,4-dihydroxy-phenylethylamine (dopamine) in the striatum of the mouse induced by drugs. Br. J. Pharmacol. *28*, 153–163 (1966)

Shore, P.A., Brodie, B.B.: Influence of various drugs on serotonin and norepinephrine in the brain. In: Psychotropic Drugs. S. Garattini, V. Ghetti, Eds., pp. 423–427, Elsevier Publishing Company, Amsterdam (1957)

Shore, P.A., Silver, S.L., Brodie, B.B.: Interaction of reserpine, serotonin and lysergic acid diethylamide in brain. Science *122*, 284–285 (1955)

Shore, P.A., Pletscher, A., Tomich, E.G., Carlsson, A., Kuntzman, R., Brodie, B.B.: Role of brain serotonin in reserpine action. Ann. N. Y. Acad. Sci. *66*, 609–617 (1957)

Sibley, D.R., Creese, I.: Guanine nucleotides regulate anterior pituitary dopamine receptors. Eur. J. Pharmacol. *55*, 341–343 (1979)

Sigg, E.B., Ochs, S., Gerard, R.W.: Effects of medullary hormones on the somatic nervous system in the cat. Am. J. Physiol. *183*, 419–426 (1955)

Sigg, E.B., Caprio, G., Schneider, J.A.: Synergism of amines and antagonism of reserpine to morphine analgesia. Proc. Soc. Exp. Biol. Med. *97*, 97–100 (1958)

Siggins, G.R., Hoffer, B.J., Bloom, F.E.: Cyclic adenosine monophosphate: possible mediator for norepinephrine effects on cerebellar Purkinje cells. Science *165*, 1018–1020 (1969)

Siggins, G.R., Hoffer, B.J., Bloom, F.E.: Studies on norepinephrine-containing afferents to Purkinje cells of rat cerebellum. III. Evidence for mediation of norepinephrine effects by cyclic 3′,5′-adenosine monophosphate. Brain Res. *25*, 535–553 (1971a)

Siggins, G.R., Oliver, A.P., Hoffer, B.J., Bloom, F.E.: Cyclic adenosine monophosphate and norepinephrine: Effects of transmembrane properties of cerebellar Purkinje cells. Science *171*, 192–194 (1971b)

Siggins, G.R., Battenberg, E.F., Hoffer, B.J., Bloom, F.E., Steiner, A.L.: Noradrenergic stimulation of cyclic adenosine monophosphate in rat Purkinje neurons: an immuno-cytochemical study. Science *179*, 585–588 (1973)

Siggins, G.R., Hoffer, B.J., Ungerstedt, U.: Electrophysiological evidence for involvement of cyclic adenosine monophosphate in dopamine responses of caudate neurons. Life Sci. *15*, 779–792 (1974)

Sigwald, J., Bouttier, D., Courvoisier, S.: Les accidents neurologiques des médications neuroleptiques. Rev. Neurol. (Paris) *100*, 31–73 (1959)

Silvestrini, B., Maffii, G.: Effects of chlorpromazine, promazine, diethazine, reserpine, hy-droxyzine, and morphine upon some mono- and polysynaptic motor reflexes. J. Pharm. Pharmacol. *11*, 224–233 (1959)

Smalstig, E.B., Sawyer, B.D., Clemens, J.A.: Inhibition of rat prolactin release by apomorphine in vivo and in vitro. Endocrinology *95*, 123–129 (1974)

Smith, C.M., Murayama, S.: Rigidity of spinal origin: quantitative evaluation of agents with muscle relaxant activity in cats. Neuropharmacology *3*, 505–515 (1964)

Sourkes, T.L.: Formation of dopamine in vivo: relation to the function of the basal ganglia. Rev. Can. Biol. *20*, 187–196 (1961)

Stadler, H., Lloyd, K.G., Gadea-Ciria, M., Bartholini, G.: Enhanced striatal acetylcholine release by chlorpromazine and its reversal by apomorphine. Brain Res. *55*, 476–480 (1973)

Stefanis, C.: Hippocampal neurons: their responsiveness to micro-electrophoretically adminis-tered endogenous amines. Pharmacologist *6*, 171 (1964)

Steg, G.: Efferent muscle innervation and rigidity. Acta Physiol. Scand. *61*, suppl. 225 (1964)

Steg, G.: Efferent muscle control and rigidity. In: Muscular Afferents and Motor Control. No-bel Symposium I, pp. 437–443, R. Granit, Ed., Almqvist & Wiksell, Stockholm and John Willy & Sons, New York, London, Sydney (1966)

Stern, J., Ward, A.A.: Supraspinal and drug modulation of the α-motor system. A. M. A. Arch. Neurol. *6*, 404–413 (1962)

Sternbach, R.A., Janowsky, D.S., Huey, L.Y., Segal, D.S.: Effects of altering brain serotonin activity on human chronic pain. In: Advances in Pain Research and Therapy, Vol. 1 J.E. Bonica, D. Albe-Fessard, Eds., pp. 601–606. New York: Raven Press 1976

Stevens, J.: An anatomy of schizophrenia. Arch. Gen. Psychiaty *29*, 177–189 (1973)

Stille, G., Hippius, H.: Kritische Stellungnahme zum Begriff der Neuroleptika (anhand von pharmakologischen und klinischen Befunden mit Clozapin). Pharmakopsychiatr. Neuro-psychopharmakol. *4*, 182–191 (1971)

Stille, G., Lauener, H., Eichenberger, E.: The pharmacology of 8-chloro-11-(4-methyl-1-pipe-razinyl)-5H-dibenzo (b,e) (1,4) diazepine (clozapine). Farmaco [Prat.] *26*, 603–625 (1971)

Struyker Boudier, H.A.J., Gielen, W., Cools, A.R., Van Rossum, J.M.: Pharmacological ana-lysis of dopamine-induced inhibition and excitation of neurones in the snail Helix aspersa. Arch. Int. Pharmacodyn. Ther. *209*, 324–331 (1974)

Svensson, T.H., Bunney, B.S., Aghajanian, G.K.: Inhibition of both noradrenergic and seroto-nergic neurons in brain by the α-adrenergic agonist clonidine. Brain Res. *92*, 291–306 (1975)

Szabo, J.: Projections from the body of the caudate nucleus in the rhesus monkey. Exp. Neurol. *27*, 1–15 (1970)

Szabo, J.: The course and distribution of efferents from the tail of the caudate nucleus in the monkey. Exp. Neurol. *37*, 562–572 (1972)

Takaori, S., Fukuda, N., Amano, Y.: Mode of action of chlorpromazine on unit discharges from nuclear structures in the brain stem of cats. Jpn. J. Pharmacol. *20*, 424–431 (1970)

Takaori, S., Nakai, Y., Matsuoka, I., Sasa, M., Fukuda, N., Shimamoto, K.: The mechanism of antagonism between apomorphine and metoclopramide on unit discharges from nuclear structures in the brainstem of the cat. Neuropharmacology *7*, 115–126 (1968)

Tarsy, D., Baldessarini, R.J.: Pharmacologically induced behavioral supersensitivity to apomorphine. Nature New Biol. *245*, 262–263 (1973)

Tedeschi, D.H., Tedeschi, R.E., Fellows, E.J.: The effects of tryptamine on the central nervous system, including a pharmacological procedure for the evaluation of iproniazidlike drugs. J. Pharm. Exp. Ther. *126*, 223–232 (1959)

Ten Cate, J., Boeles, J.T.F., Biersteker, P.A.: The action of adrenaline and noradrenaline on the knee jerk. Arch. Int. Physiol. Biochim. *67*, 468–488 (1959)

Thierry, A.M., Blanc, G., Sobel, A., Stinus, L., Glowinski, J.: Dopaminergic terminals in the rat cortex. Science *182*, 499–501 (1973)

Titeler, M., Seeman, P.: Antiparkinsonian drug doses and neuroleptic receptors. Experientia *34*, 1490–1492 (1978)

Torrey, E.F., Petersen, M.R.: Schizophrenia and the limbic system. Lancet II: 942–946 (1974)

Trabucchi, M., Cheney, D., Racagni, G., Costa, E.: Involvement of brain cholinergic mech-anisms in the action of chlorpromazine. Nature *249*, 664–666 (1974)

Trabucchi, M., Cheney, D.L., Racagni, G., Costa, E.: In vivo inhibition of striatal acetylcholine turnover by L-DOPA, apomorphine and (+)-amphetamine. Brain Res. *85*, 130–134 (1975)

Trendelenburg, U., Gravenstein, J.S.: Effect of reserpine pretreatment on stimulation of the accelerans nerve of the dog. Science *128*, 901–903 (1958)

Udenfriend, S., Weissbach, H., Bogdanksi, D.F.: Increase in tissue serotonin following administration of its precursor 5-hydroxytryptophan. J. Biol. Chem. *224*, 803–810 (1957a)

Udenfriend, S., Weissbach, H., Bogdanski, D.F.: Biochemical findings relating to the action of serotonin. Ann. N. Y. Acad. Sci. *66*, 602–608 (1957b)

Ueda, T., Maeno, H., Greengard, P.: Regulation of endogenous phosphorylation of specific proteins in synaptic membrane fractions from rat brain by adenosine 3′:5′-monophosphate. J. Biol. Chem. *248*, 8295–8305 (1973)

Ungerstedt, U.: 6-Hydroxy-dopamine induced degeneration of central monoamine neurons. Eur. J. Pharmacol. *5*, 107–110 (1968)

Ungerstedt, U.: Sterotaxic mapping of the monoamine pathways in the rat brain. Acta Physiol. Scand. [Suppl.] *367*, 1–48 (1971a)

Ungerstedt, U.: Postsynaptic supersensitivity after 6-hydroxydopamine induced degeneration of the nigrostriatal dopamine system. Acta Physiol. Scand. [Suppl.] *367*, 69–93 (1971b)

Ungerstedt, U.: Adipsia and aphagia after 6-hydroxydopamine induced degeneration of the nigro-striatal dopamine system. Acta Physiol. Scand. [Suppl.] *367*, 95–122 (1971c)

Ungerstedt, U., Pycock, C.: Functional correlates of dopamine neurotransmission. Bull. Schweiz. Akad. Med. Wiss. *30*, 44–55 (1974)

Ungerstedt, U., Butcher, L.L., Butcher, S.G., Andén, N.-E., Fuxe, K.: Direct chemical stimulation of dopaminergic mechanisms in the neostriatum of the rat. Brain Res. *14*, 461–471 (1969)

Ungerstedt, U., Avemo, A., Avemo, E., Ljungberg, T., Ranje, C.: Animal models of parkinsonism. Adv. Neurol. *3*, 257–271 (1973)

Ungerstedt, U., Ljungberg, T., Hoffer, B., Siggins, G.: Dopaminergic supersensitivity in the striatum. Adv. Neurol. *9*, 57–65 (1975)

U'prichard, D.C., Snyder, S.H.: ³H-Catecholamine binding to α-receptors in rat brain: enhancement by reserpine. Eur. J. Pharmacol. *51*, 145–155 (1978)

Valdman, A.V.: On the localization of the action of chlorpromazine and analgesics in reticular formation of the brain stem. J. Neuropharmacol. *1*, 197–200 (1962)

Van der Wende, C., Spoerlein, M.T.: Role of dopaminergic receptors in morphine analgesia and tolerance. Res. Commun. Chem. Path. Pharmacol. *5*, 35–43 (1973)

Vogt, M.: The concentration of sympathine in different parts of the central nervous system under normal conditions and after the administration of drugs. J. Physiol. (Lond.) *123*, 451–481 (1954)

Vogt, M.: Effect of drugs on metabolism of catecholamines in the brain. Br. Med. Bull. *21*, 57–61 (1965)

Vogt, M.: Functional aspects of the role of catecholamines in the nervous system. Br. Med. Bull. *29*, 168–172 (1973)

von Voigtlander, P.F., Moore, K.E.: The release of H³-dopamine from cat brain following electrical stimulation of the substantia nigra and caudate nucleus. Neuropharmacology *10*, 733–741 (1971)

von Voigtlander, P.F., Moore, K.E.: Involvement of nigrostriatal neurons in the in vivo release of dopamine by amphetamine, amantadine and tyramine. J. Pharmacol. Exp. Ther. *184*, 542–552 (1973a)

von Voigtlander, P.F., Moore, K.E.: Turning behavior of mice with unilateral 6-hydroxydopamine lesions in the striatum: effects of apomorphine, L-Dopa, amantadine, amphetamine and other psychomotor stimulants. Neuropharmacology *12*, 451–462 (1973b)

Waldmeier, P.L., Maitre, L.: On the relevance of preferential increases of mesolimbic versus striatal dopamine turnover for the prediction of antipsychotic activity of psychotropic drugs. J. Neurochem. *27*, 589–597 (1976)

Walker, J.B.; Walker, J.P.: Neurohumoral regulation of adenylate cyclase activity in rat striatum. Brain Res. *54*, 386–390 (1973)

Walters, J.R., Roth, R.H.: Dopaminergic neurons: drug-induced antagonism of the increase in tyrosine hydroxylase activity produced by cessation of impulse flow. J. Pharmacol. Exp. Ther. *191*, 82–91 (1974)

Walters, J.R., Bunney, B.S., Roth, R.H.: Piribedil and apomorphine: pre- and postsynaptic effects on dopamine synthesis and neuronal activity. Adv. Neurol. *9*, 273–284 (1975)

Walton, K.G., Liepman, P., Baldessarini, R.J.: Inhibition of dopamine stimulated adenylate cyclase activity by phenoxybenzamine. Eur. J. Pharmacol. *52*, 231–234 (1978)

Wand, P.: The response of α-motoneurons of different size to stretch and vibration of extensor muscles after injection of 5-hydroxytryptophan in spinal rats. Arch. Ital. Biol. *114*, 228–243 (1976)

Wang, S.C.: III. Emetic and antiemetic drugs. Physiol. Pharmacol. *2*, 255–328 (1965)

Wang, S.C., Borison, H.L.: A new concept of organization of the central emetic mechanism: recent studies on the sites of action of apomorphine, copper sulfate and cardiac glycosides. Gastroenterology *22*, 1–12 (1952)

Wang, S.C., Glaviano, V.V.: Locus of emetic action of morphine and hydergine in dogs. J. Pharmacol. Exp. Ther. *111*, 329–334 (1954)

Weber, E.: Ein Rauwolfiaalkaloid in der Psychiatrie: seine Wirkungsähnlichkeit mit Chlorpromazin. Schweiz. Med. Wochenschrift. *84*, 968–970 (1954)

Weber, L.J., Horita, A.: A study of 5-hydroxytryptamine formation from L-tryptophan in the brain and other tissues. Biochem. Pharmacol. *14*, 1141–1149 (1965)

Webster, R.A.: The antiadrenaline activity of some phenothiazine derivatives. Br. J. Pharmacol. *25*, 566–576 (1965)

Weight, F., Salmoiraghi, G.C.: Response of single spinal cord neurons to ACh, NE and 5-HT administered by microelectrophoresis. Pharmacologist *7*, 216 (1965)

Weight, F.F., Salmoiraghi, G.C.: Responses of spinal cord interneurons to acetylcholine, norepinephrine and serotonin administered by microelectrophoresis. J. Pharmacol. Exp. Ther. *153*, 420–427 (1966 a)

Weight, F.F., Salmoiraghi, G.C.: Adrenergic responses of Renshaw cells. J. Pharmacol. Exp. Ther. *154*, 391–397 (1966 b)

Weight, F.F., Salmoiraghi, G.C.: Motoneurone depression by norepinephrine. Nature *213*, 1229–1230 (1967)

Westerink, B.H.C., Korf, J.: Regional rat brain levels of 3,4-dihydroxyphenylacetic acid and homovanillic acid: concurrent fluorometric measurement and influence of drugs. Eur. J. Pharmacol. *38*, 281–291 (1976)

Westerink, B.H.C., Lejeune, B., Korf, J., Van Praag, H.M.: On the significance of regional dopamine metabolism in the rat brain for the classification of centrally active drugs. Eur. J. Pharmacol. *42*, 179–190 (1977)

Wilson, C.W.M., Brodie, B.B.: The absence of blood-brain barrier from certain areas of the central nervous system. J. Pharmacol. Exp. Ther. *133*, 332–334 (1961)

Wilson, C.W.M., Murray, A.W., Titus, E.: The effects of reserpine on uptake of epinephrine in brain and certain areas outside the blood-brain barrier. J. Pharmacol. Exp. Ther. *135*, 11–16 (1962)

Wilson, V.J.: Effect of intra-arterial injections of adrenaline on spinal extensor and flexor reflexes. Am. J. Physiol. *186*, 491–496 (1956)

Windle, W.F., Cammermeyer, J.: Functional and structural observations on chronically reserpinized monkeys. Science (N.Y.) *127*, 1503 (1958)

Windle, W.F., Cammermeyer, J., Joralemon, J.T., Smart, J.O., Feringa, E., McQuillen, M.: Tremor in african green monkeys. Fed. Proc. *15*, 202 (1956)

Witkin, L.B., Spitaletta, P., Plummer, A.J.: Effects of some central depressants on two simple reflexes in the mouse. J. Pharmacol. Exp. Ther. *126*, 330–333 (1959)

Witkin, L.B., Spitaletta, P., Plummer, A.J.: The effects of some central depressants on spinal reflexes of the intact anesthetized cat. Arch. Int. Pharmacodyn. Ther. *124*, 105–115 (1960)

Woodruff, G.N., McCarthy, P.S., Walker, R.J.: Studies on the pharmacology of neurones in the nucleus accumbens of the rat. Brain Res. *115*, 233–242 (1976)

Wuerthele, S.M., Moore, K.E.: Studies on the mechanisms of L-DOPA-induced depletion of 5-hydroxytryptamine in the mouse brain. Life Sci. *20*, 1675–1680 (1977)

Yaksh, T.L., Rudy, T.A.: Analgesia mediated by a direct spinal action of narcotics. Science *192*, 1357–1358 (1976)

Yaksh, T.L., Rudy, T.A.: Studies on the direct spinal action of narcotics in the production of analgesia in the rat. J. Pharmacol. Exp. Ther. *202*, 411–428 (1977)

Yaksh, T.L., Yamamura, H.I.: Depression by morphine of the resting and evoked release of [^{3}H]-acetylcholine from the cat caudate nucleus in vivo. Neuropharmacology *16*, 227–233 (1977)

Yamaguchi, N., Ling, G.M., Marczynski, T.J.: The effects of chemical stimulation of the preoptic region, nucleus centralis medialis or brain stem reticular formation with regard to sleep and wakefulness. Recent Adv. Biol. Psychiatr. *6*, 9–20 (1964)

York, D.H.: Possible dopaminergic pathway from substantia nigra to putamen. Brain Res. *20*, 233–249 (1970)

York, D.H.: Dopamine receptor blockade – a central action of chlorpromazine on striatal neurones. Brain Res. *37*, 91–99 (1972a)

York, D.H.: Potentiation of lumbo-sacral monosynaptic reflexes by the substantia nigra. Exp. Neurol. *36*, 437–448 (1972b)

York, D.H.: Motor responses induced by stimulation of the substantia nigra. Exp. Neurol. *41*, 323–330 (1973a)

York, D.H.: Antagonism of descending effects of the substantia nigra on lumbo-sacral monosynaptic reflexes. Neuropharmacology *12*, 629–636 (1973b)

Yoshida, M., Precht, W.: Monosynaptic inhibition of neurons of the substantia nigra by caudato-nigral fibers. Brain Res. *32*, 225–227 (1971)

Zieglgänsberger, W., Bayerl, H.: The mechanism of inhibition of neuronal activity by opiates in the spinal cord. Brain Res. *115*, 111–128 (1976)

Zieglgänsberger, W., Satoh, M.: The mechanism of inhibition by morphine on spinal neurones of the cat. Exp. Brain. Res. *23*, 444 (1975)

Zivkovic, B., Guidotti, A., Revuelta, A., Costa, E.: Effect of thioridazine, clozapine and other antipsychotics on the kinetic state of tyrosine hydroxylase and on the turnover rate of dopamine in striatum and nucleus accumbens. J. Pharmacol. Exp. Ther. *194*, 37–46 (1975)

CHAPTER 8

Antipsychotics:
Neurophysiological Properties (in Man)

J. ROUBICEK

Antipsychotics (neuroleptics) introduced the era of psychopharmacology and quite early on, as soon as favorable clinical activity had been ascertained, their neurophysiological properties were intensively explored. Compared to the well known EEG profiles of previously used psychoactive substances, e.g., barbiturates, opioids, stimulants, and psychodysleptics, the new antipsychotics proved to possess very clear-cut profiles.

EEG and behavioral pharmacological studies in animals are limited to gross patterned activities (seizures, motor activities, sleep) and require anthropomorphic interpretations to assess the EEG-drug effects. It has been difficult, especially in psychopharmacology, to transfer the results of observations of rabbits, rats, cats and guinea pigs – animals with great species metabolic differences – to man. Early EEG studies in phase 1 in man are necessary to identify and classify new psychoactive agents. Such studies in volunteers were introduced in the fifties by a few laboratories in Europe (Erlangen, Prague) and in the USA (St. Louis). It was established that the changes in electric brain activity in normal subjects after an oral dose of a neuroleptic corresponded with changes in the EEG of schizophrenics when treated with higher doses. Later it was shown that the EEG changes in normal volunteers and mental patients are in direct relation to the amount of neuroleptic administered. The accompanying behavioral changes are, at the same time, the results of cerebral biochemical events which are simultaneously reflected in electric cerebral activity. It was soon noticed that the changes in the EEG depend on the level of wakefulness and that higher doses of psychoactive compounds, especially during long-term treatment with larger quantities of neuroleptics, provoke some sleep patterns in the EEG. The EEG also responded very sensitively to changes in glucose, oxygen, and carbon dioxide in the blood and was in a nonspecific way dependent on the perceptive and emotional states of the examined persons. WIKLER (1954) broadly related drug effects, EEG, and behavior, stating that shifts in the direction of desynchronization in the pattern of the electroencephalogram occurred in association with anxiety, hallucinations, fantasies, illusions, or tremors and that shifts in the direction of synchronization occurred in association with euphoria, relaxation, and drowsiness. These findings and "nonspecific" EEG changes indicated the necessity to make comparisons of the EEG changes after neuroleptics (and all other psychoactive compounds) with those after placebo in mental patients. It was proposed that the patients be examined under strict comparable conditions, i.e., regarding time of examination, state of vigility, sugar in blood, etc., and this was quite feasible in studies with single doses but hardly realistic during long-term therapy with mental patients. The personality and milieu-dependent individual differences between the examinees are eradicated by averaging the results of groups of volunteers, keeping the time and environment of the experiments constant, and by making randomized examinations of persons having received an active substance or placebo. Most of the EEG studies in normal persons have been done with homogeneous groups, males aged 19–27 years, with reasonably good and constant α-activity. If one starts with a hetero-geneous group with various types of graphs, the number participating in such a study would have to be increased.

Great progress is to be seen in *EEG classification* of drugs, developed especially by FINK in the years 1961–1974, and with the development of computer techniques EEG classification became more quantitative. Studying the principal EEG changes in dominant frequency, amplitude, and variability of frequency and amplitude, burst ac-tivities and spindling, FINK (1961) proposed a set of relations of changes in some vari-ables and concomitant changes in behavior. An increase of slow activity is seen in de-creased perceptual discrimination, retarded motor activity, heightened mood, reduced thoughts, and decreased recall. When β-activity is heightened, similar behavioral ef-fects ensue with increased sleep duration and reduced affect, particularly of fear and anxiety. β-Spindling is characteristic of drugs which develop rapid tolerance, inhibit seizures, and exhibit spontaneous seizures on rapid withdrawal of medication. When β-activity is enhanced and amplitudes are decreased, mood is heightened and stimuli are perceived more acutely and more clearly. When frequent and prolonged periods of desynchronization or loss of frequencies also occur, subjects report illusions or hal-lucinations, psychomotor activity is increased, as are tremors and fears, and sleep dur-ation is reduced. When β and slow wave activity increase together, delirium occurs, with reduced perceptual acuity and recall and with psychomotor restlessness. Finally, when α-activity is enhanced in amount and amplitude, then relaxation, reveries, pleas-ant fantasies, feelings of well-being, euphoria, and heightened mood each increase. These formulations of FINK provide a basis for the EEG profile method (a systematic characterization of drug-induced cerebral effects in man) to define a clinical profile of the activity of new (or established) compounds.

For ethical reasons, it was necessary in clinical studies to compare the EEG profile of a new neuroleptic drug with a well known reference substance. Therefore chlor-promazine, the first discovered and most widely known antipsychotic substance, be-came a generally accepted reference drug for comparative clinical and electroence-phalographic studies of the later developed substances. The action of chlorpromazine and other neuroleptics with a dimethylamine-propyl side chain (e.g., promazine, triflupromazine, methopromazine), a piperidine side chain (thioridazine, mepazine), a piperazine side chain (perazine, prochlorperazine, butaperazine, perphenazine, flu-phenazine) and of the butyrophenones (haloperidol, triperidol, methylperidol), is shown in the EEG profiles to be rather uniform. These compounds produce a slowing of α-activity, sometimes with hypersynchronization and a gradual increase of the slower rhythms of the ϑ- and δ-bands, together with a decrease of fast activity in the β band (Figs. 1–6). BORENSTEIN et al. (1965) described more slow wave activity and less synchronization in sedative phenothiazines of the piperidine group and fewer slow waves with more synchronization in the piperazine group. All these substances de-crease the occurrence of parasitic extracerebral phenomena in EEG recordings be-cause the muscle artefacts especially are not so pronounced in the calmed-down men-tal patient. But there are some complications which change this uniform EEG pattern. In all pharmacological EEG studies it is necessary to take into consideration the sen-

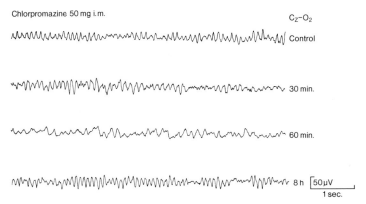

Fig. 1. Changes of EEG after 50 mg chlorpromazine i.m. in normal volunteer. Slowing of α frequency with amplitude increase in 30 min. α-Absence with dominant ϑ-rythms, 5–6 cps. Return to "control" EEG in 8 h

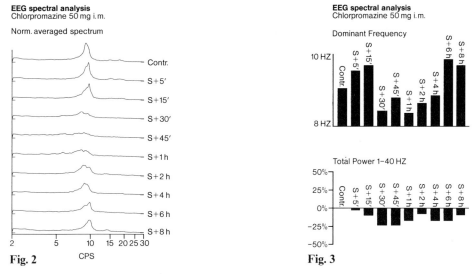

Fig. 2   Fig. 3

Fig. 2. Spectral analysis; averaged spectrum represents dynamisms of electric changes after 50 mg chlorpromazine i.m. in normal volunteer. Slowing of α-activity in 15–45 min, abolishment of α and dominancy of ϑ in 1–2 h, return to control averaged spectrum values in 8 h

Fig. 3. Instrumentally quantified changes (spectral analysis) in dominant frequency and in total electric power, 1–40 cps, in EEG after 50 mg chlorpromazine i.m. in normal volunteer in period over 8 h

sitivity of the individual. Identical doses of drugs can induce variable changes in the EEG recordings of different types of persons. It depends very much on the character and arrangement of the control recording made before the drug has been administered. The second important variable in the EEG profile when studying the effects of a drug is in the "time-dosage relationship" (ITIL, 1968). It was shown that the dopamine receptor blockade induced by a single dose of a neuroleptic agent is a dynamic

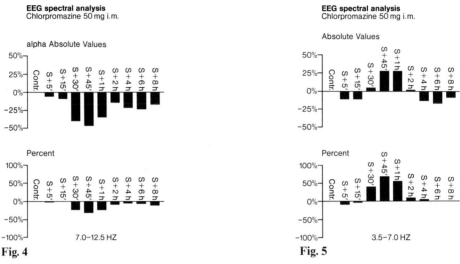

Fig. 4   **Fig. 5**

Fig. 4. Changes (decrease) in absolute and percentual values of instrumentally quantified α-activity after 50 mg chlorpromazine i.m. in normal volunteer

Fig. 5. Changes (increase) in absolute and percentual values in ϑ-activity 3.–7.0 cps, after 50 mg chlorpromazine i.m.

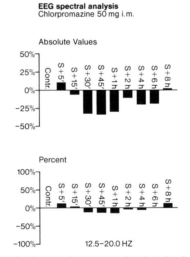

Fig. 6. Changes (decrease) in absolute and percentual values in β-activity, 12.5–20.0 cps, after 50 mg chlorpromazine i.m.

phenomenon which in the course of time is replaced by an increased sensitivity of receptor to dopamine agonists (CHRISTENSEN et al., 1976). A dopaminergic–cholinergic balance is operative in the supersensitivity situation. That means that even in a single dose study of psychoactive compounds it is necessary to have an interval of several days between the application of various, and especially of contrarily active, drugs. Further important information about the action of antischizophrenic compounds on

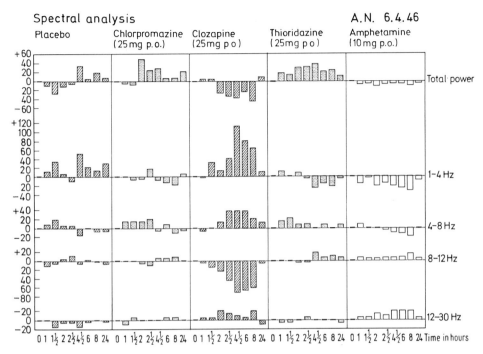

Fig. 7. Comparison of the action on EEG of three neuroleptics, chlorpromazine, thioridazine, and clozapine, in spectral analytic evaluation with placebo and with psychostimulative dex-amphetamine in the same normal examinee over period of 24 h

the EEG encouraged research in psychodysleptics, especially LSD and psilocybin. Minute doses of these drugs, which provoke a very strong desynchronization of the graph, cause an increase of frequency together with a decrease of α-amplitude and an increase of β-waves (and produce well known psychopathological phenomena at the same time), were promptly blocked in their clinical and EEG activity by chlorpromazine (ROUBICEK and SRNEC, 1955; ROUBICEK, 1961). This knowledge then led to research with experimental model psychoses. The fact that the efficient blockade of dysleptic-induced electrophysiological phenomena was achieved through neuroleptics advanced our understanding of the fundamental processes of the brain in mental disease. It is technically not possible or even necessary to show graphs and computerized profiles of all the known neuroleptics because they are mostly similar. They are alike also in their therapeutic activity and psychiatrists are increasingly skeptical about the value of extensive research with new neuroleptics, particularly if they are clinically related to those already in general use. We should show only representative groups and discuss especially the time of onset, peak and duration of EEG changes and for this purpose profiles taken over 8 or 24 h after a single dose of a neuroleptic are the most useful (Fig. 7). An examination using normal volunteers is most advantageous because there is no danger that some other drug has been recently administered which will influence the EEG profile (which is very difficult, sometimes impossible, with mental patients in today's polypragmasia). It is not easy today, for ethical and technical reasons, to get a "clean" EEG before a single dose of a neuroleptic compound in acute schizophrenia. But in the comparative EEG study with some neuroleptics it was clearly seen that it is possible to transfer the results of the EEG study with volunteers to schizophrenic patients. We know that neuroleptics do not cure the illness but primarily alleviate its symptoms. However, from various types of EEG profiles and in combination with other neurophysiological parameters, psychological tests, rating scales, behavior, even from subjective reports or examinees and from existing or nonexisting side effects, we are able to discover in which part of the CNS a neuroleptic drug is predominantly active.

Instrumentally quantified EEG – cerebral electrometry (FINK, 1975), computerized EEG (ITIL, 1975) – probably means the most important progress in psychiatry and psychopharmacology since BERGER's discovery (1929) of the EEG registration from scalp electrodes.

The classic way of analyzing rhythmic waveforms is the harmonic analysis, which is based on the *Fourier Theorem*. This theorem states that a periodic waveform is equivalent to a sum of pure sine waves – the harmonies – each one determined by its amplitude and phase. The set of harmonic amplitudes and phases is called the spectrum. The Fourier Theorem also states that the spectrum of each waveform is unique and that, given a spectrum, it is possible to reconstruct the waveform (which is called a synthesis). Calculation of Fourier spectra is made through appropriate computer programs, which display both the waveform and corresponding spectrum. It is also possible to erase some parts of the spectrum or otherwise manipulate it, and to synthetize the modified spectrum, which gives "filtered" waveform. The maxima of the spectrum indicate the dominant frequencies which characterize the periodicity of the waveform. Instead of taking the amplitude and phase, the square of the amplitudes can be calculated and the "power" spectrum is then obtained.

Various other methods of instrumental quantification, their advantages and disadvantages, will not be discussed here. They were surveyed by BRAZIER (1965) and by MATOUSEK (1967). Three principal methods of reducing analog EEG signals to numeric form are used: power spectral analysis, period analysis, and amplitude integration. It is probably not so important which method of computerization is used but that each laboratory keeps to the same method in order to be able to rationally compare the results of various studies over longer periods of time. Power spectrum analysis, predominantly used in Europe at the present time, proved that neuroleptics as a class of psychoactive compounds have an essentially different EEG profile from thymoleptic, anxiolytic, and psychodysleptic compounds. Whereas in other mentioned groups the β-activity is mostly increased, with neuroleptics the EEG changes in the instrumentally quantified graphs are mostly concentrated in the α-band and the slow δ- and ϑ-frequencies, which are slowed and increased in abundance, whereas β-activity decreases. The period analytic method, used more in the USA, gives similar results. This method especially facilitates the study of higher frequency bands. Relationships between the neurophysiological effects of centrally acting drugs and concentrations of the pharmacologically active molecules in plasma can take a wide variety of forms, ranging from simple direct relationships (e.g., those involving effects on reaction time) to extremely complex relationships (e.g., those involving clinical rating of psychopathology). Relationships between drug effects and drug concentrations in plasma are influenced (1) by features of the drug, such as its rate of distribution among the various body compartments and whether or not its metabolites are pharmacologically active, (2) by features of the effect under study, such as the frequency with which the effect can be recorded, and the sensitivity of the recording system to small changes in the effect, and (3) (when the drug is studied in association with pathologic conditions) by features of the relevant disease state, such as the speed with which the severity of the illness reacts to changes in drug concentration, and the degree to which the illness is episodic (CURRY, 1971). Some of these problems are nonexistent, or at least not so pronounced, in EEG studies with instrumental quantification in normal volunteers or in schizophrenics who have not previously received pharmacologic treatment. The main advantage of EEG is that we are able to study the changes in the target-topic organ in the brain and not in the general milieu of a whole organism. It is possible to speak of CNS bioavailability, a much more reliable factor than a blood assay. If we registered changes in brain activity we can be sure that the brain physiology has been chemically changed and that the blood–brain barrier has definitely been passed. When the EEG is not even slightly changed it is probable that the drug is not psychoactive. In active compounds we are able to examine the EEG profile of an antischizophrenic compound repeatedly at short intervals in order to understand the dynamic changes and time sequences in the CNS provoked by biochemical processes, and it is here that the 24-h studies after one dose of a drug are very useful. Certainly much easier than carrying out extensive studies regarding the changes of drug levels in cerebrospinal fluid.

The clinical separation of different classes of psychoactive compounds is certainly not a clear and rigid one. It is common empirical knowledge that the efficacious neuroleptic, thioridazine, could be used with considerable therapeutic success as a supportive thymoleptic in combination with classic antidepressives such as amitryptyline and imipramine. Even in this area the EEG profile can be used as a very sensitive screening test. With clozapine, a new antischizophrenic substance, is was possible to prove the value of EEG in prospective evaluations of clinical activity from studies in normal persons. An extraordinary quality of this neuroleptic is that it produces hardly any extrapyramidal side effects. According to the classification by the World Health Organization "neuroleptics also known as 'antipsychotics' and formerly 'major tranquillizers' or 'ataractics' have therapeutic effects on psychoses and other types of psychiatric disorders and provoke certain neurological effects such as the production of extrapyramidal symptoms." Because the therapeutic effect of clozapine is that of a strong neuroleptic with initial sedation, the idea that neuroleptic antipsychotic activity is necessarily related to extrapyramidal phenomena is not valid. Contrary to chlorpromazine and haloperidol, which increase the synthesis and turnover of dopamine, therapeutic doses of clozapine in animal experiments only increased the synthesis. The major activity of clozapine in the brain is not in the nigro-striatal system but in the limbic system and the reticular formation (CARLSSON, 1974). The results of studies by SULSER et al. (1974) and AGHAJANIAN and BUNNEY. (1974) suggest a dissociation between dopaminergic blockade and antipsychotic activity and support the idea that the main activity of clozapine is in the limbic forebrain. The mechanism by which clozapine (and in part thioridazine and sulpiride also) possibly cause a preferential activation of limbic dopamine turnover is far from being explained. It may be connected with a greater accumulation of these drugs in the limbic than in the extrapyramidal structures, possibly accounted for by a difference in the blood–brain barrier of the two areas. Alternatively, these compounds may possess, compared to haloperidol and chlorpromazine, a stronger affinity for limbic than for striatal dopamine receptors (BARTHOLINI, 1976). Clozapine in the brain from other neuroleptics is reflected in the

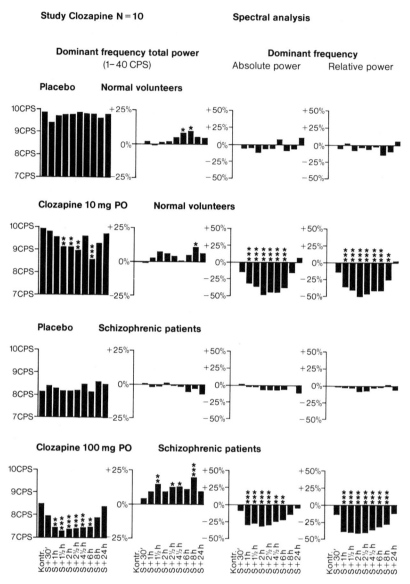

Fig. 8. Spectral analysis of total electric power and of dominant frequency in 10 normal volunteers (10 mg clozapine p.o.) and 10 schizophrenics (100 mg clozapine p.o.) over 24 h in comparison with placebo

EEG profile if this compound. Studies (ROUBICEK et al., 1975; ROUBICEK and MAJOR, 1977) in normal volunteers and schizophrenics showed that the EEG of clozapine was different from other neuroleptic compounds (and from placebo). The spectral analysis shows a gradual decrease and slowing of α-reaching a maximum after 4.5–6.0 h after administration of the drug, a highly significant increase of δ- and ϑ-activity, and a slight increase of β-frequency, especially in the 20–25 cps sub-band. The increase of

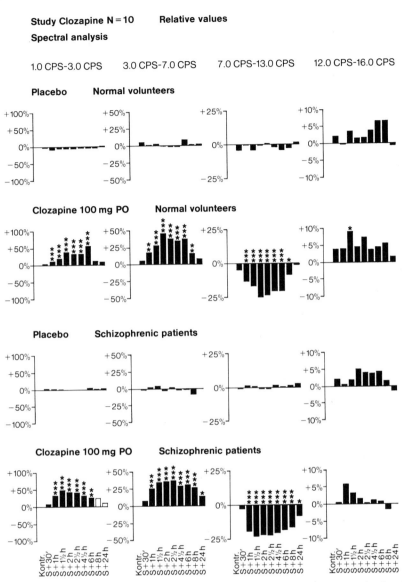

Fig. 9. Spectral analysis of δ-, ϑ-, α- and lower β-frequency (12–16 cps) in 10 normals after 10 mg clozapine p.o. and in 10 schizophrenics after 100 mg clozapine p.o. over 24 h in comparison with placebo

β-waves is more outstanding when iterative interval analysis is used for instrumental quantification in normal persons and schizophrenics (Figs. 8–10). The EEG profile of clozapine resembles, in part, the EEG changes with thymoleptics, especially impramine. The prediction that it could be used with therapeutic effect in some types of depressions was correct. Kogan and Nikolenko (1974), Nahunek et al. (1975), Klik (1976), clinically proved its antidepressive action. Clozapine seems to be particularly indicated for atypic, agitated, and anxious forms of depressive disease. *The prediction*

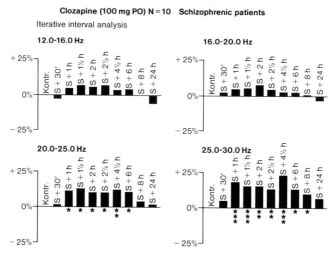

Fig. 10. Interative interval analysis of β band divided into four sub-bands after 100 mg clozapine p.o. in 10 schizophrenics

of therapeutic activity of prospective antischizophrenic and other psychoactive drugs by systematic measurements of EEG profiles is a further important step after classification. Based on the changes of symptomatology, accompanying the use of psychoactive compounds, it has been possible to formulate associations between the EEG profile changes and changes of psychopathology. With the combination of EEG and clinical criteria in a comparative study of several drugs it is possible to predict which compound will be therapeutically optimal (MATOUSEK et al., 1969). The most important items in EEG was disorganized polyfrequent recording (in visual evaluation) and variations of coefficients in ϑ- and β-frequencies (in instrumental frequency analysis). FINK and ITIL in several studies, performed in the years 1969–1975, repeatedly applied the association of EEG profile and clinical effect in the studies of presumed psychoactive compounds and proved the relation with clinical symptomatology. FINK for fenfluramine, cyclazocine and doxepin, ITIL for molindone, loxapine, and tranxene. Their experimental studies have already been confirmed by clinical trials and by long-term therapeutic experience since these drugs have been introduced in practice. ITIL (1975) proposed that computerized EEG may be helpful in the selection of the best drug for a particular patient and to subclassify schizophrenic patients. He demonstrated that therapy-resistant schizophrenic patients are sensitive to neuroleptic treatment when the synchronous "hypernormal" α-EEG patterns are transformed to low voltage, desynchronized fast EEG pattern by the administration of certain "hallucinogenic" compounds. This proposition was shown to be invalid because it is possible to see the desynchronization of schizophrenic EEG in most of the patients if an appropriately higher dose of LSD was administered. But there is another point to ITIL's (1975) proposal. Computerized EEG may certainly help to monitor drug treatment and daily doses. In addition to the clinical assessment, it is possible to apply EEG examination to evaluate the action of a drug and its dosage. In case any EEG changes occur, the single and daily dose should be increased and/or the type of neuroleptic changed. There are schizophrenic patients who do not show response to phenothiazine but improve after butyrophenone. There are chronic schizophrenics who show no response to conventional recommended doses of neuroleptics and need much higher doses. In contrast, if a patient showed marked changes with an abnormal pattern in the EEG, this could indicate a "hypersensitivity" to the drug resulting in certain side effects such as marked sedation and eventual convulsions. Earlier ITIL et al. (1966) observed an increase of low voltage fast activity and a decrease of α-waves a few days before the recurrence of a psychotic episode. With the instrumental quantification of EEG it is sometimes possible to foresee a relapse and prevent it by increasing the dosage. ITIL et al. (1974) demonstrated that children with high risk for schizophrenia (children of schizophrenic parents) have similar EEG patterns to psychotic children and schizophrenic adults. This suggests that the neurophysiological correlates of schizophrenia are present a long time before the onset of the actual illness. Speculation that the low voltage desynchronized fast EEG pattern represents a neurophysiological predisposition for schizophrenia (ITIL, 1975) and that the modification of these patterns to high voltage slow α-EEG may prevent the outbursts of schizophrenia still require further study and confirmation in larger populations of patients. Especially in studies with children, only neuroleptics without tardive dyskinesia side effects should be used.

In addition to instrumentally quantified EEG spectra, there is another neurophysiologic dynamic method developed in the last decade: the technique of extracting *potentials, evoked by sensory stimuli* from the scalp EEG, with averaging. SALETU (1974) and SHAGASS (1974) reviewed the effects of psychotropic drugs on sensory evoked activities and the contingent negative variation (CNV), discovered and introduced in research by the late WALTER-GREY et al. (1964) which have been related to such psychological responses as expectancy, attention, and motivation. Since the time of CIGANEK's (1961) survey of thiopental narcosis, many psychoactive drugs have been studied. In somatosensory evoked potentials, neuroleptic drugs provoke changes which are characterized by a latency increase in early as well as late peaks. The changes are more prominent in the late peaks and the degree of the latency change increases with increasing peak latency: the larger the peak latency, the greater the drug-induced latency increase. The amplitudes are attenuated, predominantly in the late part of the response. The amplitude changes in the primary response are rather insubstantial. This type of alteration was described by SALETU (1974, 1976) after oral administration of single doses of representatives of different neuroleptic subclasses, including chlorpromazine, thioridazine, and perphenazine in normal healthy volunteers as well as during long-term (3 months) administration of thiothixene, fluphenazine, and haloperidol in chronic schizophrenic patients. With regard to the mode of action it appears that neuroleptics affect several CNS sites in a depressant manner (DOMINO, 1962). In combination with the computer-analyzed EEG, measuring evoked potentials is a useful method to follow the development of electric changes during mental disease and pharmacologic treatment; this technique can also be utilized for the evaluation of newly developed substances.

A. Future Prospects

A possible new approach to psychopharmacologic studies could be electroencephalographic research of the anomalies of functional organization of the brain in major psy-

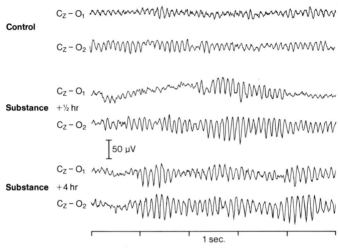

Fig. 11. EEG changes after 1 mg synthetic methionine-enkephalin i.m. (FK 33-824 Sandoz Ltd.). Slowing, increase of amplitude and hypersynchronization of α frequency, slight increase of amount of β frequency (normal volunteer)

choses. There are interhemispheral differences which could be used as a measure of EEG synchronicity in the instrumentally quantified α frequency band, eventually with concomittant research in evoked potentials. There is some evidence that the EEG indicates laterally differences in psychiatric disorders. It was shown, for example, that the dominant hemisphere of schizophrenics display "weak" nervous system dynamics and that chlorpromazine reverses a lateralized deficit. These prospects were reviewed recently by SHAW et al. (1977).

An other important innovation may be expected from an area outside neuroleptics. Antischizophrenic drugs, available today, do not therapeutically satisfy because even if neurophysiologic parameters are changed only symptomatic or regulative relief is observed in patients. Speculation on the development of some new class of compound, perhaps from the body's own substances such as hormones or biogenic amines, which are able to modify the EEG pattern has perhaps been fulfilled by the discovery of β-endorphines and the separation of a pentapeptide chain , methionine-enkephalin, with morphine-like properties from the pituitary glands (GUILLEMIN et al., 1976; KOSTERLITZ and HUGHES, 1977). Profound behavioral effects in rats suggested that these substances could be related to etiological factors in mental illness. KLINE et al. (1977) administered 3–9 mg β-endorphine to three schizophrenic patients and observed a progressive reduction or disappearance of auditory hallucinations and paranoid ideation; after administration to three depressed patients he observed improved mood in two of them. Recently we had the opportunity to study the EEG of normal volunteers with synthetic methionine-enkephalin (ROEMER et al., 1977) and found that the EEG profile differs from neuroleptics and opioids. After doses of 0.1–1.2 mg an increase of α activity, a tendency to hypersynchronization and to spindles, together with an increase of β activity was observed. Activity in the slow bands, δ and ϑ, decreased at the same time. The maximum changes occurred 2–4 h after i.m. administration of methionine-enkephalin (Figs. 11–14). These results show the very special

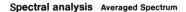

Spectral analysis Averaged Spectrum

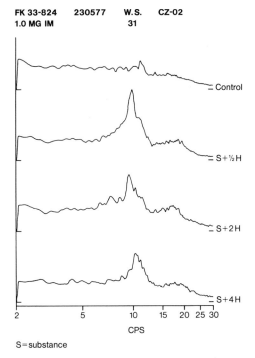

Fig. 12. Averaged spectrum EEG changes after 1 mg synthetic methionine-enkephalin i.m. Increase of electric power in 30 min with shift of peak to left side of frequency scale with maximum between 0.5–2.0 h

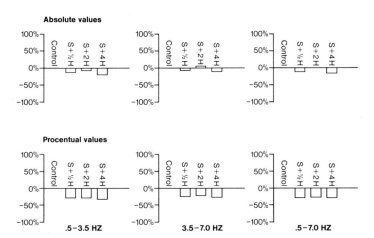

Fig. 13. Spectral analysis of EEG in δ- and 𝜗-bands after 1 mg methionine-enkephalin i.m. Decrease of absolute and percentual values (about 25 %)

EEG-Spectral analysis   FK 33-824   1.0 MG   W.S.

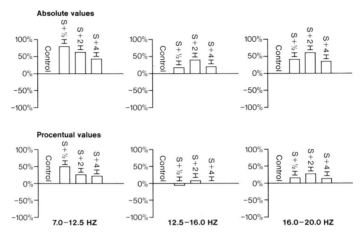

Fig. 14. Spectral analysis of EEG in α- and β-bands (up to 20 cps). Increase of absolute and percentual values in both bands

EEG profile of this substance, with no resemblance to neuroleptic and thymoleptic compounds. Further electrophysiologic and clinical studies of β-endorphines/enkephalines are the most fascinating of today's research in antischizophrenic treatment. Their relation to morphine receptors in the brain suggests the possibility of analgetic influence and this important clinical subject is another target for contemporary research in enkephaline.

B. Summary

The complex of knowledge coming from various sections of biochemical, pharmacologic, psychological and neurophysiological research bring us systematically nearer to understanding the cause and mechanisms of psychoses. In this orchestra of research the new information obtained through computerized electric activity of the brain has proved to be of value in the assessment of many psychoactive compounds. The importance of EEG examination is increased when behavioral testing is included and blood levels of drugs are simultaneously examined. However, because of the possibility of obtaining numerical quantification of events in the brain, computerized EEG provides the most important data.

References

Aghajanian, J., Bunney, B.: Dopaminergic neurons of the substantia nigra. J. Pharmacol. Exp. Ther. 5 (Suppl. 1), 58 (1974)

Bartholini, G.: Differential effect of neuroleptic drugs on dopamine turnover in the extrapyramidal and limbic system. J. Pharm. Pharmacol. 28, 429-433 (1976)

Berger, H.: Über das Electroenzephalogramm des Menschen. Arch. Psychiatr. Nervenkr. 87, 527-570 (1929)

Borenstein, P., Cujo, P., Chiva, M.: A propos de la classification des substances psychotropes selon leurs effects sur l'EEG. Ann. Med. Psychol. 2, 429–452 (1965)

Brazier, M.: The application of computers to EEG. In: Computers in Biomedical Research Brazier, M. (ed.) Vol. I, pp. 2–9. New York: Academic Press 1965

Carlsson, A.: Receptor-mediated control of dopamine synthesis. J. Pharmacol. (Suppl. 1), 5, 58 (1974)

Christensen, A., Fjalland, B., Moller-Nielsen, T.: On the supersensitivity of dopamine receptors, induced by neuroleptics. Psychopharmacology 48, 1–6 (1976)

Ciganek, L.: Die EEG Lichtreizantwort der menschlichen Hirnrinde. S.A.V. Bratislava (1961)

Curry, S.: Chlorpromazine: concentration in plasma, excretion in urine and duration effect. Proc. R. Soc. Med. 64, 285–289 (1971)

Domino, E.: Sites of action of some central nervous system depressants. Annu. Rev. Pharmacol., 215–268 (1962)

Fink, M.: EEG and behavioral effects of psychopharmacologic agents. Neuropsychopharmacology 1, 441–446 (1961)

Fink, M.: EEG and Human Psychopharmacology. Annu. Rev. Pharmacol. 9, 241–258 (1969)

Fink, M.: EEG profiles and bioavailability measures of psychoactive drugs. In: Modern Problems of Pharmacopsychiatry (Itil, T., ed.), Vol. VIII pp. 76–98. Basel: Karger 1974

Fink, M.: Prediction of clinical activity of psychoactive drugs: Application of cerebral electrometry in phase I studies. In: Predictability in Psychopharmacology (Sudilowsky, A., Gershon, S., Beer, B., eds) New York; pp. 65–88. Raven Press 1975

Guillemin, R., Ling, N., Burgus, R.: Endorphines, peptides d'origine hypothalamique et neurohypophysaire à activité morphinométique. Isolement et structure moléculaire d'α-endorphine. C.r. hebd. Séanc. Acad. Sci. Paris, Sér. D, 282, 783-785 (1976)

Itil, T.M., Keskiner, A., Fink, M.: Therapeutic studies in "therapy resistant" schizophrenic patients. Compr. Psychiatry, 7, 488–493 (1966)

Itil, T.M.: EEG and Pharmacopsychiatry. In: Clinical Pharmacology (Freyhan, F., ed.), pp. 163–194. Basel: Karger 1968

Itil, T.M., Hsu, W., Saletu, B., Mednick, S.: Computer EEG and evoked potential investigations in children of high risk for schizophrenia. Am. J. Psychiatry 131, 892–900 (1974)

Itil, T.M.,: Digital computer period analyzed EEG in psychiatry and psychopharmacology. In: Computerized EEG Analysis (Dolce, G., Künkel, H., eds.) pp. 289–308. Stuttgart: Fischer 1975

Klik, J.: Experience with clozapine in psychiatric practice. Cesk. Psychiatr. 72, 197 (1976)

Kline, N.S., Li, C.H., Lehmann, H.E., Lajtha, A., Laski, E., Cooper, T.: β-Endorphin-induced changes in schizophrenic and depressed patients. Arch. Gen. Psychiatry, in print (1977)

Kogan, W., Nikolenko, N.: New drugs and the treatment of nervous and mental diseases. Report of Leningrad Bechterev Psychoneurol. Inst. 40 (1974)

Kosterlitz, H., Hughes, J.: Peptides with morphine-like action in the brain. Br. J. Psychiatry 130, 298–304 (1977)

Matousek, M.: Automatic analysis in clinical EEG. Psychiatr. Research Inst., Prague (1967)

Matousek, M., Roubicek, J., Vinar, O., Roth, J.: Klinische und electroencephalographische Kriterien der Auswahl der optimalen Medikation. Arzneim.-Forsch. 19, 438 (1969)

Nahunek, K., Svestka, J., Misurec, J., Radova, A.: Experiences with clozapine. Cesk. Psychiatr. 71, 11 (1975)

Roemer, D., Buescher, H.H., Hill, R.C., Pless, J., Bauer, W., Cardinaux, F., Closse, A., Hauser, D., Huguenin, R.: A synthetic enkephalin analogue with prolonged parenteral and oral analgesic activity. Nature 268, 547–549 (1977)

Roubicek, J.: Experimental psychoses. Cesk. Psychiatr., 57, 420–422 (1961)

Roubicek, J., Major, I.: EEG profile and behavioral changes after a single dose of clozapine in normals and in schizophrenics. Biol. Psychiatry 12, 613–633 (1977)

Roubicek, J., Srnec, J.: Experimental psychosis LSD. Cas. Lek. Cesk. 94, 189 (1955)

Roubicek, J., Matejcek, M., Porsolt, R.: Computer analyzed EEG and behavioral changes after psychoactive drugs. Int. J. Neurol. 10, 33 (1975)

Saletu, B.: Classification of psychotropic drugs based on human evoked potentials. In: Psychotropic Drugs and the Human EEG (Itil, T., ed). Basle: Karger 1974

Saletu, B.: Psychopharmaka, Gehirntätigkeit und Schlaf. Basle: Karger 1976

Shagass, C.: Effects of psychotropic drugs in human evoked potentials. In: Psychotropic Drugs and the Human EEG (Itil, T., ed.), Vol. VIII, pp. 238–257. Basle: Karger 1974

Shaw, J., O'Connor, P., Ongley, C.: The EEG as a measure of cerebral functional organization. Br. J. Psychiatry *130*, 260–264 (1977)

Sulser, F., Stewart, R., Blumberg, T.: The limbic forebrain: The role of catecholamines in the action of antipsychotics. J. Pharmacol. Exp. Ther. *5*, (Suppl. 1), 155 (1974)

Walter-Grey, W., Cooper, R., Aldridge, V., McCallum, W., Winter, A.: Contingent negative variation. Nature *203*, 380–384 (1964)

Wikler, A.: Clinical and electroencephalographic studies on the effects of mescaline, N-allylor-morphine and morphine in man. J. Nerv. Ment. Dis. *120*, 157–175 (1954)

CHAPTER 9

Biochemical Effects of Neuroleptic Drugs

G. Bartholini and K.G. Lloyd

A. Introduction

The biochemical effects of the neuroleptic drugs can be divided according to the following criteria:

a) Changes induced by all of these compounds independently of the brain structure upon which they act. These changes, e.g., alteration of DA turnover, are qualitatively similar in all of the DA-rich brain areas and can be considered as common basic effects of neuroleptic compounds.

b) Changes induced by all of the neuroleptic drugs but specific for a given brain structure e.g., alteration of acetylcholine (ACh) or γ-aminobutyric acid (GABA) turnover. The preferential occurrence of these changes in specific brain areas is probably explained by the neuronal network proper to each region.

c) The above-mentioned effects are typical for all "classical" neuroleptic compounds which differ only in their relative potency (on biochemical and behavioural parameters) and, thus, share a similar pharmacological profile. In contrast, some compounds, which will be referred to as "atypical" neuroleptics, differ from classical drugs as they show a peculiar pharmacological spectrum.

In the following, the biochemical changes elicited by antipsychotic compounds in cerebral neurons of animals will be reviewed according to be above-mentioned criteria. In addition, the bearing of these biochemical changes on the clinical effect of neuroleptics in extrapyramidal and limbic systems will be discussed. Thus, a body of evidence suggests that neuroleptic-induced biochemical alterations in the basal ganglia are related to the extrapyramidal side-effects and, in the limbic system, to the antipsychotic action of these drugs.

B. General Biochemical Features of Neuroleptic Drugs

In all brain regions containing DA, neuroleptic compounds increase the liberation of the transmitter (Table 1). This is indirectly demonstrated by 1) increased metabolism of DA resulting in an enhanced concentration of its metabolites, 3-methoxytyramine (Carlsson and Lindqvist, 1963; Kehr, 1976), homovanillic acid and dihydroxyphenylacetic acid (Bartholini and Pletscher, 1972; Da Prada and Pletscher, 1966; Laverty and Sharman, 1965; Westerink and Korf, 1975a,b); 2) acceleration of DA utilisation following tyrosine hydroxylase inhibition by α-methyl-p-tyrosine (cf. Andén, 1969; O'Keeffe et al., 1970); 3) changes in accumulation or disappearence of labelled DA following administration of radioactive precursors (Javoy et al., 1970; Nyback and Sedvall, 1970; Persson, 1970; Pletscher et al., 1971). Direct evidence

Table 1. Effect of acute administration of various neuroleptic drugs on parameters in rat brain related to DA neurotransmission

Drug and region	Activation of tyrosine hydroxylase (ED$_{30}$ µmol/kg)[a]	Inhibition of DA-dependent adenylate cyclase K_i (µM)	Displacement of spiroperidol ($-\log IC_{50}$)[d]
A. Classical neuroleptics			
Haloperidol			
Striatum	0.6	0.037[b]	7.69
Limbic forebrain or nucleus Accumbens	2.2	0.030[b]	–
Limbic cortex	–	–	6.83
Chlorpromazine			
Striatum	2.8	0.033[b]	6.85
Limbic forebrain or nucleus accumbens	3.0	0.054[b]	–
Limbic cortex	–	–	7.21
B. Atypical neuroleptics			
Clozapine			
Striatum	30	0.060[c]	5.9
Limbic forebrain or nucleus accumbens	22	0.059[c]	–
Limbic cortex	–	–	7.32
Sulpiride			
Striatum	–	14[b]	6.06
Limbic forebrain or nucleus accumbens	–	23[b]	–
Limbic cortex	–	–	4.1

Data from: [a] Zivkovic et al., 1975; [b] Scatton et al., 1977; [c] Clement-Cormier and Robison, 1977; [d] Leysen et al., 1978

for the liberation of DA following neuroleptic administration is provided by the measurement of the enhanced neurotransmitter release in discrete brain areas by means of the push–pull cannula (Lloyd and Bartholini, 1975; Bartholini et al., 1976a).

In parallel with increased DA liberation, synthesis of the amine is also enhanced as demonstrated by the activation of tyrosine hydroxylase and the increased formation of DOPA (Zivkovic et al., 1974, 1975). Under the above conditions, the tissue concentration of DA is not changed (Andén, 1969; Gey and Pletscher, 1961) and the increased transmitter liberation reflects an enhanced turnover. The accelerated turnover of DA is connected with activation of the dopaminergic neurons as indicated by enhanced firing of DA cell bodies as seen in electrophysiological experiments (Bunney and Aghajanian, 1978).

The mechanism by which neuroleptic agents activate DA neurons and increase the liberation of transmitter is thought to be connected with the blockade of postsynaptic DA receptors, leading to impairment of dopaminergic transmission (cf. Andén, 1969; Bunney and Aghajaian, 1975). The reduced DA influence on target cells probably results in the activation of excitatory and/or diminution of inhibitory mono-/ or polysynaptic circuits reverberating on DA neurons which, as a consequence, are activated.

Evidence exists that some of the feedback circuits involved in the regulation of DA neurons are of cholinergic or GABA-ergic nature (see Sect. C.I.3.).

The hypothesis that DA receptors are blocked by neuroleptics is based on two sets of data: a) Electrophysiological results indicate that the effect of iontophoretically applied DA on identified target cells of dopaminergic neurons is blocked or reversed by locally or systemically administered neuroleptic compounds (BUNNEY and AGHAJANIAN, 1975; 1975; YORK, 1971). b) Biochemical experiments show that DA activates an adenylate cyclase which transforms ATP into cyclic AMP. All of the classical neuroleptic agents block the DA-sensitive adenylate cyclase activity whereas blockade of other cyclases (e.g., guanylate cyclase) is not a property common to all neuroleptic compounds (Table 1, CLEMENT-CORMIER and ROBISON, 1977; IVERSEN, 1977; KREUGER et al., 1975). Furthermore, neuroleptic drugs displace either DA itself or DA receptor agonists such as apomorphine from binding sites of membrane preparations from different regions of animal and human brain (SEEMAN et al., 1976a). Conversely, neuroleptics (haloperidol or spiroperidol) bind to membranes and are displaced by DA receptor agonists or by other neuroleptics (Table 1, BURT et al., 1975; CREESE et al., 1975; SEEMAN, 1977; SEEMAN et al., 1976b). The postsynaptic localization of DA receptor (on target cells) is supported by data showing that the effects of either DA receptor agonists or neuroleptics on DA-sensitive adenylate cyclase activity or on DA binding sites are not decreased (and may even be increased) by electrolytic or chemical (by 6-hydroxy DA) lesions of dopaminergic neurons (IVERSEN, 1977; SNYDER et al., 1976; VON VOIGTLANDER et al., 1973). Furthermore, injection of kainic acid into the striatum – which destroys striatal cells leaving DA terminals unaffected – leads to a reduction in both binding sites and DA-sensitive adenylate cyclase activity (COYLE et al., 1977; CREESE et al., 1977). Based on the above reported data, it is reasonable to assume that neuroleptic agents and DA act at the same receptor site located on the effector cells of DA neurons. It is also likely that the DA-sensitive adenylate cyclase is closely connected to dopaminergic transmission.

The increase in DA liberation induced by neuroleptic compounds might also be triggered by an interaction of these drugs with DA "autoreceptors" (SEEMAN and LEE, 1975). Such autoreceptors are probably localized both on the terminals (CARLSSON, 1975) and the cell bodies or dendrites (BUNNEY and AGHAJANIAN, 1975) of DA neurons. However, in the substantia nigra it appears that, if such an autoreceptor exists, it is not associated with a DA-sensitive adenylate cyclase (KEBABIAN and SAAVEDRA, 1976; PHILLIPSON et al., 1977). It is assumed that, under physiological conditions, stimulation of the autoreceptors by DA decreases DA release and synthesis. This may be mediated via changes of end product inhibition (cf. LOVENBERG and BRUCKWICK, 1975), of Ca^{++} flow through the presynaptic membranes (LOVENBERG and BRUCKWICK, 1975; ROTH et al., 1975) and/or of the availability of tyrosine or tyrosine hydroxylase cofactor (KETTLER et al., 1974; ZIVKOVIC et al., 1974). Blockade of the autoreceptors by neuroleptics is reported to enhance the liberation of DA (SEEMANN and LEE, 1975).

The evidence reviewed above for the occurrence of either mechanism involved in the activation of DA neurons by neuroleptics (long feedback or autoreceptor mediated) is mainly indirect and it is difficult to assess which component has the main bearing in vivo.

Teleologically, the neuroleptic-induced activation of dopaminergic neurons and the consequent increased liberation of DA is considered to be a homeostatic mechanism for overcoming the blockade of the postsynaptic receptors and restoring dopaminergic transmission.

C. Effects of Neuroleptic Drugs in Discrete Brain Structures

I. Extrapyramidal System

1. Acetylcholine

Neuroleptic agents enhance the turnover of ACh in the striatum of animals. The first and most direct evidence for this effect has been obtained in experiments of in vivo perfusion of the cat striatum by means of the push–pull cannula. By this technique, the liberation of neurotransmitters such as ACh (or monoamines, GABA, etc.) can be directly assessed by measuring their concentration in the perfusate. Thus, various neuroleptics of different chemical classes (chlorpromazine, haloperidol, thioridazine, clozapine) enhance the liberation of ACh from striatal neurons (cf. Bartholini et al., 1977) (Fig. 1) without altering the concentration of the neurotransmitter in the perfused tissue (Bartholini et al., 1975a). Since the activity of ACh-esterase is not changed (Bartholini et al., 1976b), the enhanced release of ACh reflects an accelerated turnover. It is unlikely that this effect is mediated by the anticholinergic properties of some neuroleptics, which might enhance the transmitter liberation via a feedback mechanism triggered by the blockade of ACh receptors. In fact, atropine, even

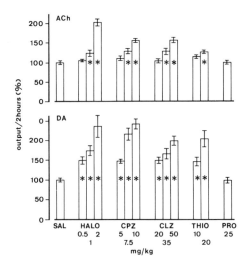

Fig. 1. Effect of neuroleptics and promethazine on the release of ACh and DA into the perfusion fluid of the cat caudate nucleus. The caudate nucleus of the gallamine-immobilized cat was perfused with Ringer solution by means of the push–pull cannula. Saline and the neuroleptic drugs (at the doses indicated) were administered iv. Output of the transmitters throughout the 2-h postinjection period in percent of the 2-h preinjection (control) period.

Abbreviations: SAL, saline; HALO, haloperidol; CPZ, chlorpromazine; CLZ, clozapine; THIO, thioridazine; PRO, promethazine. (From Bartholini et al., 1977; permission of Raven Press)

in high doses (5–25 mg/kg i.v.) causes only a moderate increase in ACh output (unpublished); in addition, haloperidol, which is one of the most potent neuroleptics in enhancing ACh turnover, is virtually devoid of anti-ACh properties (SAYERS and BURKI, 1976).

In contrast to neuroleptic agents, DA receptor agonists (e.g., apomorphine) decrease the spontaneous ACh release. These drugs (apomorphine, L-DOPA) also prevent and antagonize the neuroleptic-induced enhancement of the transmitter liberation (BARTHOLINI et al., 1976a, b). The fact that ACh release is influenced in opposite directions by DA receptor agonists and antagonists supports the hypothesis that the changes are related to the state of DA receptor activity, as altered by these drugs. As a consequence, it is likely that striatal cholinergic (inter) neurons are under the influence of an inhibitory dopaminergic input. Blockade by neuroleptics and stimulation by DA agonists of the DA receptors leads to activation and inhibition, respectively, of the target cholinergic neurons and to corresponding changes in ACh turnover (cf. BARTHOLINI et al., 1976a). Further evidence for this view is provided by the lack of effect on ACh liberation of promethazine (STADLER et al., 1973), a phenothiazine derivative which is devoid of DA receptor blocking properties as it neither influences DA turnover (ROTH et al., 1973) nor possesses antipsychotic properties (FREEDMAN et al., 1976). Similar results on tissue ACh levels (see below) have been obtained utilizing the sulphoxide derivative of chlorpromazine which is inactive as a DA receptor blocker (NYBACK et al., 1973). The DA input on cholinergic neurons appears to be of tonic nature, as acute section of the nigro-striatal DA pathway increases the utilization of ACh in the cat striatum (AGID et al., 1975). Supportive evidence for the physiological regulation of striatal cholinergic neurons by the nigro-striatal DA pathway is provided by the decrease in the striatal ACh liberation following electrical stimulation of the DA cell bodies in the pars compacta of the substantia nigra (BARTHOLINI et al., 1976b). The effect of neuroleptic drugs on striatal ACh turnover has been confirmed by several authors by measuring the changes in ACh concentration or turnover in the tissue: thus, neuroleptic agents decrease, whereas DA receptor agonists increase, the ACh levels indicating an enhanced and a reduced utilization, respectively (see e.g., CHENEY et al., 1976; CONSOLO et al., 1975; GUYENET et al., 1975; SETHY and VAN WOERT, 1974a; see LLOYD, 1978a for detailed references).

2. GABA

It seems likely that neuroleptic agents affect neurons which utilize GABA as their neurotransmitter. Thus, on acute administration, haloperidol decreases GABA levels and increases GABA turnover in the striatum and substantia nigra without altering the activity of glutamic acid decarboxylase (Table 2, KIM and HASSLER, 1975; LLOYD and HORNYKIEWICZ, 1977; MAO and COSTA, 1978 MAO et al., 1977a; MAGGI et al., 1977). It is unlikely that neuroleptics act on GABA receptors since in vitro, these drugs displace [^{3}H]-GABA from mebrane binding sites only at relatively high concentrations (greater than 50 μM) or are completely inactive (ENNA and SNYDER, 1975; LLOYD and DREKSLER, 1978). However, the situation in vivo is somewhat different as haloperidol alters [^{3}H]-GABA binding after intraperitoneal injection (LLOYD et al., 1977b; LLOYD and WORMS, unpublished data) and droperidol has been shown to exert a GABA-mimetic effect on cerebrellar Purkinje cells (MARUYAMA and KAWASAKI, 1976). In addi-

Table 2. Acute and chronic effects of neuroleptic drugs on GABA levels and turnover in different brain regions[a]

Drug	GABA levels (percent control)			GABA turnover time (percent control)		
	Striatum	S. nigra	Nucleus accumbens	Striatum	S. nigra	Nucleus accumbens
Haloperidol						
Acute	63[c]	26.1[b]	113[c]	140[d]	77[d]	80[d]
Chronic	–	131.2[b]	–	50[d]	257.8[d]	25[d]
Chlorpromazine						
Acute	86[c]	107[c]	96[c]	108[d]	130[d]	24[d]
Clozapine						
Acute	104[c]	51.2[b]	92[c]	30[d]	16[d]	62[d]
Chronic	–	69.2[b]	–	–	–	–

[a] Data from reference 2, 18 h post drug; for other data 1–2 h post drug; Data from [b] LLOYD et al., 1977b; [c] MAO and COSTA, 1978; [d] MAO et al., 1977a; [e] KIM and HASSLER, 1975

tion, it may be of relevance to note that some neuroleptics (e.g., haloperidol) contain the GABA moiety within their molecular structure (JANSSEN, 1965).

The decreased concentrations of GABA induced by neuroleptics leads to the assumption that GABA turnover is enhanced by these drugs. However, following administration of neuroleptics, measurements of the changes in transmitter accumulation after inhibition of GABA-transaminase (MAGGI et al., 1977; PEREZ DE LA MORA et al., 1975) and determination of labelled GABA accumulation from radioactive precursors (MAO et al., 1977a and b) gave discordant results. Thus, the question as to whether or not neuroleptics enhance the turnover of GABA remains as yet unanswered.

3. Neuroleptic-Induced Feedback Activation of DA Neurons: Possible Role of ACh and GABA

The neuroleptic-induced alterations in striatal ACh and GABA parallel the enhancement of DA synthesis and liberation. The latter effect, as mentioned in Sect. B, is likely to be due to at least two mechanisms, i.e., blockade of DA autoreceptors and alterations of neuronal inhibitory, and/or excitatory, inputs on the dopaminergic pathways, triggered by the blockade of postsynaptic DA receptors. Strong evidence exists, in the striatum, for the involvement of both ACh and GABA neurons in the second mechanism.

Concerning ACh, it is known that anticholinergic drugs reduce the turnover of DA synthesis and liberation (e.g., ANDÉN and BEDARD, 1971; BARTHOLINI et al., 1975b; JAVOY et al., 1975; cf. LLOYD, 1978a, b for full references). In contrast, ACh-like compounds (physostigmine, oxotremorine) enhance DA turnover (e.g., JAVOY et al., 1975; LLOYD and BARTHOLINI, 1975; cf. LLOYD, 1978a, b for full references). The influence of ACh receptor agonists and antagonists is probably exerted on both DA cell bodies and terminals but the direction of the influence (i.e., positive or negative) may differ between cell bodies and terminals (AGHAJANIAN and BUNNEY, 1973; BARTHOLINI and PLETSCHER, 1972; BUNNEY and AGHAJANIAN, 1978; JAVOY et al., 1974). Iontophoretic administration of acetylcholine excites cells in the zona reticulata but not the zona compacta of the substantia nigra, an effect which is reversed by scopolamine (AGHA-JANIAN and BUNNEY, 1975). As intranigral injection of cholinomimetics decreases (JA-VOY et al., 1974) and anticholinergics increase (BARTHOLINI and PLETSCHER, 1972) striatal DA turnover, it has been proposed that cholinergic neurons stimulate a reticu-lata-compacta nigral interneuron which is inhibitory to DA neuron activity (AGHA-JANIAN and BUNNEY, 1975). In addition to the proposed interneuron, a cholinergic ni-gral input probably originates from the formatio reticularis (SHUTE and LEWIS, 1967) and striatal afferents possibly have a thalamic origin (SIMKE and SAELENS, 1977). The cholinergic afferents to the substantia nigra do not originate from the striatum as hemitransection of the brain between these structures does not change the choline acetylase activity in the substantia nigra (KATAOKA et al., 1974; McGEER et al., 1973).

Finally, striatal cholinergic interneurons and afferents affect the DA activity pos-sibly by an input on the dopaminergic terminals; thus, perfusion of the cat caudate nucleus by Ringer solution containing ACh enhances the liberation of DA in this structure – this effect is potentiated by physostigmine and blocked by atropine (BAR-THOLINI et al., 1976 a).

A great deal of evidence exists for the involvement of GABA in the regulation of the activity of DA neurons. Thus, in electrophysiological experiments, nigral (dopa-minergic?) cells are inhibited by electrical stimulation of the caudate nucleus and this is mimicked by microiontophoretic application of GABA in the substantia nigra (CROSSMAN et al., 1974; DRAY and GONYE, 1975; DRAY and STRAUGHAN, 1976; FELTZ, 1971); both effects are blocked by picrotoxin or bicuculline (CROSSMAN et al., 1973; DRAY and GONYE, 1975). Biochemically, the turnover of striatal DA appears to be re-duced by injection of GABA in the substantia nigra (ANDÉN and STOCK, 1977 a). GA-BA receptor agonists such as muscimol or SL 76002 (see Section II.2), injected intra-peritoneally, decrease DA turnover per se or reverse the increased turnover due to neuroleptics (BIGGIO et al., 1977; KAARIAINEN, 1976; WESTERINK and KORF, 1976; LLOYD et al., 1979; BARTHOLINI et al., 1979). Infusion of picrotoxin into the cat sub-stantia nigra leads to an enhanced DA liberation in the ipsilateral caudate nucleus (CHERAMY et al., 1977). In addition, direct evidence that GABA neurons terminate on DA cell bodies and dendrites is provided by the marked loss of [³H]-GABA binding in the substantia nigra of patients with Parkinson's disease (LLOYD et al., 1977 a) where the cell loss is almost exclusively limited to the melanin-containing DA cell bodies (cf. HORNYKIEWICZ, 1966). These data strongly indicate that an inhibitory GA-BA input to the substantia nigra regulates the activity of DA neurons. Additionally, evidence exists for the occurrence of such a regulation in the caudate nucleus. Thus, in experiments with the push–pull cannula, perfusion of this structure with Ringer sol-ution containing bicuculline or picrotoxin results in an enhanced DA liberation which is prevented by concomitant addition of GABA to the perfusion fluid; finally, this amino acid, added alone to the perfusion medium, diminishes the DA release from the caudate nucleus (BARTHOLINI and STADLER, 1977; BARTHOLINI et al., 1976 a).

In conclusion, cholinergic and GABA-ergic inputs regulate the activity of nigro-striatal DA neurons and, therefore, may be involved in the neuroleptic-induced acti-vation of the latter.

4. Effects of Repeated Administration of Neuroleptics

During prolonged medication with neuroleptic drugs, the enhancement of the DA turnover is lower than that observed after a single administration of these drugs (Fig. 2). This is indicated by an attenuated increase in striatal DA synthesis (formation of DA from radioactive tyrosine, SCATTON et al., 1975) or utilization (after α-methyl-p-tyrosine, ASPER et al., 1973) and in homovanillic or dihydroxylphenylacetic acid levels (BURKI et al., 1974; BOWERS and ROZITIS, 1974; GESSA and TAGLIAMONTE, 1975; SCATTON, 1977; WALDMEIER and MAÎTRE, 1976a) in the rat and rabbit. Also, reduced accumulation of HVA has been observed in the cerebrospinal fluid of humans (GER-LACH et al., 1974; POST and GOODWIN, 1975; VAN PRAAG, 1977) or animals (BOWERS and ROZITIS, 1976) after chronic neuroleptic medication. Furthermore, in experiments with the push–pull cannula, it has been shown that after several days of treatment with haloperidol or chlorpromazine, the amounts of ACh released in the cat striatum are markedly lower than those liberated after a single administration of these compounds (BARTHOLINI et al., 1976a). This correlates well with the observation that after pro-longed haloperidol administration the enhancement of striatal choline acetylase activ-ity or ACh turnover seen after single administration is greatly reduced (LLOYD et al., 1977b; MAO et al., 1977a). In addition, the locomotor depression induced by the acute administration of physostigmine is markedly attenuated after chronic haloperidol ad-ministration (DUNSTAN and JACKSON, 1977). These changes clearly indicate a reduced cholinergic function. Also, GABA neurons seem to change their activity after re-peated neuroleptic treatment as compared to the effect observed with acute adminis-tration. Thus, the decrease in nigral GABA levels caused by a single dose of neurolep-tics in the rat substantia nigra is markedly attenuated upon chronic administration of the drugs (LLOYD and HORNYKIEWICZ, 1977). This is paralleled by an increased syn-thesis of GABA from glucose as compared to the acute situation (MAO et al., 1977a). In parallel with the biochemical changes observed during repeated treatment with neuroleptics, behavioural alterations also accur. Thus, tolerance to the cataleptogenic action of these drugs (ASPER et al., 1973; EZRIN-WATERS and SEEMAN, 1977; GESSA and TAGLIAMONTE, 1975; LLOYD et al., 1977b) as well as increased sensitivity to DA recep-tor agonists develops. This increased sensitivity is exhibited by the increased potency (lowered ED) of apomorphine (injected either intraperitoneally or intracerebrally) in inducing stereotypies or hyperactivity (ASPER et al., 1973; GIANUTSOS and MOORE, 1977; JACKSON, et al., 1975; SAYERS et al., 1975; SMITH and DAVIS, 1975; TARSY and BALDESSARINI, 1973; VON VOIGTLANDER et al., 1975). Furthermore, it has been shown recently that co-administration of a GABA agonist and haloperidol prevents the ac-quisition of tolerance to the catalepsy and markedly blocks the development of super-sensitivity to apomorphine (LLOYD and WORMS, 1980). Neurophysiologically, it has been reported that striatal cells become supersensitive to iontophoretically admin-istered DA after subacute administration of neuroleptics (YARBROUGH, 1975) and bio-chemically the apomorphine-induced reduction of DA turnover is potentiated after subacute neuroleptic treatment (GIANUTSOS and MOORE, 1977). Tolerance and super-sensitivity of the effector cells may be at least partially explained by changes at the level of the postsynaptic DA receptor. Thus, after 3 weeks of neuroleptic treatment, striatal dopamine receptor binding is significantly increased (BURT et al., 1977).

5. Functional Correlates of Neuroleptic-Induced Biochemical Alterations

a) Parkinsonian Syndrome

Parkinsonian symptoms such as rigidity and possibly tremor observed during neuroleptic medication originate from the striatal cholinergic hyperactivity which results from the reduced dopaminergic transmission; in fact, these symptoms are markedly ameliorated by anticholinergic drugs (GREENBLATT and SHADER, 1973).

However, during prolonged medication with neuroleptic drugs, the parkinsonian syndrome diminishes spontaneously (cf. DONLON and STENSON, 1976; MCCLELLAND et al., 1974; ZIRKLE and KAISER, 1974) in analogy to the progressive development of tolerance to catalepsy in rat and the reduction of ACh liberation in the cat. These effects are explained by the development of supersensitivity to DA by the target cells of the dopaminergic neurons. As discussed above, this may possibly be linked to an increased number of DA receptors or changes in their affinity. Supersensitivity development is also indicated by the enhanced behavioural and biochemical effects of DA receptor agonists after chronic neuroleptic treatment as well as by the fact that the apomorphine-induced decrease in ACh utilization is more marked in the denervated than in the intact caudate nucleus (FIBIGER and GREWAAL, 1974) and denervation enhances haloperidol binding (BURT et al., 1977).

b) Tardive Dyskinesia

This syndrome, which is reminiscent of chorea and of the choreiform movement induced in parkinsonian patients by L-DOPA, is assumed to originate from a supersensitivity of DA target cells so that the transmitter liberation overcomes the neuroleptic blockade. This results in an enhanced transmission to the postsynaptic neurons and to a decreased ACh liberation. In fact, tardive dyskinesias are ameliorated not only by switching to a more potent neuroleptic or by reserpine (which depletes the DA stores) (ZIRKLE and KAISER, 1974), but also by cholinergic drugs such as physostigmine and deanol (2-(dimethylamino)ethanol) (DAVIS et al., 1975; DE SILVA and HUANG, 1975; KLAWANS andRUBOVITS, 1974). In contrast, anticholinergic compounds aggravate the syndrome (DAVIS et al., 1975; KLAWANS and RUBOVITS, 1974; ZIRKLE and KAISER, 1974).

The role of GABA in striatal function is still obscure. The inhibitory GABA-ergic input on DA neurons suggests that GABA is involved in the regulation of the latter (see Sect. B.I.3.); therefore, GABA may play a role in the genesis of symptoms connected with altered dopaminergic transmission. In fact, a decrease of glutamic acid decarboxylase activity occurs in striatum of parkinsonian patients and is reversed by L-DOPA treatment (LLOYD and HORNYKIEWICZ, 1973). A similar diminution of the enzyme activity has been reported in Huntington's chorea (BIRD et al., 1973; McGEER et al., 1975).

II. Limbic System

1. Acetylcholine

Biochemical and histochemical results have shown that, in the limbic system, neuroleptic drugs accelerate the turnover of DA and, therefore, block DA receptors (e.g., Andén et al., 1970; Bartholini, 1976; Bowers and Rozitis, 1974; Scatton, 1977; Waldmeier and Maître, 1976b; Westerink and Korf, 1975a, b; for full references see Lloyd, 1978 c). This blockade, however, does not result in alterations of ACh turnover (as measured in experiments with the push–pull cannula by changes of the transmitter liberation into the perfusion medium) in the nucleus accumbens, the septum, or the ventral or dorsal hippocampal formation (cf. Bartholini et al., 1976b). Similar negative results have been obtained by measuring the changes in tissue levels of ACh (Guyenet et al., 1975; Ladinski et al., 1978; Sethy and Van Woert, 1974b). These data indicate that limbic cholinergic neurons of different brain areas do not receive a dopaminergic input and, therefore, do not directly mediate the effect of the blockade of DA receptors by neuroleptics. In contrast, cholinergic neurons influence the limbic dopaminergic activity, as: i) cholinomimetic compounds enhance the concentration of homovanillic and dihydroxyphenylacetic acid in limbic regions (Andén, 1974; Bartholini et al., 1975b; Westerink and Korf, 1975a, 1976) and ii) anticholinergic compounds block the neuroleptic-induced increase in limbic DA turnover (Andén, 1972; Bartholini et al., 1975b; Westerink and Korf, 1975a, b).

In contrast to the above-mentioned limbic regions, ACh turnover in cortical areas parallels changes in dopaminergic transmission. Thus, amphetamine (which liberates both DA and noradrenaline) as well as direct-acting DA agonists (e.g., apomorphine) enhance ACh liberation from the cortex (as measured by means of the cup perfusion method); this effect is blocked by haloperidol and chlorpromazine (at doses which also block noradrenaline receptors) as well as by propanolol (cf. Pepeu, 1974; Mantovani and Pepeu, 1978). In addition, DL-DOPA increases, whereas DL-threo-3,4,dihydroxyphenylserine decreases, the ACh output (cf. Pepeu, 1974). Although the data are not completely coherent and may suggest that cortical ACh neurons are influenced by a noradrenaline input, an excitatory DA action (e.g., mediated via the septum) cannot be excluded with certainty. Finally, the data available from schizophrenic patients on the effect of drugs acting on cholinergic function are contradictory (cf. Lloyd, 1978b) and suggest that limbic cholinergic neurons are not involved in the pathogenesis of the psychosis.

2. GABA

Limbic GABA neurons may be involved in the mechanism of action of neuroleptic drugs. Thus, putative direct or indirect acting GABA mimetics (e.g., SL 76002, muscimol, aminooxyacetic acid or γ-hydroxybutyric acid) diminish DA turnover in the limbic system (Andén and Wachtel, 1978; Bartholini et al., 1979; Kaariainen, 1976; Westerink and Korf, 1975b). This effect is greater in the limbic system than the striatum. SL 76002, muscimol or aminooxyacetic acid also antagonizes the neuroleptic-induced increase in DA turnover (Bartholini et al., 1979; Kaariainen, 1976; Westerink and Korf, 1975b). Histofluorimetric experiments support these findings for the nucleus accumbens and tuberculum olfactorium (Fuxe, et al., 1975). Furthermore, picrotoxin reverses the γ-butyrolactone-induced activation of tyrosine hydroxylase in the tuberculum olfactorium and increases the rate of firing of limbic DA neurons (Roth and Nowycky, 1977). It appears, therefore, that limbic DA neurons receive an inhibitory GABA input. Neuroleptic drugs may alter this input since some of these agents, e.g., haloperidol, increase the GABA turnover in the limbic system

(Table 2; MAO et al., 1977 a); in addition, pimozide blocks the apomorphine-induced enhancement of GABA accumulation after GABA-transaminase inhibitors (HÖKFELT et al., 1976). The activation of GABA neurons may originate either from the direct blockade of GABA receptors or from the primary blockade of DA receptors. Thus, butyrophenones contain the GABA moiety and, in electrophysiological experiments, droperidol has been shown to stimulate cerebrellar GABA receptors (MARUYAMA and KAWASAKI, 1976). In addition, neuroleptics of diverse chemical structures alter the [^{3}H]-GABA binding site in vitro or in vivo (LLOYD and DREKSLER, 1978). However, direct clinical evidence is against the role of GABA in schizophrenia. Thus, in spite of an initial report that baclofen, [β-(p-chlorophenyl)-GABA] a structural analogue of GABA, is useful in the treatment of psychotic patients (FREDERICKSEN, 1975), further clinical trials have proven negative (e.g., BECKMANN et al., 1977). Furthermore, it is not clear that baclofen acts specifically on GABA-receptors as interactions with substance P receptors have also been documented (HENRY and BEN-ARI, 1976; KRNJEVIC, 1977). Also, administration of SL 76002, a GABA receptor agonist and a prodrug of GABA receptor agonists (BARTHOLINI et al., 1979; LLOYD et al., 1979) or muscimol, to schizophrenic patients is without beneficial action and may even aggravate schizophrenic symptoms (CHASE and TAMINGA, 1979; MORSELLI et al., 1980). Recently, BIRD et al., 1977, have shown that glutamic acid decarboxylase (the enzyme which synthetizes GABA) activity is reduced in several limbic areas of brains taken post-mortem from schizophrenic patients. However, this finding has not been confirmed in subsequent reports (BIRD et al., 1978; MCGEER and MCGEER, 1979).

In conclusion, the antipsychotic action of neuroleptics seems to be connected to the blockade of DA receptors in the limbic system (see Sect. D). This action, however, does not seem to be mediated by limbic cholinergic neurons since the activity of the latter is not altered by blockade of dopaminergic transmission. Also, the involvement of GABA neurons in the action mechanism of neuroleptics remains an open question. Finally, the lack of action of specific compounds acting directly of GABA receptors seems to exclude the possibility that GABA neurons play a role in schizophrenia.

3. Repeated Administration of Neuroleptics: Effects in Limbic System

The antipsychotic action and the extrapyramidal side-effects of neuroleptic compounds are thought to be connected with the blockade of DA receptors in limbic areas (see Sect. D) and in striatum, see (see Sect. C.5.a.), respectively. In the striatum, target cells of DA neurons develop supersensitivity to the transmitter, explaining the reduction of the parkinsonian syndrome and the appearance of tardive dyskinesias. A similar development of supersensitivity in target cells of limbic DA neurons should lead to progressive diminution of the antipsychotic action of neuroleptic compounds. As this is not the case, it could be postulated that supersensitivity does not occur in limbic system or develops with a different pattern than in striatum. Thus, although supersensitivity to DA or apomorphine occurs in some limbic areas after chronic neuroleptic treatment (GIANUTSOS and MOORE, 1977; JACKSON et al., 1975), recent data show that during repeated administration of neuroleptics, tolerance to the increased DA turnover and synthesis occurs in striatum after lower doses of the drugs and earlier than

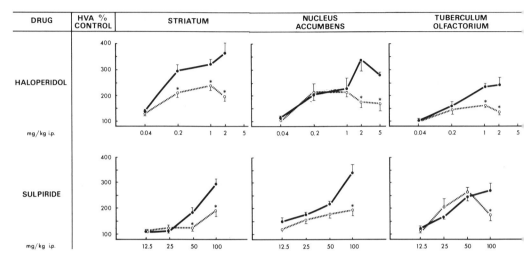

Fig. 2. The effect of acute or chronic administration of haloperidol or sulpiride on homovanillic acid levels in the striatum and limbic areas. (From Scatton, 1977)

in limbic system (Fig. 2; Julou et al., 1977; Scatton, 1977; Scatton et al., 1980), especially in the mesocortical DA neurons (Laduron et al., 1977; Scatton, 1977, Julou et al., 1977). This suggests that the sensitivity to the development of tolerance of effector cells of DA neurons is lower in limbic system than in striatum (Fig. 2 and Table 2). It may, therefore, be proposed that the concentration of neuroleptic drugs sufficient to trigger tolerance development is seldom reached in the limbic system of humans, explaining the persistence of the antipsychotics action of these compounds.

D. Atypical Neuroleptics

Since the early years of neuroleptic medication, it has appeared clear that antipsychotic action and extrapyramidal side-effects of neuroleptic agents are dissociated. Thus, some patients never exhibit extrapyramidal reactions while improving their psychotic symptoms, whereas others, in the absence of significant amelioration, develop severe striopallidal disturbances.

This dissociation is furthermore suggested by the pattern of "atypical" or "silent" neuroleptics such as clozapine, sulpiride and thioridazine, which display an antipsychotic action while causing fewer or no extrapyramidal side-effects as compared to classical neuroleptics (e.g., of butyrophenone or phenothiazine type) (for references, see Bartholini, 1976; Lloyd, 1978 b). The low incidence of extrapyramidal reaction in man (and of catalepsy in rat) suggests that striatal DA receptors are less affected by atypical than by classical neuroleptics. Indeed, clozapine and sulpiride increase DA turnover to a greater extent in the limbic system than striatum, as indicated by increases in dihydroxyphenylacetic and homovanillic acid levels (Fig. 2; Andén and Stock, 1973a; Scatton et al., 1977; Stawarz et al., 1975; Westerink and Korf, 1976). In addition, after probenecid administration (Bartholini, 1976), thioridazine as well as clozapine and sulpiride exhibit a preference for the limbic system. Furthermore, the liberation of DA measured in tissue perfusates by means of the push–pull cannula is enhanced by clozapine in the nucleus accumbens to a more pronounced extent than in the caudate nucleus of the cat; in contrast, chlorpromazine has a similar effect in the two regions (BARTHOLINI et al., 1976b). Furthermore, tyrosine hydroxylase activity is preferentially enhanced by sulpiride and clozapine in limbic areas (ZIVKOVIC et al., 1975).

Finally, the tolerance observed after chronic administration of neuroleptics is less marked in limbic regions (nucleus accumbens, tuberculum olfactorium, frontal cortex) than in the striatum (Fig. 2, BOWERS and ROZITIS, 1976; SCATTON, 1977).

The mechanism by which atypical neuroleptics induce a preferential activation of limbic DA turnover is unknown. A selective accumulation of the drugs in the limbic system cannot be excluded. Alternatively, these compounds may possess a higher affinity for limbic than for striatal DA receptors; however, the in vitro blockade of DA sensitive adenylate cyclase by these drugs is similar in limbic and striatal structures (SCATTON et al., 1977; TRABUCCHI et al., 1976). A different sensitivity of the DA effector cells in limbic and striatal structures is suggested by micro-iontophoretic experiments: thus, clozapine blocks more markedly the DA-induced depression in the nucleus accumbens than in striatum (BUNNEY and AGHAJANIAN, 1978). Finally, the less-marked activation of striatal than of limbic DA neurons may be connected with the anticholinergic properties of some of these compounds (e.g., clozapine, thioridazine) (MILLER and HILEY, 1974; SNYDER et al., 1974) which diminish the feedback activation of DA cells; although several data do not support this hypothesis (for reference see BARTHOLINI, 1976), such a mechanism cannot be completely excluded.

The possibility exists that atypical and classical neuroleptics act on different receptors. Thus, drugs of benzamide series are, at best, very weak blockers of adenylate cyclase (SCATTON et al., 1977; TRABUCCHI et al., 1976) yet some of them cause catalepsy in animals and extrapyramidal reaction in humans (cf. JENNER et al., 1978). Apparently, however, all of the derivates tested displace [^{3}H]-spiroperidol from the binding sites (BRILEY, 1978).

In conclusion, although it is still unknown by which mechanism atypical neuroleptics preferentially affect limbic DA transmission, the above data lead to two considerations:

1) The relatively weak effectiveness of these drugs on striatal DA and ACh mechanisms as compared to that of classical neuroleptics explains the lower incidence of extrapyramidal side-effects.

2) The preferential impairment of limbic DA transmission by atypical compounds supports the hypothesis that the limbic system is the anatomical substrate for the antipsychotic action of neuroleptics.

References

Aghajanian, G.K., Bunney, B.S.: Central dopaminergic neurons: neurophysiological identification and response to drugs. In: Frontiers in catecholamine research. Usdin, E., Snyder, S.H., (eds.), pp. 643–648. New York: Pergamon Press 1973

Aghajanian, G.K., Bunney, B.S.: Dopaminergic and nondopaminergic neurons in the substantia nigra: differential responses to putative transmitters. In: Neuropsychopharmacology. Boisser, J.R., Hippius, H., Pichot, P., (eds.), pp. 444–452. Amsterdam: Excerpta Medica 1975

Agid, Y., Guyenet, P., Glowinski, J., Beaujouan, J. C., Javoy, F.: Inhibitory influence of the nigrostriatal dopamine system on the striatal cholinergic neurons in the rat. Brain Res. 86, 488–492 (1975)

Andén, N.E.: Adrenergic mechanisms. Ann. Rev. Pharmacol. 9, 119–134 (1969)

Andén, N.E.: Dopamine turnover in the corpus striatum and the limbic system after treatment with neuroleptic and anti-acetylcholine drugs. J. Pharm. Pharmacol. 24, 905–906 (1972)

Andén, N.E.: Effects of oxotremorine and physostigmine on the turnover of dopamine in the corpus striatum and the limbic system. J. Pharm. Pharmacol. 26, 738–740 (1974)

Andén, N.E., Bedard, P.: Influences of cholinergic mechanisms on the function and turnover of brain dopamine. J. Pharm. Pharmacol. 23, 460–462 (1971)

Andén, N.E., Stock, G.: Inhibitory effect of γ-hydroxybutyric acid and γ-aminobutyric acid on the dopamine cells in the substantia nigra. Naunyn-Schmiedeberg's Arch. Pharmacol. 279, 890–892 (1973)

Andén, N.E., Wachtel, H.: Some effects of GABA and GABA-like drug on cerebral catecholamine mechanisms. In: Interactions between putative neurotransmitters in the brain. S. Garattini, J.F. Pujol, R. Samanin (eds.) pp.161–173, New York: Raven Press 1978

Andén, N.E., Butcher, S.G., Corrodi, H., Fuxe, K., Ungerstedt, U.: Receptor activity and turnover of brain dopamine and noradrenaline after neuroleptics. Eur. J. Pharmacol. 11, 303–314 (1970)

Asper, H., Baggiolini, M., Burki, H.R., Lauener, H., Ruch, W., Stille, G.: Tolerance phenomena with neuroleptics: catalepsy, apomorphine stereotypies and striatal dopamine metabolism in the rat after single and repeated administration of loxapine and haloperidol. Eur. J. Pharmacol. 22, 287–294 (1973)

Bartholini, G.: Differential effect of neuroleptic drugs on dopamine turnover in the extrapyramidal and limbic system. J. Pharm. Pharmacol. 28, 429–443 (1976)

Bartholini, G., Pletscher, A.: Drugs affecting monoamines in the basal ganglia. In: Advances in biochemical psychopharmacology. Costa, E., Iversen, L.L., Paoletti, R., (eds.), Vol. 6, pp.135–148. New York: Raven Press 1972

Bartholini, G., Stadler, H.: Evidence for an intrastriatal gabaergic influence on dopamine neurons of the cat. Neurophamacology 16, 343–347 (1977)

Bartholini, G. Stadler, H., Lloyd, K.G.: Cholinergicdopaminergic interregulations within the extrapyramidal system. In: Cholinergic mechanisms, P.G. Waser (Eds) pp.411–418 New York: Raven Press 1975a

Bartholini, G., Keller, H.H., Pletscher, A.: Drug-induced changes of dopamine turnover in striatum and limbic system of the rat. J. Pharm. Pharmacol. 27, 439–442 (1975b)

Bartholini, G., Stadler, H., Gadea-Ciria, M., Lloyd, K.G.: The use of the push–pull cannula to estimate the dynamics of acetylcholine and catecholamines within various brain areas. Neuropharmacology 15, 515–519 (1976a)

Bartholini, G., Stadler, H., Gadea-Ciria, M., Lloyd, K.G.: The effect of antipsychotic drugs on the release of neurotransmitters in various brain areas. In: Antipsychotic drugs: pharmacodynamics and pharmacokinetics, Sedvall, G., Uvnas, B., Zotterman, Y., (eds.), pp.105–116. Oxford: Pergamon Press 1976b

Bartholini, G., Stadler, H., Gadea-Ciria, M., Lloyd, K.G.: Interaction of dopaminergic and cholinergic neurons in the extrapyramidal and limbic systems. In: Advances in biochemical psychopharmacology. Costa, E., Gessa, G.L., (eds.), Vol. 16, pp.391–395. New York: Raven Press 1977

Bartholini, G., Scatton, B., Zivkovic, B., Lloyd, K.G.: On the mode of action of SL 76002, a new GABA receptor agonist. In: GABA-Neurotransmitters Krogsgaard, I., Larsen, P., Scheel-Krüger, J., Kofod, H. (eds.), pp. 326–339. Copenhagen: Munksgaard 1979

Beckmann, H., Frische, M., Ruther, E., Zimmer, R.: Baclofen (para-chlorophenyl-GABA) in schizophrenia. Pharmakopsychiatry 10, 26–31 (1977)

Biggio, G., Casu, M., Corda, M.G., Vernaleone, F., Gessa, G.L.: Effect of muscimol, a gabamimetic agent, on dopamine metabolism in the mouse brain. Life Sci 21, 525–532 (1977)

Bird, E.D., Mackay, A.V.P., Rayner, C.N., Iversen, L.L.: Reduced glutamic-acid-decarboxylase activity of post-mortem brain in Huntingdon's chorea. Lancet 1, 1090–1092 (1973)

Bird, E.D., Barnes, J., Iversen, L.L., Spokes, E.G., Mackay, A.V.P., Shepherd, M.: Increased brain dopamine and reduced glutamic decarboxylase and choline acetyltransferase activity in schizophrenia and related psychoses. Lancet 2, 1157–1159 (1977)

Bird, E.D., Spokes, E.G., Barnes, S., Mackay, A.V.P., Iversen, L.L., Shepherd, M.: Glutamic acid decarboxylase in schizophrenia. Lancet *1*, 156 (1978)

Bowers, M.B., Rozitis, A.: Regional differences in homovanillic acid concentrations after acute and chronic administration of antipsychotic drugs. J. Pharm. Pharmacol. *26*, 743–745 (1974)

Bowers, M.B., Rozitis, A.: Brain homovanillic acid: regional changes over time with antipsychotic drugs. Eur. J. Pharmacol. *39*, 109–115 (1976)

Briley, M.: Unpublished results (1978)

Bunney, B.S., Aghajanian, G.K.: Evidence for drug actions on both pre- and postsynaptic catecholamine receptors in the CNS. In: Pre- and postsynaptic receptors, Usdin, E., Bunney, W.E. Jr. (eds.), pp. 89–120. New York: Dekker 1975

Bunney, B.S., Aghajanian, G.K.: Mesolimbic and mesocortical dopaminergic systems: physiology and pharmacology. In: Psychopharmacology: A generation of progress. Lipton, M.A., Di Mascio, A., Killam, K.F., (eds.), pp. 159–169. New York: Raven Press 1978

Burki, H.R., Ruch, W., Asper, H., Baggiolini, ; M., Stille, G.: Effect of single and repeated administration of clozapine on the metabolism of dopamine and noradrenaline in the brain of the rat. Eur. J. Pharmacol. *27*, 180–190 (1974)

Burt, D.R., Enna, S.J., Creese, I., Snyder, S.H.: Dopamine receptor binding in the corpus striatum of mammalian brain. Proc. Natl. Acad. Sci. USA *72*, 4655–4659 (1975)

Burt, D.R., Creese, I., Snyder, S.H.: Antischizophrenic drugs: chronic treatment elevates dopamine receptors binding in brain. Science *196*, 326–328 (1977)

Carlsson, A.: Receptor-mediated control of dopamine metabolism. In: Pre- and postsynaptic receptors. Usdin, E., Bunney, W.E., Jr. (eds.), pp. 49–63. New York: Dekker 1975

Carlsson, A., Lindqvist, M.: Effect of chlorpromazine and haloperidol on formation of 3-methoxytyramine and normetanephrine in mouse brain. Acta Pharmacol. Toxicol. (Kbh.) *20*, 140–144 (1963)

Chase, T.N., Tamminga, C.A.: GABA system participation in human motor, cognitive and endocrine function. In: GABA-Neurotransmitters. Krogsgaard-Larsen, P., Scheel-Krüger, J., Kofod, H. (eds.), pp. 283–294. Copenhagen: Munksgaard 1979

Cheney, D.L., Racagni, G., Zsilla, G., Costa, E.: Differences in the action of various drugs on striatal acetylcholine and choline content in rats killed by decapitation or microwave radiation. J. Pharm. Pharmacol. *28*, 75–77 (1976)

Cheramy, A., Nieoullon, A., Glowinski, J.: Effects of peripheral and local administration of pictrotoxin on the release of newly synthesized ³H-dopamine in the caudate nucleus of the cat. Naunyn-Schmiedeberg's Arch. Pharmacol. *297*, 31–37 (1977)

Clement-Cormier, Y., Robison, G.A.: Adenylate cyclase from various dopaminergic areas of the brain and the action of antipsychotic drugs. Biochem. Pharmacol. *26*, 1719–1722 (1977)

Consolo, S., Ladinsky, H., Bianchi, S.: Decrease in rat striatum acetylcholine levels by some direct- and indirectacting dopaminergic antagonists. Eur. J. Pharmacol. *33*, 345–351 (1975)

Coyle, J.T., Schwartz, R., Bennett, J.P., Campochiaro, P.: Clinical, neuropathologic and pharmacological aspects of Huntington's disease: correlates with a new animal model. Prog. Neuropsychopharmacol. *1*, 13–30 (1977)

Creese, I., Burt, D.R., Snyder, S.H.: Dopamine receptor binding: differentiation of agonist and antagonist states with ³H-dopamine and ³H-haloperidol. Life Sci. *17*, 993–1002 (1975)

Creese, I., Schwartz, R., Coyle, J.T., Snyder, S.H.: Differential localization of dopamine receptor ³H-haloperidol binding and adenylate cyclase. Soc. Neurosci. Abstr. *3*, 454 (1977)

Crossman, A.R., Walker, R.J., Woodruff, G.N.: Picrotoxin antagonism of γ-aminobutyric acid inhibitory responses and synaptic inhibition in the rat substantia nigra. Br. J. Pharmacol. *49*, 696–698 (1973)

Crossman, A.R., Walker, R.J., Woodruff, G.N.: Pharmacological studies on single neurones in the substantia nigra of the rat. Br. J. Pharmacol. *51*, 137–138P (1974)

Da Prada, M., Pletscher, A.: On the mechanism of chlorpromazine in-induced changes of cerebral homovanillic acid levels. J. Pharm. Pharmacol. *18*, 628–630 (1966)

Davis, K.L., Hollister, L.E., Berger, P.A., Barchas, J.D.: Cholinergic imbalance hypothesis of psychoses and movement disorders: strategies f or evaluation. Psychopharmacol. Commun. *1*, 533–543 (1975)

De Silva, L., Huang, C.Y.: Deanol in tardive dyskinesia. Br. Med. J. *3*, 466 (1975)

Donlon, P.T., Stenson, R.L.: Neuroleptic induced extrapyramidal symptoms. Dis. Nerv. Syst. 37, 629–635 (1976)

Dray, A., Gonye, T.J.: Effects of caudate stimulation and microiontophoretically applied substances on neurones in the rat substantia nigra. J. Physiol. (Lond.) 246, 88–89P (1975)

Dray, A., Straughan, D.W.: Synaptic mechanisms in the substantia nigra. J. Pharm. Pharmacol. 28, 400–405 (1976)

Dunstan, R., Jackson, D.M.: The demonstration of a change in responsiveness of mice to physostigmine and atropine after withdrawal from long-term haloperidol pretreatment. J. Neurol. Transm. 40, 181–189 (1977)

Enna, S.J., Snyder, S.H.: Properties of γ-aminobutyric acid (GABA) receptor binding in rat brain synaptic membrane fractions. Brain Res. 100, 81–97 (1975)

Ezrin-Waters, C., Seeman, P.: Tolerance to haloperidol catalepsy. Eur. J. Pharmacol. 41, 321–327 (1977)

Feltz, P.: γ-aminobutyric acid and a caudato-nigral inhibition. Can. J. Physiol. Pharmacol. 49, 1113–1115 (1971)

Fibiger, H.C., Grewaal, D.S.: Neurochemical evidence for denervation supersensitivity: the effect of unilateral substantia nigra lesions on apomorphine-induced increases in neostriatal acetylcholine levels. Life Sci. 15, 57–63 (1974)

Fredericksen, P.K.: Baclofen in the treatment of schizophrenia. Lancet, 1, 702–703 (1975)

Freedman, A.M., Kaplan, H.I., Sadlock, B.J.: Modern Synopsis of Psychiatry, Vol. II, pp. 978–979 Baltimore: Williams & Wilkins 1976

Fuxe, K., Hokfelt, T., Ljungdahl, A., Agnati, L., Johansson, O., Perez de la Mora, M: Evidence for an inhibitory GABAergic control of the meso-limbic dopamine neurons: possibility of improving treatment of schizophrenia by combined treatment with neuroleptics and GABAergic drugs. Med. Biol. 53, 177–183 (1975)

Gerlach, J., Koppelhus, P., Helweg, E., Morand, A.: Clozapine and haloperidol in a single-blind cross-over trial: therapeutic and biochemical aspects in the treatment of schizophrenia. Acta Psychiatr. Scand. 50, 410–424 (1974)

Gessa, G.L., Tagliamonte, A.: Effect of methadone and dextromoramide on dopamine metabolism: comparison with haloperidol and amphetamine. Neuropharmacology 14, 913–920 (1975

Gey, K.F., Pletscher, A.: Influence of chlorpromazine and chlorprothixine on the cerebral metabolism of 5-hydroxytryptamine, norepinephrine and dopamine. J. Pharmacol. Exp. Ther. 133, 18–24 (1961)

Gianutsos, G., Moore, K.E.: Dopaminergic supersensitivity in striatum and olfactory tubercle following chronic administration of haloperidol or clozapine. Life Sci. 20, 1585–1592 (1977)

Greenblatt, D.J., Shader, R.I.: Anticholinergics. N. Engl. J. Med. 288, 1215–1219 (1973)

Guyenet, P.G., Agid, Y., Javoy, F., Beaujouan, J.C., Rossier, J., Glowinski, J.: Effects of dopaminergic receptor agonists and antagonists on the activity of the neostriatal cholinergic system. Brain Res. 84, 227–244 (1975)

Henry, J.L., Ben-Ari, Y.: Actions of the p-chlorophenyl derivative of GABA, lioresal, on nociceptive and nonnociceptive units in the spinal cord of the cat. Brain Res. 117, 540–544 (1976)

Hökfelt, T., Ljungdahl, A., Perez de la Mora, M., Fuxe, K.: Further evidence that apomorphine increases GABA turnover in the DA cell body rich and DA nerve terminal rich areas of the brain. Neurosci. Lett 2, 239–242 (1976)

Hornykiewicz, O.: Dopamine (3-hydroxytryptamine) and brain function. Pharmacol. Rev. 18, 925–962 (1966)

Iversen, L.L.: Catecholamine-sensitive adenylate cyclases in nervous tissues. J. Neurochem. 29, 5–12 (1977)

Jackson, D.M., Anden, N.E., Engel, J., Liljequist, S.: The effect of long-term penfluridol treatment on the sensitivity of the dopamine receptors in the nucleus accumbens and in the corpus striatum. Psychopharmacologia 45, 151–155 ; (1975)

Janssen, P.: Pharmacological aspects. In: Neuro-psychopharmacology. Bente, D., Bradley, P.B. (eds.), Vol.4, pp. 151–159 Amsterdam: Elsevier 1965

Javoy, F., Hamon, M., Glowinski, J.: Disposition of newly synthetized amines in cell bodies and terminals of central catecholaminergic neurons. (I) Effect of amphetamine and thioproperazine on the metabolism of CA in the caudate nucleus, the substantia nigra and the ventromedial nucleus of the hypothalamus. Eur. J. Pharmacol. 10, 178–188 (1970)

Javoy, F., Agid, Y., Boucet, D., Glowinski, J.: Changes in neostriatal DA metabolism after carbachol or atropine microinjection into the substantia nigra. Brain Res. *68*, 253–260 (1974)

Javoy, F., Agid, Y., Glowinski, J.: Oxotremorine- and atropine-induced changes of dopamine metabolism in the rat striatum. J. Pharm. Pharmacol *27*, 677–681 (1975)

Jenner, P., Elliott, P.N.C., Clow, A., Reavill, C., Marsden, C.D.: A comparison of 'in vitro' and 'in vivo' dopamine receptor antagonism produced by substituted benzamide drugs. J. Pharm. Pharmacol. *30*, 46–48 (1978)

Julou, L., Scatton, B., Glowinski, J.: Acute and chronic treatment with neuroleptics: similarities and differences in their action of nigrastriatal, mesolimbic and mesocortical dopaminergic neurons. In: Advances in biochemical psychopharmacology. Costa, E., Gessa, G.L., (eds.), Vol. 16 pp. 617–624. New York: Raven Press 1977

Kaariainen, I.: Effects of aminooxyacetic acid and baclofen on the catalepsy and on the increase of mesolimbic and striatal dopamine turnover induced by haloperidol in rats. Acta Pharmacol. Toxicol. (Kbh.) *39*, 393–400 (1976)

Kataoka, K., Bak, I.J., Hassler, R., Kim, J.J., Wagner, A.: L-glutamate decarboxylase and choline acetyltransferase activity in the substantia nigra and the striatum after surgical interruption of the strio-nigral fibres of the baboon. Exp. Brain Res. *19*, 217–227 (1974)

Kebabian, J.W., Saavedra, J.M.: Dopamine-sensitive adenylate cyclase occurs in a region of substantia nigra containing dopaminergic dendrites. Science *193*, 686–685 (1976)

Kehr, W.: 3-methoxytyramine as an indicator of impulse-induced dopamine release in rat brain in vivo. Naunyn-Schmiedeberg's Arch. Pharmacol. *293*, 209–215 (1976)

Kettler, R., Bartholini, G. and Pletscher, A.: In vivo enhancement of tyrosine hydroxylation in rat striatum by tetrahydrobioterin. Nature *249*, 476–478 (1974)

Kim, J.S., Hassler, R.: Effects of acute haloperidol on the γ-aminobutyric acid system in rat striatum and substantia nigra. Brain Res. *88*, 150–153 (1975)

Klawans, H.L., Rubovits, R.: Effect of cholinergic and anticholinergic agents on tardive dyskinesia. J. Neurol. Neurosurg. Psychiatry *27*, 941–947 (1974)

Kreuger, B.K., Forn, J., Greengard, P.: Dopamine sensitive adenylate cyclase and protein phosphorylation in the rat caudate nucleus. In: Pre- and postsynaptic receptors. Usdin, E., Bunney, W.E.Jr. (eds.), pp. 123–146. New York: Dekker 1975

Krnjevic, K.: Effects of substance P on central neurons in cats. In: Substance P. Von Euler, U.S., Perlow, B. (eds.), pp. 217–230. New York: Raven Press 1977

Laduron, P., De Bie, K., Leysen, J.: Specific effect of haloperidol on dopamine turnover in the frontal cortex. Naunyn-Schmiedeberg's Arch. Pharmacol. *296*, 183–185 (1977)

Ladinsky, H., Consolo, S., Bianchi, S., Ghezzi, D., Samanin, R.: Link between dopaminergic and cholinergic neurons in the striatum as evidenced by pharmacological biochemical and lesion studies. In: Interactions between putative neurotransmitters in the brain. Garattini, S., Pujol, J.F., Samanin, R. (eds.) pp. 3–21. New York: Raven Press 1978

Laverty, R., Sharman, D.F.: Modification by drugs of the metabolism of 3,4-dihydroxyphenylethylamine, noradrenaline and 5-hydroxytryptamine in the brain. Br. J. Pharmacol. *24*, 759–772 (1965)

Leysen, J.E., Niemegeers, C.J.E., Tollenaere, J.P., Laduron, P.M.: Serotonergic component of neuroleptic receptors. Nature *272*, 168–171 (1978)

Lloyd, K.G.: Neurotransmitter interactions related to central dopamine neurons. In: Essays in neurochemistry and neuropharmacology. Youdim, M.B.H., Lovenberg, W., Sharman, D.F., Lagnado, J.P. (eds.) Vol.III, pp. 129–207. New York: Wiley 1978a

Lloyd, K.G.: Observations concerning neurotransmitter interaction in schizophrenia. In: Cholinergic-monoaminergic interactions in the brain. Butcher, L.L. (ed.), pp. 363–392. New York: Academic Press 1978b

Lloyd, K.G.: The biochemical pharmacology of the limbic system: Neuroleptic drugs. In: Limbic mechanisms, Livingston, K.E., Hornykiewicz, O. (eds.) pp. 262–305. New York: Plenum Press 1978c

Lloyd, K.G., Bartholini, G.: The effects of drugs on the release of endogenous catecholamines into the perfusate of discrete brain areas of the cat in vivo. Experientia *31*, 560–562 (1975)

Lloyd, K.G., Dreksler, S.: ³H-GABA binding to membranes prepared from post-mortem human brain: pharmacological and pathological investigations. In: Amino acids as chemical transmitters. Fonnum, F. (ed.), pp. 457–466. New York: Plenum Press 1978

Lloyd, K.G., Hornykiewicz, O.: L-glutamic acid decarboxylase in Parkinson's disease: Effect of L-dopa therapy. Nature *243*, 521–523 (1973)

Lloyd, K.G., Hornykiewicz, O.: Effect of chronic neuroleptic or L-dopa administration on GA-BA levels in the rat substantia nigra. Life Sci. *21*, 1489–1496 (1977)

Lloyd, K.G., Worms, P.: Sustained GABA receptor stimulation and chronic neuroleptic effects. In: Long-term effects of neuroleptics. Cattabeni, F., Racagni, G., Spano, P.F. (eds.). New York: Raven Press 1980 (in press)

Lloyd, K.G., Shemen, L., Hornykiewicz, O.: Distribution of high affinity sodium-independent (3H)-γ-aminobutyric acid (3H) GABA binding in the human brain: Alterations in Parkinson's disease. Brain Res. *127*, 269–278 (1977a)

Lloyd, K.G., Shibuya, M., Davidson, L., Hornykiewicz, O.: Chronic neuroleptic therapy: Tolerance and GABA systems. In: Advances in biochemical psychopharmacology. Costa, E., Gessa, G.L. (eds.), Vol. 16, pp. 409–415. New York: Raven Press 1977b

Lloyd, K.G., Worms, P., Deportere, H., Bartholini, G.: Pharmacological profile of SL 76002, a new GABA-mimetic drug. In: GABA-Neurotransmitters. Krogsgaard-Larsen, P., Scheel-Krûger, J., Kofod, H. (eds.), pp. 308–325. Copenhagen: Munksgaard 1979

Lovenberg, W., Bruckwick, E.A.: Mechanisms of receptor mediated regulation of catecholamine synthesis in brain. In: Pre- and post-synaptic receptors. Usdin, E., Bunney, W.E.Jr. (eds.), pp. 149–168. New York: Dekker 1975

Maggi, A., Cattabeni, F., Bruno, F., Racagni, G.: Haloperidol and clozapine: specificity of action on GABA in the nigrostriatal system. Brain Res. *133*, 382–385 (1977)

Mantovani, P., Pepeu, G.: Influence of dopamine agonists on cholinergic mechanisms in the cerebral cortex. In: Interactions between putative transmitters in the brain. Garattini, S., Pujol, J.F., Samanin, R. (eds.) pp. 53–59 New York: Raven Press 1978

Mao, C.C., Costa, E.: Biochemical pharmacology of GABA transmission. In: Psychopharmacology: a generation of progress, Lipton, M.A., Di Mascio, A., Killam, K.F. (eds.) pp. 307–318 New York: Raven Press 1978

Mao, C.C., Cheney, D.L., Marco, E., Revuelta, A., Costa, E.: Turnover times of γ-aminobutyric acid and acetylcholine in nucleus caudatus, nucleus accumbens, globus pallidus and substantia nigra: effects of repeated administration of haloperidol. Brain Res. *132*, 375–379 (1977a)

Mao, C.C., Marco, E., Revuelta, A., Bertilson, L., Costa, E.: The turnover rate of γ-aminobutyric acid in the nuclei of the telencephalon: implications in the pharmacology of antipsychotics and of a minor tranquilizer. Biol. Psychiatry *2*, 359–371 (1977b)

Maruyama, S., Kawasaki, T.: Further electrophysiological evidence for the GABA-like effect of droperidol in the Purkinje cells of the cat cerebellum. Jpn. J. Pharmacol. *26*, 765–767 (1976)

McClelland, H.A., Blessed, G., Bhate, S., Ali, N., Clarke, P.A.: The abrupt withdrawal of antiparkinsonian drugs in schizophrenic patients. Br. J. Psychiatry *124*, 151–159 (1974)

McGeer, E.G., McGeer, P.L.: GABA-containing neurons in schizophrenia, Huntington's chorea and normal aging. In: GABA-neurotransmitters. Krogsgaard-Larsen, P., Scheel-Krûger, J., Kofod, H. (eds.), pp. 340–356. Copenhagen: Munksgaard 1979

McGeer, E.G., Fibiger, H.C., McGeer, P.L., Brooke, S.: Temporal changes in amine synthesizing enzymes of rat extrapyramidal system after hemitransection of 6-Hydroxydopamine administration. Brain Res. *52*, 289–300 (1973)

McGeer, P.L., McGeer, E.G., Fibiger, H.C.: Choline acetylase and glutamic acid decarboxylase in Huntington's chorea. Neurology *23*, 912–917 (1975)

Miller, R.J., Hiley, C.R.: Anti-muscarinic properties of neuroleptics and drug-induced Parkinsonism. Nature *248*, 596–597 (1974)

Morselli, P., Bossi, L., Henry, J.F., Zarifian, E., Bartholini, G.: Preliminary observations on the action of SL 76002, a new GABA mimetic compound, in neuropsychiatric disorders. In: GABA and other inhibitory neurotransmitters. Usdin, E., Fielding, S., Lal, H. (eds.). New York: Ankho Inc., in press, 1980

Nyback, H., Sedvall, G.: Further studies on the accumulation and disappearence of catecholamines formed from tyrosine-¹⁴C in mouse brain. Effect of some phenothiazine analogues. Eur. J. Pharmacol. *10*, 193–205 (1970)

Nyback, H., Wiesel, F.A., Sedvall, G.: Receptor regulation of dopamine turnover. In: Frontiers in catecholamine research, Usdin, E., Snyder, S.H. (eds.), pp. 601–604. Oxford Pergamon Press 1973

O'Keefe, R., Sharman, D.F., Vogt, M.: Effect of drugs used in psychoses on cerebral dopamine metabolism. Br. J. Pharmacol. *38*, 287–304 (1970)

Pepeu, G.: The release of acetylcholine from the brain: an approach to the study of control mechanisms. Prog. Neurobiol. *2*, 257–288 (1974)

Perez de la Mora, M., Fuxe, K., Hokfelt, T., Ljungdahl, A.: Effect of apomorphine on the GABA turnover in the DA cell group rich area of the mesencephalon. Evidence for the involvement of an inhibitory GABAergic feedback control of the ascending DA neurons. Neurosci. Lett. *1*, 109–114 (1975)

Persson, R.: Drug induced changes in ^{3}H-catecholamine accumulation after ^{3}H-tyrosine. Acta Pharmacol. Toxicol. (Kbh) *28*, 378–390 (1970)

Phillipson, O.T., Emson, P.C., Horn, A.S., Jessell, T.: Evidence concerning the anatomical location of the dopamine stimulated adenylate cyclase in the substantia nigra. Brain Res. *136*, 45–58 (1977)

Pletscher, A., Bartholini, G., Da Prada, M.: Influence of drugs on monoamines in the basal ganglia. In: Monoamines, noyaux gris et syndrome de Parkinson. De Ajuriaguerra, J. (ed.), pp. 73–84. Paris: Masson 1971

Post, R.M., Goodwin, F.K.: Time-dependent effects of phenothiazines on dopamine turnover in psychiatric patients. Science *190*, 488–489 (1975)

Roth, R.H., Nowycky, M.C.: Dopaminergic neurons: effects elicited by γ-hydroxybutyrate are reversed by pictrotoxin. Biochem. Pharmacol. *26*, 2079–2082 (1977)

Roth, R.H., Walters, J.R., Aghajanian, G.K.: Effect of impulse flow on the release and synthesis of dopamine in the rat striatum. In: Frontiers in catecholamine research. Usdin, E., Snyder, S.H. (eds.), pp. 567–574. Oxford: Pergamon Press 1973

Roth, R.H., Walters, J.R., Murrin, L.C. and Morgenroth, V.H.: Dopamine neurons: role of impulse flow and presynaptic receptors in the regulation of tyrosine hydroxylase. In: Pre- and postsynaptic receptors, Usdin, E., Bunney, W.E.Jr. (eds.), pp. 5–46 New York: Dekker 1975

Sayers, A.C., Burki, H.R.: Antiacetylcholine activity of psychoactive drugs: a comparison of the (^{3}H)-quinuclidinyl benzilate binding assay with conventional methods. J. Pharm. Pharmacol. *28*, 252–253 (1976)

Sayers, A.C., Burki, H.R., Ruch, W., Asper, H.: Neuroleptic-induced hypersensitivity of striatal dopamine receptor in the rat as a model of tardive dyskinesias. Effects of clozapine, haloperidol, loxapine and chlorpromazine. Psychopharmacologia *41*, 97–104 (1975)

Scatton, B.: Differential regional development of tolerance to increase in dopamine turnover upon repeated neuroleptic administration. Eur. J. Pharmacol. *46*, 363–369 (1977)

Scatton, B., Garret, C., Julou, L.: Acute and subacute effects of neuroleptics on dopamine synthesis and release in the rat striatum. Naunyn-Schmiedeberg's Arch. Pharmacol. *289*, 419–434 (1975)

Scatton, B., Bischoff, S., Dedek, J., Korf, J.: Regional effects of neuroleptics on dopamine metabolism and dopamine sensitive adenylate cyclase activity. Eur. J. Pharmacol. *44*, 287–292 (1977)

Scatton, B., Worms, P., Zivkovic, B., Depoortere, H., Dedek, J. and Bartholini, G.: On the neuropharmacological spectra of 'classical' (haloperidol and 'atypical' benzamide derivatives) neuroleptics. In: Sulpiride and other benzamides. Spano, P.F. (ed.), pp. 53–67. New York: Raven Press 1980

Seeman, P.: Antischizophrenic drugs – membrane receptor sites of action. Biochem. Pharmacol. *26*, 1741–1748 (1977)

Seeman, P., Lee, T.: Antipsychotic drugs: direct correlation between clinical potency and presynaptic action on dopamine neurons. Science *188*, 1217–1219 (1975)

Seeman, P., Lee, T., Chau-Wong, M., Tedesco, J., Wong, K.: Dopamine receptors in human and calf brains using (^{3}H)-apomorphine and an antipsychotic drug. Proc. Natl. Acad. Sci. USA *73*, 4354–4358 (1976a)

Seeman, P., Lee, T., Chau-Wong, M., Wong, K.: Antipsychotic drug doses and neuroleptic/dopamine receptors. Science *261*, 717–719 (1976b)

Sethy, V.H., Van Woert, M.H.: Modification of striatal acetylcholine concentration by dopamine receptor agonists and antagonists. Res. Commun. Chem. Pathol. Pharmacol. *8*, 13–28 (1974a)

Sethy, V.H., Van Woert, M.H.: Regulation of striatal acetylcholine concentration by dopamine receptors. Nature *251*, 529–530 (1974b)

Shute, C.C.D., Lewis, P.R.: The ascending cholinergic reticular system: neocortical, olfactory and subcortical projections. Brain *20*, 497–520 (1967)

Simke, J.P., Saelens, J.K.: Evidence for a cholinergic fiber tract connecting the thalamus with the head of the striatum of the rat. Brain Res. *126*, 487–495 (1977)

Smith, R.C., Davis, J.M.: Behavioral supersensitivity to apomorphine and amphetamine after chronic high dose haloperidol treatment. Psychopharmacol. Commun. *1*, 285–293 (1975)

Snyder, S.H., Greenberg, D., Yamamura, H.I.: Antischizophrenic drugs and brain cholinergic receptors. Arch. Gen. Psychiatry *31*, 58–61 (1974)

Snyder, S.H., Burt, D.R., Creese, E.: The dopamine receptor of mammalian brain: direct demonstration of binding to agonist and antagonist states. Soc. Neurosci. Symp. *1*, 28–49 (1976)

Stadler, H., Lloyd, K.G., Gadea-Ciria, M., Bartholini, G.: Enhanced striatal acetylcholine release by chlorpromazine and its reversal by apomorphine. Brain Res. *55*, 476–480 (1973)

Stawarz, R.J., Hill, H., Robison, S.E., Setler, P., Dingell, J.V., Sulser, F.: On the significance of the increase in homovanillic acid (HVA) caused by antipsychotic drugs in corpus striatum and limbic forebrain. Psychopharmacologia *43*, 125–130 (1975)

Tarsy, D., Baldessarini, R.J.: Pharmacologically induced behavioral supersensitivity to apomorphine. Nature New Biol. *245*, 262–263 (1973)

Trabucchi, M., Longoni, R., Fresia, P., Spano, R.F.: Sulpiride: a study of the effects on dopamine receptors in rat neostriatum and limbic forebrain. Life Sci. *17*, 1551–1556 (1976)

Van Praag, H.M.: The significance of dopamine for the mode of action of neuroleptics and the pathogenesis of schizophrenia. Br. J. Psychiatry *130*, 463–474 (1977)

Von Voigtlander, P.F., Boukma, S.J., Johnson, G.A.: Dopaminergic denervation supersensitivity and dopamine stimulated adenyl cyclase activity. Neuropharmacology *12*, 1081–1086 (1973)

Von Voigtlander, P.F., Losey, E.G., Trenzenberg, H.J.: Increased sensitivity to dopaminergic agents after chronic neuroleptic treatment. J. Pharmacol. Exp. Ther. *193*, 88–94 (1975)

Waldmeier, P.C., Maitre, L.: Clozapine: reduction of the initial dopamine turnover increased by repeated treatment. Eur. J. Pharmacol. *38*, 197–203 (1976a)

Waldmeier, P.C., Maitre, L.: On the relevance of preferential increases of mesolimbic versus striatal dopamine turnover for the production of antipsychotic activity of psychotropic drugs. J. Neurochem. *27*, 589–597 (1976b)

Westerink, B.H.C., Korf, J.: Turnover of acid dopamine metabolites in striatal and mesolimbic tissue of the rat brain. Eur. J. Pharmacol. *37*, 249–255 (1975a)

Westerink, B.H.C., Korf, J.: Influence of drugs on striatal and limbic homovanillic acid concentration in the rat brain. Eur. J. Pharmacol. *33*, 31–40 (1975b)

Westerink, B.H.C., Korf, J.: Regional rat brain levels of 3,4-dihydroxyphenylacetic acid and homovanillic acid: concurrent fluorometric measurement and influence of drugs. Eur. J. Pharmacol. 281–291 (1976)

Yarbrough, G.G.: Supersensitivity of caudate neurones after repeated administration of haloperidol. Eur. J. Pharmacol. *31*, 367–369 (1975)

York, D.I.: Dopamine receptor blockade – a central action of chlorpromazine on striatal neurons. Brain Res. *37*, 91–101 (1971)

Zirkle, C.L., Kaiser, C.: Antipsychotic agents (tricyclic). In: Psychopharmacological agents. Gordon, M., (ed.), pp. 39–128. New York: Academic Press 1974

Zivkovic, B., Guidotti, ; A., Costa, E.: Effects of neuroleptics on striatal tyrosine hydroxylase: changes in affinity for the pteridine cofactor. Molec. Pharmacol. *10*, 727–735 (1974)

Zivkovic, B., Guidotti, A., Revuelta, A., Costa, E.: Effects of thioridazine, clozapine and other antipsychotics on the kinetic state of tyrosine hydroxylase and on the turnover rate of dopamine in striatum and nucleus accumbens. J. Pharmacol. Exp. Ther. *194*, 36–46 (1975)

CHAPTER 10

Biochemical Effects (in Men)

M. Ackenheil

A. Introduction

The specific effects of neuroleptics in animals are well established. They interfere with the neuronal activity of the biogenic amines, dopamine (DA), noradrenaline (NA), and sometimes serotonin (5-HT). They may also influence the activity of other transmitters or mediators such as γ-aminobutyric acid (GABA), acetylcholine, and hormones, particularly prolactin. From these effects, the mechanism of antipsychotic action is concluded to be due mainly to DA-, rather than NA-receptor blockade in brain. (Carlsson and Lindqvist, 1963; van Rossum, 1966; Nybäck and Sedvall, 1968). Final evidence for this hypothesis has yet to be produced from clinical-biochemical investigations in man. Clinical-biochemical studies with neuroleptics are mainly carried out in order to answer the following questions:

1) To what extent are the biochemical effects known from animal experiments applicable for human beings?
2) Is there a relationship between antipsychotic and extrapyramidal motor system (EPMS) effects, on one hand, and biochemical effects on the other?
3) Are there differences between drugs inducing strong EPMS disturbances and others with less or no EPMS side effects?

   Generally, classical neuroleptics, e.g., chlorpromazine and haloperidol with EPMS side effects; thioridazine with few; and clozapine and sulpiride with no EPMS side effects, have been chosen for experiments.

   Biochemical studies in man present some difficulties which must be overcome:

1. The *selection of volunteers* and of patients to take the drug is critical. The neuronal activity is dependant on the personality, psychic state, age, sex, and genetics so all of these factors must be kept in mind.

2. *Application of the drug* holds problems from the pharmacologic point of view. In most cases, dose-response curves cannot be carried out and pharmacokinetic data are very seldom available. As, generally, the dosage in man is smaller than in animal experiments, the biochemical effects cannot be expected to be very pronounced.

3. The *turnover of biogenic amines* in human brain can only be measured using indirect methods in the periphery where the blood-brain barrier is an impeding hindrance. On the other hand, the therapeutic effects can be assessed more easily, for comparison with biochemical changes, in man than in animals. Psychopharmacologic drugs need days to weeks of treatment to show a therapeutic effect. For this reason, the time course of the drug, which is mostly neglected in animal experiments, has also to be considered.

4. *The investigation material available* limits the biochemical studies on drug effects. Blood, cerebrospinal fluid, and urine are obtainable from the subjects. Table 1 gives

Table 1. Survey on biochemical substances estimable in body fluids of men in relation to transmitters which are thought to be important for neuroleptic action

Transmitter system reflected	Urine	Blood	Cerebro-spinal fluid	Methods
Adrenergic	Noradrenaline	–	–	Fluorimetry, HPLC
	Adrenaline	–	–	Radioenzymatic
	Vanillinmandelic acid	–	–	Spectralphotometry
	3-Methoxy-4-hydroxy-phenyl-glycol	–	–	Spectralphotometry Gas-chromatography
	Dihydroxyphenyl-glycol	–	–	GC-Mass spectrometry
	Metanephrine			
	Normetanephrine			
		Tyrosine		Fluorimetry
		Dopamine-β-hydroxylase	?	Radioenzymatic
		Monoaminoxidase		Radioenzymatic
		Catechol-O-methyl-transferase		Radioenzymatic
Dopaminergic	Dopamine		?	Fluorimetry, radioenzymatic
	Homovanillic acid	–	–	Fluorimetry
	Dihydroxyphenyl-acetic acid	–	–	Gas-chromatography GC-Mass spectrometry
	Methoxytyramine			Fluorimetry
	Dihydroxy-phenylalanine	–		Fluorimetry HPLC
Serotonergic	5-Hydroxy-tryptamine	–		Fluorimetry
	5-Hydroxy-indoleacetic acid		–	Fluorimetry, spectral-photometry Gas chromatography GC-Mass spectrometry
		Tryptophan	–	Fluorimetry
GABAergic	γ-Aminobutyric acid		–	Fluorimetry, radioenzymatic GC-Mass spectrometry
		Hormones[a]		Radioimmunoassay

[a] Hormones which, depending on the kind of experiment, make it possible to determine activities of transmitters

a survey, without claiming to be complete, of the most important biochemical substances which can be estimated in these body fluids. They allow, to a certain extent, determination of the neuronal activity of transmitters.

B. Biochemical Findings in Urine

Urine can be obtained most easily for investigation but there are certain problems regarding the collection, particularly from psychiatric patients. With the exception of 3-methoxy-4-hydroxyphenylglycol (MHPG) which comes 30%–50% from the brain (MAAS and LANDIS, 1968) the substances measured in urine reflect peripheral rather than central effects. Furthermore, the shortest collection period is limited to a maximum of 3 h. Therefore, the estimation only indicates biochemical changes during this period, but not the brief effects which frequently occur. On the other hand, there is sufficient material so that the analytic methods do not have to be extremely sensitive.

Very few studies on urine have been reported. After haloperidol treatment, a HVA increase was found (BRUNO and ALLEGRANZA, 1965); chlorpromazine, in a single case, induced a decrease of urinary dopamine and HVA excretion (MESSIHA and TUREK, 1973). Clozapine, after a single dosage of 100 mg orally, produced a decrease of DA and an increase of both NA and A excretion (Table 2). These effects were not significant because of great individual variability. The higher NA and A excretion probably compensate for the orthostatic dysregulations induced by clozapine. Possibly, this effect is due to NA and A receptor blockade.

Treatment of schizophrenic patients with either 10 mg haloperidol or 300 mg clozapine orally per day causes slight HVA elevations after haloperidol (EBEN et al., 1974) and no clear effects after clozapine (ACKENHEIL et al., 1974 b). MHPG and HVA excretions were not changed, 5-HIAA excretion showed a tendency to higher levels.

Table 2. Catecholamine excretion in urine after clozapine

		Day I[a]		Day II[b]		Day III[c]	
DA	µg/ml	0.27	± 0.19	0.21	± 0.17	0.22	± 0.14
	µg/Vol	290	±250	257	±162	202	±111
	µg/0.1 g Creatinine	20.3	± 13	14.9	± 8	14.9	± 7
NA	µg/ml	0.021±	0.012	0.047±	0.085	0.029±	0.010
	µg/Vol	22.0	± 17.3	52.5	± 51.0	29.9	± 15.2
	µg/0.1 g Creatinine	2.0	± 1.7	3.9	± 5.2	2.3	± 1.7
A	ng/ml	8.8	± 5.6	25.0	± 40.7	10.3	± 7.9
	µg/Vol	8.6	± 6.0	31.4	± 46.0	10.0	± 6.2
	µg/0.1 g Creatinine	0.8	± 0.9	1.9	± 2.7	0.8	± 0.6
Urine volume (24 h) ml		1181	±790	1645	±907	1046	±454

[a] Day I: Before clozapine
[b] Day II: Application of clozapine (100 mg orally)
[c] Day III: After clozapine

The urinary results must be interpreted very cautiously as one cannot estimate the contribution of metabolites originating from the periphery or from the brain. According to RAESE et al. (1974), only 10% of the urinary HVA excretion originates from the brain.

C. Biochemical Findings in Blood

Blood studies offer the advantage of registering very short changes but they demand a much more sophisticated analytic and experimental methodology. The progress of analytic, e. g., radioenzymatic methods developed during the last few years have made it possible to determine noradrenaline and adrenaline in small blood samples (HENRY et al., 1975; MÜLLER, 1978). A further marker of sympathetic activity was found by discovering that dopamine-β-hydroxylase (DBH), the enzyme which converts DA to NA, was excreted together with NA from sympathetic nerves (WEINSHILBOUM and AXELROD, 1971). Finally, the development of neuroendocrinology permitted the measurement of receptor sensitivity and the reactivity of each amine system (SACHAR et al., 1977). DA receptor sensitivity can be tested by measuring growth hormone secretion after treatment with the DA receptor agonist, apomorphine (ROTROSEN et al., 1977) or with the α-receptor agonist, clonidine (MATUSSEK et al., 1977). The serotonin turnover in brain is assumed to be reflected by the level of free tryptophan in serum (TAGLIAMONTE et al., 1973, KNOTT and CURZON, 1972).

Until recently, no studies on blood have been carried out to investigate specific neuroleptic drug effects. The development of a sensitive method for measuring the DBH activity in serum and the discovery that this enzyme reflected sympathetic activity (WEINSHILBOUM and AXELROD, 1971) offered the possibility of testing such effects. Clozapine, after a single dose and after prolonged treatment, decreased DBH activity in serum (ACKENHEIL et al., 1974a). Administration of a single dose of haloperidol, as well as a 7-day treatment period, equally reduce the serum DBH activity (MARKIANOS et al., 1976). Both effects suggest an influence of the drugs on noradrenergic neurons; a fact which is known for clozapine (KELLER et al., 1973), but not so well established for haloperidol. Measurements showing a decrease of MHPG in serum after clozapine (own unpublished results) support these findings. Sulpiride, another antipsychotic drug which differs from haloperidol and clozapine by having more activating actions, showed no influence on the DBH activity after a single dose (own unpublished results).

Estimations of NA with radioenzymatic methods show increased plasma levels after clozapine which support the urinary findings (SARAFOFF et al., 1978). Longer treatment of schizophrenic patients (more than 5 years) with different neuroleptics also resulted in markedly elevated NA levels (NABER et al., 1978). There was no relationship to psychopathology and EMPS functions in these patients. After 30 days of withdrawal of neuroleptic drugs, NA plasma levels normalized and re-increased during treatment with 600 mg sulpiride per day (ZANDER et al., 1978). It can be concluded from animal experiments that these NA values indicate a noradrenergic receptor blockade. It is surprising that this effect can be seen after such a long period of treatment with neuroleptics. Other biochemical effects are diminished after this time.

During the last few years, neuroendocrinologic studies have become more and more frequent in psychopharmacology and psychiatric research. Neuroleptic drugs

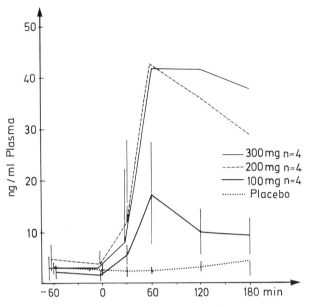

Fig. 1. Prolactin plasma levels after sulpiride (100–300 mg/day, orally). Means with standard deviations

exert an influence on the different hormones via catecholaminergic effects. Therefore, if the regulation mechanisms of hormone secretion are known, measurements of hormone levels in blood allow suggestions about the respective catecholamine system. The stimulation of catecholamine receptors with agonistic drugs, e. g., amphetamine (LANGER et al., 1976), clonidine (MATUSSEK et al., 1977), L-dopa, apomorphine (ROT-ROSEN et al., 1977), induces an increased excretion of human growth hormone. On the other hand, neuroleptic drugs block DA and NA receptors and by this effect inhibit the stimulation of growth hormone secretion (KIM et al., 1971).

Various other hormones are influenced by neuroleptic agents (BRAMBILLA et al., 1975). The infundibular DA system, which regulates prolactin secretion, has been the most important field of endocrinologic interest in neuroleptic research during the last few years. Dopaminergic neurons suppress prolactin secretion either directly or via the prolactin inhibiting factor (PIF). Therefore, conversely, DA receptor blockade increases prolactin secretion (MCLEOD et al., 1976, SHAAR and CLEMENS, 1974). Depending on the antipsychotic potency, neuroleptics increase prolactin secretion in a dose-dependant manner (LANGER et al., 1977). Figure 1 shows an example of such experiment. The increase in prolactin secretion induced by sulpiride depends on the dosage given. On the basis of the prolactin secretion, it was possible to establish an order of neuroleptics which corresponded well with their clinical effects (LANGER et al. 1977). There are two exceptions: clozapine, with strong antipsychotic activity and a small prolactin increase and sulpiride, with strong prolactin-inducing properties and not so pronounced antpsychotic effects. Nevertheless, the prolactin system has the advantage of enabling the researcher to test the DA receptor blocking activity of psychotropic drugs in man. In one study, a high correlation between the prolaction secretion

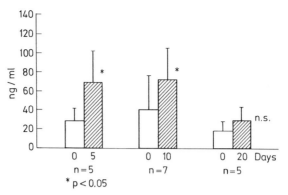

Fig. 2. CSF HVA before (open columns) and during (shaded columns) clozapine treatment (200–400 mg/day, orally). Means with standard deviations

during chlorpromazine treatment and clinical outcome could be found (WODE-HEL-GODT and SEDVALL, 1978).

In contrast to the HVA accumulation in CSF (see Sect. D), no development of tolerance occurred during the first 3–4 weeks of neuroleptic administration (SACHAR et al., 1977). Results of our group on the effects of treatment with clozapine, haloperidol, and sulpiride confirm these findings. Obviously, there is a better correlation of the time course of antipsychotic effects using the prolaction system than by measuring HVA in CSF. However, in order to examine a probable adaption of this system, prolactin secretion was measured in chronic schizophrenic patients treated for at least 5 years (maximal 20 years, mean 12 years) with different neuroleptics. Generally, the patients showed no elevated prolactin levels. Furthermore, no correlations between EPMS side effects and psychopathology could be found (NABER et al., 1978). Therefore, we assume that this system also develops tolerance and that other DA systems, (e. g., the mesolimbic or cortical system) are probably responsible for the antipsychotic effect. In spite of these latter findings, neuroendocrine measurements will remain a useful technique in psychopharmacology.

D. Biochemical Findings in CSF

One of the most direct approaches for investigating drug effects on the biochemistry of central amine metabolism is the analysis of cerebrospinal fluid (CSF). The concentration of the metabolites MHPG, homovanillic acid (HVA), and 5-hydroxyindoleacetic acid (5-HIAA) in CSF reflect, to a certain extent, the turnover of the respective amine (GULDBERG et al., 1969; MOIR et al., 1970; WILK, 1975). The metabolites are detectable by fluorimetric, gas chromatographic and mass-spectrometric methods (ANDEN et al., 1963; DZIEDCIC and GITLOW, 1974; FRI et al., 1974a, b; WILK et al., 1971; WILK, 1971; WATSON et al., 1974; WILK et al., 1972; SJÖQVIST and ÄNGARD, 1972, SWAHN et al., 1976). A somewhat better method is the "probenecid technique." By inhibiting the outflow of the acetic metabolites, probenecid causes an increase of these metabolites which reflects the biogenic amine turnover (ROOS and SJÖSTRÖM, 1969; TAMARKIN et al., 1970; KORF and VAN PRAAG, 1971; VAN PRAAG et al., 1973).

However, its use is limited because of difficulties resulting from pharmacokinetics and from the discomfort of the patient. However, like blood and urine investigations, CSF studies only give hints of the psychopharmacologic biochemical effects. Regional differences in the anatomic localization or in pre- and postsynaptic sites of action cannot be seen. Conclusions from these results have to be completed by animal experiments and vice versa.

A great deal of psychopharmacologic research has been focused on investigations of the metabolites of biogenic amines in CSF because of its close connection to the brain. Since CARLSSON and LINDQVIST postulated a DA receptor blockade to be the mechanism of action of neuroleptics, several studies have been carried out to establish this effect in man. Indeed, elevated HVA levels, indicating a DA receptor blockade, could be found with different neuroleptics. Generally, there were no differences in the degree of HVA elevation, antipsychotic potency, and induction of EPMS side effects. Therapeutic doses of haloperidol increased HVA by an average of about 70%–150% (BOWERS et al., 1965; EBEN et al., 1974; PERSON and ROOS, 1968, 1969; CHASE, 1973; RÜTHER et al., 1976; SCHILKRUT et al., 1976). Rather similar elevations were obtained with chlorpromazine (BOWERS, 1973; CHASE et al., 1970; FYRÖ et al., 1974; POST and GOODWIN, 1975), trifluoperazine (BOWERS, 1973), thiothixene, and methylperone (SEDVALL et al., 1975). Likewise, after 10 days of treatment with clozapine, HVA in CSF was increased by 83% (ACKENHEIL et al., 1974a). Oxypertine, a neuroleptic drug with a mechanism of action similar to that of reserpine (HASSLER et al., 1970) showed no effect on HVA in CSF (van PRAAG and KORF, 1975). This result was obtained with the probenecid technique, which offers the advantage of indicating more exactly the central amine turnover. Using this method, better correlations between the increase of DA turnover in man and the therapeutic effect could be found after various dosages of haloperidol (van PRAAG, and KORF, 1975). However, the majority of studies showed no clear correlations between therapeutic, biochemical, and side effects. Thioridazine, a drug with few EPMS side effects, induced a similar accumulation (43%) of HVA (BOWERS, 1975; POST and GOODWIN, 1975) as chlorpromazine, haloperidol (van PRAAG and KORF, 1975; GERLACH, 1973, GERLACH et al., 1975) and pimozide (POST and GOODWIN, 1975). According to their therapeutic response and HVA levels in CSF, BOWERS classified his patients into a group of "good prognosis" and of "poor prognosis," thus offering a biochemical subdiagnosis (BOWERS, 1973, 1974).

The estimation of 5-HIAA, which indicates the serotonin turnover, showed no significant effects of neuroleptics in most studies. According to these data, the involvement of serotonergic neurons in antipsychotic actions seems to be unlikely.

Although NA receptor blockade is also a possible mechanism of action of neuroleptics, only a few studies have measured MHPG, which reflects the central NA turnover (MAAS and LANDIS, 1968). Treatment with chlorpromazine decreases MHPG in CSF whereas oxypertine elevates MHPG (van PRAAG and KORF, 1975). The result harmonizes with the NA-depleting effect of oxypertine (HASSLER et al., 1970). After clozapine, MHPG was also decreased (ACKENHEIL et al., 1974a). Significant correlations were found between the change of MHPG levels and psychopathology throughout the treatment with chlorpromazine (WODE-HELGODT and SEDVALL, 1978). Interpretations of MHPG data are very precarious as, beside the specific pharmacologic effects, other factors play an important role, e. g., stress, type of disease, motor activity (POST et al., 1973).

The lack of good correlations between antipsychotic potency and HVA effects established in animal experiments compel the consideration of other factors which could be involved in drug action. The nature of the time course needs particular consideration. Clinical observations (EPMS side effects, sedative effects) suggest that a change in the drug action takes place, probably a development of tolerance. In the course of 5, 10, and 20 days of treatment with clozapine, the highest accumulation of HVA was found on the 5th day (Fig. 1). After 10 and 20 days of treatment, the HVA accumulation diminished indicating adaption of the DA turnover. This result in man is confirmed by animal experiments. Similar changes were observed with haloperidol (RÜTHER, 1977; GERLACH et al., 1975), chlorpromazine, thioridazine, and pimozide (POST and GOODWIN, 1975; SEDVALL et al., 1975). This effect could be responsible for the disappointing results found when trying to compare clinical effects with biochemical data. There is a dissociation between the time course of HVA levels, antipsychotic effects, and EPMS symptoms. After prolonged treatment with different neuroleptics (more than 5 years) no elevation of HVA could be found in CSF (ACKENHEIL, 1978).

Assuming that the antipsychotic effect is still present, other systems than the nigrostriatal DA system must be responsible for the antipsychotic action. Probably, the mesolimbic DA system, of which the dopaminergic activity is only reflected to a small extent by HVA in CSF, is more important. On the other hand, interactions with other transmitters must also be considered. GABA measurements in CSF, which probably indicate activity of GABAergic neurons, showed changes after prolonged treatment with neuroleptics and under sulpiride therapy (ZIMMER et al., 1978). GABAergic neurons are closely connected with dopaminergic and cholinergic neurons. Further studies will have to examine whether these effects are specifically related to the antipsychotic action.

E. Conclusions

Clinical-biochemical investigations in men, during and after treatment with neuroleptics, generally confirm the animal findings that a DA and NA receptor blockade is the mechanism of action. The best results were obtained in CSF and neuroendocrinologic studies.

No clear correlations could be found between biochemical data and EPMS effects, on one hand, and antipsychotic effects on the other. Adaption phenomena may be responsible for the lack of such a relationship.

References

Ackenheil, M.: Biochemical investigations into the mode of action of sulpiride. 11th CINP Congress, Vienna (1978)

Ackenheil, M., Beckmann, H., Greil, W., Hoffmann, G., Markianos, E., Raese, J.: Antipsychotic efficacy of clozapine in correlation to changes in catecholamine metabolism in man. In: Phenothiazines and Structurally Related Drugs. Forrest, I., Carr, C.J., Usdin, E. (eds.). New York: Raven 1974a

Ackenheil, M., Beckmann, H., Hoffmann, G., Markianos, E., Nyström, I., Raese, J.: Einfluß von Clozapin auf die MHPG-, HVS- und 5-HIES-Ausscheidung im Urin und Liquor cerebrospinalis. Arzneim. Forsch. 24, 984–987 (1974b)

Anden, N.-E., Ross, B.-E., Werdenius, B.: On the occurrence of HVA in brain and CSF and its determination by a fluorometric method. Life Sci. *2*, 448–460 (1963)

Bowers, M.B., Heninger, G.R., Gerbode, F.: Cerebrospinal fluid 5-hydroxyindoleacetic acid and homovanillic acid in psychiatric patients. Int. J. Neuropharmacol. *8*, 255–262 (1969)

Bowers, M.B.: 5-Hydroxyindoleacetic acid (5-HIAA) and homovanillic acid (HVA) following probenecid in acute psychotic patients treated with phenothiazines. Psychopharmacologia *28*, 309–318 (1973)

Bowers, M.B.: Central dopamine turnover in schizophrenic syndromes. Arch. Gen. Psychiatry *31*, 50–54 (1974)

Bowers, M.B.: Thioridazine: Central dopamine turnover and clinical effects of antipsychotic drugs. Clin. Pharmacol. Ther. *17*, 73–77 (1975)

Brambilla, F., Guerrine, A., Guastalla, A., Rovere, C., Riggi, F.: Neuroendocrine effects of haloperidol therapy in chronic schizophrenia. Psychopharmacologia *44*, 17–22 (1975)

Bruno, A., Allegranza, A.: The effect of haloperidol on the urinary excretion of dopamine, homovanillic acid, and vanilmandelic acid in schizophrenics. Psychopharmacologia *8*, 60–66 (1965)

Carlsson, A., Lindqvist, M.: Effect of chlorpromazine or haloperidol on formation of 3-methoxytyramine and normetanephrine in mouse brain. Acta Pharmacol. Toxicol. (Kbh.) *20*, 140–144 (1963)

Chase, T.N., Schnur, J.A., Gordon, E.K.: CSF monoamine catabolites in drug-induced extrapyramidal disorders. Neuropharmacology *9*, 265–268 (1970)

Chase, T.N.: Central monoamine metabolism in man. Arch. Neurol. *29*, 349–351 (1973)

Dziedzic, S.W., Gitlow, S.E.: Cerebrospinal fluid homovanillic acid and isohomovanillic acid: a gas-liquid chromatographic method. J. Neurochem. *22*, 333–335 (1974)

Eben, E., Ackenheil, M., Raese, J., Rüther, E.: Biochemische Mechanismen der extrapyramidalmotorischen Wirkung von Haloperidol am Menschen. Arzneim. Forsch. *24*, 1133–1135 (1974)

Fri, C.G., Wiesel, F.-A., Sedvall, G.: Mass fragmentographic analysis of homovanillic acid and its homoiso analogue in cerebrospinal fluid using the α-dideutero acid as internal standard. Psychopharmacologia *35*, 295–304 (1974a)

Fri, C.G., Wiesel, F.-A., Sedvall, G.: Simultaneous quantification of homovanillic acid and 5-hydroxyindoleacetic acid in cerebrospinal fluid by mass fragmentography. Life Sci. *14*, 2469–2480 (1974b)

Fyrö, B., Helgodt-Wode, B., Borg, S., Sedvall, G.: The effect of chlorpromazine on HVA levels in CSF of schizophrenic patients. Psychopharmacologia *35*, 287–294 (1974)

Gerlach, J.: Neuroleptics and cerebrospinal fluid investigations. Drugs Exptl. Clin. Res. *1*, 213–220 (1977)

Gerlach, J., Thorsen, K., Fog, R.: Extrapyramidal reactions and amine metabolites in cerebrospinal fluid during haloperidol and clozapine treatment of schizophrenic patients. Psychopharmacologia *40*, 341–350 (1975)

Guldberg, H.C.: Changes in amine metabolite concentrations in cerebrospinal fluid as an index of turnover. In: Metabolism of Amines in the Brain. Proceedings of the Symposium of the British and Scandinavian Pharmacological Societies, Edinburgh, July 1968. Hooper, G. (ed.). London: MacMillan, pp. 55–64 (1969)

Hassler, R., Bak, I.J., Kim, J.S.: Unterschiedliche Entleerung der Speicherorte für Noradrenalin, Dopamin und Serotonin als Wirkungsprinzip des Oxypertins. Nervenarzt *41*, 105–118 (1970)

Henry, D.P., Starman, B.J., Johnson, D.G., Williams, R.H.: A sensitive radioenzymatic assay for norepinephrine in tissues and plasma. Life Sci. *16*, 375–384 (1975)

Keller, H.H., Bartholini, G., Pletscher, A.: Increase of 3-methoxy-4-hydroxyphenylethylene glycol in rat brain by neuroleptic drugs. Eur. J. Pharmacol. *23*, 183–186 (1973)

Kim, S., Sherman, L., Kolodny, H., Benjamin, E., Singh, A.: Attenuation by haloperidol of human serum growth hormone (HGH) response to insulin. Clin. Res. *19*, 718 (1971)

Knott, P.J., Curzon, G.: Free tryptophan in plasma and brain tryptophan metabolism. Nature *239*, 452–453 (1972)

Korf, J., van Praag, H.M.: Amine metabolism in the human brain: Further evaluation of the probenecid test. Brain Res. *35*, 221–230 (1971)

Langer, G., Heinze, G., Reim, B., Matussek, N.: Reduced growth hormone responses in "Endogenous" depressive patients. Arch. Gen. Psychiat. *33*, 1471–1475 (1976)

Langer, G., Sachar, E.J., Gruen, P.H., Halpern, F.S.: Human prolactin responses to neuroleptic drugs correlate with antischizophrenic potency. Nature *266*, 639 (1977)

Maas, J.W., Landis, D.H.: In vivo studies of the metabolism of norepinephrine in the central nervous system. J. Pharmacol. Exp. Ther. *163*, 147–162 (1968)

McLeod, R.M.: Regulation of prolactin secretion. In: Frontiers in Neuroendocrinology. Martini, L., Ganong, W.F. (eds.). New York: Raven 1976

Markianos, E.S., Nyström, I., Reichel, H., Matussek, N.: Serum dopamine-β-hydroxylase in psychiatric patients and normals. Effect of d-amphetamine and haloperidol. Psychopharmacology *50*, 259–267 (1976)

Matussek, N., Ackenheil, A., Hippius, H., Schröder, H.-Th., Schultes, H., Wasilewski, B.: Effect of clonidine on HGH release in psychiatric patients and controls. VI. World Congress of Psychiatry. Hawaii 1977

Messiha, F.S., Turek, I.: Decreased dopamine and HVA excretion in a case with chlorpromazine-induced parkinsonism. Res. Commun. Chem. Pathol. Pharmacol. *6*, 329–330 (1973)

Moir, A.T.B., Ashcroft, G.W., Crawford, I.B.B., Eccleston, D., Guldberg, H.C.: Cerebral metabolites in cerebrospinal fluid as a biochemical approach to the brain. Brain *93*, 357–368 (1970)

Müller, Th.: Radioenzymatische Simultanbestimmung von Adrenalin und Noradrenalin im Plasma. Arzneim. Forsch. *28* (II) 1304 (1978)

Naber, D., Ackenheil, M., Fischer, G., Zander, K.: Effect of long term neuroleptic treatment on prolactin and norepinephrine levels in serum of chronic schizophrenics. 11 th CINP Congress, Vienna (1978)

Nybäck, H., Sedvall, G.: Effects of chlorpromazine on accumulation and disappearance of catecholamines formed from tyrosine-^{14}C in brain. J. Pharmacol. Exp. Ther. *162*, 294–301 (1968)

Persson, T., Roos, B.-E.: Clinical and pharmacological effects of monoamine precursors or haloperidol in chronic schizophrenia. Nature *217*, 854–856 (1968)

Persson, T., Roos, B.-E.: Acid metabolites from monoamines in cerebrospinal fluid of chronic schizophrenics. Br. J. Psychiatry *115*, 95–98 (1969)

Post, R.M., Goodwin, F.K.: Simulated behavior states: an approach to specificity in psychobiological research. Biol. Psychiatry *7*, 237–254 (1973)

Post, R.M., Goodwin, F.K.: Time-dependent effects of phenothiazines on dopamine turnover in psychiatric patients. Science *190*, 488–489 (1975)

Post, R.M., Kotin, J.K., Goodwin, F.K.: Psychomotor activity and cerebrospinal fluid amine metabolites in affective illness. Am. J. Psychiatry *130*, 67–70 (1973)

van Praag, H.M., Korf, J.: Neuroleptics, catecholamines and psychoses: A study of their interrelations. Am. J. Psychiatry *132*, 593–597 (1975)

van Praag, H.M., Flentge, F., Korf, J., Dols, L.C.W., Schut, T.: The influence of probenecid on the metabolism of serotonin, dopamine and their precursors in man. Psychopharmacologia *33*, 141–151 (1973)

Raese, J., Schmiedek, P., Ehrlich, E.: Über den Ursprung der Homovanillinsäure im Urin. Arzneim. Forsch. *24*, 1088–1093 (1974)

Roos, B.-E., Sjöström, R.: 5-hydroxyindoleacetic acid (and homovanillic acid) level in the cerebrospinal fluid after probenecid application in patients with manic-depressive psychosis. Pharmacol. Clin. *1*, 153–155 (1969)

van Rossum, J.M.: The significance of dopamine receptor blockade for the mechanism of action of neuroleptic drugs. Arch. Int. Pharmacodyn. Ther. *160*, 492 (1966)

Rotrosen, J., Angrist, B.M., Gershon, S., Sachar, E.J., Halpern, F.S.: Neuroendocrine assessment of dopaminergic activity in schizophrenia. Nonstriatal dopaminergic neurons. In: Advances in Biochemical Psychopharmacology. Costa, E., Gessa, G.L. (eds.), pp. 649–653. New York: Raven 1974

Rüther, E.: Interaction of neuroleptics: haloperidol and clozapine. Proceedings of the 10 th CINP Congress (1977)

Rüther, E., Schilkrut, R., Ackenheil, M. Hippius, H.: Clinical and biochemical parameters during neuroleptic treatment. I. Investigations with haloperidol. Pharmakopsychiatr. Neuropsychopharmacol. *9*, 33–36 (1976)

Sachar, E.J., Gruen, P.H., Altman, N., Langer, G., Halpern, F.S., Liefer, M.: Prolactin responses to neuroleptic drugs: an approach to the study of brain dopamine blockade in humans. In: Neuroregulations and Psychiatric Disorders. Udin, E., Hamburg, D.A., Barchas, J.D. (eds.). New York: Oxford University Press, 1977

Sarafoff, M., Davis, L., Rüther, E.: Clozapine induced increase of human plasma norepinephrine and its decrease by REM deprivation. Psychopharmacology (in press) (1978)

Schilkrut, R., Rüther, E., Ackenheil, M., Eben, E., Hippius, H.: Clinical and biochemical parameters during neuroleptic treatment. III. Primitive reflexes during neuroleptic treatment. Pharmakopsychiatry Neuropsychopharmacol. *9*, 43–47 (1976)

Sedvall, G., Alfredsson, G., Bjerkenstedt, L., Eneroth, B., Fyrö, B., Härnryd, C., Swahn, C.-G., Wiesel, F.-A., Wode-Helgodt, B.: Selective effects of psychoactive drugs on levels of monoamine metabolites and prolactin in cerebrospinal fluid of psychiatric patients. In: CNS and Behavioural Pharmacology. Proceedings of the 6th International Congress of Pharmacology, Helsinki, 1975. Tuomisto, J., Passonen, M.K. (eds.), pp. 255–267. Forssa: Forssan Kirjapaino Oy 1975

Shaar, C.J., Clemens, J.A.: The role of catecholamines in the release of anterior pituitary prolaction in vitro. Endocrinology *95*, 1202–1217 (1974)

Sjöqvist, B., Änggard, E.: Gas chromatographic determination of homovanillic acid in human cerebrospinal fluid by electron capture detection and by mass fragmentography with a deuterated internal standard. Anal. Chem. *44*, 2297–2301 (1972)

Swahn, C.-G., Sandgärde, B., Wiesel, F.-A., Sedvall, G.: Simultaneous determination of the three major monoamine metabolites in brain tissue and body fluids by a mass fragmentographic method. Psychopharmacology *48*, 147–152 (1976)

Tagliamonte, A., Biggio, G., Vargiu, L., Gessa, G.L.: Free tryptophan in serum, controls brain tryptophan level, and serotonin synthesis. Life Sci. *12*, 277–287 (1973)

Tamarkin, N.R., Goodwin, F.K., Axelrod, J.: Rapid elevation of biogenic amine metabolites in human CSF following probenecid. Life Sci. *9*, 1397–1408 (1970)

Watson, E., Wilk, S., Roboz, J.: Derivatization and gas chromatographic determination of some biologically important acids in cerebrospinal fluid. Anal. Biochem. *59*, 441–451 (1974)

Weinshilboum, R.M., Axelrod, J.: Serum dopamine-β-hydroxylase after chemical sympathectomy. Science *173*, 931–934 (1971)

Wilk, S.: Studies on the detection of 3-methoxy-4-hydroxy-phenylethanol in human cerebrospinal fluid. Biochem. Pharmacol. *20*, 2095–2096 (1971)

Wilk, S.: Metabolism of biogenic amines in the central nervous system of man. Proceedings of the VI. International Congress of Pharmacology, Helsinki (1975)

Wilk, S., Davis, K.L., Thacher, S.B.: Determination of 3-methoxy-4-hydroxyphenylethylene glycol (MHPG) in cerebro-spinal fluid. Anal. Biochem. *39*, 498–504 (1971)

Wilk, S., Gitlow, S.E., Bertani, L.M.: Gas liquid chromatographic methods for assay of catecholamine metabolites. In: Methods in Investigative and Diagnostic Endocrinology. Berson, S.A. (ed.). Amsterdam: North-Holland 1972, Vol. 1, pp. 452–473

Wode-Helgodt, B., Sedvall, G.: Correlations between height of subject and levels of monoamine metabolites in cerebro-spinal fluid of psychotic patients. Life Sci. (Submitted) (1978)

Zander, K.-J., Ackenheil, M., Zimmer, R.: Biochemical psychopathological features in chronic schizophrenic patients treated with sulpiride. 7th International Congress of Pharmacology, Paris (1978)

Zimmer, R., Teelken, A.W., Zander, K.-J., Ackenheil, M.: Influence of neuroleptics on the concentration of GABA in CSF of schizophrenic patients. 11th CINP Congress, Vienna (1978)

CHAPTER 11

Toxicology of Antipsychotic Agents

F. Leuschner, W. Neumann, and R. Hempel

A. Introduction

The introduction of chlorpromazine and reserpine for psychiatric use has been followed by a steady increase in the number of psychotropic agents. In the development of new compounds, there have been many attempts to improve the therapeutic indices and to vary the profile of pharmacodynamic activity in accordance with clinical requirements. The number of preparations on the market eases the work of doctors in hospital and general practice and enables them to adapt their treatment plans to individual patients. Inevitably, however, the many drugs available also increase the number and variety of possible toxic reactions and side-effects. This is at once apparent from the different spectra of activity of the individual compounds which often provoke, in man and animals, effects beyond those of their actual psychopharmacological activity. This subject will be considered in greater detail in the chapter on the side-effects of antipsychotic agents.

It would be too confusing to analyse the possible toxic aspects of all the individual modes of action of the antipsychotic agents to be discussed here. It seems more appropriate to pick out and investigate one classical representative of each of the three major groups of phenothiazines, butyrophenones and the central-acting rauwolfia alkaloids. Such an investigation will reveal that despite differences in chemical structure, and in pharmacological, biochemical and clinical efficacy, the majority of antipsychotic agents show extensive fundamental similarities in toxicological respects. We also want to stress the characteristic activities of each group.

The toxicologist's overall assessment of a substance is made up of many aspects. There are first of all the animal studies involving single and repeated doses, as well as further investigations for possible teratogenic, carcinogenic or mutagenic activities. The picture is completed by the findings from pharmacokinetic studies, and the side-effects observed in clinical trials. A complete chapter has been devoted to each of the last two subjects (Chaps. 2.12 and 2.10). So far as compounds actually on the market are concerned, the toxicologist obtains new knowledge not least from the regrettable sources of accidental or deliberate overdoses, especially those with fatal results.

Before we turn to the individual groups, it is necessary to make some basic comments on the toxicology of compounds that have been known for some time. It is not feasible to apply present-day standards to examinations of preparations that have been on the market for more than 15, and in some cases for more than 25 years.

Furthermore, the literature published on the toxic effects of drugs used to be scanty and is difficult to find. At the same time it would be wrong to take no account at all of earlier work merely because it falls short of our present-day standards. Instead, we should regard it as the first stage of a development from which we can obtain some important basic data.

Considerable problems attach to the assessment and evaluation of the toxic effects – those reported in the literature as well as those observed by the authors – of each of the three groups of neuroleptics. A pharmacological effect on the catecholamines (especially in the brain) is common to all these compounds. For instance, it is due to these pharmacological effects that administration of neuroleptics is followed by sedation and substantially reduced food consumption. This makes it extremely difficult, if not impossible, to carry out toxicity studies with high dose levels, and/or to differentiate clearly between pharmacodynamic and toxic effects. A further example to be mentioned in this context is the problem of teratological studies since it is known that teratogenic damage can be induced in rodents merely by dietary restrictions.

B. Butyrophenones

I. General

The psychotherapeutic butyrophenones currently on the market are, in terms of molecular weight, extremely efficacious. They are given in doses of a few milligrams. This group of neuroleptics is characterised by relatively low toxicity on acute as well as chronic administration. Toxic symptoms that did occur in the course of tests were often not so much expressions of direct drug effects as the results of sedation and anorexia, which are caused by these compounds and results in reduced food consumption, retarded body weight development and often also behavioral disturbances. The therapeutic index is very high: lethal doses range from 200 to 11,000 times the therapeutic levels (JANSSEN, 1968).

II. Animals

1. Acute Toxicity

Table 1 gives data on the acute toxicity of haloperidol and other butyrophenone derivatives. This shows the differences in toxicity to be slight within the chemical group apart from isolated 4-aminobutyrophenone derivatives. This also appears to apply to the animal species tested. An exception among the drugs would appear to be pimozide, and among the animals the dog, which reacted more sensitively than the rodents.

As expected, scatter was less after parenteral administration than by the oral route. Oral doses were, in particular, followed by the phenomenon of cumulative or, more correctly, late toxicity, which was first reported by JANSSEN (1968). He was able to show that the LD_{50} values changed in correlation with the follow-up period. The LD_{50} for haloperidol by the oral route was 285 mg/kg at 24 h, and 129 and 50 mg/kg at 3 and 7 days respectively. Similar findings have been described for other derivatives (see Table 1).

The median lethal doses for subcutaneous and intraperitoneal administration lie between those by the intravenous and oral routes. It would seem, however, that there are larger differences between the haloperidol derivatives (see Table 1).

Mice and rats show largely similar toxic syndromes after single doses of a butyrophenone, consisting of initial ptosis, sedation and catalepsy. Death is preceded by clonic convulsions. Death occurred in both species within hours of intravenous injection. Other routes, especially oral administration – as mentioned above – are followed by cumulative toxicity, with late deaths occurring for up to 10 days.

As mentioned at the beginning, butyrophenone derivatives are highly efficacious. The ED_{50} in pharmacological studies are in the milligram range and often below that. This, in view of the LD_{50}, means a relatively high therapeutic index for single or short-term treatments. This is reflected in, for instance, the widespread use of azaperone for the sedation of pigs for transportation (CALLEAR and VAN GESTEL, 1971), and for the handling of wild animals (MARSBOOM, 1969), with only very low drug-induced mortality (CALLEAR and VAN GESTEL, 1971; NEAVE, 1973).

MELDRUM et al. (1977) have reported on other routes. They found that typical reactions of green monkeys on 5 mg/kg haloperidol by intramuscular injection including yawning, and masticatory and atactic movements etc. Other monkeys (Car and Sooty Mangabeys), which had been given intravenous injections of haloperidol at levels ranging from 0.02 to 20.0 mg/kg, exhibited sedation, lethargy, ptosis and tremor. There were no deaths (OBERST and CROOK, 1967). SEAY and FIELD (1967) described slight to moderate local irritation after intramuscular injection in rabbits.

2. Subchronic Toxicity

The papers published on this subject are summarised in Table 2. CHRISTENSEN et al. (1965) administered oral doses of 30 mg/kg of methylperone daily to rats for 15 weeks. The weight gains were lower than those of a control group, probably due to sedation and a certain anorectic response. Blood counts, macroscopic inspection and histology revealed no pathological changes.

Similar findings were reported in respect of haloperidol by BOISSIER and PAGNY (1960), and by SEAY and FIELD (1967). Whereas there were no deaths in the other studies reported, deaths did occur in the 100-day study of BOISSIER and PAGNY. Subcutaneous doses of 1, 4, and 10 mg/kg were followed by the deaths of 4 out of 20, 5 out of 40, and 18 out of 40 animals respectively. The oral route figures were 4 out of 40 and 12 out of 20 animals respectively.

A similar reaction, with transient anorexia and sedation, was exhibited by dogs given oral haloperidol 16 mg/kg for 30 days (GAULTIER and DEROVICHE-FAHTI, 1971). The authors examined dogs treated with rising oral doses, from 10 to 20 mg/kg, of haloperidol for 100 days. They reported increased mortality; the autopsies revealed necrotic lesions in the kidneys and liver, adrenal haemorrhages and subdural haemorrhagic oedemas.

SEAY and FIELD (1967), on the other hand, found no pathological changes apart from inflammation at the injection site after administration of haloperidol to dogs (0.25 and 1.0 mg/kg i.v. for 30 days; 1.0 and 4.0 mg/kg i.m. for 4 weeks).

In monkeys, at the dose levels used (0.5 and 1.0 ml/kg of haloperidol for 2 months), the chief symptoms were neurological in the form of acute dystonia (GUNNE and BARANY, 1976).

3. Chronic Toxicity

HEYWOOD and PALMER (1974) investigated the oral toxicity of methylperone in rats and dogs. The dose levels for rats were 10, 40, and 120 mg/kg daily, administered by

Table 1. Butyrophenones: acute toxicity

Drug	Animal species	Route		LD$_{50}$ (mg/kg)[a]	Authors
Haloperidol	Mouse	i.v.		28	LECHAT et al. (1968)
Haloperidol	Mouse	i.v.		13	SEAY and FIELD (1967)
Haloperidol	Mouse	i.v.		18.9	NIEMEGEERS and JANSSEN (1974)
Haloperidol	Mouse	i.v.		30	CHRISTENSEN et al. (1965)
Haloperidol	Mouse	i.v.		13	OBERST and CROOK (1967)
Haloperidol	Mouse	i.v.		15	JANSSEN et al. (1968)
Bromperidol	Mouse	i.v.		19	NIEMEGEERS and JANSSEN (1974)
Methylperone	Mouse	i.v.		35	CHRISTENSEN et al. (1965)
Droperidol	Mouse	i.v.		20	CUISSET and ROUJAS (1976)
4-Aminobutyro-phenone derivative	Mouse	i.v.		20–200	CASCIO et al. (1976)
Azaperone	Mouse	i.v.		52	NIEMEGEERS et al. (1974)
Haloperidol	Rat	i.v.		22	SEAY and FIELD (1967)
Haloperidol	Rat	i.v.		20	CHRISTENSEN et al. (1965)
Haloperidol	Rat	i.v.		15	NIEMEGEERS and JANSSEN (1974)
Bromperidol	Rat	i.v.		25	NIEMEGEERS and JANSSEN (1974)
Azaperone	Rat	i.v.		28	NIEMEGEERS et al. (1974)
Methylperone	Rat	i.v.		40	CHRISTENSEN et al. (1965)
Haloperidol	Rabbit	i.v.		8	SEAY and FIELD (1967)
Haloperidol	Dog	i.v.		18	SEAY and FIELD (1967)
Trifluperidol	Mouse	s.c.		54 (1) 54 (3)[a] 50 (10)	HONMA et al. (1974)
Haloperidol	Rat	s.c.		60	NIEMEGEERS and JANSSEN (1974)
Haloperidol	Rat	s.c.		63	SEAY and FIELD (1967)
Haloperidol	Rat	s.c.		60	JANSSEN (1968)
Haloperidol	Rat	s.c.		75	CHRISTENSEN et al. (1965)
Azaperone	Rat	s.c.		640 (1)[a] 450 (3)	NIEMEGEERS et al. (1974)
Benperidol	Rat	s.c.		220	JANSSEN (1968)
Seperidol	Rat	s.c.		70	JANSSEN (1968)
Trifluperidol	Rat	s.c.		70	JANSSEN (1968)
Methylperidol	Rat	s.c.		60	JANSSEN (1968)
Fluanisone	Rat	s.c.		420	JANSSEN (1968)
Pipamperone	Rat	s.c.		320	JANSSEN (1968)
Haloperidol	Mouse	s.c.		54	SEAY and FIELD (1967)
Haloperidol	Mouse	s.c.		54	OBERST and CROOK (1967)
Haloperidol	Mouse	s.c.		60	CHRISTENSEN et al. (1965)
Haloperidol	Mouse	s.c.		63	NIEMEGEERS and JANSSEN (1974)
Haloperidol	Mouse	s.c.		60	JANSSEN et al. (1968)
Haloperidol	Mouse	s.c.		78	GAULTIER and DEROVICHE-FAHTI (1971)
Haloperidol	Mouse	s.c.		78	BOISSIER and PAGNY (1960)
Azaperone	Mouse	s.c.		460 (1) 179 (3)	NIEMEGEERS et al. (1974)
Bromperidol	Mouse	s.c.		114	NIEMEGEERS and JANSSEN (1974)
Methylperone	Mouse	s.c.		230	CHRISTENSEN et al. (1965)
ID-4708	Mouse	s.c.		1,600 (1) 1,200 (3) 340 (10)	HONMA et al. (1974)
Bromperidol	Rat	s.c.		84	NIEMEGEERS and JANSSEN (1974)
Methylperone	Rat	s.c.		220	CHRISTENSEN et al. (1965)
Haloperidol	Dog	s.c.	>	80	SEAY and FIELD (1967)
Azaperone	Dog	s.c.	>	40	NIEMEGEERS et al. (1974)

Table 1 (continued)

Drug	Animal species	Route	LD_{50} $(mg/kg)^a$		Authors
Pimozide	Dog	s.c.	>	5	JANSSEN et al. (1968)
Haloperidol	Mouse	i.p.		30	CARMINATI (1969)
Haloperidol	Mouse	i.p.		45	GAULTIER and DEROVICHE (1971)
Haloperidol	Mouse	i.p.		45	BOISSIER and PAGNY (1960)
Haloperidol	Mouse	p.o.		75	CHRISTENSEN et al. (1965)
Haloperidol	Mouse	p.o.		71	CASCIO et al. (1976)
Haloperidol	Mouse	p.o.		285 (1)	JANSSEN et al. (1968)
				129 (3)	
				50 (7)	
Haloperidol	Mouse	p.o.		350 (7)	NIEMEGEERS and JANSSEN (1974)
Haloperidol	Mouse	p.o.		144	SEAY and FIELD (1967)
Azaperone	Mouse	p.o.		698 (1)	NIEMEGEERS et al. (1974)
				540 (3)	
				385 (7)	
Bromperidol	Mouse	p.o.		227	NIEMEGEERS and JANSSEN (1974)
Methylperone	Mouse	p.o.		230	CHRISTENSEN et al. (1965)
Pimozide	Mouse	p.o.		5,120 (1)	JANSSEN et al. (1968)
				1,693 (3)	
				228 (7)	
Trifluperidol	Mouse	p.o.		120 (1)	HONMA et al. (1974)
				110 (3)	
				110 (10)	
ID-4708	Mouse	p.o.		800 (1)	HONMA et al. (1974)
				800 (3)	
				780 (10)	
Fenaperone	Mouse	p.o.		872–1030	GOURET et al. (1973)
Haloperidol	Rat	p.o.		75	CHRISTENSEN et al. (1965)
Haloperidol	Rat	p.o.		408	CASCIO et al. (1976)
Haloperidol	Rat	p.o.		850	SEAY and FIELD (1967)
Haloperidol	Rat	p.o.		473 (1)	JANSSEN et al. (1968)
				351 (3)	
				351 (7)	
Haloperidol	Rat	p.o.		359 (7)	NIEMEGEERS and JANSSEN (1974)
Azaperone	Rat	p.o.		300 (1)	NIEMEGEERS et al. (1974)
				270 (3)	
				245 (7)	
Methylperone	Rat	p.o.		330	CHRISTENSEN et al. (1965)
Pimozide	Rat	p.o.		5,120 (1)	JANSSEN et al. (1968)
				5,120 (3)	
				10,920 (7)	
Fenaperone	Rat	p.o.		1,080–1,150	GOURET et al. (1973)
Bromperidol	Rat	p.o.		359 (7)	NIEMEGEERS and JANSSEN (1974)
Azaperone	Guinea pig	p.o.		255 (1)	NIEMEGEERS et al. (1974)
				228 (3)	
				202 (7)	
Pimozide	Guinea pig	p.o.		245 (1)	JANSSEN et al. (1968)
				189 (3)	
				189 (7)	
Haloperidol	Hamster	p.o.		405	SEAY and FIELD (1967)
Haloperidol	Dog	p.o.		90	SEAY and FIELD (1967)
Azaperone	Dog	p.o.	>	20	NIEMEGEERS et al. (1974)
Pimozide	Dog	p.o.		40	JANSSEN et al. (1968)

[a] The figures in parentheses represent the follow-up period in days

Table 2. Butyrophenones: subchronic toxicity

Drug	Animal species	Route	Treatment period	Dosage in mg/kg	Authors
Haloperidol	Rat	i.v.	30 days	0.25, 1.0	SEAY and FIELD (1967)
Haloperidol	Rat	s.c.	100 days	1, 4, 10	BOISSIER and PAGNY (1960)
Haloperidol	Rat	i.m.	4 weeks	1, 4	SEAY and FIELD (1967)
Haloperidol	Rat	p.o.	100 days	4, 12	BOISSIER and PAGNY (1960)
Methylperone	Rat	p.o.	15 weeks	30	CHRISTENSEN et al. (1965)
Haloperidol	Dog	i.v.	30 days	0.25, 1.0	SEAY and FIELD (1967)
Haloperidol	Dog	i.m.	4 weeks	1, 4	SEAY and FIELD (1967)
Haloperidol	Dog	p.o.	30 days	16	GAULTIER and DEROVICHE (1971)
Haloperidol	Dog	p.o.	30 days	16	BOISSIER and PAGNY (1960)
Haloperidol	Dog	p.o.	100 days	10–20	GAULTIER and DEROVICHE (1971)
Haloperidol	Monkey	p.o.	2 months	0.5, 1.0	GUNNE and BARANY (1976)

Table 3. Butyrophenones: chronic toxicity

Drug	Animal species	Route	Treatment period	Dosage (mg/kg)	Authors
Haloperidol	Rat	p.o.	1 year	1, 3, 10	SEAY and FIELD (1967)
Haloperidol	Rat	p.o.	$1^1/_2$ year	3.0, 5.0, 6.5, 14.5, and 33.0	SEAY and FIELD (1967)
Haloperidol	Dog	p.o.	6 months	0.5 and 2.0	SEAY and FIELD (1967)
Haloperidol	Dog	p.o.	1 year	2, 6, 12	SEAY and FIELD (1967)
Haloperidol	Monkey	p.o.	6–10 months	0.25–1.0	WEISS et al. (1977)
Methylperone	Rat	p.o.	6 months	10, 40, 120	HEYWOOD and PALMER (1974)
Methylperone	Dog	p.o.	6 months	5, 20, 80	HEYWOOD and PALMER (1974)

gavage; the levels for dogs were 5, 20 or 80 mg/kg daily, administered in capsules. The treatment period was 26 weeks. Of the 40 rats on each dose level (20 males, 20 females) 2, 3, and 17 died, respectively, compared with 1 out of 40 in the control group. On 40 and 120 mg/kg the food consumption was reduced with correspondingly slower weight gains. The haematological, biochemical, and urinary parameters determined revealed no changes. Histological examinations revealed no drug-induced pathological changes. The data on the long-term toxicity studies are summarised in Table 3.

SEAY and FIELD (1967) report that there were no deaths among rats being given high doses of haloperidol in the food (up to 33 mg/kg) for up to 18 months. No drug-induced abnormalities were revealed by urinalysis, haematology, clinical chemistry, macroscopic inspection at the autopsy, or histopathological examinations. As expected the weights and food consumption of the test animals were below the control values, due to sedation.

In a first test series, SEAY and FIELD (1967) found no toxic effects in dogs given 0.5 and 2.0 mg/kg of haloperidol for 6 months. There were still no pathological reactions attributable to the drug after the dose levels had been raised to 2, 6 or 12 mg/kg daily, and the treatment period had been extended to one year. The body weights, haematology, urinary status and macroscopic inspections revealed no pathological changes. There were no deaths.

The only findings consisted of enlargements of the mammary glands with lactation in approximately 50% of the females between test weeks 3 and 8 – which were not dose-related and transient – and reversible increases in the SGPT at high dosages.

Dogs (3 males, 3 females) reacted more sensitively to methylperone than rats. The level of 5 mg/kg/day p.o. was still well tolerated, but 20 and still more 80 mg/kg/day p.o. were followed by sedation and fits. There were, furthermore, substantial weight losses at the highest dose and four of the six dogs died. The laboratory tests revealed no pathological changes. Macroscopic examination showed increases in the relative liver and kidney weights; there were no other changes. There was no eye damage (HEY-WOOD and PALMER, 1974).

The toxic syndrome following long-term administration of haloperidol (0.5 or 1.0 mg/kg/day p.o.) to monkeys was characterised by initial sedation, and later on transient dyskinesia, as well as uncoordinated movements after the dose (WEISS et al., 1977).

4. Fertility

The CNS effects of butyrophenones include the pituitary (hypothalamus) system and the genitals governed by the latter. Haloperidol induced permanent dioestrus in the rat (10 mg/kg p.o. for 14 days), and lower ovulation rates in the rabbit (2.5 mg/kg i.v.) (TUCHMANN-DUPLESSIS and MERCIER-PAROT, 1966, 1968; CHAND et al., 1973). In addition, the marked dose-related sedation after neuroleptics of the butyrophenone type reduces the females' readiness to conceive and the copulation drive of the males. Nevertheless litter sizes and foetal weights in the rat did not differ from those of control animals.

There were no discernible consequences of a haloperidol-induced prolongation of gestation due to delayed nidation of the fertilised ovum (rat, 3,0, 9.0 mg/kg p.o., EINER-JENSEN and SECHER, 1970; rat, 0.073, 0.65 or 1.9 mg/kg p.o., SEAY and FIELD, 1967; rat, 10 mg/kg p.o., mouse, 1.5 or 2.5 mg/kg p.o./s.c., TUCHMANN-DUPLESSIS and MERCIER-PAROT, 1967, 1968).

5. Teratology

The studies showed substantial differences between animal species. Several authors report that the administration of haloperidol (5–240 mg/kg p.o.) to gestating mice caused cleft palates which affected almost 100% of the animals; in the rat (160 mg/kg p.o.) this condition occurred in, at most, 4% (SZABO et al., 1974; SZABO and BRENT, 1974; KALTER, 1972). BERTELLI et al. (1968) found no teratogenic effects of haloperidol in mice (1.5–3.0 mg/kg p.o.), rats (2.5–10.0 mg/kg p.o.) or rabbits (5.0 or 10.0 mg/kg p.o.). EINER-JENSEN and SECHER (1970) and SEAY and FIELD (1967) likewise found no teratogenic effects in rats (3.0–9.0 mg/kg p.o.; 0.073–1.9 mg/kg p.o., and 0.6, 3.0 mg/kg i.v.); the same authors, in a dog study (1.0–4.0 mg/kg p.o.), found no malformations.

HEYWOOD and PALMER (1974) report that metylperone exhibited no teratogenic activity in rats and rabbits (15–60 mg/kg/day p.o., administration from day 6–15 (rats) and 6–18 (rabbits), respectively.

6. Perinatal and Postnatal Toxicity

The administration of haloperiol during and after gestation provoked no discernible changes in rats or dogs. There were no abnormalities; the litter sizes were within the normal ranges (0.073–1.9 mg/kg/day p.o., SEAY and FIELD, 1967). Other authors too have reported that treatment during gestation did not affect litter size, birth weights or postnatal development in mouse (1.5–3.0 mg/kg/day p.o.), rat (2.5–10.0 mg/kg/day p.o.) or rabbit (5 or 10 mg/kg/day p.o., 2.5 mg/kg/day i.v.) (TUCHMANN-DUPLESSIS and MERCIER-PAROT, 1968).

High doses (4.0 mg/kg) given by intramuscular injection shortly before parturition prolong the process of parturition in rats and increase neonatal mortality due to inadequate lactation by the sedated dams (SEAY and FIELD, 1967).

If lactating females are treated with 1.0 mg/kg/day p.o. of haloperidol or penfluridol, newborn rabbits show motor dysfunction and rats develop behavioral changes, i.e. conditioned avoidance response (cf. this chapter Sect. B.5.), (ENGEL et al., 1974; LUNDBORG, 1972; AHLENIUS et al., 1973).

ZIV et al. (1974) were able to show in cows (0.5 mg/kg/day i.m.) and ewes (1.0 mg/kg/day i.v.) that the amount of haloperidol diffused into the milk and into the foetal serum reached up to 60% or even 70% of the maternal serum level. High doses (5.0 mg/kg/day s.c.) produce toxic effects in the dam, i.e. reductions in the food and water consumption. This in turn reduces milk secretion resulting in weight losses and increasing mortality of the neonates (GIVANT et al., 1973). Intravenous doses of 0.6–1.8 mg/kg/day administered to lactating rats from day 1 to day 6 after parturition had no discernible effects on mortality, weight or development of the litters (SEAY and FIELD, 1967).

III. Human Subject

1. Acute Toxicity

There are no recorded cases of death in man caused by butyrophenone derivatives (DAVIS et al., 1968). According to GAULTIER and DEROVICHE-FAHTI (1971), the threshold doses for toxic effects range for the various derivatives from 20 to 1,200 mg/kg, and for children from 0.5 to 20.0 mg/kg. COUTSELINIS et al. (1977) measured blood levels of 42 and 68 mg/litre of haloperidol in children (4 and 5 years) at 2 h after ingestion of approximately 12–20 mg. Even 425 mg of methylperidol ingested with suicidal intent did not cause death (PETERS, 1964). PLATTS et al. (1965) describe the case of a 19-year-old male who died after taking an unknown dose of a phenelzine/trifluoperazine combination. The toxic effects included tonoclonic convulsions, hyperthermia, hyperventilation, hyperhidrosis, sialorrhoea, anuria and diarrhoea. The autopsy revealed chiefly haemorrhagic necroses.

2. Teratology

In man, ingestion of haloperidol (15 mg/kg/day) in connection with other drugs in the first months of pregnancy has in isolated instances been followed by changes in the extremities (KOPELMAN et al., 1975; SCHARDEIN, 1976). In other studies haloperidol was used in pregnancy, for instance in a dosage of 0.6 mg/kg twice daily for some days to some weeks, without harmful effects (ELERT, 1969; HANSON and OAKLEY, 1975; SCHARDEIN, 1976; TUCHMANN-DUPLESSIS, cit. by DEGKWITZ et al., 1970; VAN WAES and VAN DE VELDE, 1969).

3. Perinatal and Postnatal Toxicity

VAN WAES and VAN DE VELDE (1969) found no effects of haloperidol (0.6 mg twice daily for some days to several weeks) in woman after administration in pregnancy.

IV. Mutagenic Activity

VAN DEN BERGHE (1974) studied haloperidol in vivo (man, 1.5–4.5 mg/day for 8–10 years) and in vitro (10 mg/l), and droperidol (50 mg/l) and pipamperone (300 mg/l) in vitro to determine to what extent these compounds caused chromatid ruptures. These studies revealed no clastogenic activities. CHIOREANU and WIENER (1968) found chromosome changes in the male mouse, as represented by hypoploid or hyperploid states (0.5 mg/kg/day p.o. for 50 days). WAGNER (1971) deduced a degree of mutagenic potential for haloperidol $(1.4–5.7 \times 10^{-5})$, fluoropipamide $(6.6 \times 10^{-5}–2.7 \times 10^{-4})$ and properidol $(1.3–8.3 \times 10^{-5})$ from his in vitro studies on human lymphocytes (mol/litre).

V. Discussion of Side-Effects

The butyrophenones, like any other potent drug group, are not free from side-effects. Assessments of the latter in animal experiments are made more difficult by the fact that the higher dose levels invariably cause substantial reductions in food consumption, which give rise to symptoms that can also be caused by merely withholding food.

Although the pharmacological spectrum of activity of the butyrophenone derivatives differs substantially from those of the phenothiazines and reserpines, it can be said in general that these drug classes too act via an effect on the catecholamines, especially dopamine. This means that the chief targets are the central nervous system (CNS) and the circulation. The most dominant undesirable effects are sedation, extrapyramidal symptoms and hypotension (DEGKWITZ et al., 1970; GHATE, 1973; JANSSEN, 1968; SHADER and DiMASCIO, 1970).

It may be assumed that the neuroleptic potency of the butyrophenones is relatively closely linked to the effects on the extrapyramidal tract. Although the therapeutic index is relatively high, side effects such as parkinsonism and hyperkinetic dyskinesia may occur even at moderate doses if they are given over a prolonged period. Similar motor changes can be induced in monkeys (CHRISTENSEN et al., 1970; GAULTIER and DEROVICHE-FAHTI, 1971; GUNNE and BARANY, 1976; HEYWOOD and PALMER, 1974; JANSSEN, 1968; MELDRUM et al., 1977; PETERS, 1964; SCHIELE, 1967; WEISS et al., 1977).

The CNS effects are closely associated with actions on the endocrine system and the centres controlling the latter. This subject has been touched on in the chapters on perinatal and reproduction toxicology. At this point we shall refer only to the mammotropic effect, the antiovulatory activity and the effects on libido, potency and testes (BERTELLI et al., 1968; BORIS et al., 1970; CHAND e al., 1973; DeC.BAKER and TUCKER, 1968; GIVANT et al., 1973; MILLS, 1975; MISHKINSKY et al., 1969; PSYCHOSOS, 1968; TUCHMANN-DUPLESSIS and MERCIER-PAROT, 1966, 1968).

The adrenolytic effective component of the butyrophenone derivatives acts in a peripheral hypotensive way. This effect is less pronounced than the central activity and the effects of chlorpromazine. There are marked differences between the individual derivatives, and there have been numerous attempts to exploit the hypotensive aspect (CASCIO et al., 1976; CUISSET and ROUJAS, 1976; GAULTIER and DEROVICHE-FAHTI, 1971; JANSSEN et al., 1968).

Butyrophenones do not stand out as having undesirable effects on other organ systems (DEGKWITZ et al., 1970; GAULTIER and DEROVICHE-FAHTI, 1971; JANSSEN, 1968; SHADER and DIMASCIO, 1970). This is borne out by, for instance, the studies with azaperone of CALLEAR and VAN GESTEL (1971), and of MARSBOOM (1969) involving the use of this derivative for the sedation of pigs and wild animals. (The situation in man is covered in detail in Chap. 2.12.)

C. Phenothiazines

I. General

The phenothiazines were originally developed for different uses and it was some time before their importance as psychotropic agents came to be recognised. The parent compound, phenothiazine, was introduced in the late 1930s as an anthelminthic (MANSON-BAHR, 1940). Subsequently the compound and its derivatives were discovered to have antihistaminic, local anaesthetic and anaesthesia-potentiating activities (HALPERN et al., 1948; HALPERN and DUCROT, 1946; COURVOISIER et al., 1953; LABORIT and HUGUENARD, 1951, 1952; WINTER, 1966). In 1952 DELAY and DENIKER published their first paper on the treatment of mental disorders with chlorpromazine.

II. Animal

1. Acute Toxicity

The first data on the toxicology of the phenothiazines were published by COURVOISIER et al. (1953). These authors compared the acute toxicity of chlorpromazine and three other phenothiazine derivatives in mice, rats, rabbits, and dogs (details on the acute toxicity studies are shown in Table 4). According to these authors, the toxic effects after intravenous injection manifested themselves in rapid deterioration of the muscle tone, followed by convulsions and death from respiratory arrest. KLEINSORGE and RÖSNER (1958) stated that a total dose of 100–125 mg/kg chlorpromazine i.v. caused death in dogs due to respiratory arrest.

Later, chemical modifications of phenothiazine (cf. Table 4) resulted in slight changes in the LD_{50}. For instance, the acute toxicity was reduced by an exchange of Cl for $CO-CH_3$ in the 3-position (MERCIER et al., 1957). Other agents, e.g. promethazine, isothazine and diethazine had the same intravenous LD_{50} as chlorpromazine (COURVOISIER et al., 1953). The intravenous LD_{50} determined are, by and large, quite close to each other. The various animal species do not differ very widely in their susceptibility to the different compounds (see Table 4).

Determination of the LD_{50} for subcutaneous doses presented some initial difficulties, as the intense central sedation prevented the animals from eating for several days so that the values determined were subject to a very wide scatter. It also seems that

Table 4. Phenothiazines: acute toxicity

Drug	Animal species	Route	LD$_{50}$ (mg/kg)[a]	Authors
Chlorpromazine	Mouse	i.v.	50	COURVOISIER et al. (1953)
Chlorpromazine	Mouse	i.v.	16	JANSSEN et al. (1968)
Chlorpromazine	Mouse	i.v.	39	LECHAT et al. (1968)
Chlorpromazine	Mouse	i.v.	26	BARNES and ELTHERINGTON (1973)
Chlorpromazine	Mouse	i.v.	46	VAPAATALO and KARPPANEN (1969)
Chlorpromazine	Mouse	i.v.	16	USDIN (1970)
Chlorpromazine	Mouse	i.v.	35.5	BELILES (1972)
Acetylpheno-thiazine	Mouse	i.v.	70	MERCIER et al. (1957)
Promethazine	Mouse	i.v.	50	COURVOISIER et al. (1953)
Isothazine	Mouse	i.v.	50	COURVOISIER et al. (1953)
Diethazine	Mouse	i.v.	50	COURVOISIER et al. (1953)
Proxylpromazine	Mouse	i.v.	38	SILVESTRINI and QUADRI (1970)
Chlorprothixene	Mouse	i.v.	28	SCHECKEL (1969)
N-Alkyl-piperidyl-phenothiazine derivatives	Mouse	i.v.	35–75	NIESCHULZ et al. (1954)
Chlorpromazine	Rat	i.v.	29	BARNES and ELTHERINGTON (1973)
Chlorpromazine	Rat	i.v.	25	COURVOISIER et al. (1953)
Chlorpromazine	Rat	i.v.	25	USDIN (1970)
Promethazine	Rat	i.v.	15	COURVOISIER et al. (1953)
Chlorpromazine	Rabbit	i.v.	15	COURVOISIER et al. (1953)
Chlorpromazine	Rabbit	i.v.	16	BARNES and ELTHERINGTON (1973)
Promethazine	Rabbit	i.v.	15	COURVOISIER et al. (1953)
Isothazine	Rabbit	i.v.	15	COURVOISIER et al. (1953)
Diethazine	Rabbit	i.v.	25	COURVOISIER et al. (1953)
Chlorpromazine	Dog	i.v.	30	BARNES and ELTHERINGTON (1973)
Chlorpromazine	Dog	i.v.	100–125 (LD$_{100}$)	KLEINSORGE and RÖSNER (1954)
Chlorpromazine	Mouse	s.c.	350	BERTI and CIMA (1955)
Chlorpromazine	Mouse	s.c.	125	ZIPF and ALSTAEDTER (1954)
Chlorpromazine	Mouse	s.c.	300	BARNES and ELTHERINGTON (1973)
Chlorpromazine	Mouse	s.c.	33	JANSSEN et al. (1968)
Chlorpromazine	Mouse	s.c.	300	USDIN (1970)
Acetylpheno-thiazine	Mouse	s.c.	130	MERCIER et al. (1957)
Chlorprothixene	Mouse	s.c.	280	SCHECKEL (1969)
Pipothiazine	Mouse	s.c.	360	JULOU et al. (1973)
Thioproperazine	Mouse	s.c.	675	JULOU et al. (1973)
Fluphenozine	Mouse	s.c.	800	JULOU et al. (1973)
Chlorpromazine	Rat	s.c.	542	BARNES and ELTHERINGTON (1973)
Chlorpromazine	Rat	s.c.	280	JANSSEN (1968)
Chlorpromazine	Rat	s.c.	140	USDIN (1970)
Pipothiazine	Mouse	i.p.	108	JULOU et al. (1973)
Thioproperazine	Mouse	i.p.	130	JULOU et al. (1973)
Fluphenazine	Mouse	i.p.	117	JULOU et al. (1973)
Methdilazine	Mouse	i.p.	183	WEIKEL et al. (1960)
Thiothixene	Mouse	i.p.	100	WEISSMAN (1968)
Thioproperazine	Mouse	i.p.	115	WEISSMAN (1968)
Prochlorperazine	Mouse	i.p.	118	WEISSMAN (1968)
Chlorpromazine	Mouse	i.p.	92	BARNES and ELTHERINGTON (1973)
Chlorpromazine	Mouse	i.p.	225	FRIEBEL et al. (1954)

Table 4 (continued)

Drug	Animal species	Route	LD$_{50}$ (mg/kg)[a]	Authors
Chlorpromazine	Mouse	i.p.	115	Usdin (1970)
Chlorpromazine	Mouse	i.p.	540	Mikhailowa et al. (1969)
Fenethiazine	Mouse	i.p.	120	Friebel et al. (1954)
Diethazine	Mouse	i.p.	235	Friebel et al. (1954)
Dixyrazine	Mouse	i.p.	510	Mikhailowa et al. (1969)
Promazine	Mouse	i.p.	200	Friebel et al. (1954)
Promethazine	Mouse	i.p.	190	Friebel et al. (1954)
Thiazinamum	Mouse	i.p.	80	Friebel et al. (1954)
Chlorprothixene	Mouse	i.p.	79	Scheckel (1969)
Chlorpromazine and metabolite (substituted)	Mouse	i.p.	120 25–134	Buckley et al. (1974)
Chlorpromazine	Rat	i.p.	74	Barnes and Eltherington (1973)
Chlorpromazine	Rat	i.p.	62	Usdin (1970)
Chlorpromazine	Mouse	p.o.	319	Barnes and Eltherington (1973)
Chlorpromazine	Mouse	p.o.	75	Courvoisier et al. (1953)
Chlorpromazine	Mouse	p.o.	170	Watzman et al. (1968)
Chlorpromazine	Mouse	p.o.	550 (1) 100 (3) 23 (7)	Janssen et al. (1968)
Chlorpromazine	Mouse	p.o.	336	Usdin (1970)
Metopimazine	Mouse	p.o.	800	Guyonnet et al. (1968)
Promethazine	Mouse	p.o.	125	Courvoisier et al. (1953)
Isothazine (quaternary)	Mouse	p.o.	650	Courvoisier et al. (1953)
Chlorpromazine	Mouse	p.o.	35.5	Watzman et al. (1968)
Acetylphenothiazine	Mouse	p.o.	225	Mercier et al. (1957)
Methdilazine	Mouse	p.o.	225	Weikel et al. (1960)
Pipothiazine	Mouse	p.o.	440	Julou et al. (1973)
Thioproperazine	Mouse	p.o.	740	Julou et al. (1973)
Fluphenazine	Mouse	p.o.	380	Julou et al. (1973)
Chlorprothixene	Mouse	p.o.	179	Scheckel (1969)
Chlorpromazine	Rat	p.o.	540	Julou et al. (1968)
Chlorpromazine	Rat	p.o.	350	Usdin (1970)
Chlorpromazine	Rat	p.o.	493	Barnes and Eltherington (1973)
Chlorpromazine	Rat	p.o.	640 (1) 192 (3) 142 (7)	Janssen et al. (1968)
Methdilazine	Rat	p.o.	448	Weikel et al. (1960)
Chlorprothixene	Rat	p.o.	380	Scheckel (1969)
Methdilazine	Guinea pig	p.o.	263	Weikel et al. (1960)

[a] The figures in parentheses represent the follow-up period in days

the room (environmental) temperature has an import bearing on the result (Mercier et al., 1957).

According to Berti and Cima (1955), chlorpromazine is best tolerated by mice at 28 °C; in this case the LD$_{50}$ is 350 mg/kg. The toxicity increases up to 30 times when the room temperature is reduced to 13 °C or increased to 38 °C. Similar facts apply to other phenothiazine derivatives and may be associated with their hypothermic activities as concomitant factors. Similar conclusions were reached by ZIPF and AL-STAEDTER (1954).

The phenothiazines are far less toxic when given subcutaneously than when administered by intraperitoneal injection. So far results for both of these routes have been achieved only for the mouse and the rat (cf. Table 4). TESKE and WEICKER (1956) determined the approximate oral LD_{50} of phenothiazine in rats; they quote levels of 1–2 g/kg. The acute oral toxicity has been determined for a substantial number of phenothiazine derivatives (cf. Table 4). Overall the data indicate a moderate toxicity for the compounds. In the case of chlorpromazine, values have been published for different follow-up periods (JANSSEN, 1968). The data indicate that acute poisoning may be followed by late toxic effects.

The same authors maintain that other animal species, e.g. ruminants, rabbits, guinea pigs and golden hamsters, are non-susceptible to even relatively high doses of phenothiazine.

BREE et al. (1971) investigated the topical tolerance of intramuscular injections of chlorpromazine, 50 and 100 mg/kg, in rabbits (New Zealand Whites). The side-effects included myositis, fibroses, coagulation necroses and perineural inflammations.

It is well known that toxicity studies are affected by extraneous conditions, and this has been touched on above in connection with temperature effects. In the same way there may be deviating results in experimental studies. ASHFORD and ROSS (1968) investigated the oral toxicity of chlorpromazine and perphenazine in hyperthyroid mice. The hyperthyroid mice reacted at least three to five times more sensitively to toxic doses than did the control animals. The toxicity can furthermore be enhanced by concomitant ingestion of alcohol (VAPAATALO and KARPPANEN, 1969), or by depressed bile secretion or kidney function (BECKER et al., 1968).

2. Subchronic Toxicity

The first rat studies were reported by BERCOVITZ et al. in 1943. They administered phenothiazine in the food (0.5%) for 18 days (total dose 1,420 mg per rat, or 390 mg/kg daily; cf. Table 5). There were no deaths; the animals merely showed general depression.

HÄNEL (1950) administered phenothiazine 170 mg/kg daily by gavage for 21 days; 22 animals out of the original 30 survived the test. Daily subcutaneous administration to mice of acetylphenothiazine at dose levels of 12.5, 25.0, 50.0, and 100.0 mg/kg for 10 days provoked moderate changes in the liver cells and renal tubuli. The total dose of 400 mg/kg caused the death of 50% of the animals.

MAICKEL et al. (1970) treated rats for 30 days with chlorpromazine (4 mg/kg), promazine (10 mg/kg) or triflupromazine (2 mg/kg). The animals developed tremor, fatty infiltrations of the liver and hyperactivity of the pituitary-adrenal system. MI-TROFANOV (1974) reports haemorrhagic liver and kidney damage in rats treated with subcutaneous doses of triftazine (1.0 and 5.0 mg/kg/day) for 5 weeks.

VAPAATALO et al. (1969) treated rats with 20 mg/kg chlorpromazine – subcutaneous, intraperitoneal or oral – for 5 weeks. Eight weeks after withdrawal of treatment, X-ray checks revealed dilatation of the intestine.

JULOU et al. (1968) carried out subchronic oral toxicity studies with chlorpromazine in rats and dogs. On only 12 mg/kg/day, rats developed weight losses

Table 5. Phenothiazines: subchronic toxicity

Drug	Animal species	Route	Treatment period	Dosage (mg/kg)	Authors
Phenothiazine	Rat	p.o.	18 days	390	Bercovitz et al. (1943)
Phenothiazine	Rat	p.o.	21 days	170	Hänel (1950)
Chlorpromazine	Mouse	–	30 days	4	Maickel et al. (1970)
Chlorpromazine	Mouse	s.c. and p.o.	35 days	20	Vapaatalo et al. (1969)
Chlorpromazine	Rat	p.o.	1 month	12, 36, 54, and 81	Julou et al. (1968)
Chlorpromazine	Dog	p.o.	1 month	20	Courvoisier et al. (1953)
Chlorpromazine	Dog	p.o.	1 month	12, 36, 54, 81, 120, 180	Julou et al. (1968)
Chlorpromazine	Cat	p.o.	–	15, 30	Karkischenko (1968)
Promazine	Mouse	–	30 days	10	Maickel et al. (1970)
Promazine	Rat	–	30 days	10	Maickel et al. (1970)
Triflupromazine	Mouse	–	30 days	2	Maickel et al. (1970)
Acetylpheno-thiazine	Mouse	s.c.	10 days	12.5, 25.0, 50.0, 100.0, 400.0	Mercier et al. (1957)
Chlorpromazine	Dog	s.c.	1 month	20	Courvoisier et al. (1953)
Methiomeprazine	Mouse	p.o.	30 days	0.5–640.0	Itoh et al. (1974)
Methiomeprazine	Rat	p.o.	30 days	0.5–640.0	Itoh et al. (1974)
Mepromazine	Dog	s.c.	30 days	3, 15	Noble and Sparano (1966)
Trifluperazine	Rat	s.c.	32 days	1, 5	Mitrofanov (1974)
Metopimazine	Mouse	p.o.	1 month	10, 20	Guyonnet et al. (1968)
Metopimazine	Rat	p.o.	1 month	10, 20	Guyonnet et al. (1968)
Thioridazine	Rat	i.m.	20 days	60	Tessitore (1967)

which increased in dependence on the dose. This was accompanied by dose-related reductions in food consumption which was up to 40% lower than in the control group. External symptoms of the toxic effects were sedation and neuromuscular depression. No pathologic organ changes were detected in the survivors. A relevant reduction in lymphocytes occurred only at the highest dose level.

Daily administration of 60 mg/kg i.m. of thioridazine for 20 days to rats did not change the neurosecretory hypothalamus-pituitary system. Histologically there were indications of reduced neurosecretory activity in the supraoptic and paraventricular nuclei of the hypothalamus (Tessitore, 1967). Pathological changes in the hypothalamic region were also discernible in cats after repeated doses of 15 or 30 mg/kg (Karkischenko, 1968).

Similar changes have been reported by Itoh et al. (1974). They found that mice and rats given oral doses of levomethiomeprazine for 30 days at levels ranging from 0.5 to 640.0 mg/kg reacted with weight losses, degeneration of liver cells, changes in the epithelial cells of the renal tubules and swelling of the nerve cells in the brain, especially at the higher doses (over 80 mg/kg).

No deaths occurred among dogs treated with 20 mg/kg chlorpromazine daily orally or subcutaneously for 1 month (Courvoisier et al., 1953). Histological examination revealed no pathological findings other than slight renal changes (dilatation of glomeruli and tubuli contorti).

NOBLE and SPARANO (1966) report that 3 or 15 mg/kg levomepromazine s.c. for 30 days provoked no discernible toxic effects in dogs. Pathological changes occurred only at higher dose levels and longer treatment periods. The effects then included central depression, dysfunction associated with the extrapyramidal, autonomic and sensory nervous systems, ECG changes indicative of anoxia, inhibition of spermatogenesis, atrophy of the prostate and increase in liver weight.

Chlorpromazine exhibited relatively low toxicity in the dog studies of JULOU et al. (1968). There were no intercurrent deaths up to a dose level of 81 mg/kg daily p.o. There were no changes in the blood picture or impairments of liver or kidney function. No pathological changes were revealed by macroscopic or histological examination. On the other hand only one out of four dogs survived in the two high-dose groups (120 and 180 mg/kg). The other dogs died in the course of fits following severe sedation and neuromuscular depression. The autopsy showed haemorrhagic necroses in the liver and impaired spermatogenesis.

3. Chronic Toxicity

The papers on chronic toxicity studies are summarised in Table 6. JULOU et al. (1968) carried out long-term studies with oral doses of propericiazine and thioproperazine in rats (3.3, 10.0 or 30.0 mg/kg/day for 12 months) and dogs (3, 9, and 27 mg/kg/day for 6 months). Both the drugs proved to be relatively well tolerated. Whilst the examinations, including histological ones, showed no significant differences between the propericiazine-treated rats and the controls in respect to mortality, weight, blood picture and organs, mild toxic effects were discernible on thioproperazine and again included reduced food consumption. Each of the two compounds caused a slight weight increase in the pituitary glands.

Thioproperazine had few toxic effects in the dog studies. There were no appreciable pathological changes apart from isolated females with galactorrhoea and slight liver enlargements on the two highest dose levels. All the animals survived the study.

Table 6. Phenothiazines: chronic toxicity

Drug	Animal species	Route	Treatment period	Dosage (mg/kg)	Authors
Pericyazine	Rat	p.o.	1 year	3.3, 10.0, 30.0	JULOU et al. (1968)
Thioproperazine	Rat	p.o.	1 year	3.3, 10.0, 30.0	JULOU et al. (1968)
Methdilazine	Rat	p.o.	1 year	9.5, 19.0, 38.0, 75.0	WEIKEL et al. (1960)
Promazine	Rat	p.o.	1 year	0.1, 0.2, 0.4%	SEIFTER et al. (1957)
Chlorpromazine	Guinea pig	p.o.	1 year	30	McDONALD et al. (1966)
Pericyazine	Dog	p.o.	6 months	3, 9, 27	JULOU et al. (1968)
Thioproperazine	Dog	p.o.	6 months	3, 9, 27	JULOU et al. (1968)
Promazine	Dog	p.o.	1 year	800	SEIFTER et al. (1957)
Promazine	Dog	i.m.	1 year	25	SEIFTER et al. (1957)
Methdilazine	Dog	p.o.	1 year	1, 2, 3	WEIKEL et al. (1960)

In the case of propericiazine, 3 and 9 mg/kg daily were well tolerated. Two out of four animals on the highest dose (27 mg/kg) died after clonic convulsions. The toxic syndrome was characterised by weight loss, sedation, ataxia, and impaired liver and kidney functions (increases in SGPT and urea). The autopsy showed increased weights of liver, kidneys and adrenals. MCDONALD et al. (1966) treated guinea pigs, weight range 400–800 g, with oral doses of 30 mg/kg chlorpromazine daily for 12 months; 17 out of 36 animals died. SEIFTER et al. (1957) report on long-term tests with promazine in which the drug was administered daily for 1 year to rats in the food, at levels of 0.1%, 0.2% or 0.4%, and to dogs at doses of 800 mg/kg/day p.o. or 25 mg/kg/day i.m. These dosages provoked neither changes in the blood picture nor damage to the parenchymatous organs. Favourable results were also obtained on 1-year studies with methdilazine in rats (9.5, 19.0, 38.0 or 75.0 mg/kg/day p.o.) and in dogs (1, 2 or 3 mg/kg/day in capsules). No clearly drug-induced pathological changes were discernible.

4. Fertility

Neuroleptics affect the endocrine balance between pituitary and diencephalon to a greater or lesser degree depending on type and derivative. This results in irregularities of the menstrual cycle, gynaecomastia, galactorrhoea and changes in libido (DEGKWITZ et al., 1970; DELAY and DENIKER, 1961; DOMINO, 1962; HOLLISTER, 1964). These effects can be demonstrated in rat and dog studies with phenothiazine neuroleptics with doses up to 50 mg/kg p.o. and 10 mg/kg s.c. (DEGKWITZ et al., 1970; JULOU et al., 1968; TUCHMANN-DUPLESSIS, cit. by DEGKWITZ et al., 1970).

If male and female rats are treated for 6 weeks before and during gestation with chlorpromazine or levomepromazine in oral doses of 10 mg/kg daily, there will be fewer pregnancies or there may be none at all (JULOU et al., 1968; ALEXANDER et al., 1972). Lower implantation rates and smaller litter sizes have been recorded not only for chlorpromazine but also for other phenothiazine derivatives (dose levels up to 100 mg/kg p.o., 20 mg/kg i.m., 10 mg/kg i.p., or 30 mg/kg s.c.). The mean birth weights are lower, and there are rises in the abortion and neonate mortality rates (ALEXANDER et al., 1972; JULOU et al., 1968; KALTER, 1972; RAVINA, 1964; SINGH and PADMANABHAN, 1977; SPIETH and LORENZ, 1967; ERSHOVA, 1975; HARRINGTON et al., 1966; ITOH et al., 1976).

Rat studies have revealed several factors as possible causes of the above changes in fertility. The phenothiazines prolong the time before copulation and reduce the frequency of copulations (POMME et al., 1965; HARRINGTON et al., 1966); some animals do not copulate at all (SPIETH and LORENZ, 1967). In sheep too, chlorpromazine has a negative effect on conception and increases the mortality rate of neonates, when given intramuscularly 36 h before and after mating at a dose level of 12 mg/kg at 6 h intervals (BUTTLE and ROBERTSON, 1967; STAMP, 1967).

Impairment (blockade) of ovulation, depending on the time of the dose, has been demonstrated in rats (single administration of 5 mg/kg i.v., HARPER, 1968). Other authors report that the compound did not affect the cycle at all, or at worst only on very high doses (POMME et al., 1965; LAND, 1973; JULOU et al., 1968). Administration of phenothiazine neuroleptics invariably delayed implantation of the blastocysts in mice and rats (BINDON, 1969; CHATTERJEE and HARPER, 1970).

5. Teratology

There are virtually two solid blocks of opinions, each drawing on results and experience, concerning the teratological activity of phenothiazine and its derivatives. This illustrates better than anything else how difficult it is – if we may anticipate – to apply the results of animal experiments to man and/or to put the right interpretation on individual clinical findings. There is agreement on one fact, namely that certain animal species, most of all the mouse, are especially susceptible to teratogenic effects. SZABO et al. (1975), for instance, investigated six distinct phenothiazine derivatives and found cleft palates in mice and rats whereas these malformations did not occur in rabbits and monkeys (SZABO and BRENT, 1974, 1975). ROUX (1959) found various changes following treatment with prochlorperazine. BROCK and VON KREYBIG (1964), and WALKER and PATTERSON (1974) showed that not only the animal species but also the strain are concomitant factors in deciding the extent of teratogenic effects. SCHARDEIN (1976) maintains that the structures of individual phenothiazine derivatives play a part.

HORVATH et al. (1971) also saw embryopathies following administration of chlorpromazine, trifluoperazine, perphenazine or methophenazine to rats. The authors attribute this to drug-induced inhibitions of the flavoenzymes. All the effects seen were dependent on the day of administration during gestation. DRUGA (1974) reports the same experience after rat studies with perphenazine.

Again, other authors saw no pathological changes. JELINEK et al. (1967), for instance, and MOAYER (1967) administered chlorpromazine to gestating rats – in some cases in dose levels ranging from 10 to 60 mg/kg p.o. – without any detectable teratogenic damage. Similar results were obtained in tests with 0.5 mg/kg trifluoperazine p.o. (MORIARITY, 1963), 10 and 20 mg/kg metopimazine p.o. (GUYONNET et al., 1968) and 0.7–3.0 mg/kg fluphenazine or flupentixol p.o. (SPIETH and LORENZ, 1967). JULOU et al. (1968) likewise saw no malformation in rats, rabbits or domestic fowl.

Comprehensive synopses on the results of animal experiments have been published by KALTER (1972), NISHIMURA and TANIMURA (1976) and SCHARDEIN (1976). TUCHMANN-DUPLESSIS and MERCIER-PAROT (1968) and KALTER (1972) share the view that phenothiazine neuroleptics do not appear to have any teratogenic activity. BEALL (1972, 1973) likewise saw no teratogenic effects in rats after administration of chlorpromazine or perphenazine.

6. Perinatal and Postnatal Toxicity

Beside higher mortality and lower weights of the foetuses (ALEXANDER et al., 1972; BUTTLE and ROBERTSON, 1967; JULOU et al., 1968; KALTER, 1972; MURPHREE et al., 1962; RAVINA, 1964; SINGH and PADMANABHAN, 1977; SPIETH and LORENZ, 1967; STAMP, 1967) some authors report functional, biochemical or histological changes as well as behavioral disturbances in neonates whose dams had been treated with phenothiazine neuroleptics. Such changes in the newborn offspring of treated females cannot be ruled out in principle since phenothiazine derivatives are able to cross the placental barrier (BOULOS et al., 1971; BROOKES and FORREST, 1971; O'DONOGHUE, 1971; SJÖSTRAND et al., 1965; SMOLIYANIKOVA et al., 1976).

ORDY et al. (1966) and SAMORAJSKI et al. (1965) found ultrastructural liver changes with simultaneous effects on the enzyme pattern of the liver. TONGE (1973 a, b) demonstrated in his experiments in rats that chlorpromazine could cause lasting changes in the catecholamine metabolism of neonates.

Divergent results have been obtained in rat studies investigating the effects of phenothiazine derivatives on learning ability and behavior of dams or parents (Elis, 1975; Gauron and Rowley, 1969; Golub and Kornetzki, 1975; Hoffeld and Webster, 1965; Hoffeld et al., 1967; Werboff, 1966; Werboff and Dembicki, 1962). Prenatal administration of chlorpromazine changes the contents of biogenic amines in the brain; no such effect was detected in rabbits (10 and 30 mg/kg s.c., Nair, 1974). According to Frankova (1977), postpartum administration of 2×3 mg/kg chlorpromazine s.c. to dams changes nursing behavior, i.e. contact is shorter. On the other hand Knowles (1965) reports that administration of chlorpromazine, trifluoperazine or prochlorperazine to lactating bitches caused no discernible damage in the offspring.

III. Man

1. Acute Toxicity

Considering the large-scale world-wide use of phenothiazine preparations for approximately 30 years, fatalities in man are relatively rare. There have been repeated instances of overdosage with suicidal intent, but only 4%–5% of the attempts have been successful. In this connection it should be borne in mind that suicide attempts frequently involve the ingestion of additional drugs, e.g. barbiturates or tranquillisers. Furthermore, it sometimes happens that the clinical picture of a psychiatric illnes, with long-term treatment with psychotropic agents, is complicated by sudden death; such an outcome of mental illness is not unknown (Peele and von Loetzen, 1973).

In reviews on the subject of "poisoning", many authors have commented and/or reported in detail on the phenothiazines (Algeri et al., 1959; Almazova, 1970; Arieff and Friedman, 1973; Barry et al., 1973; Davis et al., 1968; Donnewald, 1970; Frejaville et al., 1970; Gajdos et al., 1970; Hollister, 1966; Johnson et al., 1964; Kamyanov, 1965; Kapur et al., 1977; Lapolla and Nash, 1965; Malizia et al., 1977). The acute doses ingested by patients range from a few hundred milligrams to 9.8 g; even such high doses have been survived. Low dose levels provoke drowsiness and coma, high ones tremor and convulsions. The dominant toxic symptoms are hypotension, hypothermia, extrapyramidal symptoms and changes in the respiratory tract. The ECG often reflects tachycardia, which frequently persists for 2 days after the clinical normalisation (Kurtz et al., 1971). Children are essentially more susceptible and react to lower doses. The mortality rate is higher; lethal doses range from 20 to 75 mg/kg (Davis et al., 1968; Hollister, 1966). With appropriate treatment, the toxic symptoms subside very rapidly (within 48 h).

2. Fertility

Several authors associate the ingestion of neuroleptics (at doses of 25–75 mg, for instance) with interference with the menstrual cycle, gynaecomastia, galactorrhoea changes in the libido (Degkwitz et al., 1970; Delay and Deniker, 1961; Domino, 1962; Hollister, 1964).

3. Teratology

The picture emerging from the clinical results differs from that suggested by the animal experiments. There have been isolated cases which have raised the suspicion of damage to the human embryo by phenothiazine derivatives. VINCE (1969) reports on five such cases associated with phenothiazine treatment. Other references include those by SCHARDEIN (1976), RUMEAU-ROUQUETTE et al. (1977) and ANANTH (1975); ANANTH refers particularly to the 1962 paper of the Canadian FDA on teratogenicity associated with trifluoperazine; this was not, however, unchallenged (MORIARITY, 1963).

On the other hand these isolated cases, which were not regarded as significant (SOBEL, 1960), have to be seen in the context of many publications which stress that more than a thousand times as many women have used phenothiazine products in all stages of pregnancy, and which underline the relatively good tolerance for mothers, foetuses and neonates and the absence of drug-induced malformations (AYD, 1963, 1964a, b, 1974; BAYER, 1966; ELERT, 1969; KRIS, 1965; RISE, 1976; RUMEAU-ROUQUETTE et al., 1977; SCANLAN, 1972; SHAPIRO et al., 1977; SMITHELLS, 1970; WOLF, 1968).

4. Perinatal and Postnatal Toxicity

Findings in human subjects were similar to the results of animal experiments in respect of perinatal and postnatal toxicity. Whereas RIEDER et al. (1975), STOFFER (1968) and WALSON et al. (1975) diagnosed neurological and endocrine disorders, other authors describe essentially normal neonate development (AYD, 1963, 1964a, b; ELERT, 1969; FAIRWEATHER, 1968; KRIS, 1965; SHAPIRO et al., 1977; SOBEL, 1960). O'DONOGHUE (1971, 1974) found ultrastructural liver changes with simultaneous effects on the enzyme pattern of the liver. No drug effects were detected by BLACKER et al. (1962) in children whose mothers had been treated with high doses of chlorpromazine. APGAR (1964) reports a doubtful case of neonatal hyperbilirubinaemia.

IV. Mutagenic Activities

EPSTEIN and SHAFNER (1968) found no mutagenic activity of chlorpromazine (8.3 mg/kg i.p.) in a dominant lethal factor study in mice. ROMAN (1969) studied the effects of levomepromazine on chromosomes in the rat. He found no changes in either number or structure. Similar results were obtained in studies with human chromosomes, from the blood of schizophrenic patients who had been treated with chlorpromazine or levomepromazine for periods of 1–4 years. SHAW (1970) claims that chlorpromazine exhibited clastogenic activity on lymphocytes in vitro but no changes were recorded in human subjects even at high dose levels. CHIOREANU and WIENER (1968) found hypoploid and hyperploid states in mouse chromosomes after thioperazine. ABDULLAH and MILLER (1968) found chromosomal aberrations in vitro in human fibroblasts after chlorpromazine treatment.

GEBHART (1979), in a synopsis, comments on the question of the mutagenic side-effects of phenothiazine, and discusses the conflicting results published to date. According to this author, antipsychotics should be considered as faint mutagens. Though he does not raise an objection against their administration, he thinks that further examinations are required.

V. Carcinogenicity

Studies of Wattenberg and Leong (1965) have revealed an antagonistic effect of phenothiazine derivatives on dimethylbenzantracene. The action resulted from an increase in the benzpyrene hydroxylase activity. It is possible that certain antineoplastic properties can be explained by increased enzyme activity. The complex of carcinogenic and of antineoplastic activities is discussed in a review by Julou et al. (1968). It is known from the literature that chlorpromazine and some other phenothiazine derivatives studied are more likely to exhibit antineoplastic than carcinogenic activities.

In some mouse studies, the authors administered oral doses of 5 mg/kg chlorpromazine every day for 2 years. The incidence of tumours did not differ significantly between treated and untreated mice, which confirms the findings of Lacassagne et al. (1959) and Roe (1966). The suspicion of an association between an increased incidence of breast cancer and phenothiazine treatment could be neither eliminated nor confirmed (Brugmans et al., 1973).

VI. Physical Dependence

The suspicion that they might lead to dependence attaches to all central-acting drugs used predominantly in the treatment of emotional or psychosomatic diseases, especially as long-term administration is frequently required. Deneau et al. (1969) have investigated this problem for drugs including chlorpromazine. They found no indication of any dependence-forming activity of the compound in monkeys (Macaca mulatta). Boyd (1960) obtained similar results in rats.

VII. Discussion of Side-Effects

According to the current state of knowledge, the phenothiazine neuroleptics act via effects on the catecholamine metabolism, or the catecholamine activities: phenothiazines block dopamine, they are α-antagonists to catecholamines; they inhibit the activity of serotonin neurones; in the brain they cause depletion of monoamines, or more likely, an increased turnover of amines by blocking receptors (Lipton et al., 1978). It is obvious, therefore, that given the ubiquitous distribution of these substances in the body – including the human body – not all the included effects are likely to be desirable.

As it has not so far been possible to determine definitely in animal experiments which constituent exerts the antipsychotic activity in man, it is largely left to the beholder to divide the spectrum of activity into desirable and undesirable effects. Countless papers have been published on this subject; summaries appear in Fossati (1976), Ghate (1973), Lehmann and Ban (1974), Shader and DiMascio (1970), Roizin et al. (1957) and Bobon et al. (1970), as well as in textbooks of pharmacology. (The clinical aspects have been covered in detail in Chap. 2.12.)

The most obvious side-effects are those on functions of the CNS and the endocrine system, pigmentation in the eye, photosensitisation of skin and impairments of liver function, gastrointestinal function, and of the extrapyramidal system. The most common mental changes are passivity, drowsiness and confusion. The piperazine derivatives are characterised by a marked effect on motor activity (Baruk et al., 1966; Degkwitz et al., 1970; Julou et al., 1968; Poeck, 1968; Watzman et al., 1968).

Neurological symptoms representing side-effects on the CNS include chiefly extra-pyramidal dysfunctions, Parkinson's syndrome, dystonia and dyskinesia (CHRISTEN-SEN et al., 1970; DEGKWITZ et al., 1970; BETHESDA, 1967; KLEINSORGE and RÖSNER, 1958; JULOU et al., 1968; MAICKEL et al., 1974; SCHIELE, 1967).

In this connection we would refer to a risk to drivers who may be rendered unfit to be in charge of motor vehicles (NELEMANS, 1968). Changes in brain cells have been demonstrated histologically after long-term administration; the importance of this phenomenon is at the present time still an unanswered question (DEGKWITZ et al., 1970; CAZZULLO et al., 1968; KARKISCHENKO, 1968; KLUGE et al., 1974; ROUBEIN et al., 1973).

Phenothiazine neuroleptics cause heterogeneous changes in endocrine and metabolic functions by interfering with catecholamines or the receptor system in the functional range hypothalamus-pituitary and the target organs for the pharmacological effects depending on this range. This subject has been touched on in connection with reproduction toxicology. At this point we refer to the effects on the menstrual cycle and the changes in libido (ARTELLI and CASTELLO, 1968; DEGKWITZ et al., 1970; DELAY and DENIKER, 1961; DOMINO, 1962; HOLLISTER, 1964; PSYCHOSOS, 1968; TESSITORE, 1967), and to the galactorrhoea and gynaecomastia via increased galactine release (BUCKMAN and PEAKE, 1976; MISHKINSKY et al., 1966; TALWALKER et al., 1960).

In the discussion on the side-effects of long-term therapy, a large space must be conceded to the ocular changes. Both cataracts and pigmentations of cornea or retina were observed. In the animal experiment, comparable reactions can be produced most easily in the cat, rabbit and guinea pig. They seem to be closely linked to the dose level and the duration of treatment. To what extent the phenothiazines themselves or one of their metabolites cause these changes is a question still unanswered. Continual ophthalmic check-up, therefore, is advisable if the necessity of long-term therapy at high dose levels should arise (ADAMS et al., 1974; BERNSTEIN, 1966; BOET, 1970; CERLETTI and MEYER-RUGE, 1968; DEGKWITZ et al., 1970; GERHARD et al., 1975; GORDON and BALAZS, 1967; HENKES and CANTA, 1973; JULOU et al., 1968; MASSEY, 1965; McDONALD et al., 1966; MEYER-RUGE, 1973; LINDQVIST et al., 1970; PERRY et al., 1964; SCHIELE, 1967; SHADER and DiMASCIO, 1970; ULLBERG et al., 1970; WANG et al., 1972; BETHESDA, 1967).

There are frequent references to skin changes parallel with the ocular pigmentations. It is necessary to differentiate in principle between photosensitisation and allergic reactions. The latter are very specific; they were recognised in the early stages of the use of phenothiazines when they occurred in the course of treatment as well as – in the form of a contact allergy – among workers at the production plants (APPLETON et al., 1970; KLEINSORGE and RÖSNER, 1958).

The skin pigmentations are likely to represent mainly phototoxic reactions. Animal experiments suggest bindig of phenothiazines to epidermal structures. In rare cases, long-term treatment at high dose levels has been associated with greyish metallic discolourations of the skin and/or pigmentation in organs (ALANI, 1973; ALANI and DUNNE, 1973; APPLETON et al., 1970; FORREST et al., 1970; GREINER and NICOLSON, 1964; HAYS, 1965; ISON and BLANK, 1967; JOHNSON, 1974; LJUNGGREN and MÖLLER, 1977 a, b; MASSEY, 1965; McDONALD et al., 1967; PERRY et al., 1964; SAMS and EPSTEIN, 1967; SAUNDERS et al., 1971).

The parent compound, phenothiazine, was originally used as an oxyuricide; it was recognised quite early that the drug occasionally caused anaemia. Presumably the derivatives can likewise cause an immunoallergic type of haemolytic anaemia (Bercovitz et al., 1943; Collier and Mack, 1944; Dreyfus et al., 1968; Giertz et al., 1954; Hänel, 1950; Kleinsorge and Rösner, 1958; Teske and Weicker, 1956; Thomas et al., 1938).

Changes in the white cell count are other rare side-effects of phenothiazine derivatives. Reactions seen in animals vary according to species and include transient lymphocytopenia and deviating behavior of the leucocytes. Tolerance to the test compound develops within 2–3 days of treatment (Julou et al., 1968). In man, on the other hand, there are reports of a few cases of agranulocytosis (Ananth et al., 1973; Degkwitz et al., 1970; Ebert and Shader, 1970; Kleinsorge and Rösner, 1958).

The most important cardiovascular side-effects are hypotension and arrhythmia affecting excitation. In addition, focal degenerations of myocardial fibres have occurred in animal experiments and in man. It is not yet clear whether these can be held responsible for the "sudden death" syndrome (Danner, 1971; Degkwitz et al., 1970; Deglin et al., 1977; Ebert and Shader, 1970; Gajdos et al., 1970; Moccetti, 1977; Schanda, 1977; Schiele, 1967; Bethesda, 1967).

Finally there is the drug-induced icterus, a rare side-effect but one which frequently occurs quite early in the treatment. It is probably partly of direct toxic and partly of allergic origin and manifests itself as intrahepatic cholestasis. This condition is very difficult to induce in animals. At most we can demonstrate effects on individual organ systems, e.g. damage to the lysosomal membranes. No dangerous histological changes have been demonstrated in animal experiments, even after prolonged administration (Bolton, 1968; Cordelli, 1968; Degkwitz et al., 1970; Dujovne and Zimmerman, 1969; Dujovne et al., 1968; Ebert and Shader, 1970; Julou et al., 1968; Kleinsorge and Rösner, 1958; Pisciotta and Hinz, 1965; Popov, 1967; Scholz and Kretzschmar, 1956, 1958; Torjescu, 1968; Zimmerman, 1968; Bethesda, 1967).

Apart from the more general side-effects such as nausea, vomiting, dry mouth, irregularities of defecation which may be regarded as gastrointestinal reactions, dilatations of intestinal sections have been attributed to phenothiazine treatment. In animals, similar symptoms can only be induced by intraperitoneal injection, not by any other route. Anticholinergic effects are under discussion as possible causes (Ritama et al., 1969; Shader and Harmatz, 1970; Vapaatalo et al., 1969). Promethazine has induced gastric ulcers in guinea pigs (Djahanguiri et al., 1968).

C. Reserpine

I. General

Species of rauwolfia were widely used in medicinal herbs in antiquity in their countries of origin, i.e. India, Africa and Central and South America. The more intensive chemical and pharmaceutical processing of plant extracts stimulated interest in the pharmacology of the rauwolfia alkaloids, and the latter's specific clinical use soon followed. The pharmacological data have been summarised by Bein (1956) and Plummer et al. (1954).

II. Animals

1. Acute Toxicity

The acute toxicity of reserpine and a few derivatives or alkaloids has been determined in mice, rats, rabbits, dogs, and monkeys (cf. Table 7).

In acute studies, reserpine has generally been found to be of moderate toxicity. Dogs proved particularly sensitive to intravenous administration ($LD_{50} = 0.5$ mg/kg, BARNES and ELTHERINGTON, 1973). No deaths occurred in monkeys given as high a dose as 4.0 mg/kg (PLUMMER et al., 1954; WINDLE et al., 1955). Oral administration of 1.0 g/kg to rats and of 400 mg/kg to monkeys caused no effects in either case other than transient sedation, and the animals very soon recovered from this (PLUMMER et al., 1954).

The toxic effects of reserpine include sedation, ptosis of the eyelids, falls in body temperature and blood pressure, as well as lethargy and reduced food consumption. The toxicity of reserpine is clearly affected by extraneous conditions: according to ZORYAN (1966) it is 1,200 times as high at 4 °C than at 30 °C; in mouse studies the toxicity is higher when the rooms are light than in darkness (WALKER and FRIEDMAN, 1970).

2. Subchronic Toxicity

Few papers have been published on the subchronic administration of reserpine (cf. Table 8). ROSECRANS (1967) treated rats with intraperitoneal injections of 1.0 mg/kg reserpine daily for 42 days. There were no major reactions whereas the same dose administered subcutaneously proved too toxic; even 0.5 mg/kg daily caused intolerance reactions by this route. In mice, subcutaneous doses of 0.08 mg/kg daily for 80 days induced temporary sedation and weight losses (MARKIEWICZ, 1963). Rabbits pre-

Table 7. Reserpines: acute toxicity

Drug	Animal species	Route	LD_{50} in mg/kg	Authors
Reserpine	Mouse	p.o.	500	TRIPOD et al. (1954)
Reserpine	Mouse	i.p.	16 (LD_{100})	TRIPOD et al. (1954)
Reserpine	Mouse	i.p.	70	BARNES and ELTHERINGTON (1973)
Reserpine	Mouse	i.p.	70	CARMINATI (1969)
Reserpine	Mouse	s.c.	28.5	WINTER (1966)
Reserpine	Mouse	i.v.	21	BERTHAUX and NEUMANN (1964)
Reserpine	Rat	i.v.	18	BERTHAUX and NEUMANN (1964)
Reserpine	Rat	i.v.	15.75	BEIN (1956)
Reserpine	Rabbit	i.v.	15	BEIN (1956)
Reserpine	Dog	i.v.	0.5	BARNES and ELTHERINGTON (1973)
Deserpidine	Mouse	p.o.	320	BEIN (1956)
Deserpidine	Mouse	i.p.	55	BEIN (1956)
Deserpidine	Rat	i.v.	15.7	BEIN (1956)
Rescinnamine	Rabbit	i.v.	15	BEIN (1956)
Bietaserpine	Mouse	i.v.	215	BERTHAUX and NEUMANN (1964)
Bietaserpine	Mouse	i.p.	430	BERTHAUX and NEUMANN (1964)
Bietaserpine	Mouse	p.o.	620–1,550	BERTHAUX and NEUMANN (1964)

Table 8. Reserpines: subchronic toxicity

Drug	Animal species	Route	Treatment period	Dosage (mg/kg)	Authors
Deserpidine	Rat	p.o.	30 days	1	BEIN (1956)
Reserpine	Rat	i.p.	42 days	1	ROSECRANS (1967)
Reserpine	Rat	s.c.	8 days	0,125, 0.5, 1.0	ROSECRANS (1967)

Table 9. Reserpine: chronic toxicity

Drug	Animal species	Route	Treatment period	Dosage (mg/kg)	Authors
Reserpine	Mouse	s.c.	80 days	0.08	MARKIEWICZ (1963)
Reserpine	Rat	p.o.	6 months	4	BEIN (1956)
Reserpine	Rat	p.o.	6 months	>4	PLUMMER et al. (1954)
Reserpine	Rabbit	s.c.	80 days	0.2	HÄGGENDAHL and LINDQUIST (1963)
Reserpine	Dog	p.o.	6 months	0.035	PLUMMER et al. (1954)
Reserpine	Dog	p.o.	6 months	0.035	BEIN (1956)
Reserpine	Dog	p.o.	12 months	2×0.137/day	ADAMS (1971)
Reserpine	Monkey	p.o.	6 months	3	BEIN (1956)
Reserpine	Monkey	p.o.	6 months	$\leqq 3$	PLUMMER et al. (1954)

sented a similar condition when treated for the same period with subcutaneous doses of 0.2 mg/kg (HÄGGENDAHL and LINDQUIST, 1963). The oral LD_{50} of deserpidine after 30 days was 1.0 mg/kg daily (in the food) (BEIN, 1956).

3. Chronic Toxicity

The tolerance of reserpine in long-term treatment differs between animal species. The available data are shown in Table 9. Rats tolerated oral doses of 4.0 mg/kg daily for 6 months without major complications (BEIN, 1956). BERTHAUX and NEUMAN (1964) also describe the good tolerance of reserpine, bietaserpine and methoxydeserpidine in 6-month studies. Rats received ten times the human therapeutic dose (no figures mentioned) without changes in the blood picture. Macroscopic and microscopic examination revealed no pathological changes.

The dose levels tolerated by dogs are substantially lower. BEIN (1956) quotes the tolerable oral dose as 0.035 mg/kg reserpine daily for 6 months. In a 12-month study in which each animal received 0.137 mg p.o. twice daily, the typical symptoms included permanent drawing of the nictitating membranes over the eyeballs, miosis and muscular tremor. The haematological findings were reductions in haemoglobin, haematocrit and leucocyte count but the biochemical parameters were unaffected. Eight out of 15 dogs exhibited dilatation of the right ventricles and frequent fatty infiltrations of the right side of the heart (ADAMS, 1971). Monkeys tolerated 3.0 mg/kg/ day reserpine orally for 6 months (BEIN, 1956). The animals showed marked sedation but no other major side-effects. All the blood pictures examined were normal.

4. Fertility

Like many other centrally acting drugs, reserpine affects the pituitary-gonadal system. Reserpine can inhibit ovulation in rats; the animals remain in dioestrus. Interruption or suppression of the oestrus cycle also occurred in mice and monkeys, which substantially reduces the reproductive capacity of the animals. The dosages given in these studies were 0.5–2.0 mg/kg s.c. and 0.25 mg/kg i.m. (De Feo, 1956; Gaunt et al., 1954; Harper, 1968; Martins, 1968; Pomme et al., 1965; Tuchmann-Duplessis and Mercier-Parot, 1956). Chatterjee and Harper (1970) found delayed implantation of the blastocysts in rats treated with 0.5 mg/kg reserpine subcutaneously before and after copulation. The same effect has occurred in rabbits at doses of 0.15–0.20 mg/kg p.o. or 0.04–0.16 mg/kg i.m. (Kehl et al., 1956).

Reserpine substantially affects female sexuality and the sexual behavior of males. Lower dose levels (for instance 0.5 and 1.0 mg/kg i.p.) clearly stimulate sexual excitation; they induce faster and easier copulation and shorten the interval before ejaculation (Soulairac and Soulairac, 1961, 1962; Dewsbury and Davis, 1970; Dewsbury, 1971).

Tuchmann-Duplessis and Mercier-Parot (1962) studied the effect of long term oral treatment with reserpine on rats. Males and females were given 0.1 mg/kg daily in the food for 1 year. The animals were mated at 3, 7, and 12 months. The frequency of copulations and the number of litters decreased progressively in the course of the treatment period. The number of neonates was reduced by 30%. There were, however, no malformations. The same picture, without relevant differences, continued into the third generation when the offspring were also treated with reserpine after weaning.

5. Teratology

Goldman and Yakovac (1965) found malformations in rats but these were neither significant nor dose-related (2–5 mg/kg i.m.).

In 1974, Kalter published a comprehensive review of experimental studies in mouse (0.08–2.0 mg/kg s.c.), rat (up to 0.1 mg/kg s.c., 2.5 mg/kg i.m., 2.5 mg/kg p.o. and 1.0 mg/kg i.p.) and rabbit (up to 0.2 mg/kg i.m. or p.o., approx. 0.1 parenteral). The communicated results show no teratogenic effects for reserpine. Bietaserpine likewise produced no teratogenic effects in rat studies (Berthaux and Neuman, 1964).

Other authors found retarded physical development in rats as well as changes affecting the kidneys and isolated bones after treatment with 1 mg/kg i.p. (Moriyama and Kanoh, 1976; Kanoh and Moriyama, 1977).

6. Perinatal and Postnatal Toxicity

If reserpine is given to rats or guinea pigs during gestation at dose levels of 2.5 μ –0.2 mg/kg s.c. or 1.0 mg/kg i.p., mortality is increased and the weight and number of the foetuses are reduced (Kovacic and Robinson, 1966; Towell et al., 1965; Werboff and Dembicki, 1962; West 1960). It is assumed that reserpine can cross the placenta and so act directly on the foetal catecholamine metabolism (Kovacic and Robinson, 1966; Towell et al., 1965).

Rats treated with reserpine (0.25–1.00 mg/kg i.m.) in the early stage of gestation invariably abort, but the later treatment is initiated the lower the percentage of abortions (Mayer and Meunier, 1959; Tuchmann-Duplessis and Mercier-Parot, 1956;

WEST, 1964). Similar effects have been shown in rabbits at dose levels of 0.15–0.20 mg/kg p.o. or 0.04–0.16 mg/kg i.m. (KEHL et al., 1956). Overall, the effect of reserpine on the foetus is largely dependent on the data of administration during gestation, on the dose level and on the treatment period.

The effects on neonates are covered by divergent reports. Some authors found normal development, others saw deviations. The results of animal experiments do not always correspond to observations in man. Behavioral changes in animal experiments were recorded and discussed by HOFFELD et al. (1967, 1968) and WERBOFF (1966).

A question which has attracted increasing interest of late concerns the extent to which compounds that cause no overt pathological changes in teratological studies may or may not, due to their effects on the catecholamine metabolism and their ability to cross the placenta, give rise to permanent functional disorders in neonates, especially in the brain (e.g. [³H]thymidine insertion, mitosis in cerebellum, LEWIS et al., 1977). The reactions depend on the day of gestation on which the compound is administered, on the duration of treatment and not least on the dose. BARTOLOME et al. (1976), for instance, found delayed increases in the brain weight and retarded development of the synaptosomal uptake mechanism in rats after treatment with 1 mg/kg s.c. during gestation. LAU et al. (1977) demonstrated that by contrast with administrations of reserpine in the last third of gestation, a single dose (1 mg/kg s.c.) between days 6 and 14 was sufficient for lasting biochemical changes; they report in the brain an increase, in the adrenals a retardation or reduction of the activity of thyroxine hydroxylase and a retarded general cellular and metabolic process (ornithine decarboxylase could only be demonstrated in low concentrations).

LETHINEN et al. (1972) describe changes in the sexual behavior after a single injection of reserpine during the critical stage of cerebral development (50 µg/kg i.p. on the 4th day post partum). On the other hand, female rats given 5 and 50 µg/kg reserpine s.c. on the 4th day of life did not differ in their sexual behavior from controls 3 months later (ZUCKER and FEDER, 1966). BJÖRKLUND et al. (1969) found in similar rat studies that the development of the vaginal mucosa did not differ between treated animals (5 µg/kg s.c., age 3–5 days) and controls. Further studies using animals of both sexes showed no drug-effect on the total catecholamine content of the brain or the subcellular distribution pattern. In another rat study, SIMMONS and LUSK (1969) found that reserpine administration to neonates (single or repeated injections, 30 or 6 µg/kg s.c.) had no effect on the oestrous cycle whilst the ovaries showed definite luteinisation. GERHARDT and KURCZ (1967) also showed in rats that postnatal administration of reserpine had only a temporary effect on endocrine function, influencing vaginal opening, course of oestrous cycle and pituitary LTH and STH.

III. Man

1. Acute Toxicity

Toxic effects in man have been observed after accidental ingestion in children (LOGGIE et al., 1967; PLUMMER et al., 1954) and after an overdose in a man (LANDYSHEV et al., 1969). Whereas the children (2–4 years), who had probably ingested levels of 10–15, and 200 mg respectively, recovered with suitable treatment, the dose of 5 mg plus 100 mg of hydralazine proved fatal to the man. Despite immediate treatment, death from multiple cerebral haemorrhages occured after 3 days.

2. Teratology

The literature on the use of reserpine in man contains no instance of teratogenic activity (NISHIMURA and TANIMURA, 1976). There have been isolated reports of behavioral and other changes in neonates (lethargy, bradycardia, hypothermy, nasal congestion). The clinical use of reserpine during pregnancy has given no indication of any teratogenic activity of the rauwolfia alkaloid (BAMBAS, 1971; BLOM VAN ASSENDELFT et al., 1968).

3. Perinatal and Postnatal Toxicity

The main effects in man were on the respiratory tract (rhinitis in up to 16% of the neonates) with concomitant anorexia and lethargy (APGAR, 1964; BUDNIK et al., 1955; COHLAN, 1964; DESMOND et al., 1957).

It is not yet quite clear to what extent the detrimental effects are attributable to the basic illness with concomitant hypertension and psychological disorders, e.g. eclampsia, which necessitate reserpine treatment. Until now, the use of rauwolfia alkaloids appears to have been relatively well tolerated by mothers and neonates when given for specific conditions during pregnancy (SOBEL, 1960; RAVINA, 1964; HOCHULI and WEICHE, 1972).

IV. Carcinogenicity

MARQUARDT (1975) studied reserpine for carcinogenic activity. The test model consisted of appropriate fibroblast cultures of mice, the doses were 0.3–10 µg/ml. Reserpine failed to induce any malignant transformation.

In an experimental study, KOZUKA (1970) was in fact able to show that 1 µg/kg/week s.c. reserpine exhibited antineoplastic activity in mice fed on 2,7-diacetamidofluorene.

On the other hand, a possible association between long-term administration of reserpine and an increased risk of breast cancer has of late been the subject of exhaustive discussions. Possible causes suggested include an increase in the prolactin level, but consideration has also been given to stimulation of cell growth (BISHUN et al., 1975).

V. Discussion of Side-Effects

The most common side-effects of reserpine can be explained by its mode of action. The depletion of noradrenaline and dopamine from the storage granules of the sympathetic nervous system is likely to have central as well as peripheral effects, the dominant one frequently being the resultant relative activity increase of cholinergic functions.

The pharmacological characteristics of the rauwolfia alkaloids have been summarised in a synopsis by PLUMMER et al., 1954 (see also IVEN, 1979). We would also refer to Chap. 2.12 of this Handbook.

The best known side-effects are

Sedation	Vasomotor rhinitis
Depression	Increased salivation
Parkinsonism	Bradycardia
Impairment of libido and potency	Gastric and duodenal ulcers
Hypotension	Diarrhoea

Sedation, and particularly depression and parkinsonism are more easily discernible in man than in animals. In animal experiments, comparable effects are more likely to reflect the neuroleptic activities of a compound.

Impaired libido and potency are different matters. This interference with the balance of hormonal regulations manifests itself in different forms. In female rats, for instance, dioestrus is prolonged, ovulation is impaired and the mammary glands enlarge due to increased prolactin secretion (DEGKWITZ et al., 1970; GAUNT et al., 1954; KEHL and CZYBA, 1962; LU et al., 1970; MARTINS, 1968; POMME et al., 1965; PSYCHOSOS, 1968; TUCHMANN-DUPLESSIS, 1956; ZEILMAKER, 1965).

The mammary glands also enlarge in the males. Testicular activity is reduced, and there is atrophy of the prostate and seminal vesicle (ADAMS and FUDGE, 1959; DEGKWITZ et al., 1970; DÖRING and STEPHAN, 1959; ERÄNKÖ et al., 1957; SACKLER et al., 1960; SIMILÄ et al., 1962; SOULAIRAC and SOULAIRAC, 1962; TUCHMANN-DUPLESSIS, 1956; VERNE et al., 1957).

CERNY (1970) describes a certain effect on the mating behavior of female cats. Ejaculation is impaired in male rats (FULLER, 1963), and corresponding effects are under discussion for man (MILLS, 1975). It is not yet clear whether any pathological relevance attaches to the histological cell changes found in the diencephalon by CAZZULLO et al. (1968). The effects on other endocrine glands are believed to be slight unless high doses provoke anorexia and resultant weight losses (GAUNT et al., 1954; SACKLER et al., 1960; TUCHMANN-DUPLESSIS, 1956).

Views differ on the effect of reserpine on the cardiovascular system. Single doses, or repeated doses over a few days, induce different effects – especially at high levels – than administration over a matter of months.

As reserpine is likely to be given as a long-term treatment, we are chiefly interested in reactions to chronic administration. Hypotension and bradycardia are known to occur; they are very marked at first but subside gradually. Histopathological changes of the heart muscle have not been confirmed by all authors (MARCUS and BORZELLA, 1968; synopsis of the literature quoted by JANDHYALA et al., 1974).

There have been repeated incidents of ulcers, constipation or diarrhoea as well as other dysfunctions of the gastrointestinal tract (PFEIFER et al., 1976; SHADER and DI-MASCIO, 1970; SMEJKAL, 1968). The ulcerogenic activity of reserpine has been utilised for the provocation of ulcers in experiments but the mode of action has not yet been clarified. Hyperacidity as well as hypersecretion have been described, and there have been reports of a decrease in the circulation of the blood (BLACKMAN et al., 1959; DAMRAU, 1961; DOTEUCHI, 1968; EMAS and FYRÖ, 1967; GUPTA et al., 1974; LA BARRE and DESMAREZ, 1957; NICOLOFF et al., 1961).

References

Abdullah, S., Miller, O.J.: Effect of drugs on nucleic acid synthesis and cell division in vitro. Dis. Nerv. Syst. *29*, 829–833 (1968)

Adams, A.E., Fudge, M.W.: Effects of Reserpine on the reproductive system of immature male mice. J. Exp. Zool. *142*, 337–351 (1959)

Adams, H.R.: Clinicopathologic effects of chronic reserpine administration in mongrel dogs. J. Pharm. Sci. *60*, 1134–1138 (1971)

Adams, H.R., Manian, A.A., Steenberg, M.L., Buckley, J.P.: Effects of promazine and chlorpromazine metabolites on the cornea. In: The phenothiazines and structurally related drugs. Forrest, S., Carr, C.J., Usdin, E. (eds.), pp. 281–283. New York: Raven 1974

Ahlenius, S., Brown, R., Engel, J., Lundborg, P.: Learning deficits in 4 week old offsprings of the nursing mothers treated with the neuroleptic drug penfluriol. Arch. Exp. Pathol. Pharmakol. *279*, 31–37 (1973)

Alani, M.D.: Effects of long wave ultraviolet radiation on photosensitizing and related compounds. I. Br. J. Dermatol. *89*, 361–365 (1973)

Alani, M.D., Dunne, J.H.: Effects of long wave ultraviolet radiation on photosensitizing and related compounds. II. Br. J. Dermatol. *89*, 367–372 (1973)

Alexander, G.J., Machiz, S., Alexander, R.B.: Phenothiazine tranquillizers: Effect of prolonged intake. Adv. Exp. Med. Biol. *27*, 151–160 (1972)

Algeri, E.J., Katsas, G.G., McBay, A.J.: Toxicology of some new drugs: Glutethimide, meprobamate and chlorpromazine. J. Forensic Sci. *4*, 111–135 (1959)

Almazova, I.G.: Changes in the nervous system in acute poisoning by chlorpromazine in children. Zh. Nevropathol. Psikhiatr. *70*, 1499–1501 (1970)

Ananth, J.: Congenital malformations with psychopharmacologic agents. Compr. Psychiatry *16*, 437–445 (1975)

Ananth, J., Valles, J.V., Whitelaw, J.P.: Usual and unusual agranulocytosis during neuroleptic therapy. Am. J. Psychiatry *130*, 100–102 (1973)

Apgar, V.: Drugs in pregnancy. JAMA *190*, 340–341 (1964)

Appleton, W.S., Shader, R.I., DiMascio, A.: Dermatological effects. In: Psychotropic drug side effects. Shader, R.I., DiMascio, A., (eds.), pp. 77–85. Baltimore: Williams & Wilkins 1970

Arieff, A.I., Friedman, E.A.: Coma following nonnarcotic overdosage: Management of 208 adult patients. Am. J. Med. Sci. *266*, 405–426 (1973)

Artelli, A., Castello, A.: Effetti della thioridazina sulla sfera genitale femminile nel ratto. Boll. Soc. Ital. Biol. Sper. *44*, 269–270 (1968)

Ashford, A., Ross, J.W.: Toxicity of depressant and antidepressant drugs in hyperthyroid mice. Br. Med. J. *1968 II*, 217–218

Ayd, F.J., Jr.: Prolonged administration of chlorpromazine (thorazine) hydrochloride. JAMA *169*, 1296–1301 (1959)

Ayd, F.J., Jr.: Chlorpromazine: Ten years' experience. JAMA *184*, 51–54 (1963)

Ayd, F.J., Jr.: Children born of mothers treated with chlorpromazine during pregnancy. Clin. Med. *71*, 1758–1763 (1964a)

Ayd, F.J., Jr.: Perphenazine: A reappraisal after eight years. Dis. Nerv. Syst. *25*, 311–316 (1964b)

Ayd, F.J., Jr.: Side effects of depot fluphenazines. Adv. Biochem. Psychopharmacol. *9*, 301–309 (1974)

Bambas, W.: Zur ambulanten Behandlung der Spätgestose mit Briserin. Ther. Gg. *110*, 525–536 (1971)

Barnes, C.D., Eltherington, L.G.: Drug dosage in laboratory animals. Berkeley, Los Angeles, London: University of California 1973

Barry, D., Meyskens, F.L., Becker, Ch.E.: Phenothiazine poisoning. Calif. Med. *118*, 1–5 (1973)

Bartolomé, J., Seidler, F.J., Anderson, Th.R., Slotkin, Th.A.: Effects of prenatal reserpine administration on development of the rat adrenal medulla and central nervous system. J. Pharmacol. Exp. Ther. *197*, 293–302 (1976)

Baruk, H., Launay, J., Linares, J.O., Segal, O.: Experimentation psycho – pharmacologique animale et essais clinique therapeutique de la thioridazine. Ann. Med. Psychol. (Paris) *1*, 129 (1966)

254   F. Leuschner et al.

Bayer, R.: Sedierung und Geburtenbeschleunigung mit Triflupromazin. Med. Klin. *61*, 725–728 (1966)

Beall, J.R.: A teratogenic study of chlorpromazin, orphenadrine, perphenazine, and LSD-25 in rats. Toxicol. Appl. Pharmacol. *21*, 230–236 (1972)

Beall, J.R.: A teratogenic study of four psychoactive drugs in rats. Teratology *8*, 214–215 (1973)

Becker, B.A., Hindman, K.L., Gibson, J.E.: Enhanced mortality of selected central nervous system depressants in hypoexcretory mice. J. Pharm. Sci. *57*, 1010–1012 (1968)

Bein, H.J.: The pharmacology of rauwolfia. Pharmacol. Rev. *8*, 435–483 (1956)

Beliles, R.P.: The influence of pregnancy on the acute toxicity of various compounds in mice. Toxicol. Appl. Pharmacol. *23*, 537–550 (1972)

Bercovitz, Z., Page, R.C., De Beer, E.J.: Phenothiazine: Experimental and clinical study of toxicity and anthelmintic value. JAMA *122*, 1006–1007 (1943)

Bernstein, H.N.: Ocular drug toxicities. Toxicol. Appl. Pharmacol. *8*, 334–335 (1966)

Bertelli, A., Polani, P.E., Spector, R., Seller, M.J., Tuchmann-Duplessis, H., Mercier-Parot, L.: Retentissement d'un neuroleptique, l'halopéridol, sur la gestation et le développement prénatal des rongeurs. Arzneim. Forsch. *18*, 1420–1424 (1968)

Berthaux, P., Neuman, M.: Etude pharmacologique et clinique d'un nouvel hypotenseur réserpinique: le N-diéthylanimoéthyl réserpine (DL 152 ou biétaserpine). Arzneim. Forsch. *14*, 1040–1045 (1964)

Berti, T., Cima, L.: Einfluß der Temperatur auf die pharmakologische Wirkung des Chlorpromazins. Arzneim. Forsch. *5*, 73–74 (1955)

Bethesda: Symposium on side-effects and drug toxicity, including behavioral toxicity. Psychopharmacol. Bull. *4*, 56–61 (1967)

Bindon, B.M.: The role of the pituitary gland in implantation in the mouse: Delay of implantation by hypophysectomy and neurodepressive drugs. J. Endocrinol. *43*, 225–235 (1969)

Bishun, N., Smith, N., Williams, D.: Chromosomes, mitosis and reserpine. Lancet *1975 I*, 926

Björklund, A., Falck, B., Nobin, A.: Failure of neonatally administered reserpine to affect the hypothalamic catecholamines in the adult rat. Endocrinology *85*, 788–790 (1969)

Blacker, K.H., Weinstein, B.J., Ellmann, G.L.: Mother's milk and chlorpromazine. Am. J. Psychiatry *119*, 178–179 (1962)

Blackman, J.G., Campion, D.S., Fastier, F.N.: Mechanism of action of reserpine in producing gastric haemorrhage and erosion in the mouse. Br. J. Pharmacol. *14*, 112–116 (1959)

Blom van Assendelft, P.M., Dorhout Mees, E.J., Hart, P.G., Reduction of neonatal mortality by treatment of pregnant women suffering from essential hypertension. Ned. Tijdschr. Geneeskd. *112*, 1115–1118 (1968)

Bobon, D.P.: The Neuroleptics. Basel, München, Paris, New York: Karger 1970

Boet, D.J.: Toxic effects of phenothiazines on the eye. Med. Dissertation, Gravenhage 1970

Boissier, J.-P., Pagny, J.: Etude pharmacodynamique d'un nouveau neroleptique majeur: Le halopéridol (R 1625). Thérapie *15*, 479–487 (1960)

Bolton, B.H.: Prolonged chlorpromazine jaundice. Am. J. Gastroenterol. *48*, 497–503 (1968)

Boris, A., Milmore, J., Trimal, T.: Some effects of haloperidol on reproductive organs in the female rat. Endocrinology *86*, 429–431 (1970)

Boulos, B.M., Davis, L.E., Larks, S.D., Larks, G.G., Sirtori, C.R., Almond, C.H.: Placental transfer of drugs: IV. Placental transfer of chlorpromazine, pentobarbital and phenylbutazone with fetal ECG changes as determined by direct lead tracing. Arch. Int. Pharmacodyn. Ther. *194*, 403–414 (1971)

Boyd, E.M.: Chlorpromazine tolerance and physical dependence. J. Pharmacol. Exp. Ther. *128*, 75–78 (1960)

Bree, M.M., Cohen, B.J., Abrams, G.D.: Injektion lesions following intramuscular administration of chlorpromazine in rabbits. J. Am. Vet. Med. Assoc. *158*, 1910 (1971)

Brock, N., Kreybig, T. von: Experimenteller Beitrag zur Prüfung teratogener Wirkungen von Arzneimitteln an der Laboratoriumsratte. Arch. Exp. Pathol. Pharmakol. *249*, 117–145 (1964)

Brookes, L.G., Forrest, I.S.: Chlorpromazine metabolism in sheep. I. In vivo metabolism. Agressologie *12*, 245–250 (1971)

Brugmans, J., Verbruggen, F., Dom, J., Schuermans, V.: Prolactin, phenothiazines, admission of mental hospital, and carcinoma of the breast. Lancet *1973 II*, 502–503

Buckley, J.P., Steenberg, M.L., Barry III, H., Manian, A.A.: Pharmacological and behavioral effects of mono – and disubstituted chlorpromazine derivatives. In: The phenothiazines and structurally related drugs. Forrest, I.S., Carr, C.J., Usdin, E., (eds.), pp. 617–631. New York: Raven 1974

Buckman, M.T., Peake, G.T.: Prolactin in clinical practice. JAMA 236, 871–874 (1976)

Budnick, I.S., Leikin, S., Hoeck, L.E.: Effect in the newborn infant of reserpine administered ante partum. Am. J. Dis. Child. 90, 286–289 (1955)

Buttle, H.L., Robertson, H.A.: The pharmacological blockade of the initiation but not of the maintenance of sexual receptivity of the ewe. J. Endocrinol. 39, 115–116 (1967)

Callear, J.F.F., van Gestel, J.F.E.: An analysis of the results of field experiments in pigs in the U.K. and Ireland with the sedative neuroleptic azaperone. Vet. Rec. 89, 453–458 (1971)

Carminati, G.M.: Attivita comparata di svariati farmaci in alcuni tests sperimentali di studio del compartomento. Arch. Intern. Pharmacodyn. Ther. 181, 68–93 (1969)

Cascio, G., Manghisi, E., Erba, R., Magistretti, M.J.: 4-Aminobutirofenoni ad attivita ipotensiva. Farmaco. [Sci.] 31, 442–456 (1976)

Cazzullo, C.L., Giordano, P.L., Andreola, M.L.: Etudes cytopathologiques des effets des drogues psychotropes sur la cellule nerveuse. Agressologie 9, 575–589 (1968)

Cerletti, A., Meier-Ruge, W.: Toxicological studies on phenothiazine induced retinopathy. Proc. Eur. Soc. Study Drug Toxi. 9, 170–188 (1968)

Cerny, V.A.: Influence of the hypothalamus on the mating behavior of the female cat. Diss. Abstr. Int. B 31, 3670–3671 (1970)

Chand, N., Gupta, T.K., Bhargava, K.P.: A study of anti-ovulatory activity of haloperidol in rabbits. Jpn. J. Pharmacol. 23, 827–829 (1973)

Chatterjee, A., Harper, M.J.K.: Interruption of implantation and gestation in rats by reserpine, chlorpromazine and ACTH: Possible mode of action. Endocrinology 87, 966–969 (1970)

Chioreanu, L., Wiener, F.: Die mutagene Wirkung von Haloperidol und Thioproperazil auf Mäusechromosomen. Med. Exp. 17, 417–426 (1968)

Christensen, E., Möller, J.E., Faurbys, A.: Neuropathological investigation of 28 brains from patients with dyskinesis. Acta Psychiatr. Scand. 46, 14–23 (1970)

Christensen, J.A., Hernestam, S., Lassen, J.B., Sterner, N.: Pharmacological and toxicological studies on -(4-methyl piperidino)-p-fluorobutyrophenone (FG 5111) – a new neuroleptic agent. Acta Pharmacol. Toxicol. (Copenh.) 23, 109–132 (1965)

Cohlan, S.Q.: Fetal and neonatal hazards from drugs administered during pregnancy. N.Y. State J. Med. 64, 493–499 (1964)

Collier, H.B., Mack, G.E., Jr.: Vitamin B and phenothiazine anaemia in dogs. Can. J. Res. 22, 1–11 (1944)

Cordelli, A.: Indagini sull'azione della clorpromazina sui processi di glicuroniugazione della bilirubina in fegato di ratto isolato e perfuso. Boll. Soc. Ital. Biol. Sper. 44, 1217–1219 (1968)

Courvoisier, S., Fournel, J., Ducrot, R., Kolsky, M., Koetschet, P.: Propriétés pharmacodynamiques du chlorhydrate de chloro-3 (diméthylamino-3'propyl)-10 phénothiazine (4.560 R.P.). Arch. Int. Pharmacodyn. Ther. 92, 305–361 (1953)

Coutselinis, A., Boukis, D., Kentarchou, P.: Haloperidol concentrations in blood in cases of acute intoxication. Clin. Chem. 23, 900 (1977)

Cuisset, P., Roujas, F.: Rappel de pharmacologique pratique des phénothiazines et des butyrophénones. Ann. Anesthésiol. 17, 1025–1032 (1976)

Damrau, F.: Peptic ulcers induced in white rats by reserpine and stress. Am. J. Gastroenterol. 35, 612–618 (1961)

Danner, S.: Cardiovasculaire complicaties bij gebruik van fenothiazine en imipramine-derivaten. Ned. Tijdschr. Geneeskd. 115, 1707–1708 (1971)

Davis, J.M., Bartlett, E., Termini, B.A.: Overdosage of psychotropic drugs: A review. Part I: Major and minor tranquilizers. Dis. Nerv. Syst. 29, 157–164 (1968)

DeC.Baker, S.B., Tucker, M.J.: Changes in the reproductive organs of rats and dogs treated with butyrophenones and related compounds. Proc. Eur. Soc. Study Drug Toxi. 9, 113–118 (1968)

De Feo, V.J.: Modification of the menstrual cycle in rhesus monkeys by reserpine. Science 124, 726–727 (1956)

Degkwitz, R., Heushgem, C., Hollister, L.E., Jacob, J., Julou, L., Lambert, P.A., Marsboom, R., Meier-Ruge, W., Schaper, W.K.A., Tuchmann-Duplessis, H.C.: Toxicity and side effects in man and in the laboratory animal. In: The neuroleptics. Bobon, D.P., Janssen, P.A.J., Bobon, J. (eds.), pp. 71–84. Basel, München, Paris, New York: Karger 1970

Deglin, S.M., Deglin, J.M., Chung, E.K.: Drug-induced cardiovascular diseases. Drugs *14*, 29–40 (1977)

Delay, J., Deniker, P.: C.R. du congrès des aliénists et neurologistes de langue Française, Luxembourg, p. 514. Paris: Masson 1952

Delay, J., Deniker, P.: Les nouveaux médicaments psychotropes. Paris: Masson 1961

Deneau, G., Yanagita, T., Seevers, M.H.: Self-administration of psychoactive substances by the monkey. Psychopharmacolia *16*, 30–48 (1969)

Desmond, M.M., Yanagita, T., Seevers, M.H.: Management of toxemia of pregnancy with reserpine. Obstet. Gynecol. *10*, 140–145 (1957)

Dewsbury, D.A.: Copulatory behavior of male rats following reserpine administration. Psychonomic Sci. *22*, 177–179 (1971)

Dewsbury, D.A., Davis, H.N. (1970) Effects of reserpine on the copulatory behavior of male rats. Physiol. Behav. *5*, 1331–1333 (1970)

Djahanguiri, B., Sadeghi, D., Hemmati, S.: The production of acute gastric ulcer by promethazine hydrochloride in the guinea pig. Toxicol. Appl. Pharmacol. *12*, 568–569 (1968)

Döring, G.K., Stephan, G.: Über die Beeinflussung der Genitalfunktion weißer Ratten durch das Rauwolfiaalkaloid Reserpin. Arch. Gynaekol. *191*, 570–575 (1959)

Domino, E.F.: Human pharmacology of tranquilizing drugs. Clin. Pharmacol. Ther. *3*, 599–664 (1962)

Donnewald, H.N.: L'intoxication aiguë par les phénothiazines chez l'adulte, àpropos de 112 cas. Eur. J. Toxicol. Environ. Hyg. *3*, 167–178 (1970)

Doteuchi, M.: Studies on the experimental gastrointestinal ulcers produced by reserpine and stress. II. Ulcerogenic activities of reserpine and its analogues. Jpn. J. Pharmacol. *18*, 130–138 (1968)

Dreyfus, B., Bernard, J., Josso, F., Samama, M., Pequignot, H.: Les hémolyses médicamenteuses. Presse Med. *76*, 1009–1012 (1968)

Druga, A.: Studies on the teratogenic effect of perphenazin in rats. Gyogyszereszet *18*, 462 (1974)

Dujovne, C.A., Zimmerman, H.J.: Cytotoxicity of phenothiazines on changed liver cells as measured by enzyme leakage. Proc. Soc. Exp. Biol. Med. *131*, 583–587 (1969)

Dujovne, C.A., Levy, R., Zimmerman, H.J.: Hepatotoxicity of phenothiazines in vitro as measured by loss of aminotransferases to surrounding media. Proc. Soc. Exp. Biol. Med. *128*, 561–563 (1968)

Ebert, M.H., Shader, R.I.: Hematological effects. In: Psychotropic drug side effects. Shader, R.I., DiMascio, A. (eds.), pp. 164–174. Baltimore: Williams & Wilkins 1970

Einer-Jensen, N., Secher, N.J.: Diminished weight of rat foetuses after treatment of pregnant rats with haloperidol. J. Reprod. Fertil. *22*, 591–594 (1970)

Elert, R.: Die medikamentöse perinatale Schädigung. Therapiewoche *19*, 218–221 (1969)

Elis, J.: The relationship between the stage of prenatal development and toxic effects of drugs. Proc. Eur. Soc. Toxicol. *16*, 133–137 (1975)

Emas, S., Fyrö, B.: Gastric and duodenal ulcers in cats following reserpine. Acta Physiol. Scand. *71*, 316–322 (1967)

Engel, J., Ahlenius, S., Brown, R., Lundborg, P.: Behavioral effects in offspring of nursing mothers given neuroleptic drugs. Proc. Eur. Soc. Study Drug Toxi. *15*, 20–24 (1974)

Epstein, S.S., Shafner, H.: Chemical mutagens in the human environment. Nature *219*, 385–387 (1968)

Eränkö, O.V., Hopsu, E., Kivalo, E., Telkkä, A.: Effect of prolonged administration of reserpine on the endocrine glands of the rat. Nature *180*, 1130 (1957)

Ershova, V.P.: The effect of chronic injections of chlorpromazine on the oogenesis and development of the progeny in animals (Albino mice). Farmakol. Toksikol. *38*, 473–476 (1975)

Fairweather, D.V.I.: Nausea and vomiting in pregnancy. Am. J. Obstet. Gynecol. *102*, 135–175 (1968)

Forrest, I.S., Kosek, J.C., Aber, R.C., Serra, M.T.: Rabbit as a model for chlorpromazine-induced hyperpigmentation of the skin. Biochem. Pharmacol. *19*, 849–852 (1970)

Fossati, C.: Effetti collaterali e tossici degli psicofarmaci. Clin. Ter. *76*, 265–281 (1976)

Frankova, S.: Drug-induced changes in the maternal behavior of rats. Psychopharmacology (Berlin) *53*, 83–87 (1977)

Frejaville, J.P., Guyochin, A., Gaultier, M.: Intoxications aiguës par les amines phénothiaziniques àpropos de 152 cas. Eur. J. Toxicol. Environ. Hyg. *3*, 179–187 (1970)

Friebel, H. Flick, H., Reichle, C.: Beziehungen zwischen der chemischen Konstitution und der pharmakologischen Wirkung einiger Phenothiazinderivate. Arzneim. Forsch. *4*, 171–174 (1954)

Fuller, R.: Sexual changes in the male rat following chronic administration of reserpine. Nature *200*, 585–586 (1963)

Gajdos, P., Berger, F.D., Rapin, M., Goulon, M.: Etude hemodynamique de 14 comas toxique (Barbiturique-phénothiazines-tranquillisants). Eur. J. Toxicol. Environ. Hyg. *3*, 24–35 (1970)

Gaultier, M., Deroviche-Fahti: Les intoxications par les butyrophénones. Eur. J. Toxicol. Environ. Hyg. *4*, 385–402 (1971)

Gaunt, R., Renzi, A.A., Antonchak, N., Miller, G.J., Gilman, M.: Endocrine aspects of the pharmacology of reserpine. Ann. N.Y. Acad. Sci. *59*, 22–35 (1954)

Gauron, E.F., Rowley, V.N.: Effects on offspring behavior of mother's early chronic drug experience. Psychopharmacologia *16*, 5–15 (1969)

Gauron, E.F., Rowley, V.N.: Cross-generational effects resulting from an early maternal chronic drug experience. Eur. J. Pharmacol. *15*, 171–175 (1971)

Gauron, E.F., Rowley, V.N.: Effects on offspring behavior of early drug experience and cross-fostering in parent rats. J. Pediatr. *83*, 155 (1973)

Gebhart, E.: Zur Frage der erbgutschädigenden Nebenwirkungen von psychotropen Substanzen. Fortschr. Med. *97*, 45–48, 105–106 (1979)

Gerhardt, J., Kurcz, M.: Effect of neonatal treatment with reserpine on FSH, LH and LTH production of the pituitary in rat. Acta Physiol. Acad. Sci. Hung. [Suppl. 2], *33*, 82–83 (1967)

Gerhard, J.-P., Franck, H., Sommer, S., Mack, G.: L'incidence ophthalmologique du traitement aux phénothiazines. Oto Noro Oftalmol. *47*, 71–77 (1975)

Ghate, V.R.: Antipsychotic agents. N. C. Med. J. *34*, 859–865 (1973)

Giertz, H., Hahn, F., Lange, A.: Zur Toxikologie des Phenothiazins. Klin. Wochenschr. *32*, 983–984 (1954)

Givant, Y., Shani, J., Goldhaber, G., Serebrenik, R., Sulman, F.G.: Pharmacology of three mammotropic butyrophenones in the rat. Arch. Int. Pharmacodyn. Ther. *205*, 317–327 (1973)

Goldman, A.S., Yakovac, W.C.: Teratogenic action in rats of reserpine alone and in combination with salicylate and immobilization. Proc. Soc. Exp. Biol. Med. *118*, 857–862 (1965)

Golub, M., Kornetsky, C.: Modification of the behavioral response to drugs in rats exposed prenatally to chlorpromazine. Psychopharmacologia *43*, 289–291 (1975)

Gordon, S., Balazs, T.: Cataractogenicity of various drugs in rats. Toxicol. Appl. Pharmacol. *10*, 393 (1967)

Gouret, C., Bouvet, P., Raynaud, G.: Activité psychotrope de la fénapérone et comparaison avec quelques neuroleptiques chez la souris et le rat. C.R. Soc. Biol. (Paris) *167*, 1366–1370 (1973)

Greiner, A.C., Nicolson, G.A.: Pigment deposition in viscera associated with prolonged chlorpromazine therapy. Can. Med. Assoc. J. *91*, 627–635 (1964)

Gunne, L.-M., Barany, S.: Haloperidol-induced tardive dyskinesia in monkeys. Psychopharmacology (Berlin) *50*, 237–240 (1976)

Gupta, M.B., Tangri, K.T., Bhargava, K.P.: Mechanism of ulcerogenic activity of reserpine in albino rats. Eur. J. Pharmacol. *27*, 269–271 (1974)

Guyonnet, J.C., Julou, L., Ducrot, R., Detaille, J.Y., Laffargue, B., Leau, O.: Etude des propriétés pharmacologiques générales de la méthylsulfonyl-2 (carbamoyl-4 piperidino)-3 propyl-10 phénothiazine ou métopimazine (9965 R.P.). C. R. Acad. Sci [D] (Paris) *266*, 2365–2368 (1968)

Häggendahl, J., Lindqvist, M.: Behavior and monoamine levels during longterm administration of reserpine to rabbits. Acta Physiol. Scand. *57*, 431–436 (1963)

Hänel, L.: Beitrag zur Toxikologie der gebräuchlichsten Anthelmintica. Pharmazie *5*, 18–23 (1950)

Halpern, B.-N., Ducrot, R.: Recherches expérimentales sur une nouvelle série chimique de corps loués de propriétés antihistaminiques puissantes: Les dérivés de la thiodiphénylamine. C.R. Soc. Biol. (Paris) *140*, 361–363 (1946)

Halpern, B.-N., Perrin, G., Dews, P.-B.: Pouvoir anesthésique local de quelques antihistaminiques de synthèse. Relation entre l'action anesthésique et l'action antihistaminique. J. Physiol. (Paris) *40*, 210–214 (1948)

Hanson, J.W., Oakley, G.P.: Haloperidol and limb deformity. J.A.M.A. *231*, 26 (1975)

Harper, M.J.K.: Pharmacological control of reproduction in women. Prog. Drug Res. *12*, 47–136 (1968)

Harrington, F.E., Eggert, R.G., Wilbur, R.D., Linkenheimer, W.H.: Effect of coitus on chlorpromazine inhibition of ovulation in the rat. Endocrinology *79*, 1130–1134 (1966)

Hays, G.B.: Tranquilizers may cause skin discoloration in some patients. J.A.M.A. *191*, 33 (1965)

Henkes, H.E., Canta, L.R.: Drug-induced disorders of the eye. Proc. Eur. Soc. Study Drug Toxi. *14*, 146–153 (1973)

Heywood, R., Palmer, A.K.: Prolonged toxicological studies in the rat and beagle dog with methylperone hydrochloride, with embryo toxicity studies in the rabbit and rat. Farmaco [Prat.] *29*, 586–593 (1974)

Hochuli, E., Weiche, V.: Zur Dauermedikation mit hypotensiven Substanzen in graviditate. Geburtshilfe Frauenheilkd. *1*, 32–39 (1972)

Hoffeld, D.R., Webster, R.L.: Effect of injection of tranquillizing drugs during pregnancy on offspring. Nature *205*, 1070–1072 (1965)

Hoffeld, D.R., Webster, R.L., McNew, J.: Adverse effects on offspring of tranquillizing drugs during pregnancy. Nature *215*, 182–183 (1967)

Hoffeld, D.R., McNew, J., Webster, R.L.: Effects of tranquillizing drugs during pregnancy on activity of offspring. Nature *218*, 357–358 (1968)

Hollister, L.E.: Adverse reactions to phenothiazines. J.A.M.A. *189*, 311–313 (1964)

Hollister, L.E.: Overdoses of psychotherapeutic drugs. Clin. Pharmacol. Ther. *7*, 142–146 (1966)

Honma, T., Sasajima, K., Ono, K., Kitagawa, S., Inaba, Sh., Yamamoto, H.: Synthesis and preliminary pharmacology of a novel butyrophenone derivate I D-4708. Arzneim. Forsch. *24*, 1248–1255 (1974)

Horvath, C., Druga, A., Mold, C.: The effect of phenothiazine derivatives on rat embryos. Teratology *4*, 489 (1971)

Ison, A., Blank, H.: Testing drug phototoxity in mice. J. Invest. Dermatol. *49*, 508–511 (1967)

Itoh, T., Koseki, Y., Ando, T., Saka, M., Nakaya, Sh.: Acute and subacute toxicities of levomethiomeprazine. Jpn. J. Pharmacol. *24*, 39 (1974)

Itoh, T., Ando, F., Seki, M., Nakaya, Sh.: Effect of chlorpromazine on the reproduction in rats. Jpn. J. Pharmacol. [Suppl.] *26*, 90P (1976)

Iven, H.: Nebenwirkungen von Arzneimitteln. 2. Antihypertensiva. Prakt. Arzt. *16*, 109–115 (1979)

Jandhyala, B.S., Clarke, D.E., Buckley, J.P.: Effects of prolonged administration of certain antihypertensive agents. J. Pharm. Sc. *63*, 1497–1513 (1974)

Janssen, P.A.J.: Toxicology and metabolism of butyrophenones. Proc. Eur. Soc. Study Drug Toxi. *9*, 107–112 (1968)

Janssen, P.A.J., Niemegeers, C.J.E., Schellekens, K.H.L., Dresse, A., Lenaerts, F.M., Pinchard, A., Schaper, W.K.A., Van Nueten, J.M., Verbruggen, F.J.: Pimozide, a chemically novel, highly potent and orally long-acting neuroleptic drug. Arzneim. Forsch. *18*, 261–279 (1968)

Jelinek, V., Zikmund, E., Reichlova, R.: L'influence de quelques médicaments psychotropes sur le développement du foetus chez le rat. Thérapie *22*, 1429 (1967)

Johnson, B.E.: Cellular mechanism of chlorpromazine photosensitivity. Proc. R. Soc. Med. *67*, 871–873 (1974)

Johnson, F.P., Boyd, D.A., Sayre, G.P., Tyce, F.A.J.: Sudden death of catatonic patient receiving phenothiazine. Am. J. Psychiatry *121*, 504–507 (1964)

Julou, L., Ducrot, R., Ganter, P., Maral, R., Populaire, P., Durel, J., Huttric, E., Myon, J., Pascal, S., Pasquet, J.: Toxicité à terme, effets secondaires et métabolisme des neuroleptiques phénothiaziniques. Proc. Eur. Soc. Study Drug Toxi. *9*, 11–51 (1968)

Julou, L., Bourat, G., Ducrot, R., Fournel, J., Garret, C.: Pharmacological study of pipotiazine (19.366 R.P.) and its undecylenic (19.551 R.P.) and palmitic (19.552 R.P.) esters. Acta Psychiatr. Scand. [Suppl.] *241*, 9–30 (1973)

Kalter, H.: Teratogenicity, embryolethality and mutagenicity of drugs of dependence. In: Chemical and biological aspects of drug dependence. Mulé, S.J., Brill, H. (eds.), pp. 413–448. Cleveland, Ohio: CRC Presss 1974

Kamyanov, I.M.: The clinical picture of chlorpromazine poisoning. Zh. Nevropatol. Psikhiatr. *65*, 918–919 (1965)

Kanoh, S., Moriyama, I.S.: Effects of reserpine on the pregnant rat: 2nd report. Teratology *16*, 110 (1977)

Kapur, B.M., Sellers, E.M., Marshman, J.A., MacLeod, S., Kaplan, H., Giles, H.: Predictability of emergency drug analysis. Clin. Chem. *23*, 1160 (1977)

Karkischenko, N.N.: Some morpho-physiological changes of the brain in the presence of chlorpromazine during chronic experiments. Farmakol. Toksikol. *31*, 156–159 (1968)

Kehl, R., Czyba, J.C.: Sur l'action galactogène de la réserpine chez la lapine. J. Physiol. (Paris) *54*, 356–357 (1962)

Kehl, R., Audibert, A., Gage, C., Amarger, J.: Action de la réserpine à différentes périodes de la gestation chez la lapine. C. R. Soc. Biol. (Paris) *150*, 2196–2199 (1956)

Kleinsorge, H., Rösner, K.: Toxikologie und Nebenwirkungen der Phenothiazinderivate. In: Die Phenothiazinderivate in der Medizin. Kleinsorge, H., Rösner, K. (eds.), pp. 173–190. Jena: Fischer 1958

Kluge, H., Hartmann, W., Wieczorek, V.: Begleitwirkungen von Neuroleptika aus biochemischer Sicht. Z. Ärztl. Fortbild. (Jena) *68*, 1207–1209 (1974)

Knowles, J.A.: Excretion of drugs in milk. A review. J. Pediatr. *66*, 1068–1082 (1965)

Kopelman, A.E., McCullar, F.W., Heggeness, L.: Limb malformations following maternal use of haloperidol. J.A.M.A. *231*, 62–64 (1975)

Kovacic, B., Robinson, R.L.: The effect of reserpine on catecholamine levels in the gravid rat and its offspring. J. Pharmacol. Exp. Ther. *152*, 37–41 (1966)

Kozuka, S.: Inhibiting effect of reserpine and female sensitivity in hepatic tumor induction with 2.7-diacetamidofluorene in SMA/Ms strain. Cancer Res. *30*, 1384–1386 (1970)

Kris, E.B.: Children of mothers maintained on pharmacotherapy during pregnancy and postpartum. Curr. Ther. Res. *7*, 785–789 (1965)

Kurtz, D., Feuerstein, J., Weber, M., Girardel-Reeb, M., Rohmer, F.: Intérêt de la surveillance électroencéphalographique dans le cadre de la réanimation des comas par intoxication médicamenteuse aiguë. Rev. Electroencephalogr. Neurophysiol. Clin. *1*, 171–189 (1971)

La Barre, J., Desmarez, J.-J.: A propos des phénomènes hypersécrétoires et des manifestations ulcéreuses gastriques apparaissant chez le rat traité par la réserpine. C. R. Soc. Biol. (Paris) *151*, 1451–1452 (1957)

Laborit, H., Huguenard, P.: L'hibernation artificielle par moyens pharmacodynamiques et physiques en chirurgie. Presse Med. *59*, 1329 (1951)

Laborit, H., Huguenard, P., Alluaume, R.: Un nouveau stabilisateur végétatif (Le 4560 RP). Presse Med. *60*, 206–208 (1952)

Lacassagne, A., Hurst, L., Rosenberg, A.J.: Influence de la chlorpromazine et de la réserpine sur la cancérisation expérimentale du foie chez le rat. C.R. Acad. Sci. [D] (Paris) *249*, 903–905 (1959)

Land, R.B.: Ovulation rate of finn-dorset sheep following unilateral ovariectomy or chlorpromazine treatment at different stages of the oestrous cycle. J. Reprod. Fertil. *33*, 99–105 (1973)

Landyshev, Y.S., Pronena, E.I., Markelov, I.P.: A fatal case of acute reserpine poisoning. Klin. Med. *47*, 141–142 (1969)

Lapolla, A., Nash, L.R.: Two suicide attempts with chlorpromazine. Am. J. Psychiatry *121*, 920–922 (1965)

Lau, C., Bartolomé, J., Seidler, F.J., Slotkin, T.A.: Critical periods for effects of prenatal reserpine administration on development of rat brain and adrenal medulla. Neuropharmacology 16, 799–809 (1977)

Lechat, P., Fontagné, J., Flouvat, B.: Toxicité aiguë de quelques neuroleptiques chez des animaux préalablement traités par un I.M.A.O. Proc. Eur. Soc. Study Drug Toxi. 9, 156–158 (1968)

Lehman, H.E., Ban, T.A.: Sex differences in long-term adverse effects of phenothiazine. Adv. Biochem. Psychopharmacol. 2, 249–254 (1974)

Lehtinen, P., Hyyppä, M., Lampinen, P.: Sexual behavior of adult rats after a single neonatal injection of reserpine. Psychopharmacologia 23, 171–179 (1972)

Lewis, P.D., Pathel, A.J., Bendek, G., Balázs, R.: Do drugs acting on the nervous system affect cell proliferation in the developing brain. Lancet 1977 I, 399–401 (1977)

Lindqvist, N.G., Sjostrand, S.E., Ullberg, S.: Accumulation of chorio-retinotoxic drugs in the foetal eye. Acta Pharmacol. Toxicol. (Copenh.) [Suppl. 1] 28, 64 (1970)

Lipton, M.H., DiMascio, A., Killam, K.F.: Psychopharmacology. New York: Raven 1978

Ljunggren, B.: Phenothiazine phototoxicity: Toxic chlorpromazine photoproducts. J. Invest. Dermatol. 68, 313–317 (1977)

Ljunggren, B., Möller, H.: Phenothiazine phototoxicity: An experimental study on chlorpromazine and related tricyclic drugs. Acta Derm. Venereol. (Stockh.) 57, 325–329 (1977a)

Ljunggren, B., Möller, H.: Phenothiazine toxicity: An experimental study on chlorpromazine and its metabolites. J. Invest. Dermatol. 68, 313–317 (1977b)

Loggie, J.M.H., Saito, H., Kahn, I., Fenner, A., Gaffney, Th.E.: Accidental reserpine poisoning: Clinical and metabolic effects. Clin. Pharmacol. Ther. 8, 692–695 (1967)

Lu, K.-H., Amenomori, Y., Chen, C., Meites, J.: Effects of central acting drugs on serum and pituitary prolactin levels in rats. Endocrinology 87, 667–672 (1970)

Lundborg, P.: Abnormal ontogeny in young rabbits after chronic administration of haloperidol to the nursing mothers. Brain Res. 44, 684–687 (1972)

Maickel, R.P., McGlynn, M., Snodgrass, W.R.: Some toxicological aspects of the chronic administration of phenothiazine tranquilizers. Toxicol. Appl. Pharmacol. 17, 312 (1970)

Maickel, R.P., Braunstein, M.C., McGlynn, M., Snodgrass, W.R., Webb, R.W.: Behavioral, biochemical and pharmacological effects of chronic dosage of phenothiazine tranquilizers in rats. In: The phenothiazines and structurally related drugs. Forrest, S., Carr, C.J., Usdin, E. (eds.), pp. 593–616. New York: Raven 1974

Malizia, E., Signore, L., Crimi, G.: Chlorpromazine plus thiorazidine poisoning and treatment with extracorporal dialysis. Acta Pharmacol. Toxicol. (Copenh.) [Suppl. 2] 41, 163–170 (1977)

Manson-Bahr, P.: Phenothiazine as an anthelmintic in threadworm and roundworm infections. Lancet 1940II, 808

Marcus, S.M., Borzelleca, J.F.: Observations on reserpine-induced bradycardia, Arch. Int. Pharmacodyn. Ther. 174, 12–16 (1968)

Markiewicz, L.: Biochemical and functional effects of longterm administration of reserpine in mice. Acta Physiol. Scand. 58, 376–380 (1963)

Marquardt, H.: Reserpine and chemical carcinogenesis. Lancet 1975I, 925–926 (1975)

Marsboom, R.: On the pharmacology of azaperone, a neuroleptic used for the restraint of wild animals. Acta Zool. Pathol. Antverp. 48, 155–161 (1969)

Martins, M.J.: Sur l'influence de la réserpine dans le cycle oestral du rat. C.R. Soc. Biol. (Paris) 162, 1020–1023 (1968)

Massey, L.W.C.: Skin pigmentation, corneal and lens opacities with prolonged chlorpromazine treatment. Can. Med. Assoc. J. 92, 186–187 (1965)

Mayer, G., Meunier, J.-M.: Réserpine et progestation chez la ratte. Survie des oeufs en phase latente et ovoimplantations normales ou retardées, provoquées par l'oestrègène. C. R. Acad. Sci. [D] (Paris) 248, 3355–3357 (1959)

McDonald, C.J., Creasy, W.A., Howard, R.O.: Chlorpromazine toxic ocular manifestations in guinea pigs. Clin. Res. 14, 492 (1966)

McDonald, C.J., Creasy, W.A., Howard, R.O.: Chlorpromazine oculocutaneous pigmentation. Clin. Res. 15, 252 (1967)

Meier-Ruge, W.: Eye toxicity. Proc. Eur. Soc. Study Drug Toxi. 14, 133–145 (1973)

Meldrum, B.S., Anlezark, G.M., Marsden, L.D.: Acute dystonia as an idiosyncratic response to neuroleptics in baboons. Brain *100*, 313–326 (1977)

Mercier, J., Schmitt, J., Aurousseau, J., Etzensperger, P., Bonifay, D.: Etude pharmacologique d'un nouveau neuroplégique. Le maléate acide de l'acétyl-3-diméthylamino-3, propyl-10-phénothiazine: 1.522 Cb.I -toxicité. Action sur le système nerveux central et périphérique. Arch. Int. Pharmacodyn. Ther. *113*, 53–75 (1957)

Mikhailova, T.V., Terekhina, A.I., Gilev, A.P.: Pharmacological properties of dixyrazine. A new neuroleptic of the phenothiazine series. Farmakol. Toksikol. *32*, 28–31 (1969)

Mikhailova, T.V., Terekhina, A.I., Gilev, A.P.: Chlorpromazine plus thiorazidine poisoning and treatment with extracorporal dialysis. Acta Pharmacol. Toxicol. (Copenh.) [Suppl. 2], *41*, 163–170 (1977)

Mills, L.C.: Drug-induced impotence. Amer. Fam. Physician *12*, 104–106 (1975)

Mishkinsky, J., Lajtos, Z.K., Sulman, F.G.: Initiation of lactation by hypothalamic implantation of perphenazine. Endocrinology *78*, 919–922 (1966)

Mishkinsky, J., Khazen, K., Givant, Y., Dikstein, S., Sulman, F.G.: Mammatropic and neuroleptic effects of butyrophenones in the rat. Arch. Int. Pharmacodyn. Ther. *179*, 94–105 (1969)

Mitrofanov, V.S.: Toxicity of triftazine with its repeated introduction. Farmakol. Toksikol. *37*, 462–464 (1974)

Moayer, M.: Phenothiazine im Tierexperiment und bei Hyperemesis gravidarum. Med. Klin. *62*, 1137–1141 (1967)

Moccetti, T.: Kardiotoxische Medikamente. Bern, Stuttgart, Wien: Huber 1977

Moriarity, A.J.: Trifluoperazine and congenital malformations. Can. Med. Assoc. J. *88*, 97 (1963)

Moriyama, I.S., Kanoh, S.: Effects of reserpine on the pregnant rat. Teratology *14*, 247 (1976)

Murphree, O.D., Monroe, B.L., Seager, L.D.: Survival of offspring of rats administered phenothiazines during pregnancy. J. Neuropsychiatry *3*, 295–297 (1962)

Nair, V.: Prenatal exposure to drugs: Effect of the development of brain monoamin systems. Adv. Behav. Biol. *8*, 171–211 (1974)

Neave, R.: Immobilisation and anaesthesia of the pig. Vet. Rec. *92*, 272 (1973)

Nelemans, F.A.: Psychopharmaca in traffic. Ned. Tijdschr. Geneeskd. *112*, 1862–1867 (1968)

Nicoloff, D.M., Stone, N.H., Leonard, A.S., Doberneck, R., Wangenstein, O.H.: Effect of reserpine on peptic ulceration and gastric blood flow in dogs. Proc. Soc. Exp. Biol. Med. *106*, 877–880 (1961)

Niemegeers, C.J.E., Janssen, P.A.J.: Bromoperidol, a new potent neuroleptic of the butyrophenone series. Arzneim. Forsch. *24*, 33–45 (1974)

Niemegeers, C.J.E., van Nueten, J.M., Janssen, P.A.J.: Azaperone, a sedative neuroleptic of the butyrophenone series with pronounced anti-agressive and anti-shock activity in animals. Arzneim. Forsch. *24*, 1798–1806 (1974)

Nieschulz, O., Popendiker, K., Sack, K.-H.: Pharmakologische Untersuchungen über N-Alkyl-piperidyl-phenothiazin-derivate. Arzneim. Forsch. *4*, 232–242 (1954)

Nishimura, H., Tanimura, T.: Clinical aspects of the teratogenicity of drugs. Amsterdam, Oxford: Excerpta Medica 1976

Noble, J.F., Sparano, B.M.: Some toxicologic effects of high doses of the nonaddicting analgesic agent methotrimeprazine. Toxicol. Appl. Pharmacol. *8*, 349 (1966)

Oberst, F.W., Crook, J.W.: Behavioral, physical and pharmacodynamic effects of haloperidol in dogs and monkeys. Arch. int. Pharmacodyn. Ther. *167*, 450–464 (1967)

O'Donoghue, S.E.F.: Distribution of pethidine and chlorpromazine in maternal, foetal and neonatal biological fluids. Nature *229*, 124–125 (1971)

O'Donoghue, S.E.F.: Metabolic activity in the human foetus and neonate as shown by administration of chlorpromazin. J. Physiol. (London) *242*, 105–106 (1974)

Ordy, J.M., Samorajski, T., Collins, R.L., Rolsten, C.: Prenatal chlorpromazine effects on liver, survival and behavior of mice offspring. J. Pharmacol. Exp. Ther. *151*, 110–125 (1966)

Peele, R., Loetzen, I.S.von: Phenothiazine deaths: A cortical review. Am. J. Psychiatry. *130*, 306–308 (1973)

Perry, T.L., Culling, C.F.A., Berry, K., Hansen, S.: 7-Hydroxychlorpromazine: Potential toxic drug metabolite in psychiatric patients. Science *146*, 81–83 (1964)

Peters, U.H.: Akute Intoxikationen mit Psychopharmaka. Therapiewoche *14*, 393–394 (1964)

Pfeifer, H.J., Greenblatt, D.J., Koch-Weser, J.: Clinical toxicity of reserpine in hospitalized patients: A report from the Boston collaborative drug surveillance program. Am. J. Med. Sci. *271*, 269–276 (1976)

Pisciotta, A.V., Hinz, J.H.: Inhibition of DNA synthesis by chlorpromazine. J. Lab. Clin. Med. *66*, 1011 (1965)

Platts, M.M., Usher, A., Stentiford, N.H.: Phenelzine and trifluoperazine poisoning. Lancet *1965II*, 738

Plummer, A.J., Earl, A., Schneider, J.A., Trapold, J., Barrett, W.: Pharmakology of rauwolfia alkaloids, including reserpine. Ann. N.Y. Acad. Sci. *59*, 8–21 (1954)

Poeck, K.: Schwierige diagnostische Probleme bei Arzneimittelvergiftungen. Med. Welt *47*, 2576–2585 (1968)

Pomme, B., Girard, J., Debost, M.: Troubles de la sexualité et médications psychotropes. Ann. Med. Psychol. (Paris) *1*, 551–562 (1965)

Popov, T.: Untersuchungen über die Widerstandsfähigkeit der Lysosomen-Membranen: III. Schutz der Leber-Lysosome vor der schädigenden Wirkung der Chlorpromazins durch Riboflavin in vivo. Z. Naturforsch. [B] *22*, 1157–1159 (1967)

Psychosos, A.: The effects of reserpine and chlorpromazine on sexual function. J. Reprod. Fertil. [Suppl.] *4*, 47–59 (1968)

Ravina, J.-H.: Les thérapeutiques dangereuses chez la femme enceinte. Presse Méd. *72*, 3057–3059 (1964)

Rieder, R.O., Rosenthal, D., Wender, P., Blumenthal, H.: The offspring of schizophrenics. Fetal and neonatal deaths. Arch. Gen. Psychiatry *32*, 200–211 (1975)

Rise, A.: Drug and embryo Tidsskr. Nor. Laegeforen. *96*, 446–447 (1976)

Ritama, V., Vapaatalo, H.I., Neuvonen, P.J., Idaenpaeaen. Heikkilae, J.E., Paasonen, M.K.: Phenothiazines and intestinal dilatation. Lancet *1969I*, 470

Roe, F.J.C.: The relevance of preclinical assessment of carcinogenesis. Clin. Pharmacol. Ther. *7*, 77–111 (1966)

Roizin, L., True, Ch., Knight, M.: Structural effects of tranquilizers. Proc. Assoc. Res. Nerv. Ment. Dis. *37*, 285–324 (1957)

Roman, I.C.: Rat and human chromosome studies after promazine medication. Br. Med. J. *1969IV*, 172

Rosecrans, J.A.. Effects of route of administration on the chronic toxicity of reserpine. Psychopharmacologia *10*, 452–456 (1967)

Roubein, I.F., Samuelly, M., Keup, W.: The toxicity of chlorpromazine and mescaline on mouse cerebellum and fibroblast cells in culture. Acta Pharmacol. Toxicol. (Copenh.) *33*, 326–329 (1973)

Roux, C.: Action tératogène de la prochlorpémazine. Arch. Fr. Pédiatr. *16*, 968–971 (1959)

Rumeau-Rouquette, C.: Goujard, Huel, G.: Les médicaments du systeme nerveux sont-ils tératogènes? Arch. Fr. Pédiatr. *33*, 5–10 (1976)

Rumeau-Rouquette, C., Goujard, J., Huel, G.: Possible teratogenic effect of phenothiazine in human beings. Teratology *15*, 57–64 (1977)

Sackler, A.M., Weltman, A.S., Bradshaw, M., Hielman, F.: The effects of reserpine on histamine tolerance and endocrine organs of the rat. Acta Endocrinol. (Copenh.) *34*, 619–626 (1960)

Samorajski, T., Ordy, J.M., Rolsten, C.: Prenatal chlorpromazine effects on liver enzymes, glycogen and ultrastructure in mice offspring. Am. J. Pathol. *47*, 803–831 (1965)

Sams, W.M., Jr., Epstein, J.H.: The experimental production of drug phototoxicity in guinea pigs. J. Invest. Derm. *48*, 89–94 (1967)

Saunders, D.R., Miva, T.S., Mennear, J.H.: Chlorpromazine-ultraviolet interaction on mouse ear. Pharmacologist *13*, 241 (1971)

Scanlan, F.J.: The use of thioridazine (Melleril) during the first trimester. Med. J. Aust. *1*, 1271–1272 (1972)

Schanda, H.: Kardiovaskuläre Nebenwirkungen trizyklischer Psychopharmaka unter besonderer Berücksichtigung des EKG. Fortschr. Neurol. Psychiatr. *45*, 491–500 (1977)

Schardein, J.L.: Drugs as teratogens. Cleveland, Ohio: CRC Press 1976

Scheckel, C.L.: Pharmacology and chemistry of the thioxanthenes with special reference of chlorprothixene. Mod. Probl. Pharmacopsychiatry 2, 1–14 (1969)

Schiele, B.C.: Symposium on side-effects and drugs toxicity, including behavioral toxicity. Psychopharmacol. Bull. 4, 56–61 (1967)

Scholz, O., Kretzschmar, E.: Tierexperimentelle Untersuchungen über die Megaphen-Wirkung auf die Leber. Langenbecks Arch. Chir. 283, 515–527 (1956)

Scholz, O., Kretzschmar, E.: Der cholestatische Effect des Megaphen und seine Beeinflussung durch Choleretika. Klin. Wochenschr. 36, 38–41 (1958)

Seay, P.H., Field, W.E.: Toxicological studies on haloperidol. Int. J. Neuropsychiatry [Suppl. 1] 3, 19–22 (1967)

Seifter, J., Glassman, J.M., Rauzzino, F.: Pharmacological properties of promazine. J. Pharmacol. Exp. Ther. 119, 183 (1957)

Shader, R.I., DiMascio, A.: Psychotropic drug side effects. Baltimore: Williams & Wilkins 1970

Shader, R.I., Harmatz, J.S.: Gastrointestinal effects. In: Psychotropic drug side effects. Shader, R.J., DiMascio, A. (eds.), pp. 198–205. Baltimore, Williams & Wilkins 1970

Shapiro, S., Heinonen, O.P., Siskind, V., Kaufmann, O.W., Monson, R.R., Slone, D.: Antenatal exposure to doxylamine succinate and dicyclomine hydrochloride (Bendectin) in relation to congenital malformations, perinatal mortality rate, birth weight and intelligence quotient score. Am. J. Obstet. Gynecol. 128, 480–488 (1977)

Shaw, M.W.: Human chromosome damage by chemical agents. Annu. Rev. Med. 21, 409–432 (1970)

Silvestrini, B., Quadri, E.: Investigations on the specificity of the so-called analgesic activity of non-narcotic drugs. Eur. J. Pharmacol. 12, 231–235 (1970)

Similä, S., Raijola, E., Raijola, A.: Effect of reserpine and meprobamate on the functional status of rat seminal vesicles. Ann. Med. Exp. Biol. Fenn. 40, 313–317 (1962)

Simmons, J.E., Lusk, M.: Response of neonatal female rats to reserpine and testosterone. Acta Endocrinol. (Copenh.) 61, 302–306 (1969)

Singh, S., Padmanabhan, R.: Prenatal stunting of CF rats caused by maternal administration of chlorpromazine hydrochloride. Teratology 16, 122–123 (1977)

Sjöstrand, S.E., Cassano, G.B., Hansson, E.: The distribution of 35S-chlorpromazine in mice studied by whole body autoradiography. Arch. Int. Pharmacodyn. Ther. 156, 34–47 (1965)

Smejkal, V.: Action of reserpine on the digestive tract of experimental animals. Byul. Eksp. Biol. Med. 63, 157–158 (1968)

Smithells, R.W.: Phenothiazines and teratogenicity. Practitioner 205, 836 (1970)

Smoliyanikova, N.M., Strekalova, S.N., Boiko, S.S.: Regularities governing penetration of chlorpromazine via the placental barrier. Farmakol. Toksikol. 39, 560–562 (1976)

Sobel, D.E.: Fetal damage due to ECT, insulin coma, chlorpromazine, or reserpine. Arch. Gen. Psychiatry 2, 606–611 (1960)

Soulairac, A., Soulairac, M.-L.: Action de la réserpine sur le comportement sexuel du rat mâle. C.R. Soc. Biol. (Paris) 155, 1010–1013 (1961)

Soulairac, A., Soulairac, M.-L.: Effect de l'administration chronique de réserpine sur la fonction génitale du rate mâle. Ann. Endocrinol. (Paris) 23, 281–292 (1962)

Spieth, K.D., Lorenz, D.: Untersuchungen mit Fluphenazin und Flupenthixol über die Beeinflussung der Fertilität und über die fetale Toxizität an der Ratte. Arch. Pharmakol. Exp. Pathol. 257, 338–339 (1967)

Stamp, J.T.: Perinatal loss in lambs with particular reference to diagnosis. Vet. Rec. 81, 530–534 (1967)

Stoffer, S.S.: A gynecologic study of drug addicts. Am. J. Obstet. Gynecol. 101, 779–783 (1968)

Szabo, K.T., Brent, R.L.: Species differences in experimental teratogenesis by tranquilizing agents. Lancet 1974 I, 565

Szabo, K.T., Brent, R.L.: Reduction of drug-induced cleft palate in mice. Lancet 1975 I, 1296–1297

Szabo, K.T., Difebbo, M.E., Kang, Y.J., Brent, R.L.: Teratological evaluation of tranquilizing agents in various species of laboratory animals. Preliminary report. Teratology 10, 325 (1974)

Szabo, K.T., Difebbo, M.E., Kang, Y.J., Palmer, A.K., Brent, R.L.: Comparative embryotoxicity and teratogenicity of various tranquilizing agents in mice, rats, rabbits and rhesus monkeys. Toxicol. Appl. Pharmacol. *33*, 124 (1975)

Talwalker, P.K., Meites, J., Nicoll, C.S., Hopkins, T.F.: Effects of chlorpromazine on mammary glands of rats. Am. J. Physiol. *199*, 1073–1076 (1960)

Teske, H.-J., Weicker, H.: Die Phenothiazin-Haemolyse im Tierexperiment. Ärztl. Forsch. *10*, 236–247 (1956)

Tessitore, V.: Effetti della tioridazina sul sistema neurosecernente ipotalamo-neuroipofisario. Boll. Soc. Ital. Biol. Sper. *43*, 379–381 (1967)

Thomas, J.O., McNaught, J.B., DeEds, F.: Studies on phenothiazine, VI. General toxicity and blood changes. J. Ind. Hyg. Toxicol. *20*, 419–421 (1938)

Tonge, S.R.: Permanent alterations in catecholamine concentrations in discrete areas of brain in the offspring of rats treated with methylamphetamine and chlorpromazine. Br. J. Pharmacol. *47*, 425–427 (1973a)

Tonge, S.R.: Some persistent effects of the pre- and neonatal administration of psychotropic drugs on noradrenaline metabolism in discrete areas of rat brain. Proc. Br. Pharmacol. Soc. *48*, 364–365 (1973b)

Torjescu, V.: Etude enzymo-toxicologique de la chlorpromazine. Ann. Pharm. Fr. *26*, 311–322 (1968)

Towell, M.E., Hyman, A.I., James, L.St., Steinsland, O.S., Gerst, E.C., Adamsons, K.: Reserpin administration during pregnancy. Am. J. Obstet. Gynecol. *92*, 711–716 (1965)

Tripod, J., Bein, H.J., Meier, R.: Characterization of central effects of Serpasil (reserpine, a new alkaloid of rauwolfia serpentina B.) and of their antagonistic reactions. Arch. Int. Pharmacodyn. Ther. *96*, 406–425 (1954)

Tuchmann-Duplessis, H.: Influence de la réserpine sur les glandes endocrines. Presse Méd. *64*, 2189–2192 (1956)

Tuchmann-Duplessis, H., Mercier-Parot, L.: Répercussions de la réserpine sur la gestation chez la ratte. C.R. Acad. Sci. [D] (Paris) *243*, 410–413 (1956)

Tuchmann-Duplessis, H., Mercier-Parot, L.: Influence de traitements de réserpine sur la fertilité des parents et de leurs descendants. C.R. Soc. Biol. (Paris) *156*, 587–590 (1962)

Tuchmann-Duplessis, H., Mercier-Parot, L.: Action d'un neuroleptique, le R 1625 (haloperidol) sur l'activité génitale de la ratte. C.R. Soc. Biol. (Paris) *263*, 1493–1495 (1966)

Tuchmann-Duplessis, H., Mercier-Parot, L.: Nidation retardée sous l'influence d'un neuroleptique, le R 1625 (haloperidol). C. R. Soc. Biol. (Paris) *264*, 114–117 (1967)

Tuchmann-Duplessis, H.,Mercier-Parot, L.: Retentissements endocrines de certains médicaments neurotropes. Proc. Eur. Soc. Study Drug Toxi. *9*, 119–133 (1968)

Ullberg, S., Lindquist, N.G., Sjostrand, S.E.: Accumulation of chorio-retinotoxic drugs in the foetal eye. Nature *227*, 1257–1258 (1970)

Usdin, E.: Absorption, distribution and metabolic fate of psychotropic drugs. Psychopharmacol. Bull. *6*, 4–25 (1970)

van den Berghe, H.: Clastogenic effects of haloperidol in vivo and of haloperidol, droperidol and pipamperone in vitro. Arzneim. Forsch. *24*, 2055–2058 (1974)

van Waes, A., van de Velde, E.: Safety evaluation of haloperidol in the treatment of hyperemesis gravidarum. J. Clin. Pharmacol. *9*, 224–227 (1969)

Vapaatalo, H.I., Karppanen, H.: Influence of ethanol on the toxicity of some psychotropic drugs. Scand. J. Clin. Lab. Invest. [Suppl. 108] *23*, 77 (1969)

Vapaatalo, H.I., Idänpään-Heikkila, J.E., Neuvonen, P.J.: Effects of prolonged chlorpromazine treatment on the rat intestine. Acta Pharmacol. Toxicol. (Copenh.) *27*, 262–268 (1969)

Verne, J. Tuchmann-Duplessis, H., Hébert, S.: Etude comparative de l'influence exercée par la réserpine et par l'hypophysectomie sur le testicule et la vésicule séminale du rat. Ann. Endocrinol. (Paris) *18*, 952–958 (1957)

Vince, D.J.: Congenital malformations following phenothiazine administration during pregnancy. Can. Med. Assoc. J. *100*, 223 (1969)

Wagner, M.: Die Wirkung einiger gebräuchlicher Piperidinderivate auf menschliche Chromosomen in vitro. Arzneim. Forsch. *21*, 1017–1024 (1971)

Walker, B.E., Patterson, A.: Induction of cleft palate in mice by tranquilizers and barbiturates. Teratology *10*, 159–164 (1974)

Walker, C.A., Friedman, A.H.: Twenty-four hour toxicity rhythms of sympathomimetic amines in mice. Pharmacologist *12*, 198 (1970)

Walson, P.D., Lightner, E.S., Harris, T.H., Sell, E.J.: The first reported case in a neonate of gynecomastia and lactation following the use of chlorpromazine (thorazine). Clin. Res. *23*, 143 (1975)

Wang, G.M., Wong, K.K., Dreyfuss, J., Schreiber, E.C.: Effect of tricyclic psychoactive agents on levels of K$^+$ and reduced glutathione (GSH) in rabbit lenses in vitro and on hemolysis: The implication for cataractogenicity. Clin. Pharmacol. Ther. *13*, 155 (1972)

Wattenberg, L.W., Leong, J.L.: Effects of phenothiazines on protective systems against polycyclic hydrocarbons. Cancer Res. *25*, 365–370 (1965)

Watzman, N., Manian, A.A., Barry III, H., Buckley, J.P.: Comparative effects of chlorpromazine hydrochloride and quaternary chlorpromazine hydrochloride on the central nervous system of rats and mice. J. Pharm. Sci. *57*, 2089–2093 (1968)

Weikel, J.H., Wheeler, A.G., Joiner, P.D.: Metabolic fate and toxicology of methdilazine 10-(I-methyl-3-pyrrolidylmethyl) phenothiazine. Toxicol. Appl. Pharmacol. *2*, 68–82 (1960)

Weiss, B., Santelli, S., Lusink, G.: Movement disorders induced in monkeys by chronic haloperidol treatment. Psychopharmacology *53*, 289–293 (1977)

Weissmann, A.: Psychopharmacological effects of thiothixene and related compounds. Psychopharmacologia *12*, 142–157 (1968)

Werboff, J.: Tranquilizers in pregnancy and behavioral effects on the offspring. Nature *209*, 110 (1966)

Werboff, J., Dembicki, E.L.: Toxic effects of tranquilizers administered to gravid rats. J. Neuropsychiatry *4*, 87–91 (1962)

West, G.B.: Some factors influencing histamine metabolism in rat pregnancy. Int. Arch. Allergy Appl. Immunol. *16*, 39–48 (1960)

West, G.B.: Teratogenic activity of drugs. J. Pharm. Pharmacol. *16*, 63–64 (1964)

Windle, W.F., Cammermeyer, J., Smart, J.O., Joralemon, J., Dorrill, E., McQuillan, M.P., Feringa, E.R., Pimental, L.T.: Tremor, rigidity, akinesia and associated phenomena in reserpinised african green monkeys (motion picture). Am. J. Physiol. *183*, 674 (1955)

Winter, D.: Toxizitätsveränderung neurotroper Pharmaka bei Versuchstieren mit experimentell hervorgerufener Hyperthyreoidie. Med. Pharmacol. Exp. *14*, 391–394 (1966)

Wolf, H.G.: Pränatale und neonatale Schädigungen durch Arzneimittel. Wien. Klin. Wochenschr. *80*, 498–502 (1968)

Zeilmaker, G.H.: Normal and delayed pseudopregnancy in the rat. Acta Endocrinol. (Copenh.) *49*, 558–566 (1965)

Zimmermann, H.J.: Toxic hepatopathy Am. J. Gastroenterol. *49*, 39–56 (1968)

Zipf, H.F., Alstaedter, A.: Die hypnotische Wirkung von Luminal und Evipan in Kombination mit Megaphen und anderen Phenothiazin-Derivaten. Arzneim. Forsch. *4*, 14–19 (1954)

Ziv, G., Shani, J., Givant, Y., Buchman, O., Sulman, F.G.: Distribution of triated haloperidol in lactating and pregnant cows and ewes. Arch. Int. Pharmacodyn. Ther. *212*, 154–163 (1974)

Zoryan, V.G.: Effect of reserpine on the hypothalamo-hypophysial-adrenocortical system. A review. Farmakol. Toksikol. *29*, 370–377 (1966)

Zucker, I., Feder, H.H.: The effect of neonatal reserpine treatment on female sex behavior of rats. J. Endocrinol. *35*, 423–424 (1966)

CHAPTER 12

Clinical Pharmacology (Pharmacokinetics)

B. Müller-Oerlinghausen*

A. Introduction

The present chapter describes the pharmacokinetics of antipsychotic drugs in psychiatric patients and normal human volunteers. Special consideration is given to the possible relationship between pharmacokinetic data, particularly plasma levels, and clinical effects.

The pharmacokinetic behavior of phenothiazines and other neuroleptics, i.e., highly lipophilic drugs, in humans follows the same principles as in animals and can be shortly characterized by rather rapid absorption, marked first-pass effects and a very complicated pattern of distribution and elimination of individual metabolites. In view of the high apparent volume of distribution, pharmacoanalytic methods in this area need to be extremely sensitive and specific. Unfortunately, this is often not the case, leading to a considerable lack of clear-cut and reproducible kinetic data from single dose studies. Often it is not possible to administer to previously drug-free normal volunteers doses which would be necessary in order to achieve measurable plasma levels. Even if radio-labeled compounds are used, rather high specific activities might be required. Long biologic half-lives, high serum protein binding, and the enormous interindividual metabolic variability as well as the practial impossibilities of covering the whole metabolite pattern in a single study, yield only very cautious conclusions to be drawn from available experimental data. Even greater are the difficulties with patient studies under conditions of long-term treatment, where organizational (noncompliance!), legal, and ethical problems often prevent the collection of reliable and valid data. (Ref. LADER, 1976; MAY and VAN PUTTEN, 1978; MÜLLER-OERLINGHAUSEN, 1978.)

B. Phenothiazines and Thioxanthenes

I. Chlorpromazine, Levomepromazine

1. Methods for Assessment of Chlorpromazine Concentration in Biological Fluids

Clinical pharmacology of chlorpromazine (CPZ), particularly its pharmacokinetics, could only be investigated after sensitive and reproducible methods for the determination of CPZ in plasma and other body fluids were available. (Ref. also USDIN, 1971.) Simple spectrophotometric or spectrofluorometric methods cannot be consid-

---

* In the memory of my father BERTHOLD MÜLLER-OERLINGHAUSEN, Sculptor, and my brother-in-law Prof. GERD BRAND, Philosopher, who both died during the final preparation of this manuscript

ered as reliable because of their insufficient sensitivity and specificity. (Huang and Kurland, 1961; Huang and Ruskin, 1964; March et al., 1972.) Curry (1968) introduced GLC with ECD for determination of the plasma concentrations of CPZ and three or four of the nonpolar metabolites after single dose medication, and under therapeutic conditions. Difficulties, however, seem to have occurred with the replication of this procedure by other investigators. Ether instead of heptane can be used for extraction when 7-hydroxy-CPZ (7–OHCPZ) is to be measured. (Curry and Evans, 1975.) A drawback of the ECD in contrast to the FID, however, is its nonlinearity. Modifications and improvements of the GLC method have been described by Flint et al. (1971), Christoph et al. (1972), Rivera-Calimlim et al. (1973), and Davis et al. (1977). Dahl and Strandjord (1977) tried GLC with an FID. Also TLC with or without direct densitometric evaluation has been used, particularly for separation of CPZ metabolites in urine but also in plasma. (Wechsler et al., 1967; Sakalis et al., 1973; Chan et al., 1974; Turano et al., 1974; Breyer and Villumsen, 1976.) Mass fragmentography, i. e., a combination of GLC and MS was described by Hammar and Holmstedt (1968) and by Alfredsson et al. (1976). An isotope dilution method based on GC/MS with stable isotope as internal standard was described by May et al. (1978). Another radioassay had been described earlier by Efron et al. (1971) (ref. also Knapp and Gaffne, 1972; Simpson et al., 1974). Lehr and Kaul (1975) presented a quaternization procedure with subsequent fluorometry allowing the assay of picomol quantities of CPZ. Radioimmunoassay seems not be ready yet for routine application (Spector, 1974). Laboratory error of most of these methods must be assumed to be approximately $\pm 10\%$ or considerably more. Systematic quality control of the laboratories involved does not exist. An attempt to compare the results of at least some laboratories revealed puzzling and unexplained differences in precision and reproducibility. (Turner et al., 1976.) Particular technical difficulties among many others are the losses during the extraction procedure, partly due to binding of the drug to acidic glass surface, the nonenzymatic oxydation of CPZ during processing (Turano et al., 1974; Knoll et al., 1977) and the occurrence of ghost peaks in GLC (Spirtes, 1972).

2. Pharmacokinetics of CPZ in Man

a) Absorption, Distribution, Elimination, Saliva and CSF Levels
(Single-Dose Studies)

The principle pharmacokinetic behaviour of CPZ and related phenothiazines has been outlined in the preceding chapter (Breyer-Pfaff). Extensive metabolization of CPZ is undergone with about 150 metabolites claimed to occur in human plasma, some of them probably being artifacts. Less than 1% of unchanged CPZ is excreted in the urine and still much less in the feces after a single intramuscular dose (Curry et al., 1970). There are few data on the effect of intravenous administration, which do not allow final pharmacokinetic conclusions. A half-life of 4.5 h for the slower term of the biexponential elimination curve has been calculated in an earlier study (Curry et al., 1970). In a rather recent review of the work of his own and others, Curry (1975) concludes that after single intravenous doses the half-life of the early portion of the elimination curve is 2–3 h (distribution, tissue uptake), the half-life of the "intermediate" phase approx. 15 h, and for the less steepest part approx. 61 days. This would certainly suggest the existence of a deep compartment. However, the authors' conclusions rarely appear to be based on tabulated material or statistical evidence, but rather on the interpretation of curves from single or typical cases. The apparent volume of distribution amounts to 8.1 liter/kg (MAXWELL et al., 1972). Still higher figures (V_β/F_{im}) were reported by DAHL and STRANDJORD (1977). Only minor differences of $t_{1/2\beta}$ and k_e showed in cirrhotic patients as compared to controls. (MAXWELL et al., 1972.) After a single intramuscular dose absorption takes approx. 2 h, sometimes, however, until 6 or even 8 h. The plasma levels often are stable up to 36 h. Chlorpromazine sulphoxide (CPZ-SO) could not be found, even in traces, after intramuscular doses (DAHL and STRANDJORD, 1977). The area under the curve (AUC) after an intravenous dose equals that after intramuscular application (100 mg/subject). After corresponding oral doses AUC is markedly less "to an extent ranging from 0% to 100%" (CURRY, 1975). Relative to intramuscular application the bioavailability of oral doses ranges from 10% to 69% according to DAHL and STRANDJORD (1977). This is about in the same range as the figures published by HOLLISTER et al. (1970); the latter authors compared plasma levels and urinary excretion of CPZ after four different dosage forms i.e., intramuscular, tablets, liquid, long-acting capsules, and found the poorest bioavailability with the long-acting preparation after single dose as well as under steady-state conditions. On the other hand, SUGERMAN and ROSEN (1964) investigating 24-h averaged urinary excretion were not able to find differences in absorption and excretion profile between CPZ tablets and sustained-release capsules. Also plasma levels after administration of either CPZ hydrochloride or embonate were not different in chronic schizophrenics (COOPER et al., 1973). All studies, however, demonstrate an enormous interindividual variation of plasma levels or total clearance. Particularly great, namely 100-fold, variations of peak blood levels reached between 1 and 8 h ($\tilde{x}=2.0$) were seen by MAY et al. (1978) after administration of a single liquid dose to 13 previously drug-free patients. The unusually high plasma levels could be explained by the absence of autoenzyme induction in this patient sample. A comparison between a generic and a brand-name oral CPZ preparation did not reveal any relevant differences (SIMPSON et al., 1974).

A study on the bioavailability of *levomepromazine* syrup as compared to tablets provides some evidence that presystemic metabolism, i.e., formation of sulphoxide may be more marked with a liquid preparation, which again emphasizes the importance of metabolic breakdown in the gut-wall (DAHL et al., 1977). Two interesting points are discussed in this study: (1) The lowest value of Cl/F_{po}[1], for which a 13-fold interindividual variation was demonstrated, was found in the oldest patient. (2) Values of Cl/F_{po} in two patients were 70% and 96% larger than in a previous study were CPZ tablets had been administered in the same subjects. Half-life of levomepromazine ranged between 16.5 and 77.8 h.

The CSF levels of CPZ were measured in two patients by AXELSSON et al. (1975), and a systematic study relating CSF levels and clinical outcome was performed by ALFREDSSON et al. (1976) and WODE-HELGODT et al. (1978). Levels of CSF amounting to approx. 3% of plasma levels and a high correlation with a twofold interindividual variation of the ratio C_{CSF}/C_P could be demonstrated; CPZ metabolites in CSF were below the detection limit.

---

1 Cl/F_{po} = Total clearance relative to the fraction of the oral dose that reaches systemic circulation as unchanged drug = D/A_{ss}

A comparable strong correlation seems to exist between plasma and saliva levels, the latter being surprisingly 10–100 times higher than those in plasma and peaking also earlier (May et al., 1978).

b) Multiple Dosing in Patients. Excretion Profile After Long-Term Treatment

Although plasma levels and urinary excretion of CPZ have been studied by several authors under the conditions of routine treatment in schizophrenic patients, the results are difficult to interpret and to compare, due to the differing methodologies used. (For the most detailed comment on the situation, ref. May and van Putten, 1978.)

Due to the enormous variability in CPZ absorption and metabolism, it seems self-evident that under therapeutic conditions a correlation between dosage and plasma levels might not be detectable (Wiles et al., 1976). Treatment with CPZ over several weeks possibly leads to induction of CPZ metabolizing enzymes in the liver or gut-wall. Thus, Dahl and Strandjord (1977) in agreement with earlier results of Loga et al. (1975) found plasma levels in patients, treated orally for 33 days, that were 37% lower than one had predicted from previous single dose studies. The authors could provide substantial evidence that the smaller AUC within one dosage interval after maintenance treatment was not due to increased $t_{1/2}$ or V_b, but rather increased pre-systemic breakdown. A different metabolite profile in plasma from patients as compared to previously drug-free volunteers after multiple dosage as compared to a single dose administration, has been reported by Wechsler et al. (1967), Sakurai et al. (1975), and Schooler et al. (1975, 1976). Whether the methodology introduced by Kaul et al. (1972, 1973, 1976) will lead to a more reliable assessment of conjugated and nonconjugated CPZ metabolites in plasma remains to be confirmed by other laboratories.

As to the relationship between plasma levels and administered multiple doses, the correlation seems to be particularly poor in the case of higher oral doses, which might be explained by saturation of CPZ binding to serum proteins and, thus, greater availability for metabolizing enzymes. (March et al., 1972; Wiles et al., 1976.) The assessment of urinary excretion also shows an inter- and intraindividually strongly varying metabolite pattern (Carr, 1962; West et al., 1971). Though Kelsey and Moscatelli (1974) showed in two cases that the metabolite profile may be very similar under low and high dosage. It takes about 10 days or more under continuous medication until a steady urinary excretion of hydroxilated metabolites would be achieved, the rate of excretion being related to the individual creatinine clearance (Forrest et al., 1967; Sved et al., 1971, 1972). If the biologic half-life of CPZ and its main metabolites is assumed to range between 6–9 h (Lacoursiere and Spohn, 1976), or to be approx. 30 h according to more recent data of Dahl and Strandjord (1977), it could be predicted that after discontinuation of long-term medication CPZ should have left the organism within 54–180 h. The results on the duration of the urinary excretion of CPZ after drug withdrawal are, however, rather contradictory (Cowen and Martin, 1968; Forrest et al., 1969; Sved et al., 1971; for review ref. Lacoursiere and Spohn, 1976). Storage in deep compartment like adipose tissue or high affinity binding certainly should be considered within this context.

c) Drug Binding

CPZ is bound to a high degree, more than 90%, to human plasma protein. Curry (1969) using equilibrium dialysis showed that in six patients binding varied from 91%

to 99%, and that it increased with higher pH (ref. also GABAY and HUANG, 1974). Affinity constants to human serum albumin differ somewhat according to the methodology – equilibrium dialysis, gel filtration, fluorescence quenching – the figures ranging between 7.81×10^3 and 4.33×10^5. Different binding sites seem to exist for CPZ and its more polar metabolites (JÄHNCHEN et al., 1969; GABAY and HUANG, 1974; SHARPLES, 1975) CPZ is also bound to lipoprotein and RBC membranes (MANIAN et al., 1974; BICKEL, 1976; GARVER et al., 1976; PEREL and CAFFNEY, 1977; ELFERNIK, 1978). The type of RBC binding is claimed to be the same as with rat brain synaptosomes and, thus, the RBC binding might be considered as "an important mechanism by which the drug is transported to possible receptor sites in the brain" (MANIAN et al., 1974). It is also speculated that poor response could be caused by stronger affinity or CPZ to RBC membranes than to the brain receptor.

d) Interaction of Other Drugs with CPZ Kinetics

Antiparkinsonian drugs like trihexyphenidyl or orphenadrine as well as antacids reduce the CPZ plasma levels, probably due to interference with gastrointestinal drug absorption (FANN et al., 1973; RIVERA-CALIMLIM et al., 1973, 1976; GAUTIER et al., 1977; LOGA et al., 1975). Also lithium can lead to decreased CPZ plasma levels after oral dosage in patients and normal volunteers, though the mechanism of this interaction remains to be clarified (RIVERA-CALIMLIM et al., 1978). A single dose of ethanol led to decreased urinary excretion of CPZ and its metabolites in long-term treated schizophrenics (FORREST et al., 1972). Phenobarbitone (50 mg tid, 3 weeks) as well as heavy cigarette smoking seem to lower CPZ plasma levels by enzyme induction. (FORREST et al., 1970; SWETT, 1974; LOGA et al., 1975.)

e) Relationship Between Pharmacokinetic Parameters and Clinical Effects

Pharmacokinetics in the sense of DOLLERY (1973) should be the servant, not the master, i. e., it should serve a better treatment of the patient, particularly a better prediction of what would happen if a certain drug in a definite dose is given to an individual patient (MÜLLER-OERLINGHAUSEN, 1978). It is beyond the frame of this chapter to deal in detail with the problem of whether – and to what extent – this goal has been reached regarding treatment of schizophrenic patients with CPZ and similar drugs. In their acid and merciless review MAY and VAN PUTTEN (1978) have tried to scatter the belief that any scientific evidence for a relation between steady state plasma level and treatment outcome can be gained on the ground of studies published hitherto. Instead of assessing plasma levels under (alleged) steady state conditions, they favor the idea of measuring plasma levels after administration of a single test dose before treatment onset, which is in agreement with the results of SAKURAI et al. (1975) who found a correlation between the ratio CPZ/CPZ-SO and clinical improvement. MAY and VAN PUTTEN (1978) rightly emphasize several points of weakness in clinical methodology, the most essential of which are: too small samples; poorly defined patient groups; flexible dosage and comedication; contamination by age, sex, and previous drug treatment; inadequate outcome criteria. Taking these pitfalls into consideration, the following picture of the present state of the art may be sketched.

Rather weak evidence for a "therapeutic window" of simple CPZ plasma levels arises from studies where global clinical outcome or some selected BPRS dimensions, etc., were used (CLARK and KAUL, 1975; RIVERA-CALIMLIM et al., 1976). If the metabolite pattern, particularly the ratio of CPZ to 7-OH-CPZ or CPZ-SO is taken into account, the results are contradictory. Whereas CURRY and EVANS (1975) did not find but small quantities of 7-OH CPZ in plasma of "responders" (ref. also MACKAY 1975). SAKALIS et al. (1973) and PHILIPSON et al. (1977) report on high 7-OH CPZ and CPZ levels in responders, and high CPZ-SO levels in nonresponders ($n = 8$, or 9, resp.!). In the study by WILES et al. (1976) and KOLAKOWSKA et al. (1975, 1976) global therapeutic effects were not correlated to CPZ plasma levels, whereas the appearance of parkinsonian symptoms and prolactin plasma concentrations were clearly related to CPZ concentrations under acute but not under chronic dosage conditions. SAKALIS et al. (1972) were among the first who emphasized that a correlation could be more likely detected between somatic variables than global outcome criteria and CPZ plasma levels. With regard to EPMS symptoms this could also be confirmed by GARVER et al. (1976), SAKALIS et al. (1977), and WODE-HELGODT et al. (1978). SMOLEN et al. (1975 a, b) demonstrated pupilometry to be a very sensitive tool for assessment of the comparative bioavailability of CPZ in liquid and solid preparations.

From a very systematic study with a fixed dosed regime it can be concluded that CSF levels of CPZ correlate better with clinical outcome (morbidity scores) than plasma levels; interestingly, the correlation was much poorer in males than females, and at the 4 th week as compared to the 2 nd week (WODE-HELGODT et al., 1978). AXELSSON et al. (1975) found unusually high CSF levels of CPZ-SO in one nonresponding patient.

II. Phenothiazines with Piperidine Side-Chain (Thioridazine, Mesoridazine)

1. Methods for Assessment of Thioridazine Concentration in Biologic Fluids

The development of specific methods for separating and assessing thioridazine and its main metabolites took about the same historical course as has been described for CPZ (for review ref. also BURRELL, 1977). Whereas earlier photometric and fluorometric methods partly measured thioridazine plus its metabolites (NEVE, 1960; EIDUSON and GELLER, 1963; FORREST et al., 1965; RAGLAND et al., 1965; PACHA, 1969; BUYZE et al., 1973), LC, TLC, GLC, GLC/MS, and HPLC methods provide greater specificity (CURRY and MOULD, 1969; MARTENSSON and ROSS, 1973; WEST et al., 1974; MUUSZE and HUBER, 1974; MUUSZE, 1975; GRUENKE et al., 1975; VANDERHEEREN and THEUNIS, 1976). Correlation of thioridazine plasma levels obtained with a fluorometric and a GLC method was only $r = 0.61$ in a study by GOTTSCHALK et al. (1975 a).

2. Pharmacokinetics of Thioridazine and Mesoridazine in Man

a) Single Dose Studies

The pharmacokinetic behavior of thioridazine and mesoridazine after single oral or intramuscular doses can be described as follows: GOTTSCHALK et al. (1975 b, 1976) administered 2 mg/kg mesoridazine intramuscularly to patients and normal subjects and found a wide interindividual variation of pharmacokinetic indices with peaking times ranging from 0.17 to 3.79 h, and $t_{1/2}$ ranging from 1.70 to 9.38 h ($\tilde{x} = 5.05$) except one patient with $t_{1/2} = 64.71$ h. Somewhat longer half-lives were calculated for the metabolite sulforidazine. No differences could be detected between patients and normal volunteers. After oral administration of liquid or tablet preparations of thioridazine a peaking time of 1–4 h with plasma levels ranging between 0.13 and 0.52 µg/ml (GLC) was reported by Martensson and Ross (1973). Plasma half-lives were around 10 h, which is in rough agreement with Pacha (1969), de Jonghe and van der Helm (1970) and Vanderheeren and Muusze (1977). The latter authors calculated a V_d of 3.5 liter/kg after an oral dose of 200 mg thioridazine. Gottschalk et al. (1975a) using a liquid preparation of thioridazine found peaking times of 1–4 h for thioridazine, 4–8 h for mesoridazine, and about 8 h for sulforidazine; $t_{1/2}$ was 24.0 ± 8 h, the greater variance being observed in females.

b) Multiple Dosing in Patients

After multiple dosage of 50 mg tid thioridazine over several weeks blood levels between 0.15 and 1.26 µg/ml were reported by Buyze et al. (1973); sustained release preparations were not much different from ordinary tablets. Axelsson (1975), however, found higher plasma levels with thioridazine syrup. Fluorometric determinations tend to give higher values (Mellinger et al., 1965; de Jonghe and van der Helm, 1970; for tabulated compilation of different studies ref. Vanderheeren and Muusze, 1977). Hollister et al. (1963) compared the urinary metabolite excretion after oral vs intramuscular administration of thioridazine; their results suggest that the potency of intramuscular injection is about four times higher than that of oral administration.

A highly significant interindividual variation of the metabolite pattern was shown by Vanderheeren and Muusze (1977). A correlation of the daily dose up to 6 mg/kg was found by Martensson and Roos (1973, Axelsson (1975), Axelsson and Martensson (1976), whereas at higher doses this relation levels off. Older patients appear to have higher plasma levels than younger ones (Martensson and Ross, 1973; Axelsson, 1975), which would be in agreement with an average plasma half-life of 26 h in five older patients as reported by Muusze and Vanderheeren (1977). The latter authors emphasize that also the intraindividual relative standard deviation of steady state plasma levels is high (range 9%–44%) and that it would be preferrable to measure the plasma levels several times during a clinical course, including the psychoactive metabolites mesoridazine and sulforidazine; in their study the percentage of psychoactive compounds ranged from 43%–74% of the total sum.

Contradictory results exist as regards possible interaction of other psychotropic drugs as well as alcohol and chloroquine with the absorption or metabolism of thioridazine (Buyze et al., 1973; Linnoila et al., 1974; Axelsson, 1975; Muusze and Vanderheeren, 1977; Traficante et al., 1977).

c) Drug Binding

The distribution of thioridazine metabolites between plasma and RBC was studied by Zingales (1969). The serum protein binding of thioridazine and its metabolites was investigated first by Belpaire et al. (1975) and later by Nyberg et al. (1978) using equilibrium dialysis. The mean free fraction of thioridazine in the latter study amounted to only 0.15% with serum protein, but to 2.2% with human albumin, indicating that other proteins than albumin should be relevant within this context. Free fractions of the main metabolites were around ten times higher. The free fraction of thioridazine increased with increasing serum concentrations. Evidence could be gained that common binding sites exist for the parent compound and its metabolites. The binding was influenced by sex but not by age of the patients.

d) Relationship Between Pharmacokinetic Parameters

DE JONGHE and VAN DER HELM (1970) had found a satisfactory antidepressive effect of thioridazine at an average plasma level of 2.0 µg/ml. However, in a controlled study with three different dosage groups, no correlation between plasma levels and clinical effect could be established (DE JONGHE et al. 1973). Also BERLING et al. (1975) were not able to show any relation of plasma levels (week 4 or 9, resp.) to clinical effects whereas GOTTSCHALK et al. (1975a) found some significant correlations (the correlation coefficient, however, never exceeding 0.50!) between kinetic parameters such as AUC or $t_{1/2}$ and behavioral changes 2 days after drug administration in 25 patients. Recent preliminary data of the same group (GOTTSCHALK, 1978) suggest that sophisticated statistical procedures like a stepwise discriminant analysis of a great number of clinical variables would allow to define different discriminant functions on which either placebo responders or drug responders score high and to correlate the individual scores with definite pharmacokinetic variables. NIKITOPOULOU et al. (1977) report that urinary drug excretion rate or prolactin plasma levels after single doses of thioridazine correlate better with somatic parameters such as EEG changes than thioridazine plasma levels. Whether the plasma concentration of thioridazine metabolites plays a more relevant role with regards to cardiotoxicity than the parent drug levels needs further clarification (GOTTSCHALK et al., 1978).

III. Phenothiazines with Piperazine Side-Chain
(Perazine, Butaperazine, Perphenazine, Fluphenazine)

1. Methods for Assessment of Plasma Concentrations

Sensitive methods for the assessment of piperazine side-chain phenothiazines have been developed only very recently. For butaperazine a fluorometric method is available (MANIER et al., 1974). Perazine can be determined with either TLC or GLC (BREYER and VILLUMSEN, 1976; VANDERHEEREN and THEUNIS, 1976; MÜLLER-OER-LINGHAUSEN et al., 1977; SCHLEY et al., 1978). Perphenazine and fluphenazine plasma levels, which under therapeutic conditions are very low, are measurable by GLC with or without derivatization, or by ion pair partition chromatography (LARSEN and NAESTOFT, 1973; HANSEN and KRAGH-SØRENSEN, 1973; KELSEY et al., 1973; KRAGH-SØRENSEN et al., 1973; HANSEN and LARSEN, 1974; LARSEN and NAESTOFT, 1975; HAN-SEN et al., 1976; JOHANSSON et al., 1976; WHELPTON and CURRY, 1976; RIVERA-CALIM-LIM and SIRACUSA, 1977; COOPER et al., 1978; FRANKLIN et al., 1978; DEKIRMENJIAN et al., 1978).

2. Pharmacokinetics of Piperazine Side-Chain Phenothiazines in Man

a) Single Dose Studies

After administration of single oral doses of 20 or 40 mg butaperazine, the peak serum level is reached between 1–3 h with an average peak concentration of 215 ng/ml (20 mg p. o.); very similar values were obtained under chronic administration of the same dose when blood was drawn 12 h after tablet ingestion. A linear relationship between administered dose and AUC or peak levels could be established; from the biphasic elimination curves a $t_{1/2\,b}$ ranging from 4 to 30 h was calculated. Thus, it seems that interindividual variability is less than with CPZ treatment. Steady state levels could be predicted with high accuracy from the kinetic parameters obtained after oral single dose administration (DAVIS et al., 1974). Preliminary results of single dose kinetics after administration of different forms of perphenazine were reported by HANSEN and LARSEN (1974). Higher peak blood levels were seen after single intramuscular than after divided oral doses. HANSEN et al. (1976) showed that perphenazine elimination follows apparent first-order kinetics with peak values around 4 h after oral administration. Maximum blood levels after perphenazine enanthate injection were observed after 0.5–3.5 days (VIALA, 1976).

CURRY et al. (1979) using labeled compounds studied the kinetics of fluphenazine and its esters and partly confirmed earlier results by SMULEVITCH et al. (1973). Half-lives of fluphenazine hydrochloride of approx. 15 h were comparable after oral and intramuscular administration, the bioavailability of the oral dose being much lower. For the enanthate half-lives of approx. 3.5 days, and for the decanoate of 5.3–11.7 days, were found in a small number of subjects pretreated with fluphenazine-injections for 6 months. If the concentration time curve is explained in terms of a one-compartment model, assuming a much slower absorption than elimination rate, then, the values given above can be considered as absorption half-lives; the elimination half-lives, calculated by the method of residuals for the case of enanthate, would then be in good agreement with those after fluphenazine hydrochloride administration. No evidence for the presence of the parent ester in plasma could be gained from TLC. A plasma level plateau of approx. 1 week was also seen after fluphenazine enanthate injection (DENCKER et al., 1976).

b) Multiple Dosing in Patients, and Correlation Between Plasma Levels and Clinical Effects

Butaperazine kinetics after multiple oral dosage were studied by COOPER et al. (1975) who found marked differences between an od and a tid dosage regimen, the latter producing higher plasma levels. There was some evidence of autoenzyme induction when plasma levels after a single oral dose of 40 mg in a drug-free patient were compared with those after 16 weeks treatment. GARVER et al. (1976) had shown that the incidence of dystonic reactions was related rather to the AUC or $t_{1/2\beta}$ of butaperazine in RBC than in plasma after a single oral test-dose. In a more recent and convincing study GARVER et al. (1977) could demonstrate that also the therapeutic response under repeated drug administration was correlated much better to RBC than to plasma levels when fitted to a nonlinear quadratic polynominal ($r^2 = 0.90$ vs $r^2 = 0.58$). Nonresponding chronic schizophrenic patients are reported to have lower butaperazine plasma levels than acute and better responding patients (SMITH et al., 1977).

Preliminary results on a positive relationship between perazine plasma levels and clinical response were reported by BREYER et al. (1976). Our own group has studied perazine plasma levels in 33 schizophrenic patients under the conditions of long-term treatment for at least 10 years (PIETZCKER et al., 1978). The distribution of individual plasma levels showed a wide variation, but a clear relationship between the residual psychopathologic symptoms and the plasma levels necessary for maintenance could be demonstrated. Patients with higher plasma levels had a higher incidence of slightly pathologic liver function test, and higher blood sugar levels after an oral glucose load.

HANSEN and LARSEN (1977) studied plasma levels of perphenazine and its sulphoxide after multiple oral dosage and showed that day-to-day variation of plasma levels is so great that three consecutive blood samples are needed for a reliable estimation of the steady state level. Dose per kg correlated poorly with plasma levels. In contrast, PIETZCKER et al. (1978) found a very good correlation between two consecutive determinations of perazine within a two week interval ($r_s = 0.91$), and a still very satisfactory correlation between plasma levels and body weight ($r_s = 0.76$) under the conditions of ultralong treatment.

c) Drug Binding and Drug Interactions

Serum protein binding of piperazine side-chain phenothiazines has been studied by some of the authors referred to in the Sect. B. I. 2. c). In addition, BRINKSCHULTE et al. (1978) investigated the binding of perazine to human albumin. SCHLEY et al. (1979) and SCHLEY (1979) demonstrated a specific binding of perazine to acid α_1-glycoprotein. As regards drug interaction, studies by EL-YOUSEF and MANIER (1974a–d) suggest that conjugated estrogen administration can increase plasma levels of butaperazine, whereas benztropine has no influence. Significantly higher butaperazine plasma levels occurred in subjects receiving desipramine in addition. (EL-YOUSEF and MANIER, 1974a)

IV. Pharmacokinetics of Thioxanthenes in Man

The literature of the kinetics of thioxanthenes is small and for the greater part refers to flupenthixol. According to JØRGENSEN et al. (1969) the distribution of flupenthixol in the rat is similar to that of other neuroleptic drugs such as phenothiazines with piperazine side-chain. The lowest concentration was found in the brain. Fecal excretion was four to five times higher than urinary excretion, possibly due to a marked enterohepatic circulation. JØRGENSEN and GOTTFRIES (1972) using labeled compounds studied the kinetics of flupenthixol, administered orally, and flupenthixol decanoate in oil given intramuscularly. In female patients pretreated with flupenthixol for at least 6 months a maximum of total radioactivity in plasma was reached 3–8 h after an oral dose, or 11–17 days after injection. Values within the maximum minus 20% were maintained with the decanoate for 14.1 ± 2.4 days. The radioactivity of CSF, assessed 11 days after decanoate injection, amounted to 29%–55% of the plasma concentration, which is in rough agreement with the figures reported by VRANCKX (1974). A negative linear relationship existed between individual body weight and plasma or CSF levels. According to these kinetic results, the usual injection intervals of 2 weeks might well be prolonged to 3 or 4 weeks. BERGLING et al. (1975) investigated the kinetics of thiothixene and demonstrated a clear relationship between dose and plasma levels; he also found that plasma levels decreased after treatment over 2 months. JACOBSSON et al. (1976) using a fluorometric method, studied the relationship of thiothixene plasma levels and therapeutic response in chronic schizophrenics treated orally during 4 weeks. A 20-fold interindividual variation of the plasma levels was found with a dosage at doctor's choice. Plasma levels were positively correlated to a factor comprising acute psychotic symptoms on a rating scale.

Chlorprothixene plasma levels or elimination rates do not differ in alcoholics with or without acute alcohol intoxication as compared to placebo controls according to MATTSON et al. (1974).

C. Pharmacokinetics of Clozapine and Loxapine in Man

Few data are available on the kinetics of neuroleptic drugs belonging to the group of dibenzoazepines or dibenzoxazepines. After administration of clozapine in a single oral dose, the mean half-life was calculated as 6 h. The steady state during chronic treatment was reached after 6–10 days (ACKENHEIL and HIPPIUS, 1977). Dosage per kg and plasma levels were positively correlated, but no relationship to clinical effects was found in hospitalized patients (ACKENHEIL et al. 1976). SIMPSON and COOPER (1978) provided anecdotal evidence that clozapine-induced convulsions may be more likely in patients with high plasma levels. SIMPSON et al. (1978) in a detailed and well designed clinical study compared the kinetics of oral and intramuscular loxapine. In a first stage the authors determined an individual critical single dose (ICD) for every patient. The ICD was then administered for 12 days either i. m. or p. o. The mean i. m. ICD did not differ from the mean p. o. ICD. Plasma levels of 8-OH-loxapine and 8-OH-amoxapine, however, were higher with the oral than the intramuscular form. Single dose kinetics repeated after 1 year in the same patients showed only slight differences. Under multiple dosage a greater AUC was found for intramuscular than for oral administration; this, however, did not refer to the hydroxilated metabolites. Clinical effects were similar with both preparation.

D. Pharmacokinetics of Butyrophenones in Man

The determination of butyrophenones in plasma under therapeutic conditions requires very sensitive methods (FORSMAN et al., 1974; CLARK et al., 1977). These analytic methods are suitable for calculation of kinetic parameters after single dose administration of the drug. As to haloperidol, elimination from plasma according to first-order kinetics could be established with a V_d of 17.3–29.8 liter/kg and $t_{1/2}$ of 12.6–23 h (FORSMAN et al., 1974; FORSMAN and ÖHMAN, 1975), or 12.8–35.5 h. (CRESSMAN et al., 1974), resp. The bioavailability of oral haloperidol amounted to 50%.

Steady state serum levels ranging from 0.5 to 9.5 ng/ml in 37 patients were roughly correlated to the daily dose per kg. CRESSMAN et al. (1974) from his studies with [^{3}H]-labeled haloperidol in normal volunteers predicted that it would take approx. 3–5 days to achieve the steady state level under a tid dosage regimen.

The steady state plasma levels of haloperidol reported by MARCUCCI et al. (1971) seem to be too high as compared to other authors. Only CLARK et al. (1977) and COUTSELINIS et al. (1977) found also rather high blood levels though with oral doses up to 200 mg daily, or in acute intoxications.

Penfluridol plasma levels after 4 weeks treatment showed a tenfold variation in 47 patients (JACOBSSON et al., 1976), and no correlation to clinical effects could be established. Penfluridol, a long-acting butyrophenone, has been reported to produce high blood levels, even on the 3 th day after oral administration (MJÖRNDAL et al., 1974, quoted from JACOBSSON et al., 1976).

The binding of haloperidol to human plasma and corpuscular elements of blood such as RBC was studied by FORSMAN (1976), and FORSMAN and ÖHMAN (1977). Within the range of 0.5–20 ng/ml a protein binding of 92% was calculated from studies with either equilibrium dialysis or ultrafiltration. HUGHES et al. (1976) suggest that the "cellular compartment of blood as well as the plasma compartment may act as a

12-36 h.

sink for haloperidol." As higher the free fraction in plasma as more drug is taken up by the RBC or other cellular elements.

Concomitant administration of antiparkinsonian drugs may reduce the plasma level of penfluridol without significantly changing the clinical effect (Chouinard et al., 1977).

References

Ackenheil, M., Hippius, H.: Clozapine. In: Psychotherapeutic drugs. Usdin, E., Forrest, I.S. (eds.), Part II, pp. 924–956. New York, Basel: Dekker 1977

Ackenheil, M., Brau, H., Burkhart, A., Franke, A., Pacha, W.: Antipsychotic effectiveness in relation to plasma level of clozapine. Arzneim. Forsch./Drug Res. *26*, 1156–1158 (1976)

Alfredsson, G., Woge-Helgodt, B., Sedvall, G.: A mass fragmentographic method for the determination of chlorpromazine and two of its active metabolites in human plasma and CSF. Psychopharmacology *48*, 123–131 (1976)

Axelsson, R.: On the pharmacokinetics of thioridazine in psychiatric patients. In: Antipsychotic drugs: Pharmacodynamics and pharmacokinetics. Sedvall, G., et al. (eds.), pp. 353–358. Oxford: Pergamon Press 1975

Axelsson, R., Martensson, E.: Serum concentration and elimination from serum of thioridazine in psychiatric patients. Curr. Ther. Res. *19*, 242–265 (1976)

Axelsson, S., Jönsson, S., Nordgren, L.: Cerebrospinal fluid levels of chlorpromazine and its metabolites in schizophrenia. Arch. Psychiatr. Nervenkr. *221*, 167–170 (1975)

Belpaire, F.M., Vanderheeren, F.A., Bogaert, M.G.: Binding of thioridazine and some of its metabolites to human serum protein and human albumin. Arzneim. Forsch./Drug Res. *25*, 1969–1971 (1975)

Bergling, R., Mjörndal, T., Oreland, L., Rapp, U., Wold, S.: Plasma levels and clinical effects of thioridazine and thiothixene. J. Clin. Pharmacol. *15*, 178–186 (1975)

Bickel, M.H.: Binding of chlorpromazine and imipramine to red cells, albumin, lipoproteins and other blood components. J. Pharm. Pharmacol. *27*, 733–738 (1976)

Breyer, U., Villumsen, K.: Measurement of plasma levels of tricyclic psychoactive drugs and their metabolites by UV reflectance photometry of thin layer chromatograms. Eur. J. Clin. Pharmacol. *9*, 457–465 (1976)

Breyer, U., Petruch, F., Gaertner, H.J., Pflug, B.: Dünnschichtchromatographische Bestimmung von Plasmaspiegeln tricyklischer Psychopharmaka. Arzneim. Forsch./Drug Res. *26*, 1153 (1976)

Brinkschulte, M., Jahns, I., Breyer-Pfaff, U.: A method for measuring plasma protein binding of tricyclic psychoactive drugs at therapeutic levels. 11th Spring Meeting of the German Pharmacological Society, Mainz 1978

Burrell, C.D.: Phenothiazines with piperidine side chains. In: Psychotherapeutic drugs. Usdin, E., Forrest, I.S. (eds.), Part II, pp. 795–826. New York: Dekker 1977

Buyze, G., Egberts, P.F.C., Musze, R.G., Poslavsky, A.: Blood levels of thioridazine and some of its metabolites in psychiatric patients. A preliminary report. Psychiatr. Neurol. Neurochir. *76*, 229–239 (1973)

Carr, C.J.: Metabolic studies on psychoactive drugs. Ann. N.Y. Acad. Sci. *96*, 170 (1962)

Chan, T.L., Sakalis, G., Gershon, S.: Quantitation of chlorpromazine and its metabolites in human plasma and urine by direct spectrodensitometry of thin-layer chromatograms. In: The phenothiazines and structurally related drugs. Forrest, I.S., Carr, C.J., Usdin, E. (eds.), pp. 323–333. New York: Raven Press 1974

Chouinard, G., Annable, L., Cooper, S.: Antiparkinsonian drug administration and plasma levels of penfluridol. A new long-acting neuroleptic. Comm. Psychopharmacol. *1*, 325–332 (1977)

Christoph, G.W., Schmidt, D.E., Davis, J.M., Janowsky, D.S.: A method for determination of chlorpromazine in human blood serum. Clin. Chim. Acta *38*, 265 (1972)

Clark, B.R., Tower, B.B., Rubin, R.T.: Radioimmunoassay of haloperidol in human serum. Life Sci. *20*, 319–325 (1977)

Clark, M.L., Kaul, P.N.: A preliminary report on clinical response and blood levels of chlorpromazine and its sulfoxide during chlorpromazine therapy in chronic schizophrenic patients. Psychopharmacol. Bull. *11*, 28–30 (1975)

Clark, M.L., Kaul, P.N.: A preliminary report on clinical response and blood levels of chlorpromazine and its sulfoxide during chlorpromazine therapy in chronic schizophrenic patients. In: Pharmacokinetics of psychoactive drugs. Gottschalk, L.A., Merlis, S. (eds.), pp. 191–197. New York: Spectrum Publications 1976

Cooper, S.F., Albert, J.-M., Hillel, J., Caille, G.: Plasmalevel studies of chlorpromazine following the administration of chlorpromazine hydrochloride and chlorpromazine embonate in chronic schizophrenics. Curr. Ther. Res. *15*, 73–77 (1973)

Cooper, S.F., Albert, J.-M., Dugal, R., Bertrand, M.: Separation of perphenazine, its sulphoxide and its probable phenolic metabolites by electron-capture gas-liquid chromatography. J. Chromatogr. *150*, 263–265 (1978)

Cooper, T.B., Simpson, G.M., Haber, E.J., Bergner, E.-E.E.: Butaperazine pharmacokinetics. Effect of dosage regimen on steady state blood levels. Arch. Gen. Psychiatry *32*, 903–905 (1975)

Coutselinis, A., Boukis, D., Kentarchou, P.: Haloperidol concentrations in blood in cases of acute intoxication (letter). Clin. Chem. *23*, 900 (1977)

Cowen, M.A., Martin, W.C.: Long-term chlorpromazine retention and its modification by steroids. Am. J. Psychiatry *125*, 243 (1968)

Cressman, W.A., Bianchine, J.R., Slotnick, V.B., Johnson, P.C., Plostnieks, J.: Plasma level profile of haloperidol in man following intramuscular administration. Eur. J. Clin. Pharmacol. *7*, 99–103 (1974)

Curry, S.H.: Method for the estimation of nanogram quantities of chlorpromazine and some of its relatively monopolar metabolites in plasma using gas chromatography with an electron capture detector. Anal. Chem. *40*, 1251 (1968)

Curry, S.H.: Plasma protein binding of chlorpromazine. J. Pharm. Pharmacol. *22*, 193–197 (1972)

Curry, S.H.: Metabolism and kinetics of chlorpromazine in relation to effect. In: Antipsychotic Drugs: Pharmacodynamics and Pharmacokinetics. Sedvall, G., Uvnäs, B., Zottermann, Y. (eds.), pp. 343–352. New York: Pergamon Press 1975

Curry, S.H.: Gas-chromatographic methods for the study of chlorpromazine and some of its metabolites in human plasma. Psychopharmacol. Commun. *2*, 1–15 (1976)

Curry, S.H., Mould, G.H.: Gas chromatographic identification of thioridazine in plasma and method for routine assay of the drug. J. Pharm. Pharmacol. *21*, 674–677 (1969)

Curry, S.H., Evans, S.: Assay of 7-hydroxychlorpromazine, and failure to detect more than small quantities, in plasma of responding schizophrenics. Psychopharmacol. Commun. *1*, 481–490 (1975)

Curry, S.H., Davis, J.M., Janowsky, D.S., Marshall, J.H.L.: Factors affecting chlorpromazine plasma levels in psychiatric patients. Arch. Gen. Psychiatry *22*, 209 (1970)

Curry, S.H., Whelpton, R., Schepper, P.J., de, Vranckx, S., Schiff, A.A.: Kinetics of fluphenazine after fluphenazine dihydrochloride, enanthate and decanoate administration to man. Br. J. Clin. Pharmacol. *7*, 325–331 (1979)

Dahl, S.G., Strandjord, R.E.: Pharmacokinetics of chlorpromazine after single and chronic dosage. Clin. Pharmacol. Ther. *21*, 437–448 (1977)

Dahl, S.G., Strandjord, R.E., Sigfusson, S.: Pharmacokinetics and relative bioavailability of levomepromazine after repeated administration of tablets and syrup. Eur. J. Clin. Pharmacol. *11*, 305–310 (1977)

Davis, J.M., Janowsky, D.S., Sekerke, H.J., Manier, H., El-Yousef, M.K.: The pharmacokinetics of butaperazine in serum. Adv. Biochem. Psychopharmacol. *9*, 433–443 (1974)

Davis, C.M., Meyer, C.J., Fenimore, D.C.: Improved gas chromatographic analysis of chlorpromazine in blood serum. Clin. Chim. Acta *78*, 71–77 (1977)

Dekirmenjian, H., Javaid, J.I., Duslak, B., Davis, J.M.: Determination of antipsychotic drugs by gas-liquid chromatography with a nitrogen detector using a simple acetylation technique. J. Chromatogr. *160*, 291–296 (1978)

Dencker, S.J., Johansson, R., Lindberg, D.: Correlation between plasma level and clinical response in manic psychotics given high dose fluphenazine enanthate. Acta Psychiatr. Scand. [Suppl.] *265*, 22–23 (1976)

Dollery, C.T.: Pharmacokinetics – Master or servant? Eur. J. Clin. Pharmacol. *6*, 1 (1973)

Efron, D.H., Harris, S.R., Manian, A.A., Gandette, L.G.: Radioassay of chlorpromazine and its metabolites in plasma. Psychopharmacologia *19*, 207–223 (1971)

Eiduson, S., Geller, E.: The excretion and metabolism of ^{35}S-labelled thioridazine in urine, blood, bile and feces. Biochem. Pharmacol. *12*, 1429–1435 (1963)

Elfernik, J.G.: The asymmetric distribution of chlorpromazine and its quaternary analogue over the erythrocyte membrane. Biochem. Pharmacol. *26*, 2411–2416 (1978)

El-Yousef, M.K., Manier, D.H.: Letter: Tricyclic antidepressants and phenothiazines. JAMA *229*, 1419 (1974a)

El-Yousef, M.K., Manier, D.H.: Letter: Estrogen effects on phenothiazine derivative blood levels. JAMA *228*, 827–828 (1974b)

El-Yousef, M.K., Manier, D.H.: Letter: The effect of benztropine mesylate on plasma levels of butaperazine maleate. Am. J. Psychiatry *131*, 471–472 (1974c)

El-Yousef, M.K., Manier, D.H.: Effects on conjugated estrogens on plasma butaperazine levels. Psychopharmacologia *39*, 39–41 (1974d)

Fann, W.F., Davis, J.M., Janowsky, D.S., Sekerke, H.J., Schmidt, D.M.: Chlorpromazine: Effects of antacids on its gastrointestinal absorption. J. Clin. Pharmacol. *13*, 388 (1973)

Flint, D.R., Ferullo, C.R., Levandovski, P., Hwang, B.: More sensitive gas chromatographic measurement of chlorpromazine in plasma. Clin. Chem. *17*, 830–835 (1971)

Forrest, I.S., Kanter, S.K., Sperco, J.E., Wechsler, M.B.: A comprehensive determination of thioridazine and its metabolites in urine. Am. J. Psychiatry *121*, 1049–1053 (1965)

Forrest, I.S., Forrest, F.M., Bolt, A.G., Serra, M.T.: An attempt to correlate urinary chlorpromazine excretion with clinical response to drug therapy. In: Proceedings of the Vth International Congress of Neuropsychopharmacology. Cole, J.O., Deniker, P., Hippius, H., Bradley, P.B. (eds.). Amsterdam: Excerpta Medica 1967

Forrest, I.M., Forrest, F.M., Serra, M.T.: Chlorpromazine retention. Am. J. Psychiatry *118*, 300–307 (1969)

Forrest, F.M., Forrest, I.S., Serra, M.T.: Modification of chlorpromazine metabolism by some other drugs frequently administered to psychiatric patients. Biol. Psychiatry *2*, 53–58 (1970)

Forrest, F.M., Forrest, I.S., Finkle, B.S.: Alcohol-chlorpromazine interaction in psychiatric patients. Agressologie *13*, 67–74 (1972)

Forsman, A.O.: Individual variability in response to haloperidol. Proc. R. Soc. Med. *69*, Suppl. 1, 9–12 (1976)

Forsman, A., Öhman, R.: Some aspects of the distribution and metabolism of haloperidol in man. In: Antipsychotic drugs: Pharmacodynamics and pharmacokinetics. Sedvall, G., Uvnäs, B., Zotterman, Y. (eds.), pp. 359–365. Oxford, New York, Toronto, Sydney, Paris, Frankfurt: Pergamon Press 1975

Forsman, A., Öhman, R.: Studies on serum protein binding of haloperidol. Curr. Ther. Res. *21*, 245–255 (1977)

Forsman, A., Martensson, E., Nyberg, G., Öhman, R.: A gas chromatographic method for determining haloperidol. A sensitive procedure for studying serum concentration and pharmacokinetics of haloperidol in patients. Naunyn Schmiedeberg's Arch. Pharmacol. *286*, 113–124 (1974)

Franklin, M., Wiles, D.H., Harvey, D.J.: Sensitive gas-chromatographic determination of fluphenazine in human plasma. Clin. Chem. *24*, 41–44 (1978)

Gabay, S., Huang, P.C.: The binding behavior of phenothiazines and structurally related compounds to albumin from several species. In: The phenothiazines and structurally related drugs. Forrest, I.S., Carr, C.J., Usdin, E. (eds.), pp. 175–189. New York: Raven Press 1974

Garver, D.L., Davis, J.M., Dekirmenjian, H., Jones, F.D., Casper, R., Haraszti, J.: Pharmacokinetics of red blood cell phenothiazine and clinical effects. Arch. Gen. Psychiatry *33*, 862–866 (1976)

Garver, D.L., Dekirmenjian, H., Davis, J.M., Casper, R., Ericksen, S.: Neuroleptic drug levels and therapeutic response: preliminary observations with red blood cell-bound butaperazine. Am. J. Psychiatry *134*, 304–307 (1977)

Gautier, J., Jus, A., Villeneuve, A., Jus, K., Pires, P., Villeneuve, R.: Influence of the antiparkinsonian drugs on the plasma level of neuroleptics. Biol. Psychiatry *12*, 389–399 (1977)

Gottschalk, L.A.: A preliminary approach to the problems of relating the pharmacokinetics of phenothiazines to clinical response with schizophrenic patients. Psychopharmacol. Bull. *14*, 35–39 (1978)

Gottschalk, L.A., Biener, R., Noble, E.P., Birch, H., Wilbert, D.E., Heiser, J.F.: Thioridazine plasma levels and clinical response. Compr. Psychiatry 16, 323–337 (1975a)

Gottschalk, L.A., Dinovo, E., Biener, R.: Plasma levels of mesoridazine and its metabolites and clinical response in acute schizophrenia after a single intramuscular drug dose. Psychopharmacol. Bull. 11, 33–34 (1975b)

Gottschalk, L.A., Dinovo, E., Biener, R., Birch, H., Syben, M., Noble, E.P.: Plasma levels of mesoridazine and its metabolites and clinical response in acute schizophrenia after a single intramuscular drug dose. In: Pharmacokinetics of psychoactive drugs. Gottschalk, L.A., Merlis, S. (eds.), pp. 171–189. New York: Spectrum Publications 1976

Gottschalk, L.A., Dinovo, E., Biener, R., Nandi, B.R.: Plasma concentrations of thioridazine metabolites and ECG abnormalities. J. Pharm. Sci. 67, 155–157 (1978)

Gruenke, L.D., Craig, J.C., Dinovo, E.: Identification of a metabolite of thioridazine and mesoridazine from human plasma. Res. Commun. Chem. Pathol. Pharmacol. 10, 221–225 (1975)

Hammar, C.G., Holmstedt, B.: Mass fragmentography: Identification of chlorpromazine and its metabolites in human blood by a new method. Anal. Biochem. 25, 532–548 (1968)

Hansen, C.E., Kragh-Sørensen, P.: Clinical-pharmacological aspects of measuring perphenazine in human blood. Acta Psychiatr. Scand. [Suppl.] 246, 18–22 (1973)

Hansen, C.E., Larsen, N.E.: Perphenazine concentrations in human whole blood. Psychopharmacologia (Berl.) 37, 31–36 (1974)

Hansen, C.E., Christensen, R.T., Elley, J., Hansen, B.L., Kragh-Sørensen, P., Larsen, N.E., Naestoff, J., Hvidberg, E.F.: Clinical pharmacokinetic studies of perphenazine. Br. J. Clin. Pharmacol. 3, 915–923 (1976)

Hansen, L.B., Larsen, N.E.: Plasma concentrations of perphenazine and its sulphoxide metabolite during continuous oral treatment. Psychopharmacology 53, 127–130 (1977)

Hollister, L.E., Kanter, S.L., Wright, A.: Comparison of intramuscular and oral administration of chlorpromazine and thioridazine. Arch. Int. Pharmacodyn. Ther. 144, 571–578 (1963)

Hollister, L.E., Curry, S.H., Derr, J.E., Kanter, S.L.: Studies of delayed-action medication. V. Plasma levels and urinary excretion of four different dosage forms of chlorpromazine. Clin. Pharmacol. Ther. 11, 49–59 (1970)

Huang, C.L., Kurland, A.A.: Chlorpromazine blood level in psychotic patients. Arch. Gen. Psychiatry 5, 509–513 (1961)

Huang, C.L., Ruskin, B.H.: Determination of serum chlorpromazine metabolites in psychiatric patients. J. Nerv. Ment. Dis. 139, 381–386 (1964)

Hughes, I.E., Jellett, L.B., Ilett, K.F.: The influence of various factors in the in vitro distribution of haloperidol in human blood. Br. J. Clin. Pharmacol. 3, 285–288 (1976)

Jacobsson, I., Knorring, L. von, Mattson, B., Mjörndal, T., Oreland, L., Perris, C., Rapp, W., Edenius, B., Kettner, B., Magnusson, K.E., Villemoes, P.: Penfluridol and thiothixene. Dosage, plasma levels and changes in psychopathology. Int. Pharmacopsychiatry 11, 206–214 (1976)

Jähnchen, E., Krieglstein, J., Kuschinsky, G.: Die Bedeutung der Benzolringe bei der Eiweißbindung von Promazin und Chlorpromazin. Naunyn Schmiedeberg's Arch. Pharmacol. Exp. Pathol. 263, 375–386 (1969)

Johansson, R., Borg, K.O., Gabrielsson, M.: Determination of fluphenazine in plasma by ionpair partition chromatography. Acta Pharm. Suec. 13, 193–200 (1976)

Jonghe, F.E. de, Helm, H.J. van der: Plasma concentrations of thioridazine in patients with depression. Acta Psychiatr. Scand. 46, 360–364 (1970)

Jonghe, F.E. de, Helm, H.J. van der, Schalken, H.F., Thiel, J.H.: Therapeutic effect and plasma level of thioridazine. Acta Psychiatr. Scand. 49, 535–545 (1973)

Jørgensen, A., Gottfries, C.G.: Pharmacokinetic studies on flupenthixol and flupenthixol decanoate in man using tritium labelled compounds. Psychopharmacologia 27, 1–10 (1972)

Jørgensen, A., Hansen, V., Larsen, U.D., Khan, A.R.: Metabolism, distribution and excretion of flupentixol. Acta Pharmacol. Toxicol. 27, 301–313 (1969)

Kaul, P.N., Conway, M.W., Ticku, M.K., Clark, M.L.: Chlorpromazine metabolism II: Determination of nonconjugated metabolites in blood of schizophrenic patients. J. Pharm. Sci. 61, 581 (1972)

Kaul, P.N., Conway, M.W., Ticku, M.K., Clark, M.L.: Chlorpromazine metabolism. III. Determination of conjugated metabolites in the blood of schizophrenic patients. J. Lab. Clin. Med. 81, 467 (1973)

Kaul, P.N., Whitfield, L.R., Clark, M.L.: Chlorpromazine metabolism VIII: Blood levels of chlorpromazine and its sulfoxide in schizophrenic patients. J. Pharm. Sci. *65*, 694–697 (1976)

Kelsey, M.I., Moscatelli, E.A.: Gas-liquid chromatographic analysis of phenolic and non-phenolic chlorpromazine metabolites in the urine of chronic schizophrenic patients. J. Chromatogr. *85*, 65–74 (1974)

Kelsey, M.I., Keskiner, A., Moscatelli, E.A.: Gas-liquid chromatographic analysis of fluphenazine and fluphenazine sulfoxide in the urine of chronic schizophrenic patients. J. Chromatogr. *75*, 294–297 (1973)

Knapp, D.R., Gaffney, T.E.: Use of stable isotopes in pharmacology-clinical pharmacology. Clin. Pharmacol. Ther. *13*, 307–316 (1972)

Knoll, R., Christ, W., Müller-Oerlinghausen, B., Coper, H.: Formation of chlorpromazine sulphoxide and monodesmethylchlorpromazine by microsomes of small intestine. Naunyn Schmiedeberg's Arch. Pharmacol. *297*, 195–200 (1977)

Kolakowska, T., Wiles, D.H., McNeilly, A.S., Gelder, M.G.: Correlation between plasma levels of prolactin and chlorpromazine in psychiatric patients. Psychol. Med. *5*, 214–216 (1975)

Kolakowska, T., Wiles, D.H., Gelder, M.G., McNeilly, A.S.: Clinical significance of plasma chlorpromazine levels. II. Plasma levels of the drug, some of its metabolites and prolactin in patients receiving long-term phenothiazine treatment. Psychopharmacol. Bull. *49*, 101–107 (1976)

Kragh-Sørensen, P., Larsen, N., Hansen, C.E., Naestoft, J.: Gas-chromatographic measurement of perphenazine in whole blood. Acta Psychiatr. Scand. [Suppl.] *246*, 15–17 (1973)

Lacoursiere, R.B., Spohn, H.E.: How long does chlorpromazine last? J. Nerv. Ment. Dis. *163*, 267–275 (1976)

Lader, M.: Monitoring plasma concentrations of neuroleptics. Pharmakopsychiatr. Neuropsychopharmacol. *9*, 170–177 (1976)

Larsen, N.E., Naestoft, J.: Determination of perphenazine and fluphenazine in whole blood by gas-chromatography. Med. Lab. Technol. *30*, 129–132 (1973)

Larsen, N.E., Naestoft, J.: Determination of perphenazine and its sulphoxide metabolite in human plasma after therapeutic doses by gas-chromatography. J. Chromatogr. *109*, 259–264 (1975)

Lehr, R.E., Kaul, P.N.: Chlorpromazine metabolism. IV: Quaternization as a key to determination of picomoles of chlorpromazine and other tertiary amine drugs. J. Pharm. Sci. *64*, 950–953 (1975)

Linnoila, M., Otterstroem, S., Anttila, M.: Serum chlordiazepoxide, diazepam and thioridazine concentrations after the simultaneous ingestion of alcohol or placebo drink. Ann. Clin. Res. *6*, 4–6 (1974)

Loga, S., Curry, S., Lader, M.: Interactions of orphenadrine and phenobarbitone with chlorpromazine: Plasma concentrations and effects in man. Br. J. Clin. Pharmacol. *2*, 197–208 (1975)

Mackay, A.V.P.: Assay of 7-hydroxychlorpromazine, and failure to detect more than small quantities, in plasma of responding schizophrenics – reply. Psychopharmacol. Commun. *1*, 491–492 (1975)

Manian, A.A., Piette, L.H., Holland, D., Grover, T., Leterrier, F.: Red blood cell drug binding as a possible mechanism for tranquilization. In: The phenothiazines and structurally related drugs. Forrest, I.S. et al. (eds.). New York: Raven Press 1974

Manier, D.H., Sekerke, J., Dingell, J.V., El-Yousef, M.K.: A fluorometric method for the measurement of butaperazine in human plasma. Clin. Chim. Acta *57*, 225–230 (1974)

March, J.E., Donato, D., Turano, P., Turner, W.J.: Interpatient variation and significance of plasma levels of chlorpromazine in psychotic patients. J. Med. *3*, 146–162 (1972)

Marcucci, F., Mussini, E., Airoldi, L., Fanelli, R., Frigerio, A., Nadai, F. de, Bizzi, F., Rizzo, M., Morselli, P.L., Garattini, S.: Analytical and pharmacokinetic studies on butyrophenones. Clin. Chim. Acta *34*, 321–332 (1971)

Martensson, E., Ross, B.E.: Serum levels of thioridazine in psychiatric patients and healthy volunteers. Eur. J. Clin. Pharmacol. *6*, 181 (1973)

Mattsson, B., Mjörndal, T., Oreland, L.: Plasma levels of chlorprothixene in alcoholics. Acta Psychiatr. Scand. [Suppl.] *255*, 71–74 (1974)

May, P.R.A., Putten, T. van: Plasma levels of chlorpromazine in schizophrenia. Arch. Gen. Psychiatry *35*, 1081–1087 (1978)

May, P.R.A., Putten, T. van, Jenden, D.J., Cho, A.K.: Test dose response in schizophrenia. Arch. Gen. Psychiatry *35*, 1091–1097 (1978)

Maxwell, J.D., Carrella, M., Parky, J.D., Williams, R., Mould, G.P., Curry, S.H.: Plasma disappearance and cerebral effects of chlorpromazine in cirrhosis. Clin. Sci. *43*, 143–151 (1972)

Mellinger, T.J., Mellinger, E.M., Smith, W.T.: Thioridazine blood levels in patients receiving different oral forms. Clin. Pharmacol. Ther. *6*, 486–491 (1965)

Müller-Oerlinghausen, B.: Bedeutung der Pharmakokinetik für die Therapie mit Antidepressiva. Pharmakopsychiatr. Neuropsychopharmakol. *11*, 55–62 (1978)

Müller-Oerlinghausen, B., Riedel, E., Schley, J.: Thin-layer and gas-liquid chromatographic procedures for the determination of perazine and its metabolites in human body fluids. Int. J. Clin. Pharmacol. *15*, 366–372 (1977)

Muusze, R.G.: Analysis of thioridazine and some of its metabolites in blood by liquid chromatography. Thesis, Amsterdam (1975)

Muusze, R.G., Vanderheeren, F.A.: Plasma levels and half lives of thioridazine and some of its metabolites. II. Low doses in older psychiatric patients. Eur. J. Clin. Pharmacol. *11*, 141–147 (1977)

Muusze, R.G., Huber, J.F.K.: Determination of the psychotropic drug thioridazine and its metabolites in blood by means of high pressure liquid chromatography in combination with fluorometric reaction detection. J. Chromatogr. Sci. *12*, 779–787 (1974)

Neve, H.K.: The excretion of thioridazine (Melleril, TP 21) in urine. Acta Pharmacol. Toxicol. *17*, 404–409 (1960)

Nikitopoulou, G., Thorner, M., Crammer, J., Lader, M.: Prolactin and psychophysiologic measures after single doses of thioridazine. Clin. Pharmacol. Ther. *21*, 422–429 (1977)

Nyberg, G., Axelsson, R., Martensson, E.: Binding of thioridazine and thioridazine metabolites to serum proteins in psychiatric patients. Eur. J. Clin. Pharmacol. *14*, 341–350 (1978)

Pacha, W.L.: A method for the fluorometric determination of thioridazine or mesoridazine in plasma. Experientia *25*, 103–104 (1969)

Perel, J.M., Manian, A.A.: Pharmacokinetics of therapeutic and toxic reactions: I. Phenothiazines. Neurotoxicology *1*, 9–13 (1977)

Philipson, O.T., McKeown, J.M., Baker, J., Healey, A.F.: Correlation between plasma chlorpromazine and its metabolites and clinical ratings in patients with acute relapse of schizophrenic and paranoid psychosis. Br. J. Psychiatry *131*, 172–184 (1977)

Pietzcker, A., Müller-Oerlinghausen, B., Schley, J., Chaskel, R., Poppenberg, A., Urban, R.: Beziehungen zwischen Serumkonzentration und klinischen Befunden bei langfristig mit Perazin behandelten schizophrenen Patienten. Arzneim. Forsch./Drug Res. *28*, 1302–1303 (1978)

Ragland, J.B., Kinross-Wright, V.J., Ragland, R.: Determinations of phenothiazines in biological samples. Anal. Biochem. *12*, 60–69 (1965)

Rivera-Calimlim, L., Siracusa, A.: Plasma assay of fluphenazine. Commun. Psychopharmacol. *1*, 233–242 (1977)

Rivera-Calimlim, L., Castaneda, L., Lasagna, L.: Effects of mode of management on plasma chlorpromazine in psychiatric patients. Clin. Pharmacol. Ther. *14*, 978–981 (1973)

Rivera-Calimlim, L., Nasrallah, H., Strauss, J., Lasagna, L.: Clinical response and plasma levels: Effect of dose, dosage schedules, and drug interaction on plasma chlorpromazin levels. Am. J. Psychiatry *133*, 646–652 (1976)

Rivera-Calimlim, L., Kerzner, B., Karch, F.E.: Effect of lithium on plasma chlorpromazine levels. Clin. Pharmacol. Ther. *23*, 451–455 (1978)

Sakalis, G., Curry, S.H., Mould, G.P., Lader, M.H.: Physiologic and clinical effects of chlorpromazine and their relationship to plasma level. Clin. Pharmacol. Ther. *13*, 931–946 (1972)

Sakalis, G., Chan, T.L., Gershon, S., Park, S.: The possible role of metabolites in therapeutic response to chlorpromazine treatment. Psychopharmacologia (Berl.) *32*, 279–284 (1973)

Sakalis, G., Chan, T.L., Sathananthan, G., Schooler, N., Goldberg, S., Gershon, S.: Relationships among clinical response, extrapyramidal syndrome and plasma chlorpromazine and metabolite ratios. Commun. Psychopharmacol. *1*, 157–166 (1977)

Sakurai, Y., Nakahara, T., Takahashi, R.: Prediction of response to chlorpromazine treatment in schizophrenics. Psychopharmacologia (Berl.) *44*, 195–203 (1975)

Schley, J., Riedel, E., Müller-Oerlinghausen, B.: Determination of perazine serum levels by gas liquid chromatography under clinical routine conditions. J. Clin. Chem. Clin. Biochem. *16*, 307–311 (1978)

Schley, J., Nündel, M., Riedel, E., Müller-Oerlinghausen, B.: Eine spezifische Serumproteinbindung des Neuroleptikums Perazin. Arzneim. Forsch./Drug Res. *29*, 106–108 (1979)

Schley, J.: Zur spezifischen Bindung des Neuroleptikums Perazin an Serumproteine. Naunyn-Schmiedeberg's Arch. Pharmacol. *307*, (Suppl.) R 70 (1979)

Schooler, N.R., Sakalis, G., Chan, T.L: Chlorpromazine metabolism and clinical response in acute schizophrenia: A preliminary report. Psychopharmacol. Bull. *11*, 30–33 (1975)

Schooler, N.R., Sakalis, G., Chan, T.L., Gershon, S., Goldberg, S.C., Collins, P.: Chlorpromazine metabolism and clinical response in acute schizophrenia: A preliminary report. In: Pharmacokinetics of psychoactive drugs: Blood levels and clinical response. Gottschalk, L.A., Merlis, S. (eds.), pp. 199–219. New York: Spectrum Publications 1976

Sharples, D.: The binding of chlorpromazine to human serum albumin. J. Pharm. Pharmacol. *26*, 640–641 (1975)

Simpson, G.M., Cooper, T.A.: Clozapine plasma levels and convulsions. Am. J. Psychiatry *135*, 99–100 (1978)

Simpson, G.M., Varga, E., Reiss, M. Cooper, T.B., Bergner, E.E., Lee, J.H.: Bioequivalency of generic and brand-named chlorpromazine. Clin. Pharmacol. Ther. *15*, 631–641 (1974)

Simpson, G.M., Cooper, T.B., Lee, J.H., Young, M.A.: Clinical and plasma level characteristics of intramuscular and oral loxapine. Psychopharmacology *56*, 225–232 (1978)

Smith, R.C., Dekirmenjian, H., Davis, J.M., Crayton, J., Evans, H.: Plasma butaperazine levels in long-term chronic non-responding schizophrenics. Commun. Psychopharmacol. *1*, 319–324 (1977)

Smolen, V.F., Murdock, H.R. Jr., Stoltman, W.P., Clevenger, J.W., Combs, L.W., Williams, E.J.: Pharmacological response data for comparative bioavailability studies of chlorpromazine oral dosage forms in humans: I. Pupilometry. J. Clin. Pharmacol. *15*, 734–751 (1975a)

Smolen, V.F., Murdock, H.R. Jr., Williams, E.J.: Bioavailability analysis of chlorpromazine in humans from pupilometric data. J. Pharmacol. Exp. Ther. *195*, 404–415 (1975b)

Smulevitch, A.B., Minsker, E.I., Mazayeva, N.A., Volkova, R.P., Lukanina, S.K.: The problem of clinical activity of long-acting neuroleptics. Compr. Psychiatry *14*, 227–232 (1973)

Spector, S.: Development of antibodies to chlorpromazine. In: The phenothiazines and structurally related drugs. Forrest, I.S., Carr, C.J., Usdin, E. (eds.), pp. 363–364. New York: Raven Press 1974

Spirtes, M.A.: Artifactual contamination of control serum extracts in gas chromatopraphic analyses for chlorpromazine. Clin. Chem. *18*, 317–318 (1972)

Sugerman, A.A., Rosen, R.: Absorption efficiency and excretion profile of prolonged-action form of chlorpromazine. Clin. Pharmacol. *5*, 561–568 (1964)

Sved, S., Perales, A., Palaic, D.: Chlorpromazine metabolism in chronic schizophrenics. Br. J. Psychiatry *119*, 589–596 (1971)

Sved, S., Perales, A., Houle, H.-P.: Urinary excretion in drug excretion studies in chronic schizophrenics. Br. J. Psychiatry *120*, 219–222 (1972)

Swett, C.: Drowsiness due to chlorpromazine in relation to cigarette smoking. Arch. Gen. Psychiatry *31*, 211–213 (1974)

Traficante, L.J., Hine, B., Gershon, S., Sakalis, G.: Chloroquine potentiation of thioridazine effects in rats and drugresistent schizophrenic patients: A preliminary report. Commun. Psychopharmacol. *1*, 407–419 (1977)

Turano, P., Turner, W.J., Donato, D.: Further studies of chlorpromazine metabolism in schizophrenic men. In: The phenothiazines and structurally related drugs. Forrest, I.S., Carr, C.J., Usdin, E. (eds.), pp. 315–322. New York: Raven Press 1974

Turner, W.J., Turano, P., Badzinski, S.: An attempt to establish quality control in determination of plasma chlorpromazine by a multi-laboratory collaboration. In: Pharmacokinetics of psychoactive drugs: Blood levels and clinical response. Gottschalk, L.A., Merlis, S. (eds.), pp. 33–42. New York: Spectrum Publications 1976

Usdin, E.: The assay of chlorpromazine and metabolites in blood, urine and other tissues. CRC Crit. Rev. Clin. Lab. Sci. *2*, 347–391 (1971)

Vanderheeren, F.A., Theunis, D.J.: Gas-liquid chromatographic determination of perazine, thioridazine and thioridazine metabolites in human plasma. J. Chromatogr. *120*, 123–128 (1976)

Vanderheeren, F.A.J., Muusze, R.G.: Plasma levels and half lives of thioridazine and some of its metabolites. I. High doses in young acute schizophrenics. Eur. J. Clin. Pharmacol. *11*, 135–140 (1977)

Viala, A.: Pharmacokinetic profile of perphenazine enanthate. Encéphale *2*, 273–282 (1976)

Vranckx, C.H.: Pharmacokinetics of flupentixol decanoate. Acta Psychiatr. Belg. *74*, 529–532 (1974)

Wechsler, M., Wharton, R.N., Tanaka, E., Malitz, S.: Chlorpromazine metabolite pattern in psychotic patients. J. Psychiatr. Res. *5*, 327–333 (1967)

West, N., Vogel, W.H., Boehme, D.H., Gold, S.: Urinary excretion of chlorpromazine and chlorpromazine sulfoxide in four patients on different days. J. Pharm. Sci. *60*, 953–954 (1971)

West, N.R., Rosenblum, M.P., Springe, H., Gold, S., Boehme, D.H., Vogel, W.H.: Assay procedures for thioridazine, trifluoperazine, and their sulfoxides and determination of urinary excretion of these compounds in mental patients. J. Pharm. Sci. *63*, 417–420 (1974)

Whelpton, R., Curry, S.H.: Methods for study of fluphenazine kinetics in man. J. Pharm. Pharmacol. *28*, 869–873 (1976)

Wiles, D.H., Kolakowska, T., McNeilly, A.S., Mandelbrote, B.M., Gelder, M.G.: Clinical significance of plasma chlorpromazine levels. I. Plasma levels of the drug, some of its metabolites and prolactin during acute treatment. Psychol. Med. *6*, 407–415 (1976)

Wode-Helgodt, B., Borg, S., Fyrö, B., Sedvall, G.: Clinical effects and drug concentrations in plasma and cerebrospinal fluid in psychotic patients treated with fixed doses of chlorpromazine. Acta Psychiat. Scand. *58*, 149–173 (1978)

Zingales, I.A.: Detection of chlorpromazine and thioridazine metabolites in human erythrocytes. J. Chromatogr. *44*, 547–562 (1969

CHAPTER 13

Metabolism and Kinetics

U. Breyer-Pfaff

A. Introduction

Neuroleptic drugs act principally on the central nervous system. This implies that they are lipophilic compounds which easily penetrate membranes separating single body compartments from one another. As a consequence, their excretion will ordinarily be preceded by biotransformation to more hydrophilic substances, since otherwise binding to tissues and plasma proteins and renal tubular reabsorption would lead to an extremely long persistence in the body. Thus, metabolic transformations become limiting for the elimination of the majority of these drugs.

Another reason why the metabolism particularly of tricyclic neuroleptic drugs has attracted attention is that part of their biotransformation products are still lipophilic and produce pharmacologic effects similar to those of the parent compounds (for instance Nybäck and Sedvall, 1972; Palmer and Manian, 1976; Alfredsson et al., 1977). They must therefore be regarded as potentially active and possibly contributing to therapeutic and toxic effects of the drugs in man.

B. Phenothiazines and Thioxanthenes

I. Kinetics in Animals

1. Absorption

The kinetics of the tricyclic neuroleptics are governed by their strong binding to tissue structures and by a high hepatic clearance. Therefore, drug levels in extrahepatic tissues depend on the route of administration. This has been observed upon comparison of values in rats treated orally with prochlorperazine (Phillips and Miya, 1964), chlorpromazine (Curry et al., 1971), or trifluoperazine (Schmalzing, 1977) with those obtained after intravenous injection of the drugs. Incomplete absorption seems to occur only in animals given large doses per os (see below), such that the main reason for the reduction in availability must be sought in a first-pass effect. While at least with perazine (Breyer and Winne, 1977) and trifluoperazine (Schmalzing, 1977) the intestine plays a minor role, a high hepatic extraction has been measured for chlorpromazine (van Loon et al., 1964) and trifluoperazine (Schmalzing, 1977).

Data on the rate of absorption following oral administration of phenothiazines vary largely (Zehnder et al., 1962 a, b; Curry et al., 1971; Bruce et al., 1974; Schmalzing, 1977), possibly because the drugs influence gastric motility. Chlorpromazine absorption by rats was delayed when gastric emptying was inhibited (Rivera-Calimlim, 1976). Absorption from intramuscular or subcutaneous sites was retarded only when long-chain fatty esters of fluphenazine or flupenthixol were injected as solutions in oil (EBERT and HESS, 1965; JØRGENSEN et al., 1971; DREYFUSS et al., 1976 a, b).

2. Distribution

Autoradiography of mice, rats and cats given [^{35}S]-chlorpromazine i. v. revealed during the first hours preferential localization of ^{35}S in lung, liver, adrenals, kidney, and the wall and contents of the gastro-intestinal tract, while less radioactivity was present in the brain (SJÖSTRAND et al., 1965; IDÄNPÄÄN-HEIKKILÄ et al., 1968; LINDQUIST and ULLBERG, 1972). After 2 days, radioactivity was concentrated in melanin-containing structures and here it remained detectable until 90 days after dosage (LINDQUIST and ULLBERG, 1972).

Also, chemical and radiochemical analyses in animals given phenothiazines or thioxanthenes showed the highest drug concentrations in peripheral parenchymatous organs and clearly lower levels in brain (WALKENSTEIN and SEIFTER, 1959; ZEHNDER et al., 1962 a, b; PHILLIPS and MIYA, 1964; DREYFUSS et al., 1971; JØRGENSEN et al., 1971; WEST and VOGEL, 1975; SCHMALZING, 1977; BREYER et al., 1977).

Equilibrium concentrations in blood or plasma were conspicuously low; from data measured after i. v. injection of chlorpromazine (CURRY et al., 1970; KAWASHIMA et al., 1975 b), an apparent volume of distribution of 20–25 liter/kg can be determined, while for trifluoperazine the values are 8 (SPANO et al., 1970) and 12 liter/kg (SCHMAL-ZING, 1977), respectively.

Attempts to detect specific distribution patterns of neuroleptic drugs in brain and correlating them to their pharmacologic actions have not been successful in earlier studies utilizing compounds with low specific radioactivities and doses of 10 mg/kg or more (for a review see CASSANO and PLACIDI, 1969). Autoradiography revealed that brain areas containing grey matter became labeled much faster than those rich in white matter; at later times, slightly higher concentrations were observed in the hippocampus than in other regions (CASSANO and PLACIDI, 1969; ECKERT and HOPF, 1970). These findings were partly confirmed in a study using a chemical assay method (SANDERS, 1973). Comparison of the kinetic data with histologic, biochemical and physiological data on the various brain areas did not lead to an elucidation of the mechanisms governing drug distribution (ECKERT and HOPF, 1970).

Administration of highly labeled neuroleptics of other chemical classes in low doses to rats and mice led to the detection of a specific localization in certain brain areas (LADURON and LEYSEN, 1977; HÖLLT et al., 1977) (see below). It can be anticipated that under appropriate experimental conditions a similar behavior of tricyclic neuroleptics will be observed, particularly since binding studies in vitro disclosed high affinities towards dopamine and neuroleptic receptors (CREESE et al., 1976; SEEMAN et al., 1976; LEYSEN et al., 1978).

3. Elimination

Few studies are available in which the elimination kinetics of tricyclic neuroleptics from animal tissues have been measured by specific analytic techniques. Data obtained in rats are shown in Table 1; it also contains some results measured by procedures not entirely specific for the unchanged drugs.

From the short half-lives, in conjunction with high apparent volumes of distribution (see above), it can be calculated that the plasma clearance approximately equals liver blood flow. Thus, the elimination is dependent on liver perfusion (WILKINSON and SHAND, 1975). In rats given trifluoperazine i. v. or p. o., the hepatic extraction ratio has been found to be 0.78 (SCHMALZING, 1977).

Table 1. Elimination half-lives of phenothiazine and thioxanthene drugs from tissues of rats up to 6–16 h after injection

Drug	Route	Dose (mg/kg)	Specificity of method	Tissue	Half-life (h)	Reference
Chlorpromazine	i. p.	18	Limited	Brain	7.3	MAHJU and MAICKEL
				Plasma	9.1	(1969)
	i. p.	10	Limited	Brain	2.2	CURRY et al. (1970)
	i. v.	10	High	Plasma	2.8	
	i. v.	1.34	Limited	Brain	1.7	SPANO et al. (1970)
	i. v.	13.4	Limited	Brain	3.7	
	i. v.	10	High	Brain[a]	1.8	KAWASHIMA et al.
				Plasma	3.3	(1975a)
	i. v.	5	High	Brain[a]	1.5	KAWASHIMA et al.
				Serum	3.0	(1975b)
	i. v.	2	High	Brain[a]	1.5	
				Serum	2.0	
Triflupromazine	i. p.	13.6	Limited	Brain	4.3	MAHJU and MAICKEL
				Plasma	5.1	(1969)
Trifluoperazine	i. v.	1.7	Limited	Brain	1.6	SPANO et al. (1970)
	i. v.	17	Limited	Brain	2.0	
				Plasma	2.7	
	i. v.	5	High	Brain	2.5	SCHMALZING (1977)
				Plasma	3.1	
				Lung	2.5	
				Kidney	2.5	
Fluphenazine	i. p.	8.6	Limited	Brain	4.9	MAHJU and MAICKEL
				Plasma	5.8	(1969)
Thiothixene	i. p.	2	Limited	Brain	1.8	MJÖRNDAL et al. (1976)
				Plasma	2.7	

[a] Analysis of various brain parts

The relative contribution of urinary and fecal elimination to total excretion of the drugs and their metabolites depends on the species as well as on the molecular weight of the compounds. For instance, following administration of [^{14}C]-fluphenazine, total radioactivity in feces was about 28-fold that in urine in dogs, but only four-fold in rhesus monkeys (DREYFUSS et al., 1971) and baboons (DREYFUSS et al., 1972). In rabbits, guinea pigs, and rhesus monkeys radioactivity derived from [9-^{3}H]-chlorpromazine was predominantly excreted in urine, whereas after [9-^{3}H]-prochlorperazine administration fecal ^{3}H exceeded that in urine by factors of 2.5–7.0 (FORREST et al., 1974). Sampling had to be carried out for 7–14 days in order to obtain virtually complete excretion. This is at least partly due to entero-hepatic circulation (VAN LOON et al., 1964). Bile fistula animals rapidly excreted label derived from radioactive thioridazine (ZEHNDER et al., 1962 a), thiethylperazine (ZEHNDER et al., 1962 b), prochlorperazine, trifluoperazine (VAN LOON et al., 1964; SCHMALZING and BREYER, 1978), fluphenazine (DREYFUSS et al., 1971), and perazine (BREYER et al., 1977) into bile.

II. Extent of Biotransformation in Vivo

Phenothiazines and thioxanthenes are extensively metabolized in the mammalian organism. This results from the fact that the fraction of a drug dose excreted unchanged is usually small. Maximal quantities of 2% have been reported for various phenothiazines in the urine of psychiatric patients (SALZMAN and BRODIE, 1956; ROSE et al., 1964; KANIG and BREYER, 1969; WEST et al., 1974; DE LEENHEER, 1974). Even lower amounts were found in the urine of rats given thioridazine (ZEHNDER et al., 1962 a), fluphenazine enanthate (EBERT and HESS, 1965), butaperazine (BRUCE et al., 1974), or various other piperazine-substituted phenothiazines (GAERTNER et al., 1974; WEST and VOGEL, 1975). Fecal excretion of the unmetabolized drug was low in rats treated with fluphenazine enanthate subcutaneously (EBERT and HESS, 1965) or with low doses of trifluoperazine p. o. (WEST and VOGEL, 1975). Larger fractions of the dose (up to 36%) were excreted unchanged in the feces following administration of large oral doses of butaperazine (BRUCE et al., 1974) or trifluoperazine to rats (WEST and VOGEL, 1975) or of fluphenazine to dogs or monkeys (DREYFUSS et al., 1971).

III. Metabolic Pathways

1. Reactions at the Ring System

a) Oxidation of the Ring Sulfur

The addition of one oxygen atom to form a sulfoxide was the first metabolic transformation to be detected in a phenothiazine drug (SALZMAN et al., 1955), and it is one universally occurring in vivo in phenothiazines (for reviews see EMMERSON and MIYA, 1963; WILLIAMS and PARKE, 1964) and thioxanthenes (ALLGÉN et al., 1960; KHAN, 1969; JØRGENSEN et al., 1971). Though sulfoxidation can be measured in liver microsomal preparations (KAMM et al., 1958; COCCIA and WESTERFELD, 1967), its mechanism is not fully clarified; especially it is not known whether it is catalysed by cytochrome P-450 or exclusively by a heme-free iron-containing enzyme (PREMA and GOPINATHAN, 1976).

The validity of data concerning chlorpromazine sulfoxidation in blood (MINDER et al., 1971) and brain (GORROD et al., 1974) is uncertain since artifactual oxidation of the material has not been excluded. Sulfoxidation of phenothiazines easily takes place nonenzymatically (EMMERSON and MIYA, 1963).

In the intestinal mucosa, sulfoxidation seems to be a major biotransformation reaction as can be derived from studies with [35S]-chlorpromazine in guinea pig intestinal microsomes (KNOLL et al., 1977) and with [35S]-perazine in the rat jejunum in vivo (BREYER and WINNE, 1977).

Sulfoxides mainly occur as excretory products of phenothiazines. The presence of appreciable concentrations in tissues except blood is not well established since mostly nonspecific methods have been employed for their measurement (for a discussion see BREYER and SCHMALZING, 1977).

Further oxidation of the ring sulfur to the sulfone has been observed in the rat and in man with thioridazine (ZEHNDER et al., 1962 a; MÅRTENSSON et al., 1975) and with didemethylated chlorpromazine (BREYER-PFAFF et al., 1978).

Chemical oxidation or irradiation of solutions of phenothiazine drugs led to various species of radicals some of which were relatively stable even at neutral pH (PIETTE and FORREST, 1962; GOUCHER et al., 1975). Whether the enzyme inhibition exerted by irradiated chlorpromazine solutions is due to the semiquinone free radical (AKERA and BRODY, 1968) or to other photochemical products (GOUCHER et al., 1975) cannot yet be decided. The role of radicals as intermediates in various metabolic oxidations and as agents producing therapeutic or toxic effects (FORREST and FORREST, 1963) is still hypothetical.

b) Oxidation of Ring Carbon Atoms

The only identified metabolites resulting from this pathway are phenols and their conjugation products. Introduction of the first hydroxy group primarily takes place *para* to the ring nitrogen in the yet unsubstituted ring, i. e., in the 3-position in promazine (GOLDENBERG et al., 1964) and in the 7-position in chlorpromazine (FISHMAN and GOLDENBERG, 1963; GOLDENBERG and FISHMAN, 1964) and fluphenazine (DREYFUSS and COHEN, 1971). Minor amounts of 8-hydroxychlorpromazine and of the 3.7- and 7.8-dihydroxy metabolites have been identified in patient urine (TURANO et al., 1973).

Aromatic hydroxylation of various phenothiazines can be carried out in vitro with liver microsomes (COCCIA and WESTERFELD, 1967; BECKETT et al., 1971; GAERTNER et al., 1974), its relative importance being strongly dependent on the species (BROOKES and FORREST, 1971). Introduction of a further hydroxy group into various monohydroxychlorpromazines in vitro has been observed (COCCIA and WESTERFELD, 1967; DALY and MANIAN, 1967).

Phenolic metabolites have been detected in peripheral organs of chlorpromazine-treated patients (FORREST et al., 1968) and of rats that had received trifluoperazine (SCHMALZING, 1977). In brain they were measurable when large quantities had been injected (MAICKEL et al., 1974; ALFREDSSON et al., 1977) or metabolically produced (SCHMALZING and BREYER, 1978). Their significance as metabolites in plasma is not clear. While in some laboratories considerable quantities of 7-hydroxychlorpromazine were measured in patient plasma or blood (KAUL et al., 1972) and its concentration was found to be associated with antipsychotic effect (SAKALIS et al., 1973; MACKAY et al., 1974), others were only seldom able to detect more than trace levels (MARCH et al., 1972; CURRY and EVANS, 1975; WILES et al., 1976).

No aromatic hydroxylation of thioxanthenes has been detected by previous authors (KHAN, 1969; JØRGENSEN et al., 1971) in rat, dog, and man, but recent investigations showed that dogs do excrete phenolic metabolites in feces and urine (WIEST et al., 1980).

Catechol metabolites of chlorpromazine can be O-methylated by catechol-O-methyltransferase (DALY and MANIAN, 1969), but also monohydroxy and nonvicinal dihydroxy metabolites of chlorpromazine are excreted as O-methyl derivatives (TURANO et al., 1973). The principal conjugation reaction for the phenols is glucuronidation (LIN et al., 1959; BECKETT et al., 1963; FISHMAN and GOLDENBERG, 1963; BREYER et al., 1977), a pathway which can also be measured in rat liver microsomes (DINGELL and SOSSI, 1977) and in the rat intestine (BREYER and WINNE, 1977). In addition, indications have been obtained of the occurrence of sulfates in human urine (BECKETT et al., 1963) and of the formation in monkeys of alkali-stable and acid-labile phenol conjugates which might be glucosides (FORREST et al., 1975).

In all studies with radioactively labeled phenothiazines, a considerable part of the excretory products remained unextractable with organic solvents even after enzymatic cleavage of glucuronides (EBERT and HESS, 1965; BREYER et al., 1977; SCHMALZING and BREYER, 1978). The nature of these metabolites has not been elucidated, but in analogy to the biotransformation of other xenobiotics it is assumed that they result from the reaction of a metabolic intermediate with glutathione.

As an example, reactions occurring in the ring system of chlorpromazine are depicted in Fig. 1.

c) Degradation of the Ring System

Excretion of ^{35}S from chlorpromazine as inorganic sulfate has been described to occur in the mouse; however, no experimental data were presented (CHRISTENSEN and WASE,

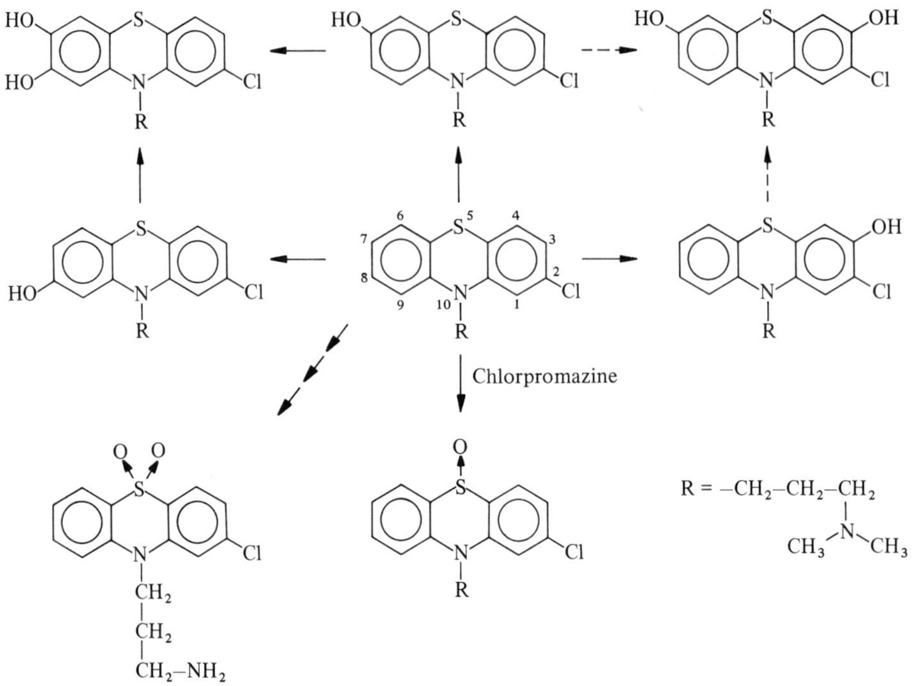

Fig. 1. Oxidative reactions at the phenothiazine ring system of chlorpromazine

Broken arrows indicate reactions which have not unambiguously been shown to occur, since alternative pathways are available for formation of the products

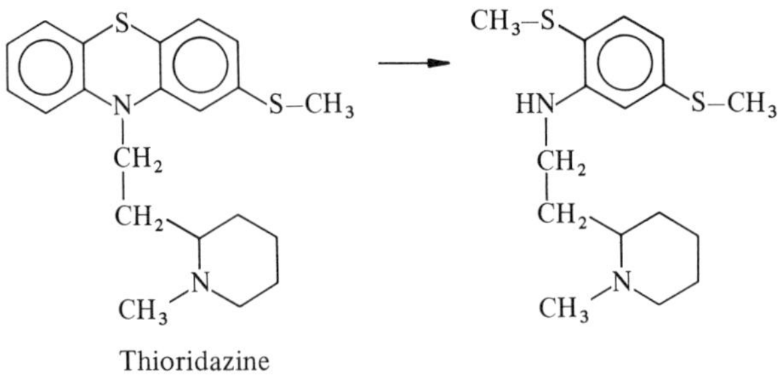

Thioridazine

Fig. 2. Degradation of the phenothiazine ring system in thioridazine

1956). No $^{35}SO_4^{2-}$ formation was found in dogs given [^{35}S]-promazine (WALKENSTEIN and SEIFTER, 1959). Cleavage of the thiazine ring with formation of a methylthioether has been observed with thioridazine (Fig. 2) (ISRAILI et al., 1977).

2. Reactions at the C-2 Substituent

The methylthio group in thioridazine was to a large extent oxidized to the sulfoxide and the sulfone in the mouse (ZEHNDER et al., 1962a). The corresponding metabolites also occurred in human plasma and urine (GRUENKE et al., 1975; MÅRTENSSON et al., 1975).

Feces of rats given butaperazine were found to contain a metabolite in which the carbonyl function of the butyryl group had been reduced to a secondary alcohol (BRUCE et al., 1974).

The identification of 3-hydroxypromazine (FISHMAN and GOLDENBERG, 1965) and 2.3-dihydroxypromazine (TURANO et al., 1973) in the urine of patients ingesting chlorpromazine suggests that the Cl atom may be removed metabolically.

3. Reactions at the N-10 Side Chain

a) N-Dealkylation

The removal of methyl groups from the dimethylamino function of chlorpromazine and promazine has been described in vivo and in vitro (for a review see WILLIAMS and PARKE, 1964). Analogously, phenothiazines carrying a piperazine ring were terminally dealkylated (EBERT and HESS, 1965; BREYER, 1969; BRUCE et al., 1974). This reaction proceeded faster in vivo and in vitro with terminal methyl than with hydroxyethyl groups (GAERTNER et al., 1974, 1975). Thioxanthenes behaved like phenothiazines, since N-dealkylation took place in dimethylamino- (RAAFLAUB, 1967) and in piperazine-substituted drugs (KHAN, 1969; JØRGENSEN et al., 1971).

N-Dealkylation products are lipophilic compounds with a distribution pattern similar to that of the parent drugs. After administration of the drugs, they were present in appreciable quantities in the organs of animals (JØRGENSEN et al., 1971; BREYER, 1972; GAERTNER et al., 1975; SCHMALZING, 1977) and in plasma (CURRY and MARSHALL, 1968; HAMMAR et al., 1968; KAUL et al., 1972; MARCH et al., 1972; SAKURAI et al., 1975; MÅRTENSSON et al., 1975; BREYER and VILLUMSEN, 1976) and in organs of patients (FORREST et al., 1968).

Further dealkylation reactions occurred in the piperazine ring of phenothiazines leading to partial or complete degradation (BREYER et al., 1974 a, b). The ethylenediamine derivatives which result from removal of one of the ethylene groups exhibit a conspicuously high affinity to membranous structures of parenchymatous organs of the rat. As a consequence, they exhibit a long half-life and they accumulate upon repeated administration of the drugs (BREYER, 1972; GAERTNER et al., 1975). The primary amines formed by complete degradation of the piperazine ring are identical with the demethylation products of dimethylamino-substituted phenothiazines (BREYER et al., 1974a).

Additional products of side-chain dealkylation are propionic acid derivatives that have been isolated from urine (RODRIGUEZ and JOHNSON, 1966; TURANO et al., 1973) and plasma (HAMMAR et al., 1968) of chlorpromazine-treated patients. Their formation via didemethylation is suggested by the fact that primary amine metabolites of chlorpromazine were deaminated upon incubation with a rat liver fraction (COCCIA and WESTERFELD, 1967). The corresponding acetic acid derivatives were also reported to be present in urine (TURANO et al., 1973).

The complete removal of the side chain by biodegradation is a matter of dispute. 2-Chlorophenothiazine and its sulfoxide have been carefully identified in urine of patients under treatment with chlorpromazine (FISHMAN and GOLDENBERG, 1965; JOHNSON et al., 1965; TURANO et al., 1973). However, they could not be detected as in vitro metabolites, and 2-chlorophenothiazine was contaminating all chlorpromazine samples and tablets that were investigated (COCCIA and WESTERFELD, 1967). Even if the side chain is removed biologically, it is not clear whether this occurs by step-wise degradation or by direct dealkylation at N-10.

b) Oxidation of the Piperazine Ring

Patients ingesting perazine excreted metabolites in which carbonyl groups had been substituted for methylene groups of the piperazine ring (KRAUSS et al., 1969; BREYER and GAERTNER, 1973). These are not intermediates in the piperazine ring degradation (RASSNER and BREYER, unpublished results).

c) N-Oxidation

The tertiary amine oxide of chlorpromazine has been detected in patient urine in small quantities (Fishman et al., 1962). Similarly small fractions of the dose were excreted as N-oxides by patients receiving perazine (Kanig and Breyer, 1969) and by rats given prochlorperazine (Gaertner et al., 1974). Evidence has also been presented for the excretion of small amounts of an alkali-labile N-oxide sulfoxide by patients treated with chlorprothixene (Raaflaub, 1967).

The small contribution of N-oxides to total excretion products is in contrast with the fact that N-oxidation of phenothiazines is a major metabolic pathway in vitro (Beckett and Hewick, 1967; Berman and Spirtes, 1971), particularly at high substrate concentrations (Breyer, 1971; Gaertner et al., 1974). The apparent discrepancy is resolved on the basis of estimates which show that in vivo drug concentrations at metabolic sites are lower than those often used in vitro; in addition, N-oxides are reduced biologically (Coccia and Westerfeld, 1967). They are, however, no intermediates in oxidative N-demethylation (Coccia and Westerfeld, 1967; Harinath and Odell, 1968).

Using trifluoperazine as substrate, Spirtes (1974) obtained indications of the formation of two isomeric N-oxides carrying the oxygen at either one of the N-atoms of the piperazine ring.

The N-oxidation of the tertiary amine drugs is not catalyzed by cytochrome P-450 (Beckett et al., 1971; Harinath and Odell, 1968), but probably by a microsomal flavine-dependent monooxygenase (Ziegler et al., 1969).

N-Hydroxy derivatives of monodemethylated chlorpromazine and of its sulfoxide have been claimed to be present in human plasma and especially in red cells following chlorpromazine ingestion (Beckett and Essien, 1973). This work seems to need confirmation by independent investigations, particularly concerning the quantitative data.

Figures 3 and 4 show oxidative biotransformations at the side chains of chlorpromazine and perazine.

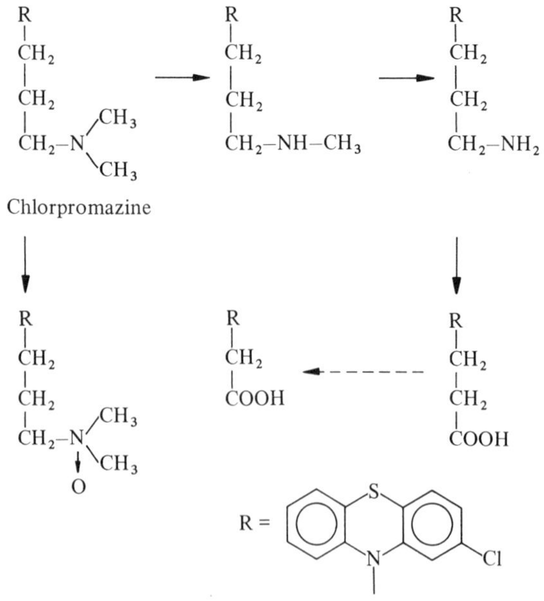

Fig. 3. Oxidative reactions at the side chain of chlorpromazine

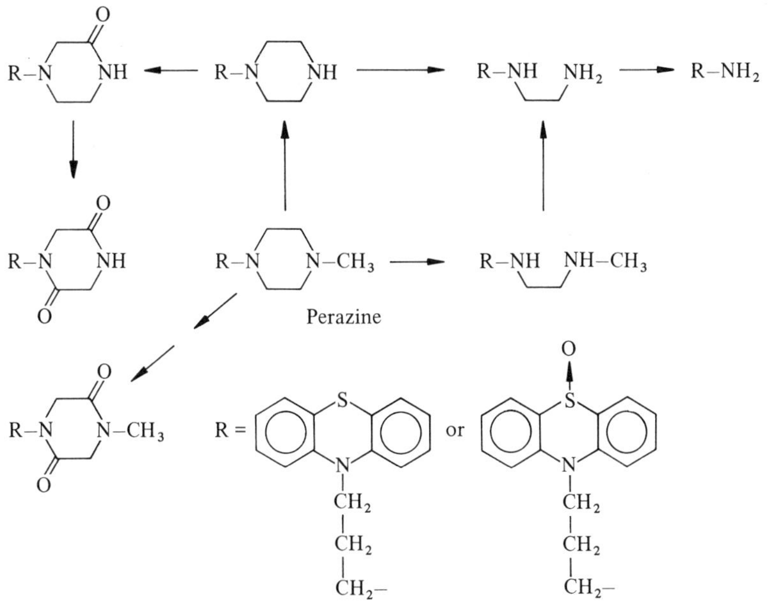

Fig. 4. Oxidative reactions at carbon atoms of the side chain of perazine

d) Hydrolysis and Conjugation Reactions

The enanthate and decanoate esters of fluphenazine and flupenthixol were hydrolyzed to the parent drugs in dogs, rats and monkeys in vivo (EBERT and HESS, 1965; DREYFUSS et al., 1971, 1976 a; JØRGENSEN et al., 1971); the reaction was also demonstrated in vitro, for instance with plasma and with homogenates from various organs (DREYFUSS et al., 1971; JØRGENSEN et al., 1971).

Fluphenazine was liberated upon incubation of urine from fluphenazine-treated patients with glucuronidase/arylsulfatase (WHELPTON and CURRY, 1976). This suggests the in vivo formation of a conjugate, possibly at the hydroxyethyl group. Indications have been obtained that in patient plasma conjugates of tertiary amine drugs and of their sulfoxides are present. The free compounds were liberated by treatment with base (ZINGALES, 1969) or with β-glucuronidase (TURANO et al., 1972).

4. Combinations of Reactions

A large part of the excretory products of phenothiazines and thioxanthenes result from a combination of various metabolic reactions, for instance from sulfoxidation preceded or followed by N-dealkylation or N-oxidation. In accordance with this, numerous reactions were undergone by chlorpromazine metabolites in vitro (COCCIA and WESTERFELD, 1967). The complex pattern of compounds produced in the metabolism of chlorpromazine has been extensively reviewed by USDIN (1971).

C. Clozapine

I. Kinetics in Animals

The distribution in the mouse organism resembled that of phenothiazines and excretion was predominantly by the fecal route (GAUCH and MICHAELIS, 1971). Orally ad-

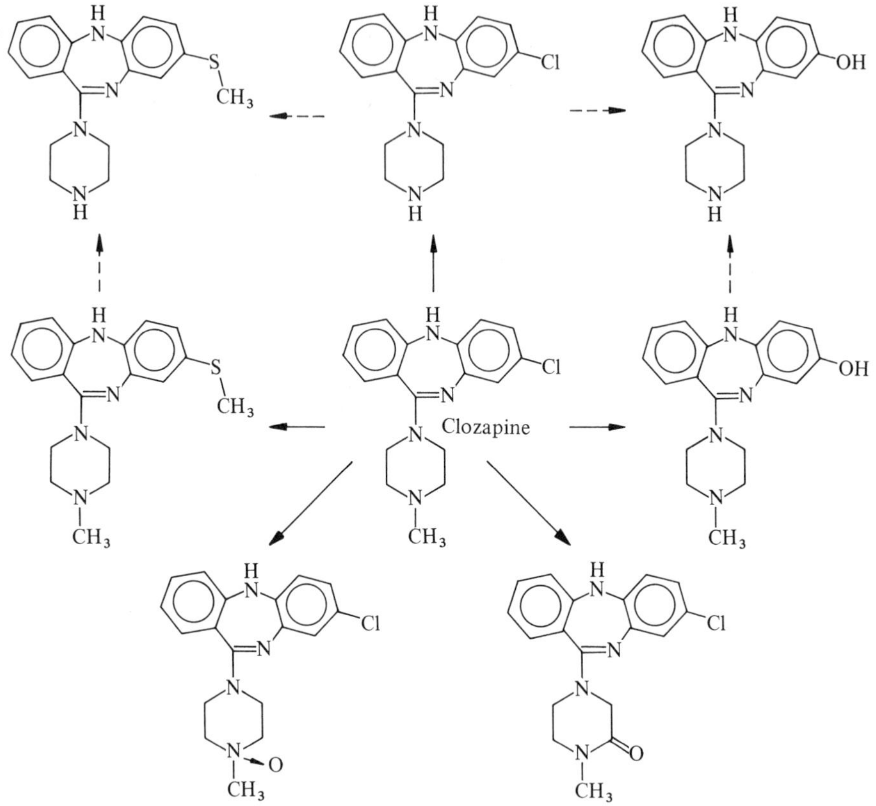

Fig. 5. Biotransformation of clozapine to products occurring in human urine

ministered clozapine was slowly absorbed in rats and largely excreted via the feces or in bile fistula rats via the bile (Tinani, 1975). However, a relatively large fraction was eliminated via the kidneys in the dog; in dog and human urine the unchanged drug represented a major compound (Gauch and Michaelis, 1971).

II. Metabolism

Substitution of a hydroxy group or a methylthio group for the chlorine atom at the ring system has been revealed upon analysis of the metabolites in human urine; a further metabolite contained a carbonyl group in the piperazine ring (Stock et al., 1977). Desmethylclozapine and clozapine-N-oxide have been detected in human and dog urine (Gauch and Michaelis, 1971) and in patient plasma (Breyer and Villumsen, 1976). Rapid reduction of the N-oxide was observed in the dog in vivo (Meier, 1975). The structures of the metabolites are shown in Fig. 5.

D. Butyrophenones and Diphenylbutylpiperidine Derivatives

I. Kinetics in Animals

The kinetic behavior of these drugs in blood, brain, and liver of rats has been carefully studied following s. c. injection of [³H]-labeled compounds. Constant brain/blood and

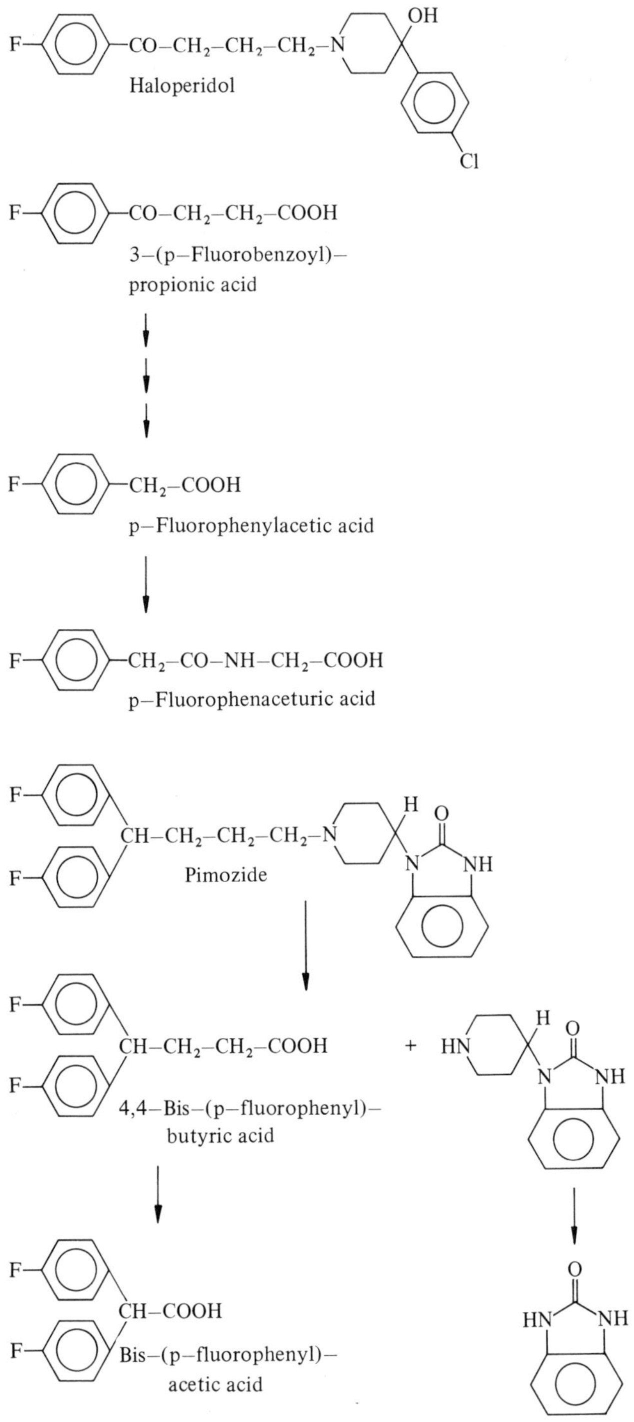

Fig. 6. Biotransformation of haloperidol and pimozide

liver/blood ratios of 1 and 7, respectively, were observed from 1 to 64 h after administration of pimozide at various doses (Janssen and Allewijn, 1968). In contrast, for drugs of the butyrophenone series the ratios were generally higher, but they depended on the dose and on the time after injection. Different kinetics in the three tissues became particularly apparent with low drug doses (Janssen and Allewijn, 1969; Lewi et al., 1970 a, b). Dose-dependent kinetics of haloperidol in rats were also observed by Öhman et al. (1977) who, moreover, obtained indications of the existence of a slowly saturable compartment in the brain. When rats or mice were injected i. v. with penfluridol, uptake into and elimination from adipose tissue was retarded in comparison with brain (Airoldi et al., 1974).

Recent studies with highly labeled [³H]-spiperone and [³H]-pimozide showed that injection of 5 or 20 µg/kg, respectively, to rats led to preferential localization of the drugs in brain areas with high dopamine content (Laduron et al., 1978a). In rats as well as in mice [³H]-spiperone bound to specific sites could be displaced by injecting unlabeled drug (Laduron and Leysen, 1977; Höllt et al., 1977; Laduron et al., 1978a). Upon differential centrifugation of rat brain homogenates, [³H]-spiperone administered in vivo was predominantly detected in the microsomal fraction which also exhibited the largest amount of specific spiperone binding in vitro (Laduron et al., 1978b).

II. Metabolism

Butyrophenones are largely metabolized prior to excretion (Braun et al., 1967; Cressman et al., 1973; Forsman et al., 1977).

The principal biodegradation observed with haloperidol in the rat was oxidative N-dealkylation resulting in the formation of p-fluorobenzoylpropionic acid. The major part of this metabolite was by a sequence of still hypothetical reactions degraded to p-fluorophenylacetic acid which was excreted as the glycine conjugate (Fig. 6) (Soudijn et al., 1967).

Analogous reactions were undergone by pimozide, 4.4-bis-(p-fluorophenyl)-butyric acid and the corresponding acetic acid being eliminated in rat urine and feces. The nitrogen-containing moiety has been detected in the free form and as the acetyl derivative; in addition, benzimidazolinone was shown to occur as a metabolite (Fig. 6) (Soudijn and Van Wijngaarden, 1969).

E. Reserpine

Kinetics and metabolism of reserpine have been comprehensively reviewed by Stitzel (1976). A short account has also been given in a previous volume of this Handbook (Rand and Jurevics, 1977).

References

Airoldi, L., Marcucci, F., Mussini, E., Garattini, S.: Distribution of penfluridol in rats and mice. Eur. J. Pharmacol. 25, 291–295 (1974)

Akera, T., Brody, T.M.: Inhibition of brain sodium- and potassium-stimulated adenosine triphosphatase activity by chlorpromazine free radical. Mol. Pharmacol. 4, 600–612 (1968)

Alfredsson, G., Wiesel, F.-A., Skett, P.: Levels of chlorpromazine and its active metabolites in rat brain and the relationship to central monoamine metabolism and prolactin secretion. Psychopharmacology *53*, 13–18 (1977)

Allgén, L.-G., Jönsson, B., Nauckhoff, B., Andersen, M.-L., Huus, I., Møller Nielsen, I.: On the elimination of chlorprothixene in rat and man. Experientia *16*, 325 (1960)

Beckett, A.H., Essien, E.E.: Chlorpromazine "hydroxylamines" in red blood cells as major metabolites of chlorpromazine in man. J. Pharm. Pharmacol. *25*, 188–189 (1973)

Beckett, A.H., Hewick, D.S.: The N-oxidation of chlorpromazine in vitro – the major metabolic route using rat liver microsomes. J. Pharm. Pharmacol. *19*, 134–136 (1967)

Beckett, A.H., Beaven, M.A., Robinson, A.E.: Metabolism of chlorpromazine in humans. Biochem. Pharmacol. *12*, 779–794 (1963)

Beckett, A.H., Gorrod, J.W., Lazarus, C.R.: The in vitro metabolism of [^{35}S]chlorpromazine. Xenobiotica *1*, 535–536 (1971)

Berman, H.M., Spirtes, M.A.: Gas chromatographic analysis of chlorpromazine and its metabolites formed by hepatic microsomes – I. Influence of magnesium. Biochem. Pharmacol. *20*, 2275–2286 (1971)

Braun, G.A., Poos, G.I., Soudijn, W.: Distribution, excretion and metabolism of neuroleptics of the butyrophenone type. Part II. Distribution, excretion and metabolism of haloperidol in Sprague-Dawley rats. Eur. J. Pharmacol. *1*, 58–62 (1967)

Breyer, U.: Urinary metabolites of 10-[3'-(4''-methyl-piperazinyl)-propyl]-phenothiazine (perazine) in psychiatric patients. I. Isolation, identification and determination of metabolites. Biochem. Pharmacol. *18*, 777–788 (1969)

Breyer, U.: Metabolism of the phenothiazine drug perazine by liver and lung microsomes from various species. Biochem. Pharmacol. *20*, 3341–3351 (1971)

Breyer, U.: Accumulation and elimination of a novel metabolite during chronic administration of the phenothiazine drug perazine to rats. Biochem. Pharmacol. *21*, 1419–1429 (1972)

Breyer, U., Gaertner, H.J.: Accumulation and elimination of metabolites in animals and man treated chronically with phenothiazines. Excerpta Med., Int. Congr. Ser. *288*, 59–66 (1973)

Breyer, U., Schmalzing, G.: Metabolism and disposition of trifluoperazine in the rat. I. A thin-layer chromatographic method for the measurement of trifluoperazine and its metabolites in rat tissues. Drug Metab. Dispos. *5*, 97–103 (1977)

Breyer, U., Villumsen, K.: Measurement of plasma levels of tricyclic psychoactive drugs and their metabolites by UV reflectance photometry of thin layer chromatograms. Eur. J. Clin. Pharmacol. *9*, 457–465 (1976)

Breyer, U., Winne, D.: Absorption and metabolism of the phenothiazine drug perazine in the rat intestinal loop. Biochem. Pharmacol. *26*, 1275–1280 (1977)

Breyer, U., Gaertner, H.J., Prox, A.: Formation of identical metabolites from piperazine- and dimethylamino-substituted phenothiazine drugs in man, rat and dog. Biochem. Pharmacol. *23*, 313–322 (1974a)

Breyer, U., Prox, A., Bertele, R., Gaertner, H.J.: Tissue metabolites of trifluoperazine, fluphenazine, prochlorperazine and perphenazine in the rat: Identification and synthesis. J. Pharm. Sci. *63*, 1842–1848 (1974b)

Breyer, U., Jahns, J., Irmscher, G., Rassner, H., Rehmer, S.: Kinetics of ^{35}S-perazine in the bile fistula rat. Naunyn Schmiedebergs Arch. Pharmacol. *300*, 47–56 (1977)

Breyer-Pfaff, U., Kreft, H., Rassner, H., Prox, A.: Formation of sulfone metabolites from chlorpromazine and perazine in man. Drug Metab. Dispos., *6*, 114–119 (1978)

Brookes, L.G., Forrest, I.S.: In vitro metabolism of ^{3}H-chlorpromazine in various mammals: a preliminary report on 13 species. Exp. Med. Surg. *29*, 61–71 (1971)

Bruce, R.B., Turnbull, L.B., Newman, J.H., Kinzie, J.M., Morris, P.H., Pinchbeck, F.M.: Butaperazine dimaleate metabolism. Xenobiotica *4*, 197–207 (1974)

Cassano, G.B., Placidi, G.F.: Penetration and distribution of neuropharmacological agents in the brain. Pharmakopsychiatr. Neuropsychopharmakol. *2*, 160–175 (1969)

Christensen, J., Wase, A.W.: Metabolism of S^{35}-chlorpromazine. Fed. Proc. *15*, 410 (1956)

Coccia, P.F., Westerfeld, W.W.: The metabolism of chlorpromazine by liver microsomal enzyme systems. J. Pharmacol. Exp. Ther. *157*, 446–458 (1967)

Creese, I., Burt, D.R., Snyder, S.H.: Dopamine receptor binding predicts clinical and pharmacological potencies of antischizophrenic drugs. Science *192*, 481–483 (1976)

Cressman, W.A., Plostnieks, J., Johnson, P.C.: Absorption, metabolism and excretion of droperidol by human subjects following intramuscular and intravenous administration. Anesthesiology *38*, 363–369 (1973)

Curry, S.H., Evans, S.: Assay of 7-hydroxychlorpromazine, and failure to detect more than small quantities, in plasma of responding schizophrenics. Psychopharmacol. Commun. *1*, 481–490 (1975)

Curry, S.H., Marshall, J.H.L.: Plasma levels of chlorpromazine and some of its relatively non-polar metabolites in psychiatric patients. Life Sci. *7*, 9–17 (1968)

Curry, S.H., Derr, J.E., Maling, H.M.: The physiological disposition of chlorpromazine in the rat and dog. Proc. Soc. Exp. Biol. Med. *134*, 314–318 (1970)

Curry, S.H., D'Mello, A., Mould, G.P.: Destruction of chlorpromazine during absorption in the rat in vivo and in vitro. Br. J. Pharmacol. *42*, 403–411 (1971)

Daly, J.W., Manian, A.A.: The metabolism of hydroxychlorpromazines by rat liver microsomes. Biochem. Pharmacol. *16*, 2131–2136 (1967)

Daly, J.W., Manian, A.A.: The action of catechol-O-methyltransferase on 7,8-dihydroxychlorpromazine – Formation of 7-hydroxy-8-methoxychlorpromazine and 8-hydroxy-7-methoxychlorpromazine. Biochem. Pharmacol. *18*, 1235–1238 (1969)

De Leenheer, A.P.: Identification and quantitative determination of phenothiazine drugs in urine samples of psychiatric patients. J. Pharm. Sci. *63*, 389–394 (1974)

Dingell, J.V., Sossi, N.: Studies on the glucuronidation of 7-hydroxychlorpromazine in vitro. Drug Metab. Dispos. *5*, 397–404 (1977)

Dreyfuss, J., Cohen, A.I.: Identification of 7-hydroxyfluphenazine as major metabolite of fluphenazine-^{14}C in the dog. J. Pharm. Sci. *60*, 826–828 (1971)

Dreyfuss, J., Ross Jr., J.J., Schreiber, E.C.: Biological disposition and metabolic fate of fluphenazine-^{14}C in the dog and rhesus monkey. J. Pharm. Sci. *60*, 821–825 (1971)

Dreyfuss, J., Beer, B., Devine, D.D., Roberts, B.F., Schreiber, E.C.: Fluphenazine-induced Parkinsonism in the baboon: Pharmacological and metabolic studies. Neuropharmacology *11*, 223–230 (1972)

Dreyfuss, J., Ross Jr., J.J., Shaw, J.M., Miller, I., Schreiber, E.C.: Release and elimination of ^{14}C-fluphenazine enanthate and decanoate esters administered in sesame oil to dogs. J. Pharm. Sci. *65*, 502–507 (1976a)

Dreyfuss, J., Shaw, J.M., Ross Jr., J.J.: Fluphenazine enanthate and fluphenazine decanoate: Intramuscular injection and esterification as requirements for slow-release characteristics in dogs. J. Pharm. Sci. *65*, 1310–1315 (1976b)

Ebert, A.G., Hess, S.M.: The distribution and metabolism of fluphenazine enanthate. J. Pharmacol. Exp. Ther. *148*, 412–421 (1965)

Eckert, H., Hopf, A.: Autoradiographic studies in the distribution of psychoactive drugs in the rat brain. IV. ^{14}C-Thioridazine. Int. Pharmacopsychiatry *4*, 98–116 (1970)

Emmerson, J.L., Miya, T.S.: Metabolism of phenothiazine drugs. J. Pharm. Sci. *52*, 411–419 (1963)

Fishman, V., Goldenberg, H.: Metabolism of chlorpromazine. IV. Identification of 7-hydroxychlorpromazine and its sulfoxide and desmethyl derivatives. Proc. Soc. Exp. Biol. Med. *112*, 501–506 (1963)

Fishman, V., Goldenberg, H.: Side-chain degradation and ring hydroxylation of phenothiazine tranquilizers. J. Pharmacol. Exp. Ther. *150*, 122–128 (1965)

Fishman, V., Heaton, A., Goldenberg, H.: Metabolism of chlorpromazine. III. Isolation and identification of chlorpromazine-N-oxide. Proc. Soc. Exp. Biol. Med. *109*, 548–552 (1962)

Forrest, I.S., Forrest, F.M.: On the metabolism and action mechanism of the phenothiazine drugs. Exp. Med. Surg. *21*, 231–240 (1963)

Forrest, I.S., Bolt, A.G., Serra, M.T.: Distribution of chlorpromazine metabolites in selected organs of psychiatric patients chronically dosed up to the time of death. Biochem. Pharmacol. *17*, 2061–2070 (1968)

Forrest, I.S., Fox, J., Green, D.E., Melikian, A.P., Serra, M.T.: Total excretion of ^{3}H-chlorpromazine and ^{3}H-prochlorperazine in chronically dosed animals: Balance sheet. Adv. Biochem. Psychopharmacol. *9*, 347–356 (1974)

Forrest, I.S., Green, D.E., Serra, M.T., Soave, O.A.: Chlorpromazine excretion in chronically dosed primates. I. Occurrence of a previously unreported class of chlorpromazine conjugates. Psychopharmacol. Commun. *1*, 51–59 (1975)

Forsman, A., Fölsch, G., Larsson, M., Öhman, R.: On the metabolism of haloperidol in man. Curr. Ther. Res. *21*, 606–617 (1977)

Gaertner, H.J., Breyer, U., Liomin, G.: Metabolism of trifluoperazine, fluphenazine, prochlorperazine and perphenazine in rats: In vitro and urinary metabolites. Biochem. Pharmacol. *23*, 303–311 (1974)

Gaertner, H.J., Liomin, G., Villumsen, D., Bertele, R., Breyer, U.: Tissue metabolites of trifluoperazine, fluphenazine, prochlorperazine, and perphenazine. Kinetics in chronic treatment. Drug Metab. Dispos. *3*, 437–444 (1975)

Gauch, R., Michaelis, W.: The metabolism of 8-chloro-11-(4-methyl-1-piperazinyl)-5H-dibenzo[b,e][1,4]diazepine (clozapine) in mice, dogs and human subjects. Farmaco [Prat.] *26*, 667–681 (1971)

Goldenberg, H., Fishman, V.: Metabolism of chlorpromazine. V. Confirmation of position 7 as major site of hydroxylation. Biochem. Biophys. Res. Commun.*14*, 404–407 (1964)

Goldenberg, H., Fishman, V., Heaton, A., Burnett, R.: A detailed evaluation of promazine metabolism. Proc. Soc. Exp. Biol. Med. *115*, 1044–1051 (1964)

Gorrod, J.W., Lazarus, C.R., Beckett, A.H.: Some aspects of the in vitro oxidation of ^{35}S-chlorpromazine. Adv. Biochem. Psychopharmacol. *9*, 191–200 (1974)

Goucher, C., Windle, J.J., Levy, L.: Stable enzyme inhibitors and stable free radical species in ultraviolet-irradiated solutions of chlorpromazine. Mol. Pharmacol. *11*, 603–612 (1975)

Gruenke, L.D., Craig, J.C., Dinovo, E.C., Gottschalk, L.A., Noble, E.P., Biener, R.: Identification of a metabolite of thioridazine and mesoridazine from human plasma. Res. Commun. Chem. Pathol. Pharmacol. *10*, 221–225 (1975)

Hammar, C.-G., Holmstedt, B., Ryhage, R.: Mass fragmentography. Identification of chlorpromazine and its metabolites in human blood by a new method. Anal. Biochem. *25*, 532–548 (1968)

Harinath, B.C., Odell, G.V.: Chlorpromazine-N-oxide formation by subcellular liver fractions. Biochem. Pharmacol. *17*, 167–171 (1968)

Höllt, V., Czlonkowski, A., Herz, A.: The demonstration in vivo of specific binding sites for neuroleptic drugs in mouse brain. Brain Res. *130*, 176–183 (1977)

Idänpään-Heikkilä, J.E., Vapaatalo, H.I., Neuvonen, P.J.: Effect of N-hydroxyethylpromethazine (Aprobit®) on the distribution of ^{35}S-chlorpromazine studied by autoradiography in cats and mice. Psychopharmacologia *13*, 1–13 (1968)

Israili, Z.H., Dayton, P.G., Kiechel, J.R.: Novel routes of drug metabolism. A survey. Drug Metab. Dispos. *5*, 411–415 (1977)

Janssen, P.A.J., Allewijn, F.T.N.: Pimozide, a chemically novel, highly potent and orally long-acting neuroleptic drug. Part II: Kinetic study of the distribution of pimozide and metabolites in brain, liver and blood of the Wistar rat. Arzneim. Forsch. *18*, 279–282 (1968)

Janssen, P.A.J., Allewijn, F.T.N.: The distribution of the butyrophenones haloperidol, trifluperidol, moperone, and clofuperol in rats, and its relationship with their neuroleptic activity. Arzneim. Forsch. *19*, 199–208 (1969)

Johnson, D.E., Rodriguez, C.F., Burchfield, H.P.: Determination by microcoulometric gas chromatography of chlorpromazine metabolites in human urine. Biochem. Pharmacol. *14*, 1453–1469 (1965)

Jørgensen, A., Fredericson Overø, K., Hansen, V.: Metabolism, distribution and excretion of flupenthixol decanoate in dogs and rats. Acta Pharmacol. Toxicol. *29*, 339–358 (1971)

Kamm, J.J., Gillette, J.R., Brodie, B.B.: Metabolism of chlorpromazine to chlorpromazine sulfoxide by liver microsomes. Fed. Proc. *17*, 382 (1958)

Kanig, K., Breyer, U.: Urinary metabolites of 10-[3'-(4"-methyl-piperazinyl)-propyl]-phenothiazine (perazine) in psychiatric patients. II. Individual metabolite patterns and their changes in the course of treatment. Psychopharmacologia *14*, 211–220 (1969)

Kaul, P.N., Conway, M.W., Ticku, M.K., Clark, M.L.: Chlorpromazine metabolism II: Determination of nonconjugated metabolites in blood of schizophrenic patients. J. Pharm. Sci. *61*, 581–585 (1972)

Kawashima, K., Dixon, R., Spector, S.: Development of radioimmunoassay for chlorpromazine. Eur. J. Pharmacol. *32*, 195–202 (1975a)

Kawashima, K., Wurzburger, R.I., Spector, S.: Correlation of chlorpromazine levels in rat brain and serum with its hypothermic effect. Psychopharmacol. Commun. *1*, 431–436 (1975b)

Khan, A.R.: Some aspects of clopenthixol metabolism in rats and humans. Acta Pharmacol. Toxicol. *27*, 202–212 (1969)

Knoll, R., Christ, W., Müller-Oerlinghausen, B., Coper, H.: Formation of chlorpromazine sulphoxide and monodesmethylchlorpromazine by microsomes of small intestine. Naunyn Schmiedebergs Arch. Pharmacol. *297*, 195–200 (1977)

Krauss, D., Otting, W., Breyer, U.: Identification of a urinary metabolite of perazine as a piperazine-2,5-dione derivative. J. Pharm. Pharmacol. *21*, 808–813 (1969)

Laduron, P., Leysen, J.: Specific in vivo binding of neuroleptic drugs in rat brain. Biochem. Pharmacol. *26*, 1003–1007 (1977)

Laduron, P.M., Janssen, P.F.M., Leysen, J.E.: Spiperone: A ligand of choice for neuroleptic receptors. II. Regional distribution and in vivo displacement of neuroleptic drugs. Biochem. Pharmacol. *27*, 317–321 (1978 a)

Laduron, P.M., Janssen, P.F.M., Leysen, J.E.: Spiperone: A lingand of choice for neuroleptic receptors. III. Subcellular distribution of neuroleptic drugs and their receptors in various rat brain areas. Biochem. Pharmacol. *27*, 323–328 (1978 b)

Lewi, P.J., Heykants, J.J.P., Allewijn, F.T.N., Dony, J.G.H., Janssen, P.A.J.: Distribution and metabolism of neuroleptic drugs. Part I: Pharmacokinetics of haloperidol. Arzneim. Forsch. *20*, 943–948 (1970 a)

Lewi, P.J., Heykants, J.J.P., Janssen, P.A.J.: On the distribution and metabolism of neuroleptic drugs. Part III: Pharmacokinetics of trifluperidol. Arzneim. Forsch. *20*, 1701–1705 (1970 b)

Leysen, J.E., Gommeren, W., Laduron, P.M.: Spiperone: A ligand of choice for neuroleptic receptors. I. Kinetics and characteristics of in vitro binding. Biochem. Pharmacol. *27*, 307–316 (1978)

Lin, T.H., Reynolds, L.W., Rondish, I.M., Van Loon, E.J.: Isolation and characterization of glucuronic acid conjugates of chlorpromazine in human urine. Proc. Soc. Exp. Biol. Med. *102*, 602–605 (1959)

Lindquist, N.G., Ullberg, S.: The melanin affinity of chloroquine and chlorpromazine studied by whole body autoradiography. Acta Pharmacol. Toxicol. *31*, Suppl. 2, 1–32 (1972)

Mackay, A.V.P., Healey, A.F., Baker, J.: The relationship of plasma chlorpromazine to its 7-hydroxy and suphoxide metabolites in a large population of chronic schizophrenics. Br. J. Clin. Pharmacol. *1*, 425–430 (1974)

Mahju, M.A., Maickel, R.P.: Accumulation of phenothiazine tranquilizers in rat brain and plasma after repeated dosage. Biochem. Pharmacol. *18*, 2701–2710 (1969)

Maickel, R.P., Fedynskyj, N.M., Potter, W.Z., Manian, A.A.: Tissue localization of 7- and 8-hydroxychloropromazines. Toxicol. Appl. Pharmacol. *28*, 8–17 (1974)

March, J.E., Donato, D., Turano, P., Turner, W.J.: Interpatient variation and significance of plasma levels of chlorpromazine in psychiatric patients. J. Med. (Basel) *3*, 146–162 (1972)

Mårtensson, E., Nyberg, G., Axelsson, R., Serck-Hansen, K.: Quantitative determination of thioridazine and nonconjugated thioridazine metabolites in serum and urine of psychiatric patients. Curr. Ther. Res. *18*, 687–700 (1975)

Meier, J.: Bioanalytical assay of clozapine and its N-oxide metabolite and the determination of their blood levels in the dog. Br. J. Pharmacol. *53*, 440P (1975)

Minder, R., Schnetzer, F., Bickel, M.H.: Hepatic and extrahepatic metabolism of the psychotropic drugs, chlorpromazine, imipramine, and imipramine N-oxide. Naunyn Schmiedebergs Arch. Pharmacol. *268*, 334–347 (1971)

Mjörndal, T., Wiesel, F.-A., Oreland, L.: Biochemical and behavioral effects of thiothixene: Relation to tissue levels of the drug. Acta Pharmacol. Toxicol. *38*, 490–496 (1976)

Nybäck, H., Sedvall, G.: Effect of chlorpromazine and some of its metabolites on synthesis and turnover of catecholamines formed from ^{14}C-tyrosine in mouse brain. Psychopharmacologia *26*, 155–160 (1972)

Öhman, R., Larsson, M., Nilsson, I.M., Engel, J., Carlsson, A.: Neurometabolic and behavioral effects of haloperidol. Relation to drug levels in serum and in brain. Naunyn Schmiedebergs Arch. Pharmacol. *299*, 105–114 (1977)

Palmer, G.C., Manian, A.A.: Actions of phenothiazine analogues on dopamine-sensitive adenylate cyclase in neuronal and glial-enriched fractions from rat brain. Biochem. Pharmacol. *25*, 63–71 (1976)

Phillips, B.M., Miya, T.S.: Disposition of S^{35}-prochlorperazine in the rat. J. Pharm. Sci. *53*, 1098–1101 (1964)

Piette, L.H., Forrest, I.S.: EPR studies of free radicals in the oxidation of drugs derived from phenothiazine in vitro. Biochim. Biophys. Acta 57, 419–420 (1962)

Prema, K., Gopinathan, K.P.: Distribution, induction and purification of a monooxygenase catalyzing sulphoxidation of drugs. Biochem. Pharmacol. 25, 1299–1303 (1976)

Raaflaub, J.: Zum Metabolismus des Chlorprothixen. Arzneim. Forsch. 17, 1393–1395 (1967)

Rand, M.J., Jurevics, H.: The pharmacology of Rauwolfia alkaloids. In: Handbuch der experimentellen Pharmakologie, Vol. XXXIX. Berlin, Heidelberg, New York: Springer 1977

Rivera-Calimlim, L.: Impaired absorption of chlorpromazine in rats given trihexyphenidyl. Br. J. Pharmacol. 56, 301–305 (1976)

Rodriguez, C.F., Johnson, D.E.: A new metabolite of chlorpromazine in human urine. Life Sci. 5, 1283–1291 (1966)

Rose, R.M., Dimascio, A., Klerman, G.L.: Non-polar urinary metabolites of chlorpromazine in male schizophrenics. J. Psychiatr. Res. 2, 299–305 (1964)

Sakalis, G., Chan, T.L., Gershon, S., Park, S.: The possible role of metabolites in therapeutic response to chlorpromazine treatment. Psychopharmacologia 32, 279–284 (1973)

Sakurai, Y., Nakahara, T., Takahashi, R.: Prediction of response to chlorpromazine treatment in schizophrenics. Psychopharmacologia 44, 195–203 (1975)

Salzman, N.P., Brodie, B.B.: Physiological disposition and fate of chlorpromazine and a method for its estimation in biological material. J. Pharmacol. Exp. Ther. 118, 46–54 (1956)

Salzman, N.P., Moran, N.C., Brodie, B.B.: Identification and pharmacological properties of a major metabolite of chlorpromazine. Nature 176, 1122–1123 (1955)

Sanders, G.T.B.: Distribution of some structurally related pharmacological agents in rat brain. Biochem. Pharmacol. 22, 601–607 (1973)

Schmalzing, G.: Metabolism and disposition of trifluoperazine in the rat. II. Kinetics after oral and intravenous administration in acutely and chronically treated animals. Drug Metab. Dispos. 5, 104–115 (1977)

Schmalzing, G., Breyer, U.: Kinetics of [^{3}H]trifluoperazine in bile fistula rats. Xenobiotica 8, 45–54 (1978)

Seeman, P., Lee, T., Chau-Wong, M., Wong, K.: Antipsychotic drug doses and neuroleptic/dopamine receptors. Nature 261, 717–719 (1976)

Sjöstrand, S.E., Cassano, G.B., Hansson, E.: The distribution of ^{35}S-chlorpromazine in mice studied by whole body autoradiography. Arch. Int. Pharmacodyn. Ther. 156, 34–47 (1965)

Soudijn, W., Van Wijngaarden, I.: The metabolism and excretion of the neuroleptic drug pimozide (R 6238) by the Wistar rat. Life Sci. 8, Part I, 291–295 (1969)

Soudijn, W., Van Wijngaarden, I., Allewijn, F.: Distribution, excretion and metabolism of neuroleptics of the butyrophenone type. Part I. Excretion and metabolism of haloperidol and nine related butyrophenone-derivatives in the Wistar rat. Eur. J. Pharmacol. 1, 47–57 (1967)

Spano, P.F., Neff, N.H., Macko, E., Costa, E.: Efflux of chlorpromazine and trifluoperazine from the rat brain. J. Pharmacol. Exp. Ther. 174, 20–26 (1970)

Spirtes, M.A.: Two types of metabolically produced trifluoperazine N-oxides. Adv. Biochem. Psychopharmacol. 9, 399–404 (1974)

Stitzel, R.E.: The biological fate of reserpine. Pharmacol. Rev. 28, 179–205 (1976)

Stock, B., Spiteller, G., Heipertz, R.: Austausch aromatisch gebundenen Halogens gegen OH- und SCH$_3$- bei der Metabolisierung des Clozapins im menschlichen Körper. Arzneim. Forsch. 27, 982–990 (1977)

Tinani, H.: Relationships between some physicochemical properties, pharmacokinetic parameters and pharmacological activities of tricyclic neurotropic agents. Thesis, Eidgenössische Technische Hochschule Zürich 1975

Turano, P., March, J.E., Turner, W.J., Merlis, S.: Qualitative and quantitative report on chlorpromazine and metabolites in plasma, erythrocytes and erythrocyte washings from chronically medicated schizophrenic patients. J. Med. (Basel) 3, 109–120 (1972)

Turano, P., Turner, W.J., Manian, A.A.: Thin-layer chromatography of chlorpromazine metabolites. Attempt to identify each of the metabolites appearing in blood, urine and feces of chronically medicated schizophrenics. J. Chromatogr. 75, 277–293 (1973)

Usdin, E.: The assay of chlorpromazine and metabolites in blood, urine, and other tissues. CRC Crit. Rev. Clin. Lab. Sci. 2, 347–391 (1971)

Van Loon, E.J., Flanagan, T.L., Novick, W.J., Maas, A.R.: Hepatic secretion and urinary excretion of three S^{35}-labeled phenothiazines in the dog. J. Pharm. Sci. *53*, 1211–1213 (1964)

Walkenstein, S.S., Seifter, J.: Fate, distribution and excretion of ^{35}S-promazine. J. Pharmacol. Exp. Ther. *125*, 283–286 (1959)

West, N.R., Rosenblum, M.P., Sprince, H., Gold, S., Boehme, D.H., Vogel, W.H.: Assay procedures for thioridazine, trifluoperazine, and their sulfoxides and determination of urinary excretion of these compounds in mental patients. J. Pharm. Sci. *63*, 417–419 (1974)

West, N.R., Vogel, W.H.: Absorption, distribution and excretion of trifluoperazine in rats. Arch. Int. Pharmacodyn. Ther. *215*, 318–335 (1975)

Whelpton, R., Curry, S.H.: Methods for study of fluphenazine kinetics in man. J. Pharm. Pharmacol. *28*, 869–873 (1976)

Wiest, E., Prox, A., Wachsmuth, H., Breyer-Pfaff, U.: Aromatic hydroxydation of chlorprothixene in man and dog. Proceedings of the Fourth International Symposium on Phenothiazines and Related Drugs. Amsterdam: Elsevier, in press 1980

Wiles, D.H., Kolakowska, T., McNeilly, A.S., Mandelbrote, B.M., Gelder, M.G.: Clinical significance of plasma chlorpromazine levels. I. Plasma levels of the drug, some of its metabolites and prolactin during acute treatment. Psychol. Med. *6*, 407–415 (1976)

Wilkinson, G.R., Shand, D.G.: Physiological approach to hepatic drug clearance. Clin. Pharmacol. Ther. *18*, 377–390 (1975)

Williams, R.T., Parke, D.V.: The metabolic fate of drugs. Annu. Rev. Pharmacol. *4*, 85–114 (1964)

Zehnder, K., Kalberer, F., Kreis, W., Rutschmann, J.: The metabolism of thioridazine (Mellaril®) and one of its pyrrolidine analogues in the rat. Biochem. Pharmacol. *11*, 535–550 (1962a)

Zehnder, K., Kalberer, F., Rutschmann, J.: The metabolism of thiethylperazine (Torecan®). Biochem. Pharmacol. *11*, 551–556 (1962b)

Ziegler, D.M., Mitchell, C.H., Jollow, D.: The properties of a purified hepatic microsomal mixed function amine oxidase. In: Microsomes and Drug Oxidations. London: Academic Press 1969

Zingales, I.A.: Detection of chlorpromazine and thioridazine metabolites in human erythrocytes. J. Chromatogr. *44*, 547–562 (1969)

CHAPTER 14

Psychometric and Psychophysiological Actions of Antipsychotics in Men

W. JANKE*

A. Introduction

I. Aims of the Review

The actions of psychotropic drugs on behavior and accompanying psychophysiological variables vary considerably with various parameters. The most basic parameters are *dose level* of the drug, *administration schedule* (single or chronic administration), *situational variables* (situation in which the drug is given), *and patient or subject parameters* (personality, initial level of arousal).

Since it is impossible to discuss completely the effects of antipsychotic drugs on men within the space of this paper, our review is based on *single-dose* studies with *healthy* subjects. The limitation to effects in normal subjects after just a single dose certainly limits the generalizability of the findings. In spite of this limitation, generalization to chronic drug administration and psychiatric patients seems possible if appropriate models are used (JANKE and DEBUS, 1975).

B. Methodological Problems in Measuring the Effects of Antipsychotic Drugs on Behavioral and Psychophysiological Parameters

I. Selection of Indicators

The quantitative assessment of the effects of antipsychotic drugs in humans is complicated by the fact that there are no measures which can be regarded as specifically valid indicators for neuroleptics. Thus, for a description of a drug's action it is usually necessary to use a multivariate experimental design with many behavioral and psychophysiological measures. These measures may be classified according to the psychological processes which are presumably being measured and the methodological approach. With regard to *psychological* functions, the measures used can be classified as perception, thinking, learning and memory, psychomotor behavior, emotion and motivation, and physiological processes. With regard to the methodological approach, the most important types of measurement techniques are self-ratings, ratings

---

* Much of the work in preparing this paper has been carried out by Miss BÄRBEL LÖLL, technical assistant at the Psychological Department of the University of Düsseldorf

My colleagues, Prof. Dr. E. WIST and Prof. Dr. G. DEBUS, read the paper and supported me with several proposals

by others, behavioral observation, and tests. Each type of measure has its advantages and disadvantages (DEBUS and JANKE, 1978).

Self-ratings have been used most frequently as indicators of emotional and motivational changes. They can easily be obtained without taking much time. On the other hand, they may not be valid for some subjects which do not have the ability to report their experience in a reliable way (e. g., schizophrenic patients with acute episodes). A serious limitation arises when a neuroleptic drug has strong somatic side effects (e. g., dry mouth) because the report of emotional behavior will be influenced by these somatic effects.

Ratings of behavior by the investigator or staff is a second technique which is used most frequently for detecting motivational and emotional changes. The sensitivity of these techniques, however, is not very high. Drug-induced changes can be demonstrated only if they are not too subtle and the observation period is not limited to a period of a few minutes. Behavior ratings are most appropriate for pharmacotherapeutic studies with chronic drug administration.

Psychophysiological methods (e. g., autonomic measures such as galvanic skin response or heart rate, and central nervous system methods such as EEG) have been applied because they seem to indicate states of arousal more validly than ratings. Serious limitations, however, arise from the fact that it is usually unknown to what extent the changes which occur under the influence of neuroleptics indicate behavioral changes or simply physiological changes which do not have any relationship to behavioral changes.

Psychological tests constitute another important group of assessment techniques. They are often regarded as the "real" psychometric indicators because they are usually constructed according to the principles of psychometrics. Psychological tests in drug evaluation are applied mostly for the measurement of performance in the various areas of psychological functioning (perception, thinking, memory and learning, psychomotor behavior). In spite of the widespread use of performance tests in drug evaluation studies it should be clear that these techniques also involve serious difficulties (JANKE, 1972; JANKE, 1979; DEBUS and JANKE, 1978). The outstanding problems with performance tests are: (1) Dependency of results upon motivation (e.g., need for achievement), (2) dependency of results upon level of unspecific arousal, and (3) factorial complexity of results: Most tests tap very different abilities so that it is difficult to explain drug induced changes as a result of a specific ability.

The score of any performance test is the result of specific abilities (e. g., space or verbal) and the motivation to cooperate and to get good results. A decrease of performance may thus be the result of decreased abilities and decreased motivation. On the other hand, an increase of performance under the influence of a psycholeptic drug may be the result of compensatory motivational changes and not due to increased abilities. Several authors report that relatively high dose levels of hypnotics, tranquilizers or neuroleptics did not reveal the expected decrease of performance in specific tests (DÜKER, 1963; JANKE, 1964a).

Performance and arousal are related by an inverted U-function. Whether a psycholeptic drug will result in a decrease or increase of performance is dependent on the initial arousal level of the subject. Many discrepancies reported in the literature on the effect of neuroleptics may probably be explained by the performance-arousal model.

II. Selection of Situational Conditions

The effects of neuroleptics usually change with the environmental and situational conditions under which the drugs are given (reviews by JANKE et al., 1979; JANKE and DEBUS, 1978; DEBUS and JANKE, 1978). Many authors have pointed to many factors which should be taken into account. There is, however, no systematic knowledge of (a) which factors lead to which results and (b) to which extent the various factors contribute to drug response variance. At the present time it may be concluded from findings with drugs such as haloperidol, pimozide, promazine, and promethazine (BOUCSEIN and JANKE, 1974; JANKE, 1964a; JANKE and DEBUS, 1972) that positive effects (emotional relaxation, no deactivation) of neuroleptics can be demonstrated most easily under the following two conditions: (1), the situation should shift the initial level of arousal to a higher level, e. g., by noise (stress conditions). (2), the tasks to be performed should not be too strenous or the work load of the situation should be low.

III. Selection of Subjects

It is commonplace to emphasize that the effects of neuroleptics differ between normal subjects and psychiatric patients. It should not be forgotten, however, that there are also huge drug response differences *within* the group of psychiatric patients (for summary RICKELS, 1968) and within the group of normal subjects (for summary JANKE et al., 1979). Which subjects should participate in the behavioral evaluation of neuroleptics, in order to get an exhaustive drug action profile, has not been thoroughly investigated up to now. From the findings on the relationship between the experimental situation and drug response it might be concluded that subjects who are in a state of high physiological and behavioral arousal are best suited. Up to now, however, most studies have been carried out with unselected subjects, both normal and abnormal subjects. Since unselected normal subjects are on average in a state of lesser arousal than psychiatric patients, it should be expected that the action of an antipsychotic drug would differ for the two groups. The differences, however, might disappear if subjects in a high state of arousal are selected.

IV. Time Course of Action

It is well known from clinical observations that the effects of neuroleptics change during the course of treatment. It is maintained that the antipsychotic effects do not appear immediately whereas sedative effects (subjective and objective deactivation) are most intense in the initial period of the treatment and eventually disappear.

The evidence for this statement from experimental and well-controlled studies is rather limited and contradictory (KORNETSKY et al., 1959; SERAFETINIDES and CLARK, 1973; JANKE, 1965). KORNETSKY et al. (1959) found that chlorpromazine reduced performance only after acute administration; SERAFETINIDES and CLARK (1973) used chlorpromazine, clopenthixol and haloperidol, and JANKE (1965) fluphenazine, and could not find performance decrement after acute or after chronic administration.

In spite of these contradictory results, it may be necessary to regard the effects of neuroleptics only with respect to the measurement time. This, however, does not mean that the effects measured with acute administration do not allow predictions concerning the effects observed during chronic administration.

C. Review of Antipsychotic Drugs on Different Areas of Psychological Functioning

The following review is arranged according to various areas of psychological functioning. Because of the drug response variability discussed earlier, and the limits of space, the verbal comments are supplemented by tables of results extracted from the literature. It should be taken into consideration in reading these tables that the scoring of the result of a study is only partly objective. As far as possible a "plus" or "minus" was scored if the difference between drug and placebo was statistically significant ($p \leq 0.05$). To a considerable degree the scoring method is based on subjective criteria because the statistical levels of significance are frequently not given in detail. The scoring is based on those results which were obtained at the peak of action, usually some hours after administering the drugs.

I. Effects of Antipsychotic Drugs on Perception

1. Assessment Approaches

In explaining the effects of drugs on perception one has to be aware of the fact that successful perception is usually only possible with participation of motivation processes (readiness for stimulus input, concentration, and attention) and thinking and memory processes (structuring of information). This implies that a given change in a perception test may not only be due to changes in perceptual processes but also to changes of motivation and thinking as well.

The basic attributes of perceptual processes may concern (1) sensitivity, (2) speed of perception, (3) selectiveness of perception, and (4) structuring and gestalt forming.

Within this paper it is only possible to discuss a rather limited part of the whole topic. The reason for this is not only the lack of space but the fact that the number of experimental studies is too small for most areas (for summaries on the effects of drugs on perception Malitz and Kanzler, 1970; Robinson and Sabat, 1975).

2. Determination of Thresholds

Thresholds are the most important measures for perceptual sensitivity. They can be determined in all sensory modalities.

a) Critical Flicker Fusion Frequency

Critical flicker fusion frequency (CFF) is one of the most investigated performance measures (review on the drug effect: Smith and Misiak, 1976). CFF seems to be a good indicator of general activation. Thus, by measuring CFF one hopes to get a global impression of the deactivating effects of drugs.

Table 1. Effects of antipsychotic drugs in normal subjects after single-dose administration: *Flicker fusion frequency*

Drug	Dose (mg)	Number of studies +	Number of studies 0	Number of studies −	References
Butaperazine	3.5	0	1	0	GRAUPNER and KALMAN (1972) (0)
	6	0	1	0	GRAUPNER and KALMAN (1972) (0)
	10	0	1	0	GRAUPNER and KALMAN (1972) (0)
Chlorpromazine	25–50	0	1	3	TURNER (1966) (−); GRAUPNER and KALMAN, (1972) (0, −); BESSER and DUNCAN (1967) (−)
	100	0	0	2	LEHMANN and CSANK (1957) (−); HOEHN-SARIC et al. (1964) (−)
Floropipamide	20	0	0	1	IDESTRÖM and CADENIUS (1963) (−)
	40	0	0	1	IDESTRÖM and CADENIUS (1963) (−)
Fluphenazine	1	0	2	0	JANKE (1965) (0), TURNER (1966) (0)
	2	0	1	0	LIND and TURNER (1968) (0)
Homofenazine	3	0	1	0	JANKE (1966) (0)
Perphenazine	2	0	1	0	BESSER et al. (1966) (0)
	4	0	1	0	BESSER et al. (1966) (0)
Prochlorperazine	10	0	1	0	IDESTRÖM (1960) (0)
	20	0	0	1	IDESTRÖM (1960) (−)
	30	0	0	2	IDESTRÖM (1960) (−); LEHMANN and CSANK (1957) (−)
Promazine	50	0	1	0	JANKE (1964a) (0)
	75	0	0	1	JANKE (1964a) (−)
Promethazine	25	0	2	0	BOUCSEIN and JANKE (1974) (0); GRAUPNER and KALMAN (1972) (0)
Reserpine	1–2	0	1	0	LEHMANN and CSANK (1957) (0)
Thioridazine	50	0	1	0	GEHRING et al. (1971) (0)

+ = Increase (compared to placebo), 0 = No difference (between drug and placebo), − = Decrease (compared to placebo)

As Table 1 shows, it can be concluded for several drugs that they decrease CFF at small dose levels, e. g., chlorpromazine (50 mg) or prochlorperazine (10 mg). There are some neuroleptics which have not yet been shown to decrease CFF, e.g., fluphenazine (1 and 2 mg). Whether the picture would change with higher dose levels remains to be seen. The differences between neuroleptics and other types of psycholeptics are slight: Tranquilizing agents and hypnotics behave very similar to neuroleptics (JANKE and DEBUS, 1968; MCNAIR, 1973). *Lower* dose levels of tranquilizers (e. g., meprobamate, 400–800 mg; chlordiazepoxide, 10–20 mg) do not decrease CFF. They may be compared to very low doses of neuroleptic drugs (e. g., chlorpromazine 25 mg) and of barbiturates (e. g., amobarbital and secobarbital 100 mg). *Higher* dose levels than those mentioned lead to a decrease of flicker fusion frequency with all three drug types. Antipsychotic and tranquilizing drugs, however, seem to decrease CFF to a lesser degree than barbiturates.

b) Other Thresholds

From the findings available, no systematic effects of neuroleptics on various thresholds (pain, tactual, auditive, visual) could be found (BENJAMIN et al., 1957, for 10 mg prochlorperazine; Kornetsky et al., 1957, for 200 and 400 mg chlorpromazine; Ideström and Cadenius, 1963, for 20 and 40 mg floropipamide; Shurtleff et al., 1962, for 25–200 mg chlorpromazine, 25–200 mg promethazine, 2–16 mg perphenazine, 2–16 mg trifluoperazine).

3. After-Effects

It is thought that aftereffects are the expression of central excitatory and inhibitory processes (e. g., Eysenck, 1963). Several kinds of aftereffects have been studied, e. g., kinesthetic and figural aftereffects or the negative afterimage. The findings with various neuroleptics differ considerably. The main tendency for these drugs is to have no effects at all (Janke and Debus, 1972, for 2 mg haloperidol and 2 mg pimozide) or to inhibit of aftereffects (Lehmann and Csank, 1957, for 100–150 mg chlorpromazine and 30–60 mg prochlorperazine; Janke and Debus, 1972, for 1 mg haloperidol and 1 mg pimozide). Increase of afterimage sensitivity after 1 mg reserpine and perphenazine was reported by Lehmann and Csank (1957). Altogether the number of studies is too small to draw a final conclusion. The effects of antipsychotics, at the dose levels discussed in this paper, are comparable to those of tranquilizers.

4. Perceptual Speed

Perceptual speed seems to be very sensitive to drug-induced alterations. The usual measurement technique is to present stimuli (e. g., digits) tachistoscopically and determine the recognition threshold. As can be seen from the findings summarized in Table 2 there is little influence of low doses of neuroleptics on perceptual speed. Only the high dose 200 mg of chlorpromazine reduced perceptual speed significantly. In

Table 2. Effects of antipsychotic drugs in normal subjects after single-dose administration: *Perceptual speed*

Drug	Dose (mg)	Number of studies			References
		+	0	−	
Chlorpromazine	100	0	1	0	Kornetsky and Humphries (1958) (0)
	200	0	0	1	Kornetsky and Humphries (1958) (−)
Fluphenazine	1	0	0	1	Janke (1966) (−)
Haloperidol	1	0	1	0	Janke and Debus (1972) (0)
	2	0	1	0	Janke and Debus (1972) (0)
Homofenazine	3	0	0	1	Janke (1966) (−)
Pimozide	1	0	1	0	Janke and Debus (1972) (0)
	2	0	1	0	Janke and Debus (1972) (0)
Promazine	50	0	1	0	Janke (1964a) (0)
	75	0	0	1	Janke (1964a) (−)
Promethazine	25	0	1	0	Boucsein and Janke (1974) (0)

+ = Increase (compared to placebo), 0 = No difference (between drug and placebo), − = Decrease (compared to placebo)

comparison to other psycholeptics it seems that perceptual speed is more negatively influenced by barbiturates than by neuroleptics (JANKE, 1964a).

5. Other Areas of Perception

Beside the areas of perception discussed in the last section, other tests have been employed occasionally but the amount of data is too small to justify any comments. This lack of data is regrettable regarding the importance some theories attribute to the perceptual processes of schizophrenics. A very promising method is the *detection of signals from noise* or the *recognition of embedded figures*. Some studies with schizophrenic patients under the influence of phenothiazines have been carried out which showed that the thresholds for detecting signals from noise may be altered by neuroleptics (KOPELL and WITTNER, 1968; RAPPAPORT et al., 1972). This, however, has not been found in studies with normal subjects. Other important aspects of perception are tapped by measurements of *time perception* or *perception of movement*. Low doses of neuroleptics have no effects on time perception (BENJAMIN et al., 1957, for 10 mg prochlorperazine). Perception of movement has not been investigated.

6. Conclusions on the Effects of Antipsychotic Drugs on Perceptual Processes

The effects of antipsychotic drugs administered in low doses to normal subjects appear to be slight. They do not support hypotheses which maintain that this type of drug has specific effects on sensory input. Intensity and quality of the effects of antipsychotic drugs, in the dose levels which are of interest in this context, do not differ very much from those of other psycholeptics; they are most comparable to tranquilizers. Sedatives (e. g., barbiturates) normally induce even in low doses more impairment of perceptual performance than the antipsychotic drugs.

II. Effects of Antipsychotic Drugs on Thinking and Intelligence (Cognitive Processes)

1. Assessment Approaches

The most widely used methods of assessment are subtests taken from the classical intelligence test batteries (e. g., Wechsler Test). Most sensitive to psycholeptic drugs are those tests which demand fast operation with verbal material, e. g., word fluency tests. Tests which refer to complex reasoning problems and problem-solving behavior have rarely been used.

2. General Intelligence Tests

General intelligence has been investigated mainly with psychiatric patients. With these subjects, it could be shown that pharmacotherapy with reserpine, chlorpromazine, and other neuroleptics leads to improvement of general intelligence scores in a number of studies.

Single doses of neuroleptics reveal remarkably few effects in normal and psychiatric subjects. Insignificant effects of neuroleptics on intelligence test batteries have been reported for 1 mg fluphenazine (JANKE, 1965) or 5 mg methylperidol (JANKE, 1964b).

3. Reasoning

The few studies which have been carried out with reasoning tests show no significant changes after administration of 75 and 100 mg chlorpromazine (Davis et al., 1969; Delay et al., 1959), 1 mg fluphenazine (Janke, 1965, 1966) or 5 mg methylperidol (Janke, 1964 b).

4. Word Fluency

Word fluency is measured by tests in which the subjects have to enumerate as many words as possible within a given class (e. g., all words beginning with E). Those rare experiments (see Table 3) which report findings in this area demonstrate for several neuroleptics (fluphenazine, haloperidol, homofenazine, promethazine) no impairment of the ability to perform verbal associations quickly. Interestingly enough, Janke (1966) found significant impairment with 10 mg chlordiazepoxide while 3 mg homofenazine and 1 mg fluphenazine did not induce significant changes. In one study, word fluency performance was even improved by 1 and 2 mg pimozide.

Table 3. Effects of antipsychotic drugs in normal subjects after single-dose administration: *Word fluency*

Drug	Dose (mg)	Number of studies			References
		+	0	−	
Fluphenazine	1	0	1	0	Janke (1966) (0)
Haloperidol	1	0	1	0	Janke and Debus (1972) (0)
	2	0	1	0	Janke and Debus (1972) (0)
Homofenazine	3	0	1	0	Janke (1966) (0)
Moperone	5	0	0	1	Janke and Debus (1962) (−)
Pimozide	1	1	0	0	Janke and Debus (1972) (+)
	2	1	0	0	Janke and Debus (1972) (+)
Promazine	25	0	0	1	Janke and Debus (1962) (−)
Promethazine	25	0	1	0	Boucsein and Janke (1974) (0)

+ = Increase (compared to placebo), 0 = No difference (between drug and placebo), − = Decrease (compared to placebo)

5. Verbal Thinking

There are only a few experiments available which show that verbal thinking is relatively resistant to the influence of neuroleptics. Nonsignificant results in tests of verbal thinking have been demonstrated with chlorpromazine (25–200 mg), promethazine (25–200 mg), perphenazine (2–16 mg) and trifluoperazine (2–8 mg) (DiMascio et al., 1963b), 75 mg chlorpromazine (Davis et al., 1969), 1 mg fluphenazine (Janke, 1965), and 5 mg methylperidol (Janke 1964 b). On the other hand, even a small dose of chlorpromazine (50 mg) decreased verbal thinking (Brimer et al., 1964).

6. Conclusions on the Effects of Antipsychotic Drugs on Cognitive Processes

Antipsychotic drugs, at the dose levels discussed in this paper, do not influence thinking and intellectual performance to a considerable degree. This is comparable to the effects of tranquilizers (for reviews: BERGER and POTTERFIELD, 1969; JANKE and DEBUS, 1968; MCNAIR, 1973). The dose levels for inducing impairment are relatively high (e. g., more than 200 mg chlorpromazine).

III. Learning

1. Assessment Approaches

Learning in humans has been explored to a far lesser degree than the other behavioral functions. If the literature is classified according to the kind of learning tasks, it can be seen that some tasks have rarely been studied. Most studies refer to associative learning with verbal material. There is a gap with regard to conditioning, in particular with operant behavior, and nonverbal behavior. Since the animal studies use almost conditioning exclusively, especially operant conditioning, human and animal studies can hardly be compared.

2. Verbal Learning

Some studies with normal subjects show that higher doses of neuroleptics impair verbal learning (MCPEAKE and DIMASCIO, 1964, 1965; HENINGER et al., 1965, for 100 and 200 mg chlorpromazine, 8 and 16 mg trifluoperazine; DAVIS et al., 1969, for 75 mg chlorpromazine; LEHMANN and CSANK, 1957, for 100–150 mg chlorpromazine). The effects are apparently related to motivational changes since large drug–personality interactions have been observed (MCPEAKE and DIMASCIO, 1964, 1965). Lower doses of neuroleptics seem to have no influence on verbal learning, even after administration for 1 week, which has been shown for 10 and 20 mg thioridazine, 50 mg chlorpromazine and 50 mg sulpiride by LILJEQUIST et al. (1975).

3. Classical Conditioning

In spite of the fact that conditionability of patients under the influence of drugs is very important for psychotherapeutic treatment, there are only a few well-controlled studies with neuroleptics. Classical *autonomic* conditioning to electric shocks has been found to be impaired by 50 mg chlorpromazine (DUREMAN, 1959; SCHNEIDER and COSTILOE, 1957), and 50 mg thioridazine (SLOANE et al., 1969), but not by 20 mg prochlorperazine (UHR et al., 1961). Moreover, the latter drug did not change autonomic conditioning to positive stimuli (UHR et al., 1961). Impaired classical conditioning of autonomic reactions is not necessarily the result of impaired conditionability but may be due to reduced responsivity to unconditioned stimuli (ALEXANDER, 1959). Classical *verbal* conditioning seems to be impaired by 100 mg chlorpromazine (GUPTA, 1973).

4. Operant Conditioning

Investigators in behavioral animal pharmacology have frequently emphasized that operant conditioning techniques are very sensitive in differentiating several types of drugs. It has been maintained (e. g., for reviews: COOK and SEPINWALL, 1975; COOK and Davidson, 1978) that antipsychotic drugs specifically block conditioned avoidance response at doses that have no appreciable effects on escape response. The potency of the avoidance blocking property of a drug in animals seems to be related to its antipsychotic potency in schizophrenics (Cook and Davidson, 1978). Regrettably, the human literature has almost completely omitted this area. The reason for this is the difficulty in realizing operant learning under laboratory conditions.

5. Conclusions Concerning the Effects of Antipsychotic Drugs on Learning

At the present time, the available empirical material permits only preliminary conclusions in some restricted areas of learning: Verbal learning and classical conditioning is impaired by higher dose levels (e. g., 100 mg and more chlorpromazine).

IV. Memory Processes

From the very few empirical studies on memory processes there is no clear evidence for any disturbing effects on short or long term memory (Liljequist et al., 1975; Heimann et al., 1968) even in high dose levels (100–150 mg chlorpromazine, Lehmann and Csank, 1957). One study even reported improvement of short term memory (Stone et al., 1969). Another study showed that the improvement or decrease of nonsense syllable retention induced by chlorpromazine (100 and 200 mg) and trifluoperazine (8 and 16 mg) was dependent on personality traits (McPeake and DiMascio, 1964, 1965). It is to be supposed that these effects are due to motivational drug actions and not to specific memory changes.

V. Effects of Antipsychotic Drugs on Psychomotor Performance

1. Assessment Approaches

Psychomotor tests refer to a broad range of different abilities which correlate only modestly. A rough classification is possible according to the following main characteristics:

Kind of movement: According to this, the tests can measure strength, speed, persistance, precision, or coordination of movement.

Part of the body involved in the movement: The movement can be performed by finger, hand, arm, or the whole body.

Participation of sensory systems: Some movements can be performed only with participation of sensoric components. These measures are often referred to as sensorimotor abilities.

2. Psychomotor Speed

Speed of oscillating movements as measured by the *tapping test* (see Table 4) is reduced by most antipsychotic drugs at relatively high dose levels (chlorpromazine 100 mg, promazine 75 mg). Promethazine, however, demonstrates negative effects at a very low dose level (25 mg).

Table 4. Effects of antipsychotic drugs in normal subjects after single-dose administration: *Tapping speed*

Drug	Dose (mg)	Number of studies			References
		+	0	−	
Chlorpromazine	25	0	2	0	DiMascio et al. (1963b) (0); Wenzel and Rutledge (1962) (0)
	50	0	2	0	DiMascio et al. (1963b) (0); Wenzel and Rutledge (1962) (0)
	100	0	3	4	DiMascio et al. (1963b) (0); Heninger et al. (1965) (−, −); Kornetsky and Humphries (1958) (−); Kornetsky et al. (1959) (−); Lehmann and Csank (1957) (0); Wenzel and Rutledge (1962) (0)
	200	0	0	4	DiMascio et al. (1963b) (−); Heninger et al. (1965) (−); Kornetsky and Humphries (1958) (−); Kornetsky et al. (1959) (−)
Floropipamide	20	0	1	0	Iderström and Cadenius (1963) (0)
	40	0	1	0	Iderström and Cadenius (1963) (0)
Haloperidol	1	0	1	0	Janke and Debus (1972) (0)
	2	0	1	0	Janke and Debus (1972) (0)
Perphenazine	2	0	1	0	DiMascio et al. (1963b) (0)
	4	0	1	0	DiMascio et al. (1963b) (0)
	8	0	1	0	DiMascio et al. (1963b) (0)
	16	0	1	0	DiMascio et al. (1963b) (0)
Pimozide	1	0	2	0	Janke and Debus (1972) (0, 0)
	2	0	2	0	Janke and Debus (1972) (0, 0)
Prochlorperazine	10	0	2	0	Benjamin et al. (1957) (0); Iderström (1960) (0)
	20	0	1	0	Iderström (1960) (0)
	30	0	2	0	Iderström (1960) (0); Lehmann and Csank (1957) (0)
Promazine	50	0	2	0	Janke (1964a) (0, 0)
	75	0	1	1	Janke (1964a) (0, −)
Promethazine	25	0	0	3	Boucsein and Janke (1974) (−, −); DiMascio et al. (1963b) (−)
	50	0	0	1	DiMascio et al. (1963b) (−)
	100	0	0	1	DiMascio et al. (1963b) (−)
	200	0	0	1	DiMascio et al. (1963b) (−)
Reserpine	5	0	1	0	DiMascio et al. (1958) (0)
Trifluoperazine	2	0	1	0	DiMascio et al. (1963b) (0)
	4	0	1	0	DiMascio et al. (1963b) (0)
	8	0	2	0	DiMascio et al. (1963b) (0); Heninger et al. (1965) (0)
	16	0	2	0	DiMascio et al. (1963b) (0); Heninger et al. (1965) (0)

+ = Increase (compared to placebo), 0 = No difference (between drug and placebo), − = Decrease (compared to placebo)

3. Sensorimotor Speed

Speed of motor reactions to sensory stimuli as measured by *reaction time* tests is at least as sensitive as motor speed (see Table 5). The low dose of 50 mg chlorpromazine had impairing effects in several experiments. Again some phenothiazines seem to have only slight effects. Altogether, the number of studies is too small to reach conclusions for most drugs.

Table 5. Effects of antipsychotic drugs in normal subjects after single-dose administration: *Reaction time*

Drug	Dose (mg)	Number of studies			References
		+	0	−	
Chlorpromazine	25	0	2	0	CHESSICK et al. (1966) (0), WENZEL and RUTLEDGE (1962) (0)
	50	0	1	3	EVANS and JEWETT (1962) (−); LOOMIS and WEST (1958) (−); TECCE et al. (1975) (−), WENZEL and RUTLEDGE (1962) (0)
	100	0	3	1	BRODIE (1967) (0); LEHMANN and CSANK (1957) (0); MILNER and LANDAUER (1971) (−)[a]; WENZEL and RUTLEDGE (1962) (0)
	200	0	0	1	ZIRKLE et al. (1959) (−)
Floropipamide	20	0	1	0	IDESTRÖM and CADENIUS (1963) (0)
	40	0	1	0	IDESTRÖM and CADENIUS (1963) (0)
Fluphenazine	1	0	2	0	JANKE (1965) (0), (1966) (0)
Homofenazine	3	0	1	0	JANKE (1966) (0)
Moperone	5	0	1	0	JANKE and DEBUS (1962) (0)
Perphenazine	10	0	1	0	HEIMANN et al. (1968) (0)
Prochlorperazine	10	0	1	1	BENJAMIN et al. (1957) (−); IDESTRÖM (1960) (0)
	20	0	1	0	IDESTRÖM (1960) (0)
	30	0	1	0	IDESTRÖM (1960) (0)
	30–60	0	0	1	LEHMANN and CSANK (1957) (−)
	0.15/kg	0	1	0	NAKRA et al. (1975) (0)
	0.30/kg	0	1	0	NAKRA et al. (1975) (0)
Promazine	25	0	1	0	JANKE and DEBUS (1962) (0)
	50	0	1	0	JANKE (1964a) (0)
	75	0	3	0	JANKE and DEBUS (1963) (0), JANKE (1964a) (0)
Promethazine	25	0	0	1	BOUCSEIN and JANKE (1974) (−)
Sulpiride	40 ml	0	1	0	LEWRENZ and KEMPE (1974) (0)
Thioridazine	50	0	1	0	GEHRING et al. (1971) (0)
	100	0	0	2	PÖLDINGER (1965) (−); MILNER and LANDAUER (1971) (−)[a]

+ = Increase (compared to placebo), 0 = No difference (between drug and placebo), − = Decrease (compared to placebo), [a] Dose level estimated

4. Complex Psychomotor and Sensory Coordination

The most used measure in this area is the pursuit rotor test (see Table 6). In this test the subject has to maintain a pen on a rotating disc. In other tests the subjects have to perform complex movements with both hands. These movements are controlled visually. Several studies show that promethazine and chlorpromazine, in dose levels of 50 mg and more, decrease performance measured by the pursuit rotor test. Perphenazine and trifluoperazine do not have impairing actions in the usual dose levels. No studies exist for other types of neuroleptics.

Table 6. Effects of antipsychotic drugs in normal subjects after single-dose administration: *Complex psychomotor and sensomotor coordination*

Drug	Dose (mg)	Number of studies			References
		+	0	−	
Chlorpromazine	25	0	2	0	DiMascio et al. (1963b) (0); Wenzel and Rutledge (1962 (0)
	50	0	2	0	DiMascio et al. (1963b) (0); Wenzel and Rutledge (1962) (0)
	100	0	2	3	DiMascio et al. (1963b) (0); Heninger et al. (1965) (−); Kornetsky and Humphries (1958) (−); Milner and Landauer (1971) (−)[a]; DiMascio et al. (1963b) (−); Heninger et al. (1965) (−); Kornetsky et al. (1957) (−); Kornetsky and Humphries (1958) (−); Wenzel and Rutledge (1962) (0)
Fluphenazine	1	0	1	0	Janke (1965) (0)
Perphenazine	2	0	1	0	DiMascio et al. (1963b) (0)
	4	0	1	0	DiMascio et al. (1963b) (0)
	8	0	1	0	DiMascio et al. (1963b) (0)
	10	0	1	0	Heimann et al. (1968) (0)
	16	0	1	0	DiMascio et al. (1963b) (0)
Prochlorperazine	10	0	0	1	Benjamin et al. (1957) (−)
Promazine	50	1	0	0	Janke (1964a) (+)
	75	0	1	0	Janke (1964a) (0)
Promethazine	25	0	1	0	DiMascio et al. (1963b) (0)
	50	0	0	1	DiMascio et al. (1963b) (−)
	100	0	0	1	DiMascio et al. (1963b) (−)
	200	0	0	1	DiMascio et al. (1963b) (−)
Reserpine	5	1	0	0	DiMascio et al. (1958) (+)
Thioridazine	100[a]	0	0	1	Milner and Landauer (1971) (−)
Trifluoperazine	2	0	1	0	DiMascio et al. (1963b) (0)
	4	0	1	0	DiMascio et al. (1963b) (0)
	8	0	2	0	DiMascio et al. (1963b) (0); Heninger et al. (1965) (0)
	16	0	2	0	DiMascio et al. (1963b) (0); Heninger et al. (1965) (0)

+ = Increase (compared to placebo), 0 = No difference (between drug and placebo), − = Decrease (compared to placebo), [a] Dose level estimated

5. Finger, Hand, and Arm Dexterity

Dexterity can be assessed by tests in which small objects have to be manipulated (see Table 7). Single doses of neuroleptics seem to increase or decrease the performance score in dexterity tests according to the dose level of the drug and personality structure of the subjects. Small dose levels in emotionally labile subjects tend to have positive effects, possibly because of their tension-reducing properties (e. g., Janke, 1964 a). On the other hand, higher levels of neuroleptics probably produce a decrease in performance.

Table 7. Effects of antipsychotic drugs in normal subjects after single-dose administration: *Dexterity in fine motor tests* (e. g., Purdue peg board)

Drug	Dose (mg)	Number of studies			References
		+	0	−	
Chlorpromazine	200	0	1	0	Zirkle et al. (1959) (0)
Floropipamide	20	0	1	0	Ideström and Cadenius (1963) (0)
	40	0	1	0	Ideström and Cadenius (1963) (0)
Fluphenazine	1	0	2	0	Janke (1965) (0), (1966) (0)
Homofenazine	3	0	1	0	Janke (1966) (0)
Moperone	5	0	1	0	Janke and Debus (1962) (0)
Prochlorperazine	10	0	1	0	Benjamin et al. (1957) (0)
Promazine	25	0	1	0	Janke and Debus (1962) (0)
	50	1	0	0	Janke (1964a) (+)
	75	0	1	0	Janke (1964a) (0)

+ = Increase (compared to placebo). 0 = No difference (between drug and placebo), − = Decrease (compared to placebo)

6. Finger and Hand Steadiness

Steadiness is measured by a variety of methods, e. g., threading a needle or using acceleration transducers (see Table 8). Single small doses of neuroleptics reduce static and intentional tremor in emotionally labile subjects (promazine 50 and 75 mg, Janke, 1964 a; promethazine, Boucsein and Janke, 1974). The positive effects seem to vanish at higher dose levels.

7. Precision of Small Movements of Fingers, Hands, and Arms

This type of test is represented by aiming and dotting (see Table 9). In these tasks the subject has to aim with a pencil and place a dot inside a small circle. The few studies available show that this type of performance is relatively insensitive to the influence of neuroleptics.

8. Other Types of Psychomotor Abilities

Other types of psychomotor tests refer to static ataxia, body coordination, mirror tracing, or other specific abilities. The findings of the small number of experiments conducted are not conclusive.

Table 8. Effects of antipsychotic drugs in normal subjects after single-dose administration: *Finger and hand steadiness*

Drug	Dose (mg)	+	0	−	References
Chlorpromazine	25	0	1	0	DiMascio et al. (1963b) (0)
	50	0	1	0	DiMascio et al. (1963b) (0)
	100	0	1	2	DiMascio et al. (1963b) (0); Heninger et al. (1965) (−); Kornetsky and Humphries (1958) (−)
	200	0	0	3	DiMascio et al. (1963b) (−); Heninger et al. (1965) (−); Kornetsky and Humphries (1958) (−)
Floropipamide	20	0	1	0	Ideström and Cadenius (1963) (0)
	40	0	1	0	Ideström and Cadenius (1963) (0)
Fluphenazine	1	0	1	0	Janke (1965) (0)
Haloperidol	1	0	1	0	Janke and Debus (1972) (0)
	2	0	1	1	Janke and Debus (1972) (0, −)
Moperone	5	0	1	0	Janke and Debus (1962) (0)
Perphenazine	2	0	1	0	DiMascio et al. (1963b) (0)
	4	0	1	0	DiMascio et al. (1963b) (0)
	8	0	1	0	DiMascio et al. (1963b) (0)
	10	0	1	0	Heimann et al. (1968) (0)
	16	0	1	0	DiMascio et al. (1963b) (0)
Pimozide	1	0	1	0	Janke and Debus (1972) (0)
	2	0	1	0	Janke and Debus (1972) (0)
Prochlorperazine	0.15/kg	0	1	0	Nakra et al. (1975) (0)
	0.30/kg	0	1	0	Nakra et al. (1975) (0)
Promazine	25	0	1	0	Janke and Debus (1962) (0)
	50	1	0	0	Janke (1964) (+)
	75	1	0	0	Janke (1964) (+)
Promethazine	25	1	1	0	Boucsein and Janke (1974) (+); DiMascio et al. (1963b) (0)
	50	0	1	0	DiMascio et al. (1963b) (0)
	100	0	1	0	DiMascio et al. (1963b) (0)
	200	0	1	0	DiMascio et al. (1963b) (0)
Reserpine	5	1	0	0	DiMascio et al. (1958) (+)
Trifluoperazine	2	0	1	0	DiMascio et al. (1963b) (0)
	4	0	1	0	DiMascio et al. (1963b) (0)
	8	0	2	0	DiMascio et al. (1963b) (0); Heninger et al. (1965) (0)
	16	0	2	0	DiMascio et al. (1963b) (0); Heninger et al. (1965) (0)

+ = Increase (compared to placebo), 0 = No difference (between drug and placebo), − = Decrease (compared to placebo)

Table 9. Effects of antipsychotic drugs in normal subjects after single-dose administration: *Precision of small movements* (e. g., aiming, dotting tests)

Drug	Dose (mg)	Number of studies			References
		+	0	−	
Fluphenazine	1	0	1	0	JANKE (1966) (0)
Homofenazine	3	0	1	0	JANKE (1966) (0)
Promazine	50	0	1	0	JANKE (1964) (0)
	75	0	1	1	JANKE (1964) (−); JANKE and DEBUS (1963) (0)
Promethazine	25	0	1	0	BOUCSEIN and JANKE (1974) (0)

+ = Increase (compared to placebo), 0 = No difference (between drug and placebo), − = Decrease (compared to placebo)

9. Conclusions About the Effects of Antipsychotic Drugs on Psychomotor Abilities

Single doses of antipsychotic drugs influence psychomotor behavior differently at lower and higher dose levels. Low doses may improve psychomotor performance tests if the score is dependent on steadiness but not strongly influenced by speed. High dose levels of antipsychotic drugs impair psychomotor performance, particularly if the test scores are determined by sensorimotor speed factors. The differentiation of neuroleptics from other types of psycholeptics by psychomotor tests is difficult. The conclusions which have been drawn for antipsychotic drugs can be generalized to tranquilizers and barbiturates (JANKE and DEBUS, 1968).

VI. Concentration and Vigilance

1. Assessment Approaches

Concentration is defined operationally as the ability to perform simple cognitive tasks with maximal speed over a longer time period. The tasks may be simple arithmetic calculations, cancelling specific symbols (e. g., letters or numbers within a list) or coding of symbols according to a key. The best known coding test is the digit symbol test (DST).

Vigilance means the ability to direct the attention to signals (auditory, visual, symbolic) which occur irregularly within other stimuli. The tests to measure vigilance demand *continuous attention to external stimuli*. One of the most known tests in this area is the continuous performance test (CPT) devised by ROSVOLD et al. (1956). The task of the subject is to detect specific combinations of letters which occur at irregular intervals.

2. Vigilance

Only a few studies (see Table 10) demonstrate that chlorpromazine at dose levels higher than 50 mg reduces vigilance. Most of the studies have been carried out by KORNETSKY and his associates. A number of years ago, MIRSKY and KORNETSKY (1964) proposed a model according to which phenothiazines should influence CPT scores. Digit symbol test scores, however, should be influenced to a lesser degree. As

Table 10. Effects of antipsychotic drugs in normal subjects after single-dose administration: *Vigilance* (e. g., continuous performance test)

Drug	Dose (mg)	Number of studies			References
		+	0	−	
Chlorpromazine	25	0	1	0	RAPPAPORT and HOPKINS (1971) (0)
	50	0	1	1	LOEB et al. (1965) (−); RAPPAPORT and HOPKINS (1971) (0)
	100	0	1	1	KORNETSKY and ORZACK (1964) (0); MIRSKY et al. (1959) (−)
	200	0	0	2	KORNETSKY and ORZACK (1964) (−); MIRSKY et al. (1959) (−)

+ = Increase (compared to placebo), 0 = No difference (between placebo and drug), − = Decrease (compared to placebo)

far as the CPT is concerned, the number of studies at the present is still too small to support the hypothesis that the test is an especially sensitive measure for detecting the effects of antipsychotic drugs. It seems safe, however, to predict that vigilance is one of the most important functions for understanding the actions of neuroleptics on schizophrenics (GOLDBERG, 1972; RAPPAPORT et al., 1972).

3. Concentration as Measured by Coding Tests (Digit Symbol Test)

Quite a number of experiments (see Table 11, p. 322) demonstrate that chlorpromazine lowers digit symbol test scores at dose levels of 100 mg and more. Other phenothiazines have remarkably little effect. This is true even for promethazine which has impairing effects on other performance areas at low dose levels.

4. Concentration Measured by Continuous Arithmetic Calculations

Performance scores in the usual concentration tests are notably insensitive to neuroleptics (see Table 12, p. 323). It can be seen that only high dose levels of neuroleptics produce impairment. Possibly these results do not reflect the sedating effects of the drugs but may be explained by increased mental effort to overcome impairing effects (DÜKER, 1963). The low sensitivity of continuous arithmetic performance to antipsychotic drugs has been found with other types of psycholeptic drugs (MCNAIR, 1973; JANKE and DEBUS, 1968).

5. Concentration Measured by Cancellation Tests

The conclusions drawn regarding arithmetic calculations (see Table 13, p. 324) are valid for the performance measured by cancellation tests: Only higher dose levels of antipsychotic drugs are efficient at all.

6. Conclusions Concerning the Effects of Antipsychotic Drugs on Concentration and Vigilance

The effects of antipsychotic drugs on *vigilance* are negative in relatively low doses (chlorpromazine 50 mg). The empirical evidence, however, is very small regarding

Table 11. Effects of antipsychotic drugs in normal subjects after single-dose administration: *Digit symbol test*

Drug	Dose (mg)	Number of studies			References
		+	0	−	
Chlorpromazine	25	0	1	0	DiMascio et al. (1963b) (0)
	50	0	1	0	DiMascio et al. (1963b) (0)
	100	0	3	2	DiMascio et al. (1963b) (0); Heninger et al. (1965) (−); Kornetsky and Humphries (1958) (0); Kornetsky et al. (1959) (−); Kornetsky and Orzack (1964) (0)
	200	0	0	6	DiMascio et al. (1963b) (−); Heninger et al. (1965) (−); Kornetsky et al. (1957) (−); Kornetsky and Humphries (1958) (−); Kornetsky et al. (1959) (−); Kornetsky and Orzack (1964) (−)
Perphenazine	2	0	1	0	DiMascio et al. (1963b) (0)
	4	0	1	0	DiMascio et al. (1963b) (0)
	8	0	1	0	DiMascio et al. (1963b) (0)
	16	0	1	0	DiMascio et al. (1963b) (0)
Prochlorperazine	0.15/kg	0	1	0	Nakra et al. (1975) (0)
	0.30/kg	0	1	0	Nakra et al. (1975) (0)
Promethazine	25	0	1	0	DiMascio et al. (1963b) (0)
	50	0	1	0	DiMascio et al. (1963b) (0)
	100	0	0	1	DiMascio et al. (1963b) (−)
	200	0	0	1	DiMascio et al. (1963b) (−)
Trifluoperazine	2	0	1	0	DiMascio et al. (1963b) (0)
	4	0	1	0	DiMascio et al. (1963b) (0)
	8	0	2	0	DiMascio et al. (1963b) (0); Heninger et al. (1965) (0)
	16	0	2	0	DiMascio et al. (1963b) (0); Heninger et al. (1965) (0)

+ = Increase (compared to placebo), 0 = No difference (between drug and placebo), − = Decrease (compared to placebo)

other antipsychotic drugs since studies in this area are lacking at the present time. *Concentration* measured by various procedures (arithmetic calculations, coding tests, cancellation tests) is influenced only by higher dose levels of antipsychotic drugs.

VII. Effects of Antipsychotic Drugs on Psychophysiological Parameters

1. Problems of Psychophysiological Measures

Psychophysiological variables refer to those physiological functions which have been demonstrated to vary with psychological states such as emotion, general arousal, and motivation. They are often regarded as *objective* indicators of emotional and arousal changes. Physiological measures in exploring the effects of psychotropic drugs are applied in different experimental designs. Different conclusions are possible depending

Table 12. Effects of antipsychotic drugs in normal subjects after single-dose administration: *Arithmetic calculations*

Drug	Dose (mg)	Number of studies			References
		+	0	−	
Chlorpromazine	25	1	2	0	CHESSICK et al. (1966) (0); DiMASCIO et al. (1963b) (0); HAWKINS et al. (1961) (+)
	50	0	1	0	DiMASCIO et al. (1963b) (0)
	100	0	1	2	DiMASCIO et al. (1963b) (0); FORREST et al. (1967) (−); HENINGER et al. (1965) (−)
	200	0	0	4	DiMASCIO et al. (1963b) (−); HENINGER et al. (1965) (−); KORNETSKY et al. (1957) (−); ZIRKLE et al. (1959) (−)
Fluphenazine	1	0	1	0	JANKE (1965) (0)
Haloperidol	1	0	1	0	JANKE and DEBUS (1972) (0)
	2	0	1	0	JANKE and DEBUS (1972) (0)
Perphenazine	2	0	1	0	DiMASCIO et al. (1963b) (0)
	4	0	1	0	DiMASCIO et al. (1963b) (0)
	8	1	0	0	DiMASCIO et al. (1963b) (+)
	16	0	1	0	DiMASCIO et al. (1963b) (0)
Pimozide	1	0	1	0	JANKE and DEBUS (1972) (0)
	2	0	1	0	JANKE and DEBUS (1972) (0)
Prochlorperazine	20	0	1	0	UHR et al. (1960) (0)
Promazine	50	0	1	0	JANKE (1964a) (0)
	75	0	1	0	JANKE (1964a) (0)
Promethazine	25	0	1	0	DiMASCIO et al. (1963b) (0)
	50	0	1	0	DiMASCIO et al. (1963b) (0)
	100	0	1	0	DiMASCIO et al. (1963b) (0)
	200	0	0	1	DiMASCIO et al. (1963b) (−)
Trifluoperazine	2	0	1	0	DiMASCIO et al. (1963b) (0)
	4	1	0	0	DiMASCIO et al. (1963b) (+)
	8	1	1	0	DiMASCIO et al. (1963b) (+); HENINGER et al. (1965) (0)
	16	0	2	0	DiMASCIO et al. (1963b) (0); HENINGER et al. (1965) (0)

+ = Increase (compared to placebo), 0 = No difference (between drug and placebo), − = Decrease (compared to placebo)

upon the design. The basic experimental designs are (a) physiological changes to emotion and/or arousal-inducing stimuli, e. g., auditory or visual neutral or nonneutral stimuli and (b) basic physiological activity in standardized waking or sleeping situations. One specific design for (a) is the habituation experiment in which the responses to repetitive stimuli are measured.

Experimental design (a) is the only one which leads to results which can be interpreted in behavioral terms. Changes of physiological response which are measured by experimental design (b) cannot be explained unequivocally. They may not really indicate a psychological state but only peripheral or central physiological functioning. The reason for this is that drugs often lead to behavioral–somatic dissociations. Dis-

W. JANKE

Table 13. Effects of antipsychotic drugs in normal subjects after single-dose administration: *Cancellation tests*

Drug	Dose (mg)	Number of studies			References
		+	0	−	
Chlorpromazine	100	0	1	0	LEHMANN and CSANK (1957) (0)
Fluphenazine	1	0	1	0	JANKE (1965) (0)
Prochlorperazine	10	0	1	0	BENJAMIN et al. (1957) (0)
	0.15/kg	0	1	0	NAKRA et al. (1975) (0)
	0.30/kg	0	1	0	NAKRA et al. (1975) (0)
	30–60	0	0	1	LEHMANN and CSANK (1957) (−)
Reserpine	5	0	1	0	LEHMANN and CSANK (1957) (0)
Sulpiride	4 ml	0	1	0	LEWRENZ and KEMPE (1974) (0)
Thioridazine	100	0	0	1	PÖLDINGER (1965) (−)

+ =Increase (compared to placebo), 0=No difference (between drug and placebo), − =Decrease (compared to placebo)

sociations can be easily obtained with measures of skin conductance when a drug has anticholinergic effects. It has to be supposed that many autonomic variables are influenced directly by many neuroleptic drugs. Thus, these variables are of little value as indicators of behavioral changes if the ingested drug has strong autonomic influences.

Taking the limitations discussed above into account, it seems useful to emphasize those physiological effects which have been measured by means of experimental design (a).

2. Measures of Central Nervous System

a) Assessment Approaches

Most drug research with CNS measures is based on computer-analysed spontaneous electroencephalogram (EEG) in the waking state. To a lesser degree, the EEG during sleep has been explored. In the recent years much interest has been directed to changes of electric brain activity to sensory stimulation. The main variables in these studies were evoked potentials and the so-called contingent negative variation. At the present time all measurement approaches to electric brain activity changes are at their beginnings because many of the problems arising in drug studies have not been solved. One of these problems is the statistical treatment of the data. Some authors use conventional univariate statistics with multivariate data. Thus, the reported statistical levels of significance are very often misleading.

b) Spontaneous Electric Activity

Several investigators have warned against considering individual characteristics of the EEG without taking structural relationships into account (see Table 14). Reviews on the effects of neuroleptics on EEG variables state some common characteristics (SALETU, 1976; FINK, 1969, 1978; ITIL, 1968) such as the increase of slow frequencies (increase of δ- and ϑ-waves, decrease of β-frequencies).

Table 14. Types of reaction to psychotropic drugs with examples (scheme proposed by FINK, 1969)

I.   Slowing of EEG frequencies
   a) Increased frequency slowing
      Many phenothiazines
      Some butyrophenones
   b) Increased frequency slowing + increased alpha + decreased seizure activity
      Piperazinylphenothiazines
   c) Increased seizure activity
      Reserpine

II. Increased fast activity
   a) Increased amplitude
      Hypnotics of the barbiturate type
      Tranquilizers of the benzodiazepine type
      Meprobamate
   b) Decreased amplitude
      Central stimulants
      Psychotomimetics (e. g., LSD)

III. Increased slow and fast activity
   a) Maximum amplitude decrease
      Anticholinergics
   b) Little amplitude decrease
      Tricyclic antidepressants

IV. Alpha variation
   a) Alpha increase
      Alcohol
      Heroin
      Morphine
   b) Alpha decrease
      MAO Inhibitors

Many writers try to classify psychotropic agents according to their main EEG effects (e. g., FINK, 1969; ITIL, 1968, 1974). Best known is the proposed classification by FINK and ITIL. The schedule by FINK (1969) is shown in Table 14.

Much of the work on the actions of psychotropic drugs on the EEG is based on single drug administration in normal subjects. All kinds of antipsychotics have been investigated under these conditions. The possibility of drawing final conclusions, however, is limited because the range of drugs and dose levels is very small. At the present time, differences between the various antipsychotic agents have not been firmly established. One of the problems is that some differences reported may be the result of dose-level variations. In spite of this it cannot be denied that there are differences between the various subclasses. Very interesting is the fact that clozapine showed effects which differed from classic antipsychotics in several investigations (ROUBICEK et al., 1975; ROUBICEK and MAJOR, 1977).

c) Evoked Potentials

Evoked potentials (EP) are changes of electric brain activity as a result of sensory stimulation. These changes are extracted by computer techniques from the background EEG activity. In the recent years a number of drugs have been explored (reviews: BAUST et al., 1977; SALETU, 1974). Single doses of different types of antipsychotics lead, according to SALETU (1974), to the following changes: (1) an increase of the latency of the early and late peaks and (2) a tendency towards attenuated amplitudes in the late part of the response. These conclusions, however, cannot be generalized since findings incompatible with these conclusions have been reported as well (e.g., BAUST et al., 1977).

d) Contingent Negative Variation

The contingent negative variation (CNV) is an event-related electric potential which occurs between the presentation of two stimuli. It is supposed that CNV is related to attention and/or to arousal. TECCE (TECCE and COLE, 1972; TECCE et al., 1978) proposed that CNV can be explained by two models: (1) Magnitude of CNV has a positive monotonic relationship to attention (Attention hypothesis), and (2) CNV is related to arousal level according to the inverted U-curve (Arousal hypothesis). At the present time, experimental results with neuroleptics are rare. With the necessary caution, it might be concluded that neuroleptics in normal subjects decrease CNV (TECCE et al., 1978). Some findings with schizophrenics seem to show that the effects of drugs are dependent on the arousal of the subjects (TECCE et al., 1978).

3. Autonomic Nervous System Measures

a) Assessment Approaches

Many different measures assessing autonomic nervous system function have been applied in drug studies (reviews or general discussions: TECCE and COLE, 1972; LADER and WING, 1966; LADER, 1975). The most important ones involve:
Cardiovascular system: Heart rate, blood pressure, peripheral blood volume
Thermoregulation: Body and finger temperature
Electrical properties of the skin: Basal skin conductance, spontaneous fluctuations of skin conductance, galvanic skin response to stimuli
Respiratory system: Respiration rate
Other systems: Pupillary diameter.

The basic problem in the use of autonomic parameters as indicators of psychic state with antipsychotic drugs was discussed earlier. It should be stressed again that the explanation of autonomic changes in terms of behavioral processes is always problematic.

b) Tonic Autonomic Level

A number of studies revealed the tendency of neuroleptics to change the autonomic balance to the direction of lower sympathetic arousal. This shift has been shown most frequently with chlorpromazine (25–200 mg) for *galvanic skin resistance* (e.g., DUREMAN, 1959; FORREST et al., 1967; SCHOLANDER, 1961). Other neuroleptics have also been investigated in single or multivariable experiments (e.g., KELLY et al., 1958, for prochlorperazine; BENJAMIN et al., 1957; DIMASCIO et al., 1958, for reserpine; DIMASCIO et al., 1963 a, b, for several neuroleptics; GEHRING et al., 1971, for thioridazine; HENINGER et al., 1965, for chlorpromazine and trifluoperazine; HEIMANN et al., 1968, for perphenazine).

A remarkable exception to this shift in the direction of reduced sympathetic arousal is heart rate change. It has been shown for several phenothiazines that heart rate is increased even by low dose levels (e.g., DUREMAN, 1959, for 50 mg chlorpromazine).

c) Autonomic Responsiveness to Arousal-Inducing Stimuli

α) *Response to emotionally loaded stimuli.* Physiological responsiveness to tones – unconditioned as well as conditioned to shocks – is reduced by phenothiazines (e. g., ALEXANDER, 1959; BENJAMIN et al., 1957; DUREMAN, 1959; GLIEDMAN and GANTT, 1956; cited by ALEXANDER, 1959; SLOANE et al., 1969). There are, however, contradictory findings. SCHNEIDER and COSTILOE (1957) did not find a significant decrease of galvanic skin resistance amplitude with a dose of 50 mg chlorpromazine. Regarding the differentiation of various types of psycholeptic drugs, the empirical findings do not allow much generalization. On the other hand, it has been reported that sedatives and tranquilizers reduced physiological responsiveness by the same amount as neuroleptics.

β) *Habituation of physiological responses.* It has been established by a number of studies that the speed and rate of habituation is related to the degree of unspecific arousal (for summary see LADER and WING, 1966; LADER, 1975). The autonomic measures in habituation experiments are usually galvanic skin conductance and heart rate. At the present time there are only a few findings available which show indeed that habituation is facilitated by antipsychotics (SCHOLANDER, 1961, for 50 mg chlorpromazine). These changes, however, are not specific to this type of drug since sedatives such as amobarbital and tranquilizers such as chlordiazepoxide (LADER and WING, 1966) lead to the same effects.

VIII. Emotional Processes

1. Assessment Approaches

Emotional processes refer to constructs which are based to a large extent on introspection, at least as far as the terminology is concerned (e. g., anxiety, anger, joy). Usually a number of emotions are distinguished. Only some of these emotions can be operationally defined. Most drug research has been directed toward the study of anxiety, to a lesser degree to anger and least to other emotions such as joy. Factor analytic research has repeatedly demonstrated that each emotion can be characterized by its intensity on an activation dimension and a pleasure dimension (agreeable – unagreeable).

Each emotion may be indicated by different measures: Self-report of experience, measurement of behavior (e. g., approach, escape, and avoidance) and physiological data. Most drug studies have used self-report data. These are frequently supplemented by physiological data as discussed in a previous section. A very promising approach for studying emotions may be realized by inducing emotions in an experimental situation (*situational* tests). Situational tests may become very useful for studying anxiety or conflicts (DEBUS and JANKE, 1980).

At the present time, the quantitative differentiation of various emotional changes is only in its early stages. For this reason only two emotional "qualities," namely emotional stability and anxiety, are considered in the following section. *Emotional stability* is a very broad concept which is defined at its positive pole by a positive feeling-tone (well-being, self-confident, no emotional tension). *Anxiety* is taken, in this context, to be a more specific emotional quality which is defined by the feeling of apprehension.

2. Emotional Stability

The findings of the studies using objectively scored self-report measures lead to the following conclusions on the effect of single doses of antipsychotic drugs in normal subjects (see Table 15):

a. There is no unitary effect of the cited drugs in discussion as to the intensity or direction of their effects. Antipsychotic drugs may induce emotional stabilization or

Table 15. Effects of antipsychotic drugs in normal subjects after single-dose administration: *Subjective emotional stability (self-report)*

Drug	Dose (mg)	Subjects	Conditions	Result	References
Chlorpromazine	25	unsel.	stress	−	CHESSICK et al. (1966)
	37.5	unsel.	normal	0	VINCENT (1955)
	75	unsel.	normal	+	DAVIS et al. (1969)
	100	unsel.	normal	0	DiMASCIO et al. (1963b)
	100	unsel.	normal	0	DELAY et al. (1959)
	200	unsel.	normal	−	HENINGER et al. (1965)
	200	unsel.	normal	−	DiMASCIO et al. (1963b)
	200	extr., stab.	normal	−	HENINGER et al. (1965)
	200	intr., lab.	normal	+	HENINGER et al. (1965)
Fluphenazine	1	lab.	normal	0/+	SCHÄFER-PLOG (1968)
	1	stab.	normal	0	SCHÄFER-PLOG (1968)
	1	lab.	normal	+	JANKE (1965)
	1	lab.	normal	0	JANKE (1966)
Haloperidol	1	unsel.	h.w.l.	−	JANKE and DEBUS (1972)
	1	unsel.	l.w.l.	+	JANKE and DEBUS (1972)
	2	unsel.	h.w.l.	−	JANKE and DEBUS (1972)
	2	unsel.	l.w.l.	+	JANKE and DEBUS (1972)
Homofenazine	3	lab.	normal	+	JANKE (1960)
Moperone	5	lab.	normal	+	JANKE and DEBUS (1962)
Perphenazine	8	unsel.	normal	−	DiMASCIO et al. (1963b)
	10	unsel.	normal	0	HEIMANN et al. (1968)
Pimozide	1	unsel.	h.w.l.	0	JANKE and DEBUS (1972)
	1	unsel.	l.w.l.	+	JANKE and DEBUS (1972)
	2	unsel.	h.w.l.	0	JANKE and DEBUS (1972)
	2	unsel.	l.w.l.	0	JANKE and DEBUS (1972)
Prochlorperazine	20	unsel.	normal	0	UHR et al. (1961)
Promazine	25	lab.	normal	+	JANKE and DEBUS (1962)
	50	lab.	normal	+	JANKE (1964a)
	50	stab.	normal	−	JANKE (1964a)
	75	lab.	normal	0	JANKE (1964a)
	75	stab.	normal	−	JANKE (1964a)
Promethazine	25	unsel.	stress	+	BOUCSEIN and JANKE (1974)
	25	unsel.	normal	0	BOUCSEIN and JANKE (1974)
Sulpiride	4	unsel.	normal	0	LEWRENZ and KEMPE (1974)
Trifluoperazine	16	extr., stab.	normal	0	HENINGER et al. (1965)
	16	intr., lab.	normal	0	HENINGER et al. (1965)

Unsel. = Unselected, extr. = Extraverted, intr. = Introverted, lab. = Emotionally labile, stab. = Emotionally stable, h.w.l. = High work load, l.w.l. = Low work load, + = Increased (compared to placebo), 0 = No difference (between drug and placebo), − = Decrease (compared to placebo)

emotional relaxation. Whether the one or the other direction is obtained is dependent on the dose level, personality of the subject and situational factors.

   b. The probability of emotional stabilization seems to increase when the following conditions are met: (1) The dose level should be low. As can be seen in several studies where more than one dose level was used, the high dose level did not induce emotional stabilization (JANKE and DEBUS, 1972, for pimozide; JANKE, 1964a, for promazine). (2) The subjects should be emotionally labile (anxious) and introverted because emotionally stable and extraverted subjects tend to show emotional labilization (JANKE, 1964a; DIMASCIO et al., 1963 a, b).

   c. The situation in which the drug is administered should not demand that the subject has to perform difficult tasks ("high work load"). Several studies revealed that emotional stabilization which occurred under low work load conditions was not demonstrated under high work load conditions (JANKE, 1964a, for promazine; JANKE and DEBUS, 1972, for pimozide and haloperidol).

   d. Stress conditions seem to facilitate the induction of emotional stabilization (BOUCSEIN and JANKE, 1974, for promethazine).

   e. Tranquilizers are usually more efficient than antipsychotic drugs in inducing emotional stability. The greater efficiency of tranquilizers can be concluded from the fact that with antipsychotic drugs, emotional stabilization occurs only with very low doses under specific conditions while effects of tranquilizers can be shown under many more conditions (JANKE, 1964a; JANKE and DEBUS, 1968; JANKE et al., 1979; DEBUS and JANKE, 1979). A characteristic effect of antipsychotics which has been reported rarely for tranquilizers and sedatives is that the experience is unpleasant.

3. Anxiety

Anxiety has been assessed mainly by self-report techniques. Some investigators, however, found anxiety-reducing properties in experimental anxiety-inducing situations (e.g., SLOANE et al., 1969). There is no evidence that antipsychotic drugs reduce anxiety specifically beyond their actions on emotional stability or general emotional tension (BRODIE, 1967; LEHMANN and BAN, 1971). This unspecifity, however, seems to hold also for the anti-anxiety drugs (see critical review by DEBUS and JANKE, 1980).

IX. Motivational Processes

1. Assessment Approaches

Motivational processes as they are defined in this paper are constructs involving the individual's tendency or readiness to perform certain actions or achieve certain goals. According to these goals different motives are distinguished, e.g., hunger and thirst, sexual motivation, social motivation and need for achievement. A construct basic to motivation is *activation*. Activation is a basic concept because it is involved in all specific motivations. Activation in this general sense has been found in a number of factor analytic studies with adjective check lists (for summaries see JANKE and DEBUS, 1978) and was designated "energy," "activation," "wakefulness," "vigor," "leistungsorientierte Aktivität" (achievement oriented activation). Assessment methods used for motivation measurement are self-report techniques, projective tests (e. g., TAT = Thematic Apperception Test), preference behavior, and physiological methods.

2. Activation

Activation is a concept which is defined so broadly that it is usually measured at different levels (physiological, subjective experience, performance). In the following section activation changes measured by psychometric self-report ratings will be discussed (see Table 16). This limitation is necessary because the simultaneous discussion of findings from different levels would exceed the scope of this paper. In order to avoid semantic confusion, self-reported activation is labeled "subjective activity".

A relatively large number of studies show that neuroleptic drugs decrease subjective activity even at small dose levels. As with the emotions the effects, however, may vary with dose level, personality, and situational conditions. Emotionally labile or neurotic subjects under low work load conditions may respond to low doses of some antipsychotic drugs not with the expected *decrease* of activity but rather with an increase (Janke and Debus, 1972; Janke, 1966).

The results of the experimental studies on the effects of single doses of antipsychotic drugs on the subjective activity of normal subjects may be summarized as follows:

1. Mental activity of unselected normal subjects is influenced negatively by most antipsychotic drugs at relatively low dose levels, e. g., chlorpromazine (50 mg), haloperidol (2 mg), perphenazine (8 mg), pimozide (2 mg), promethazine (50 mg), promazine (50 mg), reserpine (5 mg).

2. Under some conditions, subjective activity assessed by self-report measures is not decreased but increased by some antipsychotic drugs. The conditions which lead to an increase of mental activity are not fully known. Some studies suggest that an increase in activity may occur in emotionally unstable subjects under situational conditions which do not demand the accomplishment of difficult tasks (Janke, 1966; Schäfer-Plog, 1968, for fluphenazine; Janke and Debus, 1972, for haloperidol and pimozide). At the present time it is not known whether all neuroleptic drugs can lead to "paradoxical" increments of subjective activity since it has been observed, up to now, only with nonphenothiazines (with the exception of fluphenazine). The best explanation of the activity increments is in terms of activation theory. Such an account has been used for pimozide and haloperidol (Janke and Debus, 1972). It is not possible here to explain the model employed. That part of the model which is important in this context assumes that subjective activity is related to arousal by an inverted U-curve. By reducing their high level of arousal, emotionally unstable subjects feel that their subjective mental activity is increased. The model proposed has to be checked in further experiments. It probably is too simple because for some drugs (e. g., chlorpromazine) increments of performance have never been shown.

3. Regarding the differentiation of antipsychotic drugs from tranquilizers and sedatives (e. g., barbiturates), a number of experiments have shown that the deactivating effects of antipsychotic drugs are comparably smaller than those of sedatives but greater than those of tranquilizers.

3. Other Motivational Aspects

The effects of antipsychotic drugs on specific motives has very rarely been experimentally investigated. Most motives have not been regarded at all (e. g., sexual motivation,

Table 16. Effects of antipsychotic drugs in normal subjects after single-dose administration: *Subjective mental activity* (self-report)

Drug	Dose (mg)	Subjects	Conditions	Result	References
Chlorpromazine	25	unsel.	normal	−	Bäumler (1975)
	25	unsel.	normal	0	DiMascio et al. (1963b)
	50	unsel.	normal	0	DiMascio et al. (1963b)
	100	unsel.	normal	−	Delay et al. (1959)
	100	unsel.	normal	0	DiMascio et al. (1963b)
	200	unsel.	normal	−	DiMascio et al. (1963b)
Floropipamide	20	unsel.	normal	(−)	Ideström and Cadenius (1963)
	40	unsel.	normal	−	Ideström and Cadenius (1963)
Fluphenazine	1	lab.	normal	+	Janke (1965)
	1	lab.	normal	+	Janke (1966)
	1	lab.	normal	+	Schäfer-Plog (1968)
	1	stab.	normal	(+)	Schäfer-Plog (1968)
Homofenazine	3	lab.	normal	0	Janke (1966)
Haloperidol	1	lab.	h.w.l.	−	Janke and Debus (1972)
	1	lab.	l.w.l.	0	Janke and Debus (1972)
	2	lab.	h.w.l.	−	Janke and Debus (1972)
	2	lab.	l.w.l.	+	Janke and Debus (1972)
Perphenazine	2	unsel.	normal	0	DiMascio et al. (1963b)
	4	unsel.	normal	0	DiMascio et al. (1963b)
	8	unsel.	normal	−	DiMascio et al. (1963b)
	10	unsel.	normal	0	Heimann et al. (1968)
	16	unsel.	normal	−	DiMascio et al. (1963b)
Moperone	5	lab.	normal	0	Janke and Debus (1962)
Pimozide	1	lab.	h.w.l.	0	Janke and Debus (1972)
	1	lab.	l.w.l.	+	Janke and Debus (1972)
	2	lab.	h.w.l.	0	Janke and Debus (1972)
	2	lab.	l.w.l.	−	Janke and Debus (1972)
Promethazine	25	unsel.	normal	0	DiMascio et al. (1963b)
	25	unsel.	normal	−	Boucsein and Janke (1974)
	50	unsel.	normal	0	DiMascio et al. (1963b)
	100	unsel.	normal	−	DiMascio et al. (1963b)
	200	unsel.	normal	−	DiMascio et al. (1963b)
Promazine	25	lab.	normal	0	Janke and Debus (1962)
	50	lab.	normal	0	Janke (1964a)
	50	stab.	normal	−	Janke (1964a)
	75	lab.	normal	−	Janke (1964a)
	75	stab.	normal	−	Janke (1964a)
Reserpine	5	unsel.	normal	−	DiMascio et al. (1958)

Unsel. = Unselected, lab. = Emotionally labile, stab. = Emotionally stable, h.w.l. = High work load, l.w.l. = Low work load, + = Increase (compared to placebo), 0 = No difference (between drug and placebo), − = Decrease (compared to placebo)

hunger, thirst). *Need for achievement* was investigated by Bäumler by means of the Thematic Apperception Test for 25 mg chlorpromazine. The drug lowered the achievement motivation in general and especially the "fear of failure" (Bäumler, 1975). Schäfer-Plog (1968) found changes in the level of aspiration which were better adjusted to actual performance in unstable subjects medicated with 1 mg fluphenazine.

Social motivation has not been explored systematically. From "symptom lists" or "adjective check lists" it seems possible to conclude that social motivation is reduced by antipsychotic drugs (e. g., JANKE, 1964a, 1966; DiMASCIO et al., 1963 a, b). Reduced social motivation is probably one of the reasons for the impaired social interactional behavior which has been shown for 50 mg chlorpromazine by LENNARD et al. (1967).

References

Alexander, L.: Effects of psychotropic drugs on conditional responses in man. Neuropsychopharmacology *2*, 93–123 (1959)

Bäumler, G.: Beeinflussung der Leistungsmotivation durch Psychopharmaka: I. Die 4 bildthematischen Hauptvariablen. Z. Exp. Angew. Psychol. *22*, 1–14 (1975)

Baust, W., Wortmann, J.J., Zimmermann, A.: Untersuchungen zur Beeinflussung kortikaler somatosensorischer Reizantwortpotentiale durch Pharmaka. Arzneim.-Forsch. *27*, 440–445 (1977)

Benjamin, F.B., Ikai, K., Clare, H.E.: Effect of proclorperazine on psychologic, psychomotor, and muscular performance. U.S. Armed Forces Med. J. *8*, 1433–1440 (1957)

Berger, F.M., Potterfield, J.: The effect of antianxiety tranquilizers on the behavior of normal persons. In: The psychopharmacology of the normal human. Evans, W.O., Kline, N.S. (eds.), 38–113. Springfield: Thomas 1969

Besser, G.M., Duncan, C.: The time course of action in single doses of diazepam, chlorpromazine and some barbiturates as measured by auditory flutter threshold and visual flicker fusion thresholds in man. Br. J. Pharmacol. Chemother. *30*, 341–348 (1967)

Besser, G.M., Duncan, C., Quilliam, J.P.: Modification of the auditory flutter fusion threshold by centrally acting drugs in man. Nature *211*, 751 (1966)

Boucsein, W., Janke, W.: Experimentalpsychologische Untersuchungen zur Wirkung von Propiramfumarat und Promethazin unter Normal- und Streßbedingungen. Arzneim. Forsch. *24*, 675–693 (1974)

Brimer, A., Schnieden, H., Simon, A.: The effect of chlorpromazine and chlordiazepoxide on cognitive functioning. Br. J. Psychiatry *110*, 723–725 (1964)

Brodie, C.M.: Chlorpromazine as anxiety-reducer: Effects on complex learning and reaction time. J. Exp. Res. Personality *2*, 160–167 (1967)

Chessick, R.D., McFarland, R.L., Clark, R.K., Hammer, M., Bassan, M.I.: The effect of morphine, chlorpromazine, pentobarbital and placebo on anxiety. J. Nerv. Ment. Dis. *141*, 540–548 (1966)

Cook, L., Davidson, A.B.: Behavioral pharmacology: animal models involving aversive control of behavior. In: Psychopharmacology. Lipton, M.A., DiMascio, A., Killam, K.F. (eds.), 563–568. New York: Raven Press 1978

Cook, L., Sepinwall, J.: Psychopharmacological parameters of emotions. In: Emotions. Levi, L. (ed.). New York: Raven Press 1975

Davis, K.E., Evans, W.O., Gillis, J.S.: The effects of amphetamine and chlorpromazine on cognitive skills and feelings in normal adult males. In: The psychopharmacology of the normal human. Evans, W.O., Kline, N.S. (eds.), 126–161. Springfield: Thomas 1969

Debus, G., Janke, W.: Psychologische Aspekte der Psychopharmakotherapie. In: Handbuch der Psychologie. Pongratz, L.S. (ed.), 2161–2227, Vol. 8/2. Göttingen: Hogrefe 1978

Debus, G., Janke, W.: Methods and methodological considerations in measuring antianxiety effects of tranquilizing drugs. Prog. Neuropsychopharmacol. *3*, (1980)

Delay, J., Pichot, P., Nicolas-Charles, D., Peerse, J.: Etude psychométrique des effects de l'amobarbital (amytal) et de la chlorpromazine sur des sujects normeaux. Psychopharmacologia *1*,, 48–58 (1959)

DiMascio, A., Klerman, G.L., Rinkel, M., Greenblatt, M., Brown, J.: Psycho-physiologic evaluation of phenyltoloxamine, a new phrenotropic agent. Am. J. Psychiatry *115*, 301–318 (1958)

DiMascio, A., Havens, L.L., Klerman, G.L.: The psychopharmacology of phenothiazine compounds: A comparative study of the effects of chlorpromazine, promethazine, trifluoperazine and perphenazine in normal males. I: Introduction, aims and methods. J. Nerv. Ment. Dis. *136*, 15–28 (1963a)

DiMascio, A., Havens, L.L., Klerman, G.L.: The psychopharmacology of phenothiazine compounds: A comparative study of the effects of chlorpromazine, promethazine, trifluoperazine, and perphenazine in normal males. II: Results and discussion. J. Nerv. Ment. Dis. *136*, 168–186 (1963b)

Düker, H.: Über reaktive Anspannungssteigerung. Z. Exp. Angew. Psychol. *10*, 46–72 (1963)

Dureman, E.I.: Drugs and autonomic conditioning. Stockholm: Almqvist & Wiksell 1959

Evans, W.O., Jewett, A.: The effect of some centrally acting drugs on disjunctive reaction time. Psychopharmacologia *3*, 124–127 (1962)

Eysenck, H.J. (ed.): Experiments with drugs. Oxford: Pergamon Press 1963

Fink, M.: EEG and human psychopharmacology. Rev. Pharmacol. *9*, 241–259 (1969)

Fink, M.: Psychoactive drugs and the waking EEG, 1966–1976. In: Psychopharmacology. Lipton, M.A., DiMascio, A., Killam, K.F. (eds.), 691–698. New York: Raven Press 1978

Forrest, G.L., Bortner, T.W., Bakker, C.B.: The role of personality variables in response to chlorpromazine, dextroamphetamine and placebo. J. Psychiatr. Res. *5*, 281–288 (1967)

Gehring, A., Blaser, P., Spiegel, R., Pöldinger, W.: Bericht über eine pharmakopsychologische Testuntersuchung. Arzneim. Forsch. *21*, 15–20 (1971)

Gliedman, L.H., Gantt, W.H.: The effects of reserpine and chlorpromazine on orienting behavior and retention of conditioned reflexes. South. Med. J. *49*, 880–883 (1956)

Goldberg, S.C.: Behavioral mechanisms of drug action in schizophrenia. Psychopharmacologia *24*, 1–5 (1972)

Graupner, O.K., Kalman, E.V.: Die Flimmer-Verschmelzungs-Frequenz unter dem Einfluß verschiedener Pharmaka. II: Phenothiazinderivate. Psychopharmacologia *27*, 343–347 (1972)

Gupta, B.S.: The effects of stimulant and depressant drugs on verbal conditioning. Br. J. Psychol. *64*, 553–557 (1973)

Hawkins, D.R., Pace, R., Pasternack, B., Sandifer, M.G.: A multivariant psychopharmacologic study in normals. Psychosom. Med. *23*, 1–17 (1961)

Heimann, H., Reed, C.F., Witt, P.N.: Some observations suggesting preservation of skilled motor acts despite drug-induced stress. Psychopharmacologia *13*, 287–298 (1968)

Heninger, G., DiMascio, A., Klerman, G.L.: Personality factors in variability of response to phenothiazines. Am. J. Psychiatry *121*, 1091–1094 (1965)

Hoehn-Saric, R., Bacon, E.F., Gross, M.: Effects of chlorpromazine on flicker fusion. J. Nerv. Ment. Dis. *138*, 287–292 (1964)

Ideström, C.M.: Experimental psychologic methods applied in psychopharmacology. Acta Psychiatr. Neurol. Scand. *35*, 302–313 (1960)

Ideström, C.M., Cadenius, B.: Chlordiazepoxide, dipiperon and amobarbital. Dose effect studies on human beings. Psychopharmacologia *4*, 235–246 (1963)

Itil, T.M.: Electroencephalography and pharmacopsychiatry. In: Clin. Psychopharmacology. Mod. Probl. Pharmacopsychiatry, Itil, T.M. (ed.), Vol. *1*, 163–194. Basel: Karger 1968

Itil, T.M.: Quantitative electroencephalography. In: Psychotropic drugs and the human EEG. Mod. Probl. Pharmacopsychiatr. Vol. *8*,. Itil, T.M. (ed.), 43–75. Basel: Karger 1974

Janke, W.: Experimentelle Untersuchungen zur Abhängigkeit der Wirkung psychotroper Substanzen von Persönlichkeitsmerkmalen. Frankfurt: Akademische Verlagsgesellschaft 1964a

Janke, W.: Untersuchungen mit Psychopharmaka als Hilfsmittel der psychologischen Grundlagenforschung. Neuropsychopharmacology *3*, 166–169. Amsterdam: Elsevier (1964b)

Janke, W.: Untersuchungen zur Frage von Wirkungsunterschieden von Fluphenazin nach erst- und mehrmaliger Applikation. Psychopharmacologia *7*, 349–365 (1965)

Janke, W.: Über psychische Wirkungen verschiedener Tranquilizer bei gesunden, emotional labilen Personen. Psychopharmacologia *8*, 340–374 (1966)

Janke, W.: General considerations on the use of performance tests in drug therapy. Psychopharmacologia *26*, (Suppl.), 40 (1972)

Janke, W.: Einführung in die Pharmakopsychologie. Stuttgart: Kohlhammer 1979

Janke, W., Debus, G.: Bericht über experimentalpsychologische Untersuchungen über die Wirkung von Methylperidol 5 mg, Chlordiazepoxyd 10 mg, Meprobamat 400 mg, Promazin 25 mg und Placebo auf gesunde Personen. Marburg: Institut für Psychologie 1962

Janke, W., Debus, G.: Experimental studies on antianxiety agents with normal subjects: Methodological considerations and review of the main effects. In: Psychopharmacology: a review of progress 1957–1967. 205–230. Efron, D.H. (ed.). Washington: U.S. Government Printing Office 1968

Janke, W., Debus, G.: Double-blind psychometric evaluation of pimozide and haloperidol versus placebo in emotionally labile volunteers under two different work load conditions. Pharmakopsychiatr. Neuropsychopharmakol. *5*, 34–51 (1972)

Janke, W., Debus, G.: Pharmakopsychologische Untersuchungen an gesunden Probanden zur Prognose der therapeutischen Effizienz von Psychopharmaka. Arzneim. Forsch. *25*, 1185–1195 (1975)

Janke, W., Debus, G.: Die Eigenschaftswörterliste. Göttingen: Hogrefe 1978

Janke, W., Debus, G., Longo, N.: Differential psychopharmacology of tranquilizing and sedating drugs. In: Differential psychopharmacology of anxiolytics and sedatives. Mod. Probl. Pharmacopsychiatr. Boissier, J.R. (ed.), Vol. 14, 13–98. Basel: Karger 1979

Kelly, E.L., Miller, J.G., Marquis, D.G., Gerard, R.W., Uhr, L.: Personality differences and continued meprobamate and proclorperazine administration. Arch. Neurol. Psychiatry *80*, 241–252 (1958)

Kopell, B.S., Wittner, W.K.: The effects of chlorpromazine and methamphetamine on visual signal-from-noise detection. J. Nerv. Ment. Dis. *147*, 418–424 (1968)

Kornetsky, C., Humphries, O.: Psychological effects of centrally acting drugs in man: Effects of chlorpromazine and secobarbital on visual and motor behavior. J. Ment. Sci. *104*, 1093–1099 (1958)

Kornetsky, C., Humphries, O., Evarts, E.V.: Comparison of psychological effects of certain centrally acting drugs in man. Arch. Neurol. Psychiatr. *77*, 318–324 (1957)

Kornetsky, C., Orzack, M.H.: A research note on some of the critical factors on the dissimilar effects of chlorpromazine and secobarbital on the digit symbol substitution and continuous performance tests. Psychopharmacologia *6*, 79–86 (1964)

Kornetsky, C., Vates, T.S., Kessler, E.K.: A comparison of hypnotic and residual psychological effects of single doses of chlorpromazine and secobarbital in man. J. Pharmacol. Exp. Ther. *127*, 51–54 (1959)

Lader, M.H.: Psychophysiological aspects of psychopharmacology. In: Neuropsychopharmacology 168–175. Boissier, J.R., Hippius, H., Pichot, P. (eds.). Amsterdam: Excerpta Medica 1975

Lader, M.H., Wing, L.: Physiological measures, sedative drugs, and morbide anxiety. Oxford: University Press 1966

Lehmann, H.E., Ban, T.A.: Effects of psychoactive drugs on conflict avoidance behavior in human subjects. Activitas Nervosa Superior *13*, 82–85 (1971)

Lehmann, H.E., Csank, J.: Differential screening of phrenotropic agents in man: Psychophysiologic test data. J. Clin. Exp. Psychopathol. *18*, 222–235 (1957)

Lennard, H.L., Epstein, L.J., Katzung, B.G.: Psychoactive drug action and group interaction process. J. Nerv. Ment. Dis. *145*, 69–78 (1967)

Lewrenz, H., Kempe, P.: Psychologische Untersuchungen nach Dogmatil[+]-Applikation. Münch. Med. Wochenschr. *116*, 583–584 (1974)

Liljequist, R., Linnoila, M., Mattila, M.J., Saario, I., Seppälä, T.: Effect of two weeks' treatment with thioridazine, chlorpromazine, sulpiride and bromazepam, alone or in combination with alcohol, on learning and memory in man. Psychopharmacologia *44*, 205–208 (1975)

Lind, N.A., Turner, P.: The effect of chlordiazepoxide and fluphenazine on critical flicker frequency. J. Pharm. Pharmacol. *20*, 804 (1968)

Loeb, M., Hawkes, G.R., Evans, W.O., Alluisi, E.A.: The influence of d-amphetamine, benactyzine, and chlorpromazine on performance in an auditory vigilance task. Psychon. Sci. *3*, 29–30 (1965)

Loomis, T.A., West, T.C.: Comparative sedative effects of a barbiturate and some tranquilizer drugs on normal subjects. Pharmacol. Exp. Ther. *122*, 525–531 (1958)

Malitz, S., Kanzler, M.: Effects of drugs on perception in man. Res. Publ. Ass. Nerv. Ment. Dis. *48*, 35–53 (1970)

McNair, D.M.: Antianxiety drugs and human performance. Arch. Gen. Psychiatry *29*, 611–617 (1973)

McPeake, J.D., DiMascio, A.: Drug-personality interaction in the learning of a nonsense syllable task. Psychol. Rep. *15*, 405–406 (1964)

McPeake, J.D., DiMascio, A.: Drug personality interaction in the learning of a nonsense syllable task. J. Psychiatr. Res. *3*, 105–111 (1965)

Milner, G., Landauer, A.A.: Alcohol, thioridazine and chlorpromazine effects on skills related to driving behavior. Br. J. Psychiatry *118*, 351–352 (1971)

Mirsky, A., Kornetsky, C.: On the dissimilar effects of drugs on the digit symbol substitution and continuous performance tests. Psychopharmacologia *5*, 161–177 (1964)

Mirsky, A., Primac, D.W., Bates, R.: The effects of chlorpromazine and secobarbital on the C.P.T. J. Nerv. Ment. Dis. *128*, 12–17 (1959)

Nakra, B.R.S., Bond, A.J., Lader, M.H.: Comparative psychotropic effects of metoclopramide and prochlorperazine in normal subjects. J. Clin. Pharmacol. *15*, 449–454 (1975)

Pöldinger, W.: Vergleichende Untersuchungen antidepressiv wirkender Psychopharmaka an gesunden Versuchspersonen. Neuropsychopharmakologie *4*, 416–420 (1965)

Rappaport, M., Hopkins, H.K.: Signal detection and chlorpromazine. Hum. Factors *13*, 387–390 (1971)

Rappaport, M., Hopkins, H.K., Silverman, J., Hall, K.: Auditory signal detection in schizophrenics. Psychopharmacologia *24*, 6–28 (1972)

Rickels, K. (Ed.): Nonspecific factors in drug therapy. Springfield: Thomas 1968

Rickels, K., Weise, C.C., Clark, E.L., Wheeler, B., Rose, C.K., Rosenfeld, H., Gordon, P.E.: Thiothixene and thioridazine in anxiety. Br. J. Psychiatry *125*, 79–87 (1974)

Robinson, D.N., Sabat, S.R.: Sensory psychopharmacology. In: Current development in psychopharmacology. Essman, W.B., Valzelli, L. (eds.), Vol. 2, 185–204. New York: Wiley 1975

Rossvold, H.E., Mirsky, A.F., Sarason, I., Bransome, E.B., Beck, L.H.: A continuous performance test of brain damage. J. Consult. Psychol. *20*, 343–350 (1956)

Roubicek, M., Major, I.: EEG profile and behavioral changes after a single dose of clozapine in normals and schizophrenics. Biol. Psychiatry *12*, 613–633 (1977)

Roubicek, J., Matejcek, M., Porsolt, R.: Computer analysed EEG and behavioral changes after psychoactive drugs. Int. J. Neurol. *10*, 33–40 (1975)

Saletu, B.: Classification of psychotropic drugs based on human evoked potentials. In: Mod. Probl. Pharmacopsychiatr., Vol. 8. Psychotropic drugs and the human EEG. Itil, T.M. (ed.), 258–285. Basel: Karger 1974

Saletu, B.: Psychopharmaka, Gehirntätigkeit und Schlaf. München: Karger 1976

Schäfer-Plog, U.: Die Wirkung von Fluphenazin auf das Testverhalten von Versuchspersonen unter Berücksichtigung der vegetativen Labilität und des Einflusses des Versuchsleiters. Arzneim. Forsch. *18*, 443–447 (1968)

Schneider, R.A., Costiloe, J.P.: Effect of centrally active drugs on conditioning in man: The inhibiting and facilitating effects of chlorpromazine, amobarbital and methylphenidylacetate on the conditioned galvanic skin response. Am. J. Med. Sci. *233*, 418–423 (1957)

Scholander, T.: The effects of amphetamine and chlorpromazine on the habituation of autonomic response elements. Ann. Acad. Reg. Scient. Upsaliensis *5*, 35–62 (1961)

Serafetinides, E.A., Clark, M.L.: Psychological effects of single-dose antipsychotic medication. Biol. Psychiatry *7*, 263–267 (1973)

Shurtleff, D., Mostofsky, D., DiMascio, A.: The effects of some phenothiazine derivates on the discrimination of auditory clicks. Psychopharmacologia *3*, 153–165 (1962)

Sloane, R.B., Payne, R.W., Willett, R.A.: The effect of thioridazine on autonomic conditioning and arousal in normal subjects. Int. Pharmacopsychiatry *2*, 206–214 (1969)

Smith, J.M., Misiak, H.: Critical flicker frequency (CFF) and psychotropic drugs in normal human subjects: A review. Psychopharmacology *47*, 175–182 (1976)

Stone, G.C., Callaway, E., Jones, R.T., Gentry, T.: Chlorpromazine slows decay of visual short-term memory. Psychon. Sci. *16*, 229–230 (1969)

Tecce, J.J., Cole, J.O.: Psychophysiologic responses of schizophrenics to drugs. Psychopharmacologia *24*, 159–200 (1972)

Tecce, J.J., Cole, J.O., Savignano-Bowman, J.: Chlorpromazine effects on brain activity (contingent negative variation) and reaction time in normal women. Psychopharmacologia *43*, 293–295 (1975)

Tecce, J.J., Savignano-Bowman, J., Cole, J.O.: Drug effects on contingent negative variation and eyeblinks. In: Psychopharmacology. Lipton, M.A., DiMascio, A., Killam, K.F. (eds.), 745–758. New York: Raven Press 1978

Turner, P.: A comparison of fluphenazine and chlorpromazine on critical flicker fusion frequency. J. Pharm. Pharmacol. *18*, 836 (1966)

Uhr, L., Platz, A., Miller, J.G.: A pilot experiment on the effects of meprobamate and of prochlorperazine on tests of cognition and perception. Percep. Mot. Skills *11*, 90 (1960)

Uhr, L., Clay, M., Platz, A., Miller, J.G., Kelly, E.L.: Effects of meprobamate and of prochlorperazine on positive and negative conditioning. J. Abnorm. Soc. Psychol. *63*, 546–551 (1961)

Vincent, H.B.: The effect of largactil on Rorschach test results. Diss. Halifax: Dalhousie Univers. 1955

Wenzel, D.G., Rutledge, C.: Effects of centrally acting drugs on human motor and psychomotor performance. J. Pharmac. Sci. *51*, 631–644 (1962)

Zirkle, G.A., King, P.D., McAtee, O.B., v. Dyke, R.: Effects of chlorpromazine and alcohol on coordination and judgment. J.A.M.A. *14*, 1496–1499 (1959)

CHAPTER 15

Endocrine Effects of Neuroleptics[*]

F.G. SULMAN and Y. GIVANT

A. History

Psychotherapeutic drugs have been reported to interfere with a variety of endocrine functions, including lactation in man and experimental animals. In 1954, WILKINS reported the development of gynecomastia following treatment with Rauwolfia alkaloids. WINNIK and TENNENBAUM showed in 1955 that treatment with chlorpromazine (Largactil, Thorazine or Megaphen) could lead to milk secretion in women. SULMAN and WINNIK, and WINNIK and SULMAN, studying this problem in 1956, described spontaneous lactation in women and animals, and other endocrine disturbances after treatment with chlorpromazine. Our experience with psychopharmaca was confirmed and lactation was reported to occur in women who received either reserpine or chlorpromazine (MARSHALL and LEIBERMAN, 1956, and PLATT and SEARS, 1956). Animal experiments also confirmed our findings, treatment with reserpine resulted in milk secretion in rabbits (MEITES, 1957, SAWYER, 1957). Administration of various other phenothiazine derivatives also produced mammary differentiation and milk secretion in rats (SULMAN et al., 1970). These endocrine disturbances were presumed to result from the action of major tranquilizers on the reticular formation and hypothalamic regions which regulate the releasing and inhibiting functions of the pituitary. The name "hypothalamic tranquilizers" has, therefore, been given to those agents which cause endocrine disturbances such as lactation or suppression of gonadotropins and STH.

Abbreviations

ACTH	= Adrenocorticotropic hormone	MAO	= Monoamine oxidase
ADH	= Antidiuretic hormone, vasopressin	MSH	= Melanophore stimulating hormone (intermedin)
FSH	= Follicle stimulating hormone	PIF	= Prolactin inhibiting factor
ICSH	= Interstitial stimulating hormone (in the male)	PRF	= Prolactin releasing factor
		STH	= Somatotropic hormone, growth hormone
LH	= Luteinizing hormone (in the female)		
		TSH	= Thyrotropic hormone
LTH	= Luteotropic hormone, lactotropic hormone (prolactin)	UCH	= Uterus contracting hormone (oxytocin)

Many other drugs and nonspecific agents have been shown to elicit mammary growth and secretion in estrogen-primed rats and rabbits when the priming dose was set high, or to maintain secretory activity in postpartum rats after litter removal. The

---

[*] This article contains only a short survey of the endocrine effects of psychotherapeutic drugs. For more comprehensive information earlier publications should be consulted: DIKSTEIN and SULMAN (1966), DE WIED (1967), GIVANT and SULMAN (1976)

drugs appearing effective in rats included – in addition to chlorpromazine and reserpine – meprobamate, adrenaline, noradrenaline, serotonin, atropine, dibenamine, eserine, pilocarpine, amphetamine, morphine, 3-methylcholanthrene, 3,4-benzyprene, 9,10-dimethyl-1,2-benzanthracene, and 10% formaldehyde (Meites, 1963). Stress (e. g., cold, heat, restraint, and electrical stimulation) releases prolactin to a lesser degree. However, the above "extra-hypothalamic" psychopharmaca will only provoke lactation if estrogen priming has been too high, e. g., 10 μg/rat/day for 10 days. We have shown that meprobamate, hydroxyzine, ethinamate, phenobarbital, and benactyzine are devoid of any prolactin-releasing effect in rats primed for 10 days with subthreshold doses (8 μg/day) of estrogen (Ben-David et al., 1965). On the other hand, when high threshold doses of estrogen (10 μg/day) were used for priming, many nonspecific stressful stimuli, as reported above, released prolactin and initiated mammary secretion.

Phenothiazine derivatives have a broad spectrum of pharmacologic effects: antiemetic, analgetic, antihistamine, adrenergic blocking, anticholinergic, antipsychotic, antipruritic, antitussive, antinauseant, antispasmotic, tranquilizing, and mammotropic. Their general endocrine involvement is, therefore, not surprising.

Rules of the structure-activity relationship of phenothiazines with regard to their mammotropic effect were published by us (Khazan et al., 1966; Khazen et al., 1968) and confirmed by other authors, mostly as secondary parameters of chemical and pharmacologic interaction. A special section (cf. D) will therefore be devoted to the biochemical mechanisms of the endocrine side effects of psychopharmaca.

B. Psychotherapeutic Drugs Affecting the Endocrine System

I. Phenothiazines

Chlorpromazine [Thorazine, Largactil, Megaphen, 4560 RP, 2-chloro-10-(dimethylaminopropyl)-phenothiazine] is an extremely interesting drug with regard to its effect on endocrine function. The observation of its hypothermic and hypometabolic effects by Laborit and Huguenard in 1951 provided the first stimulus to investigate its effects on endocrine activity.

The development of the drug as a major tranquilizer and its subsequent widespread clinical use led to the discovery of side effects such as galactorrhea (Winnik and Tennenbaum, 1955) and amenorrhea (Kulcsar et al., 1957). These drew the interest of many clinicians to its effect on endocrine functions. The influence of chlorpromazine and other phenothiazines on the activity of the endocrine glands controlled by the pituitary is important for the understanding of the action of these drugs on the hypothalamus, and, more generally, of the mechanism of the central nervous control of pituitary function (De Wied, 1967).

The fact that release of several of the pituitary hormones is blocked, while at the same time that of others is stimulated, was explained by assuming that phenothiazines stimulate or depress the facilitatory and inhibitory areas in the brain which are involved in the regulation of pituitary function. However, in vitro experiments by Danon et al. (1963), showed that phenothiazines act via the hypothalamus, enhancing prolactin release by suppressing the output of the prolactin-inhibiting factor (PIF). This property appears to be shared by all drugs of the neuroleptic class, including Rauwolfia derivatives and butyrophenones. Phenothiazine derivatives depress hypothalamic activity and hypothalamic energizers cannot prevent this effect (KHAZAN et al., 1966). It is specific and cannot be induced by tranquilizers or sedatives which are not active at hypothalamic level.

Direct evidence that perphenazine stimulates prolactin secretion from the pituitary by suppressing PIF is found in the work of DANON et al. (1963): the addition of perphenazine to a pituitary-hypothalamus combined organ culture abolishes the inhibitory effect of the hypothalamic fragments upon prolactin secretion by the pituitary. The blocking action of perphenazine on PIF appears to be reversible and temporary, as diestrus in rats – a concomitant of its administration – terminates 7 days after treatment with the drug with resumption of a normal estrus cycle (BEN-DAVID, 1968).

Treatment with phenothiazine derivatives, such as perphenazine, results in a prompt release of prolactin from the pituitary into the blood, followed by a rate of production and release of the hormone which first increases and later levels off at a stage significantly above that of the controls. The elevated steady-state production and release of the hormone is accompanied by increased weight of the pituitary and by mammary gland growth and secretion (SHANI et al., 1976).

In summary, phenothiazines suppress ACTH, STH, TSH, FSH, LH, and ICSH, but stimulate LTH and MSH. Therefore, lactation appears as a side effect of short phenothiazine treatment as does the eye pigmentation (cornea, vitreous fluid, and retina) which occurs after protracted phenothiazine treatment (SULMAN, 1964). A list of 170 prolactin-releasing phenothiazines has been given by us (SULMAN et al., 1970).

II. Butyrophenones

The clinical use of many butyrophenones as neuroleptics is accepted today in psychiatry, obstetrics and anesthesiology (JANSSEN et al., 1959). As butyrophenones can be conceived as "opened" phenothiazines, they have phenothiazine-like properties and can influence endocrine functions. Some butyrophenones have been reported to elicit central hormonal effects in animals, such as suppression of gonadotropin secretion (JANSSEN, 1967) and prolactin release (DICKERMAN et al., 1974). It is, therefore, obvious that the butyrophenones may affect endocrine functions by central interference with the hypothalamus pituitary axis.

We have compared the endocrine effects of butyrophenone in rats with its psychopharmacologic action, as measured by fall in body temperature, catatonic behavior, and eye ptosis (MISHKINSKY et al., 1969). The aim of that study was to establish structure-activity rules for the mammotropic effect of butyrophenones. It was found that small polar substituents in a position para to the piperidine ring increase the neuroleptic potency and are equally important for the mammotropic effect. Lengthening of this group, however, impairs the lactogenic activity of the substance. A close correlation seems to exist between the mammotropic effect and the effect an body temperature which is used to assess the sedative effect. No definite correlation was found to exist between the mammotropic and the cataleptic and ptotic effects of these drugs (Table 1). In summary, butyrophenones suppress ACTH, FSH, and LH; their effect on STH, TSH, MSH, ADH, and UCH is unknown. They stimulate LTH.

Table 1. Comparison of psychopharmacologic and endocrine effects of 23 butyrophenones[a]

Code name	Generic name (Manufacturer)	Psychopharma-cologic effect	Endocrine effect
R-2498	Trifluperidol (Janssen)	+ +	+ + +
R-1658	Moperone (Janssen)	+ +	+ + +
R-5147	Spiroperidol (Janssen)	+ + +	+ + +
R-4749	Droperidol (Janssen)	+ +	+ +
R-9298	Clofluperol (Janssen)	+	+ +
R-4584	Benzperidol (Janssen)	+	+ +
R-1625	Haloperidol (Janssen)	+	+ +
R-6238	Pimozide (Janssen)	−	+ +
R-2028	Fluanison (Janssen)	+ +	+ +
R-3201	Haloperidide (Janssen)	+	+
R-4457	(Code No.) (Janssen)	+	+
R-3345	Floropipamide (Janssen)	+	+
R-2963	Methylperidide (Janssen)	+	+
R-2962	Amiperone (Janssen)	+	+
R-1892	Butyropipazone (Janssen)	+ +	+
FR-02	(Code No.) (Sandoz)	−	+
R-1647	Anisoperidone (Janssen)	+	+
R-4082	Floropipeton (Janssen)	+ +	+
R-4006	(Code No.) (Janssen)	+ +	+
R-1929	Azaperone (Janssen)	+ + +	+
R-3264	(Code No.) (Janssen)	+ +	−
FR-33 R-7158	(Sandoz) (Janssen)	+ +	−
R-3248	Aceperone (Janssen)	+	−

[a] Psychopharmacologic effects include decrease in body temperature, catalepsy, and ptosis. Test were conducted in female rats (200 ± 10 g). Butyrophenone treatment: 1, 5, and 40 mg/kg/ day for 5 days. Preparations are listed in descending order of their prolactin-releasing and FSH-LH-suppressing effect

III. Rauwolfia Derivatives

The endocrine effects of reserpine are well known. They are mediated by the hypothalamus (Khazan et al., 1961). Rauwolfia derivatives suppress ACTH, TSH, FSH, LH, ICSH, but stimulate release of LTH, STH, MSH, and ADH. With regard to TSH suppression which can result in a complete regression of exophthalmus, there exists an interesting observation from our group (Assael et al., 1960a) showing that 5×10 mg reserpine injected i.m. in a female paranoic patient relieved her severe exophthalmus.

The fact that reserpine can stimulate LTH and STH (Table 2) should be taken into account when judging the reports of the Boston Collaborative Drug Surveillance Group (1974), an Oxford group (Armstrong et al., 1974), and a Helsinki group (Heinonen et al., 1974), all of them reporting an increased incidence of mammary cancer in reserpine-treated female patients. The controversy raging now on this subject shows that reserpine need not be relevant in all cases, but it should warn everybody to reduce the use of reserpine and its derivatives because there is no doubt that many – if not all – mammary cancers are LTH or STH-dependent.

Table 2. Comparison of psychopharmacologic and endocrine effects of 16 reserpine derivatives[a]

Generic name	Proprietary name (Manufacturer)	Psychopharma-cologic effect	Endocrine effect
1. Deserpidine	Harmonyl (Abbott)	+ + +	+ + +
2. Reserpine	Serpasil (CIBA)	+ + +	+ + +
3. Rescinnamine	Moderil (Pfizer)	+ + +	+ + +
4.	SU-10,704 (CIBA)	+ + +	+ +
5.	SU-9,064 (CIBA)	+ + +	+ +
6. Tetrabenazine	Nitoman (Roche)	+ +	+ +
7.	SU-7,064 (CIBA)	+ +	+
8.	SU-11,279 (CIBA)	+	+
9.	SU-9,673 (CIBA)	+	+
10.	SU-10,092 (CIBA)	+	−
11. Benzquinamide	Quantril (Pfizer)	+	−
12. Yohimbine	Quebrachine	+	−
13. Ajmaline	Cardiorythmine (Servier)	+	−
14.	SU-9,300 (CIBA)	+	−
15. Methoserpidine	Cecaserpyl (Roussel)	+	−
16. Ajmalicine	Raubasin (C.H. Boehringer)	+	−

[a] The endocrine effect was assessed by suppression of FSH-LH and prolactin release. Data from BEN-DAVID et al. (1968)

IV. Benzodiazepines

Benzodiazepines are not very active endocrine psychopharmaca, as their effect is due to internuncial blocking which rarely affects the hypothalamus. The appetite-increasing effect of chlordiazepoxide (Librium) is well known; it seems to be connected with STH release due to the presence of a secondary amine group in its molecule. ACTH, FSH, LH, LTH, MSH, and ADH do not seem to be influenced, whereas the possibility should be entertained that benzodiazepines can slightly suppress TSH and UCH. Recently, diazepam (Valium) abuse (80–140 mg/day) has been reported to release prolactin and to induce gynecomastia (MOERCK and MAGELUND, 1979).

V. Barbiturates

Barbiturates given in a single dose may stimulate ACTH, ADH, and STH, but when administered chronically they depress ACTH and STH. They can inhibit TSH, FSH, LH, ICSH, and LTH when given in large doses. MSH and UCH do not seem to be affected by barbiturates. FSH and LH release in rats is inhibited by pentobarbital (EVERETT et al., 1964). This has become a standard method for gonadotropic inhibition.

VI. Lithium

Lithium increases ACTH (LAZARUS and BENNIE, 1972). Its effect on STH, FSH, LH, ICSH, LTH, and MSH is negligible, but it may suppress ADH. Its most important endocrine effect, however, is the immediate suppression of TSH and thyroxine release, visible within 24 h of a dosage of $1-3 \times 250$ mg lithium carbonate. This effect was observed in 1968 by SCHOU et al. and has since then been confirmed by many psychiatrists. Its use for short-term treatment of hyperthyroidism is now well established. We use it as a valuable tool for the treatment of "intermittent hyperthyreosis" which occurs as a reaction to stress, especially heat stress. The clinician may diagnose such cases as "masked" or "apathetic" hyperthyroidism or "forme fruste" hyperthyreosis or thyroid autonomy. When high excretion of urinary thyroxine (TAL and SULMAN, 1972) shows the etiology of the psychic complaints of a patient (insomnia, irritability, tension, palpitations, precordial pains, flushes, pollakisuria, exhaustion, depression, confusion), lithium therapy can adduce speedy relief (SULMAN et al., 1975).

VII. Thalidomide

Thalidomide is still used today – in spite of its teratogenic side effects – for alleviating the allergic, neuritic, and psychic reactions of leprotic patients. The endocrine effect of thalidomide and some of its derivatives was, therefore, studied by our group in rats (LOCKER et al., 1971). Thalidomide increases ACTH and decreases TSH. Its congeners behave differently. The ACTH-releasing effect of thalidomide explains its antiallergic, antineuritic and psychic effect in leprotic patients which is due to cortisone stimulation.

VIII. Antidepressants

MAO inhibitors and tricyclic antidepressants have not been reported to elicit endocrine side effects when given in appropriate dosage.

MAO inhibitors increase adrenaline and noradrenaline at low doses (1–2 tablets per day in man), yet serotonin only at higher doses (SULMAN et al., 1973). MAO inhibitors stimulate ACTH release in rats (ZOR et al., 1965a) and potentiate the effect of insulin (ZOR et al., 1965b). They can also inhibit STH release; thus, nialamide (Niamide), isocarboxazid (Marplan), phenelzine (Nardil), mebanazine (Actomol), pargyline (Eutonyl), pheniprazine (Catron), and tranylcypromine (Parnate) suppress STH, whereas iproniazid (Marsilid), etryptamine (Monase), amphetamine, and norpargyline do not suppress STH (ZOR et al., 1965c). TSH seems not to be affected. FSH and LH are supppressed (ZOR et al., 1968). These suppressive effects are due to interference of MAO inhibitors with the phosphogluconate oxidative pathway in the pituitary (ZOR et al., 1967a, b). On the other hand, LTH is suppressed by iproniazid (Marsilid), pargyline (Eutonyl), and phenelzine (Nardil), probably by potentiating the effect of dopamine which stimulates PIF release (HORROBIN, 1973).

Tricyclic antidepressants elevate plasma LTH in man. It is unlikely that they work via their catecholamine-releasing effect. Our work has shown that their tricyclic structure suppresses PIF (KHAZEN et al., 1968). If amitriptyline or imipramine are given to depressive patients with high initial prolactin levels (because of psychic stress), LTH release may be reduced (HORROBIN, 1974). This effect seems to be due to catecholamine release of the tricyclic antidepressants when given over a protracted period. It is well known that all sympathomimetic substances suppress LTH release.

Sulpiride (Dogmatil) is a powerful LTH releaser in women (*L'Hermite* et al., 1972) and rats (CALAF, 1973). This has been confirmed by DEBELJUK et al., (1974) and by our group in rats which received 5 mg/kg, i.p. LTH release begins within 15 min, reaches its peak after 30 min and remains high for 60 min (unpublished results).

IX. Hydroxyzine

Hydroxyzine was studied by our group in six patients with various psychologic disturbances, ranging from hysteria to melancholia, anxiety, depression, phobia, and con-
versive reactions. Generally, this drug has a tranquilizing effect which is not sufficient
for treatment of psychotic conditions. Thus, one psychotic patient did not respond.
In minor disturbances, mainly neuroses, hydroxyzine may be considered efficient. All
responding patients showed marked decrease of 17-Ketosteroid excretion pointing to
the tranquilizing effect of this drug. No other decrease in endocrine activity was noted:
17-hydroxysteroids, ACTH, as well as estrogen and gonadotropin excretion remained
unchanged (ASSAEL et al., 1960 b).

X. Ergot Derivatives

Ergot preparations have become of practical interest due to the introduction of 2-Br-
α-ergocryptine (CB-154); general name bromocriptine, proper name Parlodel (DEL
POZZO and FLUECKIGER, 1973). As this preparation suppresses LTH release from the
pituitary, it will probably become of practical interest for the prevention of iatrogenic
lactation when phenothiazine, butyrophenone and reserpine treatment is given to psychiatric cases. The human dose is 2.5 mg 1–3 times daily. In higher doses it suppresses
TSH, LH, and STH release from the pituitary (MASHITER et al., 1977).

C. Mechanisms of Endocrine Effects

It is obvious that there must be more than one mechanism of endocrine action for so
many different psychopharmaca, which often display diverse actions on the
neuroendocrine centers and receptors. The following three theories, which do not con-
tradict each other, can explain the endocrine effects of psychopharmaca.

I. The Mediator Theory (SULMAN et al., 1970) (Fig. 1)

Catecholamine-releasing psychopharmaca depress the hypothalamic-inhibiting centers and can suppress pituitary tropins. Serotonin-releasing psychopharmaca have the
opposite effect and can release pituitary tropins. Cholinergic mediators do not seem
to display special endocrine effects, except on ACTH release (HEDGE and SMELIK,
1968). Psychopharmaca which release both catecholamines and serotonin – such as
the MAO inhibitors and the tricyclic antidepressants – have unpredictable endocrine
effects: small doses increase only catecholamine release but large doses also increase
release of 17-KS, 17-OHS, and serotonin (SULMAN et al., 1973).

II. The Tropin Balance Theory (SULMAN and WINNIK, 1956) (Fig. 1 and 2)

This theory was developed by us when we noticed that the treatment of psychiatric
patients and laboratory animals with chlorpromazine produced different endocrine
results (WINNIK and SULMAN, 1956). Figure 1 shows that there exist balanced pituitary
tropins regulated by the feedback system of their secondary hormones: ACTH, STH,
TSH, FSH, LH (and ICSH). On the other hand, there also exist unbalanced pituitary

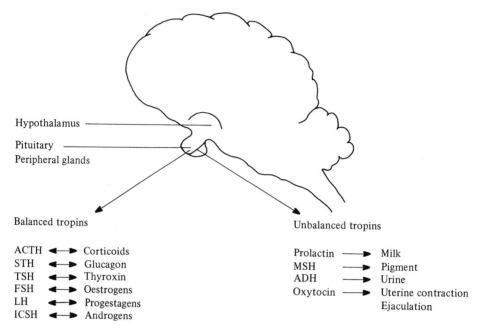

Fig. 1. Endocrine effects of psychopharmaca explained by the Tropin Balance Theory. Balanced tropins can withstand hypothalamic suppression

Balanced tropins	Week				Unbalanced hormones	
	1	2	3	4		
Hypothalamus	↓	↓	↓	↓	LTH↑:	Milk↑
Pituitary	–	↓	↓	–	MSH↑:	Pigment↑
					ADH↑:	Urine↓
Peripheral hormones	–	–	↓	–	Oxytocin↑:	Uterine contraction↓ Ejaculation↓

Fig. 2. Reaction of balanced and unbalanced tropins to hypothalamic depression. Endocrine effects of psychopharmaca can be explained by the "tropin balance theory". Unbalanced tropins react with a rebound reaction of "overshoot" when their inhibiting factor is suppressed by psychopharmaca

tropins which are not subject to a feedback system as they do not produce secondary hormones: LTH, MSH, ADH , and UCH. We further showed (SULMAN, 1956) that balanced tropins are regulated by selective accumulation of their secondary hormones in their governing centers of the pituitary (and the hypothalamus). This is a mechanism which obviously cannot exist for unbalanced tropins which produce only milk, pigment etc. In Fig. 2 it is shown that hypothalamic inhibition by chlorpromazine suppresses the hypothalamus in the first week; this suppression affecting the pituitary in the second week and the peripheral hormones in the third week. In the fourth week

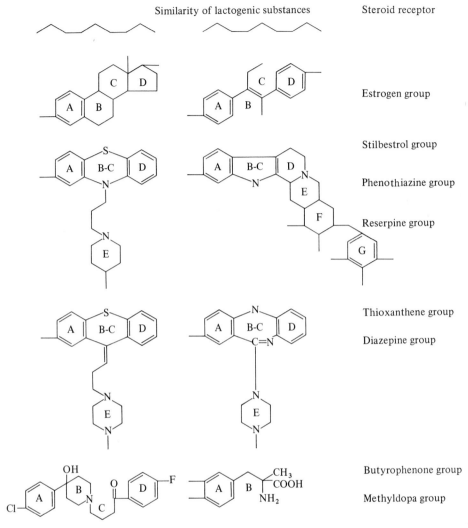

Fig. 3. Endocrine effects of psychopharmaca explained by the steroid receptor theory. Cyclic structures containing 3–5 rings compete for the steroid receptors. They can act when they have a polar group on an aromatic ring A and an unbranched side chain protruding from ring B–C which can simulate half a hexane ring

the suppression is overcome by the feedback of the balanced tropins and the hormonal imbalance is readjusted. Again, this cannot hold for the unbalanced tropins which are subject to the action of both inhibiting and releasing factors. In this case, an overshoot reaction of the suppressed inhibiting centers results in increased release of LTH, MSH, ADH, and UCH (oxytocin). Chlorpromazine, therefore, suppresses ACTH, STH, TSH, FSH, and LH (and ICSH) but stimulates LTH, MSH, ADH, and UCH (SULMAN, 1959). This would hold for all drugs of the phenothiazine, reserpine, and butyrophenone groups.

III. The Steroid Receptor Theory (SULMAN et al., 1970) (Fig. 3)

This theory was developed by us when we furnished proof that estradiol and phenothiazine derivatives compete for the same brain receptor (SHANI et al., 1971). Labeled
and unlabeled phenothiazine derivatives injected i. v. into rats prevented the uptake
of labeled estrogen derivatives in the hypothalamus and the pituitary – not however
in other brain sites. Figure 3 shows the different ring systems which fit into a typical
steroid receptor as, e. g., the estrogen group, stilbestrol group, phenothiazine group,
reserpine group, thioxanthene group, diazepine group, and butyrophenone group.
Methyldopa works on another principle mentioned earlier – the mediator theory –
whereby as a "false transmitter" it prevents catecholamine release. The steroid receptor can be blocked by steroids or 3–5 ring structures alike; it is related to the hypothalamic PRF and PIF since clinical experience has shown that it is stimulated by
small doses of estrogen and suppressed by larger ones. A side chain protruding from
the three-cyclic psychopharmaca allows them to become hormonally active only if it
is an unbranched 3C-membered chain which can fold and imitate half a hexane ring.
This explains why certain substituted three-cyclic rings are hormonally active whereas
others are not. Figure 3 shows also the importance of a polar substitution on the psychopharmaca which corresponds to the C-3 position of the steroids. More details can
be found in earlier publications (SULMAN et al., 1970; GIVANT and SULMAN, 1976).

D. Conclusions

The present short survey clearly indicates that psychopharmaca acting via the hypothalamus are the most liable to produce endocrine side effects. This is due to the presence of releasing and inhibiting hormones in the hypothalamus and the reaction of
hypothalamus and pituitary to autonomous mediators such as dopamine, adrenaline,
noradrenaline, serotonin, and acetylcholine. It can be safely stated that a psychophar-
macon eliciting endocrine side effects has its main target in the hypothalamus,
whereas psychopharmaca devoid of endocrine side effects act at internuncial synapses. This holds especially true for the benzodiazepines and the carbamides (meprobamate). Still, there exist many drugs which may elicit endocrine side effects by receptor
mechanisms not yet sufficiently elucidated. A typical case is the galactorrhea, elicited
occasionally by cimetidine (Tagamet), a H_2-receptor antagonist used for the treatment
of gastric and duodenal ulcers (BATESON et al., 1977).

References

Armstrong, B., Stevens, N., Doll, R.: Retrospective study of the association between use of rau-
    wolfia derivatives and breast cancer in English women. Lancet 2, 672–675 (1974)
Assael, M., Gabai, F., Winnik, H.Z., Khazan, N., Sulman, F.G.: Recession of exophthalmos
    after massive doses of reserpine. Lancet 1, 499–500 (1960a)
Assael, M., Sulman, F.G., Winnik, H.Z.: Clinical and endocrinological effects of hydroxyzine.
    J. Ment. Sci. 106, 1027–1030 (1960b)
Bateson, M.C., Browning, M.C.K., Maconnachie, A.: Galactorrhoea with cimetidine. Lancet
    2, 247–248 (1977)
Ben-David, M.: The role of the ovaries in perphenazine-induced lactation. J. Endocrinol. 41,
    377–385 (1968)
Ben-David, M., Dikstein, S., Sulman, F.G.: Production of lactation by non-sedative phenothi-
    azine derivatives. Proc. Soc. Exp. Biol. Med. 118, 265–270 (1965)
Boston Collaborative Drug Surveillance Program: Reserpine and breast cancer. Lancet 2, 669–
    671 (1974)

Calaf, J.: Prolactin release. Proc. Int. Symp. Human Prolactin. Brussels: Exc. Med. Int. Congr. Ser. *308*, 221–222 (1973)

Danon, A., Dikstein, S., Sulman, F.G.: Stimulation of prolactin secretion by perphenazine in pituitary-hypothalamus organ culture. Proc. Soc. Exp. Biol. Med. *114*, 366–368 (1963)

Debeljuk, L., Dashal, H., Rozados, R., Guitelman, A.: Effect of sulpiride on prolactin release by rat pituitaries *in vitro*. Experientia *30*, 1355–1356 (1974)

Del Pozo, E., Flueckiger, E.: Prolactin inhibition: experimental and clinical studies. Proc. Int. Symp. Human Prolactin. Brussels: Exc. Med. Int. Congr. Ser. *308*, 291–301 (1973)

De Wied, D.: Chlorpromazine and endocrine function. Pharmacol. Rev. *19*, 251–288 (1967)

Dickerman, S., Kledzik, G., Gelato, M., Chen, H.J., Meites, J.: Effect of haloperidol on serum and pituitary prolactin, LH and FSH, and Hypothalamic PIF and LRF. Neuroendocrinology *15*, 10–20 (1974)

Dikstein, S., Sulman, F.G.: Drugs acting on the hypothalamus-pituitary axis. Obstet. & Gyncl. Survey *21*, 531–547 (1966)

Everett, J.W., Radford, H.M., Holsinger, J.: Hormonal steroids. In: Steroids. Martini, L., Pecil, A. (eds.). New York: Academic Press 1964, Vol. 1, pp. 235–246

Givant, Y., Sulman, F.G.: Endocrine effects of psychotherapeutic drugs. In: Psychotherapeutic Drugs. Usdin, E., Forrest, I.S. (eds.). New York: Marcel Dekker 1976, pp. 387–436

Hedge, G.A., Smelik, P.G.: Corticotropin release: Inhibition by intrahypothalamic implantation of atropine. Science *159*, 891–892 (1968)

Heinonen, O.P., Shapiro, S., Tuominen, L., Turunen, M.I.: Reserpine use in relation to breast cancer. Lancet *2*,, 675–677 (1974)

Horrobin, D.F.: Prolactin Physiology and Clinical Significance. London: Medical and Technical Publishing Co. MTP 1973

Horrobin, D.F.: In: Prolactin 1974. Horrobin, D.F. (ed.). London: Medical and Technical Publishing Co. MTP 1974

Janssen, P.A.J.: The pharmacology of haloperidol. Int. J. Neuropsychiatry *3* [Suppl. 1], 10–18 (1967)

Janssen, P.A.J., Van den Westeringh, C., Jageneau, A.H.M., Demoen, P.J.A., Hermans, B.K.F., Van Daele, G.H.P., Schellekens, K.H.L., Van der Eycken, G.A.M., Niemegeers, C.J.E.: Chemistry and pharmacology of CNS depressants related to 4-(4-hydroxy-4-phenylpiperidino) butyrophenone. Part I: Synthesis and screening data in mice. J. Med. Pharm. Chem. *1*, 281–297 (1959)

Khazan, N., Sulman, F.G.: Melanophore-dispersing activity of reserpine in Rana frogs. Proc. Soc. Exp. Biol. Med. *107*, 282–284 (1961)

Khazan, N., Sulman, F.G., Winnik, H.Z.: Activity of pituitary-adrenal cortex axis during acute and chronic reserpine treatment. Proc. Soc. Exp. Biol. Med. *106*, 579–581 (1961)

Khazan, N., Ben-David, M., Mishkinsky, J., Khazen, K., Sulman, F.G.: Dissociation between mammotropic and sedative effects of nonhormonal hypothalamic tranquilizers. Arch. Int. Pharmacodyn. Ther. *164*, 258–271 (1966)

Khazen, M., Mishkinsky, J., Ben-David, M., Sulman, F.G.: Lactogenic effect of phenothiazine-like drugs. Arch. Int. Pharmacodyn. Ther. *174*, 428–441 (1968)

Kulcsar, S., Polishuk, W., Rubin, L.: Aspects endocriniens du traitement à la chlorpromazine. Presse Méd. *65*, 1288–1290 (1957)

Laborit, H., Huguenard, P.: L'hibernation artificielle par moyens pharmacodynamiques et physiques. Presse Méd. *64*, 1329–1331 (1951)

Lazarus, J.H., Bennie, E.H.: Effect of lithium on thyroid function in man. Acta Endocrinol. *70*, 266–272 (1972)

L'Hermite, M., Delroye, P., Nokin, J., Vekemans, M., Robyn, C.: IV th Tenovus Workshop on Prolactin. Cardiff: Alpha Omega Alpha 1972

Locker, D., Superstine, E., Sulman, F.G.: The mechanism of the Push and Pull Principle. VIII: Endocrine effects of thalidomide and its analogues. Arch. Int. Pharmacodyn. Ther. *194*, 39–55 (1971)

Marshall, W.K., Leiberman, D.M.: A rare complication of chlorpromazine treatment. Lancet *1*, 162–163 (1956)

Mashiter, K., Adams, E., Beard, M., Holley, A.: Bromocriptine inhibits prolactin and growth-hormone release by human pituitary tumours in culture. Lancet *2*, 197–198 (1977)

Meites, J.: Induction of lactation in rabbits with reserpine. Proc. Soc. Exp. Biol. Med. *96*, 728–730 (1957)

Meites, J.: Neurohumoral and pharmacological control of prolactin secretion. Scientific group on the physiology of lactation. Geneva: WHO 1963

Meites, J., Nicoll, C.S., Talwalker, P.K.: Effect of reserpine and serotonin on milk secretion and mammary growth in the rat. Proc. Soc. Exp. Biol. Med. *101*, 563–565 (1959)

Mishkinsky, J., Khazen, K., Givant, Y., Dikstein, S., Sulman, F.G.: Mammotropic and neuroleptic effects of butyrophenones in the rat. Arch. Int. Pharmacodyn. Ther. *179*, 94–105 (1969)

Moerck, H.J., Magelund, G.: Lancet *1*, 1344–1345 (1979)

Platt, R., Sears, H.T.N.: Reserpine in severe hypertension. Lancet *1*, 401–403 (1956)

Sawyer, C.H.: Induction of lactation in the rabbit with reserpine. Anat. Rec. *127*, 362–363 (1957)

Schou, M., Amdisen, A., Jensen, S.E., Olsen, T.: Occurrence of goitre during lithium treatment. Br. Med. J. *3*, 710–713 (1968)

Shani (Mishkinsky), J., Givant, Y., Sulman, F.G., Eylath, U., Eckstein, B.: Competition of phenothiazines with oestradiol for oestradiol receptors in rat brain. Neuroendocrinology *8*, 307–316 (1971)

Shani, J., Givant, Y., Goldhaber, G., Sulman, F.G.: Multi-phasic prolactin release in mammary development in virgin rats after prolonged treatment with perphenazine or perphenazine sulfoxide. J. Endocrinol. *70*, 311–312 (1976)

Sulman, F.G.: Experiments on the mechanism of the "Push and Pull" principle. J. Endocrinol. *14*, 27–28 (1956)

Sulman, F.G.: The mechanism of the "Push and Pull" principle. II. Endocrine effects of hypothalamus depressants of the phenothiazine group. Arch. Int. Pharmacodyn. Ther. *118*, 298–307 (1959)

Sulman, F.G.: Skin pigmentation following chlorpromazine treatment. Lancet *2*, 592–593 (1964)

Sulman, F.G., Winnik, H.Z.: Hormonal effects of chlorpromazine. Lancet *1*, 161–162 (1956)

Sulman, F.G., Ben-David, M., Danon, A., Dikstein, S., Givant, Y., Khazen, K., Mishkinsky-Shani, J., Nir, I., Weller, C.P.: Hypothalamic Control of Lactation. Monograph. Gross, F., Labhart, A., Mann, T., Samuels, L.T., Zander, J. (eds.). Berlin, Heidelberg, New York: Springer 1970

Sulman, F.G., Pfeifer, Y., Superstine, E.: Adrenal medullary exhaustion from tropical winds and its management. Isr. J. Med. Sci. *8*, 1022–1027 (1973)

Sulman, F.G., Tal., E., Pfeifer, Y., Superstine, E.: Intermittent hyperthyreosis – a heat stress syndrome. Horm. Metab. Res. *7*, 424–428 (1975)

Tal, E., Sulman, F.G.: Urinary thyroxine. Lancet *1*, 1291–1292 (1972)

Wilkins, R.W.: Clinical usage of rauwolfia alkaloids, including reserpine (Serpasil). Ann. N.Y. Acad. Sci. *59*, 36–44 (1954)

Winnik, H.Z., Sulman, F.G.: Hormonal depression due to treatment with chlorpromazine. Nature *178*, 365–366 (1956)

Winnik, H.Z., Tennenbaum, L.: Apparition de galactorrhée au cours du traitement de largactil. Presse Méd. *63*, 1092–1093 (1955)

Zor, U., Dikstein, S., Sulman, F.G.: The effect of monoamine oxidase inhibitors on growth and the rat tibia test. J. Endocrinol. *32*, 36–44 (1965a)

Zor, U., Dikstein, S., Sulman, F.G.: The effect of monoamine oxidase inhibitors on growth: Mechanism of the potentiating effect on corticosteroids. J. Endocrinol. *33*, 211–222 (1965b)

Zor, U., Mishkinsky, J., Sulman, F.G.: The hypoglycaemic effect of mebanazine (Actomol) and its mechanism. Biochem. Pharmacol. *14*, 1059–1064 (1965c)

Zor, U., Locker, D., Schleider, M., Sulman, F.G.: Effect of monoamine oxidase inhibitor (Mebanazine) on brain glucose-6-phosphate dehydrogenase activity. Eur. J. Pharmacol. *2*, 193–195 (1967a)

Zor, U., Shore, J., Locker, D., Sulman, F.G.: Metabolic effects of monoamine oxidase inhibitors on the rat pituitary. J. Endocrinol. *39*, 1–6 (1967b)

Zor, U., Locker, D., Schleider, M., Sulman, F.G.: Metabolic and enzymatic effects of monoamine oxidase inhibitors with and without hydrocortisone on the accessory sex glands of the rat. Eur. J. Pharmacol. *3*, 81–83 (1968)

Antidepressants
Chemistry (Structure and Effectiveness)

CHAPTER 16

Chemistry (Structure and Activity)

F.J. ZEELEN

Antidepressant activity in the human has been described for a large number of compounds and it is difficult to organize the available data in a systematic way. Here they are grouped not into strict chemical classes but according to major research topics. Although some of the tricyclic major tranquillizers described in Chap. 1 such as Thioridazine (OVERALL et al., 1964) and Flupenthixol (YOUNG et al., 1976) also show clinically useful antidepressant activity, the chapter on thymoleptics (Chap. 16) starts with a discussion of imipramine, which was the first thymoleptic compound not to show additional neuroleptic activity.

As described in Chap. 23, large variations in the rate at which different individuals metabolize imipramine and its analogs are known to occur which, together with the narrow therapeutic margin of these drugs, make it difficult to estimate the optimum dosage for any particular patient. Attention is first focused on the possibility of finding derivatives of imipramine with a reduced rate of metabolism, since such derivatives might prove to be safer and more reliable. The analogs derived from imipramine by the introduction of nonessential modifications (e. g., isosteric replacements) are briefly reviewed, followed by a description of those studies which define the key features of the imipramine molecule. It should be realized that the imipramine structure is, in all probability, not the optimum structure for antidepressant activity. To illustrate this point, after a brief discussion of some antidepressants which only retain a number of the key features of the imipramine molecule there follows an extensive discussion of structures unrelated to imipramine which have been shown to be effective antidepressants in the clinic. The latter structures have been developed on the basis of screening studies performed in animals.

The question then arises as to whether the "ideal" antidepressant should have both noradrenaline and serotonin reuptake blocking activity or be selective. Only clinical studies with compounds having a selective action can give the answer, and thus a review of the most selective compounds available is given followed by a discussion of those antidepressants having another mechanism of action. A separate chapter has been reserved for the monoamine oxidase inhibitors (Chap. 17).

A. Thymoleptics

I. Imipramine

KUHN (1957) reported the clinical observation that Imipramine, a compound originally described as having histamine antagonizing and spasmolytic activity (SCHIND-
LER and HÄFLIGER, 1954), showed useful thymoleptic activity.

The bioavailability of orally administered imipramine is good (29%–77%); it is,
however, rapidly metabolized, partly explaining the high doses (75–300 mg daily)
needed to obtain good clinical effects (GRAM and CHRISTIANSEN, 1975). Large individual variations are seen; in patients receiving 150 mg daily, plasma levels varied from
28 to 374 nmol/liter (NAGY and TREIBER, 1973). As both the thymoleptic effect and
the occurrence of side-effects (anticholinergic and cardiac effects) are related to plasma levels (WALTER, 1971), one might hope that derivatives more resistant to metabolism will be more potent and reliable. The major pathways of metabolism are N-demethylation and oxidation of the benzene ring at the 2 position, para to the activating
amino group (GRAM and CHRISTIANSEN, 1975). The hydroxylated metabolites do not
penetrate into the brain so that this pathway is inactivating. The demethylated analog
Desimipramine was shown in the clinic to be as potent as imipramine, although with
less sedative effect (BRODIE et al., 1961; GILLETTE et al., 1961).

The major pharmacologic effects of imipramine and desimipramine are the inhibition of noradrenaline and serotonin reuptake into the neuronal synaptosomes. CARLS-
SON (1966) and CARLSSON et al. (1969) have suggested that the blockade of serotonin
reuptake in the brain might be related to the mood-elevating effects seen after treatment with these compounds, whereas the inhibition of noradrenaline reuptake might
be correlated with the increase in drive. In in vitro tests imipramine has a stronger effect on serotonin uptake than desimipramine, whereas the latter compound has a
stronger effect on noradrenaline uptake (CARLSSON et al., 1969; TODRICK and TAIT,
1969; HORN and TRACE, 1974; TUOMISTO, 1974). In view of the metabolism of imipramine to desimipramine the differences in vivo are less pronounced. More selective
compounds will be needed to test the Carlsson hypothesis.

Blockade of the inactivating hydroxylation by the introduction of methyl groups
was of no practical use as these compounds were less active (BICKEL and BRODIE,
1964). Better results were obtained by replacing the central ring-N by CH, thus removing most of the activation of the benzene nuclei.

Structure-activity relationships for the dibenzocycloheptane and dibenzocyclo-heptene series have been discussed by ENGELHARDT et al. (1968). In contrast to imi-pramine, where the introduction of a 10,11-double bond gives Balipramine, which is no more potent than imipramine (THEOBALD et al., 1964), the dibenzocycloheptenes

were slightly more active than the dibenzocyclohepanes in the tetrabenazine antago-nism test. The decreased metabolism makes Protriptyline, although its intrinsic activ-ity is somewhat lower than imipramine (TODRICK and TAIT, 1969), one of the most potent analogs (CHARAMPOUS and JOHNSON, 1967; MOODY et al., 1973), with a clini-cally effective dose of 10–60 mg daily (HOLLISTER, 1972).

The 10,11-double bond in these compounds has introduced another metabolic pathway since it can be oxidized to the epoxide (HUCKER et al., 1975). This makes

SC 27123, in which the double bond has been replaced by a cyclopropyl ring, an in-teresting analog. In animal experiments, after oral administration this compound was indeed a potent antagonist of the reserpine-induced syndrome (COYNE and CUSIC, 1974).

II. Imipramine Analogs

The unexpected and important finding of the thymoleptic activity of imipramine stim-ulated research in this area. Unfortunately some time elapsed before reliable animal tests were developed, so that in the first decade after the discovery of imipramine chemists looking for patentable compounds had to rely heavily on intuition and made only minor changes to the imipramine molecule.

The replacement of the ring-N by an sp_3-C leading to the protriptyline series has already been discussed. Replacement by an sp_2-C gives Amitriptyline and Nortripty-line, both as active as imipramine and desimipramine (KLERMAN and COLE, 1965; ÅSBERG et al., 1971).

It also proved possible to replace one or both of the bridge carbon atoms by nitrogen (Monro et al., 1963; Winthrop et al., 1962a; Sparatore et al., 1974), sulfur (Winthrop et al., 1962b; Metyšová et al., 1965) or oxygen (Yale and Sowinsky, 1964; Ribbentrop and Schaumann, 1965) without losing the thymoleptic activity. Two of these, Doxepine and Dothiepin, are marketed as antidepressants.

Doxepine is a mixture of 82%–85% of the *trans*-isomer and 15%–18% of the *cis*-isomer (Devriendt et al., 1973). In man, however, part of the *trans*-isomer is converted to the *cis*-isomer (Pinder et al., 1977a). In pharmacologic experiments the *trans*-isomer proved a much more potent serotonin uptake inhibitor than the *cis*-isomer (Buczko et al., 1974), whereas the *cis*-isomer was more potent in decreasing spontaneous motor activity (Otsuki et al., 1973). The oxygen substituent activates the benzene nucleus so that hydroxylation of that ring is one of the metabolic pathways (Hobbs, 1969). Dothiepin is the pure *trans*-isomer; its sulfur atom is subject to metabolic oxydation (Brodie et al., 1977; Nakra et al., 1977). Despite this increased metabolism both doxepine and dothiepin are as potent as amitriptyline (Doxepine Review, 1971); Lambourn and Rees, 1974; Pinder et al., 1977a).

Substitution in the aromatic nucleus tends to decrease activity. Only monosubstitution with a small electron-withdrawing group seems to increase the serotonin uptake inhibiting activity without greatly influencing the noradrenaline uptake inhibiting activity (Todrick and Tait, 1969). The 3-chloro derivative, Chlorimipramine, is marketed as an antidepressant.

One of the benzene rings of imipramine and its analogs can be replaced by other aromatic rings such as thiophen (Bastian et al., 1966, 1971; Bastian and Weber, 1971), pyridine (Villani and Mann, 1968; Villani et al., 1972) or pyrimidine (Kobayashi, 1973) without losing too much of the activity. IB-503, a 2:1 mixture of *trans*- and *cis*-isomers, was investigated in the clinic and found to have antidepressant activity (Vencovský et al., 1969).

The length of the side chain seems to be critical; shorter side chains being less active in animal experiments and the longer side chains inactive as antidepressant and more toxic. Again, some of the carbon atoms can be replaced by oxygen (STELT et al., 1966), sulfur (DOSTERT and JALFRE, 1974) or by nitrogen and oxygen (AICHINGER et al., 1969). Noxiptilen is marketed as an antidepressant (Agedal Symposium, 1969).

Substitution of the side chain tends to decrease the serotonin uptake blocking activity. Two derivatives with a methyl substituent on the β-carbon atom of the side chain, Trimipramine and Butriptyline, are marketed (LAMBERT and GUYOTAT, 1961; Butriptyline review, 1971). Both compounds are marketed as the racemates, although pharmacologic investigations have shown small but significant differences in the profile on the two optical antipodes (JULOU et al., 1961).

The antidepressant activity decreases with decreasing basicity of the amino side chain (LAPIN et al., 1970). Opipramol has both weak thymoleptic and tranquillizing activity (ROGERS et al., 1969; MURPHY et al., 1970). However, Lofepramine was found in the clinic as active as amitriptyline (ERICSOO and ROHTE, 1970; WRIGHT and HERRMANN, 1976; LEHMANN and HOPES, 1977).

III. Search for the "Active" Conformation of Imipramine and Its Analogs

X-Ray crystal structure analysis of imipramine has shown the existence of two different conformations (POST et al., 1974) which were different from the conformation found in aqueous solution (ABRAHAM et al., 1974, 1977). This indicates that imipramine is a flexible molecule, which may explain why it can interact with a number of biologic systems. One may hope that more rigid analogs will show more selectivity.

Most of the work described here, has been performed within the last 5 years and only a few biologic results have been reported.

In view of the hypothesis of Wilhelm (1972), which states that for thymoleptic activity the side chain should occur in a bent conformation, the following two derivatives with rigid side chains are important:

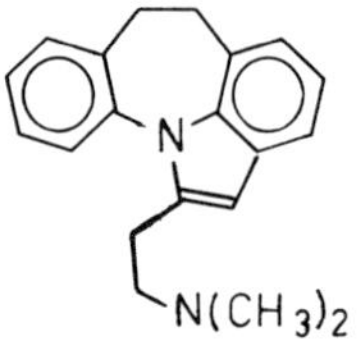

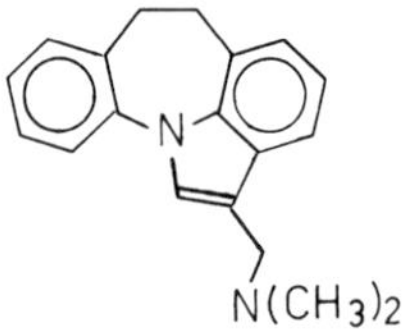

The first compound with an extended side chain was as active as imipramine in the reserpine antagonism test, whereas the second compound was inactive, thus refuting the Wilhelm hypothesis (Toscano et al., 1976). Azipram is the N-benzyl analog of the first-mentioned compound. A related structure, interestingly enough lacking the traditional 3-carbon side chain, is Quinupramine. Its serotonin and noradrenaline uptake blocking activity is comparable to that of desimipramine (Uzan and LeFur, 1975).

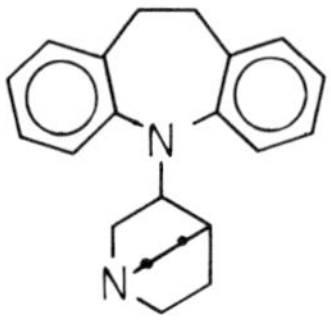

Another way to render the side chain rigid is to introduce a cyclopropyl or an allenyl group:

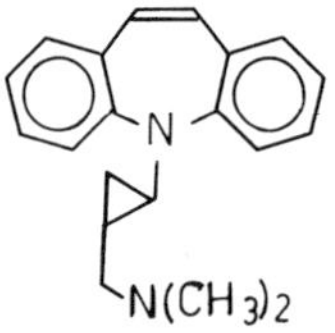

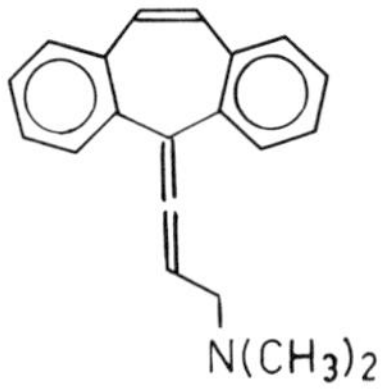

Studies in animals have shown that these modifications hardly affected the activity of the nonrigid parent compound (Kaiser et al., 1971; Roszkowski et al., 1975).

Ring closure of the side chains in the following modifications also gave derivatives with serotonin and noradrenaline uptake blocking activity comparable to that of the imipramine series (Carnmalm et al., 1974; Moncovic et al., 1973).

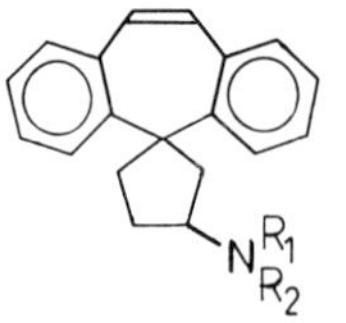

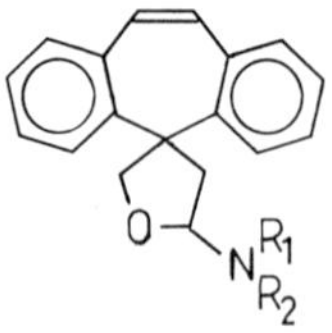

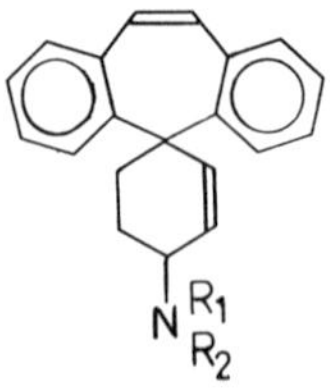

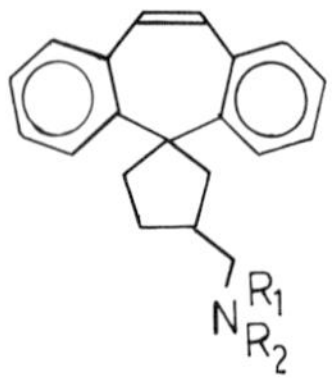

Whether these derivatives show selectivity has not yet been reported. More results are available from the series of which Cyproheptadine is an example.

The most important activities of cyproheptadine are its serotonin and histamine antagonizing activity with some anticholinergic and orexigenic properties (ENGEL-HARDT et al., 1965). During in vitro experiments the serotonin and noradrenaline uptake inhibiting activity of cyproheptadine was less than that of imipramine (UZAN and LeFUR, 1975). In imipramine and amitriptyline the central 7-membered ring exists in

different conformations. The interconversion of these conformations is very rapid (ABRAHAM et al., 1974); in cyproheptadine however, due to the steric hindrance between the protons in the 4 and 6 positions of the aromatic rings and the allylic protons of the piperidine ring, no inversion of the 7-membered ring occurs. When a substituent is present in cyproheptadine and the symmetry of the original compound is destroyed, the substituted cyproheptadine can be resolved into two isomers. It was then shown for the 3-methoxy derivative of cyproheptadine that the (+) isomer was responsible for the anticholinergic activity, whereas the antiserotonin and antihistamine activity resided in the (−) isomer (REMY et al., 1977).

In Pizotifen, a thiophen analog of cyproheptadine, the barrier to inversion may be lower. This compound also shows serotonin and histamine antagonizing activity and it is used for the treatment of migraine. Preliminary clinical studies have also indicated antidepressant activity in a dose of 5 mg daily, a very low dose for an imipramine analog (SPEIGHT and AVERY, 1972). In the RO-4-1284 antagonism test in mice, the activity of pizotifen was only of the same order of magnitude as that of imipramine and its analogs (COLPAERT et al., 1975).

The investigations mentioned above need to be extended, but nevertheless they clearly show that part of the lack of selectivity of action of imipramine and its analogs is related to the flexibility of these systems, enabling these compounds to adapt to the steric requirements of the different receptors.

Fixation of the conformation of the central ring is possible by the introduction of a 5,10-oxide bridge. This led to a potent series, the *trans* 11-hydroxy derivative MK-940 having the strongest oral tetrabenazine antagonizing effect in mice (CHRISTY et al., 1970).

This modification may not be the only factor, however, since LU-3009, in which the 7-membered ring has been opened, seems to be as potent as MK-940 (PETERSEN et al., 1966; UZAN and LEFUR, 1975). Other isobenzofurans were also found to be active in the tetrabenazine antagonism test (BAUER et al., 1976; KLIOSE et al., 1977). In clinical investigations, the EEG changes observed after MK-940 administration were different from those seen after amitriptyline administration (GANNON et al., 1970).

The side chain of LU-3009 may not have the optimum length, because in the structurally related phenylindene series, Indrilene, having a side chain with one methylene group less, was found to be the most potent derivative (DIJKSTRA et al., 1967).

IV. Further Exploration of Structure-Activity Relationships

The penetration of imipramine and its analogs into the brain is excellent (CHRISTIANSEN and GRAM, 1973) although plasma levels have to be high in order to see a clinical effect, e. g., imipramine 2×10^{-7} mol/liter (WALTER, 1971; NAGY and TREIBER, 1973), protriptyline 7×10^{-7} mol/liter (MOODY et al., 1973), and amitriptyline 4×10^{-7} mol/ liter (BRAITHWAITE et al., 1972). On the other hand compounds with comparable molecular weight are active at much lower plasma levels, e.g., progesterone 1×10^{-9} mol/ liter or ketobemidone $\sim 8 \times 10^{-9}$ mol/liter. This suggests that imipramine and its analogs do not have a high complimentarity to the receptor(s), which would also explain the low selectivity of these compounds. In other words, with imipramine and its analogs, the optimum structures have not been found and further research is needed.

In order to explain the differences in activity of the structurally related neuroleptics and thymoleptics, STACH and PÖLDINGER (1966) and WILHELM (1972) suggested that the angle between the two aromatic nuclei would be decisive. This hypothesis was based on molecular models, but REBOUL and CRISTIAU (1977 a, b) failed to confirm it using measured X-ray crystallographic data. Because several of the compounds studied occur in more than one conformation no definite proof was possible, although the predicted trend was observed. Maprotiline is an interesting example of a compound not having an imipramine-like structure but, due to the presence of the ethylene bridge, fulfilling the above mentioned structural requirements for thymoleptic activity (WILHELM and SCHMIDT, 1969). It was shown to be an antidepressant in the clinic (KIELHOLZ, 1972; MURPHY, 1975; Ludiomil Symposium, 1977; PINDER et al., 1977 b). In animal experiments maprotiline did not, in contrast to imipramine, influence the uptake of serotonin (Maître et al., 1975; GORDEN, 1977).

The pharmacologic profile of ID-9206 was comparable to that of maprotiline (FU-
KUSHIMA et al., 1977).

V. Compounds Found in Screening

The following compounds, all with structures strikingly different from imipramine,
have been found in random screening. Although none is more potent than imipramine, this range of structurally unrelated compounds, all showing antidepressant activity, illustrates that the optimum structures for antidepressant activities have not yet
been found.

The tetrahydroisoquinoline, Nomifensine, was shown to be a potent antagonist of
the reserpine-induced syndrome (HOFFMANN et al., 1971). In contrast to imipramine,
it not only inhibited the uptake of noradrenaline but also that of dopamine (HUNT
et al., 1974; RANDRUP and BRAESTRUP, 1977). In clinical trials it proved to be as potent
an antidepressant as imipramine and desimipramine (ACÉBAL, 1976), and rapidly
metabolized (HEPTNER et al., 1978). Further studies will be necessary to evaluate the
clinical significance of its dopamine reuptake blocking activity.

An initial pharmacokinetic study in volunteers with Ciclazindol, a compound having a somewhat related structure has been reported (SWAISLAND et al., 1977). Fe-
moxitine was also found in screening. The first clinical trials with the (+) isomer
showed antidepressant activity at the high dose of 300–600 mg daily (BUUS-LASSEN
et al., 1975).

Imafen showed an antidepressant profile in the RO-4-1284 antagonism test in mice
(COLPAERT et al., 1975). It has some structural relationship with Dexamisole which
was shown in the clinic to have antidepressant activity. (NIEMEGEERS, 1972; BRUGMANS
et al., 1972). For both compounds the d-enantiomer showed the strongest activity.

When an oxazine, synthesized as a closed ring analog of propranolol, was
screened, activity was found in the reserpine antagonism test suggesting antidepressant activity (GREENWOOD et al., 1975). A study of the relationship between
chemical structure and reserpine-antagonizing activity led to the 60-fold more potent
analog, Viloxazine (MALLIOU et al., 1972). Compared with imipramine its serotonin
uptake inhibiting activity is somewhat lower, but its noradrenaline uptake inhibiting
activity higher (UZAN and LEFUR, 1975). Its metabolism is fast so that its clinical

potency is only half that of imipramine (Vivalan Symposium, 1975; PINDER et al., 1977c). The compound is a racemate. The S-enantiomer at least 10-fold more potent than the R-enantiomer in animal experiments (HOWE et al., 1976). However, no dissociation was found between antidepressant and sedative activity with these two isomers.

The tetrahydrothiapyranoindoles form another series showing promising activity when screened for reserpine-antagonizing activity. Tandamine was selected for further study (JIRKOVSKY et al., 1977). It has been resolved into its optical antipodes and the laevorotatory enantiomer was found to be more active than the racemate. Tandamine was more active than imipramine in inhibiting the tyramine pressor response after a single oral dose in man, confirming the strong noradrenaline reuptake blocking activity found in animal experiments (EHSANULLAH et al., 1977). In a clinical study in depressed patients using a dose of 75–200 mg/day, a weak antidepressant activity was seen; activating/stimulatory effects were more pronounced (SALETU et al., 1977).

A series of analogs has been synthesized and tested, and it was shown that the sulfur atom can be replaced by oxygen or a methylene group without serious loss of activity (ASSELIN, 1976).

Dibenzepin was originally reported to be an antihistaminic (HUNZIKER et al., 1963) but is currently used as an antidepressant. However, high doses leading to high plasma levels are needed to see a clinical effect (MODESTIN, 1973).

The large variety of structures with antidepressant activities shows that we have not yet reached the optimum structures as far as potency and selectivity of action are concerned.

VI. Search for Compounds with Greater Specificity

Imipramine and its analogs show a series of activities among which the noradrenaline and serotonin reuptake inhibiting activities are the best studied. Some dissociation between these two activities has been achieved with desimipramine, the strongest noradrenaline reuptake inhibitor, and chlorimipramine, the strongest serotonin reuptake inhibitor. The separation is, however, too low to definitely establish the clinical significance of these activities. Thus, compounds with a greater specificity are needed to provide pharmacology with the necessary feed-back from the clinic. Of the newer compounds we have already mentioned maprotiline and tandamine, which mainly affect the central noradrenergic system. Recently, a number of more selective inhibitors of the serotonin reuptake system have been reported. These are Zimelidine (SIWERS et al., 1977), a close analog of the antihistaminic clorpheniramine, and Fluoxetine (WONG et al., 1975; FULLER et al., 1975; FULLER and PERRY, 1977; LEMBERGER et al., 1978).

Chlorimipramine is metabolized to the desmethyl derivative, which has a noradrenaline reuptake blocking effect (THOMAS and JONES, 1977). It is logical to expect that zimelidine and fluoxetine can also be metabolized by N-demethylation to other active compounds. This is not possible with Org 6582 which, in in vivo studies in the rat, was found to be a potent and selective serotonin reuptake inhibitor (GOODLET et al., 1976).

VII. Compounds with a Mechanism of Action Different From that of Imipramine and Its Analogs

Iprindol is an antidepressant having a structure and mechanism of action different from that of the imipramine series (RICE et al., 1964). It does not inhibit noradrenaline or serotonin uptake (BEVAN et al., 1975; SANGHOI and GERSHON, 1975), but further studies are necessary to define its mechanism of action. From the few clinical studies which have been reported with this compound it can be concluded that it is as effective as, but slightly less potent than, imipramine (RICKELS et al., 1973).

Much more detailed investigations have been reported for Mianserin, a compound originally synthesised for antiserotonin activity (V.D.BURG et al., 1970). A study of the changes in EEG induced by the drug in healthy volunteers pointed to antidepressant activity (ITIL et al., 1972; ITIL, 1973). This was confirmed in further clinical trials in which it proved to be a potent antidepressant as effective as the classic antidepressants such as imipramine and amitriptyline (COPPEN et al., 1976; MURPHY et al., 1976; JASKARI et al., 1977).

The X-ray structure analysis of mianserin (VAN RIJ and FEIL, 1973) shows striking differences from imipramine and IB-503, e. g., in the angles between the aromatic rings (REBOUL and CRISTAU, 1977a). This agrees with the differences in pharmacologic profile, indicating that mianserin has a different mechanism of action. It has no reserpine-antagonizing effect in the mouse, rat, or cat and, in in vivo animal studies, no effect on brain monoamine uptake (PEET and BEHAGEL, 1978). In contrast to amitriptyline, mianserin had no effect on the pressor response after tyramine administration, indicating that in man also this drug does not inhibit noradrenaline reuptake (COPPEN et al., 1978). Its mechanism of action may be that mianserin increases synaptosomal serotonin release (RAITERI et al., 1976) and that mianserin increases noradrenaline release by blocking presynaptic α-receptors (BAUMANN and MAÎTRE, 1977; BERENDSEN et al., 1978). The difference between mianserin and the classic antidepressants is demonstrated in the clinic by the absence of the anticholinergic effects and cardiotoxicity seen during treatment with amitriptyline (JASKARI et al., 1977; KOPERA, 1978). Compared with maprotiline, and also to a lesser extent with amitriptyline, the risk of suicidal ideation was less with mianserin (MONTGOMERY et al., 1978).

B. Conclusion

Looking back over more than 20 years of research in the antidepressant field, it is evident that the lack of suitable animal test models has slowed down progress in this area. It took some 10 years before such models were available and generally accepted. Only then could a systematic exploration of structure-activity relationships start. The first reported studies are promising but much more work will have to be done before we achieve the final target of making available to the medical profession a series of safe, reliable, potent, and specific compounds with different mechanisms of action for the treatment of depressive illnesses.

References

Abraham, R.J., Kricka, L.J., Ledwith, A.: The nuclear magnetic resonance spectra and conformations of cyclic compounds. J. Chem. Soc. [Perkin II], 1648 (1974)

Abraham, R.J., Lewtas, K., Thomas, W.A.: A nuclear magnetic resonance investigation of complex formation between imipramine and related psychotropic drugs with benzylalcohol and other aromatic solutes. J. Chem. Soc. [Perkin II], 1964 (1977)

Acébal, E., Subirá, S., Spatz, J., Falent, R., Merzberger, B., Gales, A., Moizeszowicz, J.: A double blind comparative trial of nomifensine and desimipramine in depression. Eur. J. Clin. Pharmacol. *10*, 109 (1976)

Agedal: Bericht über das Symposium anläßlich der Einführung des Antidepressivums. Arzneim. Forsch. *19*, 833 (1969)

Aichinger, G., Behner, O., Hoffmeister, F., Schütz, S.: Basische tricyclische Oximinoaether und ihre pharmacologische Eigenschaften. Arzneim. Forsch. *19*, 838 (1969)

Åsberg, M., Crönholm, B., Sjöqvist, F., Tuck, D.: Relationship between plasma level and therapeutic effect of nortriptyline. Br. Med. J. *3*, 331 (1971)

Asselin, A.A., Humber, L.G., Komlossy, J., Charest, M.P.: Cycloalkanindols. J. Med. Chem. *19*, 792 (1976)

Bastian, J.M., Ebnöther, A., Jucker, E., Risse, E., Stoll, A.P.: 4H-Benzo[4,5]-cyclohepta[1,2-b]thiophene. Helv. Chim. Acta *49*, 214 (1966)

Bastian, J.M., Ebnöther, A., Jucker, E., Risse, E., Stoll, A.P.: Beiträge zur Chemie des 4,5-Dihydro-10H-benzo[5,6]cyclohepta[1,2-b]thiophens. Helv. Chim. Acta *54*, 277 (1971)

Bastian, J.M., Weber, H.P.: Die molekulare und kristalline Struktur von 9,10-Dihydro-4-(3-dimethylamino-propyliden)-4H-benzo[4,5]cyclohepta[1,2-b]thiophen-hydrochlorid. Helv. Chim. Acta *54*, 293 (1971)

Bauer, V.J., Duffy, B.J., Hoffman, D., Klioze, S.S., Kosley, R.W., McFadden, A.R., Martin, L.L., Org, H.H., Geyer, H.M.: Synthesis of Spiro[isobenzofuran-1(3H),4'-piperidines] as potential central nervous system agents. J. Med. Chem. *19*, 1315 (1976)

Baumann, P.A., Maître, L.: Blockade of presynaptic α-receptors and of amine uptake in the rat brain by the antidepressant mianserine. Naunyn-Schmiedeberg's Arch. Pharmacol. *300*, 31 (1977)

Berendsen, H., de Graaf, J., Nickolson, V., Schönbaum, E.: Mianserin affects thermoregulation bimodally via 5-HT and NA. Abs. of paper 7th Int. Congr. Pharmacol., Paris (1978).

Bevan, P., Bradshaw, C.M., Szabadi, E.: Effects of iprindol on responses of single cortical and caudate neurones to monoamines and acetylcholine. Br. J. Pharmacol. *55*, 17 (1975)

Bickel, M.H., Brodie, B.B.: Structure and antidepressant activity of imipramine analogues. Int. J. Neuropharmacol. *3*, 611 (1964)

Braithwaite, R.A., Goulding, R., Theano, G., Bailey, J., Coppen, A.: Plasma concentration amitriptyline and clinical response. Lancet *I*, 1297 (1972)

Brodie, B.B., Dick, P., Kielholz, P., Poeldinger, W., Theobold, W.: Preliminary pharmacological and clinical results with desmethylimipramine, a metabolite of imipramine. Psychopharmacologia *2*, 467 (1961)

Brodie, R.B., Chasseaud, L.F., Crampton, E.L., Hawkins, D.R., Risdall, P.C.: High performance liquid chromatographic determination of dothiophen and northiaden in human plasma and serum. J. Int. Med. Res. *5*, 388 (1977)

Brugmans, J., van Lommel, R., Baro, F.: Clinical aspects of tetramisol, an anthelmintic with antidepressant activity. Psychopharmacologia *26*, 85S (1972)

Buczko, W., de Gaetano, G., Garattini, S.: Influence of some tricyclic antidepressive drugs on the uptake of 5-hydroxytryptamine by rat blood platelets. J. Pharm. Pharmacol. *26*, 814 (1974)

v.d. Burg, W.J., Bonta, I.L., Delobelle, J., Ramon, C., Vergaftig, B.: A novel type of substituted piperazine with high antiserotonine potency. J. Med. Chem. *13*, 35 (1970)

Butriptyline, International Symposium on J. Med. (Basel) *2*, 250 (1971)

Buus-Lassen, J., Squires, R.F., Christiansen, J.A., Molander, L.: Neurochemical and pharmacological studies on a new 5HT-uptake inhibitor, FG 4363, with potential antidepressant properties. Psychopharmacologia *42*, 21 (1975)

Carlsson, A.: Drugs which block the storage of 5-hydroxytryptamine and related amines. In: Handbook of Experimental Pharmacology, Vol. XIX. Berlin, Heidelberg, New York: Springer 1966, p. 529

Carlsson, A., Corrodi, H., Fuxe, K., Hökfelt, T.: Effect of antidepressant drugs on the depletion of intraneuronal brain 5-hydroxytryptamine stores caused by 4-methyl-α-ethyl-meta-tyramine. Eur. J. Pharmacol. *5*, 357 (1969)

Carnmalm, B., Jacupovic, E., Johansson, L., de Paulis, T., Rämsby, S., Stjernström, N.E., Renyi, A.L., Ross, S.B., Ogren, S.O.: Antidepressive agents. J. Med. Chem. *17*, 65 (1974)

Charampous, K.D., Johnson, P.C.: Studies of C¹⁴-Protriptyline in man: plasma levels and excretion. J. Pharmacol. *7*, 93 (1967)

Christiansen, J., Gram, L.F.: Imipramine and its metabolites in human brain. J. Pharm. Pharmacol. *25*, 604 (1973)

Christy, M.E., Boland, C.C., Williams, J.G., Engelhardt, E.L.: Antidepressants. J. Med. Chem. *13*, 191 (1970)

Colpaert, F.C., Lenaerts, F.M., Niemegeers, C.J.E., Janssen, P.A.J.: A critical study on RO-4-1284 antagonism in mice. Arch. Int. Pharmacodyn. Ther. *215*, 40 (1975)

Coppen, A., Gupta, R., Montgomery, S., Ghose, K., Baily, J., Burns, B., deRidder, J.J.: Mianserin hydrochloride, a novel antidepressant. Br. J. Psychiatr. *129*, 342 (1976)

Coppen, A., Ghose, K., Swade, C., Wood, K.: Effect of mianserin hydrochloride on peripheral uptake mechanisms for noradrenaline and 5-hydroxytryptamine in man. Br. J. Clin. Pharmacol. *5*, 13S (1978)

Coyne, W.E., Cusic, J.W.: Aminoalkyldibenzo[a,e]cyclopropa[c]cycloheptene derivatives, a series of potent antidepressants. J. Med. Chem. *17*, 72 (1974)

Devriendt, E., Weemaes, J., Jansen, F.H.: Colorometric, ultra violet spectrometric and spectrofluorometric determination of doxepine and some of its metabolites in serum and urine. Arzneim. Forsch. *23*, 863 (1973)

Dijkstra, S.J., Berdahl, J.M., Campbell, K.N., Coombs, C.M., Lankin, D.G.: Phenylindenes and phenylindanes with antireserpine activity. J. Med. Chem. *10*, 418 (1967)

Dostert, P., Jalfre, M.: Tricyclic compounds with an alkylaminoalkylthio chain. Eur. J. Med. Chem. *9*, 259 (1974)

Doxepine, a review. Drugs *1*, 194 (1971)

Ehsanullah, R.S.B., Ghose, K., Kirby, M.J., Turner, P., Witts, D.: Clinical pharmacological studies of tandamine, a potential antidepressive drug. Psychopharmacology *52*, 73 (1977)

Engelhardt, E.L., Zell, H.C., Saari, W.S., Christy, M.E., Colton, C.D., Stone, C.A., Stavorski, J.M., Wenger, H.C., Luddon, C.T.: Structure-activity relationships in the cyproheptadine series. J. Med. Chem. *8*, 829 (1965)

Engelhardt, E.L., Christy, M.E., Colton, C.D., Friedman, M.B., Boland, C.C., Halpern, L.M., Vermeer, V.C., Stone, C.A.: Antidepressants. J. Med. Chem. *11*, 325 (1968)

Eriksoo, R., Rohte, O.: Chemistry and pharmacology of a new potential antidepressant. Arzneim. Forsch. *20*, 1561 (1970)

Fukushima, H., Nakamura, M., Yamamoto, H.: Pharmacology of 9-γ-Methylaminopropyl-9,10-methanoanthracene. HCl (ID-9206.HCl), a new potent antidepressant. Arch. Int. Pharmacodyn. Ther. *229*, 163 (1977)

Fuller, R.W., Perry, K.W.: Increase of pineal noradrenaline concentrations in rats by desimipramine but not fluoxetine: implications concerning the specificity of these uptake inhibitors. J. Pharm. Pharmacol. *29*, 710 (1977)

Fuller, R.W., Perry, K.W., Molloy, B.B.: Effect of 3-(p-trifluoromethylphenoxy)-N-methyl-3-phenylpropylamine on the depletion of brain serotonin by 4-chloramphetamine. J. Pharmacol. Exp. Ther. *193*, 796 (1975)

Gannon, P., Itil, T., Keskiner, A., Hsu, B.: Clinical and quantitative encephalographical effects of MK 940. Arzneim. Forsch. *20*, 971 (1970)

Gillette, J.R., Dingelt, J.V., Sulser, F., Kuntzman, R., Brodie, B.B.: Isolation from rat brain of a metabolic product, desmethylimipramine, that mediates the antidepressant activity of imipramine. Experientia *17*, 417 (1961)

Goodlet, I., Mireylees, S.E., Sugrue, M.F.: The selective inhibition of 5-hydroxytryptamine re-uptake by Org 6582. Br. J. Pharmacol. *56*, 367 (1976)

Gordon, A.M.: The biochemistry of depression. J. Int. Med. Res. *5*, Suppl. 4, 81 (1977)

Gram, L.F., Christiansen, J.: First-pass metabolism of imipramine in man. Clin. Pharmacol. Ther. *17*, 555 (1975)

Greenwood, D.T., Malliou, K.B., Todel, A.H., Turner, R.W.: 2-Aryloxymethyl-2,3,5,6-tetrahydr-1,4-oxazines, a new class of antidepressants. J. Med. Chem. *18*, 573 (1975)

Heptner, W., Hornke, J., Cavagna, F., Fehlhaber, H.W., Rupp, W., Neubauer, H.P.: Metabolism of nomifensin in man and animal species. Arzneim. Forsch. *28*, 58 (1978)

Hobbs, D.C.: Distribution and metabolism of doxepin. Biochem. Pharmacol. *18*, 1941 (1969)

Hoffmann, I., Ehrhart, G., Schmitt, K.: 8-Amino-4-phenyl-1,2,3,4-tetrahydroisochinoline, eine neue Gruppe antidepressiver Psychopharmaka. Arzneim. Forsch. *21*, 1045 (1971)

Hollister, L.E.: Clinical use of psychotherapeutic drugs. Drugs *4*, 361 (1972)

Horn, A.S., Trace, R.C.A.M.: Structure-activity relations for the inhibition of 5-hydroxytryptamine uptake by tricyclic antidepressants into synaptosomes from serotonergic neurones in rat brain homogenates. Br. J. Pharmacol. *51*, 399 (1974)

Howe, R., Leigh, T., Rao, B.S., Todd, A.H.: Optical isomers of 2-(2-ethoxyphenoxymethyl)tetrahydro-1,4-oxazine (Viloxazine) and related compounds. J. Med. Chem. *19*, 1074 (1976)

Hucker, H.B., Balletto, A.J., Demetriades, J., Arison, B.H., Zacchei, A.G.: Expoxide metabolites of protriptyline in rat urine. Drug Metab. Dispos. *3*, 80 (1975)

Hunt, P., Kannengiesser, M.H., Raynaud, J.P.: Nomifensine, a new potent inhibitor of dopamine uptake into synaptosomes from rat brain corpus striatum. J. Pharm. Pharmacol. *26*, 370 (1974)

Hunziker, F., Lauener, H., Schmutz, J.: Zur Chemie und Pharmakologie von in 10 Stellungen basisch substituierten 5-Dibenzo-[b,e][1,4]diazepin Derivaten. Arzneim. Forsch. *13*, 324 (1963)

Itil, T.M., Polvan, N., Hsu, W.: Clinical and EEG effects of GB-94,a "tetracyclic" antidepressant. Curr. Ther. Res. *14*, 395 (1972)

Itil, I.M.: Drug developments in Europe: discovery of "tetracyclic" psychotropic drugs. Psychopharmacol. Bull. *9*, 41 (1973)

Jaskari, M.O., Ahlfors, U.G., Ginman, L., Lydeken, K., Tienari, P.: Three double-blind comparative trials of Mianserine (Org GB-94) and Amitriptyline in the treatment of depressive illness. Pharmakopsychiatr. Neuropsychopharmacol. *10*, 101 (1977)

Jirkovsky, I., Humber, L.G., Voith, K., Charest, M.P.: Synthesis and primary pharmacological sceening of tandamine and related tetrahydrothiopyranoindoles with potential antidepressant properties. Arzneim. Forsch. *27*, 1642 (1977)

Julou, L., Leau, O., Ducrot, R., Fournel, J., Bardone, M.C.: Propriétés pharmacodynamiques générales du (dimethylamino-3'methyl-2'propyl-1')-5-iminodibenzyl et de ses isomères optiques, droit et gauche. Compt. Rend. Soc. Biol. *155*, 307 (1961)

Kaiser, C., Tedeschi, D.H., Fowler, P.J., Pavloff, A.M., Lester, B.M., Zirkle, C.L.: Analogues of phenothiazines. J. Med. Chem. *14*, 179 (1971)

Kielholz, P.: Depressive Zustände. Bern: Hans Huber Verlag 1972

Klerman, G.L., Cole, J.O.: Clinical pharmacology of imipramine and related antidepressant compounds. Pharmacol. Rev. *17*, 101 (1965)

Kliose, S.S., Bauer, V.J., Geyer, H.M.: Synthesis of Spiro[isobenzofuran-1(3H),4'-piperidines] as potential central nervous system agents. J. Med. Chem. *20*, 610 (1977)

Kobayashi, S.: Synthesis of pyrimidines and condensed pyrimidines. Bull. Chem. Soc. Japan *46*, 2835 (1973)

Kopera, H.: Anticholinergic and blood pressure effects of mianserin, amitriptyline and placebo. Br. J. Clin. Pharmacol. *5*, 29S (1978)

Kuhn, R.: Über die Behandlung depressiver Zustände mit einem Iminodibenzylderivat. Schweiz. Med. Wochenschr. *87*, 1135 (1957)

Lambert, P.A., Guyotat, J.: Un nouvel antidépresseur sédatif. Presse Medicale *31*, 1425 (1961)

Lambourn, J., Rees, J.A.: A general practioner study of dothiopin and amitriptyline. J. Int. Med. Res. *2*, 210 (1974)

Lapin, J.P., Ksenofontova, T.A., Ya Kvitko, I., Porai-Koshits, B.A.: Central neurotropic activity of aminopropyl and aminopropionyl derivatives of iminodibenzyl and diphenylamine and its relation to their ionisation constants. Farmakol. Toksikol. (Moscow) *33*, 8 (1970) in Chem. Abstracts *73*, 12760t (1970)

Lehmann, E., Hopes, H.: Experimentelle Untersuchung der psychophysiologischen Wirkung eines neuen Antidepressivums (Lofepramin) im Vergleich zu Imipramin und Plazebo. Arzneim. Forsch. *27*, 1100 (1977)

Lemberger, L., Rowe, H., Carmichael, R., Oldham, S., Horng, J.S., Bijmaster, F.P., Wong, D.T.: Pharmacologic effects in man of a specific serotonin-reuptake inhibitor. Science *199*, 436 (1978)

Ludiomil in general practise, a symposium. J. Int. Med. Res. *5*, Suppl. 4, (1977)

Maître, L., Waldmeier, P.C., Greengrass, P.M., Jackel, J., Sedlacek, S., Delini-Stula, A.: Maprotiline-Its position as an antidepressant in the light of recent neuropharmacological and neurobiochemical findings. J. Int. Med. Res. *3*, Suppl. 2, 2 (1975)

Malliou, K.D., Todd, A.H., Turner, R.W., Bainbridge, J.G., Greenwood, D.T., Madinaveitia, J., Sommerville, A.R., Whittle, B.A.: 2-(2-Ethoxyphenoxymethyl)-tetrahydro-1,4-oxazine hydrochloride, a potential psychotropic agent. Nature *238*, 157 (1972)

Metyšová, J., Metyš, J., Votava, Z.: Pharmakologische Eigenschaften der 6,11-Dihydrodibenz-(b,e)thiepin Derivate. Arzneim. Forsch. *15*, 524 (1965)

Modestin, J.: Über die Abhängigkeit der klinischen Wirksamkeit des Dibenzepins (Noveril) von seiner Plasma-Konzentration. Pharmakopsychiatr. *6*, 29 (1973)

Moncovic, I., Perran, Y.G., Martel, R., Simpson, W.J., Gylys, J.A.: Substituted tetrahydrofurfurylamines as potential antidepressants. J. Med. Chem. *16*, 403 (1973)

Monro, A.M., Quinton, R.M., Wrighley, T.J.: Some analogues of imipramine. J. Med. Chem. *6*, 255 (1963)

Montgomery, S., Cronholm, B., Åsberg, M., Montgomery, D.B.: Differential effects on suicidal ideation of mianserin, maprotiline and amitriptyline. Br. J. Clin. Pharmacol. *5*, 77S (1978)

Moody, J.S., Whyte, S.F., Naylor, G.J.: A simple method for the determination of protriptyline in plasma. Clin. Chim. Acta *43*, 355 (1973)

Murphy, J.E., Donald, J.F., Beaumont, G.: Opipramol and chlordiazoepoxide in the treatment of anxiety in general practise. Practitioner *205*, 677 (1970)

Murphy, J.E.: Ludiomil symposium. J. Intern. Med. Res. *3*, Suppl. 2 (1975)

Murphy, J.E., Donald, J.F., Molla, A.L.: Mianserin in the treatment of depression in general practise. Practitioner *217*, 135 (1976)

Nagy, A., Treiber, L.: Quantitative determination of imipramine and desimipramine in human blood plasma by direct densitometry of thin layer chromatograms. J. Pharm. Pharmacol. *25*, 599 (1973)

Nakra, B.R.S., Class, R.C., Rees, J.A.: Steady-state serum concentrations of Dothiepin and northiaden after two dosage regimes of dothiepin hydrochloride. J. Int. Med. Res. *5*, 391 (1977)

Niemegeers, C.J.E.: On the pharmacology of tetramisole, an anthelmintic with antidepressant activity in man. Psychopharmacologia *26*, Suppl. 84 (1972)

Otsuki, J., Ishiko, J., Sakai, M., Shimahara, K., Momiyama, T.: Pharmacological activities of doxepine hydrochloride in relation to its geometrical isomers. Chem. Abstracts *78*, 131954 (1973)

Overall, J.E., Hollister, L.E., Meyer, F., Kimbell, I., Shelton, J.: Imipramine and Thioridazine in depressed and schizophrenic patients. J. Am. Med. Assoc. *189*, 605 (1964)

Peet, M., Behagel, H.: Mianserin, a decade of scientific development. Br. J. Clin. Pharmacol. *5*, 5S (1978)

Petersen, P.V., Lassen, N., Hansen, V., Huld, T., Hjortkjaer, J., Holmblad, J., Møller-Nielsen, I., Nijmark, M., Pedersen, V., Jørgensen, A., Hongs, W.: Pharmacological studies of a new series of bicyclic thymoleptics. Acta Pharmacol. Toxicol. *24*, 121 (1966)

Pinder, R.M., Brogden, R.N., Speight, T.M., Avery, G.S.: Doxepin, a review. Drugs *13*, 161 (1977a)

Pinder, R.M., Brogden, R.N., Speight, T.M., Avery, G.S.: Maprotiline, a review. Drugs *13*, 321 (1977b)

Pinder, R.M., Brogden, R.N., Speight, T.M., Avery, G.S.: Viloxazine, a review. Drugs *13*, 401 (1977c)

Post, M.L., Kennard, O., Horn, A.S.: Possible pharmacological and theoretical implications of X-ray structure of the tricyclic antidepressant imipramine. Nature *252*, 493 (1974)

Raiteri, M., Angelini, F., Bertollini, A.: Comparative study of the effects of mianserin, a tetracyclic antidepressant, and of imipramine on uptake and release of neurotransmitters in synaptosomes. J. Pharm. Pharmacol. *28*, 483 (1976)

Randrup, A., Braestrup, C.: Uptake inhibition of biogenic amines by newer antidepressant drugs. Psychopharmacology *53*, 309 (1977)

Reboul, J.P., Cristau, B.: Analyse pharmacochimique des données fournies par la radiocristallographie des amines psychotropes polycycliques. I. Définition et calcul des paramètres conformationnels. Eur. J. Med. Chem. *12*, 71 (1977a)
    II. Confrontation des valeurs paramétriques. Eur. J. Med. Chem. *12*, 76 (1977b)

Remy, D.C., Rittle, K.E., Hunt, C.A., Anderson, P.S., Engelhardt, A.L., Clineschmidt, B.V., Scriabine, A.: (+) and (−)-3methoxy cyproheptadine. J. Med. Chem. *20*, 1681 (1977)

Ribbentrop, A., Schaumann, W.: Pharmakologische Untersuchungen mit Doxepin, einem Antidepressivum mit zentral anticholinerger und sedierender Wirkung. Arzneim. Forsch. *15*, 863 (1965)

Rice, L.M., Hertz, E., Freed, M.E.: Antidepressive Agents. J. Med. Chem. *7*, 313 (1964)

Rickels, K., Chung, H.R., Csanolosi, I., Sablosky, L., Simon, J.H.: Iprindole and imipramine in non-psychotic depressed out-patients. Br. J. Psychiatr. *123*, 329 (1973)

Rogers, S.C., Davies, F.J., Galbraith, A.W.: A study of depression in two general practises, including a double blind comparison of desimipramine and opipramol. Clin. Trials J. *6*, 5 (1969)

Roszkowski, A.P., Schuler, M.E., Marx, M., Edwards, J.A.: A central nervous system depressant-antidepressant. Experientia *31*, 960 (1975)

van Rij, C., Feil, D.: The molecular and crystal structure of (+)mianserin hydrobromide. Tetrahedron *29*, 1891 (1973)

Saletu, B., Krieger, P., Grünberger, J., Schanda, H., Sletten, I.: Tandamine – a new norepinephrine reuptake inhibitor. Int. Pharmacopsychiatr. *12*, 137 (1977)

Sanghoi, I., Gershon, S.: Effect of acute and chronic iprindole on serotonin turnover in mouse brain. Biochem. Pharmacol. *24*, 2103 (1975)

Schindler, W., Häfliger, F.: Über Derivate des Iminodibenzyls. Helv. Chim. Acta *37*, 472 (1954)

Siwers, B., Ringberger, V.A., Tuck, J.R., Sjöqvist, F.: Initial clinical trial based on biochemical methodology of zimelidine (a serotonin uptake inhibitor) in depressed patients. Clin. Pharmacol. Ther. *21*, 194 (1977)

Sparatore, F., Sommovigo, P.G., Boida, V.: Research on nitrogen-containing seven-atom heterocycles of pharmacologic interest. Boll. Chim. Farm. *113*, 219 (1974)

Speight, T.M., Avery, G.S.: Pizotifen: a review. Drugs *3*, 159 (1972)

Stach, K., Pöldinger, W.: Strukturelle Betrachtungen der Psychopharmaka: Versuch einer Korrelation von chemischer Konstitution und klinischer Wirkung. Prog. Drug Res. *9*, 129 (1966)

v.d. Stelt, C., Funcke, A.B.H., Tersteege, H.M., Nauta, W.Th.: The effect of alkyl substitution in drugs. Arzneim. Forsch. *16*, 1342 (1966)

Swaisland, A.I., Franklin, R.A., Southgate, P.J., Coleman, A.J.: The pharmacokinetics of ciclazindol (Wy 23409) in human volunteers. Br. J. Clin. Pharmacol. *4*, 61 (1977)

Theobald, W., Bück, O., Kunz, H.A., Morpurgo, C., Stenger, E.G., Wilhelmi, G.: Vergleichende Pharmakologische Untersuchungen mit Tofranil, Pertofran und Insidon. Arch. Int. Pharmacodyn. Ther. *148*, 560 (1964)

Thomas, P.C., Jones, R.B.: The effects of clomipramide and desmethylclomipramine on the in vitro uptake of radiolabelled 5-HT and noradrenaline into rat brain cortical slices. J. Pharm. Pharmacol. *29*, 562 (1977)

Todrick, A., Tait, A.C.: The inhibition of human platelet 5-hydroxytryptamine uptake by tricyclic antidepressive drugs. The relation between structure and potency. J. Pharm. Pharmacol. *21*, 751 (1969)

Toscano, L., Grisanti, G., Fionello, G., Seghetti, E., Bianchetti, A., Bossoni, G., Riva, M.: Basic derivatives of 6,7-dihydroindolo[1,7-a,b][1]benzazepine and 6H-indolo[7,1-c,d][1,5]benzoxazepine as potential antidepressant agents. J. Med. Chem. *19*, 208 (1976)

Tuomisto, J.: A new modification for studying 5-HT uptake by blood platelets: a re-evaluation of tricyclic antidepressants as uptake inhibitors. J. Pharm. Pharmacol. *26*, 92 (1974)

Uzan, A., LeFur, G.: Effets de différents hétérocycles sur l'incorporation de 5-hydroxytryptamine et de noradrenaline par une préperation de cerveau de rat. Ann. Pharm. Fr. *33*, 345 (1975)

Vencovský, E., Šedivec, Vl., Peterová, E., Baudis, P.: Vorläufige Mitteilung über die Behandlung der Manien mit IB-503 Sandoz. Arzneim. Forsch. *19*, 491 (1969)

Villani, F.J., Mann, T.A.: The synthesis and pharmacological properties of dibenz[b,c][1,4]oxazepin-11(5H)-ones. J. Med. Chem. *11*, 894 (1968)

Villani, F.J., Daniels, P.J.L., Ellis, C.A., Mann, T.A., Wang, K.C., Wefer, E.A.: Derivatives of 10,11-dihydro-5H-dibenzo[a,d]cycloheptene and related compounds. J. Med. Chem. *15*, 750 (1972)

Vivalan: International Symposium. J. Int. Med. Res. *3*, Suppl. 3 (1975)

Walter, C.J.S.: Clinical significance of plasma imipramin levels. Proc. R. Soc. Med. *64*, 282 (1971)

Wilhelm, M., Schmidt, P.: Synthese und Eigenschaften von 1-Aminoalkyldibenzo[b,c]bicyclo[2,2,2]octadienen. Helv. Chim. Acta *52*, 1385 (1969)

Wilhelm, M.: Die Chemie polyzyklischer Psychopharmaka. In: Depressive Zustände, P. Kielholz (ed.). Bern: Hans Huber Verlag 1972, p. 129

Winthrop, S.O., Davis, M.A., Herr, F., Stewart, J., Gaudry, R.: New Psychotropic Agents. J. Med. Pharm. Chem. *5*, 1199 (1962 a)

Winthrop, S.O., Davis, M.A., Herr, F., Stewart, J., Gaudry, R.: New psychotropic agents. J. Med. Pharm. Chem. *5*, 1207 (1962 b)

Wong, D.T., Bijmaster, F.P., Horng, J.S., Molloy, B.B.: A new selective inhibitor for uptake of serotonin into synaptosomes of rat brain-3-(p-trifluomethylphenoxy)-N-methyl-3-phenylpropylamine. J. Pharmacol. Exp. Ther. *193*, 804 (1975)

Wright, S., Herrmann, L.: Doppelblindversuch zum Wirkungsvergleich von Lofepramin und Amitriptylin bei ambulant behandelten Patienten mit depressiven Zustandsbildern. Arzneim. Forsch. *26*, 1167 (1976)

Yale, H.L., Sowinski, F.: Novel polycyclic Heterocycles. J. Med. Chem. *7*, 609 (1964)

Young, J.P.R., Hughes, W.C., Lader, M.H.: A controlled comparison of flupenthixol and amitriptyline in depressed out patients. Br. Med. J. *1*, 1116 (1976)

CHAPTER 17

Monoamine Oxidase Inhibitors as Antidepressants

N.S. KLINE and T.B. COOPER

A. Introduction

The history of monoamine oxidase inhibitor (MAOI) use in psychiatry is a curious one and far from complete. The inspiration for our own use derived from the work of CHESSIN et al. (1956) who found that "marsalinizing" (treating with Marsilid, i.e., iproniazid) an animal before administering reserpine produced a paradoxical effect[1]. The animal rather than becoming sedated became hyperalert and active. SCOTT described these findings during a visit to Warner Laboratories as part of a discussion which dealt with the mode of action of reserpine. The possibility of using this combination to activate retarded schizophrenic patients and to treat depression suggested itself.

The senior author started a clinical investigation of the iproniazid-reserpine combination (SAUNDERS et al., 1959) and shortly thereafter began trials with iproniazid alone (LOOMER et al., 1958). The second investigation was completed before the first and the results were presented in April 1957 at a Regional Research Conference of the American Psychiatric Association. The first published report was an unlikely "journal" (KLINE, 1957) – the Hearings Before the Senate, May 1957. The report of the Syracuse meetings appeared in 1958 (LOOMER et al., 1958).

Prior to our own work, SMITH (1953) had given iproniazid to a group of 11 patients with various diagnoses at doses of 2 mg per kg of body wt. His trial was for a period of only 3 weeks and, although he noted some slight improvement in two of the depressed patients, he concluded that overall the drug was ineffectual. KAMMAN et al. in a double-blind study found definite improvement in ward behavior of a group of 30 patients given 1 mg per pound of body wt. for a period of 8 weeks and then 2 mg per pound for an additional 8 weeks. The patients showed significantly more improvement than a group of placebo treated patients, but not so much as a third group of 30 patients on a "total push program." He did not feel the drug investigation was worth pursuing. The descriptions of SELIKOFF et al. (1952) in iproniazid treatment of tuberculosis were of "subjective feeling of improvement ... not warranted by the roentgenographic findings." This finding was compatible with the use of iproniazid to activate patients and improve their mood. We, like many others, missed the clinical implications for psychiatry when these "side effects" were first described.

The first reference to iproniazid specifically used for the treatment of patients diagnosed as "depressions" is in our April 1957 presentation and a number of case histories are given in the May 1957 presentation before a US Congressional Commitee (KLINE, 1957). CRANE (1956) at this same conference reported on a follow-up of his

---

1 The experiments are in line with those of PLETSCHER et al. (1956)

description of iproniazid side effects. The new study involved 20 psychiatric patients. In his summary, no specific reference is made to the effect on depressed patients. Of the three depressed patients included in his study, only one improved (a case of involutional psychosis).

Subsequently AYD (1957) reported on patients to whom he had been giving iproniazid for a number of years, including some depressed patients. He had not published his results until he was satisfied as to their validity.

The specific dates are of interest since they were subsequently of importance in a law suit brought by one of the co-authors of the original publication (LOOMER et al., 1958) claiming that several years before he alone had originated the idea of treating retarded and depressed patients with MAOI[2]. Very much earlier (1938) GADDUM and KWIATKOWSKY had advanced the theory that ephedrine produced its stimulant effect by acting as an amine oxidase inhibitor; by competing with epinephrine for the receptor substance in the affector cells, ephedrine retarded the breakdown of epinephrine so that it had a more sustained action. Similarly, GOODMAN and GILMAN (1965), in their standard textbook of pharmacology had, for many years, suggested this same mode of action for the "psychomotor stimulants" including amphetamines. More recently ZELLER and BARSK (1952) had shown that iproniazid was a potent MAOI and BRODIE et al. (1956) had demonstrated that iproniazid resulted in increased brain monoamine levels. The senior author was probably the first to suggest that the antidepressant effect of iproniazid was due to the rise in brain 5-hydroxytryptamine (serotonin) (5-HT) and norepinephrine levels (KLINE, 1977).

The report of the senior author's results in 1957 prompted extensive clinical use of MAOIs in the treatment of depression. It was estimated by both the Federal Drug Administration (FDA) and Hoffmann-LaRoche that approximately 600,000 patients were treated in the subsequent year. Gradually MAOI use became less prevalent because they were considered unpredictable. This together with the risk of hypertensive attacks precipitated by ingestion of foods rich in tyramine, interactions with drugs such as some of the decongestants and parenteral amphetamines, and the introduction to the market of tricyclic antidepressant drugs (TCA) accelerated the decrease in the use of MAOIs. Recently there has been a marked revival and MAOI use is now on the increase.

B. Pharmacology – Background

Several detailed reviews of the MAOI literature have been published in recent years (e.g., USDIN, 1974; BERGER and BARCHAS, 1977; BALDESSARINI, 1977).

I. Pharmacology of MAOIs

This enzyme is localized in the mitochondria of cells of the kidney, lung, spleen, placenta, thymus, thyroid gland, muscle, heart, and central nervous tissue with high

---

2 A crucial point in the "defense" was substantiation that the work derived from iproniazid-reserpine investigations. If this were not the case there would have been no rationale for starting this combination on patients even before iproniazid alone was used. Further, KLINE's reference to patients treated in private practice was the first report of patients specifically treated because they were diagnosed as depressives

concentrations found in liver and intestine (FRANZEN and EYSELL, 1969). MAO is also found in the blood platelet and blood plasma although the latter differs in substrate specificity for MAO from other tissues (MURPHY and DONNELLY, 1974).

II. Function

Any drug which interferes with the function of MAO is by definition an MAOI regardless of other pharmacologic properties which that particular molecule may possess. Because of this heterogeneity it is convenient to distinguish between those substances which inhibit MAO only in vitro from those which are also active in vivo. Substances which are only effective in vitro require high concentrations to produce inhibition and such substances include amphetamine, cocaine, and diphenylhydramine. None of these agents have been used clinically for their MAO inhibiting properties and it is not now generally believed that the pharmacologic activities of cocaine or amphetamine are significantly related to their ability to inhibit MAO. The MAOI can be further subdivided into short-acting or reversible inhibitors and the long-lasting (mainly irreversible) inhibitors. The substituted indole-alkylamines and B-carbolines are short-acting MAOI while long-acting inhibitors include the hydrazine derivatives; propargylamines, cyclopropylamines, and aminopyrazines (VON BRUECKE et al., 1969).

The function of MAO in general metabolism is not fully understood. MAO deaminates several biologically important amines, e. g., dopamine, tyramine, 5-HT, and, to some extent, noradrenaline and adrenaline. The biochemical actions of MAOIs, therefore, are not restricted to a single substrate but involve multiple substrates. The importance of these biochemical effects is determined by the concentration, activity and turnover rates of the different amines in various tissues and the occurrence of "alternative metabolizing enzymes", e. g., catechol-0-methyltransferase (COMT). Monoamine oxidase probably regulates the tissue metabolism of catecholamines, e. g., serotonin (SPECTOR et al., 1963) while COMT inactivates noradrenaline and adrenaline after they are released into the circulation (KOPIN and AXELROD, 1963).

In recent years multiple forms of mitochondrial MAO have been described (YOUDIM, 1973; FULLER, 1972; JOHNSTON, 1968; YAUG and NEFF, 1973) although some investigators question whether these forms are artifacts of the extraction and purification process or else suggest that the MAO itself is not different but merely bound in different membrane environments (HOUSLAY et al., 1974, 1976). Despite these disagreements the concept of at least two forms of MAO (A and B) has been sustained. Typical representative inhibitors of each group are clorgyline (type A) which selectively eliminates 5-HT and norepinephrine and deprenyl (type B) which selectively degrades phenylethylamine. Specific and mixed type MAOIs are listed in Table 1.

Whatever the outcome of the use of this binary classification it is clear that attempts to extrapolate from organ to organ or species to species are questionable. Further caution must be taken concerning the demonstration of selective inhibition in vitro because many studies have indicated that these inhibitors may not be specific in vivo (FOWLER et al., 1978). It has been further suggested that particular inhibitors may have only short-lived specificity in vivo, due either to the nature of the localization of the enzyme within the target organ, to the elevated amine concentration acting as a reversible inhibitor of the alternate form of the enzyme or to biotransformation of

Table 1. Some inhibitor drugs and substrates of Type A and B monoamine oxidase (NEFF and YANG, 1974)

	Monoamine oxidase	
	Type A	Type B
Preferred substrates	Serotonin norepinephrine normetanephrine	Benzylamine b-phenyl- ethylamine
Specific inhibitor drugs (substituted amines)	Clorgyline Lilly 51641	Deprenyl pargyline
Common substrates	Dopamine tyramine tryptamine	
Nonspecific inhibitor drugs (Hydrazines)	Isocarboxazid Phenelzine iproniazid	Nialamine pheniprazine
(Simple amines)	Alpha ethyl tryptamine	Tranylcypromine

the selective inhibitor producing less specific inhibition (FOWLER et al., 1978). Clearly the ideal would be an inhibitor which would decrease the breakdown of a target amine in a given brain area without inhibiting the metabolism of other amines in that or other areas of the brain (or elsewhere in the body), since such accumulation may be responsible for toxic side effects. The recent promising use of (–) deprenyl in Parkinson's disease is an example of such an approach (BIRKMAYER and YAHR, 1978). Prospective studies involving the use of such selective inhibitors could give additional impetus to the revived use of MAOIs in clinical psychiatric practice (FULLER, 1978).

III. Structure and Biologic Action

The structural formulae of typical MAOI and amphetamines are shown in Fig. 1. The structure of amphetamine is included to emphasize the similarity between amphetamine, tranylcypromine, and to a lesser extent pheniprazine and phenelzine. These three inhibitors also have amphetaminelike properties which are unrelated to their effect on MAO. In animals, inhibition of MAO prolongs and potentiates the action of tyramine but not that of adrenaline or noradrenaline (BURN et al., 1954), which are both inactivated by O-methylation (AXELROD, 1957). HORWITZ et al. (1960) demonstrated that the pressor effect of dopamine (another substrate of MAO) was markedly augmented and prolonged in patients receiving pheniprazine, nialamide, or tranylcypromine and they also have reported marked potentiation of the pressor effect of tyramine given orally or intravenously to patients treated with pargyline (HORWITZ et al., 1964). Sympathomimetic amines act either directly by combining with a receptor or indirectly by causing release of noradrenaline from nerve terminals. After MAO inhibition a variety of amines (tyramine, amphetamine, etc.) may evoke enhanced effects whether they are substrates of MAO or not because they now may release larger amounts of transmitter amines than normally. This mechanism can operate peripherally as well as centrally.

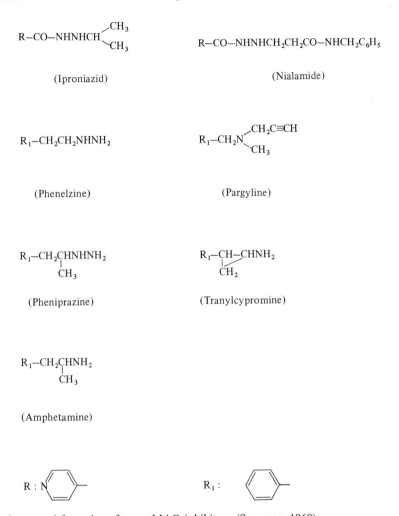

Fig. 1. Structural formulae of some MAO-inhibitors (SJOQVIST, 1968)

IV. Mode of Action

It is rather widely believed that the MAOIs mode of action as an antidepressant involves the inhibition of MAO. It seems logical to assume this when one considers the chemical heterogeneity of these compounds with apparently only MAOI as a common property. HENDLY and SNYDER (1968) have suggested, however, that MAOI may in fact act as an antidepressant by blocking neuronal reuptake of central amines, i.e., the same mechanism suggested for the mode of action of TCA (SCHILDKRAUT, 1965; BUNNEY and DAVIS, 1965). Some support for this hypothesis is to be found in the data from the controlled experiments of ESCOBAR et al. (1974), when optical isomers of tranylcypromine were given to patients, the L-isomer was the more effective antidepressant. The L-isomer has been shown to be a more potent blocker of amine reuptake than the D-isomer whereas the latter is a more effective MAOI.

In addition to MAOI and amine reuptake blockade, increases in other amines and production of false transmitters have been suggested (BIEL and BOPP, 1974) as possible modes of action. Further complicating the picture is the growing list of compounds with demonstrable antidepressant activity in man which neither inhibit MAO nor block reuptake of central amines (ROSLOFF and DAVIS, 1974; LEONARD, 1978). Finally, postsynaptic mechanisms are also being explored as possibly relevant to the antidepressant effect.

Thus, although MAOIs have antidepressant activity, the mechanism of action is not necessarily that of MAO inhibition. Elucidation of the mode of action may contribute to an understanding of the biologic basis of depressive illness.

V. MAOIs Used Clinically

Clinical use of MAOIs include the hydrazine derivatives, phenelzine and isocarboxiazid, the nonhydrazine derivatives, cyclopropylamine, tranylcypromine, and pargyline, the latter marketed for the treatment of hypertension rather than depression. It is of interest to note, that despite widespread use of these compounds in the United States the FDA has seen fit to rate phenelzine as the only MAOI effective in the treatment of depression.

These particular MAOI themselves are rapidly metabolized but the enzyme inhibition they produce is essentially irreversible, thus small daily doses of MAOI will be cumulative. Inhibition therefore persists after the disappearance of the MAOI and its metabolites from the body. MAO activity can only be restored by resynthesis of the enzyme which is a slow process.

Increases in brain amines do not show a dose-response relationship of the MAOIs; MAO must be almost completely inhibited before brain amine content rises. This is not surprising when one considers the massive preponderance of glial cells in the brain and that it is presumably neuronal MAO which is involved. The time lag before

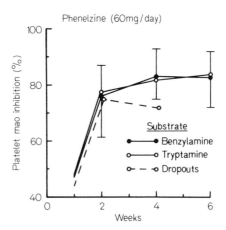

Fig. 2. Mean platelet MAOI ± SD of 55 depressed patients at 2, 4, and 6 weeks of treatment with phenelzine 60 mg/day with benzylamine and tryptamine as substrates. Reproduced with permission of the editor, Arch. Gen. Psychiatry *35*, 629–635 (1978)

antidepressant effect is well known in clinical practice and MACLEAN et al. (1965) have reported that, in a study of terminally ill depressed patients treated with MAOIs, brain levels of the biogenic amines were not maximal until 4 weeks of therapy. A similar time course of platelet MAOI has been shown by ROBINSON et al. (1978) (Fig. 2).

Early on we gave very large doses of MAOI, but were unable to lessen the time required for the antidepressant effect to appear. We even used intravenous preparations without any observable differences. The delay in response might be a result of the time necessary for monoamine to accumulate once this became possible when the enzyme that catabolized them was blocked. If this were the case, the direct administration of monoamines possibly could speed up the response. We reported this to be the case (KLINE and SACKS, 1963; KLINE et al., 1964) and recently reviewed the subject again (KLINE and SACKS, 1979). In January, 1979, a conference under the direction of Arvid Carlsson was held in London on *Biogenic Amines and Affective Disorders*. The papers presented at that meeting describing the actions of tryptophane, 5-HT, 5-hydroxytryptophan (5-HTP), etc., are compatible with this hypothesis.

VI. Biochemical Markers – Usefulness in Practice

The discovery that platelets are rich in MAO activity (type B) and the development of a convenient blood platelet MAO assay (ROBINSON et al., 1968) has led to a series of detailed and systematic studies of the efficacy of MAOIs in the treatment of depression using the blood platelet assay as a monitoring technique (ROBINSON et al., 1978; DAVIDSON et al., 1978). ROBINSON, NIES, and colleagues (1978) have clearly demonstrated that in patients treated with phenelzine, clinical response is related to platelet MAO inhibition and dosage per unit body wt. A suitable dose was determined to be 1 mg/kg body wt. in these studies. The difference in findings when patients were separated by the % MAO inhibition achieved are particularly striking (Fig. 3). Studies published by other groups (DAVIDSON et al., 1978) confirm that patients who achieve

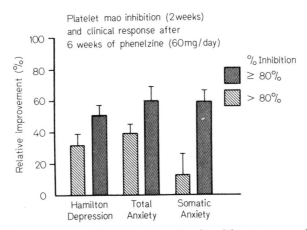

Fig. 3. Relative % improvement ± SEM after 6 weeks phenelzine treatment (60 mg/day) in groups of patients with low platelet MAO inhibition (< 80%) at 2 weeks and 36 patients with high inhibition (> 80%) with tryptamine as substrate. Reproduced with permission of the editor, Arch. Gen. Psychiatry *35,* 629–635 (1978)

a high level of platelet MAOI show greater clinical improvement. Of interest is the observation that some patients receiving 90 mg phenelzine/day did not achieve adequate inhibition and these authors suggested that even higher doses may be indicated.

It is very clear from these studies that many previous studies of MAOIs used less than adequate dosage. When dosage of 60 mg/day or higher are used, then the MAOIs compare favorably with the tricyclic antidepressants though there may be a subgroup of patients who benefit most from MAOI treatment (see Sect. E).

VII. Acetylation Phenotype

Phenelzine is believed to have a major metabolic pathway involving acetylation, a process under polymorphous control, with the gene for slow acetylation being recessive (EVANS et al., 1960). Using sulfamethezine it is possible to determine whether a patient is a slow or fast acetylator. It was suggested that slow acetylators respond better to phenelzine (JOHNSTONE and MARSH, 1973) or else they may suffer from more side effects (EVANS et al., 1965). Studies carried out in recent years, however, have not confirmed these earlier findings, and determinations of acetylation phenotype is not recommended as a predictor of outcome (ROBINSON et al., 1978; DAVIDSON et al., 1978; MARSHALL et al., 1978). DAVIDSON et al. (1978) point out that the rapid rate of elimination of phenelzine and the extended duration of MAO inhibition make it unlikely that the rate of acetylation would predict the degree to which phenelzine inhibits MAO. These authors were unable to demonstrate any correlation between acetylation phenotype and platelet MAOI after 3 weeks of therapy.

C. Evaluation of MAOI Antidepressant Efficacy

I. Experimental Design Problem

1. Spontaneous Remission

There is little question that the majority of depressions will remit spontaneously even without treatment. At times this has been mistakenly or meretriciously used to raise questions about the effectiveness of antidepressant medications including MAOIs. It is highly unusual for spontaneous remissions or placebo responses to occur in a majority of the patients within 3 weeks of the start of evaluation. It is not unusual for such placebo responses as do occur to begin within a few days, followed by relapse a week or two later. This failure to take into account the timing of the placebo response, and the much longer period usually required for spontaneous remission has made it difficult to demonstrate the effectiveness of antidepressant drugs. Double-blind, placebo-controlled studies seem an obvious way to obtain an answer but there are real problems with this approach. Since in the United States those patients with depression who are admitted to the hospital are usually either very severe cases or have some additional disorder, they are not the best group for evaluation. On the other hand, patients seen in private practice who are *not* given antidepressant medication may lead to an even greater problem: *not* to administer antidepressant medication when it is indicated constitutes a breach of medical ethics and, in addition, may involve the psychiatrist in legal action, should the patient commit suicide. Incidentally, suicide is the most frequent cause of psychiatrists being sued in the United States.

II. Controlled and Open Studies

Question as to the value of the MAOI arose in part because of the negative report in a Medical Research Council trial carried out in Britain. An adequate dose of 60 mg of phenelzine was used, but the patients were hospitalized and largely suffered from endogenous depression and other psychoses. The work of ROBINSON et al. (1978) and DAVIDSON et al. (1978) indicates that nonendogenous depressions appear to respond significantly better than endogenous depressions when given the MAOI phenelzine.

PAYKEL (1971) found that in endogenous depressions characterized by guilt, retardation, and diurnal rhythm, phenelzine was effective in only 18% of the cases. In an indeterminant group of cases of depression, phenelzine was effective in 33%, however in cases of reactive and depressive neuroses characterized by irritability, but low in respect to retardation and guilt, the drug was effective 70% of the time.

WEST and DALLY (1959) report that the best response to MAOIs is in atypical depressions characterized by anxiety and phobias, with the absence of guilt, chronicity, fatigue, somatic complaints, weight loss, and sleep disturbances.

III. Time Lapse Before Response

ROBINSON et al. (1978) found that 60% of ultimate improvement had occurred by the end of the 2nd week, which confirms the senior author's clinical experience (NSK). In this clinician's (NSK) experience a minimum of 3 weeks administration is necessary to evaluate the patient. The previously cited experiments of MACLEAN et al. (1965) indicated that brain amines were maximal 4 weeks after commencement of MAOI medication.

DUNLEAVY and OSWALD (1973) showed that MAOIs were effective only when doses were high enough to significantly alter REM and paradoxical sleep.

There have been a number of other double-blind, placebo-controlled studies, the majority of which report favorably on the MAOIs. In some of the studies (usually on the hospitalized patients), MAOIs were not significantly more effective than placebo, but there exists no study in which placebo did better than MAOIs. BERGER and BARCHAS (1977), among others, have summarized these data. As to the effect of iproniazid they referred, in turn, to the reviews of KILOH et al. (1960); to MORRIS and BECK (1974), in respect to phenelzine (which was superior to placebo in five of nine studies). Tranylcypromine was superior to placebo in three of four studies, and isocarboxyzid and nialamide were active, but not quite so effective as the other MAOIs. Phenelzine was found equal in effectiveness to TCAs.

Another demonstration of the effectiveness of tranylcypromine was carried out by SCHIELE (1965) who located 600 patients who had deteriorated when tranylcypromine was withdrawn (in response to FDA actions) and responded when it was again administered (when the FDA reversed itself).

D. Practicum for Clinical Use

I. How to Select Patients for a MAOI

Although the MAOI are usually classified as antidepressants, the designation given them by KLINE and associates (LOOMER et al., 1958) as "psychic energizers" seems to more adequately describe their action. They seem particularly useful in those cases of depression characterized by reduced energy and drive. These are sometimes referred to in the European literature as "vital-depression." A clear differentiation between the types of patients best responding to TCA and those responding to MAOIs has yet to be made. It seems highly likely that a biochemical test to differentiate the preferred medication should be available in the relatively near future. In the senior author's experience, the bipolar depressives and those characterized by disturbances of biologic function (early morning awakening, anorexia, vasomotor liability, etc.) do respond well to treatment with MAOIs.

II. Patient Compliance

Most, though not all, of the studies on depressed patients are done in a hospital whereas most patients are treated on an ambulatory basis. As a consequence, in certain respects there is a marked discrepancy between conclusions or inferences that may be drawn from the published literature in contrast to successful clinical usage.

The major problem encountered in private practice is that patients discontinue treatment or do not comply with instructions as to usage. One reason is that other patients, or even an over-informative pharmacist may describe the "perils" of a medication in such a way that the patient decides that the risk is too great. Following the withdrawal of iproniazid from the market in the United States because of putative liver damage and the withdrawal followed by reintroduction of tranylcypromine (Parnate), there were quite a number of self-appointed authorities who advised against the use of MAOI. Iproniazid (Marsilid) was introduced as an antidepressant in April of 1957. There was substantial agreement between the FDA and the pharmaceutical company that, during its first year of use for this purpose, approximately 600,000 patients were treated in the United States. The drug was already on the market for its use, in the treatment of tuberculosis so that it was readily available. In those patients who developed jaundice, the condition was indistinguishable from infectious hepatitis. In retrospect, it is not clear whether the incidence of hepatitis was higher in patients on iproniazid than those in the general population. There is also some clinical evidence that there was a mild epidemic of infectious hepatitis during that period. In any case, the risk of a high incidence of hepatitis from using MAO inhibitors has not materialized.

Another reason for noncompliance is the side effects of a medication. There are a few patients who find the side effects of MAOI to be so unpleasant that they discontinue treatment. Actually the side effects (to be discussed subsequently) are relatively rare and mild.

A third possible reason for noncompliance is confusion about which foods, drinks, and medications should be avoided. This uncertainty should be relieved by providing the patient with a printed list. It is also important to have someone spend a few minutes to reassure the patient about the side effects, to explain how to determine whether a reaction to the medication is occurring, and also to discuss how any emergency should be handled.

III. When to Use a Monamine Oxidase Inhibitor

The first decision to be reached is that an antidepressant medication is needed. This requires that a distinction be made between existential depression and pathologic depression. In the case of existential depressions, there is a relevant and recent external event that predates the depression. It is important to inquire about this in some detail. Should any of us wake up tomorrow morning for the first time with a severe depression, we would be able to enumerate up to a dozen reasons as the "cause" of our depression. Since all of those factors exist now, but without "causing" depression, it is much more likely that in this case the depression is pathologic. In such conditions we tend to fasten on to all sorts of life events and to view them not only tragically but to regard them as contributory factors.

Thus, if the patient is asked to relate his reasons for being depressed, care should be taken to make certain that the reported cause is of recent origin and of sufficient importance to warrant an existential depression. There are usually some differences in the nature of the depression itself. An existential depression is usually relieved to at least some degree by pleasant or hopeful events in the environment. Usually such patients can be temporarily distracted and during such periods appear to be essentially normal. By way of contrast, the patient with pathologic depression tends more frequently to be consistently depressed and it is much more difficult to provide sufficient distractions to obtain relief. Often encouraging or happy environmental events fail to provoke an appropriate response. A rough rule of thumb would be that 3 days of unrelieved depression would be a good reason to suspect that the condition is pathological rather than existential.

IV. Secondary Causes of Depression

The next step is to make certain that the depression is not secondary to some other condition. Most viral infections have as an accompaniment, and frequently as a sequelae, mild-to-moderate depression lasting for several months. The same is true with most liver disorders such as infectious mononucleosis or infectious hepatitis. The same is reported to be true of pancreatic infections.

There are a variety of neurologic conditions which have the same effect, e. g., Wilson's disease. It is not unusual for operative procedures to be followed by depression, and several studies estimate that 80% of women give some evidence of depression a few weeks before and/or a few weeks after delivery. There are a variety of drugs also capable of inducing depression. The best known of these is reserpine where the incidence of depression is probably 15%–20%. Hormone preparations, including oral contraceptives, may induce both depressed and manic states. The phenothiazines, and even slightly more, the minor tranquilizers may be accompanied or followed by mild depression. Obviously if the depression is secondary to drugs or other procedures, the offending agent should be discontinued and a reasonable period allowed for the effect to wear off. However, just as obviously, if the condition is acute and severe, treatment may be necessary. Sometimes under these circumstances, amphetamines are the medication of choice. However, if they do not work within a few days or if tolerance begins to develop, there should be no hesitancy about using antidepressant medications.

Once having decided that the depression is pathologic, the next question would be whether electroconvulsive (ECT) therapy was indicated. There are strong advocates for widespread use of ECT, but most practitioners at present restrict the use of ECT to those patients who are acutely suicidal and particularly for those they cannot hospitalize. The other major use would be for patients who have failed to respond to reasonably extensive pharmacotherapy. There are a number of studies which claim superior results for ECT and in an interesting way these illustrate the fact that determination as to which treatment will be used is not based entirely on "demonstrated" therapeutic response. That is, ECT is a relatively inconvenient type of treatment in that, as currently used, it requires an intravenous injection, an attendant or nurse, possibly an anesthetist, and a recovery room. In many cases, it also involves the patient going to a hospital. The patient, the doctor and the equipment must all be together in one place at one time. This is in contrast to pharmacotherapy which does not require equipment and in which adjustments and changes can be made over the telephone if necessary. Whether it is true or not, most patients perceive the risks of ECT to be greater than those of pharmacotherapy. In general, the procedure is also more expensive. There also exists a question as to whether the recovery is as long-lasting.

The next important question is whether a TCA or a MAOI should be used. Rather than the indications, the contraindications for one or the other should be considered first.

All of the contraindications are relative and require the exercise of clinical judgement. Contraindications to the use of TCA are thrombophlebitis present or in the recent past, increased intraocular pressure, recent myocardial infarct, and cardiac irregularities. Contraindications to the MAOI are the existence of a pheochromocytoma, marked hypotension, or the presence of liver malfunction.

The MAOIs do not have the wide spread from sedative to stimulating properties as is the case with the tricyclics. Tranylcypromine (Parnate), however, is definitely the most stimulating of the group. Phenelzine (Nardil), as a rule, is not overly stimulating. Isocarboxyazid is the mildest of the group both in respect to side effects and therapeutic action. Paradoxically, however, high doses of any of the MAOIs or even smaller doses in sensitive individuals may produce definite sleepiness requiring a reduction in dose. Pargyline (Eutonyl) marketed as an antihypertensive agent is also a potent MAOI and a very satisfactory antidepressant preparation. It is of the same order of potency as phenelzine and tranylcypromine. Many years ago, we evaluated pargyline (Eutonyl) as an antidepressant and found it to be quite acceptable, but the pharmaceutical company which owned the patent decided not to market it for this purpose. It is particularly useful if patients have to be discontinued from reserpine, because of possible depressant effect, and a potent hypotensive agent is still needed. It is at least slightly paradoxical to find hypertension listed as a contraindication to the use of the MAOI depressants and, at the same time, to find that FDA approval has been given for more than a decade to pargyline for use as an agent *against* hypertension. As with other contraindications the hypertension is relative as long as care is exercised not to cause too abrupt a decrease in blood pressure.

V. Indications for the Monoamine Oxidase Inhibitors

The MAOIs are indicated if the patient has previously been treated with one of these medications and had successful results. There is also evidence that members of the same family respond to the same medication so that, if a close relative has successfully recovered with the use of an MAOI, it is probably sensible to begin treatment with a member of this group. There are a number of studies which would indicate that the atypical depressions do better on MAOIs than patients treated with tricyclics. Contrariwise, the more typical depressions are claimed to respond better to tricyclics.

Patients who tolerate the side effects of tricyclics poorly are candidates for treatment with the MAOIs. Also, those patients for whom the tricyclics are "contraindicated" should be considered as candidates.

E. Use in Phobic Anxiety

Another major use of MAOIs is in the treatment of phobic anxiety, as well as in obsessive compulsive reactions. Its use for this purpose fits in with our (NSK) description of MAOIs as psychic energizers. A presentation on this subject was given as early as 1958 (LOOMER et al., 1958). In more recent papers, LADER (1976) as well as TYRER et al. (1973) described the treatment of patients with phobic anxiety states. According to LADER, "the antianxiety effects of these drugs appears to be independent of any antidepressant action." In psychodynamic terms, the phobias, obsessions, and compulsions may be "short circuits" to avoid experiencing dysphoria, as well as to conserve psychic energy. If the reservoir of psychic energy is increased, it may become possible for the patient to deal with the symptoms. Frequently, under these circumstances, psychotherapy is useful in conjunction with the medication. The concept of psychic energy is derived from Freud whose universe is divided into (1) psychotopology (2) psychoenergetics, and (3) psychodynamics. Since until recently there was no way of manipulating psychic energy, relatively little has been written on the subject. The earliest presentation derived from an attempt to reconcile psychodynamic and physiologic theories with drug action (OSTOW and KLINE, 1959).

F. Achievers' Depression

One of the rewards (and headaches) of practice in New York City is that it can involve the treatment of a most unusual group of patients. Perhaps the best term for them is that they are "achievers." New York is one of the most competitive cities in the world and most of these special patients are ones who have migrated there because New York is "where it's at." Most of them possess experience, intelligence, drive, and creativity. They perform consistently at or near the peak of their potential. Virtually no outsiders can detect the difference on a particular occasion between a 96% performance on their part and a 99% one. But the insider (they themselves) often suffer severely because of this relative "inadequacy" or "deterioration." Over a period of time this difference may become detectable by others. The group includes some of the country's foremost political, literary, artistic, and scientific research personalities. Most of them come with a history of extensive psychotherapy, which has given them "insight" but has failed to sharpen the cutting edge which had initially differentiated them from a host of competitors and aspirants.

In these individuals a dose of one or two 10 mg tablets of isocarboxazid is often sufficient to restore them to full capacity. At this low dose it is usually not necessary to observe rigid dietary restrictions. Additions of 2–3 g of L-tryptophan divided throughout the day (or given at one time hs if there is insomnia) may be a useful addition if there is no response or if the response is favorable but there is a relapse.

I. Posology

Although it has not been clearly demonstrated, the belief exists that MAOIs given late in the day may be more productive of insomnia than if they are given earlier. Instead of a three times a day dose, many clinicians will therefore give two-thirds of the dose in the morning and one-third at midday. As initial treatment, therefore, 10 mg of tranylcypromine or 15 mg of phenelzine are given with two tablets in the morning and one at midday, making an initial starting dose of 30 mg of tranylcypromine or 45 mg of phenelzine. In milder cases or where the patient may be unusually sensitive to medication, it is probably useful to start with two of the 10 mg of isocarboxazid (Marplan) in the morning and a third at midday. Within a week this can usually be doubled. It is often necessary to go to 60 mg of tranylcypromine or 90 mg of phenelzine. An upper dose of 90 mg or even 120 mg of isocarboxazid is not unusual. For retarded depressions, tranylcypromine would be the drug of choice whereas phenelzine is indicated for other types of severe depression, including the agitated or anxious ones.

On occasion, if there is only partial response and there is no indication of a severe drop in blood pressure, the dose of tranylcypromine may be increased to 90 mg and that of phenelzine to 135 mg.

There is interesting evidence to indicate that the dose of MAOI should be pushed until at least mild hypotension occurs. There is a theoretical as well as practical rationale for this procedure.

Medications should be continued for approximately 2–3 months *after* the patient has achieved maximal improvement although in most cases they can be decreased by about 25%. Experience has shown that discontinuance too soon after improvement leads to rapid relapse. At the end of the 2–3 month period, the amount of the medication being administered should be reduced by approximately 50% and continued for another month. If there is no relapse, the medication should then be cut in half and continued for a 2nd month. If there is no relapse at the end of this period, the drug can be discontinued.

For long-term treatment and prophylaxis against recurrence, lithium is usually the medication of choice. In certain cases, however, a low dose of one of the antidepressants (such as an MAOI) has to be continued. In other cases, the lithium prevents the patient from having a severe recurrence but periodically the depression may recur in milder form and, if the patient had initially responded to an MAOI, it is reasonable to use it again. Usually a somewhat lower dose is satisfactory than that which was required initially and often the time is abbreviated, although this is not always the case.

II. Toxicity and Side Effects

Therapy with MAOIs can be associated with numerous side effects and adverse reactions.

In an overdose situation, acute toxic effects are manifest within a few hours. Overdose produces agitation, hallucinations, hyperpyrexia, hyperreflexia, blood pressure changes, and convulsions. Treatment of resultant hypertension with sympathomimetic amines, or administration of barbiturates for agitation is contraindicated because of the adverse interactions of these drugs with MAOIs. JARVIK (1970) has recommended conservative management of blood pressure, temperature, and electrolytes.

Central nervous system effects include insomnia, irritability, agitation, and motor restlessness. On occasion MAOIs have been shown to convert a retarded into an agitated depression. Hypomania or precipitation of psychosis in patients with a history of schizophrenia also has been reported.

Autonomic side effects include dry mouth, constipation, dizziness, orthostatic hypotension, impotence, and delayed ejaculation.

Liver toxicity resulted in the withdrawal of iproniazid as an antidepressant. NELSON et al. (1976) have recently demonstrated that isopropylhydrazine, a metabolite of iproniazid, was oxidized by cytochrome P-450 enzyme in human liver microsomes to highly reactive acylating and alkylating agents. Covalent bonding of these metabolites to liver macromolecules paralleled hepatic cellular necrosis. The clinical syndrome involves jaundice, hepatocellular damage, elevated liver enzymes and biliary stasis. These reactions were much more prevalent with iproniazid and pheniprazine than with the MAOIs in current use.

Side effects which are rarely seen include blood dyscrasias and pathologic skin reactions.

III. Interactions

The tyramine (cheese reaction) is probably the most widely recognized and important incompatibility.

BLACKWELL et al. (1964) were the first to report on the "cheese" reaction. A patient who had headaches following consumption of cheese wrote to Professor LINFORD REES at St. Bartholomew's Hospital in London and Dr. BARRY BLACKWELL was assigned to investigate. He found that a number of patients on phenelzine or tranylcypromine developed symptoms after consuming mature cheeses. The symptoms usually consisted of severe headache frequently in the evening when the patient was at rest. Blood pressure was markedly elevated (dependent upon the amount of cheese consumed); there was increased pulse rate at times and EKG anomalies. In addition, nausea and vomiting were common. We now know that the reaction can occur within a few minutes but may be delayed several hours. It is usually over in anywhere from 10 to 150 min. Most of the patients recover but occasionally there has been angina, cardiac failure, pulmonary edema, intracranial hemorrhage, and it is possible, that the most frequent are subarachnoid hemorrhages.

The effect can be antagonized by administration of α-adrenoceptor antagonists such as phentolamine. Some clinicians recommend 200–300 mg of chlorpromazine if other treatment is not available. There has also been a verbal report that nitroglycerin is useful in an emergency.

Later, in 1963, after the initial report, ASATOOR et al. (1963) surmised that tyramine was the responsible agent. However, since phenethylamine and tryptamine were both present in the cheese as well, these could not be totally eliminated. According to MARLEY (1977), approximately 30% of the hypertensive crisis are unrelated to food and may constitute a form of autopotentiation. These patients, according to MARLEY, are usually on tranylcypromine which may produce both the MAO inhibition and the hypertensive crisis. This makes it difficult to evaluate the occasional cases reported as resulting from food products other than those with tyramine since they may be only coincidental to the autopotentiation which would have occurred in any case. BLACKWELL has one case where hypertension occurred following bananas (unpublished and referred to by MARLEY).

KRIKLER and LEWIS (1965) reported a rise in blood pressure following chocolate (which contains phenethylamine but not tyramine). Broad beans have also been indicated (HODGE et al., 1964) (containing dopa but not tyramine).

There is some wisdom in limiting the number of restricted foods to as few as possible with the hope that patients will then adhere to the regimen! Even for tyramine-containing food SHAW (1977) states that 5–7 mg are needed to increase blood pressure and 25 mg can precipitate a hypertensive crisis. BALDESSARINI (1977) states "Realistically, because more than 10 mg tyramine is required to produce hypertension, the foods most likely to produce adverse reactions are the cheeses and certain yeast products used as food supplements." There is apparently a factor, in addition to the food, indicating the state of our ignorance since, not infrequently, patients will accidentally take one of the restricted foods and find that there is no unpleasant reaction. They will then begin utilizing cheese, wine, etc., more frequently and in increasingly larger doses. Then suddenly, and rather unaccountably, in view of their apparent immunity, there may be a sudden hypertensive crisis. There has been no satisfactory explanation of why events should follow this course. It is wise to caution the patient, however, that this is a real possibility and the only way to be safe is to abstain from the restricted foods conclusively shown to cause reactions.

It is believed that the tyramine acts by (a) vasoconstriction, (b) increased stroke and minute volume, and (c) increased amount of circulating blood. Under ordinary circumstances, tyramine is not absorbed from the gut because of the presence of substantial amounts of MAO in the intestinal wall. Even if some were absorbed, it would be destroyed by the hepatic microsomal enzyme in the liver. When a MAOI is administered breakdown during absorption does not occur and liver action is limited so that the effect is almost equivalent to a massive intravenous injection.

MIELKE (1976) claims that at times the reaction to foods may be delayed 12 h or longer so that a careful history is necessary. The onset is almost always with headache, but in addition to other symptoms (already listed) there may be chest pain, hyperactivity, confusion, delusions, hallucinations, and even coma.

1. With Tricyclic Antidepressants

Combining MAOI and tricyclics is one of the most potent treatments for resistant cases of depression. There is now general agreement as to how this combination should be used. Summarizing our own experience with the investigations of others (SPIKER and PUGH, 1976; ANANTH and LUCHINS, 1977; SCHUCKIT et al., 1971) it is clear that the combination seemingly is safe if both types of medication are started simultaneously. It is also possible to add an MAOI to the regimen of a patient on a tricyclic. *Great caution,* however, must be exercised in adding a TCA in the treatment of a patient who is already on a MAOI. This can be done but the initial dosage should be extremely small, e. g., 10 mg of impramine or amitriptyline and increase in dose should be gradual. It has been found that moderate to high doses of imipramine may cause severe reactions and imipramine is more likely to precipitate a hypertensive crisis than is amitriptyline. CARLSSON (personal communication, 1979) has pointed out that the reason for hypertensive crisis is that the tricyclics may cause a sudden release of biogenic amines from their storage sites, some of which remain active since MAO is blocked. The reason why the reverse process (MAOI added to TCA) is safer results from the fact that MAO inhibition takes place only gradually. The general use of different MAOIs seems safe. SHAW (1977) is in agreement with this conclusion.

2. With Narcotic Analgesics

It has been found that pethidine and meperidine given to patients receiving MAOIs may produce restlessness, muscular rigidity, enhanced tendon reflexes, extensor plantar responses, and Cheyne-Stokes respiration and coma. This possibly results from a release of 5-HT from peripheral tissue. If narcotic analgesics are necessary, the opiates are probably the safest ones to use.

3. With Insulin

Monoamine oxidase inhibitors appear to lower fasting blood sugar even to the point of hypoglycemia. The effect also leads to potentiation of insulin and hence diabetics who are placed on MAOIs should be carefully followed until a new equilibrium has been reached (COOPER and ASHCROFT, 1966).

4. With Other Prescription Medications

Unless used in massive doses, oral amphetamines in our experience do not appear to have a significant effect on blood pressure although there are cautions on the package insert about avoiding all anorexiants. Parenteral administration should be assiduously avoided. Reactions can also appear with the intravenous administration of adrenaline or noradrenaline. On the other hand, ephedrine appears to be relatively safe.

Levodopa as used in antiparkinsonian treatment should be avoided if possible.

Reserpine, α- and narcotic antagonists must be used with very great caution. Alcohol, chloral hydrate, and barbiturates may be occasionally potentiated.

There is some question, based on animal work, that antiparkinsonian agents may interact. It is not a major problem in humans.

One very real danger is that a patient on an MAOI may be in an accident or require emergency surgery. If the surgeon or anesthetist is unaware that the patient is on a MAOI, serious problems can arise from the parenteral administration of a number of preoperative medications in addition to the narcotics. Some form of atropine, or a synthetic equivalent, is frequently used to dry up mucous membranes. Such medication should be strictly avoided. There is real value in having patients on MAOI carry some indication that they are receiving an MAOI so that, if they forget, are confused or in coma, they do not inadvertently jeopardize their lives.

5. With Over-the-Counter Medications

Probably the most common danger is that patients on MAOIs forget that certain decongestants such as "Contac" are contraindicated since they sometimes do not regard such preparations as really being a "medication." Any decongestant which contains atropine, scopolamine, or phenylpropanolamine is almost certain to produce a marked rise in blood pressure.

G. Potential for Drug Abuse

SHOPSIN and KLINE (1976) report both the amphetamines and MAOIs share common clinical and pharmacologic properties, namely (a) to clinically induce euphoriant stimulating response and psychotomimetic effects in certain individuals, and (b) to increase, albeit by different mechanisms, the amount of functionally available neurotransmitter (catecholamines and indolamines) at the receptor site. The present data now indicate that, like the amphetamines, the use of MAOIs can be clinically associated with dependence and tolerance. Reference is made to four cases of such dependence.

I. Behavioral Toxicity

There is evidence that behavioral alterations (MURPHY et al., 1974; NIES et al., 1973, 1974; MURPHY, 1977) might result from genetically controlled variation in endogenous MAO activity.

Iproniazid. Twenty-seven percent of 507 patients on iproniazid in a variety of studies were found to have psychotic reactions. The incidence was six times as great in patients on 150 mg/day as opposed to 75 mg/day. There was no report of such a psychotic reaction in less than 3 weeks. Manic and hypomanic episodes occurred in patients who previously had had spontaneous episodes of this sort. The incidence of psychotic reaction was higher in endogenous depressives than in reactive, atypical, or neurotic depressions. On the other hand, both paranoid and schizophrenic reactions were highest in the cases of atypical depressions. In a study by FRIEND et al. (1958), eight of ten normal volunteers obtained a euphoric response when given 10 mg/kg of iproniazid. Withdrawal of iproniazid treatment frequently produced insomnia, excessive dreaming, headaches, irritability, and depression (CRANE, 1956; FISHER et al., 1952).

Phenelzine. Based on a review of the literature, MURPHY (1977) found an average of 11% reported as having behavioral side effects. This rose slightly to 15% in the placebo-controlled studies. The changes were similar to those for iproniazid, namely, hypomanic and manic episodes, increased restlessness, hyperactivity, agitation, and irritability with occasional confusional states. An important point is made that some of these reactions may be due to the patient's condition rather than the medication. MURPHY (1977) cites a paper by RASKIN (1972) reporting a 21%–23% incidence of "agitation or excitement" in 110 depressed patients *prior* to double-blind study, and a 9% incidence of the same behavior during treatment with either phenelzine or placebo. In many of the studies no reference is made to behavioral toxicity so that it is impossible to evaluate this effect.

BAILEY et al. (1959) treated 29 schizophrenics characterized by depression, withdrawal, disinterest, apathy using 60 mg/day of phenelzine for 6–9 months with an increase to 100 mg/day for the last month in the nonresponders. Activity was increased in all patients and 70% developed exacerbations of psychopathology.

Tranylcypramine. In the reported studies an overall incidence of 13% was found. Increased restlessness and overstimulation were common but only one patient was reported as becoming hypomanic, although four others were judged to be "on the verge" of such reactions.

Pargyline. This nonhydrazine MAOI is used primarily in antihypertensive therapy. Side effects are similar to the other MAOIs.

Isocarboxazid. Insufficient data is available to draw conclusions.

Procarbazine. Is a methylhydrazine used as an antitumor agent. Mood lability has been described among treated patients.

Nialamide. Hyperactivity has also been reported.

Pheniprazine. In this study, individuals were reported as having increases in visual imagery correlated with urinary tryptamine increases.

MURPHY (1977) concludes that MAOI treatment in man and animals can turn the depressant effects of reserpine into stimulant ones and can markedly enhance the effect of biogenic amine precursors such as L-Dopa. He states:

The potential for the adverse behavioral effects of the MAOIs (can) result from an interaction with endogenous or even dietary factors ... an organized principle for effects of this type is the interpretation that MAO, unlike many catabolic enzymes, has indirect regulatory functions on biogenic amine storage and synthesis that are impaired by MAO inhibiting drugs. Thus, these MAOIs render the organism more vulnerable to other events which can alter amine functions and which may have behavioral consequences.

Deprenyl. Deprenyl which inhibits MAO type B is remarkable in that no cheese type reactions have been reported. In a recent volume on the subject, the hyperactivity appeared to be less malignant than with other MAOIs. In an article by MENDLEWICZ and YOUDIM (cit. under BIRKMAYER and YAHR, 1978) they state:

The hyperactivity syndrome which occurs in rats due to accumulation of brain 5-HT following administration of monoamine oxidase inhibitor with tryptophan on 5-HTP is dependent on the inhibition of MAO activity by more than 85%. Apparently the enzyme is present in the brain grossly in excess of normal requirement. This has been suggested to be the reason why successful therapy of depressive illness by MAOIs sometimes may be difficult to achieve. Evidence for this hypothesis received support from the present study where four patients who did not respond to the 5-HTP plus deprenyl combination showed platelet MAO inhibition far below the 85% mark. As previously cited, the work of ROBINSON et al. (1978) and DAVIDSON et al. (1978) indicate that at least 60% and preferably 80% inhibition must be achieved for clinical effects.

Procaine hydrochloride. In the rat brain or liver, procaine was more effective in inhibiting serotonin oxidation than phenylethylamine oxidation and had an intermediate effect on tryptamine oxidation (FULLER and ROUSH, 1977). However, it did not alter brain norepinephrine levels and only slightly elevated brain serotonin levels, nor did it protect against the degradation of exogenous radioactive tryptamine. It would thus appear that procaine is a very *weak* MAOI although possibly in high doses it may inhibit MAO. If its reported usefulness in treating geriatric patients is confirmed and is dependent upon MAO inhibition, then more effective inhibitors would seem to be available.

H. Management of Overdosage and Side Effects

Specific treatment is immediate by slow intravenous injection of a potent α adrenergic blocking agent such as phentolamine (Regitine) in doses of 5 mg as needed.

BALDESSARINI (1977) states: In an emergency, if a specific alpha blocking agent is not at hand, parenteral injections of chlorpromazine, 50–100 mg intramuscular can be used while appropriate medical treatment is arranged. Some physicians even ask patients undertreatment with an MAO inhibitor to carry several chlorpromazine tablets with instructions to take from 100 to 300 mg if a sudden severe throbbing headache occurs and to seek immediate emergency medical aid.

Table 2. Instructions to patients on a monoamine oxidase inhibitor.

Patients on an MAOI (monoamine oxidase inhibitor) must beware of using certain substances while on this medication and for two weeks after stopping.

The MAOI antidepressant medications are:

Marplan (trade name) – isocarboxazid (generic name)
Nardil (trade name)   – phenelzine (generic name)
Parnate (trade name) – tranylcypromine (generic name)

There are a few MAOI medications used for other purposes:

Eutonyl (trade name) – pargyline (generic name)
Eutron (trade name)   – contains pargyline
Furoxone (trade name) – furazolidone
Matulane (trade name) – procarbazine

Food (and Drink):

Tyrosine is an amino acid found in some foods. When the food ages, ferments and under certain other conditions, it breaks down to produce tyramine. Normally tyramine in turn is destroyed by an enzyme, monoamine oxidase, but when an MAOI is given the tyramine may accumulate and cause an increase of blood pressure. A great deal depends on how much of the food is eaten and how it is prepared. A review of the literature plus our own experience has resulted in the recommendations which follow. We have not included foods when the evidence against them seemed questionable. We strongly recommend therefore that you adhere to these regulations since we have made them as liberal as possible.

Do *not* eat cheeses except

Cream and cottage cheese, yogurt and cheeses labelled "processed" (those in which fermentation has been stopped).

One or two slices of pizza made with no more than the usual amount of Mozzarella is the limit.

Do *not* consume gravies, stews or drinks made with meat extracts or yeast extracts

Meat itself (including stews) and natural gravies are safe.

Bakery products and other foods containing cooked yeast are safe.

Do *not* eat:
Pickled herring chicken liver, goose liver and paté de foie gras

Food which has been aged without refrigeration (particularly meat and poultry)

Freshly prepared frozen or canned food is safe.

Broad bean pods and snow pea pods (as served in some Chinese dishes)

The beans themselves are safe.

Do *not* use alcohol except in small amounts. Do *not* take more than a single glass of Port or Sherry.

In any 3 hour period limit yourself to 2 glasses of white wine (4 ounces each *or* 2 glasses ($1^1/_2$ ounces each) of whiskey, scotch, vodka, etc.

Do *not* take other red wines and especially *not* Chianti. Beer and ale should *not* be used.

Wine used in cooking is safe.

Avoid food or drink which has made you uncomfortable in the past or to which you are allergic.

Several patients have asked about bananas. They are safe. The one negative report is about a patient who boiled the bananas and ate the peel. Chocolate in reasonable amounts is safe in our experience.

Table 2 (continued)

Medicines

Non-prescription drugs

Do *not* take any over-the-counter preparations unless you obtain your doctor's approval except those listed in the other column.

Particularly avoid

Nasal and pulmonary decongestants such as Contac (and its generic equivalents). Also do *not* use tablets, drops or sprays used to treat asthma, coughs, colds, sinus conditions, hay fever unless you check with your doctor. The same is true for sleeping medications, pep-up pills, anti-appetite and anti-weight preparations and LO-MOTIL.

Prescribed medications

*Be absolutely certain that each and every doctor treating you for *any* condition is aware that you are on an MAOI. Some medications such as Rauwolfia (reserpine), L-Dopa, Ismelin (guanethidine), and drugs for diabetes are usually not used or require adjustment of dosage.

Caution

Aspirin, Tylenol, Bufferin (and their generic equivalents) are safe. So are vitamins, citrate or milk of magnesia and enemas.

Medications such as Gelusil and Metamucil used to reduce gastric acidity tend to interfere with the absorption of other medications if taken at the same time. Take the medications separately an hour or two apart.

If an operation is needed, the MAOI is usually discontinued a week or two in advance. In case of emergency surgery be certain that the doctors know you are on an MAOI.

Injections for dental work are safe.

Except for Demerol (meperidine) and possibly morphine, most narcotics used for medical purposes are safe.

Your doctor (aware that you are on MAOI) may prescribe oral amphetamines and related substances in low doses but usually will *not* give these preparations by injection.

If you DO ingest some of the foods or medications listed above, the probability is that nothing will happen if the amount is small (except for over-the-counter medications, Chianti and certain cheeses when there will almost certainly be a reaction).

Do *not* regard this as an indication that you won't get the reaction *next* time. We are not certain why but sometimes the reaction occurs and sometimes it does not. As a rule the reaction which occurs is a severe pounding headache (usually within a few hours).

If this or some other severe side-effect should occur, GO TO THE EMERGENCY ROOM AT A HOSPITAL. They are much better prepared to treat you than is your doctor at your home or even his office. Usually prompt treatment can quickly relieve the condition.

To serve as additional protection you will be given a card to remind you about which foods and medications to avoid, and also what to do in case of an emergency.

Reminder for patients on an MAOI

Be certain to tell ALL doctors who treat you that you are on an MAOI.

Table 2 (continued)

AVOID:

Pickled herring, liver, aged meat or poultry, yeast or meat extracts	Over-the-counter medications, except aspirin (and similar substances), vitamins, citrate and milk of magnesia.
Broad bean and snow pea pods	
Cheese except cottage and cream cheese and yogurt	Particularly avoid Contact and similar preparations such as nasal and pulmonary decongestants for asthma, colds, stuffy nose, sinus conditions, hay fever. Also sleeping medications, anti-appetite and anti-weight drugs unless your doctor has approved.
Beer, ale, wine (especially Chianti). Alcohol in other forms except in very limited amounts	

In case of a reaction (such as a severe pounding headache) go to the EMERGENCY ROOM at a Hospital.

This table can be reproduced by permission of N.S. KLINE and T.B. COOPER (1980). In: Handbook of Experimental Pharmacology, Vol. 55/I, Eds. G. STILLE and F. HOFFMEISTER

Based on our own experience we have devised a fairly comprehensive series of recommendations (Table 2). Similar tables have been devised by SHAW (1977).

Our own recommendations for recognizing the clinical signs and for the treatment of monoamine oxidase inhibitor overdosage are shown in Table 3.

The most common side effect which requires management is the drop in blood pressure which occurs in some patients. As a rule, unless the drop is quite marked, patients rarely have complaints. Many patients with blood pressures in the 100/60 range produce more side effects in the physician than in the patient. Unless there are specific complaints, it does not seem advisable to recommend corrective measures. Patients should be cautioned about climbing stairs or standing up too precipitously. This is particularly true after the patient has been sleeping. Particular caution is needed in men who arise in the middle of the night to urinate. Standing relatively motionless before the toilet bowl may cause a drop in blood pressure. It is recommended that under these circumstances the patient *sit* on the toilet rather than stand before it. Another way of managing this condition is by moving from one foot to another and keeping the blood flowing by contraction of muscles. The same technique can be used prior to standing up. It is a good idea to have patients arising from a prone position to sit on the bed at least half a minute and then move arms and legs to increase cerebral blood flow.

Another technique which can be used is an elastic corset belt as well as supportive hosiery. Patients who have difficulty with dizziness or with staggering, even without subjective dizziness at times, often show dramatic improvement if the abdominal wall is supported.

Another technique is the utilization of fluorocortisone acetate (Fluorinef) at oral doses of 0.1 mg/day. It usually takes the medication several days to work and precautions should be followed as to close observation and appropriate discontinuance where it is indicated. This cortisone derivative is used in the treatment of idiopathic hypotension and works in most cases equally well with the hypotension induced by monoamine oxidase inhibitors.

As a precaution, in those patients with a history of hypomanic or manic episodes in the past, it is strongly advisable to start the patient on lithium. This as a rule will

Table 3. Manual for emergency management of overdosage: monoamine oxidase inhibitors (KLINE et al., 1974)

Clinical signs:
Weakness, dizziness, postural hypotension, excitability, hypertonia, spasticity eventuating in convulsions
Dry mouth
Nausea, vomiting
Mydriasis (dilated pupils) photophobia (abnormal sensitivity to light)
Stupor
Mental confusion and incoherence progressing to stupor, even coma
Neck stiffness
Ataxia, sluggish reflexes
Convulsions
Coma
Hypotension/shock
Hypertensive crisis as manifested by
    flushed face
    occipital headache radiating frontally
    neck stiffness
    nausea, vomiting
    photophobia
Hyperpyrexia
    sweating with fever or with cold, clammy hands
Hypertension and fever are accompanied at times by twitching and myoclonic fibrillation of skeletal muscles, sometimes progressing to generalized rigidity and coma
Rapid heartbeat or slow heartbeat associated with dilated pupils and constricted chest pains
Very rapid breathing and congestion and occasional rhythm problems
Respiratory depression
Death may occur from
    respiratory failure
    circulatory failure
    intracranial bleeding
Watch out for hypertensive crisis appearing concurrently with postural hypotension.
Clinical signs of overdosage may not appear for up to 12 h after drug ingestion allowing for early treatment. Overdosage signs may continue 8–10 days after ingestion of drug. (The action of certain amines is markedly potentiated, since MAOIs block the enzyme which usually leads to amine catabolism. This is particularly so if amines are given parenterally.)

Dangerous combinations
1. With drugs that may precipitate a hypertensive crisis. (This may be fatal, the result of circulatory collapse or intracranial bleeding.)
   Parenteral use of sympathomimetic drugs, such as
       amphetamine
       epinephrine
       norepinephrine
   Methyldopa or dopamine
   Large/parenteral doses of dibenzazepine derivatives, such as desipramine (Pertofrane, Norpramine), amitriptyline (Elavil itself or found in Etrafon or Triavil)
   Large doses of certain proprietary drugs such as those used for cold, hay fever, or dieting which may contain a sympathomimetic agent
   Food high in tyramine, such as beer, wines (especially Chianti), fermented cheeses, pickled herring, chicken livers, yeast extract
   Food high in tryptophan, such as broad beans
2. With drugs possibly causing serious hypotension if used in high doses
   Barbiturates
   Narcotics

Table 3 (continued)

Analgesics
Alcohol
Thiazide diuretics
Phenothiazine compounds

Treatment

1. Maintain open airway, support respirations if necessary with oxygen or artificial respiration
2. Attempt removal of drug by vomiting, gastric lavage, catharsis, and forced diuresis
3. Maintain hydration and electrolyte balance with intravenous fluids, record intake and output
4. Therapy for convulsions
   Correct shock or hypotension if present
   Barbiturates help relieve myoclonic reactions; administer cautiously
   Give intravenous phenothiazine for sedation
   Administer 10–15 mg succinylcholine chloride intravenously, very slowly, and under strict
       controlled ventilation
   Reduce fever with external cooling
5. Hypotension/shock/coma therapy
   Treat conventionally bearing in mind that MAOIs potentiate
   Watch rate of infusion; avoid sudden variations in blood pressure
   Plasma and plasma expanders are most valuable, since MAOIs block vascular bed response
   Vasopressors may be given very cautiously and only when all other measures have been
       used and found inadequate
   Binders and pressure bandages may be used to support blood pressure
6. Hypertension
   Use phentolamine (Regitine) 5 mg intravenously
       OR pentolinium (Ansolysen) 3 mg subcutaneously
       administer slowly to prevent excessive hypotension
       do not give parenteral reserpine
   Continue treatment till homeostasis is restored; follow for at least 10 days; toxic effects may
       be prolonged
   Liver function tests should be performed initially and repeated in 4–6 weeks, if not sooner
       on indication

Special notes

Use cautiously and only if necessary the following drugs.
   Barbiturates. Their use may result in apnea. A phenothiazine is better if sedation is needed.
   Vasopressors/stimulants. Remember tissues are already saturated with epinephrine.
   CNS depressants such as narcotics, Demerol, ethanol, anesthetics, atropine, papaverine,
       scopolamine, etc.
   Cocaine or local anesthetics containing sympathomimetic vasoconstrictors.

---

prevent or at least modify any induced manic or hypomanic episodes. There is also
some evidence that it helps to abort schizophrenic symptoms as well. In the milder
cases where there is slight agitation and medication has already been changed to the
least stimulant of the MAOIs, the benzodiazepines and related substances are sometimes helpful.

   In those patients in whom the MAOIs induce sleepiness 5–10 mg of amphetamine
or a related substance is sometimes sufficient when given in the morning to relieve the
lethargy without interfering with the eventual therapeutic results. On occasion, it may
be necessary to repeat this once or twice during the day. As is frequently the case with

psychotropic drugs, during the first few days the patient may feel somewhat odd and "spaced out." If possible, it is useful to have the patient persist in order to determine whether these symptoms do not disappear. Unless the case is acute and severe, it is often useful to begin at a low dose and increase the MAOI every 2–3 days, thus avoiding some of the side effects.

Another occasional symptom is constipation. Under these circumstances, either enema or saline cathartic is recommended, as well as a stool softener. Laxatives can be used but it is advisable to start with a quarter to half of the usual dose to be on the alert for idiosyncratic action. In elderly patients, intestinal anergia must be looked for and asked about since otherwise it may not be reported.

Occasionally patients will develop edema, particularly of the peripheral type. There is no contraindication to the use of diuretics under these circumstances. It is wise to make certain that the patient is receiving an adequate protein intake to be certain that the edema is not due to protein deficiency.

Weight gain is a frequent complaint of patients on almost any type of psychotropic drug. Not infrequently the weight gain is the result of the patient beginning to feel better and consuming more calories than he or she is aware or willing to report. In most cases, after the initial weight gain, if patients are placed on a diet, any excess weight can be reduced. Cautious use of *oral anorexiant* agents may be necessary for a week or two.

Rarely patients will develop a dermatologic reaction. Under these circumstances, a different MAOI should be tried. In our experience, the recommended waiting period between MAOIs is not necessary and at times different MAOIs may even be combined. On occasion, the same MAOI may be started subsequently without recurrence of the skin reaction.

I. Summary

The MAOIs have been used as antidepressant drugs for the past two decades. Despite carefully controlled studies demonstrating clinical efficacy and the relative safety of such medications no new MAOI has been introduced to the United States drug market since 1964. Our understanding of MAO as an enzyme and its substrate and inhibitor specificity has increased substantially since 1964 and these data should permit the development of highly selective MAOIs with the clinically desirable features of high potency with minimal side effects.

References

Ananth, J., Luchins, D.: A review of combined tricyclic and MAOI therapy. Compr. Psychiatry *18*, 221–230 (1977)

Asatoor, A.M., Levi, A.J., Milne, M.D.: Tranylcypromine and cheese. Lancet *2*, 733–734 (1963)

Axelrod, J.: O-methylation of epinephrine and other catechols in vitro and in vivo. Science *126*, 400 (1957)

Ayd, F.J.: A preliminary report on marsilid. Am. J. Psychiatry *114*, 459 (1957)

Bailey, S.D., Bucci, L., Gosline, E., Kline, N.S., Park, I.H., Rochlin, D., Saunders, J.C., Vaisberg, M.: Comparison of iproniazid with other amine oxidase inhibitors, including W-1544, JB-516, R04-1018, and R05-0700. Ann. N.Y. Acad. Sci. *80*, 652–668 (1959)

Baldessarini, R.J.: Mood drugs. In: Disease-A-Month.Dowling, H.F. (ed.), Vol. 24, *2*,. Chicago: Year Book Medical Publishers 1977

Berger, P.A., Barchas, J.D.: Monoamine oxidase inhibitors. In: Psychotherapeutic drugs. Usdin, E., Forrest, I. (eds.). New York: Dekker 1977

Biel, J.H., Bopp, B.: Monoamine oxidase inhibitor antidepressants. In: Psychopharmacological agents. Gordon, M. (ed.), pp. 302–309. New York: Academic Press 1974

Birkmayer, W., Yahr, M. (eds.): Deprenyl, an inhibitor of MAO-type B in the treatment of Parkinsonism. J. Neural. Transm. *43*, 3–4 (1978)

Blackwell, B., Marley, E., Ryle, A.: Hypertensive crisis associated with monoamine-oxidase inhibitors. Lancet *1*, 722–723 (1964)

Brodie, B.B., Pletscher, A., Shore, P.A.: Possible role of serotonin in brain function and in reserpine action. J. Pharmacol. Exp. Ther. *116*, 9 (1956)

Bunney, W.E., Davis, J.M.: Norepinephrine in depressive reactions. A review. Arch. Gen. Psychiatry *13*, 483–494 (1965)

Burn, J.H., Philpot, F.J., Trendelenburg, U.: Effect of denervation on enzymes in iris and blood vessels. Br. J. Pharmacol. *9*, 423–428 (1954)

Chessin, M., Dubnick, B., Kramer, E.R., Scott, C.C.: Modifications of pharmacology of reserpine and serotonin by iproniazid. Fed. Proc. *15*, 409 (1956)

Cooper, A.J., Ashcroft, G.: Potentiation of insulin hypoglycaemia by MAOI antidepressant drugs. Lancet *1*, 407–409 (1966)

Crane, G.E.: Further studies on iproniazid phosphate. Isonicotinil-isopropylhydrazine phosphate Marsilid. J. Nerv. Ment. Dis. *124*, 322–331 (1956)

Crane, G.E.: The psychiatric side-effects of iproniazid. Am. J. Psychiatry *112*, 494–501 (1956)

Davidson, J., McCleod, M.N., Blum, M.R.: Acetylation phenotype, platelet monoamine oxidase inhibition, and the effectiveness of phenelzine in depression. Am. J. Psychiatry *135*, 467–469 (1978)

Dunleavy, D.L.F., Oswald, I.: Phenelzine, mood response and sleep. Arch. Gen. Psychiatry *28*, 353–356 (1973)

Escobar, J.I., Schiele, B.C., Zimmermann, R.: The tranylcypromine isomers: A controlled clinical trial. Am. J. Psychiatry *131*, 1025–1026 (1974)

Evans, D.A.P., Manley, K.A., McKusick, V.A.: Genetic control of isoniazid metabolism in man. Br. Med. J. *2*, 485–491 (1960)

Evans, D.A.P., Davison, K., Pratt, R.T.C.: The influence of acetylator phenotype on the effects of treating depression with phenelzine. Clin. Pharmacol. Ther. *6*, 430–435 (1965)

Fisher, M.M., Mammlok, E.R., Tendlau, A., Tebrock, H.E., Drumm, A.E., Spiegelman, A.: Isonicotinic acid hydrazide and its derivatives in tuberculosis: An evaluation of the side-effects in relation to peripheral circulation; preliminary report. *52*, 1519–1527 (1952)

Fowler, C.J., Callingham, B.A., Mantle, T.J., Tipton, K.F.: Monoamine oxidase A and B: A useful concept? Biochem. Pharmacol. *27*, 97–101 (1978)

Franzen, F., Eysell, K. (eds.): Biologically active amines found in man. Oxford: Pergamon Press 1969

Friend, D.G., Zileli, M.S., Hamlin, J.T., Reutter, F.W.: The effect of iproniazid on the inactivation of norepinephrine in the human. J. Clin. Exp. Psychopathol. *19*, 61–71 (1958)

Fuller, R.W.: Selective inhibition of monoamine oxidate. Adv. Biochem. Psychopharm. *5*, 339–354 (1972)

Fuller, R.W.: Selectivity among monoamine oxidase inhibitors and its possible importance for development of antidepressant drugs. Prog. Neuropsychopharmacol. *2*, 303–311 (1978)

Fuller, R.W., Roush, B.W.: Procaine hydrochloride as a monoamine oxidase inhibitor: Implications for geriatric therapy. J. Am. Geriatr. Soc. *25*, 90–93 (1977)

Gaddum, J.H., Kwiatkowski, H.: The action of ephedrine. J. Physiol. (Lond.) *94*, 87–100 (1938)

Goodman, L.S., Gilman, A.: The pharmacological basis of therapeutics. 2 nd ed., p. 517. New York: Macmillan 1965

Hendley, E.D., Snyder, S.H.: Relationship between the action of monoamine oxidase inhibitors on the noradrenaline uptake system and their antidepressant efficacy. Nature *220*, 1330–1331 (1968)

Hodge, J.V., Nye, E.R., Emerson, G.W.: Monoamine-oxidase inhibitors, broad beans, and hypertension. Lancet *1*, 1108 (1964)

Horwitz, D., Goldberg, L.I., Sjoerdsma, A.: Increased blood pressure responses to dopamine and norepinephrine produced by monoamine oxidase inhibitors in man. J. Lab. Clin. Med. *56*, 747–753 (1960)

Horwitz, D., Lovenberg, W., Engelman, K., Sjoerdsma, A.: Monoamine oxidase inhibitors, tyramine, and cheese. J. Am. Med. Assoc. *188*, 1108 (1964)

Houslay, M.D., Garrett, N.J., Tipton, K.F.: Mixed substrate experiments with human brain monoamine oxidase. Biochem. Pharmacol. *23*, 1937–1944 (1974)

Houslay, M.D., Tipton, K.F., Youdim, M.B.H.: Minireview Multiple forms of monoamine oxidase: Fact and artefact. Life Sci. *19*, 467–478 (1976)

Jarvik, M.: Drugs used in the treatment of psychiatric disorders. In: The pharmacological basis of therapeutics. 5th ed. Goodman, L.S., Gilman, A. (eds.), pp. 151–203. New York: MacMillan 1970

Johnston, J.P.: Some observations upon a new inhibitor of monoamine oxidase in brain tissue. Biochem. Pharmacol. *17*, 1285–1297 (1968)

Johnstone, E.C., Marsh, W.: Acetylator status and response to phenelzine in depressed patients. Lancet *1*, 567–570 (1973)

Kamman, G.R., Freeman, J.G., Lucero, R.J.: The effect of 1-isonicotynil-2-isopropyl hydrazine (IIH) on the behavior of long-term mental patients. J. Nerv. Ment. Dis. *118*, 391–407 (1953)

Kiloh, L.G., Child, J.P., Latner, G.: A controlled trial of iproniazid in the treatment of endogenous depression. J. Ment. Sci. *106*, 1139–1144 (1960)

Kline, N.S.: Present status of psychopharmacological Research: Includes Loomer, H., Saunders, J.C., Kline, N.S.: Iproniazid, an amine oxidase inhibitor, as an example of a psychic energizer. Hearings before the subcommittee of the Committee on Appropriations, United States Senate, 85th Congress, 1st Session on H.R. 6287, pp. 1372–1390, May 9, 1957. Washington, D.C.: U.S. Government Printing Office 1957

Kline, N.S.: Quoted in: Berger, P.A., Barchas, J.D. In: Psychotherapeutic drugs. Usdin, E., Forrest, I. (eds.), p. 1175. New York: Dekker 1977

Kline, N.S., Sacks, W.: Relief of depression within one day using an M.A.O. inhibitor and intravenous 5-HTP. Am. J. Psychiatry *120*, 274–275 (1963)

Kline, N.S., Sacks, W.: Treatment of depression with an MAO inhibitor followed by 5-HTP – an unfinished research project. Presented at Symposium on Biogenic Amines and Affective Disorders. London. Jan. 18–21, 1979

Kline, N.S., Alexander, S.F., Chamberlain, A.: In: Psychotropic drugs. Manual for emergency management overdosage. New Jersey: Medical Economics Company 1974

Kline, N.S., Sacks, W., Simpson, G.M.: Further studies on: One day treatment of depression with 5-HTP. Am. J. Psychiatry *121*, 379–381 (1964)

Kopin, I.J., Axelrod, J.: The role of monoamine oxidase in the release and metabolism of norepinephrine. Ann. N.Y. Acad. Sci. *107*, 848 (1963)

Krikler, D.M., Lewis, B.: Dangers of natural foodstuffs. Lancet *1*, 1166 (1965)

Lader, M.: Antianxiety drugs: Clinical pharmacology and therapeutic use. Drugs *12*, 362–373 (1976)

Leonard, B.E.: Some effects of mianserin on monoamine metabolism in the rat brain. Br. J. Clin. Pharmacol. *5*, 11S–12S (1978)

Loomer, H.P., Saunders, J.C., Kline, N.S.: A clinical and pharmacodynamic evaluation of iproniazid as a psychic energizer. Psychiatr. Res. Rep. *8*, 129–141 (1958)

Maclean, R., Nicholson, W.J., Pare, C.M.B., Stacey, R.S.: Effect of monoamine-oxidase inhibitors on the concentrations of 5-hydroxytryptamine in the human brain. Lancet *2*, 205–208 (1965)

Marley, E.: Monoamine oxidase inhibitors. In: Drug interactions. Grahame-Smith, D.G. (ed.), pp. 178–194. Baltimore: University Park Press 1977

Marshall, E.F., Mountjoy, C.O., Campbell, I.C., Garside, R.F., Leitch, I.M., Roth, M.: The influence of acetylator phenotype on the outcome of treatment with phenelzine, in a clinical trial. Br. J. Clin. Pharmacol. *6*, 247–254 (1978)

Mielke, D.H.: Adverse reactions of thymoleptics. In: Depression: Behavioral, biochemical, diagnostic and treatment concepts. Gallant, D.M., Simpson, G.M. (eds.), pp. 273–308. Stuttgart: Spectrum Publications 1976

Morris, J.B., Beck, A.T.: The efficacy of antidepressant drugs. A review of research (1958 to 1972). Arch. Gen. Psychiatry *30*, 667–674 (1974)

Murphy, D.L.: The behavioral toxicity of monoamine oxidase-inhibiting antidepressants. Adv. Pharmacol. Chemother. *14*, 71–105 (1977)

Murphy, D.L., Donnelly, C.H.: Monoamine oxidase in man: enzyme characteristics in platelets, and other human tissue. In: Neuropsychopharmacology of monoamines and their regulatory enzymes. Usdin, E. (ed.), pp. 71–85. New York: Raven Press 1974

Murphy, D.L., Belmaker, R., Wyatt, R.J.: Monoamine oxidase in schizophrenia and other behavioral disorders. J. Psychiatr. Res. *11*, 221–247 (1974)

Neff, N.H., Yang, H.-Y.T.: Life Sci. *14*, 2061–2074 (1974)

Nelson, S.D., Mitchell, J.R., Timbrell, J.A., et al.: Isoniazid and iproniazid: Activation of metabolites to toxic intermediates in man and rat. Science *193*, 901–903 (1976)

Nies, A., Robinson, D.S., Lamborn, K.R., Lampert, R.P.: Genetic control of platelet and plasma monoamine oxidase activity. Arch. Gen. Psychiatry *28*, 834–838 (1973)

Nies, A., Robinson, D.S., Harris, L.S., Lamborn, K.R.: Comparison of monoamine oxidase substrate activity in twins, schizophrenics, depressives, and controls. In: Advances in biochem. psychopharmacol. Neuropsychopharmacology of monoamine and their regulatory enzymes. Usdin, E. (ed.). New York: Raven Press 1974

Ostow, M., Kline, N.S.: The psychic action of reserpine and chlorpromazine. In: Psychopharmacology frontiers. Kline, N.S. (ed.), Appendix, pp. 481–513. Boston, Mass.: Little, Brown & Co. 1959

Paykel, E.S.: Classification of depressed patients: A cluster analysis derived grouping. Br. J. Psychiatry *118*, 275–288 (1971)

Pletscher, A., Shore, P.A., Brodie, B.B.: Serotonin as a mediator of reserpine action in brain. J. Pharmacol. Exp. Ther. *116*, 84–89 (1956)

Raskin, A.: Adverse reactions to phenelzine: Results of a nine-hospital depression study. J. Clin. Pharmacol. *12*, 22–25 (1972)

Robinson, D.S., Lovenberg, W., Keiser, H., Sjoerdsma, A.: Effects of drugs on human blood platelet and plasma amine oxidase activity in vitro and in vivo. Biochem. Pharmacol. *17*, 109–119 (1968)

Robinson, D.S., Nies, A., Ravaris, C.L., Ives, J.O., Bartlett, D.: Clinical psychopharmacology of phenelzine: MAO activity and clinical response. In: Psychopharmacology: A generation of progress. Lipton, M.A., DiMascio, A., Killam, K.F. (eds.). New York: Raven Press 1978

Rosloff, B.N., Davis, J.M.: Effect of iprindole on norepinephrine turnover and transport. Psychopharmacologia (Berl.) *40*, 53–64 (1974)

Saunders, J.C., Radinger, N., Rochlin, D., Kline, N.S.: Treatment of depressed and regressed patients with iproniazid and reserpine. Dis. Nerv. Syst. *20*, 1–8 (1959)

Schiele, B.C.: The parnate specific patient. Minn. Med. *48*, 355–357 (1965)

Schildkraut, J.J.: The catecholamine hypothesis of affective disorders: A review of supporting evidence. Am. J. Psychiatry *122*, 509–522 (1965)

Schuckit, M., Robins, E., Feighner, J.: Tricyclic antidepressants and monoamine oxidase inhibitors: Combination therapy in the treatment of depression. Arch. Gen. Psychiatry *24*, 509–514 (1971)

Selikoff, I.J., Robitzvek, E.H., Ornstein, G.G.: Toxicity of hydrazine derivatives of isonicotinic acid in the chemotherapy of human tuberculosis. Q. Bull. Sea View Hosp. *13*, 17–26 (1952)

Shaw, D.M.: The practical management of affective disorders. Br. J. Psychiatry *130*, 432–451 (1977)

Shopsin, B., Kline, N.S.: Monoamine oxidase inhibitors: Potential for drug abuse. Biol. Psychiatry *11*, 451–456 (1976)

Sjoqvist, F.: In: Monoamine oxidase inhibitors: Relationship between pharmacological and clinical effects. Cheymol, J., Boissier, J.R., Vol. 10. New York: Pergamon Press 1968

Smith, J.A.: The use of the isopropyl derivative of isonicotinylhydrazine (marsilid) in the treatment of mental disease; A preliminary report. Am. Practitioner *4*, 519–520 (1953)

Spector, S., Hirsch, C.W., Brodie, B.B.: Association of behavioral effects of pargyline, a non-hydrazide monoamine oxidase inhibitor with increase in brain norepinephrine. Int. J. Neuropharmacol. *2*, 81–93 (1963)

Spiker, D.G., Pugh, D.D.: Combining tricyclic and monoamine oxidase inhibitor antidepressants. Arch. Gen. Psychiatry *33*, 828–830 (1976)

Tyrer, P., Candy, J., Kelly, D.: Phenelzine in phobia anxiety: A controlled trial. Psychol. Med. *3*, 120–124 (1973)

Usdin, E. (ed.): Neuropsychopharmacology of monoamines and their regulatory enzymes. Advances in biochemical psychopharmacology, Vol. *12*. New York: Raven Press 1974

Von Bruecke, F., Hornykiewicz, O., Sigg, E.B.: Monoamine oxidase inhibitors. In: The pharmacology of psychotherapeutic drugs. pp. 78–102. Berlin, Heidelberg, New York: Springer 1969

West, E.D., Dally, P.J.: Effects of iproniazid in depressive syndromes. Br. Med. J. *1*, 1491–1494 (1959)

Yang, H.-Y.T., Neff, N.H.: B-phenylethylamine: A specific substrate for type B monoamine oxidase of brain. J. Pharmacol. Exp. Ther. *187*, 365–371 (1973)

Youdim, M.B.: Multiple forms of mitochondrial monoamine oxidase. Br. Med. Bull. *29*, 120–122 (1973)

Zeller, E.A., Barsky, J.: In vivo inhibition of liver and brain monoamine oxidase by 1-isonicotinyl-2-isopropyl hydrazine. Proc. Soc. Exp. Biol. Med. *81*, 459–461 (1952)

CHAPTER 18

Tricyclic Antidepressants: General Pharmacology

I. Møller Nielsen

A. Introduction

The antidepressant effect of the first tricyclic antidepressant was not predicted by pharmacologists. In fact, a series of analogs to antihistaminics were screened for central depressant effect (Domenjoz and Theobald, 1959) and first tried clinically as tranquilizers. The recognition of the antidepressant activity of imipramine was due to the serindipity of Kuhn (1957). Following that, pharmacologists began the search for proper animal models to characterize this property of drugs and investigate for possible modes of action. Since then a large number of derivatives have been synthesized, most of which belong to the group of tricyclic antidepressants; a few nontricyclic compounds with antidepressant activity and with largely the same pharmacologic profile of action will be included in the discussion.

B. Behavioral Effects

Thymoleptics possess mild central depressant activity in normal animals. They reduce spontaneous motor activity in doses considerably higher than those of neuroleptic compounds. Although spontaneous motor activity is reduced the animals may show increased excitability (Stille, 1964; Stille, 1968). Thymoleptics reduce the activity of rats in an open field (Kinnard et al., 1967). In cats and dogs imipramine induces sedation in a dose of 5–10 mg/kg (Sigg, 1959). With higher doses a state of flexibilitas cerea is induced (Domenjoz and Theobald, 1959). In studying the effects of imipramine on electrocortical activity and wakefulness in cats, Horovitz and Chow (1962) found no indication of stimulating effect; EEG arousal was not blocked but there was an increase in behavioral arousal threshold with higher doses. On the other hand, Himwich (1959) reported a blockade of arousal reaction to sound with 2.5 mg imipramine/kg. Larger doses blocked arousal to pain as well. In a discriminated avoidance behavior test in rats, Morpurgo (1965) found a rather weak inhibition of active avoidance with imipramine and desipramine, which were much less active than neuroleptics. Discrimination ability was only slightly impaired. Development of secondary conditioned response was increased with imipramine, 5–10 mg/kg p. o. The effect was reduced with higher doses. This was taken as an indication of central stimulant properties (Maxwell and Palmer, 1961). In a Sidman avoidance procedure, Hanson (1961) studied amitriptyline and imipramine at dose levels of 5–20 mg/kg p. o. No indication of increased response was seen at any dose, loss of avoidance was seen at moderate doses, and escape was decreased at higher doses. Chlorpromazine was active at lower dose levels.

Antidepressants selectively block the mouse-killing (muricidal) behavior in rats. They were active in doses that did not affect rotarod performance or inhibit conditioned avoidance response. Selective blockade was also shown by other classes of drugs such as amphetamines and some antihistamines. Muricidal effect was abolished by lesions in centro medial amygdala (Horovitz et al., 1966).

Although mild tranquilizer effects are the immediately observed effects of thymoleptics, one compound shows overt stimulant effects, namely nomifensin. This compound increases spontaneous motor activity and induces stereotyped activity (Hoffman, 1973; Costall et al., 1975; Bræstrup and Scheel-Krüger, 1976). The effect is not blocked by α-MT (α-methyltyrosine) 2 h before nomifensin but by α-MT 5 h before or by reserpine. Thus nomifensin, in contrast to other thymoleptics, is considered a dopamine-releasing compound of the methylphenidate type (Bræstrup and Scheel-Krüger, 1976).

C. Interaction with Other Drugs

The central stimulating properties of thymoleptics may come to light in combination with other centrally acting drugs. Thymoleptics antagonize the various symptoms of the reserpine syndrome. Already in 1959 Domenjoz and Theobald showed that imipramine in a dose of 50 mg/kg counteracted the potentiating effect of 2 mg reserpine/kg on anesthesia produced by 2-M-4A (2-methoxy-4-allylphenoxyacetic acid N,N diethylamide). Likewise they found that the reduction of spontaneous motor activity by 2 mg reserpine/kg was antagonized by imipramine, 50 mg/kg. Furthermore, imipramine in doses of 50–100 mg antagonized the reserpine-induced ptosis. These were rather high doses but later studies have shown antidepressants to be active at more reasonable dose levels (Sulser et al., 1962). In a routine screening of thymoleptics for antagonism against reserpine-induced ptosis (Table 1, column 1) imipramine was active at a dose level of 3.5 mg/kg and amitriptyline at 13 mg/kg. The most active compounds were the secondary amines, protriptyline, desipramine, and litracen. Instead of reserpine, synthetic benzquinolizines have also been used, e. g., Ro 4-1284 or tetrabenazine. The antagonistic effects of thymoleptics against tetrabenazine-induced ptosis are listed in Table 1, column 2. A rather close correlation to the effect against reserpine ptosis may be noted. The immobility and catalepsy induced by tetrabenazine is also antagonized by thymoleptics at about the same dose level (Table 1, column 3). The antagonistic effect of thymoleptics against the sedative effect of tetrabenazine is reversed with higher doses (Vernier et al., 1962).

Reserpine-induced hypothermia is antagonized by thymoleptics. Imipramine, desipramine, and nortriptyline given *before* reserpine enhance the hyperthermic phase of reserpine and prevent the subsequent hypothermic phase (Jori and Garattini, 1965; Garattini and Jori, 1967). Imipramine, desipramine, amitriptyline, and nortriptyline given *after* reserpine elicit a marked rise in body temperature above the reserpine-induced hypothermic level (Vernier et al., 1962; Morpurgo and Theobald, 1965; Votava et al., 1965; Garattini and Jori, 1967). Reserpine-induced gastric ulcers are prevented by rather large doses of imipramine, desipramine, amitriptyline, or nortriptyline (Garattini et al., 1962; Votava et al., 1965).

These effects of thymoleptics are most likely a result of potentiation of central noradrenergic mechanisms (see below). The same mechanism may be responsible for the

Table 1. Various pharmacologic effects of a series of thymoleptics

	1	2	3	4	5	6	7	8	9	10
	Reserpine ptosis ED 50 mg/kg	Tetrabenazine ptosis ED 50 mg/kg	Tetrabenazine motility ED 50 mg/kg	Apomorphine gnawing ED 50 mg/kg	5-HTP potentiation ED 50 mg/kg	NA uptake inhibition in vitro IC 50 x10^{-8}M	5-HT uptake inhibition IC 50 x10^{-7}M	DA uptake inhibition IC 50 x10^{-6}M	Anticholinergic effect IC 50 x10^{-7}M	[^{3}H]-PrBCM binding IC 50 x10^{-7}M
Amitriptyline	13	7	3	3.6	21	13	3.0	5.4	1.2	0.47
Nortriptyline	5	2.5	0.4	4.9	>20	2.9	15	3.6	4.5	4.8
Protriptyline	0.4	0.2	0.3	7.9	>20	0.08	13	3.3	4.5	1.2
Imipramine	3.5	3	1–2	3.7	20	7.5	3.2	18	4.3	4.8
Desipramine	0.8	0.6	0.5	6.9	>20	0.14	18	9.1	15	34
Imipramine N-oxide	2.5	3	2	49	>20	61	150	–	>240	–
Chlorimipramine	3.5	4	1.5	5.0	8.8	27	0.33	4.3	6.9	3.1
Opipramol	>40	>40	>40	62.6	>40	480	>420	3.0	50	–
Trimeprimine	>20	>20	>20	22.8	>20	770	260	6.6	4.2	–
Melitracen	6	6	2	7.6	>40	23	55	8.2	1.2	0.95
Litracen	2	2	1	16	>40	–	99	8.0	19	6.4
Dibenzepin	15	2	11	22.2	>20	55	140	>100	31	–
Doxepin	42	48	>40	4.0	54	370	39	13	5.2	5.4
Iprindol	41	45	22	>40	>20	–	440	14	59	200
Maprotiline	15	6	7	5.6	>20	–	360	10	19	24
Nomifensin	–	2	0.3	28.4	>20	0.80	160	0.05	>110	500
Viloxazine	–	>10	–	18.1	>20	140	>640	56	>150	>500
Mianserin	≫10	≫10	–	>20	>20	81	>640	–	48	13
Atropine	10								0.07	0.05

potentiating effect of thymoleptics on the central action of amphetamines. Imipramine, desipramine, amitriptyline, and nortriptyline enhanced and prolonged the hyperthermic effect of amphetamine in rats (Morpurgo and Theobald, 1965; Valzelli et al., 1967). In a Sidman avoidance test, Carlton (1961) found no effect of imipramine, 10 mg/kg, on response rate but 5–10 mg/kg increased the effect of 1 mg amphetamine/kg, producing greater peak response and prolongation of the period of supernormal responding. Similarly Scheckel and Boff (1964) found that tricyclic antidepressants in rather low doses potentiated the effect of amphetamine and cocaine in a Sidman continuous avoidance procedure. Anticholinergics were also active but, in contrast to these drugs, tricyclic antidepressants also produced stimulant effect when combined with a small, nondepressant dose of tetrabenazine. While imipramine had no effect per se on selfstimulation in the medial forebrain bundle it greatly augmented the effect of metamphetamine (Stein and Seifter, 1961; Stein, 1967). It should be mentioned, however, that imipramine and desipramine inhibit the parahydroxylation of amphetamine so that the potentiation and prolongation of amphetamine effects may be partly, if not entirely, due to increased brain levels of amphetamine (Valzelli et al., 1967).

The effect of the catecholamine precursor Dopa (dihydroxyphenylalanine) is also potentiated by thymoleptics. Desipramine enhanced the hyperthermic effect of Dopa (Jori and Garattini, 1965). In mice pretreated with an MAOI (monoamine oxidase inhibitor) thymoleptics enhance the behavioral effect of Dopa producing a syndrome of piloerection, salivation, increased excitability, jumping, squeaking, and aggressive fighting (Everett, 1967).

In mice, tricyclic antidepressants modify and intensify the behavioral effect of apomorphine, causing an intense gnaw compulsion syndrome (Ther and Schramm, 1962; Pedersen, 1967). Similarly thymoleptics potentiate the gnawing in mice induced by Dopa following the decarboxylase inhibitor Ro 4-4602 (Molander and Randrup, 1976). The potency of thymoleptics in provoking apomorphine-induced compulsive gnawing is given in Table 1, column 4. It may be seen that amitriptyline and imipramine are among the most potent compounds. When thymoleptics are given in higher doses the effect is reversed. Pretreatment with α-MT, a tyrosinehydroxylase inhibitor, but not diethyldithiocarbamate (dopamine-β-hydroxylase inhibitor) abolished the gnaw compulsion indicating that catecholamines, probably dopamine plays an important role for the gnaw compulsion syndrome (Pedersen, 1968).

The effects of 5-HT (5-hydroxytryptamine) precursors tryptophan and 5-HTP (5-hydroxytryptophan) in mice and rats are potentiated by some tricyclic antidepressants. In mice, 5-HTP given after a thymoleptic compound which blocks the reuptake of 5-HT in central serotoninergic neurones (see later) results in an intense syndrome consisting of excitation, lordosis, and abduction of the hind limbs (Hyttel and Fjalland, 1972). This syndrome is not seen after 5-HTP alone. Mice treated with an MAOI elicits a similar syndrome when a 5-HT uptake inhibitor is given before tryptophan. The ED50 values for 5-HTP potentiation of a series of thymoleptics are listed in Table 1, column 5. Among the established tricyclic antidepressants, chlorimipramine was the most potent drug in this respect. The tertiary amines, imipramine and amitriptyline, were also active although much weaker than chlorimipramine. Secondary amines were inactive. Some newer nontricyclic 5-HT uptake inhibitors have also been tested. Femoxetine (FG 4963) was slightly less potent than chlorimipramine, fluoxetine (Lilly 110140) three times more potent and citalopram (Lu 10-171) six times more potent than chlorimipramine (CHRISTENSEN et al., 1977).

When given to rabbits after an MAOI, thymoleptics cause an often fatal syndrome characterized by hyperthermia and excitation (NYMARK and MØLLER NIELSEN, 1963; LOVELESS and MAXWELL, 1965; CARLSSON et al., 1969 c, d; GONG and ROGERS, 1971). Following administration of the MAOI, brain levels of NA (noradrenaline), DA (dopamine), and 5-HT are elevated. However, pretreatment with α-MT which abolishes the increase in NA and DA did not prevent the hyperthermic reaction. On the other hand, pretreatment with PCPA (parachlorophenylalanine), a 5-HT synthesis inhibitor, prevents the increase in brain 5-HT and the hyperthermic reaction does not occur (GONG and ROGERS, 1971). Furthermore, citalopram which is a bicyclic specific 5-HT uptake inhibitor (HYTTEL, 1977) causes marked hyperthermia after an MAOI. This effect is completely inhibited by pretreatment with PCPA (CHRISTENSEN et al., 1977).

D. Interaction with Biogenic Amines

Thymoleptics potentiate the effects of catecholamines. These effects are most readily demonstrated on peripheral organs. The pressor effect of NA in the pithed rat preparation is potentiated (MØLLER NIELSEN et al., 1966). A quantitative assessment of a series of tricyclic antidepressants is given in Table 2. Again the most active compounds in this respect were the secondary amines, protriptyline and desipramine, while nortriptyline was surprisingly weak. Due to the α-blocking effect, the pressor response may be reversed when higher doses are given. In the ganglion-blocked dog, amitriptyline potentiated the pressor effect of NA (VERNIER et al., 1962; CAIRNCROSS, 1965), while the pressor effect of the indirectly acting sympathomimetic amine, phenylethylamine, was blocked dose dependently in the dose range 0.1–3.0 mg/kg, i. v. (VERNIER et al., 1962). Also, in cats the potentiating effect on NA-induced pressor response has been shown (SIGG, 1959; SCHAEPPI, 1960; STILLE, 1964; CAIRNCROSS et al., 1965; Møller Nielsen et al., 1966; HOFFMEISTER, 1969). The pressor effect of NA is increased and prolonged immediately after injection of imipramine, the action is maximal 1–2 h after injection and lasts for several hours (SCHAEPPI, 1960).

Table 2. Potentiation of the NA pressor response in pithed rats

	ED 50 mg/kg
Amitriptyline	4.0
Nortriptyline	2.1
Imipramine	0.35
Desipramine	0.07
Imipramine N-oxide	0.56
Chlorimipramine	3.5
Opipramol	>4
Protriptyline	0.025
Melitracen	2.5
Litracen	0.78
Mianserin	>5

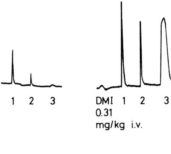

1 = Pre   2 = Post   3 = NA

Fig. 1. Potentiation by desipramine (DMI) of the contraction of the cat nictitating membrane to pre- and postganglionic stimulation of the cervical sympathetic trunk and exogenous NA

The contraction of the nictitating membrane of the cat to exogenous NA and stimulation of the cervical sympathetic trunk is a convenient model for the study of the effect of tricyclic antidepressants on adrenergic mechanisms. The intact and acutely denervated membrane contracts upon intravenous injection of NA, this effect was intensified by previous treatment with thymoleptics (Cairncross et al., 1965; Greenwood, 1975; Sigg, 1959; Schaeppi, 1960; Møller Nielsen et al., 1966; Sigg et al., 1963 b). Also the contraction to 5-HT injection was strongly potentiated (Sigg et al., 1963 b). Contractions elicited by submaximal electric stimulation of the pre-ganglionic or postganglionic cervical sympathetic trunk were potentiated by thy-moleptics (Fig. 1) (Cairncross et al., 1965; Hoffmeister, 1969; Sigg et al., 1963 b; Ryall, 1961) although Schaeppi (1960) found a decrease in the pre- and post-ganglionic elicited contraction after 6 mg imipramine/kg. The effect of supramaximal stimulation was not enhanced but somewhat prolonged (Cairncross et al., 1965). The chronically denervated nictitating membrane, where the superior cervical ganglion has been removed 3 weeks before the experiment, becomes supersensitive to NA, but the effect is not further enhanced by the administration of thymoleptic drugs. This preparation on the other hand is well suited to demonstrate the α-receptor blocking effect of higher doses. In experiments where one nictitating membrane is denervated and the other is left intact it can be shown that amitriptyline at a dose of 0.3 mg/kg possesses potentiating effect on the intact membrane and α-blocking effect on the de-nervated membrane. This means that the effect seen on the intact membrane is the net result of two competing effects, facilitation of transmission and α-blockade.

While the effect of directly acting NA agonists is enhanced, that of indirectly ac-ting agonists such as tyramine and phenylethylamine is antagonized. This was shown in blood pressure experiments with dogs where amitriptyline antagonized the pressor effect of phenylethylamine (Vernier et al., 1962). In cats the pressor effect as well as the contraction of the nictitating membrane to intravenous injection of tyramine were antagonized by protriptyline (Cairncross et al., 1965).

The enhancing effect of thymoleptics on NA effects may also readily be shown in isolated organ preparations sensitive to this neurotransmitter. In the isolated guinea pig hypogastric nerve–vas deferens preparation, Cairncross (1965) showed that ami-triptyline in a concentration of 1 µg/ml enhanced the contraction evoked by electric stimulation of the nerve; higher concentrations inhibited the contraction.

Table 3. Inhibition of the tyramine-induced chronotropism in guinea pig auricles in vitro

	IC 50 μM
Amitriptyline	6.4
Nortriptyline	11.7
Imipramine	6.3
Desipramine	3.6
Chlorimipramine	> 32
Melitracen	> 31
Litracen	9.6
Iprindol	> 34

The isolated perfused renal artery of the rat is another experimental model suitable to show the influence of thymoleptics on the NA response. BONACCORSI and HRDINA (1967) showed that desipramine in a concentration of $6.6 \times 10^{-8} M$ potentiated the contractile effect of NA. Due to an α-adrenolytic effect, higher doses inhibited NA response.

In the isolated guinea pig auricle, thymoleptics potentiate the positive inotropic effect of NA (STILLE, 1968). Desipramine was very active in this respect, nortriptyline, imipramine, and dibenzepine were also quite active while no effect was seen with amitriptyline. In contrast, the chronotropic effect of the indirectly acting sympathomimetic amine, tyramine, is antagonized by the tricyclic antidepressants. The inhibitory effect of a series of antidepressants against the chronotropic effect of 4 μg tyramine/ml are listed in Table 3. Desipramine was most active while the other secondary amines nortriptyline and litracen were less active; chlorimipramine, melitracen, and iprindol were without activity at reasonable concentrations. In experiments with the guinea pig atria, GREEFF and WAGNER (1969) found that, in contrast to other tricyclic antidepressants which reduced the positive inotropic effect of tyramine, melitracen increased this effect.

The isolated perfused spleen constitutes an excellent model for the study of the influence on noradrenergic function since it allows recording of the contractile response as well as the efflux of catecholamines. THOENEN et al. (1964) have performed some elegant experiments on the effects of imipramine and R 4-6011, a nortriptyline analog, on the perfused cat spleen. Both compounds in suitable concentrations increased and prolonged the contractile response of the spleenic trabecular muscle and at the same time increased the NA output as a result of stimulation of the spleenic nerve. Higher doses reduced spleenic contraction while the output of NA was still enhanced.

E. Amine Uptake Inhibition

The results described so far all indicate that thymoleptics in some way interfere with the disposition of transmitters in NA and 5-HT neurone systems. The first indication that this might be the case was put forward by SIGG (1959) who on the basis of peripheral effects (potentiation of NA pressor effect and nictitating membrane studies) suggested that the antidepressant effect might be caused by a sensitization of central adrenergic synapses. Based on similar experimental evidence, SCHAEPPI (1960) suggested that the potentiating effect of thymoleptics (as that of cocaine) might be caused by an inhibition of the inactivation of the transmitter NA at the level of the synapse, perhaps through inhibition of an inactivating enzyme. Almost simultaneously it was shown that binding of catecholamines was an important mechanism of inactivation of these neurohormones (AXELROD et al., 1959). Removal of the superior cervical ganglion in cats 5 days or more before the experiment prevented the uptake of [³H]-NA in tissues innervated by the sympathetic nerve (HERTTING et al., 1961). Studying the uptake of [³H]-NA in the isolated perfused rat heart, IVERSEN (1963) found that the rate of NA uptake obeyed Michaelis–Menten kinetics. Cocaine reduced the uptake of circulating catecholamines by various tissues (WHITBY et al., 1960; IVERSEN, 1963). Likewise it was shown that imipramine reduces the uptake of [³H]-NA in heart, spleen, and adrenals and increases the level of circulating NA in plasma (AXELROD et al., 1961). In the perfused rat heart, imipramine and desipramine inhibited the uptake of [¹⁴C]-NA in low concentrations, desipramine being seven times more active than imipramine (IVERSEN, 1965). In the brain, imipramine and desipramine were found to have no influence on the level of catecholamines (SULSER et al., 1962). In studies with intraventricular injection of tritiated NA, the uptake of this amine into the brain was reduced by imipramine, desipramine, and amitriptyline (GLOWINSKI and AXELROD, 1964). While the neuroleptic, chlorpromazine, inhibited uptake of NA in peripheral adrenergically innervated tissues (AXELROD et al., 1961) it did not do so in brain tissue where only tricyclic antidepressants were active (GLOWINSKI and AXELROD, 1964).

Since then, numerous studies have been concerned with the effect of tricyclic antidepressants on the uptake in nerve endings in the central nervous system of NA, DA, and 5-HT. The uptake mechanism is a saturable energy requiring process (DENGLER et al., 1961; MAXWELL et al., 1969) designated the amine pump. Tricyclic antidepressants inhibit the uptake of NA in cortical slices from mice in vitro (ROSS and RENYI, 1967, 1975) and in synaptosomal preparations from the hypothalamic region (ROSS and RENYI, 1975). The inhibition was competitive. Desipramine was the most potent inhibitor with a K_i value of 4.7 nM, followed by nortriptyline, imipramine, chlorimipramine, and amitriptyline. When given systemically prior to sacrifice, desipramine and imipramine inhibited the uptake of [³H]-NA into cortical slices of mice (ROSS and RENYI, 1967). Using synaptosomal preparations from different brain areas, HORN et al. (1971) found tricyclic antidepressants competitive inhibitors of NA uptake in cerebral cortex and in hypothalamus while a non-competitive inhibition was seen in striatum. In hypothalamus desipramine was 20 times as potent as imipramine while in striatum imipramine was more potent than desipramine. The reason for this difference may be that hypothalamus is rich in NA neurones which are sensitive to uptake inhibition by desipramine, while the striatal synaptosomal preparation is rich in DA synaptosomes which take up NA by an amine pump not readily blocked by desipramine (SQUIRES, 1974).

Using [³H]-metaraminol as an indicator of the amine pump function CARLSSON and WALDECK (1965) studied a large number of different substances for uptake inhibition in mouse hearts. Tricyclic antidepressants were very active with protriptyline and desipramine as the most potent compounds, but also other substances such as guanethidine, amphetamine, cocaine, and chlorpromazine showed some activity. A series of tricyclic and other antidepressants have been tested for inhibition of [³H]-NA uptake in mouse atria in vitro (HYTTEL, 1977). The results are given in Table 1, column 6 and confirmed the very potent effect of secondary amines as compared to their tertiary analogs. Opipramol, trimeprimine, and iprindol had very low activity. The very weak effect of iprindol was also reported by GLUCKMAN and BAUM (1969). In spite of this lack of uptake inhibition iprindol did potentiate the pressor effect of NA in anesthetized dogs and in contrast to amine pump inhibitors it also potentiated the pressor effect of tyramine. Using the rabbit aortic strip as source of the amine pump the structure activity relationship of tricyclic and related compounds was studied by MAXWELL et al. (1969). It was found that maximal inhibition was obtained with tricyclic compounds in which the two phenyl rings were held at an angle to one another by an ethyl bridge. Furthermore they confirmed that secondary amines were more active than tertiary amines. However, among a series of bicyclic compounds described by PETERSEN et al. (1966) the phthalane Lu 3-010 (talopram) was an even more potent blocker of NA uptake in mouse cerebral cortical slices than desipramine (ROSS and RENYI, 1967). Most of the studies mentioned were based on in vitro measurements. A technique based on the displacement of NA by the amine H 77/77 (4,α-dimethylmeta-tyramine) enabled the assessment of amine pump inhibition by thymoleptics given systemically (CARLSSON et al., 1969b). This effect was effectively prevented by protriptyline and desipramine while imipramine and amitriptyline were less active.

Tricyclic antidepressants also inhibit the uptake of 5-HT. Brain tissue was shown to accumulate 5-HT by a saturable active transport mechanism (ROSS and RENYI, 1969; FUXE and UNGERSTEDT, 1967; CARLSSON et al., 1968; BLACKBURN et al., 1967; AGHAJANIAN and BLOOM, 1967; IVERSEN, 1974). The uptake of [^{3}H]-5-HT by mouse brain slices was inhibited by cocaine, imipramine, and amitriptyline, and to a lesser extent by nortriptyline and desipramine (ROSS and RENYI, 1969). Chlorimipramine was found to be the most potent inhibitor of 5-HT uptake in brain tissue (CARLSSON et al., 1969 a, c; HORN, 1976). It has been shown that thrombocytes accumulate 5-HT by an uptake mechanism very similar to that of nervous tissue and that thymoleptics inhibit this uptake (BORN and GILLSON, 1959; STACEY, 1961). This method is very convenient for the screening of a large number of compounds for 5-HT uptake inhibition (Table 1, column 7). Chlorimipramine is by far the most potent of the known tricyclic antidepressants and it may be seen that in contrast to NA uptake inhibition, tertiary amines are more potent than their secondary analogs. Similar results were reported by TODRICK and TAIT (1969) and HORN and TRACE (1974). Recently some new and more specific 5-HT uptake inhibitors have been reported, femoxetine (BUUS LASSEN et al., 1975), fluoxetine (WONG et al., 1974), and citalopram (HYTTEL, 1977).

The influence of thymoleptics on DA uptake is weak. In rat striatal homogenates incubated with [^{3}H]-DA, amitriptyline was a noncompetitive inhibitor of DA uptake (HORN et al., 1971). Of the tricyclic antidepressants, amitriptyline, nortriptyline, protriptyline, chlorimipramine, and opipramol were among the most active inhibitors of uptake by rat striatal synaptosomes (Table 1, column 8) (HALARIS et al., 1975; HALARIS and FREEDMAN, 1975; HYTTEL, 1978). Nomifensine is among the most potent inhibitors of DA uptake (Table 1, column 8), even more potent than benztropine (HUNT et al., 1974; HYTTEL, 1977; RANDRUP and BRÆSTRUP, 1977).

Being originally derived from antihistaminic drugs it is not surprising that many thymoleptics are quite potent anticholinergic and antihistaminergic compounds. In Table 1 are listed the antagonistic effects of various thymoleptics against the acethylcholine-induced contraction of the guinea pig ileum preparation (column 9) and the muscarinic affinity determined as the ability to displace [^{3}H]-propylbenzilylcholine mustard ([^{3}H]-PrBCM) in whole rat brain synaptosomal suspensions (column 10). There is a good correlation between the affinity of these compounds to central muscarinic receptors and the peripheral anticholinergic effect as measured in the guinea pig ileum model. Amitriptyline and melitracen were the most potent anticholinergic thymoleptics, while nomifensin, viloxazine and iprindol were quite weak. Measured in the guinea pig ileum preparation the antihistaminic effect of amitriptyline was twice as potent as diphenhydramine while imipramine was a third as potent.

F. Cardiovascular Effects

One of the major drawbacks of tricyclic antidepressants is their influence on cardiovascular function which plays a role mainly in the case of acute overdosage (THORSTRAND, 1975), although cardiovascular side effects may also be seen in the therapeutic dose range (review see JEFFERSON, 1975). In normotensive anesthetized dogs, imipramine lowered blood pressure dose dependently and the carotid occlusion reflex was inhibited. Cardiac output was reduced while total peripheral resistance increased (SIGG et al., 1963 a). This effect was confirmed by JANDHYALA et al. (1977) who studied imipramine and its metabolites, desipramine, 2-OH-imipramine, and 2-OH-desipramine. These drugs in lower doses caused increased heart rate and reduced cardiac output at times when index of contractility ($dP/dt/i.p.$) was unaffected. Higher doses caused depressed heart rate, index of contractility and cardiac output. In anesthetized cats, amitriptyline at successive intravenous injections of small to large doses (0.08–5 mg/kg) caused progressive and pronounced reduction of contractility, preload, right ventricular pressure, and carotic blood flow with unchanged afterload. During a 10 min intravenous infusion of amitriptyline corresponding to 1.7 mg/kg, slight tachycardia, increased contractility and decreased carotid flow occurred, probably reflecting slight myocardial stimulation due to increased sympathetic tone possibly combined with an anticholinergic effect. Infusion of higher doses caused changes as described for intravenous injections.

Electrocardiographic changes are induced by tricyclic antidepressants at toxic dose levels. BOISSIER et al. (1965) published a study with imipramine, desipramine, amitriptyline, and nortriptyline on guinea pigs in which they reported ECG changes in the following sequence: right axial rotation, repolarization disturbances, intraventricular conduction disturbances and rhythm disturbances (atrio-ventricular conduction disturbances). ELONEN and co-workers have studied in detail the cardiotoxic effect of amitriptyline, nortriptyline, protriptyline, and doxepin (ELONEN et al., 1974; ELONEN, 1974; ELONEN, 1975; ELONEN and MATTILA, 1975; ELONEN et al., 1975). Doxepin and amitriptyline produced the most marked ECG changes while nortriptyline and protriptyline were less active. Mild changes included flattened or inverted T waves, diminished R wave voltage and slightly deepened S wave. Severe changes were deepened and broadened S wave with ST changes and severely deformed QRS complexes. With an intracardiac electrode, progressive prolongation of the PQ interval was seen until one ventricular beat dropped out. Broadening of the QRS complex was then observed. Thus, atrioventricular block and subsequently intraventricular block occurred. The occurrence of ECG changes does not seem to correlate with the potency of inhibition of the NA uptake mechanism. Thus, NA potentiation does not seem to be the main reason for cardiotoxic effect. Doxepin injected in fractional intravenous doses to mice produced arrhytmia followed by bradycardia which gradually developed into asystole and death. β-blockers decreased the severity of arrhytmia dose dependently but in larger doses they worsened doxepin bradycardia and accelerated death. This latter effect may be due to other effects (membrane effects) rather than to β-blockade. Thus β-blockers may be used in the treatment of thymoleptic-induced arrhytmia but the therapeutic ratio is narrow. During in vitro studies with perfused rabbit hearts, stimulation of the sympathetic nerve caused arrhythmias in hearts exposed to desipramine and doxepin but not to iprindol (BARTH and MUSCHOLL, 1974). Inhibition of NA uptake, however, does not seem to be responsible since cocaine was ineffective. Nerve stimulation per se caused increased heart rate but no arrhythmia. It seemed that the combination of increased ventricular rate by nerve stimulation and decreased atrioventricular conduction induced by the thymoleptic could lead to irregular ventricular contraction.

G. Concluding Remarks

In view of the many pharmacologic actions of tricyclic antidepressants the question arises what might be the mode of action by which these compounds exert their antidepressant effect. The first suggestion to answer this question was put forward by SIGG (1959) who, having shown that imipramine in peripheral noradrenergic systems potentiated the effect of exogenous NA or NA released by nerve stimulation, indicated that imipramine might exert its antidepressant effect by sensitization of central adrenergic synapses. The subsequent finding that tricyclic antidepressants inhibit the uptake of NA into presynaptic nerve endings (GLOWINSKI and AXELROD, 1964; ROSS and RENYI, 1967, 1975; HORN et al., 1971) strengthened this hypothesis. However it was soon discovered that tricyclic antidepressants also inhibited the neuronal uptake of 5-HT (ROSS and RENYI, 1969; TODRICK and TAIT, 1969; HORN and TRACE, 1974). Considering the relative potencies of tricyclic antidepressants with respect to inhibition of NA and 5-HT uptake in relation to their clinical efficacy and profile of action CARLSSON advanced the hypothesis that 5-HT uptake inhibition is related to mood elevation whereas NA uptake inhibition is related to increase in drive (CARLSSON et al., 1969a; CARLSSON, 1976). KIELHOLZ and PÖLDINGER (1968) have pointed out that secondary amines (desipramine, nortriptyline and protriptyline), which are the most potent NA uptake inhibitors, have more pronounced psychomotor-activating effect in relation to their mood elevating effect while the reverse seems to be the case for tertiary amines (imipramine and amitriptyline). The theory that the antidepressant effect is related to 5-HT uptake inhibition is supported by the finding that the mood elevating effect of imipramine is suppressed by PCPA, an inhibitor of 5-HT synthesis, but not by α-MT, an inhibitor of catecholamine synthesis (SHOPSIN et al., 1975). RANDRUP and BRÆSTRUP (1977) have challenged this hypothesis on the grounds that most antidepressants are active clinically in about the same dose range, although uptake inhibition of NA and 5-HT vary up to 1000 times. These authors point out that, although weaker, the inhibition of DA uptake was almost equal for all antidepressants, an observation which is confirmed in our laboratory, and, therefore, facilitation of DA transmission should be considered as a possible mode of action of antidepressants. In this connection it is of interest that MODIGH (1975, 1976) has shown that repeated ECT and prolonged treatment with protriptyline sensitize DA receptors. Treatment with neuroleptics have also been shown to cause supersensitivity of DA receptors (CHRISTENSEN et al., 1976; MØLLER NIELSEN et al., 1978). This again might explain why some neuroleptics seem to have antidepressant effect (YOUNG et al., 1976; SHAW, 1977). CORSINI et al. (1975) have taken advantage of the neuroleptic-induced supersensitivity of the DA receptors in clinical experiments in which they treated depressed patients with a combination of haloperidol and chlorimipramine. After 1 week, haloperidol was discontinued while chlorimipramine therapy continued. Within 2 days a dramatic remission of depressive symptoms was seen.

From the above it follows that all three transmitters have been implicated in explaining the antidepressant effect of tricyclic antidepressants. However, it is entirely possible that depression is not a single entity and that all three transmitters and their interaction may be involved in depressive illness.

References

Aghajanian, G.K., Bloom, F.E.: Localization of tritiated serotonin in rat brain by electron-microscopic autoradiography. J. Pharmacol. Exp. Ther. *156*, 23–30 (1967)

Axelrod, J., Weil-Malherbe, H., Tomchick, R.: The physiological disposition of H^3-epinephrine and its metabolite metanephrine. J. Pharmacol. Exp. Ther. *127*, 251–256 (1959)

Axelrod, J., Whitby, L.G., Hertting, G.: Effect of psychotropic drugs on the uptake of H^3-norepinephrine by tissues. Science *133*, 383–384 (1961)

Barth, N., Muscholl, E.: The effects of the tricyclic antidepressants desipramine, doxepin and iprindole on the isolated perfused rabbit heart. Naunyn-Schmiedeberg's Arch. Pharmacol. *284*, 215–232 (1974)

Blackburn, K.J., French, P.C., Merrils, R.J.: 5-hydroxytryptamine uptake by rat brain in vitro. Life Sci. *6*, 1653–1663 (1967)

Boissier, J.-R., Simon, P., Witchitz, S.: Étude chez le cobaye de la toxicité cardiaque de l'imipramine, de l'amitriptyline et de leurs dérivés monodesméthylés. Thérapie *XX*, 67–75 (1965)

Bonaccorsi, A., Hrdina, P.: Interactions between desipramine and sympathomimetic agents on the cardiovascular system. In: Proceedings of the First International Symposium on Antidepressant Drugs. Garattini, S. (ed), pp. 149–157. Amsterdam: Excerpta Medica Foundation 1967

Born, G.V.R., Gillson, R.E.: Studies on the uptake of 5-hydroxytryptamine by blood platelets. J. Physiol. *146*, 472–491 (1959)

Bræstrup, C., Scheel-Krüger, J.: Methylphenidate-like effects of the new antidepressant drug nomifensine (HOE 984). Eur. J. Pharmacol. *38*, 305–312 (1976)

Buus Lassen, J., Squires, R.F., Christensen, J.A., Molander, L.: Neurochemical and pharmacological studies on a new 5-HT-uptake inhibitor, FG 4963, with potential antidepressant properties. Psychopharmacology *42*, 21–26 (1975)

Cairncross, K.D.: On the peripheral pharmacology of amitriptyline. Arch. Int. Pharmacodyn. Ther. *154*, 438–448 (1965)

Cairncross, K.D., McCulloch, M.W., Mitchelson, F.: The action of protriptyline on peripheral autonomic function. J. Pharmacol. Exp. Ther. *149*, 365–372 (1965)

Carlsson, A.: The contribution of drug research to investigating the nature of endogenous depression. Pharmakopsychiatr. Neuropsychopharmacol. *9*, 2–10 (1976)

Carlsson, A., Waldeck, B.: Inhibition of ^{3}H-metaraminol uptake by antidepressive and related agents. J. Pharm. Pharmacol. *17*, 243–244 (1965)

Carlsson, A., Fuxe, K., Ungerstedt, U.: The effect of imipramine of central 5-hydroxytryptamine neurons. J. Pharm. Pharmacol. *20*, 150–151 (1968)

Carlsson, A., Corrodi, H., Fuxe, K., Hökfelt, T.: Effect of antidepressant drugs on the depletion of intraneuronal brain 5-hydroxytryptamine stores caused by 4-methyl-α-ethyl-meta-tyramine. Eur. J. Pharmacol. *5*, 357–366 (1969a)

Carlsson, A., Corrodi, H., Fuxe, K., Hökfelt, T.: Effects of some antidepressant drugs on the depletion of intraneuronal brain catecholamine stores caused by 4,α-dimethyl-meta-tyramine. Eur. J. Pharmacol. *5*, 367–373 (1969b)

Carlsson, A., Jonason, J., Lindqvist, M.: On the mechanism of 5-hydroxytryptamine release by thymoleptics. J. Pharm. Pharmacol. *21*, 769–773 (1969c)

Carlsson, A., Jonason, J., Lindqvist, M., Fuxe, K.: Demonstration of extraneuronal 5-hydroxytryptamine accumulation in brain following membrane-pump blockade by chlorimipramine. Brain Res. *12*, 456–460 (1969d)

Carlton, P.L.: Potentiation of the behavioral effects of amphetamine by imipramine. Psychopharmacology *2*, 364–376 (1961)

Christensen, A.V., Fjalland, B., Møller Nielsen, I.: On the supersensitivity of dopamine receptors, induced by neuroleptics. Psychopharmacology *48*, 1–6 (1976)

Christensen, A.V., Fjalland, B., Pedersen, V., Danneskiold-Samsøe, P., Svendsen, O.: Pharmacology of a new phthalane (Lu 10-171), with specific 5-HT uptake inhibiting properties. Eur. J. Pharmacol. *41*, 153–162 (1977)

Corsini, G.U., Masala, C., Del Zompo, M., Piccardi, M.P., Mangoni, A.: Potentiation of the antidepressant effect of chlorimipramine following haloperidol withdrawal. 6th Int. Congr. Pharmacol. Abs. *1080*. Helsinki Juli 1975

Costall, B., Kelly, D.M., Naylor, R.J.: Nomifensine: A potent dopaminergic agonist of antiparkinson potential. Psychopharmacology *41*, 153–164 (1975)

Dengler, H.J., Spiegel, H.E., Titus, E.O.: Uptake of tritium-labeled norepinephrine in brain and other tissues of cat in vitro. Science *133*, 1072–1073 (1961)

Dengler, H.J., Titus, E.O.: The effect of drugs on the uptake of isotopic norepinephrine in various tissues. Biochem. Pharmacol. *8*, 64 (1961)

Domenjoz, R., Theobald, W.: Zur Pharmakologie des Tofranil [N-(3-dimethylaminopropyl)-iminodibenzyl-hydrochlorid]. Arch. Int. Pharmacodyn. Ther. *CXX*, 450–489 (1959)

Elonen, E.: Correlation of the cardiotoxicity of tricyclic antidepressants to their membrane effects. Med. Biol. *52*, 415–423 (1974)

Elonen, E., Mattila, M.J., Saarnivaara, L.: Cardiovascular effects of amitriptyline, nortriptyline, protriptyline and doxepin in conscious rabbits. Eur. J. Pharmacol. *28*, 178–188 (1974)

Elonen, E.: Effect of β-adrenoceptor blocking drugs, physostigmine, and atropine on the toxicity of doxepin in mice. Med. Biol. *53*, 231–237 (1975)

Elonen, E., Mattila, M.J.: Cardiovascular effects of amitriptyline, nortriptyline, protriptyline and doxepin in conscious rabbits after subacute pretreatment with protriptyline. Med. Biol. *53*, 238–244 (1975)

Elonen, E., Linnoila, M., Lukkari, I., Mattila, M.J.: Concentration of tricyclic antidepressants in plasma, heart and skeletal muscle after their intravenous infusion to anaesthetized rabbits. Acta Pharmacol. Toxicol. (Kbh.) *37*, 274–281 (1975)

Everett, G.M.: The dopa response potentiation test and its use in screening for antidepressant drugs. In: Proceedings of the First International Symposium on Antidepressant Drugs. Garattini, S. (ed.), pp. 164–167. Amsterdam: Excerpta Medica Foundation 1967

Fuxe, K., Ungerstedt, U.: Localization of 5-hydroxytryptamine uptake in rat brain after intraventricular injection. J. Pharm. Pharmacol. *19*, 335–336 (1967)

Garattini, S., Giachetti, A., Jori, A., Pieri, L., Valzelli, L.: Effect of imipramine, amitriptyline and their monomethyl derivatives on reserpine activity. J. Pharm. Pharmacol. *14*, 509–514 (1962)

Garattini, S., Jori, A.: Interactions between imipramine-like drugs and reserpine on body temperature. In: Proceedings of the First International Symposium on Antidepressant Drugs. Garattini, S. (ed.), pp. 179–193. Amsterdam: Excerpta Medica Foundation 1967

Glowinski, J., Axelrod, J.: Inhibition of uptake of tritiated-noradrenaline in the intact rat brain by imipramine and structurally related compounds. Nature *204*, 1318–1319 (1964)

Gluckman, M.I., Baum, T.: The pharmacology of iprindole, a new antidepressant. Psychopharmacology *15*, 169–185 (1969)

Gong, S.N.C., Rogers, K.J.: Role of brain monoamines in the fatal hyperthermia induced by pethidine or imipramine in rabbits pretreated with pargyline. Br. J. Pharmacol. *42*, 646 P (1971)

Greeff, K., Wagner, J.: Cardiodepressive und lokalanaesthetische Wirkungen der Thymoleptica. Vergleichende Untersuchungen mit Imipramin, Desipramin, Amitriptylin, Nortriptylin und Melitracen. Arzneim. Forsch. *19*, 1662–1664 (1969)

Greenwood, D.T.: Animal pharmacology of viloxazine (vivalan). J. Int. Med. Res. *3*, 18–30 (1975)

Halaris, A.E., Freeman, D.X.: Psychotropic drugs and dopamine uptake inhibition. Res. Publ. Assoc. Res. Nerv. Ment. Dis. *54*, 247–258 (1975)

Halaris, A.E., Belendiuk, K.T., Freedman, D.X.: Antidepressant drugs affect dopamine uptake. Biochem. Pharmacol. *24*, 1896–1898 (1975)

Hanson, H.M.: The effect of amitriptyline, imipramine, chlorpromazine and nialamide on avoidance behavior. Fed. Proc. *20*, 396 (1961)

Hertting, G., Axelrod, J., Kopin, I.J., Whitby, L.G.: Lack of uptake of catecholamines after chronic denervation of sympathetic nerves. Nature *189*, 66 (1961)

Himwich, H.E.: Stimulants. In: The effect of pharmacological agents on the nervous system. Braceland, F.J. (ed.), pp. 356–383. Baltimore: Williams & Wilkins Company 1959

Hoffmann, I.: 8-amino-2-methyl-4-phenyl-1,2,3,4-tetrahydroisoquinoline, a new antidepressant. Arzneim. Forsch. *23*, 45–50 (1973)

Hoffmeister, F.: Zur Frage pharmakologisch-klinischer Wirkungsbeziehungen bei Antidepressiva, dargestellt am Beispiel von Noxiptilin. Arzneim. Forsch. *19*, 458–462 (1969)

Horn, A.S.: The interaction of tricyclic antidepressants with the biogenic amine uptake systems in the central nervous system. Postgrad. Med. J. *52*, 25–30 (1976)

Horn, A.S., Trace, R.C.A.M.: Structure-activity relations for the inhibition of 5-hydroxytryptamine uptake by tricyclic antidepressants into synaptosomes from serotoninergic neurones in rat brain homogenates. Br. J. Pharmacol. *51*, 399–403 (1974)

Horn, A.S., Coyle, J.T., Snyder, S.H.: Catecholamine uptake by synaptosomes from rat brain. Structure-activity relationships of drugs with differential effects on dopamine and norepinephrine neurons. Mol. Pharmacol. *7*, 66–80 (1971)

Horovitz, Z.P., Chow, M.-I.: Effects of centrally acting drugs on the correlation of electrocortical activity and wakefulness of cats. J. Pharmacol. Exp. Ther. *137*, 127–132 (1962)

Horovitz, Z.P., Piala, J.J., High, J.P., Burke, J.C., Leaf, R.C.: Effects of drugs on the mouse-killing (muricide) test and its relationship to amygdaloid function. Int. J. Neuropharmacol. *5*, 405–411 (1966)

Hunt, P., Kannengiesser, M.-H., Raynaud, J.P.: Nomifensine: a new potent inhibitor of dopamine uptake into synaptosomes from rat brain corpus striatum. J. Pharm. Pharmacol. *26*, 370–371 (1974)

Hyttel, J.: Neurochemical characterization of a new potent and selective serotonin uptake inhibitor: Lu 10-171. Psychopharmacology *51*, 225–233 (1977)

Hyttel, J.: Inhibition of [³H]-dopamine accumulation in rat striatal synaptosomes by psychotropic drugs. Biochem. Pharmacol. *27*, 1063–1068 (1978)

Hyttel, J., Fjalland, B.: Central 5-HTP decarboxylase inhibiting properties of RO 4-4602 in relation to 5-HTP potentiation in mice. Eur. J. Pharmacol. *19*, 112–114 (1972)

Iversen, L.L.: The uptake of noradrenaline by the isolated perfused rat heart. Br. J. Pharmacol. *21*, 523–537 (1963)

Iversen, L.L.: Inhibition of noradrenaline uptake by drugs. J. Pharm. Pharmacol. *17*, 62–64 (1965)

Iversen, L.L.: Uptake mechanisms for neurotransmitter amines. Biochem. Pharmacol. *23*, 1927–1935 (1974)

Jandhyala, B.S., Steenberg, M.L., Perel, J.M., Manian, A.A., Buckley, J.P.: Effects of several tricyclic antidepressants on the hemodynamics and myocardial contractility of the anesthetized dogs. Eur. J. Pharmacol. *42*, 403–410 (1977)

Jefferson, J.W.: A review of the cardiovascular effects and toxicity of tricyclic antidepressants. Psychosom. Med. *37*, 160–179 (1975)

Jori, A., Garattini, S.: Interaction between imipramine-like agents and catecholamine-induced hyperthermia. J. Pharm. Pharmacol. *17*, 480–488 (1965)

Kielholz, P., Pöldinger, W.: Die Behandlung endogener Depressionen mit Psychopharmaka. Dtsch. Med. Wochenschr. *93*, 701–704 (1968)

Kinnard, W.J., Barry, H., III, Watzman, N., Buckley, J.P.: Methods of evaluation of antidepressant activity. In: Proceedings of the First International Symposium on Antidepressant Drugs. Garattini, S. (ed.), pp. 89–98. Amsterdam: Excerpta Medica Foundation 1967

Kuhn, R.: Über die Behandlung depressiver Zustände mit einem Iminodibenzylderivat (G 22355). Schweiz. Med. Wochenschr. *35/36*, 1135–1140 (1957)

Loveless, A.H., Maxwell, D.R.: A comparison of the effects of imipramine, trimipramine, and some other drugs in rabbits treated with a monoamine oxidase inhibitor. Br. J. Pharmacol. *25*, 158–170 (1965)

Maxwell, D.R., Palmer, H.T.: Demonstration of anti-depressant or stimulant properties of imipramine in experimental animals. Nature *191*, 84–85 (1961)

Maxwell, R.A., Keenan, P.D., Chaplin, E., Roth, B., Eckhardt, S.B.: Molecular features affecting the potency of tricyclic antidepressants and structurally related compounds as inhibitors of the uptake of tritiated norepinephrine by rabbit aortic strips. J. Pharmacol. Exp. Ther. *166*, 320–329 (1969)

Modigh, K.: Electroconvulsive shock and postsynaptic catecholamine effects: Increased psychomotor stimulant action of apomorphine and clonidine in reserpine pretreated mice by repeated ECS. J. Neural Transm. *36*, 19–32 (1975)

Modigh, K.: Correlation between clinical effects of various antidepressive treatments and their effects on monoaminergic receptors in the brain. XV Scandinavian Congress of Physiology and Pharmacology, Århus 1976. Acta Physiol. Scand., Suppl. *440*, 37 (1976)

Molander, L., Randrup, A.: Effects of thymoleptics on behaviour associated with changes in brain dopamine. I. Potentiation of dopa-induced gnawing of mice. Psychopharmacology *45*, 261–265 (1976)

Morpurgo, C.: Drug-induced modifications of discriminated avoidance behavior in rats. Psychopharmacology *8*, 91–99 (1965)

Morpurgo, C., Theobald, W.: Influence of imipramine-like compounds and chlorpromazine on the reserpine-hypothermia in mice and the amphetamine-hyperthermia in rats. Med. Pharmacol. Exp. *12*, 226–232 (1965)

Møller Nielsen, I., Nymark, M., Hougs, W., Pedersen, V.: The pharmacological properties of melitracen (N 7001) and litracen (N 7049). Arzneim. Forsch. *16*, 135–140 (1966)

Møller Nielsen, I., Christensen, A.V., Hyttel, J.: Adaptational phenomena in neuroleptic treatment. In: Advances in Biochemical Psychopharmacology, Vol. 19. Dopamine. Roberts, P.J., Woodruff, G.N.M., Iversen, L.L. (eds.), pp. 267–274. New York: Raven Press 1978

Nymark, M., Møller Nielsen, I.: Reactions due to the combination of monoamineoxidase inhibitors with thymoleptics, pethidine, or methylamphetamine. Lancet Sept. *7*, 524–525 (1963)

Pedersen, V.: Potentiation of apomorphine effect (compulsive gnawing behaviour) in mice. Acta Pharmacol. Toxicol. (Kbh.) *25*, 63 (1967)

Pedersen, V.: Role of catecholamines in compulsive gnawing in mice. Br. J. Pharmacol. *34*, 219P (1968)

Petersen, P.V., Lassen, N., Hansen, V., Huld, T., Hjortkjær, J., Holmblad, J., Møller Nielsen, I., Nymark, M., Pedersen, V., Jørgensen, A., Hougs, W.: Pharmacological studies of a new series of bicyclic thymoleptics. Acta Pharmacol. Toxicol. (Kbh.) *24*, 121–133 (1966)

Randrup, A., Bræstrup, C.: Uptake inhibition of biogenic amines by newer antidepressant drugs: Relevance to the dopamine hypothesis of depression. Psychopharmacology *53*, 309–314 (1977)

Ross, S.B., Renyi, A.L.: Inhibition of the uptake of tritiated catecholamines by antidepressant and related agents. Eur. J. Pharmacol. *2*, 181–186 (1967)

Ross, S.B., Renyi, A.L.: Inhibition of the uptake of tritiated 5-hydroxytryptamine in brain tissue. Eur. J. Pharmacol. *7*, 270–277 (1969)

Ross, S.B., Renyi, A.L.: Tricyclic antidepressant agents. I. Comparison of the inhibition of the uptake of ^{3}H-noradrenaline and ^{14}C-5-hydroxytryptamine in slices and crude synaptosome preparations of the midbrain-hypothalamus region of the rat brain. Acta Pharmacol. Toxicol. (Kbh.) *36*, 382–394 (1975)

Ryall, R.W.: Effects of cocaine and antidepressant drugs on the nictitating membrane of the cat. Br. J. Pharmacol. *17*, 339–357 (1961)

Schaeppi, U.: Die Beeinflussung der Reizübertragung im peripheren Sympathicus durch Tofranil. Helv. Physiol. Acta *18*, 545–562 (1960)

Scheckel, C.L., Boff, E.: Behavioral effects of interacting imipramine and other drugs with d-amphetamine, cocaine and tetrabenazine. Psychopharmacology *5*, 198–208 (1964)

Shaw, D.M.: The practical management of affective disorders. Br. J. Psychiatr. *130*, 432–451 (1977)

Shopsin, B., Gershon, S., Goldstein, M., Friedman, E., Wilk, S.: Use of synthesis inhibitors in defining a role for biogenic amines during imipramine treatment in depressed patients. Psychopharmacol. Commun. *1*, 239–249 (1975)

Sigg, E.B.: Pharmacological studies with Tofranil. Can. Psychiatr. Assoc. J. *4*, S75–S85 (1959)

Sigg, E.B., Osborne, M., Korol, B.: Cardiovascular effects of imipramine. J. Pharmacol. Exp. Ther. *141*, 237–243 (1963a)

Sigg, E.B., Soffer, L., Gyermek, L.: Influence of imipramine and related psychoactive agents on the effect of 5-hydroxytryptamine and catecholamines on the cat nictitating membrane. J. Pharmacol. Exp. Ther. *142*, 13–20 (1963b)

Squires, R.F.: Effects of noradrenaline pump blockers on its uptake by synaptosomes from several brain regions; additional evidence for dopamine terminals in the frontal cortex. J. Pharm. Pharmacol. *26*, 364–367 (1974)

Stacey, R.S.: Uptake of 5-hydroxytryptamine by platelets. Br. J. Pharmacol. *16*, 284–295 (1961)

Stein, L.: Psychopharmacological substrates of mental depression. In: Proceedings of the First International Symposium on Antidepressant Drugs. Garattini, S. (ed.), pp. 130–140. Amsterdam: Excerpta Medica Foundation 1967

Stein, L., Seifter, J.: Possible mode of antidepressive action of imipramine. Science *134*, 286–287 (1961)

Stille, G.: Zur pharmakologischen Prüfung von Antidepressiva am Beispiel eines Dibenzodiazepins. Arzneim. Forsch. *14*, 534–537 (1964)

Stille, G.: Pharmacological investigation of antidepressant compounds. Pharmakospychiatr. Neuropsychopharmakol. *1*, 92–106 (1968)

Sulser, F., Watts, J., Brodie, B.B.: On the mechanism of antidepressant action of imipramine-like drugs. Ann. N. Y. Acad. Sci. *96*, 279–288 (1962)

Ther, L., Schramm, H.: Apomorphin-Synergismus (Zwangsnagen bei Mäusen) als Test zur Differenzierung psychotroper Substanzen. Arch. Int. Pharmacodyn. Ther. *138*, 302–310 (1962)

Thoenen, H., Huerlimann, A., Haefely, W.: Mode of action of imipramine and 5-(3'-methylaminopropyliden)-dibenzo[a,e]cyclohepta[1,3,5]trien hydrochloride (Ro 4-6011) a new antidepressant drug, on peripheral adrenergic mechanisms. J. Pharmacol. Exp. Ther. *144*, 405–414 (1964)

Thorstrand, C.: Cardiovascular effects of poisoning by hypnotic and tricyclic antidepressant drugs. Acta Med. Scand., Suppl. *583*, 1–34 (1975)

Todrick, A., Tait, A.C.: The inhibition of human platelet 5-hydroxytryptamine uptake by tricyclic antidepressive drugs. The relation between structure and potency. J. Pharm. Pharmacol. *21*, 751–762 (1969)

Valzelli, L., Consolo, S., Morpurgo, C.: Influence of imipramine-like drugs on the metabolism of amphetamine. In: Proceedings of the First International Symposium on Antidepressant Drugs. Garattini, S. (ed.), pp. 61–69. Amsterdam: Excerpta Medica Foundation 1967

Vernier, V.G., Hanson, H.M., Stone, C.A.: The pharmacodynamics of amitriptyline. In: Psychosomatic medicine. The first Hahnemann symposium. Nodine, J.H., Moyer, J.H. (eds.), pp. 683–690. Philadelphia: Lea & Febiger 1962

Votava, Z., Metysová, J., Metys, J., Benesová, O., Bohdanecký, Z.: Comparison of pharmacological effects of some antidepressants of imipramine type and their desmethyl derivatives. In: Neuro-psychopharmacology, Vol. 4. Bente, D., Bradley, P.B. (eds.), pp. 395–401. Amsterdam: Elsevier Publishing Company 1965

Whitby, L.G., Hertting, G., Axelrod, J.: Effect of cocaine on the disposition of noradrenaline labelled with tritium. Nature *187*, 604–605 (1960)

Wong, D.T., Horng, J.S., Bymaster, F.P., Hauser, K.L., Molloy, B.B.: A selective inhibitor of serotonin uptake: Lilly 110140, 3-(p-trifluoromethylphenoxy)-N-methyl-3-phenylpropylamine. Life Sci. *15*, 471–479 (1974)

Young, J.P.R., Hughes, W.C., Lader, M.H.: A controlled comparison of flupenthixol and amitriptyline in depressed patients. Br. Med. J. *1*, 1116–1118 (1976)

CHAPTER 19

Neurophysiological Properties (in Animals)

G. Gogolák

Many results on the pharmacological effects of antidepressant agents have been obtained by means of neurophysiological, especially electroencephalographic (EEG) methods. In establishing the effects of various psychotherapeutic drugs on the central nervous system (CNS), neurophysiological techniques alone, however, are of limited value. In fact, no appropriate experimental (animal) models are as yet available for psychiatric disorders, and according to Hoffmeister, (1969 b); Hoffmeister et al. (1969) a possible antidepressant potency of a given agent can only be based on its entire pharmacological profile rather than on results obtained by either neurophysiological, biochemical or behavioral techniques alone. On the other hand, a recent review on the EEG effects of antidepressant agents (Florio et al., 1977) points out that so far no correlation has been found between the data of neurophysiological and those of biochemical experiments. Although the pharmacological studies on these drugs have increasingly centered on biochemical investigations, their results have also remained inconclusive as far as the explanation of the antidepressants' action in mental depression is concerned (cf. Luchins, 1976; Shopsin et al., 1974).

A. Tricyclic Antidepressants (ADs)

I. Effects of ADs on the Electrical Activity of the Brain

Similarities between classic ADs (imipramine for example) and classical neuroleptics (chlorpromazine for example) are reflected by their chemical structures as well as by many common pharmacological effects. Similar to chlorpromazine (CPZ), imipramine (IMI) and its related compounds have also been reported to induce high-voltage slow wave activity and spindling in the neocortical tracings, and a disintegration of the hippocampus (HC) theta activity. These changes of the bioelectrical activities have repeatedly been found in various species, following the administration of ADs with doses ranging from 0.5 to 10.0 mg/kg. A synopsis of these results is presented in Table 1[1].

Reports on the "spontaneous" EEG activity under the influence of ADs are, however, not concordant: DIMI (see Table 1 for a list of abbreviations) unlike IMI failed to induce any EEG synchronization up to 10 mg/kg (Jaramillo and Greenberg, 1975); Hishikawa et al. (1965) found no changes of the HC activity after IMI or AMI

---

1 Data on some investigational ADs (Plotnikoff et al., 1972; Shimizu et al., 1974 a, b; Stille et al., 1968 b) are not listed in this table. Because of the previous completion of this paper, the recent EEG study on the effects of viloxazine, IMI, AMI, and DIMI (Neal and Bradley, 1978) could not referred to.

Table 1. Reports on resting EEG patterns induced by various ADs

Species	Method	Agent	Dose (mg/kg)	References
Rabbit	Non--immobilized	DIB	20.0–40.0	Stille et al. (1965, 1968a)
		CLOD	> 10.0	
		DOX	1.0– 5.0	Moore and White (1975)
		IMI	3.0–10.0	Gianelli and Marinato (1960)
		IMI	9.0	Monnier and Krupp (1959)
		IMI	5.0–10.0	White et al. (1969)
		IMI	2.5– 5.0	Benešová et al. (1962, 1964b)
		AMI	1.25– 2.50	
		PRT	1.25– 5.00	
		PRP	5.0	
		IMI, AMI, DIB, NOX	2.5–10.0	Hoffmeister et al. (1969)
		IMI, AMI, DOX, BUT	1.0– 5.0	Jaramillo and Greenberg (1975)
		IMI, AMI DAMI, CIMI DIMI	2.0– 5.0 20.0	Schmitt and Schmitt (1966a)
		IMI, AMI, LOP	1.0– 5.0 10.0–20.0	Watanabe et al. (1976)
	Immobilized	AMI	2.0– 8.0	Mercier et al. (1963)
		IMI	2.5–10.0	van Meter et al. (1959)
		IMI, AMI, DIMI	1.0– 3.0	Steiner and Himwich (1963a)
Cat	Non--immobilized	AMI, DIB, NOX	5.0	Hoffmeister et al. (1969)
		IMI	2.5–10.0	Horowitz and Chow (1962)
		IMI, AMI, DIMI	5.0–15.0	Wallach et al. (1969a)
	Immobilized	AMI	1.0– 9.0	Mercier et al. (1963)
		AMI	0.2–10.0	Vernier (1961)
		IMI	0.5– 4.0	Dasberg and Feldman (1968)
		IMI	1.0–10.0	Plas and Naquet (1961)
		IMI	1.0–10.0	Sigg (1959a, b)
	Encéphale isolé,	IMI	2.0–20.0	Bradley and Key (1959)
	Cerveaux isolé, Immobilized	IMI	0.3– 5.0	Crepax et al. (1961a, b, d)
Dog	Immobilized	IMI	10.0	Himwich (1962)
Monkey	Non--immobilized	AMI	0.1– 3.0	Vernier (1961)
		IMI	0.1– 7.0	
	Immobilized	AMI	2.0	Mercier et al. (1963)

AMI	= Amitriptyline	DIB	= Dibenzepine	NT	= Northiadene
BUT	= Butriptyline	DIMI	= Desipramine	PRH	= Proheptatriene
CDIMI	= Chlordesipramine	DOX	= Doxepin	PRO	= Protriptyline
CIMI	= Chlorimipramine	IMI	= Imipramine	PRP	= Propazepine
CLOD	= Clodazone	LOP	= Lopramine	PRT	= Prothiadene
DAMI	= Nortriptyline	NOX	= Noxiptiline	TRI	= Trimepramine

at doses of 2 and 4 mg/kg; with chronic administration, IMI was reported either to produce in the neocortical EEG a slight decrease of the amplitude with a frequency displacement to the higher range (FERLINI and PERBELLINI, 1963), or to change the spontaneous resting EEG activity to an arousal pattern (HIMWICH, 1965). Apparently, ADs have both central depressant and some central stimulant properties (HOFFMEISTER, 1969b; MAXWELL and PALMER, 1961; STILLE, 1965; STILLE et al., 1965); the latter effects, however, are rather difficult to prove by EEG methods only.

ADs given to experimental animals in high doses induced hypersynchronization (GIANELLI and MARINATO, 1960), single spikes and generalized spiking (DASBERG and FELDMANN, 1968; HIMWICH, 1965; LANGE et al., 1976; STEINER and HIMWICH, 1963a; STILLE and SAYERS, 1964; TRIMBLE et al., 1977; VAN METER et al., 1959; WALLACH et al., 1969a, among others). These "seizure-like" EEG activities were reported to have their origin in limbic structures (HIMWICH et al., 1962; STEINER and HIMWICH, 1963a; VAN METER et al., 1959) and to be accompanied by peripheral epileptogenic manifestations in experiments on non-immobilized animals (TRIMBLE et al., 1977; WALLACH et al., 1969a). STEINER and HIMWICH (1963a), investigating the effect of several compounds such as phenothiazines, antihistaminic agents, and ADs on the rabbit, found that ADS especially were able to elicit spiking in the HC, amygdala, and olfactory bulb. Such an action has been proved for IMI, AMI, DAMI, and opipramol, but not for DIMI. Depending on the individual agent and, of course, on the experimental conditions, the doses of ADs which induce EEG spiking range from 10 to 30 mg (LANGE et al., 1976; STEINER and HIMWICH, 1963a; STILLE and SAYERS, 1964).

The effects of ADs on the "spontaneous" EEG in animal experiments may be summarized as follows: In general, depending on the dose applied, these drugs can either induce an enhancement of the resting EEG patterns or seizure-like activity in rhinencephalic structures. It should, however, be mentioned that a synchronization of neocortical activity can be induced not only by tricyclic psychopharmacological agents but also by centrally acting cholinolytic drugs and by appropriate doses of several central depressants (e.g., general anaesthetics, hypnotics, or minor tranquilizers). Consequently, these EEG changes observed under the influence of many ADs are largely unspecific. Moreover, spiking in the limbic structures could also be observed in the cat after high CPZ doses (20–40 mg/kg) (PRESTON, 1956); in the rabbit the effective convulsant doses were found to be around 50 mg/kg (STEINER and HIMWICH, 1963a).

Although no investigations were aimed at revealing the relative potency of ADs for the induction of both the EEG synchronization and rhinencephalic spiking, there might be some correlation between these properties. AMI, for example, having a high EEG-synchronizing potency, was found also to be very effective in inducing limbic spiking. DIMI, on the other hand, proved to be fairly inactive in eliciting either of these effects. Although the effects of ADs on the "spontaneous" EEG reported so far have failed to offer any evidence for their action in mental depressions, these findings may indicate central depressant, anticholinergic and convulsive properties. Studies dealing with these actions of ADs will be discussed in the following sections.

II. Actions of ADs on the Excitability of the CNS

ADs have been reported to influence the brain excitability by a biphasic action. These drugs have both anticonvulsant properties with low doses and, as mentioned in the preceding chapter, significant convulsant properties with high dose levels (cf., LANGE et al., 1976). Different chemically or electrically induced epileptiform discharges have served as experimental models for the evaluation of the effects of ADs on the excitability of various brain areas. A great deal of these investigations was carried out on rhinencephalic structures by means of electrically induced afterdischarges. Reviews dealing with the neurophysiological effects of ADs (FLORIO et al., 1977; RINALDI, 1967; SCHMITT, 1967; SIGG, 1968), however, stress that the action of these agents on the limbic structures are rather controversial.

Amygdaloid afterdischarges, induced by electrical stimulation of this same structure in the rabbit, were found to be enhanced following the i. v. administration of IMI or DIMI (2 mg/kg) as well as AMI or DAMI (1 mg/kg); under the influence of these drugs, the duration and the amplitude of the afterdischarges were increased and the threshold for eliciting these discharges was decreased. On the other hand, AMI or DAMI at 2–5 mg/kg, IMI at 10 mg/kg and, to a lesser extent, DIMI at 10 mg/kg affected the duration, amplitude and threshold of these afterdischarges contrary to those caused by the lower doses (SCHMITT, 1967; SCHMITT and SCHMITT, 1966b).

An initial depression, followed by a sustained enhancement of limbic afterdischarges induced by electrical stimulation of amygdaloid and hippocampal structures, was observed in the rabbit under the influence of IMI (1–5 mg/kg) and AMI (2–5 mg/kg); in the same experiments LOP (10–20 mg/kg) caused only little enhancing effect (WATANABE et al., 1976). An increase in the amplitude and duration of amygdaloid afterdischarges was also found in the cat after administration of IMI (10 mg/kg) (SCHALLEK et al., 1962).

However, other studies report only depressant effects of ADs on the amygdaloid afterdischarges: AMI with doses ranging from 2 to 10 mg/kg shortened the afterdischarge duration in the cat (MERCIER et al., 1963). The threshold necessary for the elicitation of these discharges (BARRAT and PRAY, 1965; HOROVITZ, 1967; HOROVITZ et al., 1963) or of temporal seizures (PEÑALOZA-ROJAS et al.,1961), brought about by amygdaloid stimuli in the cat, was shown to be raised by thiazesim and IMI, respectively. In rats with chronically implanted electrodes, the amygdaloid afterdischarges were shortened, following the i. p. administration of IMI or AMI (50 mg/kg) (SHIMIZU et al., 1974a). By means of similar experimental procedures, KAMEI et al. (1975) listed AMI, IMI, and DAMI in decreasing order of their potency to shorten the duration of these discharges.

Afterdischarges elicited by *septal* stimulation could neither be influenced by IMI, AMI, DIMI, DAMI (SCHMITT, 1967; SCHMITT and SCHMITT, 1966b), nor by thiazesim (HOROVITZ et al., 1963) in non-immobilized rabbits and cats; the duration of these discharges, however, was shortened by the application of IMI in the immobilized cat (SCHALLEK and KUEHN, 1960; SCHALLEK et al., 1962).

Afterdischarges induced by stimulation of the *HC* were not significantly influenced by thiazesim (HOROVITZ et al., 1963), AMI, IMI, DIMI, or DAMI (MONNIER and KRUPP, 1959; SCHMITT, 1967; SCHMITT and SCHMITT, 1966b; STILLE and SAYERS, 1964). DIB had a slight depressant effect (STILLE et al., 1965) and LOP produced a slight enhancement (WATANABE et al., 1976) of these afterdischarges. IMI and AMI were found to cause an initial depression, followed by sustained enhancement of hippocampal afterdischarges (WATANABE et al., 1976).

BAKER and KRATKY (1967) investigated the effects of IMI and CPZ on hippocampal foci which were established by topical application of strychnine or picrotoxin; IMI and CPZ were given intravenously as well as topically. The authors assume that these tricyclic agents have both a weak excitatory action on the HC itself and an inhibitory action on extra-hippocampal structures, whereby the latter effect could be more dominant with parenteral applications of these drugs.

An elevation of the threshold necessary for the induction of *neocortical afterdischarges* was found after administrations of IMI, AMI, DAMI, and DIB; DIMI in doses up to 20 mg/kg failed to cause such an effect (MONNIER and KRUPP, 1959; STILLE et al., 1965; STILLE and SAYERS, 1964). MERCIER et al. (1963) reported on some enhancement of the neocortical epileptogenic reactivity after application of AMI (1–2 mg/kg).

IMI was found to cause a triphasic alteration of the EEG spike-wave discharges induced by estrogen (JULIEN et al., 1975). This agent produced an increase of the discharge amplitudes (5 mg/kg), a slight or no reduction of the discharges (10–15 mg/kg), and a significant enhancement of the epileptogenic activity (20 mg/kg). To find a relationship between the anticonvulsant doses and convulsant doses of IMI, the effect of this drug was studied on various models of experimental epilepsy (LANGE et al., 1976). The neurophysiological experiments dealt with neocortical discharges which were elicited either by topical application of benzylpenicillin, conjugated estrogen, or by electrical stimulation. Doses of IMI ranging from 2.5 to 15.0 mg/kg, produced a reduction of the chemically induced spiking as well as a shortening of the duration and an elevation of the threshold of the electrically induced afterdischarges. IMI, with doses higher than 20 mg/kg, however, elicited spontaneous cortical discharge patterns and intensified both the chemically and electrically induced discharging. These findings once again demonstrate a bisphasic effect of IMI on the neocortical excitability, and suggest similarities between ADs and local anaesthetics with regard to both anticonvulsant and convulsant properties. Moreover, on the basis of both their own findings and the collected data (cf., Table 1 in LANGE et al., 1976), the authors point out that the antiepileptic potency of IMI was to be observed particularly in those experiments that serve as models for major motor seizures in human beings.

III. Action of ADs on the EEG Arousal Response

The influence of ADs on the EEG arousal response (AR) has been repeatedly studied in the cat and the rabbit by using different experimental procedures (immobilized, nonimmobilized, encéphale isolé preparations); this response was induced by various electrical and/or sensory stimuli. In general, ADs were found to have an inhibitory effect on the EEG-AR with doses in the range 2–10 mg/kg. A great deal of these investigations was carried out with IMI and AMI (BRADLEY and KEY, 1959; CREPAX et al., 1961 a, b; DASBERG and FELDMAN, 1968; HIMWICH, 1959; HIMWICH et al., 1962; ITO and SHIMIZU, 1976; MERCIER et al., 1963; MONNIER and KRUPP, 1959; SIGG, 1959 a, b; STEINER and HIMWICH, 1963 a, b; VAN METER et al., 1959; VERNIER, 1961; WHITE et al., 1969; cf. CRISMON, 1967). These tertiary amines were considered to be more potent in blocking the EEG-AR than their corresponding desmethyl-derivatives (SIGG, 1968). Moreover, the effectiveness of ADs seems to depend also on the stimulus applied. According to HIMWICH (1959), for example, the AR elicited by "sound" was inhibited by IMI (2.5 mg/kg), but higher doses had to be given to achieve an inhibition of the response induced by pain. In experiments carried out on the immobilized rabbit,

Table 2. Effects of ADs on the EEG arousal reaction induced by electrical stimulation of the mesencephalic reticular formation in the rabbit

Drug	Dose (mg/kg) causing an elevation of the threshold			
	by 50%[a]	by 100%[a]	by 50%[b]	by 100%[c]
AMI	0.8	2.7	4.8	2.0
IMI	4.5	8.0	5.1	>5.0
DIMI	>8.0		>20.0	
DAMI	>8.0		7.7	
PRO	>8.0			
DIB	>8.0		15.8	>5.0
TRI			5.1	
NOX				2.0
CLOD			>20.0	

Data were compiled from the following publications:
[a]   Herz (1965) (immobilized)
[b]   Stille et al. (1968a) (non-immobilized)
[c]   Hoffmeister et al. (1969) (non-immobilized)

DIMI and DAMI were shown to be more active than IMI and AMI in depressing the EEG-AR elicited by "hand clap." These tertiary derivatives, on the other hand, affected the pain-induced response more than their corresponding secondary derivatives (Steiner and Himwich, 1963 b). In both tests, AMI proved to be more potent than IMI.

The relative potency of various ADs in inhibiting the EEG-AR may be estimated by means of the data compiled for Table 2. In immobilized as well as in non-immobilized rabbits, AMI was shown to have the highest inhibitory effect on the EEG-AR. Comparable data on this effect of several other ADs were also found in the three different laboratories.

However, it should be noted that in some cases IMI was also reported to have only a weak or no inhibitory effect at all on the EEG-AR (Ferlini and Perbellini, 1963; Gianelli and Marinato, 1960; Horovitz and Chow, 1962; Plas and Naquet, 1961) LOP, at least with doses up to 20 mg/kg, failed to inhibit the AR elicited by electrical or sensory stimuli, while in the same experiments IMI or AMI (1–5 mg/kg) were found to be effective (Watanabe et al., 1976). Arousal discharges in the olfactory bulb, elicited by electrical stimulation of the mesencephalic reticular formation or by sensory stimuli, were also enhanced following the administration of low IMI doses (Rubio-Chevannier et al., 1961). These results may be indicative of some stimulating properties of ADs (Himwich, 1965; Peñalozas-Rojas et al., 1961; Stille, 1965, 1968) which often seem to be covered by actions producing EEG synchronization and inhibition of the EEG-AR.

IV. Drug-Interaction Studies on ADs

ADs having a wide spectrum of pharmacological activities also interfere with cholinergic, adrenergic and serotoninergic mechanisms. Especially the central anti-cholinergic actions of these agents are well documented in a variety of experiments.

By means of EEG studies the effect of ADs on both the "spontaneous" bioelectrical activity and the EEG-AR has been attributed – at least partly – to a central *cholinolytic action* of these drugs (cf., FLORIO et al., 1977; RINALDI, 1967). Under the influence of cholinergic drugs – eserine or arecoline – an arousal pattern that can be antagonized by ADs appears in the EEG. Of the many publications those papers will primarily be discussed which also consider the relative anticholinergic potency of ADs.

In the rabbit, HERZ (1965) evaluated the arecoline doses which were able to change the resting EEG induced by a standard dose of various ADs into an arousal pattern. AMI, and to a lesser extent IMI, showed high anti-arecoline activity. Rather insignificant effects were found for PRO, DIMI, DAMI, and DIB. In cats with lesion of the pontomesencaphalic junction, AMI was similarly found to be more effective than DAMI in inhibiting the eserine- or arecoline-induced neocortical desynchronization; the authors (RATHBURN and SLATER, 1963) suggest a close relation of this activity to an inhibition of muscarinic phenomena.

The antagonistic action of four ADs upon the EEG-AR – produced in the rabbit by arecoline or nicotine – was reported by STILLE (1968): AMI was found to be the most potent agent; DIMI up to 10 mg/kg did not exert any anticholinergic activity; IMI and DIB showed less activity than AMI. Similar to DIMI, two investigational ADs also failed to have any anticholinergic properties (SCHMITT and STILLE, 1968). By means of different experimental procedures, BENEŠOVÁ and co-workers (BENEŠOVÁ, 1967; BENEŠOVÁ et al., 1962, 1963, 1964 a, b) also proved anticholinergic effects of ADs. These agents were listed in decreasing order of their potency in antagonizing the effects of eserine, tremorine and nicotine: AMI, PRH, PRT, DIB, IMI, DAMI, NT, DIMI (BENEŠOVÁ and NAHUNEK, 1971). In preventing the cortical desynchronization caused by eserine, ADs were graded according to their potency in the following order: AMI, BUT, DOX, IMI, and DIMI (JARAMILLO and GREENBERG, 1975).

While the AR induced by eserine could be antagonized by IMI (2–5 mg/kg) or AMI (1–2 mg/kg), LOP in doses up to 20 mg/kg remained ineffective (WATANABE et al., 1976). Discussing the characteristic atropine-like effect of several ADs, MOORE and WHITE (1975) have also shown a dose-dependent antagonistic effect of DOX and IMI against eserine. In studies on the interaction of eserine and IMI, DASBERG, and FELDMAN (1968) suggested different effects of IMI on reticular and cortical structures.

In connection with the cholinolytic property of ADs, we should refer to investigations on the antimuscarinic actions of these drugs, which have been proved by different experimental methods (REHAVI et al., 1977; SIGG et al., 1965; WEINSTOCK and COHEN, 1976). Whether the anti-cholinergic effects of ADs do contribute to their clinical actions in mental depressions is still open to discussion (HERZ, 1963, 1965; HOFFMEISTER, 1969 a, b; HOFFMEISTER et al., 1969; SIGG, 1968).

The interactions of ADs and *adrenergic mechanisms* were studied mainly by biochemical methods. Some EEG data were obtained on the interaction of ADs and amphetamine-like agents. STEINER et al. (1963 a) proved AMI's and IMI's ability to antagonize EEG-AR by d-amphetamine in the rabbit, whereas less activity was shown for DIMI and DAMI. Similar results were reported for IMI in the cat (BRADLEY and KEY, 1959). DOX was also found to antagonize the methamphetamine-induced EEG-AR in rabbits (MOORE and WHITE, 1975); this AD, however, failed to effect the behavioral arousal induced by amphetamine.

ADs were reported to enhance amphetamine effects in various experimental models (cf., Sigg, 1968). The methamphetamine effect on the evoked potential was promoted by AD agents (Plotnikoff and Everett, 1965). Dasberg and Feldman's (1968) experiments, for example, show that the amphetamine-induced cortical desynchronization was enhanced by IMI, and the effect of IMI in inducing limbic discharges could also be enhanced by amphetamine.

The influence of ADs on *monoaminergic neurons* has been investigated also by means of single unit recordings. In studies on transmitter dynamics (Nybäck et al., 1975; Sheard et al., 1972) both 5-HT-containing neurons in the midbrain raphe nucleus and NE-containing neurons in the locus coeruleus were shown to be inhibited in their firing rate under the influence of ADs. In agreement with biochemical studies, secondary amines were found to be more potent than their tertiary amine derivatives in inhibiting the firing rate of noradrenergic neurons. The order of potency was: DIMI, CDIMI, IMI, DAMI, AMI, and CIMI. Iprindol had only insignificant effects. On the other hand, the firing of the cells containing 5-HT was depressed especially by tertiary amines; the secondary amines were much less effective. Due to their potency in inhibiting serotoninergic neurons, ADs were graded as follows: CIMI, IMI, DIMI; AMI = IMI; AMI > PRO. The firing rate of dopaminergic neurons in the substantia nigra was not influenced by either IMI or DIMI (Bunney et al., 1973).

Bramwell (1972, 1974) also found raphe units to respond to IMI with slackening or cessation of their firing; the effect of DIMI, however, was reported to result either in excitation or inhibition of the raphe unit activity. A number of publications (Bradshaw et al., 1971, 1973, 1974; Bevan et al., 1973) deals with the iontophoretic application of IMI and DIMI on cortical neurons: When applied for short periods, these ADs did not influence the firing rate of the majority of cortical units. In addition, the interaction studies showed that both IMI and DIMI, depending on the doses applied, were able either to antagonize or to potentiate the effects of NE, 5-HT, and acetylcholine. The authors suggest that "a given concentration of the antidepressant has a differential effect on different systems: while the effects of one potential neurotransmitter are potentiated, the effects of another transmitter may be antagonized."

Avanzino et al. (1971) found that both IMI and NE applied microiontophoretically to single neurons of the brain stem have similar – mostly inhibitory – effects on the neuronal firing. With simultaneous application, these agents acted synergistically; IMI, applied before NE, however, caused a slight reduction of the NE effect. A synergistic effect of NE and DIMI was also reported by Hoffer et al. (1971) who found cerebellar Purkinje cells responding to microelectrophoretic NE application with a reduction of their firing rate.

Since monoamines were shown to be involved in the regulation of *sleep-wakefulness cycles,* and ADS, on the other hand, interfere with the re-uptake of NE and 5-HT, ADs have been also employed in several studies dealing with sleep mechanisms (for a detailed information of the neurophysiology and neurochemistry of sleep and wakefulness cf., Jouvet, 1972; Moruzzi, 1972).

Many of these investigations were carried out by means of EEG and electromyographic recordings, which proved to be convenient methods for the recognition and differentiation of sleep stages.

Considerable alteration of sleep patterns was observed in animal experiments under the influence of various ADs (Baxter and Gluckman, 1969; Bert et al., 1977;

HISHIKAWA et al., 1965; JARAMILLO and GREENBERG, 1975; JOUVET, 1968; KHAZAN et al., 1967; KHAZAN and SULMAN, 1966; KORÁNYI et al., 1976; WALLACH et al., 1969 a, b). These drugs were reported to cause a prolongation of the non-REM-(NREM)-sleep time and a suppression of the REM-sleep periods (cf., FLORIO et al., 1977). Comparative studies show, however, that ADs do not influence the sleep pattern in a uniform manner. Investigating the effects of various ADs in the rat, JARAMILLO and GREENBERG (1975) listed DIMI, IMI, AMI, and BUT in decreasing order of their REM-suppressing potency; the NREM-sleep was shortened by DIMI, but was rather enhanced by AMI and BUT. In this study as well as in another one carried out on the cat (BAXTER and GLUCKMAN, 1969), iprindol failed to affect the sleep-pattern at all. The REM-sleep suppressant effect of both IMI and DIMI and their relative potency have been confirmed also by other investigations (KHAZAN and BROWN, 1970; LOEW and SPIEGEL, 1976, among others). However, in the cat, CIMI and IMI were found to be more potent than DIMI in suppressing the REM-sleep phases (HAEFELY et al., 1976). Data concerning the IMI-effect on the NREM-sleep periods are rather controversial (BENEŠOVÁ, 1975; JARAMILLO and GREENBERG, 1975; KHAZAN and BROWN, 1970).

It is interesting to note that TRI, a potent AD agent, while increasing the total sleep time, failed to influence the REM-sleep at all (KHAZAN and BROWN, 1970). This example also shows that so far no relationship has been found between the antidepressant potency of these psychotherapeutic agents and their effectiveness in influencing the sleep pattern.

Ponto-geniculo-occipital (PGO) waves, which are known to be associated with REM-sleep periods, were also shown to be influenced by AD agents. In the baboon, a daily administration of CIMI (1.7 mg/kg) caused both a suppression of the REM-sleep periods and a decrease of the frequency, amplitude, and total number of PGO waves during the treatment period (BERT et al., 1977).

Pharmacological studies on the drug-induced PGO waves are based on the findings (DELORME et al., 1965, 1966) that these waves can be elicited either by reserpine or p-chlorophenylalanine (PCPA). In pharmacological experiments (HAEFELY et al., 1973, 1976; JALFRE et al., 1970, 1973, 1974; RUCH-MONACHON et al., 1976 a–d) PGO waves were induced in the cat either by PCPA or by Ro 4-1284 (a benzoquinolizine derivative with reserpine-like actions) whereby depletion was achieved predominantly of either 5-HT or NE. ADs, among many other drugs, were able to depress the PGO activity induced by Ro 4-1284. Moreover, a correlation was found between the effectiveness of ADs in reducing the occurence of these PGO waves and their inhibitory potency on the 5-HT uptake. ADs, having inhibitory actions also on the NE uptake, were shown to affect the occurence of those PGO waves which were induced by PCPA treatment. Details on doses and relative potency of many ADs are presented in the papers quoted above. These data are in accordance with the findings on the effects of some ADs on the reserpine-induced PGO waves (VAN RIEZEN et al., 1976). Since ADs also have anticholinergic properties, mention should be made of the influence of cholinergic mechanisms on the PGO waves activity. Atropine, for example, was able to inhibit the PGO waves induced by both PCPA or reserpine (cf. RUCH-MONACHON et al., 1976 d; VAN RIEZEN et al., 1976).

Although these studies dealing with the effects of ADs on the PGO wave activity do not explain the actions of ADs in affective disorders, they do, however, demonstrate an excellent correlation between neurophysiological and biochemical findings.

V. Additional Neurophysiological Studies on the Effects of ADs

Under the influence of IMI, *evoked potentials* elicited in the neocortex by auditory or sciatic nerve stimulation were found to be augmented in the rabbit (VAN METER et al., 1959), and to be either unaffected or slightly enhanced in the cat (SIGG, 1959b). Fairly low doses (0.2–0.8 mg/kg) of IMI, AMI, DAMI, and DIMI potentiated the enhancing effects of methamphetamine on the neocortical evoked potentials (PLOTNIKOFF and EVERETT, 1965). The ADs themselves promoted these potentials only slightly.

The effects on limbic evoked responses of IMI, AMI, DIMI, and DAMI (with doses of 2–10 mg/kg) were investigated by SCHMITT (1967). These findings may be summarized as follows: A significant amplitude increase of the evoked potential induced in the septum by stimulation of the dorsal HC; a slight increase of the hypothalamic potentials evoked from the HC; a transient increase of the hippocampal evoked potential following amygdala stimulation, and finally, no changes of these potentials induced either in the HC or in the amygdala by septal stimulation.

In addition, several other evoked response studies with ADs (CREPAX et al., 1961 a, c; HEISS et al., 1967, 1969a, b; HOROVITZ et al., 1967; JALFRE et al., 1971; PLAS et al., 1960; PLAS and NAQUET, 1961) were carried out under different experimental conditions. A standardized evoked potential method, recently suggested for the classification of psychotropic drugs (POLLOCK et al., 1976) might also be appropriate for the classification of various AD agents.

Only few investigations were carried out on the effects of ADs by means of other classic neurophysiological methods such as, *caudate spindles* (ITO and SHIMIZU, 1976), and *recruiting* or *augmenting responses* (CREPAX et al., 1961 a, c; FERLINI and PERBELLINI, 1963; MONNIER and KRUPP, 1959; PLAS and NAQUET, 1961; SIGG, 1959; WATANABE et al., 1976).

No significant changes of either the mono- or polysynaptic *reflexes* were observed in the cat with high spinal transection under the influence of IMI (SIGG, 1959). Reductions of the patellar, flexor, and linguomandibular reflexes were found following IMI administration. This effect was less pronounced in the spinal cat than in the anaesthetized preparation. Similar effects were proven for DIMI, with the exception of the flexor reflex which was enhanced by this drug in both experimental set-ups (THEOBALD et al., 1964). An enhancement of polysynaptic reflexes by DIB was only to be observed in animals with an intact spinal cord, but not in the spinal preparation (STILLE et al., 1965). TAN and HENATSCH (1968, 1969 a, b) found that in the decerebrate cat, the activity of the extensor motor system was generally increased following the application of low IMI doses (0.5–2.0 mg/kg). This effect was due to a reduction of inhibitory mechanisms, whereby supraspinal structures were suggested to be the site of this IMI action.

Long-lasting and marked reduction of mono- and polysynaptic reflexes was found in the anaesthetized rat following the application of IMI (12.5 mg/kg) (SHIMIZU et al., 1974a).

The effect of ADs on the central 5-HT neurotransmission was studied on the extensor hind limb reflex of the spinal rat; this reflex was reported to be enhanced by an increase of 5-HT receptor activity (MEEK et al., 1970). IMI and CIMI were found to be effective in potentiating the action of 5-HTP, tryptophan, and nialamide on the hind limb reflex; the secondary amine derivatives DIMI and PRO remained ineffective.

The *neuromuscular transmission* was found not to be influenced by IMI (THEOBALD et al., 1964) in the gastrocnemius preparation of the anaesthetized rat. SINHA et al. (1966), on the other hand, reported on the neuromuscular blocking action of IMI, AMI, and DIMI. These experiments were carried out on the sciatic nerve gastrocnemius preparation of the anaesthetized cat, on the isolated rectus muscle of the frog, and on the phrenic nerve–diaphragma preparation of the rat. AMI proved to be most potent, DIMI the least potent agent. The block induced by ADs in the cat sciatic nerve preparation could be completely reversed by eserine; in the other preparations, however, this block proved to be neither competitive nor depolarizing. Both the nerve conduction and the contractile mechanisms of the muscles were not changed by these ADs. The experiments of CHANG and CHUANG, 1972, however, showed that both IMI DIMI caused a relaxation primarily by a direct action on the muscle. DIMI, in addition, inhibited the axonal conduction as well as the synaptic transmission. IMI, on the other hand, affected the axonal conduction more than DIMI. Analysis of the ADs action led to the conclusion that these drugs act on the excitable membrane in a different manner to local anaesthetics or CPZ. LERMER et al. (1971) assumed AMI to cause an inhibition of the neuromuscular transmission in the frog sartorius preparation primarily by a presynaptic site of action; the postsynaptic effect was found to be of minor importance.

B. Monoamine Oxidase Inhibitors (MAOIs)

I. Effects of MAOIs on the Electric Activity of the Brain

Unlike the large number of biochemical studies published on MAOIs, only few and rather controversial data are available on the EEG effects of these agents. Some MAOIs were reported to induce two periods of EEG arousal patterns. Following drug administration, the first period occurred with a short latency and was attributed to an amphetamine-like action; the more persistent second period of activation pattern appeared with a long latency (1–2 h), and was suggested to be dependent on the inhibition of brain MAO. These EEG periods were observed in various species following acute or chronic administration of *tranylcypromine* (COSTA et al., 1960; LING, 1962; HIMWICH, 1965; HIMWICH and PETERSEN, 1961; MELDRUM et al., 1972). The occurrence of the delayed activation pattern was suggested to be related to an accumulation of 5-HT and/or NE in the CNS. However, in the experiments of FUNDERBURK et al. (1961) the chronic administration of tranylcypromine (2 mg/kg/day for 12 days and 5 mg/kg/day for the consecutive 5 days) to cats resulted in an increase of EEG synchronization, which was also accompanied by a significant elevation of the brain 5-HT level.

Detailed investigations on the effects of *pheniprazine* were carried out on both the rabbit and cat (COSTA et al., 1960; SHIMIZU et al., 1964). Like tranylcypromine, pheniprazine also induced both an early and a late phase of EEG arousal pattern. The latter period was shown to be accompanied by an accumulation of catecholamines, β-phenylethylamine (SHIMIZU et al., 1964), and especially of 5-HT (COSTA et al., 1960).

Similar EEG-AR periods were obtained under the influence of both *etryptamine* and *methyltryptamine* (HIMWICH, 1961; MATTHEWS et al., 1961; STEINER et al., 1963 b,c; VAN METER et al., 1961). The experiments of STEINER et al. (1963 b) indicate that the delayed EEG activation pattern induced by these drugs was not necessarily due to changes of the brain monoamine level. VANE et al. (1961), however, found both methyltryptamine and etryptamine to induce in the cat a long lasting period of resting EEG patterns following the short period of EEG-AR.

Findings on the EEG effects of *iproniazide* are particularly inconsistent: In the rabbit, cat, and dog no changes of the bioelectrical activities were found following administration of either single or repeated doses of this drug (COSTA et al., 1960; KUEHN and SCHALLEK, 1958; LING, 1962; SCHALLEK, 1960; SCHALLEK and KUEHN, 1959). Other experiments showed EEG activation patterns either in the rabbit after extremely high iproniazide doses (500–900 mg/kg) (HIMWICH et al., 1958), or in cats with lesion in the pontile reticular formation following a pretreatment with iproniazide (19–20 mg/kg/day) for 5 consecutive days (SCHALLEK, 1960). Finally, spindles and slow cortical waves were found in cats with chronically implanted electrodes, which had been given iproniazide (20 mg/kg/day) for 5 days (FUNDERBURK et al., 1961). Similar EEG-changes were observed in the rabbit 20 h after administration of iproniazide (80 mg/kg) (TISSOT and MONNIER, 1958). It is interesting to note that both COSTA et al. (1960) and FUNDERBURK et al. (1961) reported an elevation of the brain 5-HT level under the influence of iproniazide, but, at the same time, found different EEG effects.

Both *isocarboxazide* and *nialamide* were shown to induce a synchronization of the neocortical activity accompanied by an increase in brain 5-HT; these agents were administered to cats in daily doses of 10 mg/kg for 3 days (FUNDERBURK et al., 1961). Gradual changes from low-voltage fast activity to slow wave patterns were observed in the cat and the monkey under the influence of nialamide (20–30 mg/kg) (MANCHANDA et al., 1963).

The EEG effects of *pargyline* were studied in the rabbit and monkey (EVERETT, 1961). These investigations proved that the accumulation of brain catecholamines was concomitant with the appearance of both the EEG- and the behavioural-AR.

The neurophysiological effects of *harmaline* and its related agents (FUENTES and LONGO, 1971; GOGOLÁK et al., 1977; SCHMITT, 1966; TRUJILLO et al., 1977) will be not discussed in this review; harmaline has been a useful agent for studies on tremor mechanisms (cf., LAMARRE and WEISS, 1973).

In connection with the controversial data reported above, mention should be made of an interesting publication (STEINER et al., 1963c) which points out the determining role of the experimental methods for findings on the effects of etryptamine or reserpine.

II. Additional Neurophysiological Results on the Effects of MAOIs

Not only the investigations mentioned above, but also other neurophysiological studies have led to controversial results on the effects of MAOIs.

Data reported on the effects of various MAOIs on the EEG-AR, induced by either sensory stimuli or electrical stimulation of the ascending reticular formation, may be summarized as follows: A decrease of the stimulus threshold for the induction of EEG-AR was found in the cat after application of pheniprazine (SHIMIZU et al., 1964). An elevation of this threshold followed administration of both methyltryptamine in the cat's encéphale isolé preparation (VANE et al., 1961), and iproniazide in the non-immobilized rabbit (TISSOT and MONNIER, 1958). No significant changes of this arousal response were observed under the influence of nialamide, tranylcypromine, isocarboxazide, or iproniazide in cats either with chronically implanted electrodes (FUNDERBURK and DRAKONTIDES, 1960; FUNDERBURK et al., 1961; MACHANDA et al., 1963) or in the encéphale isolé preparation (KUEHN and SCHALLEK, 1958; SCHALLEK and KUEHN, 1959).

Amygdaloid afterdischarges were found to be enhanced in the cat (SCHALLEK and KUEHN, 1960; SCHALLEK et al., 1962) and in the monkey (WADA, 1962) under the influence of iproniazide. Isocarboxazide caused similar effects (SCHALLEK et al., 1962). Pheniprazine, on the other hand, did not influence these afterdischarges at all (SHIMIZU et al., 1964).

The duration of hippocampal afterdischarges was shortened after the application of nialamide, isocarboxazide, tranylcypromine, and iproniazide in various species (FUNDERBURK et al., 1961; MACHANDA et al., 1963; WADA, 1962).

The effect of tranylcypromine on the limbic excitability were found to be inconsistent (COSTA et al., 1961); the hippocampal evoked potentials were inhibited by this agent in the "acute preparation" (fulguration of the mesencephalic tegmentum) only, but significant effects were observed in the cat with chronically implanted electrodes. Iproniazide was shown to diminish the response on transcallosal stimulations (GLUCKMAN et al., 1957; MARRAZZI, 1957). In the baboon, myoclonic and EEG paroxismal responses to photic stimulation were reduced after i. v. administration of tranylcypromine (15–30 mg/kg). This protective effect was achieved by means of relatively high tranylcypromine doses which also caused autonomic and behavioural, as well as EEG effects (MELDRUM et al., 1972).

The spontaneous firing rate of midbrain raphe units was shown to decrease under the influence of various MAOIs in the anaesthetized rat (AGHAJANIAN et al., 1970). The firing of these neurons containing 5-HT could equally be depressed by MAOIs with amphetamine-like action (tranylcypromine and phenelzine) and by those without this additional effect (pargyline and iproniazide). This action of MAOIs was prevented by a pretreatment with PCPA, while a prior treatment with α-methyl-p-tyrosine remained ineffective. These findings may suggest a relation of both MAOIs effects, i. e., the accumulation of 5-HT in the CNS and the inhibition of raphe neurons containing 5-HT.

Most of the MAOIs were found to suppress both the REM and the NREM sleep periods. In the case of tranylcypromine and harmaline, the effect was attributed to an amphetamin-like action. Iproniazide, phenylisopropylhydrazine, pargyline, and nialamide, however, were assumed to have a specific and selective effect on the REM sleep phases (for detailed informations cf., JOUVET, 1968). Although not under discussion here, MAOIs were also applied in neurophysiological experiments concentrating on mechanisms of REM-sleep periods, PGO-wave activity and their modification by various neurotransmitters (GERSHON and BROOKS, 1976; RUCH-MONACHON et al., 1976c).

This short summary shows how little information is available on the neurophysiological effects of MAOIs. Most investigations were carried out in the early sixties. Concurrently with the decline of the clinical use of MAOIs there has been a considerable decrease in the number of publications dealing with the pharmacological effects of these agents.

C. Concluding Remarks

The aim of this paper was to collect data on the effects of antidepressant agents such as obtained by neurophysiological methods. Particularly those publications have been pointed out which allow for a comparison of the individual effects of various antidepressants. Owing to the variety of experimental procedures employed in the investigations presented here, many results could only be commented on with reservation or not be commented on at all; in some cases only relevant references have been quoted.

The significance of various laboratory studies for the discovery of psychotherapeutic agents has been repeatedly discussed (cf., HOFFMEISTER, 1969 a, b; SCHMITT and SCHMITT, 1966a; STILLE, 1964, 1968, 1974; WUTTKE and HOFFMEISTER, 1969). How far do the neurophysiological investigations have any predictory value for the discovery of anti-depressant drugs? The results reported in this review show that these agents can influence the EEG activity of various brain areas, the EEG-AR, the firing pattern of monoaminergic neurons, or various other electrobiological phenomena. It has, however, not been possible to study the effect of antidepressant agents on those unknown mechanisms which might be related to emotional states or affective disorders in human beings. Moreover, it should be mentioned that most of the neurophysiological investigations were carried out in "acute" experiments; with depressed patients, however, antidepressants have to be given over a period of some weeks to achieve any therapeutic effects.

Since antidepressants have manifold pharmacological actions, (i. e., peripheral and central) which may or may not be of significance for their therapeutic effects in mental depression, some experimental findings might be regarded as an indication of side effects of these agents and/or their interactions with other drugs.

Acknowledgements. The author wishes express gratitude to Mrs. ANDREA MOTEJLEK and Mrs. MANFREDA SATZINGER for their competent assistance. Thanks are due to Professor H. COPER and Professor F. HOFFMEISTER for their kind help in gathering the literature. Apprecation is due to Professor CH. STUMPF, Dr. S. HUCK, and Dr. R. JINDRA for reading the manuscript.

References

Aghajanian, G.K., Graham, M.H., Sheard, M.H.: Serotonin containing neurons in brain: depression of firing by monoamine oxidase inhibitors. Science *169*, 1100–1102 (1970)

Avanzino, G.L., Ermirio, R., Zummo, C.: Effects of microiontophoretic application of imipramine on single neurons in the brain stem. Neuropharmacology *10*, 661–664 (1971)

Baker, W.W., Kratky, M.: Acute effects of chlorpromazine and imipramine on hippocampal foci. Arch. Int. Pharmacodyn. Ther. *165*, 265–275 (1967)

Barrat, E.S., Pray, S.L.: Effect of a chemically depressed amygdala on the behavioral manifestation produced in cats by LSD-25. Exp. Neurol. *12*, 173–178 (1965)

Baxter, B.L., Gluckman, M.I.: Iprindole: an antidepressant which does not block REM sleep. Nature *223*, 750–752 (1969)

Benešová, O.: The relation of imipramine-like drugs to the cholinergic system. In: Antidepressant drugs. Garattini, S., Dukes, M.N.G. (eds.), pp. 247–254. Amsterdam: Excerpta Medica Foundation 1967

Benešová, O.: The effect of maprotiline and imipramine on sleep cycles in rats. Act. Nerv. Sup. (Praha) *17*, 4 (1975)

Benešová, O., Nahunek, K.: Correlation between the experimental data from animal studies and therapeutical effects of antidepressant drugs. Psychopharmacologia *20*, 337–347 (1971)

Benešová, O., Bohdanecký, Z., Votava, Z.: Electrophysiological comparison of the action of imipramine and propazepine. Psychopharmacologia *3*, 423–431 (1962)

Benešová, O., Bohdanecký, Z., Votava, Z.: Über einige zentrale Wirkungen von Prothiaden – einer neuen Substanz mit antidepressiver Wirkung. Naunyn-Schmiedeberg's Arch. Pharmacol. *245*, 124–125 (1963)

Benešová, O., Bohdanecký, Z., Grofova, I.: Electrophysiological analysis of the neuroleptic and antidepressant actions of psychotropic drugs in rabbits. Int. J. Neuropharmacol. *3*, 479–488 (1964a)

Benešová, O., Bohdanecký, Z., Votava, Z.: Über einige zentrale Wirkungen von Prothiaden. Arzneim. Forsch. *14*, 100–103 (1964b)

Bert, J., Saier, J., Tognetti, P., Toure, F.: Effect de la chlorimipramine sur l'activité de pointes „Ponto-géniculo-occipitales" (PGO) du babouin Papio hamadryas. Psychopharmacology *51*, 301–304 (1977)

Bevan, P., Bradshaw, C.M., Roberts, M.H.T., Szabadi, E.: The dual action of tricyclic antidepressant drugs on responses of single cortical neurons to acetylcholine. Br. J. Pharmacol. *49*, 173P–174P (1973)

Bradley, P.B., Key, B.J.: A comparative study of the effects of drugs on the arousal system in the brain. Br. J. Pharmacol. *14*, 340–349 (1959)

Bradshaw, C.M., Roberts, M.H.T., Szabadi, E.: Effect of tricyclic antidepressants on monoamine responses of single cortical neurones. Br. J. Pharmacol. *41*, 394P–395P (1971)

Bradshaw, C.M., Roberts, M.H.T., Szabadi, E.: Comparison of the effects of imipramine and desimipramine on single cortical neurones. Br. J. Pharmacol. *48*, 358P–359P (1973)

Bradshaw, C.M., Roberts, M.H.T., Szabadi, E.: Effects of imipramine and desimipramine on responses of single cortical neurones to noradrenaline and 5-hydroxytryptamine. Br. J. Pharmacol. *52*, 349–358 (1974)

Bramwell, G.J.: Effect of imipramine on unit activity in the midbrain raphé of rats. Br. J. Pharmacol. *44*, 345–346 (1972)

Bramwell, G.J.: The effect of antidepressants on unit activity in the midbrain raphé of rats. Arch. Int. Pharmacodyn. Ther. *211*, 24–33 (1974)

Bunney, B.S., Walters, J.R., Roth, R.H., Aghajanian, K.: Dopaminergic neurons: Effects of antipsychotic drugs and amphetamine on single cell activity. J. Pharmacol. Exp. Ther. *185*, 560–571 (1973)

Chang, C.C., Chuang, S.-T.: Effects of desipramine and imipramine on the nerve, muscle, and synaptic transmission of rat diaphragms. Neuropharmacology *11*, 777–788 (1972)

Costa, E., Morpurgo, C., Revzin, A.M.: Theoretical implications of the chemotherapy of depressions. Recent Adv. Biol. Psychiatr. *3*, 122–139 (1961)

Costa, E., Pscheidt, G.R., Van Meter, W.G., Himwich, H.: Brain concentrations of biogenic amines and EEG patterns of rabbits. J. Pharmacol. Exp. Ther. *130*, 81–88 (1960)

Crepax, P., Fadiga, E., Massarini, A., Volta, A.: Ricerche sull'azione neurofarmacologica della imipramina. Arch. Sci. Biol. *45*, 201–235 (1961a)

Crepax, P., Fadiga, E., Volta, A.: Syncronizzazione elettroencefalografica e modifizioni della soglia del risveglio corticale provocate della somnimistrazione di imipramina nal gatto. Boll. Soc. Ital. Biol. Sper. *37*, 66–69 (1961b)

Crepax, P., Fadiga, E., Volta, A.: Effetti della imipramina su fenomeni elettrici cerebrali dovuti all'attivazione di circuiti talamo-corticali, transcallosali e intracorticali, nel gatto. Boll. Soc. Ital. Biol. Sper. *37*, 180–183 (1961c)

Crepax, P., Fadiga, E., Volta, A.: Modificazioni dell'attività elettrica rinencefalica, osservate nel gatto per effetto del trattamento con imipramina. Boll. Soc. Ital. Biol. Sper. *37*, 378–381 (1961d)

Crismon, C.: Chlorpromazine and imipramine: parallel studies in animals. Psychopharmacol. Bull. *4*, 1–151 (1967)

Dasberg, H., Feldman, S.: Effect of imipramine, physostigmine and amphetamine on the electrical activity of the brain in the cat. Psychopharmacologia *13*, 129–139 (1968)

Delorme, F., Jeannerod, M., Jouvet, M.: Effects remarquables de la réserpine sur l'activité EEG phasique ponto-géniculo-occipitale. C.R. Soc. Biol. *159*, 900–903 (1965)

Delorme, F., Froment, J.L., Jouvet, M.: Suppression du sommeil par la p-chlorométamphétamine et la p-chlorophénylalanine. C.R. Soc. Biol. *160*, 2347–2351 (1966)

Everett, G.M.: Some electrophysiological and biochemical correlates of motor activity and aggressive behavior. In: Neuropharmacology. Rothlin, E. (ed.), Vol. 2, pp. 479–484. Amsterdam: Elsevier Publ. Comp. 1961

Ferlini, G., Perbellini, D.: Rilievi elettroencefalografici in animali trattati con imipramina. Riv. Patol. Nerv. Ment. *84*, 232–240 (1963)

Florio, V., Longo, V.G., Verdeaux, G.: EEG effects of antipsychotics, tranquilizers and antidepressants. In: Handbook of electroencephalography and clinical neurophysiology, Vol. 7, Part C, Longo, V.G. (ed.), pp. 7C–53 – 7C–56. Amsterdam: Elsevier Publ. Comp. 1977

Fuentes, J.A., Longo, V.G.: An investigation on the central effects of harmine, harmaline, and related β-carbolines. Neuropharmacology *10*, 15–23 (1971)

Funderburk, W.H., Drakontides, A.B.: Effects of nialamide on the electroencephalogram. Fed. Proc. *19*, 278 (1960)

Funderburk, W.H., Finger, K.F., Drakontides, A.B., Schneider, J.A.: EEG and biochemical findings with MAO inhibitors. Ann. N.Y. Acad. Sci. *96*, 289–302 (1961)

Gershon, M.D., Brooks, D.C.: Monoamine oxidase inhibition and the induction of pontogeniculo-occipital waves activity by reserpine in the cat. J. Pharmacol. Exp. Ther. *197*, 556–566 (1976)

Gianelli, A., Marinato, J.: Modificazioni indotte dalla imipramina sull'attivita bioelettrica cerebrale nel coniglio. In: Le sindromi depressive, Fazio, G. (ed.), pp. 531–533. Torino: Edizioni Minerva Medica 1960

Gluckman, M.I., Hart, E.R., Marazzi, A.S.: Cerebral synaptic inhibition by serotonin and iproniazid. Science *126*, 448–449 (1957)

Gogolák, G., Jindra, R., Stumpf, Ch.: Effect of harmaline on the cerebellorubral system. Experientia *33*, 1352–1354 (1977)

Haefely, W., Jalfre, M., Monachon, M.A.: NE-neurons and phasic sleep phenomena. In: Frontiers in catecholamine research. Usdin, E., Snyder, S.H. (eds.), pp. 773–775. Oxford: Pergamon Press 1973

Haefely, W., Ruch-Monachon, M.A., Jalfre, M., Schaffner, R.: Interaction of psychotropic agents with central neurotransmitters as revealed by their effects on PGO waves in the cat. Arzneim. Forsch. *26*, 1036–1039 (1976)

Heiss, W.-D., Heilig, P., Hoyer, J.: Retinale Impulsaktivität und Elektroretinogramm unter dem Einfluß von Imipramin. Experientia *23*, 728–729 (1967)

Heiss, W.-D., Heilig, P., Hoyer, J.: Die Wirkung von Psychopharmaka auf die Aktivität retinaler Neurone. Vision Res. *9*, 493–506 (1969a)

Heiss, W.-D., Hoyer, J., Heilig, P.: Die Wirkung von Psychopharmaka auf visuell evozierte Potentiale der Katze. Vision Res. *9*, 507–513 (1969b)

Herz, A.: Excitation and inhibition of cholinoceptive brain structures and its relationship to pharmacological induced behaviour changes. Int. J. Neuropharmacol. *2*, 205–216 (1963)

Herz, A.: Central cholinolytic activity and antidepressive effect. In: Neuro-Psychopharmacology. Bente, D., Bradley, B. (eds.), Vol. 4, pp. 402–404. Amsterdam: Elsevier Publ. Comp. 1965

Himwich, H.E.: Stimulants. In: The effect of pharmacological agents on the nervous system. Braceland, F.J. (ed.), Vol. 37, pp. 356–383. Baltimore: Williams & Wilkens Comp. 1959

Himwich, .H.E.: Experiments with alpha-methyltryptamine. J. Neuropsychiatry 2, [Suppl.] S136–S140 (1961)

Himwich, W.A.: Interaction of monoaminooxydase inhibitors with imipramine and similar drugs. Rec. Adv. Biol. Psychiatry *4*, 257–265 (1962)

Himwich, H.E.: Anatomy and physiology of the emotions and their relation to psychoactive drugs. In: The scientific basis of drug therapy in psychiatry. Marks. J., Pare, C.M. (eds.), pp. 3–24. Oxford: Pergamon Press 1965

Himwich, W.A., Petersen, J.C.: Effect of the Combined administration of imipramine and a monoamine oxidase inhibitor. Am. J. Psychiatry *117*, 928–929 (1961)

Himwich, H.E., Costa, E., Pscheidt, G.R., Van Meter, W.G.: Discussion. Ann. N.Y. Acad. Sci. *80*, 614–616 (1958)

Himwich, H.E., Morillo, A., Steiner, W.G.: Drugs affecting rhinencephalic structures. J. Neuropsychiatry *3*, 515–526 (1962)

Hishikawa, Y., Nakai, K., Øida, H., Kanako, Z.: The effect of imipramine, desmethylimipramine and chlorpromazine on the sleep-wakefulnesscycle of the cat. Electroencephalogy Clin. Neurophysiol. *19*, 518–521 (1965)

Hoffer, B.J., Siggins, G.R., Bloom, F.E.: Studies on norepinephrine containing afferents to Purkinje cells of rat cerebellum. II. Sensitivity of Purkinje cells to norepinephrine and related substances administered by microiontophoresis. Brain Res. *25*, 523–534 (1971)

Hoffmeister, F.: Zur Frage pharmakologisch-klinischer Wirkungsbeziehungen bei Antidepressiva, dargestellt am Beispiel von Noxiptilin. Arzneim. Forsch. *19*, 458–462 (1969a)

Hoffmeister, F.: Methodische Probleme der Psychopharmakologie, dargestellt am Beispiel der Antidepressiva. Arzneim. Forsch. *19*, 808–810 (1969b)

Hoffmeister, F., Wuttke, W., Kroneberg, G.: Zur Pharmakologie des Thymoleptikum Noxiptilin (BAY 1521). Arzneim. Forsch. *19*, 846–858 (1969)

Horovitz, Z.P.: The amygdala and depression. In: Antidepressant drugs, Garattini, S., Duke, M.N.G. (eds.), pp. 121–129. Amsterdam: Excerpta Medica Foundation 1967

Horovitz, Z.P., Chow, M.: Effects of centrally acting drugs on the correlation of electrocortical activity and wakefulness of cats. J. Pharmacol. Exp. Ther. *137*, 127–132 (1962)

Horovitz, Z.P., Furgiuele, A.R., Brannick, L.J., Burke, J.C., Craver, B.N.: A new chemical structure with specific depressant effects on the amygdala and on the hyper-irritability of the "septal rat." Nature *200*, 369–370 (1963)

Ito, T., Shimizu, M.: Effect of psychotropic drugs on caudate spindle in the cat. Jp. J. Pharmacol. *26*, 527–534 (1976)

Jalfre, M., Monachon, M.A., Haefely, W.: Pharmacological modifications of benzoquinolozine-induced geniculate spikes. Experientia *26*, 691 (1970)

Jalfre, M., Monachon, M.A., Haefely, W.: Effects on the amygdalo-hippocampal evoked potential in the cat of four benzodiazepines and some other psychotropic drugs. Naunyn-Schmiedeberg's Arch. Pharmacol. *270*, 180–191 (1971)

Jalfre, M., Monachon, M.A., Haefely, W.: Drug and PGO waves in the cat. In: 1st Can. Int. Sympos. on Sleep, pp. 155–185. Montreal 1972. Montreal: Roche Scientific Service 1973

Jalfre, M., Ruch-Monachon, M.A., Haefely, W.: Methods for assessing the interaction of agents with 5-HT neurons and receptors in the brain. Adv. Biochem. Psychopharmacol. *10*, pp. 121–134 (1974)

Jaramillo, J., Greenberg, R.: Comparative pharmacological studies on butriptyline and some related standard tricyclic antidepressants. Can. J. Physiol. Pharmacol. *53*, 104–112 (1975)

Jouvet, M.: Neuropharmacology of sleep. In: Psychopharmacology, a review of progress. Efron, D.H. (ed.), pp. 523–540. Washington, DC: US Government Printing Office 1968

Jouvet, M.: The role of monoamines and acetylcholine-containing neurons in the regulation of the sleep-waking cycle. In: Reviews of physiology, biochemistry and experimental pharmacology, Vol. 64, pp. 166–307. Berlin, Heidelberg, New York: Springer 1972

Julien, R.M., Fowler, G.W., Danielson, M.G.: The effects of antiepileptic drugs on estrogen-induced electrographic spike-wave discharge. J. Pharmacol. Exp. Ther. *193*, 647–656 (1975)

Kamei, Ch., Masuda, Y., Oka, M., Shimizu, M.: Effects of antidepressant drugs on amygdaloid afterdischarges in rats. Jpn. J. Pharmacol. *25*, 359–365 (1975)

Khazan, N., Brown, P.: Differential effects of three tricyclic antidepressants on sleep an REM sleep in the rat. Life Sci. *9*, 279–284 (1970)

Khazan, N., Sulman, F.G.: Effect of imipramine on paradoxical sleep in animals with reference to dreaming and enuresis. Psychopharmacologia *10*, 89–95 (1966)

Khazan, N., Bar, R., Sulman, F.G.: The effect of cholinergic drugs on paradoxical sleep in the rat. Int. J. Neuropharmacol. *6*, 279–282 (1967)

Korányi, L., Tamásy, V., Lissák, K., Király, I., Borsy, J.: Effect of thyrotropin-releasing hormone (TRH) and antidepressant agents on brain stem and hypothalamic multiple unit activity in the cat. Psychopharmacology *49*, 197–200 (1976)

Kuehn, A., Schallek, W.: Effects of drugs on resting and activated EEG of cat. Fed. Proc. *17*, 368 (1958)

Lamarre, Y., Weiss, M.: Harmaline-induced rhythmic activity of alpha and gamma motoneurons in the cat. Brain Res. *63*, 430–434 (1973)

Lange, S.C., Julien, R.M., Fowler, G.W.: Biphasic effects of imipramine in experimental models of epilepsy. Epilepsia *17*, 183–195 (1976)

Lermer, H., Avni, J., Bruderman, I.: Neuromuscular blocking action of amytryptiline. Eur. J. Pharmacol. *13*, 266–268 (1971)

Ling, G.M.: Some effects of tranylcypromine and triflupromazine on electrocortical activity. Can. Psychiatr. Assoc. J. *7*, [Suppl.] S44–S54 (1962)

Loew, D., Spiegel, R.: Polygraphic sleep studies in rats and humans. Their use in psychopharmacological research. Arzneim. Forsch. *26*, 1032–1035 (1976)

Luchins, D.: Biogenic amines and affective disorders. A critical analysis. Int. Pharmacopsychiatry *11*, 135–149 (1976)

Manchanda, S.K., Subberwal, U., Anand, B.K., Singh, B.: Effect of nialamide on the electroencephalographically recorded activity of the brain. Arch. Int. Pharmacodyn. Ther. *143*, 408–420 (1963)

Marrazzi, A.S.: The effects of certain drugs on cerebral synapses. Ann. N.Y. Acad. Sci. *66*, 496–507 (1957)

Matthews, R.Y., Roberts, B.J., Atkins, P.K.: Neuropharmacological studies on d-1-alphaethyltryptamine acetate. J. Neuropsychiatry *2*, [Suppl.], 151–158 (1961)

Maxwell, D.R., Palmer, H.T.: Demonstration of antidepressants or stimulant properties of imipramine in experimental animals. Nature *191*, 84–85 (1961)

Meek, J., Fuxe, K., Anden, N.E.: Effects of antidepressant drugs of the imipramine type on central 5-hydroxitryptamine neurotransmission. Eur. J. Pharmacol. *9*, 325–332 (1970)

Meldrum, B.S., Balzamo, E., Wada, J.A., Vuillon-Cacciuttolo, G.: Effects of 1-tryptophan, 1–3,4, di-hydroxyphenylalanine and trancylpromine on the electroencephalogram and photically induced epilepsy in the baboon, Papio Papio. Physiol. Behav. *9*, 615–621 (1972)

Mercier, J., Etzensperger, P., Dessaigne, S.: Essai de localisation et d'interprétation de l'action de l'amytryptiline au niveau du système nerveux. J. Physiol. (Paris) *55*, 581–609 (1963)

Monnier, M., Krupp, P.: Elektrophysiologische Analyse der Wirkung verschiedener Neuroleptica (Chlorpromazin, Reserpin, Tofranil, Meprobamat). Schweiz. Med. Wochenschr. *89*, 430–433 (1959)

Moore, R.H., White, R.P.: Central anticholinergic actions of Doxepin in rabbits. Arch. Int. Pharmacodyn. Ther. *213*, 113–120 (1975)

Moruzzi, G.: The sleep-waking cycle. In: Reviews of physiology, biochemistry and experimental pharmacology, Vol. 64, pp. 1–165. Berlin, Heidelberg, New York: Springer 1972

Neal, H., Bradley, P.B.: Electrophysiological studies with a new antidepressant drug: comparison of the effects of viloxazine (ICI 58,834) with three tricyclic antidepressants in the encéphale isolé. Neuropharmacology *17*, 835–849 (1978)

Nybäck, H.V., Walters, J.R., Aghajanian, G.K., Roth, R.H.: Tricyclic antidepressants: Effects of the firing rate of brain noradrenergic neurons. Eur. J. Pharmacol. *32*, 302–312 (1975)

Peñaloza-Rojas, J.H., Bach-Y-Rita, G., Rubio-Chevannier, H.F., Hernández-Peon, R.: Effects of imipramine upon hypothalamic and amygdaloid excitability. Exp. Neurol. *4*, 205–213 (1961)

Plas, R., Naquet, R.: Contribution à l'étude neurophysiologique de l'imipramine. C.R. Soc. Biol. (Paris) *155*, 840–843 (1961)

Plas, R., Barrabino, J.H., Naquet, R.: Approche neurophysiologique du problème de la spécifité d'action therapeutique des drogues tranquillisantes. Rev. Neurol. *103*, 363–364 (1960)

Plotnikoff, N., Everett, G.M.: Potentiation of evoked cortical responses in the rabbit by methamphetamine and antidepressants. Life Sci. *4*, 1135–1147 (1965)

Plotnikoff, N., Will, F., Evans, A., Meekma, P.: PS-2747, a new antidepressant agent. Arch. Int. Pharmacodyn. Ther. *195*, 330–342 (1972)

Pollock, B., Bock, P.R., Fuchs, A.M., Lohaus, R.: Visually evoked potentials in cortical and subcortical brain structures of conscious rabbits with chronically implanted electrodes. Arzneim. Forsch. *26*, 327–334 (1976)

Preston, J.B.: Effects of chlorpromazine on the central nervous system of the cat: a possible neural basis for action. J. Pharmacol. *118*, 100–115 (1956)

Rathbun, R.C., Slater, I.H.: Amitryptiline and nortryptiline as antagonists of central and peripheral cholinergic activation. Psychopharmacologia *4*, 114–125 (1963)

Rehavi, M., Maayani, S., Sokolovsky, M.: Tricyclic antidepressants as antimuscarinic drugs: in vivo and in vitro studies. Biochem. Pharmacol. *26*, 1559–1567 (1977)

Rinaldi, F.: Effects of antidepressant drugs on the electrical activity of the brain. In: Antidepressant drugs. Garattini, S., Dukes, M.N.G. (eds.), pp. 99–103. Amsterdam: Excerpta Medica Foundation 1967

Rubio-Chevannier, H., Bach-Y-Rita, G., Peñaloza-Rojas, J., Hernández-Peón, R.: Potentiating action of imipramine upon reticular arousal. Exp. Neurol. *4*, 214–220 (1961)

Ruch-Monachon, M.A., Jalfre, M., Haefely, W.: Drugs and PGO waves in the lateral geniculate body of the curarized cat. I. PGO wave activity induced by Ro 4-1284 and by p-chlorophenylalanine (PCPA) as a basis for neuropharmacological studies. Arch. Int. Pharmacodyn. Ther. *219*, 251–268 (1976a)

Ruch-Monachon, M.A., Jalfre, M., Haefely, W.: Drugs and PGO waves in the lateral geniculate body of the curarized cat. II. PGO wave activity and brain 5-hydroxytryptamine. Arch. Int. Pharmacodyn. Ther. *219*, 269–286 (1976b)

Ruch-Monachon, M.A., Jalfre, M., Haefely, W.: Drugs and PGO waves in the lateral geniculate body of the curarized cat. III. PGO wave activity and brain catecholamines. Arch. Int. Pharmacodyn. Ther. *219*, 287–307 (1976c)

Ruch-Monachon, M.A., Jalfre, M., Haefely, W.: Drugs and PGO waves in the lateral geniculate body of the curarized cat. IV. The effects of acetylcholine, GABA and benzodiazepines on PGO wave activity. Arch. Int. Pharmacodyn. Ther. *219*, 308–325 (1976d)

Schallek, W.: Neurophysiological studies with monoamine oxidase inhibitors. Dis. Nerv. Syst. *21*, 1–3 (1960)

Schallek, W., Kuehn, A.: Effects of drugs on spontaneous and activated EEG of cat. Arch. Int. Pharmacodyn. Ther. *120*, 319–333 (1959)

Schallek, W., Kuehn, A.: Effects of psychotropic drugs in limbic system of cat. Proc. Soc. Exp. Biol. Med. *105*, 115–117 (1960)

Schallek, W., Kuehn, A., Jew, N.: Effects of chlordiazepoxid and other psychotropic agents on the limbic system of the brain. Ann. N.Y. Acad. Sci. *96*, 303–312 (1962)

Schmitt, H.: Action de l'harmine et de l'harmaline sur l'électro-encéphalogramme du lapin. Arch. Int. Pharmacodyn. Ther. *162*, 84–92 (1966)

Schmitt, H.: Selective action of antidepressant drugs on some rhinencephalic and related structures. In: Antidepressant drugs. Garattini, S., Dukes, M.N.G. (eds.), pp. 104–115. Amsterdam: Excerpta Medica Foundation 1967

Schmitt, H., Schmitt, H.: Valeur de la pharmacologie prévisionnelle dans le domaine des antidépresseurs dérivés de l'iminodibenzyle. Thérapie *21*, 653–674 (1966a)

Schmitt, H., Schmitt, H.: Action de l'imipramine, de l'amitryptiline et de leurs dérivés monodéméthyles sur les postdécharges provoquées par l'excitation de certaines structures rhinencéphaliques chez le lapin. Thérapie *21*, 675–684 (1966b)

Schmitt, W., Stille, G.: Beziehungen zwischen pharmakologischen und klinischen Untersuchungsergebnissen mit neuen antidepressiv wirksamen Substanzen. Exc. Med. Int. Congr. Series *180*, VI. Int. Congr. C.I.N.P. Tarragona: April 1968 pp. 541–544

Sheard, M.H., Zolovick, A., Aghajanian, G.K.: Raphe neurons: Effect of tricyclic antidepressant drugs. Brain Res. *43*, 690–694 (1972)

Shimizu, A., Hishikawa, Y., Matsumoto, K., Kaneko, S.: Electroencephalographic studies on the action of monoamine oxidase inhibitor. Psychopharmacologia *6*, 368–387 (1964)

Shimizu, M., Hirooka, T., Karasawa, T., Masuda, Y., Oka, M., Ito, T., Kamei, C., Sohji, Y., Hori, M., Yoshida, K., Kaneko, H.: Pharmacological evaluation of 3-(N-3,3-diphenylpropyl-N-methyl)-aminopropran-1-d-hydrochloride (PF-82), a new type of antidepressant drug. Arzneim. Forsch. *24*, 166–173 (1974a)

Shimizu, M., Yoshida, K., Karasawa, T., Masuda, M., Oka, M., Ito, T., Kamei, C., Hori, M., Sohji, Y., Furukawa, K.: 1,2-Benzisoxazole-3-acetamidoxime hydrochloride, a new psychotropic agent. Experientia *30*, 405 (1974b)

Shopsin, B., Wilk, S., Sathananthan, G., Gershon, S., Davis, K.: Catecholamines and affective disorders revised: A critical assessment. J. Nerv. Ment. Dis. *158*, 369–383 (1974)

Sigg, E.B.: Neuropharmacological assessment of tofranil (imipramine), a new antidepressant agent. Fed. Proc. *18*, 144 (1959a)

Sigg, E.B.: Pharmacological studies with tofranil. Can. Psychiatr. Assoc. J. *4*, Spec. Suppl. *74*, S75–S85 (1959b)

Sigg, E.B.: Tricyclic thymoleptic agents and some newer antidepressants. In: Neuropsychopharmacology. A Review of Progress. Efron, D.H. (ed.), pp. 655–669. Washington D.C.: U.S. Government Printing Office 1968

Sigg, E.B., Drakontides, A.B., Day, C.: Muscarinic inhibition of dendritic postsynaptic potentials in cat cortex. Int. J. Neuropharmacol. *4*, 281–289 (1965)

Sinha, J.N., Dixit, K.S., Srimal, R.C., Chandra, O., Bhargava, K.P.: Effect of amitryptiline and related drugs on neuromuscular transmission. Arch. Int. Pharmacodyn. Ther. *162*, 79–83 (1966)

Steiner, W.G., Himwich, H.E.: Effects of antidepressant drugs on limbic structures of rabbit. J. Nerv. Ment. Dis. *137*, 277–284 (1963 a)

Steiner, W.G., Himwich, H.E.: An electroencephalographic study of the blocking action of selected tranquilizers as functions of terminal methyl amine group. Biochem. Pharmacol. *12*, 678–691 (1963 b)

Steiner, W.G., Bost, K., Himwich, H.E.: An electroencephalic study of some structural aspects of d-amphetamine antagonism in phenothiazine and related compounds. Int. J. Neuropharmacol. *2*, 327–335 (1963 a)

Steiner, W.G., Pscheidt, G.R., Costa, E., Himwich, H.E.: α-Ethyltryptamine (etryptamine): an electroencephalographic, behavioral and neurochemical analysis. Psychopharmacologia *4*, 354–366 (1963 b)

Steiner, W.G., Pscheidt, G.R., Himwich, H.E.: Influence of methodology on electroencephalographic sleep and arousal: studies with reserpine and etrytamine in rabbits. Science *141*, 53–55 (1963 c)

Stille, G.: Zur pharmakologischen Prüfung von Antidepressiva am Beispiel eines Dibenzodiazepines. Arzneim. Forsch. *14*, 534–537 (1964)

Stille, G.: Discussion Working Group 5. In: Neuropsychopharmacology 4. Bente, D., Bradley, B. (eds.), pp. 211–214. Amsterdam: Elsevier Publ. Corp. 1965

Stille, G.: Pharmacological investigation of antidepressant compounds. Neuropsychopharmacology *1*, 92–106 (1968)

Stille, G.: Einfluß psychotroper Substanzen auf neurophysiologische Parameter bei Versuchstieren. Arzneim. Forsch. *24*, 1051–1057 (1974)

Stille, G., Sayers, A.: The effect of antidepressant drugs on the convulsive excitability of brain structures. Int. J. Neuropharmacol. *3*, 605–609 (1964)

Stille, G., Lauener, H., Eichenberger, E.: Ein pharmakologischer Vergleich klinisch gebräuchlicher Antidepressiva unter besonderer Berücksichtigung von Noveril (HF-1927 Wander). Schweiz. Med. Wochenschr. *95*, 366–372 (1965)

Stille, G., Lauener, H., Eichenberger, E.: Ein Antidepressivum aus der Gruppe der 2-Benzimidazoline. Int. Pharmakopsychiatry *1*, 214–220 (1968 a)

Stille, G., Lauener, H., Eichenberger, E., Matussek, N., Pöldinger, W.: Observations concerning adrenergic functions and antidepressant activity. Pharmakopsychiat. Neuro-Psychopharmakology *1*, 123–135 (1968 b)

Tan, Ü., Henatsch, H.-D.: Unterdrückung von rekurrenter und präsynaptischer Hemmung spinaler Motoneurone durch das Antidepressivum Imipramin (Tofranil). Pflüger's Arch. *300*, R 89-R 90 (1968)

Tan, Ü., Henatsch, H.-D.: Wirkungen von Imipramin auf die spinal motorischen Extensor- und Flexorsysteme der Katze. Naunyn-Schmiedeberg's Arch. Pharmacol. *262*, 337–357 (1969 a)

Tan, Ü., Henatsch, H.-D.: Differenzierung supraspinaler und spinaler Abgriffspunkte der Imipramin Wirkungen auf spinale Hemmungs- und Erregungssysteme. Pflüger's Arch. *307*, R120–R121 (1969 b)

Theobald, W., Büch, O., Kunz, H.A., Morpurgo, C., Stenger, E.G., Wilhelmi, G.: Vergleichende Pharmakologische Untersuchungen mit Tofranil®, Pertofran® und Insidon®. Arch. Int. Pharmacodyn. Ther. *148*, 560–596 (1964)

Tissot, R., Monnier, M.: Suppression de l'action de la réserpine sur le cerveaux par ses antagonistes: Iproniazid et L.S.D. Helv. Physiol. Acta *16*, 268–276 (1958)

Trimble, M., Anlezark, G., Meldrum, B.: Seizure activity in photosensitive baboons following antidepressant drugs and the role of serotonergic mechanisms. Psychopharmacologia *51*, 159–164 (1977)

Trujillo, G.D. de, Scotti de Carolis, A., Longo, V.G.: Influence of diazepam, l-dopa and dopa-mine on the cerebellar and spinal electrical patterns induced by harmine in the rabbit. Neuropharmacology *16*, 31–36 (1977)

Vane, J.R., Collier, H.O.J., Corne, S.J., Marley, E., Bradley, P.B.: Tryptamine receptors in the central nervous system. Nature *191*, 1068–1069 (1961)

Van Meter, W.G., Costa, E., Ayala, G.F., Himwich, H.E.: Behavioural, EEG and biochemical variations after the administration of alphamethyltryptamine (IT 403). Rec. Adv. Biol. Psy-chiatry *3*, 166–177 (1961)

Van Meter, W.G., Owens, H.F., Himwich, H.E.: Effects of tofranil, an antidepressant drug on electrical potentials of rabbit brain. Can. Psychiatr. Assoc. J. *4*, Spec. Suppl. S113–S118 (1959)

Van Riezen, H., Van Proosdij, J., Schönbaum, E.: Effects of various drugs supposed to interact with serotonin on PGO frequency changes induced by reserpine and 5-hydroxytrypto-phane. Monogr. Neurol. Sci. *3*, 37–44 (1976)

Vernier, V.G.: The pharmacology of antidepressant agents. Dis. Nerv. Syst. *22*, 7–13 (1961)

Wada, J.A.: Discussion. Ann. N.Y. Acad. Sci. *96*, 313 (1962)

Wallach, M.B., Winters, W.D., Mandell, A.J., Spooner, Ch.E.: A correlation of EEG, reticular multiple unit activity and cross behavior following various antidepressant agents in the cat. IV. Electroencephal. Clin. Neurophysiol. *27*, 563–573 (1969a)

Wallach, M.B., Winters, W.D., Mandell, A.J., Spooner, Ch.E.: Effect of antidepressant drugs on wakefulness and sleep in the cat. Electroencephal. Clin. Neurophysiol. *27*, 574–580 (1969b)

Watanabe, S., Ueki, S., Kawasaki, H.: Electroencephalographic effects of lopramine. Folia Pharmacol. Jpn. *72*, 153 (1976)

Weinstock, M., Cohen, D.: Tricyclic antidepressant drugs as antagonists of muscarinic recep-tors in sympathetic ganglia. Eur. J. Pharmacol. *40*, 321–328 (1976)

White, R.P., Drew, W.G., Fink, M.: Neuropharmacological analysis of agonistic actions of cyclazocine in rabbits. Biol. Psychiatry *1*, 317–330 (1969)

Wuttke, W., Hoffmeister, F.: Zur Frage pharmakologisch-klinischer Wirkungsbeziehungen bei Antidepressiva, dargestellt am Beispiel von Noxiptilin. 2. Mitteilung. Arzneim. Forsch. *19*, 462–464 (1969)

Supplementary References

Reference is not made to the following literature, which has appeared subsequently:

Koella, W.P., Glatt, A., Klebs, K., Dünst, T.: Epileptic phenomena induced in the cat by the antidepressants maprotiline, imipramine, clomipramine, and amitriptyline. Biol. Psychiatr. *14*, 485–497 (1979)

Montigny, C. de, Aghajanian, G.K.: Tricyclic antidepressants: long-term treatment increases responsibility of rat forebrain neurons to serotonin. Science *202*, 1303–1306 (1978)

Neal, H., Bradley, P.B.: Electrocortical changes in the encéphale isolé cat following chronic treatment with antidepressant drugs. Neuropharmacology *18*, 611–615 (1979)

Scuvée-Moreau, J.J., Dresse, A.: Effect of various antidepressant drugs on the spontaneous fir-ing rate of locus coeruleus and dorsal raphe neurons in the rat. Europ. J. Pharmacol. *57*, 219–225 (1979)

Wolfe, B.B., Harden, T.K., Sporn, J.R., Molinoff, P.B.: Presynaptic modulation of beta adren-ergic receptors in rat cerebral cortex after the treatment with antidepressants. J. Pharmacol. exp. Therap. *207*, 446–457 (1978)

CHAPTER 20

Clinical Neurophysiological Properties of Antidepressants

T.M. ITIL and C. SOLDATOS

A. Introduction

Electroencephalography (EEG), the major method of clinical neurophysiology has widely been used in psychopharmacology. It has led to the discovery of "drug-specific" neurophysiological profiles which reflect the changes of brain bioelectric activity induced by a CNS-active drug. Every substance which has a significant effect on human brain function also produces systematic and significant effects on EEG. The changes seen after administration of a CNS-active substance are invariably different from placebo-induced changes; and, what is more important, these are replicable. They follow the same general pattern after repeated administration in the same or even in different populations. Of course, there are intra- and interindividual differences in the neurophysiological response to a certain CNS-active substance, depending obviously on several factors, with the more prominent being the intra- and interindividual "biologic variability." The group response of several individuals to a therapeutically effective psychotropic drug, however, invariably shows a similar profile on repeated trials (ITIL, 1974).

It has been convincingly shown that drugs with similar CNS action produce similar neurophysiological profiles in humans. Even drugs belonging to different chemical groups, but having similar clinical (psychotropic) effects, show similar profiles. It appears that the kind of neurophysiological property determines the kind of clinical effect, i.e., the specific psychoactive property of a psychotropic drug. The hypothesis that the "physiological equivalency" is indicative of "therapeutic equivalency" has been validated in recent years by the discovery of psychotropic properties of a series of compounds by EEG alone (ITIL, 1972, 1978).

In the very early period of the development of psychiatric EEG research, it was observed that a certain psychological–behavioral state is accompanied by characteristic EEG changes. Thus, it is a common observation that a relaxed state is accompanied by more "synchrony" of brain rhythms, tension and excitability by "desynchronization" and faster rhythms, and a lower level of consciousness by appearance of slower rhythms. This is confirmed through drug studies using EEG analysis. For example, a drug having, or expected to have, sedative effects also produces, in general, an increase of slow EEG activity.

B. EEG Classification of Psychotropic Drugs

Through visual (eyeball or qualitative) EEG analysis, it was possible to adequately distinguish between drugs belonging to separate classes (ITIL, 1961, 1964). This is illustrated in Fig. 1.

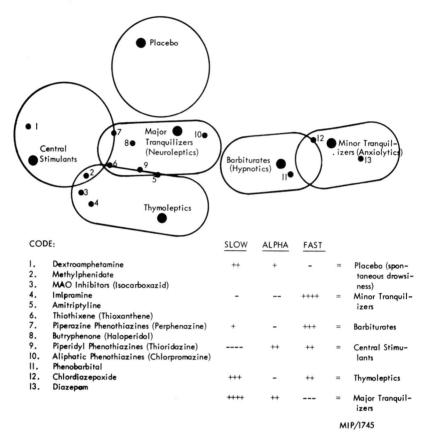

Fig. 1. According to visual classification, there is some overlap between major tranquilizers, central stimulants, and thymoleptics. Also, some of the minor tranquilizers showed effects similar to barbiturates, and vice versa

Nevertheless, some limited overlap between thymoleptics, major tranquilizers, and psychostimulants is also apparent. Drugs that are in the "border areas" in terms of their EEG properties also have clinical properties that are common to their class and to the adjacent class. For instance, thioridazine, which is basically a neuroleptic, also has thymoleptic properties and, its EEG profile, is closer to those of thymoleptics than, for example, that of chlorpromazine. Amitriptyline, a potent antidepressant, has more sedative properties than imipramine; based on its EEG profile, it is closer to sedative compounds than to stimulants.

Using the analog frequency analyzer, the qualitative EEG findings could indeed be confirmed. It was possible to discriminate the CNS effects of chlorpromazine (a neuroleptic), imipramine (an antidepressant) and chlordiazepoxide (an anxiolytic) from placebo (saline) and from each other in normal volunteers (Itil et al., 1968) (Fig. 2), and in schizophrenic patients (Itil et al., 1969).

The introduction of quantitative pharmaco-EEG (QPEEG™) using computer-analyzed EEG (CEEG™) further improved the EEG classification of drugs (Itil et al., 1971). Based on period analysis of the primary wave and the first derivative, it was

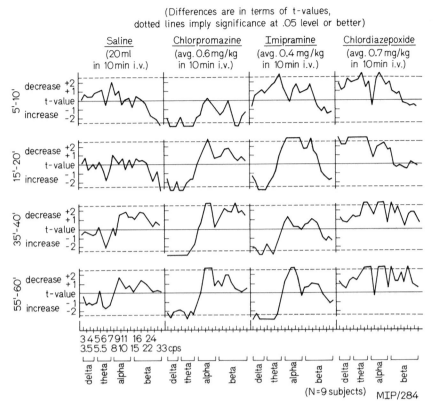

Fig. 2. EEG Drug profiles of chlorpromazine, imipramine, and chlordiazepoxide based on analog power spectra. The abscissa shows the frequency ranges of the analog frequency analyzer; the ordinate, the differences between pre- and post-drug (four different time periods) in terms of t-values. Downward deflection is increase of values and upward decrease of values in comparison to pre-drug measurements. After saline i.v., only one of 24 frequency bands showed, in two of four time periods, statistically significant changes in comparison to pre-drug values (increase of 33 cps activity). After 0.6 mg chlorpromazine/kg (administered in 10 min i.v.), a statistically significant increase of delta and theta frequencies in all time periods was observed. Fast activity increased only during 5–10 min after administration, while fast α activity decreased in three of the four time periods. After imipramine (0.4 mg/kg in 10 min i.v.) slow waves also statistically increased, and there was an increase of fast activities (without reaching the level of statistical significance) in all four time periods. Chlordiazepoxide (administered 0.7 mg/kg in 10 min, i.v.) showed significantly different EEG profiles from those of imipramine and chlorpromazine. Slow waves and α activity decreased and fast waves showed some increase in the first two time periods. (From ITIL, T.M., et al.: Agressologie 9 (2), 267–280, (1968)

possible to discriminate between four basic groups of psychotropic drugs: Neuroleptics (major tranquilizers), anxiolytics (minor tranquilizers), psychostimulants, and thymoleptics (antidepressants) (Fig. 3) (ITIL, 1974).

Repeated studies with drugs having similar clinical effects gave similar CEEG profiles. The antidepressant CEEG profile for the primary wave of the digital computer period analysis is remarkably characterized by an increase of slow activity, a decrease of alpha activity, and an increase of fast frequency levels. In the first derivative

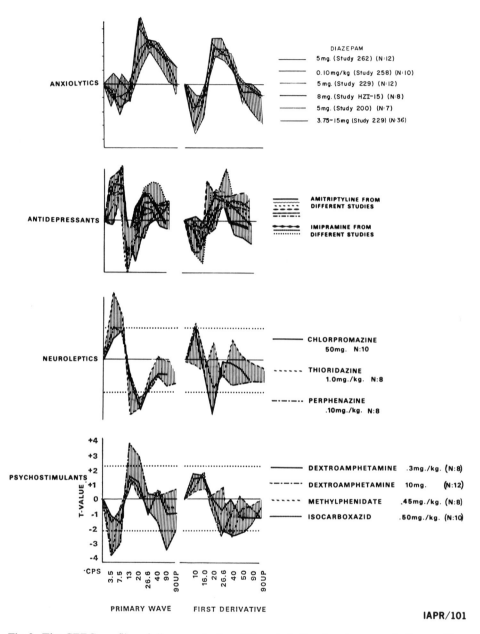

Fig. 3. The CEEG profiles of diazepam in five different studies showing very similar profiles. Amitriptyline in nine studies and imipramine in three studies show similar profiles. Thus, the characteristic CEEG profile of antidepressants is established (increase of fast and slow activities, decrease of α waves in the primary wave measurements, and decrease of slow and increase of faster potentials in the first derivative measurements)

Neuroleptics, such as chlorpromazine, thioridazine, and perphenazine, produce similar CEEG profiles in three different studies. Psychostimulants (dextroamphetamine in two studies, methylphenidate and isocarboxazide) produce similar profiles as typical for psychostimulant compounds

measurements a decrease of slow and increase of fast waves were observed. All tricyclic antidepressants showed similar EEG pattern. Drugs belonging to other classes, but having some antidepressant action, also had similarities to that profile. New drugs that were not expected to be antidepressants from animal pharmacology, but which showed an "antidepressant" CEEG profile, were confirmed through clinical studies to have antidepressant properties.

C. Method of EEG Analysis

Three different methods of EEG quantifications were used in psychopharmacology: Digital computer period analysis, power spectrum, and amplitude integration. The effects of most of the psychotropic drugs on EEG were studied using period analysis (BURCH et al., 1964). Recently, computer programs were developed which permit simultaneous analysis by both period analysis and power spectral density analysis (ITIL et al., 1971). In general, period analysis seems to be more illustrative in detecting the type of psychotropic properties of drugs, partly because most psychotropic drug experiences were gathered with this method, and a large computer data base is available. Power spectrum analysis is a powerful method for discriminating drug effects from placebo.

Another EEG analytical method is the one that focuses on amplitude rather than frequency measurements of the brain activity (DROHOCKI, 1937). Some investigators (GOLDSTEIN, 1974; MARJERRISON, 1974) have very successfully used the mean integrated amplitude (MIA) in drug studies. In the new computer analysis systems, the EEG amplitude measurements are included as another parameter to the frequency measurements of the primary wave and the first derivative in both period analysis and power spectrum.

D. EEG Findings in Depression

LEMERE (1941) was the first to report that manic-depressive patients tend to have a large amplitude, strongly dominant α rhythm. DAVIS (1941, 1942) confirmed LEMERE's finding showing that manic-depressed individuals have more α-type EEGs compared with schizophrenics, that predominantly depressed patients have more α-type and mixed α and slow activity EEGs, whereas predominantly manic patients have more mixed α and fast activity EEGs. GREENBLATT et al., 1944, further discriminated the manic patients, based on the large amount of fast activity found in his manic group. HURST et al. (1954) also found that manic patients have higher α frequencies than the depressed patients, but they did not show a shift in α frequency accompanying the phase change whenever a manic-depressive patient shifted from mania to depression or from depression to mania. On the contrary, HARDING et al. (1966) observed an increase in α frequency during manic episodes of two manic-depressive patients.

Through visual analysis of the EEGs of 73 schizophrenics and 100 endogenous depressed patients, it was shown that there is a significant relationship between alpha dominance and depression, and β dominance and schizophrenia (ITIL, 1964). BREZINOVA et al. (1966) reported a greater abundance of α rhythm in patients with endogenous depression. VOLAVKA et al. (1967) compared the EEGs of five depressed patients during the episodes of depression and during remission. The patients showed significantly more α and β activities during the depressive phase.

Several investigators tried to relate the occurrence of clinical EEG abnormalities with depression. The results are contradictory; in spite of the fact that this is partly due to the application of different criteria of EEG abnormality by various investigators, it appears that there are no confirmed specific, clinically abnormal EEG findings for depression, at least at a gross visual analysis level. If an increased incidence of EEG abnormalities in depression could be definitely established, it would be an indication of brain dysfunction. However, the clinical significance of the "abnormal" EEG would still be doubtful since the various abnormalities reported in depressed patients are rather minor and nonspecific. FEHLOW (1974), reporting a high incidence of EEG "abnormality" in 200 depressed patients (45.5%), and an even higher incidence in 100 schizophrenics (57%), includes in the "abnormalities" an unspecified dysrhythmia and even a reduction of α rhythm. This exemplifies the above-mentioned methodological considerations and the validity of reported EEG findings in terms of their clinical significance.

In conclusion, although there is no pathognomonic EEG pattern in depression, it appears that depression is generally related to an increased amount of α activity. This is the common finding of various studies both comparative and serial. This, if confirmed in a large study using quantitative EEG analysis, is a very important finding since many well-controlled studies demonstrate that the EEG pattern of schizophrenia is characterized by a decrease of the amount of α waves (ITIL et al., 1972c; ITIL, 1977a). Accordingly, the EEG patterns of schizophrenia and depression may almost be diametrically opposite. This indicates that the electrophysiological correlates of both illnesses are different, suggesting different biochemical bases of schizophrenia and depression. These findings support the fact that drugs effective in depressive illness are ineffective in schizophrenia patients, and they may even exacerbate the schizophrenic symptomatology. From all existing evidence, it seems likely that the decrease of α activity, induced by the antidepressants, has a corrective function, given the commonly found abundance of α waves in depression.

E. EEG Findings with Antidepressants

The EEG findings on the effects of antidepressants have been obtained using either visual or computer analysis of the EEGs. Visual EEG analysis is usually qualitative, producing information on the abnormal wave-forms and only to a limited extent is it quantitative. Computer EEG analysis, using analog or digital systems, is almost exclusively quantitative and does not usually provide information on pathological EEG findings of clinical relevance. Ideally both qualitative and quantitative aspects of the EEG analysis should be thoroughly covered in any drug study. In our studies we invariably combine the precision of computerized quantification of the EEG with the clinical usefulness of the qualitative (visual) EEG interpretation.

I. Drugs Commonly Used as Antidepressants

This group includes drugs widely used in clinical practice for their antidepressant effects, and they may be known primarily as antidepressants (e.g., tricyclics) or as belonging to other drug classes but having antidepressant action in addition to their primary effects (e.g., antidepressant MAO inhibitors, thioridazine, etc.).

1. Tricyclic Antidepressants

a) Imipramine

Imipramine was found by FINK (1959) to increase slow waves as well as superimposed fast activity in the EEG. Using an analog frequency analyzer, FINK (1961) described the differences in EEG alterations between chlorpromazine, a major tranquilizer, and imipramine, an antidepressant. Later in another study he showed that imipramine produces, in addition to slow waves, a decrease of α activity and an increase of fast β (FINK, 1965).

According to investigations using analog power spectra after acute intravenous administration of imipramine, it was observed that the basic characteristics of imipramine-induced alterations are an increase of power in slow frequencies, a decrease of α and slow β frequencies, and an increase of faster activities (Fig. 2) (ITIL, 1968). The chlorpromazine-induced alterations in normal volunteers were similar to imipramine in all time periods (15–20, 35–40, 55–60 min) except 5–10 min after i. v. administration. Chlordiazepoxide produced EEG alterations, based on analog frequency analyzer, that were very different from those induced by chlorpromazine and imipramine. Similar findings were obtained when imipramine and chlorpromazine were intravenously administered in a group of schizophrenic patients (Fig. 4) (ITIL et al., 1969).

According to our studies with digital computer period analysis, the CEEG profiles of imipramine are characterized by an increase of slow waves as well as fast β activity and a decrease of α waves in the primary wave measurements, along with a decrease of slow and an increase of fast activity in the first derivative measurements (Fig. 5).

This CEEG profile is quite similar to the one of amitriptyline. In comparison to amitriptyline, however, it was observed that imipramine in some populations decreases, not increases, very slow activity (1.3–3.5 cps), while increasing fast activities. CEEG profiles of imipramine are also similar at different time periods. In general, the changes lessen 6 h after oral drug administration. The CEEG changes induced by imipramine are significantly time and dose related. This suggests the CEEG is an accurate method of determining the bioavailability of antidepressive compounds and of studying the pharmacodynamics of psychotropic drugs at the CNS level (FINK, 1974; ITIL, 1977 b). As mentioned above, CEEG alterations induced by imipramine could be statistically discriminated not only from diazepam, but also from amitriptyline. Imipramine, compared mg per mg to amitriptyline, produces fewer slow waves but more fast activities, supporting the clinical findings that imipramine has more "stimulatory" and fewer "sedative" properties than does amitriptyline.

Although, as is known, imipramine was initially investigated as an antiepileptic compound, an increase in epileptic potentials was reported in some subjects during treatment with imipramine (BORENSTEIN and DABBAH, 1959 a; DELAY et al., 1959; MENGOLI and MACCAGNANI, 1959; KUGLER, 1960). Due to the increase of epileptic activity in the EEG, it was suggested that caution be exercized in giving imipramine to epileptic patients (VAN METER et al., 1959; ZAPPOLI, 1959; HARRER, 1960). Even with relatively low doses (50 mg, i. m.) BORENSTEIN and DABBAH (1959 a) observed activation of sharp waves, spikes, and paroxysmal patterns in epileptic patients (in 75%) as well as in nonepileptic patients (in 50%). KILOH et al. (1961) reported an increase of epileptic potentials after relatively high single doses (75 mg) in 18 of 36 epileptics; however, not one case was found in 24 nonepileptic patients.

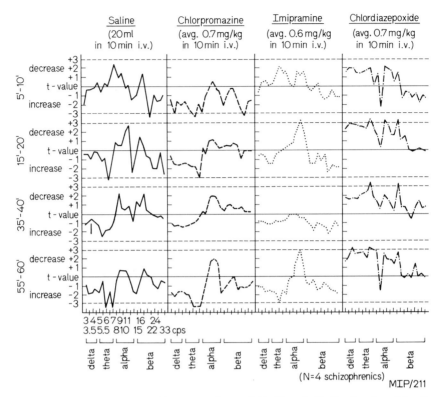

Fig. 4. Changes 55–60 min after chlorpromazine and 15–20 and 55–60 min after chlordiazepoxide in EEG power spectra in a group of schizophrenic patients. After saline and imipramine changes in single frequency bands are observed. (Differences are in terms of t-values. Dotted lines imply significance at 0.04 level.)

Actual epileptic seizures were increased with doses of imipramine much larger than the usual therapeutic dose, e. g., with 800 mg (Brooke and Weatherly, 1959), 1250 mg (Levene and Lasceles, 1959), 2500 mg (Moll, 1959). According to Kiloh et al. (1961), although imipramine may provoke epileptic attacks even in therapeutic doses, treatment of epileptic patients with depression is not contradictory. Increasing the daily dosage of the antiepileptic medication is in most cases a sufficient prophylactic measure.

More recently, the antiepileptic properties of imipramine are once again stressed. Zurabashvili (1969), in his review of animal tests and human clinical observations on the pharmacological action and therapeutic efficacy of imipramine, claims that the positive effect of this drug on depression of almost any possible etiology resides ultimately in its ability to "normalize" the EEG. Fromm et al. (1972) reported the value of imipramine in the treatment of petit mal epilepsy. Fowler and Julien (1974) investigated the effect of imipramine on experimental petit mal in cats. They found that 1.0–5.0 mg imipramine/kg effectively blocks the 3 Hz spike-wave discharges induced by estrogen. Doses above 5.0 mg/kg did not produce further improvement; on the contrary, they elicited a polyspike EEG pattern. Even higher doses were associated

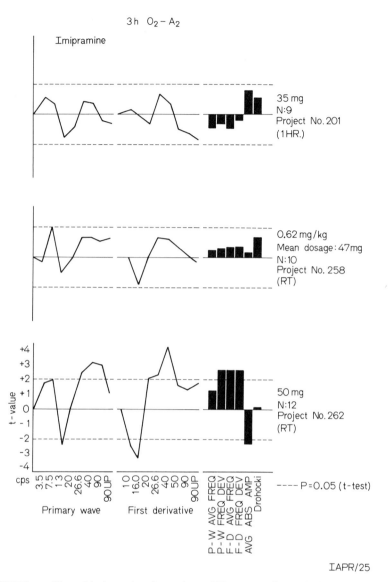

Fig. 5. CEEG profiles of imipramine from three different studies. All three CEEG profiles show similarity in shape both in primary wave and first derivative measurements (the lower the dosage, the lesser the quantity of the changes)

with major seizures. It appears that low doses of imipramine, comparable to the ones used in clinical practice, do not have the serious epileptogenic properties of the higher doses. There is even some evidence that low doses of imipramine can be beneficial to petit mal epilepsy. However, special caution is necessary when the drug is given to children, in terms of not reaching higher doses and not extending the treatment over prolonged periods of time.

b) Amitriptyline

Quantitative EEG analysis demonstrated that amitriptyline not only decreases α
rhythms and increases slow potentials, as reported earlier by BORENSTEIN et al. (1962)
and DAVISON (1965), but also produces high frequency nonrhythmical fast activity
(FINK and ITIL, 1968). These changes are similar in most respects to those of imipramine ("thymoleptic EEG reaction type") (ITIL, 1964, 1968); however, amitriptyline induces less fast activity than does imipramine.

According to a series of studies, after single oral dosages of 10–75 mg, amitriptyline produced statistically significant alterations in EEG within 1 h of oral administration which lasted up to at least 6 h. The computer EEG profile of amitriptyline is characterized by an increase of slow waves (1.3–3.5 and 3.5–7.5 cps bands), decrease of α

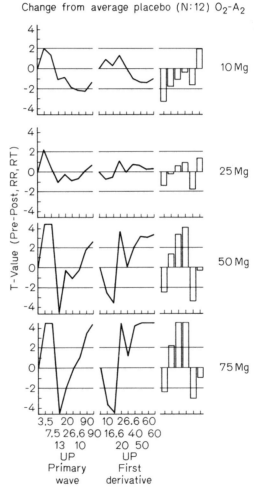

Fig. 6. Amitriptyline computer EEG profiles at different time periods. The abscissa and ordinate are the same as in Fig. 1. Amitriptyline-induced changes are very similar during the first,
third, and sixth hours after oral administration. (From ITIL, T.M.: Psychotropic Drugs and the
Human EEG, S. Karger A.G., Basel, New York)

activity (7.5–13 cps), and increase of fast waves over 20 cps (Fig. 6). The first derivative measurements (superimposed activities on top of the primary wave) show a decrease of activities up to 16 cps and increase up to 90 cps. There is a decrease of zero cross average frequency and average absolute amplitude, an increase of zero cross frequency deviation, first derivative average frequency and frequency deviation, and amplitude variability (DROHOCKI, 1937). The computer EEG profiles of amitriptyline show remarkable similarities at different time periods after administration and after different dosage, particularly in primary wave measurements.

Also, in different studies (populations) amitriptyline computer EEG profiles showed outstanding similarities (Fig. 7).

The consistency of the quality as well as the increasing quantity of CEEG profiles after increasing dosages of amitriptyline again indicates that this method is a useful tool for determining the bioavailability of psychotropic drugs at the CNS level.

During chronic multiple oral dose administration, the computer EEG profile of amitriptyline is similar to that of single dose except that instead of an increase, a decrease of fast activities was observed in the primary wave measurements.

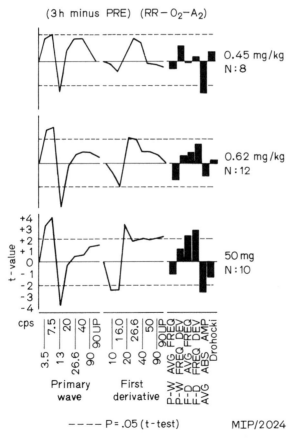

Fig. 7. The abscissa and ordinate are the same in Fig. 1. Although there are some differences in dosages, amitriptyline produces very similar CEEG profiles in different populations

Activation of paroxysmal activity in the EEG during amitriptyline treatment was seen particularly in epileptic patients (Davison, 1965). The occurrence of epileptic seizures during amitriptyline medication (particularly in high dosages) has also been reported (Davies and Allaye, 1963). Betts et al. (1968) reported seven patients who had grand mal epileptic fits in relation to amitriptyline treatment. All but one of the patients experienced seizures only while on the drug and always within a few days of either starting medication or changing to a higher dose: the other patient did have a previous epileptic history, but had not had fits for many years. Two patients had EEG findings of epileptogenic activity, but no clinical evidence. A further two patients had slight brain damage. In addition, we found (Gannon et al., 1970) that a grand mal seizure may occur after discontinuation of amitriptyline treatment. This particular patient had no history of epilepsy and showed no epileptic activity in his EEG either before and during the treatment, or after the grand mal seizure.

Amitriptyline appears to be more epileptogenic than imipramine. This is obviously due to its more sedative properties. It has been our general observation that psychotropic drugs with more sedative properties are also more epileptogenic. In clinical practice, however, these epileptogenic properties should be considered as negligible, unless the drug is going to be given to patients with seizure disorders or lowered convulsive thresholds. In these cases, psychotropic drugs with sedative properties (e. g., amitriptyline) can be given only if necessary and with special caution, particularly during the initial period of the treatment and shortly after discontinuation. Large doses and sudden dose changes should be avoided.

c) Protriptyline

Similar dosages of amitriptyline and imipramine produce almost identical CEEG profiles even in different populations such as U.S. and Turkish subjects (Itil, 1975), indicating not only extreme sensitivity of the method but also relative "specificity" of these tricyclic antidepressants as far as their effect on brain function is concerned. However, protriptyline's CEEG profile depends very much on the types of subjects studied (biologic variability). Our investigations demonstrated that subjects with fast β EEGs before protriptyline administration showed different CEEG profiles than did those subjects with α or slow EEGs. We found that protriptyline's CEEG profile in low dosages (5–10 mg) seems to resemble imipramine (fewer slow waves and more fast activity than imipramine), while in higher dosages (20 and 40 mg) protriptyline's profile shows more similarity to psychostimulant compounds (decrease of slow waves, increase of α and slow β activity (Fig. 8).

Protriptyline-induced CEEG changes are most marked during 1 h (with amitriptyline during 3 h) after oral administration. Statistically significant dose-related alterations (dose response curves) with protriptyline were seen only at 1 h after oral administration and only in four of 22 EEG measurements. In dosage ranges of 5–40 mg (mean 18.7 mg) protriptyline could be significantly differentiated from amitriptyline (dose ranges 10–75 mg, mean 40 mg) but not from imipramine (50 mg).

d) Nortriptyline

Nortriptyline showed in our studies definite antidepressant profiles similar to the ones of amitriptyline and imipramine. One hour after administration of nortriptyline, the quantitative changes were less that after 3 h. The 3-h EEG recording showed an increase of slow waves, decrease of α, and increase of fast activities in primary wave

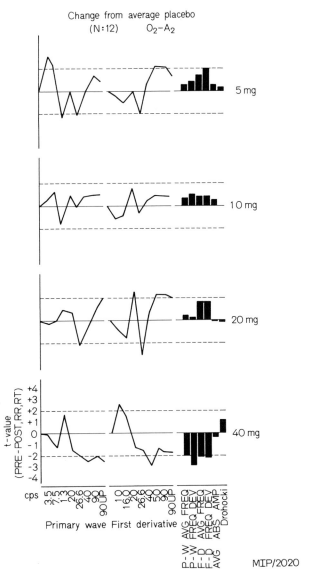

Fig. 8. The CEEG profiles of protriptyline showed similarity to psychostimulant compounds when it was administered in 40 mg dosages. However, after 5 mg and, to a lesser degree, after 10 mg, an increase of slow waves are seen which are indicative of the CNS inhibitory properties of this compound

measurements and decrease of slow and increase of fast activity in the first derivative measurements (Fig. 9).

e) Desmethylimipramine

Desmethylimipramine is a metabolite of imipramine that has also been found to be an effective antidepressant. It generally has more stimulatory effects than imipramine. The CEEG profile of desmethylimipramine corresponds to its clinical action. It does

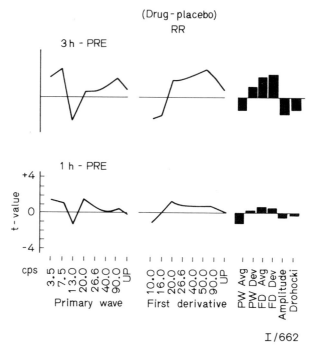

I/662

Fig. 9. There are no systematic changes 1 h after nortriptyline. However, 3 h after administration there is the characteristic antidepressant CEEG drug profile

produce less slow waves than imipramine, which means that it has less sedative properties and more fast activity and which is an indication of its stimulatory effect.

Our investigations with high dosage of desmethylimipramine (400 mg) showed an increase of sharp waves and spikes but no grand mal seizures when the drug was given to schizophrenic patients. Mᴀɴɴ (1962) and Mᴇᴅᴜɴᴀ et al. (1961) advised caution when this drug is used in epileptic patients.

f) Doxepine

According to Fɪɴᴋ (1974) a quantitative EEG study of doxepine revealed CEEG alterations similar to imipramine's. Since this compound also produces changes in frequency ranges similar to the ones produced by diazepam and other anxiolytic compounds, the anxiolytic properties of doxepine, in addition to its antidepressant effects, were predicted. This is in accordance with the clinical findings of depressive patients with anxiety (Sɪᴍᴇᴏɴ et al., 1969).

2. MAO Inhibitors

a) Tranylcypromine

Of the MAO inhibiting antidepressants, tranylcypromine has CEEG profiles in quality similar to the tricyclic antidepressants. After the administration of 10 mg tranylcypromine to a group of normal healthy volunteers, typical EEG alterations were observed 3 h after oral administration and lasted up to 24 h. Computer EEG profiles of

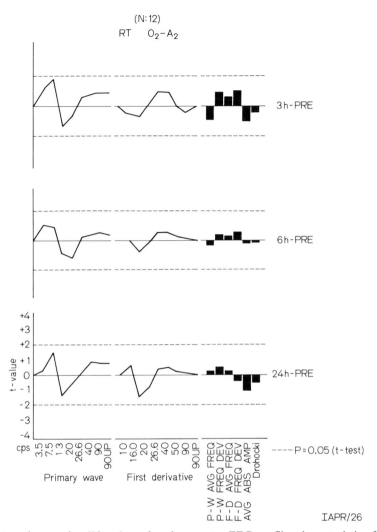

Fig. 10. Oral tranylcypromine (10 mg) produced computer EEG profiles characteristic of tricyclic antidepressants with increase of slow and fast waves and decrease of α activities. Changes in this population did not reach the level of statistical significance in any of the time periods. However, even 24 h after a single-dose oral administration, there is a typical CEEG profile, similar to 3 and 6 h after drug administration

tranylcypromine are characterized by an increase of slow waves, decrease of α, and increase of fast activities in the primary wave measurements and decrease of slow and increase of 20–40 cps activities in the first derivative measurements (Fig. 10).

The response to tranylcypromine is very much subject dependent. In comparison to amitriptyline or even imipramine, a lesser number of subjects respond to tranylcypromine with "typical" CEEG profiles of tricyclic antidepressants (high biologic variability). This results in less quantitative changes (changes do not always reach the level of statistical significance).

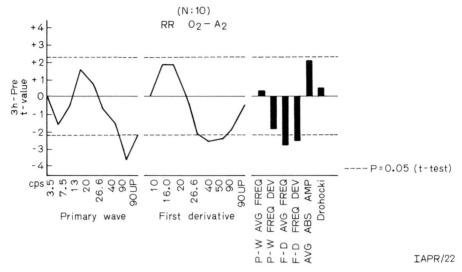

Fig. 11. A single oral dose of 0.5 mg isocarboxazid/kg produced an increase of activities in 13–20 cps in both primary wave and first derivative measurements. There was a decrease of very slow waves in the primary wave measurements and a decrease of very fast activity in both primary wave and first derivative measurements. Isocarboxazid, although an MAO inhibitor, showed computer EEG profiles similar to psychomotor stimulants

b) Isocarboxazide

Our investigations demonstrated that isocarboxazide produces statistically significant EEG alterations after single oral dosages of 0.5 mg/kg. The CEEG profiles of isocarboxazide are characterized by an increase of the 13–20 cps activities but decrease of slower and faster frequencies in the primary wave measurements (Fig. 11).

The superimposed activities up to 16 cps showed an increase, and at the higher frequencies, a decrease. According to CEEG profiles, isocarboxazide does indeed show alterations more similar to the central stimulant compounds than to the tricyclic antidepressants or the other antidepressant MAO inhibitor, tranylcypromine.

c) Iproniazid

Iproniazid produces a slight increase of slow potentials and a marked increase of fast activity in the EEG. Pisanty (1959), Grisoni et al. (1959), and Santanelli et al. (1961) reported the suppression of epileptic activity in the EEG and a decrease in the number of grand mal seizures during iproniazid treatment of epileptic patients. Neither a significant increase of epileptic potentials in the EEG nor the occurrence of epileptic seizures has been reported during treatment of depressive patients with iproniazid.

d) Nialamide

Nialamide, another antidepressive MAO inhibitor, produces fast β activity and some 5–7 cps theta waves in the EEG. Sharp (1960) found an increase of epileptic seizures during nialamide treatment, whereas Benassi and Bertolotti (1960) suggested using it in combination with anti-epileptics for the control of grand mal seizures in patients with uncontrolled epilepsy.

3. Inorganic Salts

a) Lithium

Lithium carbonate is extensively used in the treatment of manic-depressive psychosis. It reduces manic symptomatology and it has a prophylactic effect in the occurrence of both manic and depressive episodes.

We studied the EEG effects of lithium with the analog frequency analyzer in manic patients, and with computer period analysis in normal volunteers. It was established that lithium produces marked alterations in brain function in daily dosages of 800 mg. Lithium-induced EEG alterations are characterized by a decrease of α activity and an increase of slow waves with superimposed fast activities. These EEG findings resemble those seen after anticholinergic thymoleptics, and particularly, anticholinergic hallucinogens (ITIL and AKPINAR, 1971). The major differences from anticholinergic drugs were a marked increase of epileptic potentials and an increase of synchronization and rhythmical activity after lithium; these are some of the characteristic changes seen after chlorpromazine. A shift of EEG energy patterns to slow frequencies is reported by SATTERFIELD (1974). HENIGER (1974), using a neuropsychological testing strategy in studying 40 patients receiving lithium carbonate, found an increase of EEG theta intensity along with several other changes in the performance tests. Based on his findings, he hypothesized that a unique type of cortical synchronization serves as an important mechanism involved in the therapeutic effect of lithium on manic symptomatology.

There are striking similarities between the EEG patterns produced by lithium and the ones seen after E.C.T. Activation of latent epileptic foci has been found during lithium treatment and KALINOWSKY and HOCH (1961) reported epileptic seizures in patients taking the drug. An EEG pattern of high amplitude, slow and sharp waves, or even spike and wave complexes, was not an infrequent finding in some of our patients while on lithium treatment (Fig. 12).

REILLY et al. (1973) studied 12 healthy subjects given placebo for 2 weeks, and lithium carbonate for 2 subsequent weeks. Six of the subjects showed EEG abnor-

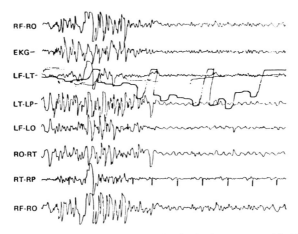

Fig. 12. Occurrence of generalized paroxysmal dysrhythmic groups with high voltage slow waves and sharp waves. No epileptic seizures

malities with lithium. Two of the six had normal, and four abnormal, pre-lithium EEG. The dominant frequency underwent a significant slowing, whereas it appeared that previously existing abnormalities were accentuated. Gottschalk and Sack (1973) found an increased percentage of EEG pathology and a frequent activation of very slight EEG changes in patients during lithium treatment. They could not determine a relationship between the degree of EEG changes and the serum levels of lithium. Okuma et al. (1974) reported that about half of their 23 manic-depressive patients with normal pretreatment EEGs developed EEG abnormalities after taking lithium carbonate for a period varying from 3 days to 2 years. It has been suggested that lithium-induced EEG changes may reflect the presence of therapeutic effect. However, Bily et al. (1973) who studied 27 manic-depressive patients, could not correlate the treatment outcome with the EEG findings.

In spite of the commonly accepted epileptogenic properties of lithium, a beneficial effect of the drug on epileptic seizures has also been reported (Gershon, 1968). Erwin et al. (1973) studied 17 patients with epileptic EEGs in a 6 week lithium treatment (serum level 0.6–1.25 mcg/litre) and found a clear reduction of discharge rate in 9 patients, no change in 7, and a tremendous increase in one only. The clinical changes paralleled the EEG findings. Jus et al. (1973) did not observe any change of the EEG patterns of 18 patients with temporal lobe epilepsy after single dose lithium administration. In a second phase of their study, they randomly selected 8 patients to whom they started giving 600 mg lithium daily. They had to interrupt the treatment 2 weeks later because the number of seizures increased in 3 patients, the behavior was impaired in 4, and the EEG pathology augmented in 5. The issue of the therapeutic effect of lithium in epilepsy still remains controversial. It would be safer to avoid use of lithium in epileptic patients until judgment can be based on definitive studies.

The CEEG profiles of lithium according to the computer period analysis showed an increase of slow and fast activities decrease of α waves in primary wave measurements, decrease of slow and increase of fast activity in the first derivative measurements. Accordingly, the CEEG profiles of lithium resemble those of tricyclic antidepressants. Lithium differed from tricyclic antidepressants in that lithium-induced slow waves were slower and fast waves were faster than those of tricyclic antidepressants.

4. Miscellaneous Antidepressants

a) Dibenzepin

EEG changes during dibenzepin treatment include synchronization of α activity, intensification of pathological changes existing prior to treatment, and appearance of paroxysmal potentials and slow wave activity (Zakowska-Dabrowska and Strzyzewski, 1972).

b) Opipramol

Opipramol was found comparable to imipramine in its therapeutic action as well as in its influence on the EEG (Ekiert et al., 1973). The EEG changes, however, did not correlate with clinical improvement. Patients with CNS lesion or abnormal pretreatment EEGs showed more EEG changes with opipramol.

II. Drugs Belonging to Other Classes but Having Some Antidepressant Properties

1. Neuroleptics with Antidepressant Properties

a) Thioridazine ✓ Mellaril

Thioridazine is unique among the neuroleptics for its antidepressant properties at the clinical level. In our studies after single dosages of 50 mg, the computer EEG profile of thioridazine in primary wave measurements is typical for major tranquilizers (antipsychotics) (ITIL, 1974). In the first derivative measurements, however, there are obvious similarities to the thymoleptic drugs with decrease of slow waves and increase of superimposed fast activities. Accordingly, we stated that among the antipsychotic phenothiazines, thioridazine is probably the one which shows the closest similarities in CEEG profiles to those of antidepressant drugs. In an earlier study using thiopental-activated EEG, the significant differences between perphenazine and thioridazine were demonstrated (ITIL, 1964).

There have been relatively few reports of an increase of epileptic activity in the EEG during thioridazine treatment (MAYER, 1959). In our various studies, we have observed grand mal seizures in only two patients with thioridazine and these seizures promptly disappeared after daily doses of 400 mg were discontinued. Thioridazine has been reported to be effective in epileptic patients with behavior disorders without markedly increasing epileptic seizures (FRAIN, 1960; PAUIG et al., 1961). A decrease of epileptic potentials in the EEG was observed when thioridazine was given in combination with chlordiazepoxide (ITIL et al., 1967a). During combined treatment, involving thioridazine with diphenylhydantoin, a decrease of epileptic potentials and improvement in behavior were observed in behaviorally disturbed children and adolescents (ITIL et al., 1967b).

b) Thiothixene

Thiothixene, a potent antipsychotic, was reported to have central stimulatory properties based on clinical trials. In our investigations using digital computer analysis of the EEG, we reported that thiothixene produces slow activities in addition to superimposed fast activities (similar to tricyclic antidepressants) during resting EEG (ITIL et al., 1972b). Although thiothixene EEG profiles in primary wave measurements are very similar to the major tranquilizers, in the first derivative measurements there is an increase of superimposed fast activities (decrease of fast activity with major tranquilizers). In our studies with thiothixene, not a single case of clinical seizure was observed and the EEG patterns did not include epileptiform potentials.

c) Molindone

Molindone, an oxygenated indole derivative, has been found to be effective in acute and chronic schizophrenic patients. Our EEG investigations (ITIL et al., 1970) have confirmed that this compound has an EEG profile similar to the "major tranquilizer reaction type", primarily because of the increase of very slow and decrease of fast activity. Strong similarities to the psychostimulant CEEG profile also became obvious because of the increase of α waves in combination with the decrease of β and the slight decrease of theta. Stimulating properties of the drug were confirmed clinically. Clinical antidepressive properties of molindone were suggested in depressive patients with psychomotor retardation.

2. Psychostimulants

Psychostimulants in general have mood-elevating properties. Both dextroamphetamine and methylphenidate have been given to patients with psychopathology that includes depression.

a) Dextroamphetamine

Our series of investigations have clearly shown that dextroamphetamine, after single oral dosages of 10–20 mg, produces statistically significant alterations in the brain function of normal healthy volunteers. The CEEG profiles of dextroamphetamine are characterized by a decrease of slow waves, an increase of activities in the ranges of 13–26 cps, and a decrease of faster frequencies in the primary wave measurements.

The CEEG alterations in general are more obvious in the primary wave measurements than in the first derivative. The effects of dextroamphetamine are seen within 1 h of oral administration and last at least up to 6 h.

b) Methylphenidate

The CEEG profiles of methylphenidate in dosages of 0.45 mg/kg are very similar to those seen after dextroamphetamine. In comparison to 0.3 mg dextroamphetamine/kg, methylphenidate in this dosage produces more α activity and slow β waves, but a lesser degree of theta and delta activity. The marked effects of methylphenidate on computer EEG are seen relatively late (6 h after oral administration).

III. Drugs Predicted as Antidepressants Based on their CEEG Profiles

1. Drugs Predicted by Animal Pharmacology as Antidepressants, and Confirmed Based on CEEG Profiles

a) Sedative Type

α) *Amoxapine.* Amoxapine, a compound chemically and pharmacologically similar to imipramine and amitriptyline, was predicted to be an antidepressant. In a quantitative pharmaco-EEG study, we found that amoxapine in dosages of 6.25 mg, 12.5 mg, 25 mg, 50 mg, and 75 mg, but particularly in dosages of 25 and 50 mg, showed CEEG profiles similar to those seen after 25 mg imipramine (Fig. 13). However, interestingly, amoxapine did not produce very fast activities in either primary wave or first derivative measurements in any of the dosages between 6.25 and 75 mg. In contrast, the 75 mg amoxapine profile showed alterations very similar to thioridazine, a major tranquilizer. Accordingly, based on CEEG profiles, we predict that amoxapine in dosages of 25–50 mg would have imipramine-like clinical effects, while in 75 mg and higher dosages it may act similar to the sedative effective major tranquilizers such as thioridazine.

β) *Fluvoxamine.* Fluvoxamine has been predicted by animal pharmacology to have antidepressant properties in humans. It is quite effective in inhibiting serotonin

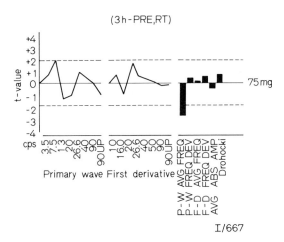

(3h-PRE,RT)

Fig. 13. After 75 mg amoxapine there was a decrease of α and slow β activity and an increase of slow waves and fast potentials in the primary wave measurement, and increase of 20–40 cps activities in the first derivative measurements

uptake by blood platelets and brain synaptosomes whereas, in contrast to tricyclic antidepressants, it has little effect, if any, on the norepinephrine uptake processes. In our studies, the CEEG profiles of fluvoxamine, particularly in the 50 mg and 75 mg dosages, were found to be similar to the CEEG profile of imipramine (Fig. 14).

According to its CEEG profile that was characterized by more fast activity and less slow waves compared with imipramine, we noted that fluvoxamine shows more similarity to "stimulant" antidepressants such as protriptyline (ITIL et al., 1977a).

γ) *Fluotracen.* Fluotracen, a unique chemical entity, has a pharmacologic profile indicative of both antidepressant and neuroleptic activity. We have shown that in lower dosage fluotracen has a sedative type of CEEG profile, whereas in higher doses its CEEG profile is very similar to that of amitriptyline (ITIL et al., 1977b) (Fig. 15).

The clinical trials demonstrate the potent antidepressant properties of fluotracen in depressed patients. Fluotracen was found to produce slightly more EEG abnormalities than amitriptyline, mainly in the form of irregular paroxysmal groups. This may be related to the sedative effects of the drug. No clinical seizure activity was observed.

δ) *Viloxazine.* Viloxazine is a β receptor blocker analog, found effective in depressive patients. The CEEG profiles of low dosages of viloxazine are similar to the CEEG profiles of "psychostimulant" compounds such as desipramine and dextroamphetamine (Fig. 16a).

In higher dosages the CEEG profile of viloxazine resembled more the CEEG profile of the "sedative" type of antidepressant such as amitriptyline (Fig. 16b). Therefore, we predicted that viloxazine in low doses is expected to have a more stimulatory, and in higher doses a more sedative, type of antidepressant effect. No irregularities were produced by viloxazine in normal volunteers during our study.

ε) *Sulpiride.* Sulpiride is a compound of a new chemical structure with unusual pharmacologic effects. Based on several clinical studies, it was found to have the same effect on schizophrenic patients as neuroleptics without extrapyramidal side effects

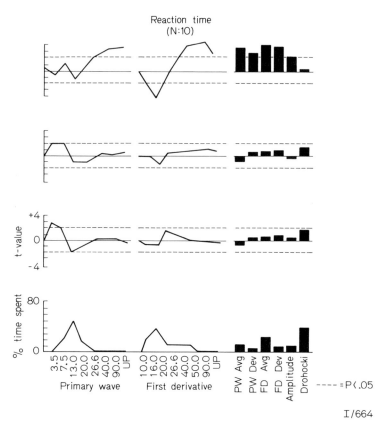

Reaction time
(N:10)

I/664

Fig. 14. According to the group profiles in the fourth hour recording, fluvoxamine in dosages of 50 mg produces CEEG profiles which show some similarity to those of imipramine from this study and from the computer data base. However, fluvoxamine CEEG profiles were characterized by a lesser increase of slow waves in the primary wave measurements. Thus, the CEEG profiles of fluvoxamine show more similarity to protriptyline and desipramine than to imipramine and amitriptyline. The CEEG profiles of fluvoxamine, particularly in higher dosages, after 4 h of drug administration, were more "typical" than those of earlier time periods, suggesting delayed onset effects

and similar therapeutic effects on depressive patients as the tricyclic antidepressants. However, its mode of action has not been determined. According to our studies, the CEEG profiles of sulpiride are similar to those seen after amitriptyline, and to a lesser degree, to those seen after thioridazine (Fig. 17). Some of the antidepressant-like CEEG profiles of sulpiride showed an increase of slow and fast activities, and a decrease of α activity.

b) Stimulant Type

α) *Thyrotropin Releasing Hormone (TRH)*. TRH was found to have therapeutic effects in depression (Prange et al., 1972) which stimulated us to carry out a study with the hormone. In a group of depressive patients, 1,000 Mcgm. TRH administered i. v. produced noticeable changes in computer-analyzed EEG measurements (Fig. 18).

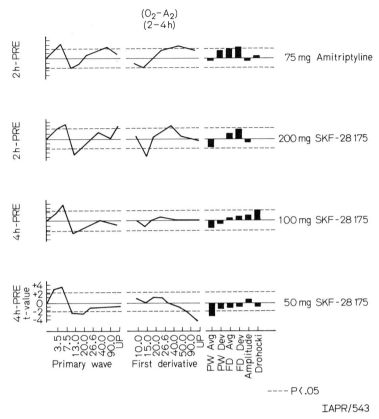

Fig. 15. The CEEG profiles of 100 mg, but particularly 200 mg fluotracen (SKF28175) show striking resemblance to those of 75 mg amitriptyline (antidepressant type of CEEG profiles). Fluotracen at 50 mg produced more slow and less fast activity in both primary and first derivative measurements (neuroleptic type CEEG profile) (N:10)

An increase of the frequencies between 13–26.6 cps and a decrease in faster and slower activities in the primary wave measurements, and increase of frequencies up to 10 cps and decrease above 10 cps in the first derivative measurements were seen in CEEG profiles. Five of the 16 CEEG measurements reached the level of statistical significance ($P < 0.05$). CEEG profiles of TRH resemble protriptyline and, more closely, dextroamphetamine (ITIL et al., 1975).

2. Drugs Predicted to be Antidepressants by CEEG Alone, But Not by Animal Pharmacology

α) *Mianserin*. In the search for potent antiserotonin/antihistamine compounds, without side effects, to investigate in manic patients, we were offered a compound GB-94 (mianserin hydrochloride), which belongs to a known group of "tetracyclic" compounds. Based on chemical structures, mianserin has been predicted to be a potent antihistamine and a potent antiserotonin, which was confirmed by animal pharmacology. Accordingly, mianserin was investigated in clinical trials in the treatment of al-

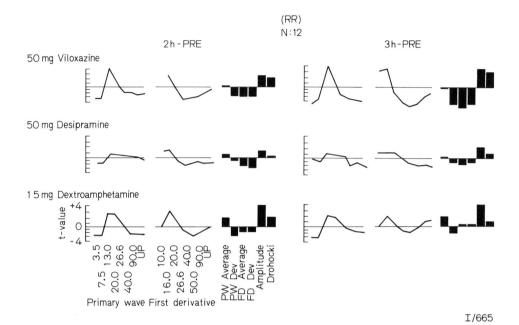

Fig. 16 a. Dextroamphetamine showed typical psychostimulant type CEEG profiles 2 and 3 h after administration of 15 mg. In quality, desipramine can produce similar CEEG profiles. Viloxazine (50 mg) produced, in quality and quantity, similar CEEG profiles to psychostimulant compounds

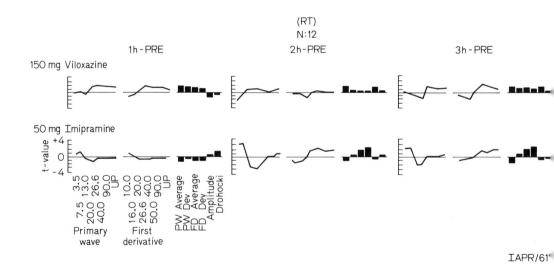

Fig. 16 b. Imipramine produces typical antidepressant CEEG profiles 2 and 3 h after oral administration of 50 mg. Viloxazine (150 mg) produced profiles similar to 50 mg Imipramine during the third hour. However, viloxazine does not produce slow waves as much as imipramine in the primary wave measurements

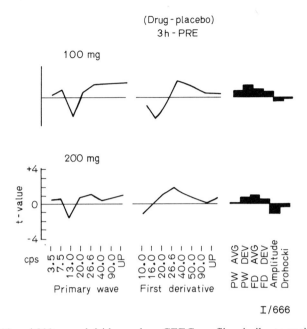

Fig. 17. Both 100 and 200 mg sulpiride produce CEEG profiles similar to antidepressant compounds

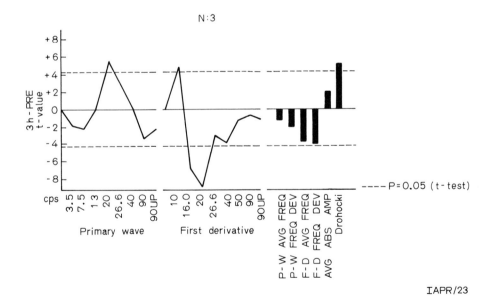

Fig. 18. TRH (10 mg i. v.) produces a decrease of very slow waves, increase of activities in 20–26 cps, and decrease of high frequency activity in the primary wave measurements, as well as an increase of slow waves and decrease of fast activities in the first derivative measurements. The CEEG profile of TRH showed some similarity to psychostimulants and "stimulatory" tricyclic antidepressants such as desipramine and protriptyline

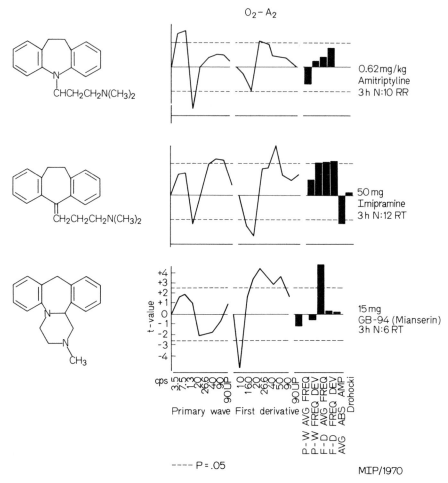

Fig. 19. GB-94 (15 mg) produced CEEG profiles similar to imipramine, but particularly to amitriptyline

lergic conditions, hay fewer, asthma, and migraine. Since, however, the clinical testing did not reveal any superiority to existing antihistamines, clinical trials were discontinued.

Before clinical trials in manic patients, we investigated the effects of mianserin in normal volunteers using the methods of quantitative pharmaco-EEG. In the pilot dose-finding trials we were able to determine that mianserin produced noticeable changes in the EEG. In a double-blind controlled quantitative pharmaco-EEG study, we observed that the types of EEG changes induced by mianserin were similar to those which we described as "antidepressant" EEG reaction-type (ITIL, 1964, 1968). These were characterized by a decrease of α activity and an increase of slow waves, with an increase of superimposed fast β activity (Fig. 19). Because of the similarity of the CEEG profiles of mianserin to amitriptyline, we predicted the clinical effects of mianserin would be similar to those of amitriptyline (ITIL, 1972, 1973).

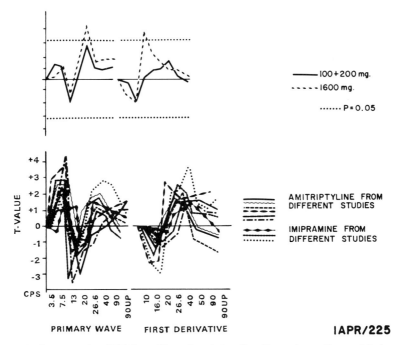

Fig. 20. At the bottom, the CEEG profiles of amitriptyline from six studies and imipramine from three different studies. At the top, the CEEG profiles of 100–200 mg mesterolone as well as 1600 mg mesterolone. The quality (shape) of the CEEG changes after mesterolone showed striking similarity to tricyclic antidepressants. However, tricyclic antidepressants produced more slow waves and lesser fast activities in the primary wave measurements than mesterolone, indicating mesterolone has more "stimulatory" properties

A double-blind controlled clinical study with amitriptyline indicated that GB-94 is indeed a potent antidepressive compound, very similar to amitriptyline in the treatment of depressive syndromes (ITIL et al., 1972a). Subsequent clinical trials in five countries confirmed our clinical findings (KOPERA, 1973). FINK, using his methods of digital computer period-analyzed EEG, could also demonstrate that GB-94 produces alterations in brain function similar to antidepressant thymoleptics (FINK, 1977). The onset of the therapeutic effects of GB-94 is faster than that of amitriptyline, although not at the level of statistical significance. To date, no pharmacologic or biochemical properties of GB-94 have been found to explain its antidepressive effects (VAN RIEZEN et al., 1975).

β) *Mesterolone.* Mesterolone, an androgenic hormone (17-hydroxy-1-methyl-5-androstane-3-1) was predicted to have psychotropic properties because of clinical observations of increase of mental alertness, mood elevation, and improvement of memory and concentration. Quantitative pharmaco-EEG trials demonstrated that mesterolone in single oral dosages of 100–1.600 mg has noticeable CNS effects, which are different (at the level of statistical significance) from those of placebo. Computer EEG profiles of higher dosages are characterized by an increase of slow waves and fast activities, with decrease of α waves in the primary wave measurements and decrease of slow and increase of fast activities in the first derivative measurements (Fig. 20).

Since these profiles are similar to those of tricyclic antidepressants, we predicted that mesterolone would be effective in depressive syndromes with and without androgen deficiency. Our further investigations showed that mesterolone indeed has significant CNS effects, even after 10 mg single oral dosage, which has less endocrinological effect. Preliminary clinical trials demonstrated that mesterolone has indeed antidepressive effects in some depressive patients (Itil et al., 1974).

F. Summary and Conclusion

All drugs which have therapeutic effects on depressive syndromes produce significant effects on human brain function which can be observed by scalp-recorded EEG. Quantitative analysis of EEG, particularly using digital computer methods demonstrated that these effects are dose and time related. The effects of the same drugs even in different populations are replicable. The antidepressant-induced EEG changes can be categorized in two groups:

1) The majority of "classic" antidepressants produce "thymoleptic" EEG reaction-type (Itil, 1968). These EEG alterations are characterized by an increase of very slow and very fast activities and a decrease of α waves in the primary wave measurements of the computer period analysis, and a decrease of slow and increase of fast activities in the first derivative measurements (Itil, 1975). Compounds producing these kinds of CEEG changes are the tricyclic antidepressants (e. g., amitriptyline, nortriptyline, imipramine), some MAO inhibitors (e. g., tranylcypromine), and certain members of other antidepressant groups (i. e., amoxapine, fluvoxamine, fluotracen, [SK + F-28,175], sulpiride, viloxazine in high dosages, mianserin, and mesterolone in high dosage). These changes are established within 3 h of single-dose oral administration of these compounds in normal volunteers and in depressed patients. During chronic multiple dosage treatment of patients with these drugs, an increase of slow waves and a decrease of fast activities were observed, along with an appearance of sharp waves, spikes, paroxysmal groups and irregularities.

From the neurophysiological point of view, the appearance of slow waves is indicative of a CNS depression, possibly due to the result of the inhibitory effects on the reticular activating system of the brain stem. The increase of fast activity, on the other hand, suggests a CNS stimulation. Accordingly, thymoleptics produce a dual action in CNS, both central stimulatory and inhibitory processes are activated.

2) Some antidepressants produce CEEG effects similar to those seen after "psychostimulant" compounds such as dextroamphetamine. These changes are characterized by an increase of α and slow β activities, and decrease of slower and faster potentials in the primary wave measurements of the computer period analysis, and increase of slower and decrease of fast potentials in the first derivative measurements. Drugs producing such psychostimulant EEG effects are, among the MAO inhibitors, isocarboxazide, iproniazid, nialamide; among the psychostimulants, dextroamphetamine and methylphenidate; among the tricyclic antidepressants, desipramine and in some populations, protriptyline; and among other compounds, the low dosages of viloxazine, thyrotropin-releasing hormone; and in low dosages the androgen, mesterolone.

3) The third group of compounds, some of them neuroleptics (e. g., thioridazine, molindone, thiothixene), which may have some antidepressant effects, produce slow

waves and some superimposed fast activities in EEG. These changes are similar to those produced by tricyclic antidepressants but more slow and, to a lesser degree, more fast activities were apparent.

Although some psychostimulants and some neuroleptics may have antidepressant effects in some patients, the potent antidepressant compounds such as amitriptyline and imipramine produce the "typical" antidepressant (thymoleptic) CEEG effects. The type (quality) of the changes as established by CEEG profiles after drug administration is indicative of the therapeutic value of a compound. Any drug which produces a typical antidepressant CEEG profile in normal volunteers will also have antidepressant effects in patients. If a compound does not produce an antidepressant CEEG profile, it does not have potent clinical antidepressant effects even if these were predicted by animal pharmacology. On the other hand, based on the CEEG profiles alone, the antidepressant properties of a series of compounds (cyclazocine, FINK et al., 1969, 1970; mianserin, ITIL et al., 1972a; mesterolone, ITIL et al., 1974) were discovered which have no typical antidepressant pharmacologic and/or biochemical profiles.

The systematic changes in human CEEG within a few hours of oral administration of a single dose of antidepressants suggest a specific type of biochemical alteration, probably in the reticular activating system of the brain stem. The CEEG changes may last up to 6 h, as in the case of amitriptyline and fluotracen, indicating long lasting biochemical changes. Despite intra- and interindividual variabilities, in quality, the CEEG profiles of antidepressants are very similar in different populations even in different countries. According to the CEEG findings, the common biochemical changes of antidepressants cannot be explained by their effects on known biogenic amines. Although they produce almost identical CEEG profiles, amitriptyline and fluvoxamine have inhibitory effects predominantly 5 HT re-uptake, fluotracen and viloxazine have predominant effects on the norepinephrine re-uptake, imipramine has somewhat equal effects on both norepinephrine and 5 HT re-uptake, and mianserin has no systematic effects on any of the well-known biogenic amines. Accordingly, one can hypothesize that the common CEEG changes for antidepressant drugs are the results of common biochemical changes. These biochemical changes are closely related to the therapeutic action of antidepressants. These biochemical changes are not primarily related to the central serotonin or catacholamine systems. Patients with depression must have a deficiency in a biochemical substrate which are restored by the antidepressant compounds. If one could establish the biochemical correlates of the electrophysiological changes induced by antidepressants in the human brain, one would eventually establish the biochemical substrate of the therapeutic process in depression. Subsequently, it may be possible to determine the pathogenesis of the depressive illness.

Acknowledgement. The authors would like to express their gratitude to Ms. PHYLLIS SEAMAN, assistant chief coordinator, to Mrs. AILEEN KUNITZ, administrative director, and to Mrs. BARBARA CLARK, secretary, for their assistance in the organization and typing of this manuscript.

References

Benassi, P., Bertolotti, P.: Serotonina e inibitori della monoaminoossidasi: studio EEG negli epilettici. Riv. Sper. Freniat. *84*, 351–367 (1960)

Betts, T.A., Kalra, P.L., Cooper, R., Jeavons, P.M.: Epileptic fits as a probable side-effect of amitriptyline. Lancet *1*, 390–392 (1968)

Bily, J., Hametova, M., Hanus, H., Polackovaj, L.: Prognosis of Lithium prophylaxis. Activ. Nerv. Super. (Praha) *15*, 88–89 (1973)

Borenstein, P., Dabbah, M.: Action du Tofranil (G 22.355) sur l'electroencephalogramme. Ann. Med. Psycho. (Paris) *117*, 923–931 (1959 a)

Borenstein, P., Dabbah, M., Bles, G., Roussel, A.: L'aminotriptyline dans les epilepsies. Etude clinique et electroencephalographique. Ann. Med. Psychol. (Paris) *120*, 153–167 (1962)

Brezinova, V., Novorna, E., Plzak, M., Soucek, K., Zaviral, J.: A contribution to the longitudinal study of manic depressive psychosis. Electroencephalogr. Clin. Neurophysiol. *20*, 284 (1966)

Brooke, G., Weatherly, J.R.C.: Imipramine. Lancet *2*, 568–569 (1959)

Burch, N.R., Nettleton, W.H., Sweeney, J., Edwards, R.J.: Period analysis of the electroencephalogram on a general purpose digital computer. Ann. N.Y. Acad. Sci. *115*, 827 (1964)

Davies, D.M., Allaye, R.: Amitriptyline poisoning. Lancet *2*, 543–643 (1963)

Davis, P.A.: Electroencephalograms of manic-depressive patients. Am. J. Psychiatry *98*, 430–433 (1941)

Davis, P.A.: A comparative study of the EEGs of schizophrenic and manic-depressive patients. Am. J. Psychiatry *99*, 210–217 (1942)

Davison, K.: EEG activation after intravenous amitriptyline. Electroencephalogr. Clin. Neurophysiol. *19*, 298–300 (1965)

Delay, J., Deniker, P., Lemperiere, T., Ropert, M., Colin, W., Ogrizek, B.: Etude de l'efficacité de l'imipramine (G 22.355) dans le traitement des etats depressifs. Ann. Med. Psychol. (Paris) *117*, 531–535 (1959)

Drohocki, Z.: Die spontane elektrische Spannungsproduktion der Großhirnrinde. Pflügers Arch. Ges. Physiol. *239*, 658–679 (1937)

Ekiert, H., Gogol, Z., Welbel, L., Buchowska, I.: Electroclinical aspect of insidon treatment in patients with neurotic symptoms. Psychiat. Polska (Warszawa) *7*, 169–177 (1973)

Erwin, C.W., Gerber, C.J., Morrison, S.D., James, J.F.: Lithium carbonate and convulsive disorders. Arch. Gen. Psychiatry *28*, 646–648 (1973)

Fehlow, P.: EEG-Befunde bei Psychosen mit besonderer Berücksichtigung des depressiven Syndroms. Psychiatr. Neurol. Med. Psychol. (Leip.) *26*, 409–415 (1974)

Fink, M.: Electroencephalographic and behavioral effects of Tofranil. Can. Psychiatr. Assoc. J. [Suppl.] *4*, 166–171 (1959)

Fink, M.: Quantitative electroencephalography and Human psychopharmacology: Frequency spectra and drug action. Med. Exp. *5* , 364–369 (1961)

Fink, M.: Quantitative EEG and human psychopharmacology. III. Changes on acute and chronic administration of chlorpromazine, imipramine and placebo (saline). In: Applications of Electroencephalography in Psychiatry. Wilson, W.P. (ed.), pp. 226–240. Durham, N.C.: Duke Univ. Press 1965

Fink, M.: EEG profiles and bioavailability measures of psychoactive drugs. In: Psychotropic Drugs and the human EEG. Itil, T.M. (ed.), pp. 76–98. Basel, New York: Karger 1974

Fink, M., Itil, T.M.: EEG and human psychopharmacology. IV. Clinical antidepressants. In: Psychopharmacology: Review of progress 1957–1967. Efron, D.H., Cole, J.O., Levine, J., Wittenborn, R.O. (eds.), pp. 671–682. Washington, D.C.: U.S. Govt. Printing Office 1968

Fink, M., Itil, T.M., Zaks, A., Freedman, A.M.: EEG patterns of cyclazocine, a narcotic antagonist. In: Neurophysiological and behavioral aspects of psychotropic drugs. Karczmar, A., Koella, W. (eds.), pp. 62–71. Springfield, Ill.: Thomas 1969

Fink, M., Simeon, J., Itil, T.M., Freedman, A.M.: Clinical antidepressant activity of cyclazocine – a narcotic antagonist. Clin. Pharmacol. Ther. *11*, 41–48 (1970)

Fink, M.: Strategies of new psychotropic drugs development. Presented at the scientific meeting on the occasion of the 50 th anniversary of Organon. Amsterdam, October 27, 1977

Fowler, G.W., Julien, R.M.: Imipramine and the experimental petit mal epilepsy. Neurology *24*, 369 (1974)

Frain, M.M.: Preliminary report on Mellaril in epilepsy. Am. J. Psychiatry *117*, 547–548 (1960)

Fromm, G.H., Amores, C.Y., Thies, W.: Imipramine in epilepsy. Arch. Neurol. *27*, 198–204 (1972)

Gannon, P., Itil, T.M., Keskiner, A., Hsu, B.: Clinical and quantitative electroencephalographical effects of MK940. Arzneim. Forsch. *20*, 971–974 (1970)

Gershon, S.: Use of Lithium salts in psychiatric disorders. Dis. Nerv. Syst. *1*, 51–55 (1968)

Goldstein, L.: Psychotropic drug-induced EEG changes as revealed by the amplitude integration method. In: Psychotropic drugs and the human EEG. Mod. probl. Pharmacopsychiat. Itil, T.M. (ed.), Vol. 8, pp. 131–148. Basel, New York: Karger 1974

Gottschalk, H., Sack, G.: EEG Untersuchungen unter Lithiumbehandlung. Psychiatr. Neurol. Med. Psychol. (Leip.) *25*, 297–300 (1973)

Greenblatt, M., Healy, M.M., Jones, G.A.: Age and electroencephalographic abnormality in neuropsychiatric patients: A Study of 1593 Cases. Am. J. Psychiatry *101*, 82–90 (1944)

Grisoni, R., Canali, G., Pacini, L.: The action of iproniazid on the epileptic patterns of the EEG in man. Neuropsychopharmacology. Bradley, P.B., Deniker, P., Radouco-Thomas, C. (eds.), Vol. 1, pp. 584–586. Amsterdam, New York: 1959

Harding, G.F.A., Jeavons, P.M., Jenner, F.A., Drummond, P., Sheridan, M., Howells, G.W.: The electroencephalogram in three cases of periodic psychosis. Electroencephalogy. Clin. Neurophysiol. *21*, 20–37 (1966)

Harrer, G.: Zur Chemotherapie der Depression. Wien. Med. Wochenschr. *11*, 255–259 (1960)

Heninger, G.R.: Neuropsychologic mechanisms of Lithium Therapy. J. Psychiatr. Res. *10*, 157–158 (1974)

Hurst, L.A., Mundy-Castle, A.C., Beerstecher, D.M.: The electroencephalogram in manic-depressive psychosis. J. Ment. Sci. *100*, 220–240 (1954)

Itil, T.M.: Elektroencephalographische Befunde zur Klassifikation Neuro- und Thymoleptischer Medikamente. Med. Exp. *5*, 347–363 (1961)

Itil, T.M.: Elektroencephalographische Studien bei endogenen Psychosen und deren Behandlung mit Psychotropen Medikamenten unter besonderer Berücksichtigung des Pentothalelektroencephalogramms. Istanbul: Ahmet Sait Matbaasi 1964

Itil, T.M.: Electroencephalography and pharmacopsychiatry. In: Modern problems of pharmacopsychiatry. Petrilowitsch, N., Freyhan, F.A., Pichot, P. (eds.), pp. 163–194. Basel, New York: Karger 1968

Itil, T.M.: Quantitative pharmaco-encephalography in the discovery of a new group of psychotropic drugs. Dis. Nerv. Syst. *33*, 557–559 (1972)

Itil, T.M.: Quantitative pharmaco-EEG – A new approach to the discovery of a psychotropic drug. In: Psychopharmacology, sexual disorders and drug abuse. Ban, T.A., Boissier, J.R., Gessa, G.J., Heimann, H., Hollister, L., Lehmann, H.E., Munkvad, I., Steinberg, H., Sulser, F., Sundwall, A., Vinar, O. (eds.), pp. 13–30. Amsterdam, London: North Holland 1973

Itil, T.M.: Quantitative pharmaco-electroencephalography. In: Psychotropic drugs and the human EEG, mod. probl. pharmacopsychiat. Itil, T.M. (ed.), Vol. 8, pp. 43–75. Basel, New York: Karger 1974

Itil, T.M.: Computer EEG profiles of antidepressants: quantitative pharmaco-EEG in the development of new antidepressive drugs. In: Antidepressants (Industrial Pharmacology). Fielding, S., Lal, H. (eds.), Vol. *II*,, pp. 319–359. Mt. Kisco, New York: Futura 1975

Itil, T.M.: Qualitative and quantitative EEG findings in schizophrenia. Schizophrenia Bull. *3*, 61–79 (1977a)

Itil, T.M.: Bioavailability and bioequivalence of psychotropic drugs based on computerized EEG measurements. Drugs Exptl. Clin. Res. *1 (1–2)*, 251–257 (1977b)

Itil, T.M.: Quantitative electroencephalography in psychopharmacology – quantitative pharmaco-electroencephalography in the discovery of psychotropic properties of drugs. In: Deniker, P., Radouco-Thomas, C., Villeneuve, A. (eds.), Neuropsychopharmacology, Vol. 2, pp. 1183–1190. New York: Pergamon Press 1978

Itil, T.M., Patterson, C.D., Polvan, N., Mehta, D., Bergey, B.: Clinical and CNS effects of oral and i.v. thyrotropin releasing hormone (TRH). Dis. Nerv. Syst. *36*, 529–536 (1975)

Itil, T.M., Akpinar, S.: Lithium effect on human electroencephalogram. Clin. Electroencephalogr. *2*, 89–102 (1971)

Itil, T.M., Güven, F., Cora, R., Hsu, W., Polvan, N., Ucok, A., Sanseigne, A., Ulett, G.A.: Quantitative pharmaco-electroencephalography using frequency analyzer and digital computer methods in early drug evaluations. In: Drugs, development, and brain functions. Smith, W.L. (ed.), pp. 145–166. Springfield, Ill.: Thomas 1971

Itil, T.M., Holden, J.M.C., Fink, M., Shapiro, D.M., Keskiner, A.: Treatment of chronic psychotic patients with combined medications. In: Proc. Vth Int. Congr. Neuropsychopharmacology, Int. Congr. Series No. 129. Brill, H., Cole, J.O., Deniker, P., Hippius, H., Bradley, P.B. (eds.), pp. 1016–1020. Amsterdam, New York: Excerpta Medica 1967a

Itil, T.M., Rizzo, A.E., Shapiro, D.M.: Quantitative study of behavior and EEG correlation during treatment of disturbed children and adolescents. Dis. Nerv. Syst. 28, 731–736 (1967b)

Itil, T.M., Shapiro, D., Fink, M.: Differentiation of psychotropic drugs by quantitative EEG analysis. Agressologie 9, 267–280 (1968)

Itil, T.M., Shapiro, D., Fink, M., Kiremitci, N., Hickman, C.: Quantitative EEG studies of clordiazepoxide, chlorpromazine and imipramine on volunteer and schizophrenic subjects. In: The Psychopharmacology of the normal human. Evans, W.O., Kline, N.S. (eds.), pp. 219–237. Springfield, Ill.: Thomas 1969

Itil, T.M., Polvan, N., Ucok, A., Eper, E., Güven, F., Hsu, W.: Comparison of the clinical and electroencephalographical effects of molindone and trifluoperazine in acute schizophrenic patients. Physicians' Drug Manual 2, 80–87 (1970)

Itil, T.M., Polvan, N., Hsu, W.: Clinical and EEG effects of GB-94, a "tetracyclic" antidepressant (EEG model in the discovery of a new psychotropic drug). Curr. Ther. Res. 14, 395–413 (1972a)

Itil, T.M., Saletu, B., Coffin, C., Klingenberg, H.: Quantitative EEG changes during thiothixene treatment of chronic schizophrenics. Clin. Electroencephalogy. 3, 109–117 (1972b)

Itil, T.M., Saletu, B., Davis, S.: EEG findings in chronic schizophrenics based on digital computer period analysis and analog power spectra. Biol. Psychiatry 5, 1–13 (1972c)

Itil, T.M., Cora, R., Akpinar, S., Herrmann, W.M., Patterson, C.: "Psychotropic" action of sex hormones: computerized EEG in establishing the immediate CNS effects of steroid hormones. Curr. Ther. Res. 16, 1147–1170 (1974)

Itil, T.M., Bhattacharyya, A., Polvan, N., Huque, M., Menon, G.N.: Fluvoxamine (DU-23,000), a new antidepressant. Quantitative pharmaco-electroencephalography and pilot clinical trials. Progress in Neuro-Psychopharmacology, Vol. 1, pp. 309–322. Oxford/New York: Pergamon Press 1977a

Itil, T.M., Polvan, N., Engin, L., Guthrie, M.B., Huque, M.F.: Fluotracen (SKF-28175), a new thymo-neuroleptic with rapid action and long-acting properties (quantitative pharmaco-EEG and clinical trials in the development of fluotracen (SKF-28175). Curr. Ther. Res. 21, 343–360 (1977b)

Jus, A., Villeneuve, A., Gautier, J., Pires, A., Cote, J.M., Jus, K., Villeneuve, R., Perron, D.: Influence of lithium carbonate on patients with temporal epilepsy. Can. Psychiatr. Assoc. J. 18, 77–78 (1973)

Kalinowsky, L.B., Hoch, P.H.: Somatic treatments in psychiatry – pharmacotherapy, convulsive, insulin, surgical, and other methods. New York: Grune and Stratton 1961

Kiloh, L.G., Davison, K., Osselton, J.W.: An electroencephalographic study of the analeptic effects of imipramine. Electroencephal. Clin. Neurophysiol. 13, 216–223 (1961)

Kopera, H.: Aspects of clinical pharmacology and clinical experiences with ORG GB-94. Paper presented at the 50th anniversary meeting on Organon. Amsterdam, October 26, 1973

Kugler, J.: Chemotherapie der Depression und EEG. Wien. Klin. Wochenschr. 72, 465–468 (1960)

Lemere, F.: Cortical energy production in the psychoses. Psychosom. Med. 3, 152–156 (1941)

Levene, L.J., Lascelles, C.F.: Imipramine. Lancet 2, 675 (1959)

Mann, A.M.: Desmethylimipramine (G35020) in the treatment of depression: pilot study in a general hospital and outpatient setting. Can. Med. Assoc. J. 86, 495–498 (1962)

Marjerrison, G.: Effects of minor tranquilizers on the EEG. In: Psychotropic Drugs and the Human EEG. Mod. probl. pharmacopsychiat. Itil, T.M. (ed.), Vol. 8, pp. 149–157. Basel, New York: Karger 1974

Mayer, K.: Klinische und pharmakopsychologische Untersuchungen zur therapeutischen Wirkung von Phenotiazine. Medizinische Klinik 15, 733–736 (1959)

Meduna, L.J., Abood, L.G., Biehl, J.H.: (3) N (1-methyl-aminopropyl) iminodibenzyl: a new antidepressant. Preliminary report. J. Neuropsychiatry 2, 232–237 (1961)

Mengoli, G., Maccagnani, G.: Modificazioni elettroencefalografiche indotte dal derivato iminodibenzilico G22355 (Tofranil). Ipotesi fisio-patogenetiche sul meccanismo d'azione. Rass. Studi. Psichiat. 48, 899–921 (1959)

Moll, A.E.: Indications for electroshock, Tofranil and psychotherapy in the treatment of depression (discussion). Can. Psychiatr. Assoc. J. [Suppl.] 4, 989–996 (1959)

Okuma, T., Takeshita, H., Nakao, T., Uchida, Y., Kishimoto, A., Fukuhara, T., Matsushima, Y.: The effect of lithium carbonate on the electroencephalogram of manic-depressive psychotics. Clin. Psychiatry (Tokyo) 16, 397–408 (1974)

Pauig, P.M., Deluca, M.A., Osterheld, R.G.: Thioridazine hydrochloride in the treatment of behavior disorders in epileptics. Am. J. Psychiatry 117, 832–833 (1961)

Pisanty, J.: Algunos efectos curioses de la iproniazida. I. Effecto anticonvulsivante en epilepsias de tipo gran mal. Medicina (Mex.) 39, 141–143 (1959)

Prange, A.J. Jr., Wilson, I.C., Lara, P.P., Alltop, L.B., Breese, G.R.: Effects of thyrotropin releasing hormones on depression. Lancet 2, 299–1002 (1972)

Reilly, E., Halmi, K.A., Noyes, R. Jr.: Electroencephalographic responses to Lithium. Int. Pharmacopsychiatry 8, 208–213 (1973)

Santanelli, R., Municchi, L., Serra, C.: Modificazioni elettroencefalografiche indotte in sogetti epilettici dal trattamento prolungato con iproniazide. Riv. Neurol. 31, 467–478 (1961)

Satterfield, J.H.: EEG Changes with Lithium in depressed patients. Psychopharmacol. Bull. 10, 157–158 (1974)

Sharp, W.L.: Convulsions associated with antidepressant drugs. Am. J. Psychiatry 117, 458–459 (1960)

Simeon, J., Spero, M., Fink, M.: Clinical and EEG studies of doxepin: interim report. Psychosomatics 10, 14–17 (1969)

Van Meter, W.G., Owens, H.F., Himwich, H.E.: Effects of Tofranil, an antidepressant drug, on electrical potentials of rabbit brain. Can. Psychiatr. Assoc. J. [Suppl.] 4, 113–119 (1959)

Van Riezen, H., Behagel, I.R.H., Chafic, M.: Development of psychotropic drugs. Psychopharmacol. Bull. 11, 10–15 (1975)

Volavka, J., Grof, P., Mrklas, L.: EEG frequency analysis in periodic endogenous depressions. Psychiatr. Neurol. (Basel) 153, 384–390 (1967)

Zappoli, R.: Rilievi elettroencefalografici in pazienti affetti da distima depressiva trattato con Tofranil (derivato iminodibenzilico G22355). Riv. Sper. Freniat. 83, 1–20 (1959)

Zakowska-Dabrowska, T., Strzyzewski, W.: The action of Noveril on the bioelectric activity of the brain. Psychiat. Polska (Warszawa) 6, 523–528 (1972)

Zurabashvili, A.D.: Some data on the neuropharmacodynamics and the therapeutic efficacy of Tofranil (imipramine). In: Voprosy Psikhiatrii. Zurabashvili, A. (ed.), pp. 243–274. Tbilisi, U.S.S.R.: Sabchota Sakartvelo 1969

CHAPTER 21a

Biochemical Effects of Antidepressants in Animals*

F. SULSER and P.L. MOBLEY

A. Introduction

Antidepressant drugs with proven clinical efficacy include inhibitors of monoamine oxidase (MAO), tertiary and secondary amines of tricyclic antidepressants, and a number of other drugs which affect monoaminergic systems in brain (e. g., maprop-tiline, nomifensine, iprindole, mianserin). It is the aim of this chapter to discuss biochemical effects of these drugs with emphasis on the possible relevance to their antidepressant action.

B. Monoamine Oxidase Inhibitors

I. Multiple Forms of MAO and Selective MAO Inhibitors

The clinical use of MAO inhibitors as antidepressants has been seriously restricted because of severe side effects such as the precipitation of hypertensive crises resulting from the interaction with dietary factors, e. g., tyramine (HORVITZ et al., 1964; MARLEY and BLACKWELL, 1970). The possible existence of multiple forms of MAO with different substrate specificity offers, however, the possibility to synthesize more specific and probably safer MAO inhibitors which retain antidepressant activity.

Based on the biphasic inhibition pattern of the metabolism of tyramine by clorgyline, JOHNSTON (1968) proposed two forms of MAO, type A, and type B; type A being selectively inhibited by clorgyline. Serotonin (5HT) is preferentially metabolized by type A MAO while tyramine and tryptamine appear to be substrates for both forms. Multiple bands of MAO activity have been separated electrophoretically (YOUDIM et al., 1969; KIM and D'IORIO, 1968) though their relation to type A and B is unknown. There is also some question as to whether or not the multiple bands may result from attached phospholipids (HOUSLAY and TIPTON, 1973). Thus, the significance of the observed multiplicity of MAO using electrophoretic techniques remains equivocal (SANDLER and YOUDIM, 1972; NEFF and YANG, 1974; HOUSLAY et al., 1976).

In vitro evidence suggests that norepinephrine (NE), in addition to 5HT is also selectively metabolized by the A form (GORIDIS and NEFF, 1971) while phenylethylamine (PEA) (YANG and NEFF, 1973) and benzylamine (HALL et al., 1969) are substrates for type B MAO. Dopamine (DA), like tryptamine and tyramine, is metabolized by both forms (HALL et al., 1969). Besides clorgyline, other selective inhibitors of the A form include Lilly 51641 (FULLER, 1968) and harmaline (FULLER, 1972); deprenyl appears to be a selective inhibitor of the B form (KNOLL and MAGYAR, 1972). However, the

* Supported by USPHS grants MH-11468, MH-29228, MH-08107 and by the Tennessee Department of Mental Health and Mental Retardation

concept of multiple forms of MAO has been questioned recently (HOUSLAY et al., 1976; JAIN, 1977). Whether the observed multiplicity is due to multiple enzymes, one enzyme in different lipid environments, or one enzyme with multiple sites is not yet clear. In addition, it is possible that the A and B forms are themselves heterogeneous (SQUIRES, 1972; FOWLER et al., 1978).

Although the nature of the multiplicity is unknown, evidence based on experiments in vivo supports the concept of functionally different types of MAO. For example, in preparations containing brain mitochondria isolated from rats pretreated with type A inhibitors (clorgyline, Lilly 51641, NSD 2023), the metabolism of 5HT was found to be selectively inhibited whereas pretreatment with deprenyl preferentially inhibited the metabolism of PEA and benzylamine (CHRISTMAS et al., 1972; YANG and NEFF, 1974). Also, the endogenous levels of 5HT, NE and DA have been reported to increase after clorgyline while the concentration of 5-hydroxyindoleacetic acid and 3,4-dihydroxyphenylacetic acid decreased. Conversely, after the administration of deprenyl only the level of DA was found to increase with a corresponding decrease of 3,4-dihydroxyphenylacetic acid (YANG and NEFF, 1974). While these results indicate that DA is a substrate for both A and B forms of MAO, in accord with in vitro evidence, other in vivo work indicates that DA is a preferential substrate for the A form. According to WALDMEIER et al. (1976), clorgyline increased the levels of NE and DA in whole brain over a 24-h period while deprenyl had no effect on either amine. Also, in animals pretreated with clorgyline, [³H]-Dopa elicited large increases in labeled DA, methoxytyramine, NE, and normetanephrine whereas deprenyl exerted only a weak effect. Moreover, the formation of homovanillic acid, 3,4-dihydroxyphenylacetic acid and 3-methoxy-4-hydroxyphenylglycol appear to be selectively inhibited following the administration of clorgyline (BRAESTRUP et al., 1975; WALDMEIER et al., 1976).

II. Physiologic Consequences of MAO Inhibition

One consequence of the increase of intraneuronal amines – and presumably of the availability of physiologically active amines at their corresponding receptor sites following MAO inhibition – is a decrease in the synthesis of catecholamines apparently due to feedback inhibition of tyrosine hydroxylase (NEFF and COSTA, 1966; NGAI et al., 1968; SPECTOR et al., 1967). Recent work also indicates the possibility of the regulation of amine biosynthesis through changes in the rate of synthesis and/or disposition of the nonfolate pterins (MANDELL and KNAPP, 1978).

MAO inhibitors are known to effect the uptake and release of neurotransmitters. IVERSEN (1965) has shown that MAO inhibitors can inhibit the uptake of NE. However, this inhibition of uptake appears not to be a common property of all MAO inhibitors. Thus, tranylcypromine and deprenyl decrease the uptake of [³H]-NE into brain tissue while pargyline and nialamide have no effect (KNOLL and MAGYAR, 1972). HENDLEY and SNYDER (1968) found that blockade of uptake of tritiated metaraminol by MAO inhibitors correlated better with their antidepressant efficacy than did their ability to block the activity of MAO. Clinical evidence suggests that (−)-tranylcypromine is a more effective antidepressant than the corresponding (+)-enantiomer (ESCOBAR et al., 1974). This is of interest since the (+)-isomer is a more potent MAO inhibitor than the (−)-isomer (ZIRKLE et al., 1962) while the (−)-isomer is a more potent inhibitor of catecholamine uptake into brain synaptosomes (HORN and SNYDER, 1972).

MAO inhibitors exert various effects on the efflux of monoamines from nerve tissue. For example, under certain experimental conditions, these drugs can decrease the release of NE associated with nerve stimulation (DAVEY et al., 1963) and the efflux of [³H]-NE accumulated in heart tissue (AXELROD et al., 1961). Moreover, it has been reported that pargyline can retard the efflux of [³H]-metaraminol from brain tissue whereas pheniprazine increases its release. However, both MAO inhibitors increase the release of metaraminol from heart tissue (BREESE et al., 1970).

Experimental data obtained by employing methods to study the release of biogenic amines from brain in vivo (perfusion through push–pull cannulas) indicate that MAO inhibitors increase the availability of biogenic amines at presumptive aminergic receptor sites. Thus, following MAO inhibition, a marked increase in the amount of extraneuronal NE and normetanephrine occurred in the perfusate from the rat hypothalamus (STRADA and SULSER, 1972). MAO inhibition also caused an increase in the concentration of 5HT in the effluent from perfused cerebral ventricles (GOODRICH, 1969). This being the case, one would expect a desensitization of the noradrenergic receptor since alterations in transmitter–receptor interactions lead to compensatory changes in receptor sensitivity. VETULANI et al. (1976a) have demonstrated that chronic treatment with MAO inhibitors significantly decreased the cyclic AMP response to NE in slices from the limbic forebrain of rats (see Sect. D).

C. Tricyclic Antidepressants and Other Drugs Which Affect Monoaminergic Systems in Brain

I. Effects of Tricyclic Antidepressants on MAO Activity

It has been suggested that tricyclic antidepressants owe their activity, at least in part, to inhibition of MAO. Unlike MAO inhibitors, the administration of these drugs to animals does not increase the levels of catechol and/or indolealkylamines in brain (PLETSCHER and GEY, 1959; SULSER et al., 1962, 1964). However, in vitro studies indicate that many of the tricyclic antidepressants, including iprindole, can inhibit MAO (GABAY and VALCOURT, 1968; ROTH and GILLIS, 1975 a, b; USDIN and USDIN, 1961). Tricyclic antidepressants can also inhibit human platelet MAO in vitro (EDWARDS and BURNS, 1974) and in vivo (SULLIVAN et al., 1977).

Since the B form of MAO appears to be more sensitive to inhibition by tricyclic antidepressants, in vivo inhibition of the metabolism of PEA might be expected. In the rabbit, acute and chronic administration of imipramine has been reported to increase the level of PEA in brain while iprindole given either acutely or chronically failed to significantly alter the level of PEA (MOSNAIM et al., 1974). Von VOIGTLANDER and LOSEY (1976) determined whether tricyclic antidepressants alter the metabolism of [C¹⁴]-PEA in vivo. These workers found that neither acute nor chronic treatment for 7 days with imipramine, amitriptyline, or iprindole blocked the disappearance of [C¹⁴]-PEA whereas the MAO inhibitors, pargyline, tranylcypromine, and nialamide, caused a marked increase in labeled PEA in brain. It thus appears that in the absence of confirmation of this effect in vivo, the pharmacologic and therapeutic significance of the in vitro inhibition of MAO by tricyclic antidepressants is difficult to assess.

II. Blockade by Tricyclic Antidepressants
of the Uptake of Biogenic Amines

Since neuronal reuptake mechanisms for biogenic amines are involved in the termination of their action (e. g., Iversen, 1974), the demonstrated inhibition of this uptake by imipramine-like drugs has been widely accepted as the predominant mode of action of this type of antidepressant drug. Kinetically, the inhibition of the uptake of NE by tricyclic antidepressants is competitive in nature and, generally, secondary amines are more potent than the corresponding tertiary amines in blocking the uptake of NE through the neuronal membrane (Table 1) whereas tertiary amines of tricyclic antidepressants are more potent inhibitors of the reuptake of 5HT than the corresponding secondary amines (Carlsson et al., 1969; Ross and Renyi, 1967, 1969; Maxwell et al., 1969; Salama et al., 1971; Todrick and Tait, 1969; Ahtee and Saarnivara, 1971; Koe, 1976). Tricyclic antidepressants act as competitive inhibitors of the high affinity uptake (uptake 1) of NE (Berti and Shore, 1967; Maxwell et al., 1969) and evidence has been provided that this type of drug exerts a blocking action on the uptake of NE in brain in vivo (Sulser et al., 1969). Uptake 1 is a saturable process, stereochemically selective for (R)-NE and involves a Na^+/K^+-dependent carrier system which depends on metabolic energy and on the functioning of the Na^+/K^+-stimulated ATPase (Bogdanski et al., 1968; Bogdanski and Brodie, 1969; Iversen, 1973).

Blockade of the high affinity uptake of NE through the neuronal membrane in peripheral and central noradrenergic neurons increases the availability of the physiologically active amine at noradrenergic receptor sites. This effect explains many of the pharmacologic actions of tricyclic antidepressants, e. g., the potentiation of exogenous NE or of NE released by nerve stimulation and the antagonism of the reserpine-like syndrome. Moreover, tricyclic antidepressants reduce the spontaneous activity of the NE-containing cells of the locus coeruleus; antidepressants having a secondary amine in the side chain are more potent than their corresponding tertiary amine analogs (Nybäck et al., 1975).

While the effects of tricyclic antidepressants on uptake mechanisms through the neuronal membrane represent the main site of action in adrenergic neurons, some studies have also indicated an impairment by these drugs of the intraneuronal amine concentrating mechanism of storage vesicles. Thus, when slices of various brain areas (except caudate nucleus) were incubated with [³H]-tyramine, desipramine given in vivo or added in vitro inhibited the synthesis of [³H]-octopamine but not the uptake, retention, or the oxidative deamination of [³H]-tyramine (Steinberg and Smith, 1970). Since desipramine does not inhibit dopamine β-hydroxylase, the data may indicate that the drug prevented the uptake of [³H]-tyramine into the storage granules where tyramine is converted to octopamine. Leitz (1970) studied the effect of desipramine on the metaraminol induced release of NE from slices of the heart and found that the tricyclic antidepressant reduced the release of NE to a much greater extent than it blocked the uptake of metaraminol. Since the release of NE and the uptake of metaraminol were stoichiometrically related, the results indicate that desipramine not only reduced the uptake of metaraminol but acted within the neuron to prevent metaraminol from releasing NE.

The blockade of the reuptake of 5HT by tricyclic antidepressants results in an accumulation of 5HT at postsynaptic 5HT receptors. Negative feedback mechanisms

Table 1. Inhibition of monoamine uptake by phenylbutylamine- and phenoxypropylamine-related drugs in synaptosomal preparations of rat brain[a]

Compound	IC_{50}[b] (μM)					
	Corpus Striatum				Hypothalamus	
	DA		5-HT		NE	
CP-24,441 (1R, 4S)[c]	S	0.15	S	0.84	S	0.018
CP-24,442 (1S, 4R)[c]	M	1.4	I	14	M	0.37
CP-22,186 (trans pair)[c]	S	0.39	S	0.83	S	0.029
CP-22,185 (cis pair)[c]	W	7.6	M	3.8	I	1.2
EXP-561	S	0.51	P	0.038	S	0.028
Mazindol (protonated)	S	0.15	S	0.24	P	0.0015
Nomifensine	S	0.41	W	5.4	S	0.020
Nefopam	M	1.6	S	0.33	S	0.022
Tofenacine	I	19	M	1.2	M	0.41
PR-F-36-C1	M	2.4	S	0.52	M	0.17
WY-5244	W	6.5	S	0.41	W	0.80
Desipramine	I	21	M	3.4	P	0.0056
Imipramine	I	20	S	0.81	S	0.066
Chlorimipramine	W	8.1	P	0.099	M	0.11
Protriptyline	I	12	M	2.6	S	0.018
Nortriptyline	I	11	M	1.7	S	0.025
Amitriptyline	I	13	M	1.2	M	0.13
Doxepin	I	24	M	2.9	M	0.12
Amedalin	I	101	W	8.6	S	0.011
Daledalin	I	13	M	3.1	S	0.079
Lu 3-010	I	41	W	7.4	S	0.011
Chlorpromazine	I	12	M	3.9	S	0.022
Thioridazine	M	3.5	W	5.5	I	4.0
Cyproheptadine	I	11	I	13	M	0.44
Iprindole	I	20	I	18	I	3.1
Cocaine	M	1.7	S	0.85	M	0.27
Pseudococaine	I	73	I	26	I	8.6
Benztropine	S	0.54	I	14	M	0.45
Viloxazine	I	180	I	82	W	0.66
Lilly 94939 Nisoxetine	M	2.9	M	1.2	P	0.0079
Lilly 100140 Fluoxetine	I	12	S	0.27	W	0.74
FG 4963	W	5.4	S	0.22	W	0.61

[a] Uptake of 0.1 μM [^{14}C] Labeled DA, 5-HT, or NE was measured by method of WONG et al. (1973)

[b] P = potent, S = strong, M = moderate, W = weak, I = "inactive." These designations are arbitrarily defined in terms of IC_{50} values. For DA uptake: S, $IC_{50} < 1 \mu M$; M, IC_{50} 1–5 μM; W, IC_{50} 5–10 μM; I, $IC_{50} > 10 \mu M$. For 5-HT uptake: P, $IC_{50} < 0.1 \mu M$, S, IC_{50} 0.1–1.0 μM; M, IC_{50} 1–5 μM; W, IC_{50} 5–10 μM; I, $IC_{50} > 10 \mu M$. For NE uptake: P, $IC_{50} < 0.01 \mu M$; S, IC_{50} 0.01–0.10 μM; M, IC_{50} 0.1–0.5 μM; W, IC_{50} 0.5–1.0 μM; I, $IC_{50} > 1.0 \mu M$

[c] CP-24,441 and CP-24,442 are the enantiomers of racemic trans-N-methyl-4-phenyl-1,2,3,4,-tetra-hydro-1-naphthylamine (CP-22,186). CP-22,185 is the racemic cis-N-methyl-4-phenyl-1,2,3,4-tetrahydro-1-naphthylamine. (From KOE, 1976)

might then be activated resulting in a decreased turnover of cerebral 5HT (Corrodi and Fuxe, 1969; Meek and Werdinius, 1970). It is noteworthy in this regard that the tertiary amines, chlorimipramine, imipramine, and amitriptyline, depressed the firing rate of raphé neurons whereas secondary amines, e. g., desipramine and protriptyline, exerted either minimal or no depressant effect in equivalent doses (Sheard et al., 1972). The data obtained with tricyclic antidepressants on flexor and extensor reflex activity in the rat also support the view that the tertiary amines of tricyclic antide-pressants preferentially inhibit the uptake of 5HT whereas the secondary amines pref-erentially inhibit the uptake of NE (Lidbrink et al., 1971; Meek et al., 1970). The tri-cyclic antidepressants and other currently available antidepressants do, however, not appreciably inhibit the uptake of DA into dopaminergic neurons (Horn et al., 1971; Fuxe and Ungerstedt, 1968; Koe, 1976) with the exception of nomifensine (Table 1) which, in addition to being an effective inhibitor of NE re-uptake also exerts potent blocking properties on the uptake of DA (Hunt et al., 1974; Koe, 1976; Tuomisto, 1977). While blockade of DA re-uptake might be in part responsible for anti-Parkin-son activity of drugs, its relevance to antidepressant efficacy is unknown.

While previous hypotheses on the molecular basis of blockade of monoamine up-take have attempted to overlap the phenyl and nitrogen of tricyclic antidepressants with the extended phenethylamine moiety of catecholamines (Maxwell et al., 1969, 1970; Horn, 1973), a direct overlap of inhibitor structure with the phenethylamine skeleton at the neuronal membrane amine pump need not be assumed, except for phenethylamine-related inhibitors. A comprehensive study on the molecular geome-try of inhibitors of the uptake of catecholamines and 5HT has recently been published (Koe, 1976).

The question arises whether the clinical antidepressant activity of antidepressant drugs is more closely related to their biochemical effect on noradrenergic or on sero-tonergic neurons. At present, this question is difficult to answer because MAO in-hibitors increase the availability of both monoamines and tricyclic antidepressants af-fect transport mechanisms of both amines or are in vivo converted by microsomal en-zymes to metabolites which in concert with the parent drug will inhibit both transport systems. If differences in the relative degree of blocking uptake of NE or 5HT are in-deed of clinical significance in the modulation of mood, the availability of and con-trolled clinical trials with more selective uptake inhibitors such as maproptiline (Maître et al., 1971, 1974) and nisoxetine [Fuller et al., 1975 (preferential inhibitors of NE reuptake), and FG-4963 (Buus Lassen et al., 1975), Lu 10-171 (Hyttel, 1977)] and fluoxetine (preferential inhibitors of 5HT uptake) should provide more definite answers to this problem. Studies with fluoxetine will be of particular interest because this drug is a selective inhibitor of 5HT uptake into specific brain regions in vivo and N-demethylation does not alter either its potency or selectivity toward inhibiting the uptake of 5HT (Wong et al., 1975). The selectivity of nisoxetine in blocking NE-reup-take is interesting in view of its structural similarity to fluoxetine. Thus, replacing the p-trifluoromethyl group of fluoxetine with an 0-methoxy group converts the molecule from a specific inhibitor of 5HT uptake to a specific inhibitor of NE uptake (Fuller et al., 1975).

Although it cannot be assumed that all tricyclic antidepressants have to elicit their therapeutic effect via one common mechanism, the clinical efficacy of iprindole has nevertheless raised some questions on the validity of the current catecholamine hypothesis of affective disorders. Iprindole does not block the neuronal uptake of NE nor of 5HT and does not alter the metabolism nor the turnover of NE and 5HT (LAHTI and MAICKEL, 1971; ROSS et al., 1971; FREEMAN and SULSER, 1972; ROSLOFF and DAVIS, 1974; SANGHVI and GERSHON, 1975). Moreover, NYBÄCK et al. (1975) demonstrated that iprindole, unlike other tricyclic antidepressants, did not suppress the spontaneous firing rate of NE cells in the locus coeruleus, thus, also indicating that this antidepressant did not increase the availability of NE at post synaptic receptor sites. The therapeutic efficacy of mianserin appears also not related to inhibition of monoamine uptake (COPPEN et al., 1976; GOODLET et al., 1977). Obviously, an acute increase in the availability of catechol- and/or indolealkylamines is not directly related to therapeutic efficacy and the blockade of neuronal tranport mechanisms for biogenic amines is not an absolute prerequisite for antidepressant efficacy.

III. Interaction of Tricyclic Antidepressants with Other Drugs

CARLSSON and WALDECK (1965 a, b) have demonstrated that tricyclic antidepressants interfere with the uptake of hydrophilic amines (e. g., guanethidine and metaraminol) by blocking the rather unspecific transport system in neuronal membranes. Such an effect can explain the prevention by tricyclic antidepressants of the adrenergic neurone blockade and the depletion of catecholamines caused by guanethidine (STONE et al., 1964). It also explains the reduction by tricyclic antidepressants of the 6-hydroxydopamine-induced depletion of NE and DA as well as the reduction in 5HT depletion caused by p-chloroamphetamine because the biochemical effects of 6-hydroxydopamine and p-chloroamphetamine depend on their neuronal uptake (EVETTS and IVERSEN, 1970; MEEK et al., 1971; FULLER et al., 1975). Indeed, one method of evaluating uptake inhibition by potential antidepressants in vivo uses amine depleting drugs which require active transport into monoaminergic neurons (Table 2).

Table 2. ED_{50} values for various uptake inhibitors as antagonists of 6-hydroxydopamine or p-chloroamphetamine. (From FULLER et al., 1975)

Uptake inhibitor	Antagonism of 6-hydroxydopamine (ED_{50} mg/kg, i.p.)[a]	Antagonism of p-chloroamphetamine (ED_{50} mg/kg, i.p.)[a]
Protriptyline	0.12	~32
Desmethylimipramine	0.25	N.E.
EXP 561	0.50	0.25
Nisoxetine	0.9	N.E.
Nortriptyline	1.2	>32
Chlorpheniramine	1.3	8.1
Desmethylchlorimipramine	1.6	>32
Imipramine	3.4	N.E.
Doxepin	4.7	N.E.
Amitriptyline	5.4	N.E.
Chlorimipramine	6.0	10
Fluoxetine (Lilly 110140)	N.E.	0.40
Desmethylfluoxetine (Lilly 103947)	N.E.	1.6

[a] The ED_{50} values represent the doses giving 50% protection against depletion of heart NE (6-hydroxydopamine) or brain 5-HT (p-chloroamphetamine). N.E.: Not effective

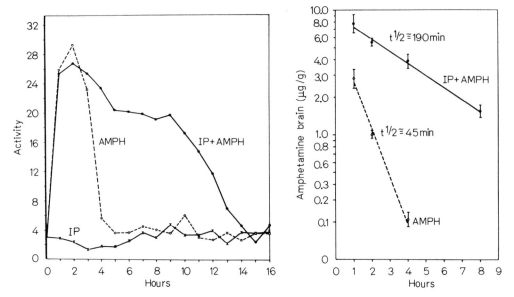

Fig. 1. Effect of iprindole on CNS stimulation elicited by d-amphetamine (left) and on the half-life of [³H]-d-amphetamine in brain (right). CNS stimulation (locomotor and stereotyped activity) was measured in Williamson activity cages and is expressed as mean counts per hour. Vertical bars represent the standard deviation of the mean. N = 4–6. Iprindole was given i. p. 30 min before d-amphetamine or [³H]-d-amphetamine. IP = iprindole (10 mg/kg); AMPH = d-amphetamine (5 mg/kg). (From FREEMAN and SULSER, 1972)

The blockade by tricyclic antidepressants of the rather unspecific transport system in neuronal membranes has clinical consequences. For example the antihypertensive effect of guanethidine, bethanidine, and debrisoquin can be nullified by tricyclic antidepressants (LEISHMAN et al., 1963; MITCHELL et al., 1970).

Tricyclic antidepressants enhance and/or prolong various behavioral effects of amphetamine (CARLTON, 1961; STEIN and SEIFTER, 1961; SCHECKEL and BOFF, 1964). This action of tricyclic drugs is the consequence of an inhibition of para-hydroxylation of amphetamine (SULSER et al., 1966; CONSOLO et al., 1967; VALZELLI et al., 1967; GROPPETTI and COSTA, 1969; LEWANDER, 1969; FREEMAN and SULSER, 1972). A typical example of this drug interaction is depicted in Fig. 1.

In contrast to the enhancement by tricyclic antidepressants of many central actions of amphetamine, peripheral effects of this indirectly acting sympathomimetic amine are reduced or blocked by tricyclic antidepressants (SIGG, 1959). Since imipramine-like drugs inhibit the metabolism of amphetamine to p-hydroxyamphetamine and p-hydroxynorephedrine, it was conceivable that these hydroxylated metabolites could mediate the peripheral effects of amphetamine. This hypothesis has been disproven however, since iprindole, which is a potent inhibitor of the aromatic hydroxylation of amphetamine (FREEMAN and SULSER, 1972), did not block the blood pressure response to amphetamine in the rat (FREEMAN and SULSER, 1975).

Tricyclic antidepressants have since been shown to inhibit the metabolism of a number of other drugs, e. g., guanethidine (MITCHELL et al., 1970), tremorine, oxotremorine, pentobarbital, and hexobarbital (KATO et al., 1963; SJÖQVIST et al., 1968; SHAH and LAL, 1971), propranolol (SHAND and OATES, 1971), and methadone (LIU and WANG, 1975).

IV. Effect of Tricyclic Antidepressants Following Their Prolonged Administration on Adaptive Presynaptic Regulation

The pharmacologic findings that tricyclic antidepressants failed to antagonize the reserpine-like syndrome (model depression) in rats whose brains had been selectively depleted of catecholamines (SULSER et al., 1964; SCHECKEL and BOFF, 1964) and the early demonstration that NE re-uptake by noradrenergic neurons is inhibited by this type of drug (AXELROD et al., 1961; DENGLER et al., 1961; GLOWINSKI and AXELROD, 1965) have contributed to the experimental basis of the clinically relevant catecholamine hypothesis of affective disorders (SCHILDKRAUT, 1965; BUNNEY and DAVIS, 1965). However, this hypothesis is chiefly based on studies of acute biochemical effects elicited by a number of clinically effective psychotropic drugs and does not take into consideration the discrepancy in the time course between biochemical and pharmacologic effects elicited by, e.g., tricyclic antidepressants within minutes and their clinical therapeutic action which requires treatment for several weeks.

SEGAL et al. (1974) have first reported adaptive changes in the activity of tyrosine hydroxylase following the chronic administration of reserpine and/or tricyclic antidepressants. Thus, repeated administration of desipramine for 8 days produced a significant decrease in the activity of tyrosine hydroxylase in the locus coeruleus and hippocampus cortex area, but only a marginal decrease in the activity of the enzyme in the caudate nucleus, a predominantly dopaminergic area (Fig. 2). No significant change in enzyme activity was observed 24 h following the administration of desipramine. Such adaptive changes in the biosynthetic capacity can explain the decrease in the level of NE observed following chronic (SCHILDKRAUT et al., 1970, 1971; ROFFLER-TARLOV et al., 1973) but not acute administration of tricyclic antidepressants (SULSER et al., 1962, 1964). A decreased activity of tyrosine hydroxylase is also compatible with the finding of a decreased turnover rate of NE following chronic administration of tricyclic antidepressants (ROSLOFF, 1975; NIELSEN and BRAESTRUP, 1977). However, ROFFMAN et al. (1977) reported that the acute administration of imipramine or desipramine decreased while chronic administration of these tricyclic antidepressants increased the level of 3-methoxy-4-hydroxyphenylglycol sulfate in brain suggesting that chronic treatment with these drugs may enhance the turnover of NE. The reason for this discrepancy in results is not known. Since amitriptyline and nortriptyline did not elicit similar effects on the turnover of NE, it is unlikely that these effects on turnover reflect a mechanism for the delayed therapeutic activity of tricyclic antidepressants.

V. Miscellaneous Biochemical Effects of Antidepressant Drugs

Most tricyclic antidepressants share with the structurally related phenothiazines and antihistaminic agents peripheral and central anticholinergic properties (DOMENJOZ and THEOBALD, 1959; HALLIWELL et al., 1964). Biochemically, desipramine has been reported to decrease the "bound" acetylcholine fraction in brain while reserpine significantly increased the amount of "bound" acetylcholine in whole brain (HRDINA and

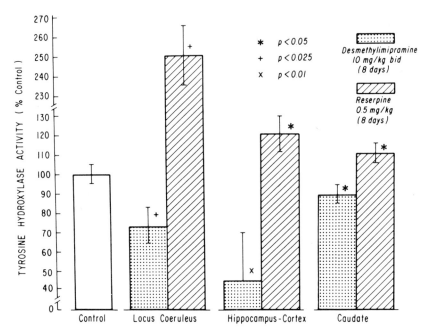

Fig. 2. Opposite effects of repeated administration of desmethylimipramine and of reserpine on tyrosine hydroxylase activity in discrete brain regions of the rat. Each bar represents the mean percent ± standard error of the mean of corresponding controls. There were at least eight animals per group. Significance was determined by the Mann-Whitney U-test. (From SEGAL et al., 1974)

LING, 1973). While the anticholinergic properties of tricyclic antidepressants can explain many of the autonomic side effects such as dry mouth and difficulty in accommodation, their contribution to the antidepressant efficacy is not known.

Tricyclic antidepressants block histamine H_2 receptors in brain (GREEN and MAAYANI, 1977). While some of the pharmacologic effects of tricyclic antidepressants may be related to blockade of H_2 receptors, the antihistamine potency of these and other drugs does not seem to parallel their clinical efficacy.

Tricyclic antidepressants have also been shown to inhibit DA-sensitive adenylate cyclase in homogenates of rat brain striatum, with amitriptyline and doxepin being particularly potent (KAROBATH, 1975). Obviously, there exists a discrepancy between the rather potent effects of some tricyclic antidepressants on DA sensitive adenylate cyclase in vitro and the low or absent antipsychotic activity of these drugs in vivo. Tricyclic antidepressants also inhibit the activity of cyclic nucleotide phosphodiesterase in brain (ROBERTS and SIMONSEN, 1970; ABDULLA and HAMADAK, 1970). The physiological significance of this biochemical effect is difficult to assess as it is shared by many other agents, e.g., benzodiazepines and promethazine (MUSCHEK and MCNEILL, 1971; BEER et al., 1972; BERNDT and SCHWABE, 1973), and because no class of drugs has yet been shown to act physiologically via their effect on cyclic nucleotide phosphodiesterases in either peripheral organs or in the CNS.

U'PRICHARD et al. (1978) have recently reported that tricyclic antidepressants display a high affinity for α-noradrenergic receptor sites in brain as determined by competition for the binding of the α-antagonist [³H]-WB-4101 (2-[2′,6′-dimethoxy]-phenoxyethylamine methylbenzodioxan) to membrane fractions of rat brain. The relative affinities of tertiary and secondary amines of tricyclic antidepressants as determined in such binding assays may be correlated with some of the side effects of these drugs. It is doubtful, however, whether such binding data reflect a mechanism for therapeutic efficacy in man as these in vitro effects occur almost instantly and are shared by a wide variety of other drugs (e. g., neuroleptics, phentolamine).

D. Effect of Antidepressant Drugs on the Sensitivity of the NE-Receptor-Coupled Cyclic AMP Generating System in the Limbic Forebrain and in Other Structures of the Brain

Recently, evidence has accumulated for a postsynaptic regulatory mechanism involving the NE-receptor-coupled adenylate cyclase system in the CNS. Following the administration of drugs which can precipitate despair in primates or severe depressive reactions in man (e. g., 6-hydroxydopamine, reserpine), an increased responsiveness of the cyclic AMP generating system to NE occurs in cortical slices (PALMER, 1972; WEISS and STRADA, 1972; HUANG et al., 1973; KALISKER, 1973), in slices from the hypothalamus and brain stem (PALMER et al., 1973) and from the limbic forebrain area (VETULANI et al., 1976a). Conversely, antidepressant drugs when administered on a clinically relevant time basis, decreased the responsiveness of the limbic cyclic AMP generating system to NE (VETULANI and SULSER, 1975; VETULANI et al., 1976 a, b; SCHMIDT and THORNBERRY, 1977). While MAO inhibitors, given acutely, caused an

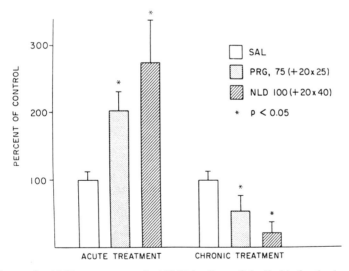

Fig. 3. Relative cyclic AMP responses to 5 μM NE in slices of the limbic forebrain of rats following acute and chronic treatment with MAO inhibitors. Animals were killed 18 h after the last injection. Pargyline *(PRG)* was administered at a dose of 75 mg/kg followed by daily doses of 25 mg/kg for 20 days; nialamide *(NLD)* was given at a dose of 100 mg/kg i. p. followed by daily doses of 40 mg/kg for 20 days. *SAL* = Saline. The data are expressed as a percentage of the control response to NE ± SEM. (From SULSER and VETULANI, 1977)

Table 3. Effect of long-term (4–8 weeks) treatment with desipramine or iprindole on the response of the cyclic AMP generating system in the rat limbic forebrain to N.E. (From VETULANI et al., 1976b)

	Time of sacrifice[a] (h)	N	Basal level of cyclic AMP (pmol/mg protein±SEM)	Cyclic AMP response to NE[b] (pmol/mg protein±SEM)	Percent of control response
Control	1 or 24	15	17.8±2.6	20.4±2.7	100
Desipramine	1	12	20.5±2.7	9.9±3.5[c]	49
Desipramine	24	14	16.6±1.6	6.9±2.1[e]	34
Iprindole	1	13	22.3±3.6	9.4±4.7[c]	46
Iprindole	24	15	16.9±1.5	7.9±2.4[d]	38

[a] Time after the last injection
[b] Difference in the level of cyclic AMP between the preparation exposed to 5 μM NE and that of the control preparation
[c] $p<0.05$
[d] $p<0.01$
[e] $p<0.001$ (difference from control response; Student t-test)

enhanced cyclic AMP response to NE, treatment with the MAO inhibitors for 3 weeks resulted in a significant desensitization of the NE-receptor-coupled adenylate cyclase system (Fig. 3). This change in the reactivity was unrelated to the actual size of the store of the catecholamine and depended solely on time (VETULANI et al., 1976a). Clinically effective tricyclic antidepressants such as desipramine (potent blocker of NE uptake) and iprindole (no effect on neuronal uptake of NE) also reduced the reactivity of the system to (R)-NE following their chronic but not acute administration (Table 3). The reduction in the neurohormonal response is not related to the concentration of the antidepressant drugs in brain tissue but again depends on time (VETULANI et al., 1976b). Tricyclic antidepressants, regardless of their action on presynaptic sites, thus share this delayed action on the limbic NE-receptor-coupled adenylate cyclase system with MAO inhibitor-type antidepressants. The development of delayed subsensitivity following chronic administration of tricyclic antidepressants has been confirmed in cortical slices (SCHULTZ, 1976; FRAZER and MENDELS, 1977) and in slices of the limbic forebrain (SCHMIDT and THORNBERRY, 1977).

The question arises about how one distinguishes between blockers of the NE-receptor-coupled adenylate cyclase system and drugs which reduce the sensitivity of the system following their chronic administration. Some of the pharmacodynamic differences between the two classes of drugs are summarized in Table 4.

The reduced sensitivity of the NE-receptor-coupled adenylate cyclase system resulting from prolonged administration of different prototypes of clinically effective antidepressant drugs suggests that the therapeutic action may be related to this common delayed postsynaptic change in noradrenergic receptor function in the limbic forebrain and in other brain areas with noradrenergic projections rather than to the acute and inconsistent action at presynaptic sites. It is doubtful, however, that blockade of reuptake of NE is the sole factor in causing subsensitivity of the NE-receptor-coupled adenylate cyclase system because iprindole does not block the neuronal reup-

Table 4. Pharmacologic distinction between blockade and desensitization of central noradrenergic receptor function by psychotropic drugs. (From Sulser and Robinson, 1977)

Central NE receptor blockade by drug	Desensitization of central NE-receptor-coupled cyclic AMP generating system by drug
1. Blockade is easily demonstrated in vitro	1. No blockade in vitro (in reasonable molar concentration)
2. Blockade depends on concentration of drug in tissue	2. Desensitization is not dependent on concentration of drug in tissue but instead depends on time

3. Drug activates interneuronal feedback mechanisms:
  a) Increase in the activity of tyrosine hydroxylase
  b) Increase in the rate of turnover of catecholamines
	3. Drug does not activate interneuronal feedback mechanisms:
	  a) No increase in the activity of tyrosine hydroxylase
	  b) No increase in the rate of turnover of catecholamines

4. Usually, drug also blocks markedly DOPAMINE receptors	4. No blockade of DOPAMINE receptors

Table 5. Effect of chronic administration of antidepressants on specific dihydroalprenolol binding. (From Banerjee et al. 1977)

Drug treatment	Specific [^{3}H]-dihydroalprenolol binding pmol/g protein
None	70.0 ± 3.5
Desipramine	24.2 ± 1.5 $(p < 0.001)$
Iprindole	40.4 ± 2.8 $(p < 0.001)$
Doxepin	48.6 ± 2.4 $(p < 0.001)$

Desipramine, iprindole, and doxepin were injected intraperitoneally in male Sprague-Dawley rats (180–220 g) at a dose of 10 mg/kg daily for 6 weeks. Specific binding, defined as the difference between total and nonspecific binding, was 60–70% of the total binding. Values are means $\pm$ S.E.M.

take of the catecholamine but nevertheless causes desensitization upon chronic administration (Vetulani et al., 1976b). Moreover, nisoxetine which is a potent and selective inhibitor of the reuptake of NE has recently been reported not to reduce the neurohormonal responsiveness of the system (Schmidt and Thornberry, 1977). Studies aimed at the elucidation of the molecular basis of reduced noradrenergic receptor function have provided data suggesting that – at least with regards to β adrenergic receptors – the resistant state of adenylate cyclase towards NE after chronic administration of tricyclic antidepressants is linked to a decrease in the actual number of β-adrenergic receptors (Table 5). The possible therapeutic consequences of such drug-induced postsynaptic adaptive changes in the NE-receptor-coupled adenylate cyclase system and their implications for a molecular pathology of depressive illness have recently been discussed (Sulser, 1978).

References

Abdulla, Y.H., Hamadak, K.: 3'5'-cyclic adenosine monophosphate in depression and mania. Lancet *1*, 378–381 (1970)

Ahtee, L., Saarnivara, L.: The effect of drugs upon the uptake of 5-hydroxytryptamine and metaraminol by human platelets. J. Pharm. Pharmacol. *23*, 495–501 (1971)

Axelrod, J., Hertting, G., Patrick, R.W.: Inhibition of H³-norepinephrine release by monoamine oxidase inhibitors. J. Pharmacol. Exp. Ther. *134*, 325–328 (1961)

Banerjee, L.P., Kung, L.S., Riggi, S.T., Chanda, S.K.: Development of β-adrenergic receptor subsensitivity by antidepressants. Nature *268*, 455–456 (1977)

Beer, B., Chasin, M., Clody, D.E., Vogel, J.R., Horovitz, Z.P.: Cyclic adenosine monophosphate phosphodiesterase in brain: Effect on anxiety. Science *176*, 428–430 (1972)

Berndt, S., Schwabe, U.: Effect of psychotropic drugs on phosphodiesterase and cyclic AMP levels in rat brain in vivo. Brain Res. *63*, 303–312 (1973)

Berti, F., Shore, P.A.: A kinetic analysis of drugs that inhibit the adrenergic neuronal membrane amine pump. Biochem. Pharmacol. *16*, 2091–2094 (1967)

Bogdanski, D.F., Brodie, B.B.: The effects of inorganic ions on the storage and uptake of H³-norepinephrine by rat heart slices. J. Pharmacol. Exp. Ther. *165*, 181–189 (1969)

Bogdanski, D.F., Tissari, A., Brodie, B.B.: The effects of inorganic ions on uptake, storage and metabolism of biogenic amines in nerve endings. In: Psychopharmacology – A review of Progress. Efron, D.H. (ed.), pp. 17–26. Washington: U.S. Government Printing Office 1968

Braestrup, C., Andersen, H., Randrup, A.: The monoamine oxidase B inhibitor deprenyl potentiates phenylethylamine behavior in rats without inhibition of catecholamine metabolite formation. Eur. J. Pharmacol. *34*, 181–187 (1975)

Breese, G.R., Chase, T.N., Kopin, I.J.: Effect of monoamine oxidase inhibitors on the disposition of intracisternally administered metaraminol – ³H. Biochem. Pharmacol. *19*, 525–532 (1970)

Bunney, W.E., Davis, J.M.: Norepinephrine in depressive reactions. Arch. Gen. Psychiatry *13*, 483–494 (1965)

Buus Lassen, J., Squires, R.F., Christensen, J.A., Molander, L.: Neurochemical and pharmacological studies on a new 5 HT uptake inhibitor FG4963, with potential antidepressant properties. Psychopharmacologia *42*, 21–26 (1975)

Carlsson, A., Waldeck, B.: Inhibition of ³H-metaraminol uptake by antidepressive and related agents. J. Pharm. Pharmacol. *17*, 243–244 (1965a)

Carlsson, A., Waldeck, B.: Mechanism of amine transport in the cell membranes of the adrenergic nerves. Acta Pharmacol. Toxicol. *22*, 293–300 (1965b)

Carlsson, A., Corrodi, H., Fuxe, K., Hökfelt, T.: Effect of antidepressant drugs on the depletion of intraneuronal brain 5-hydroxytryptamine stores caused by 4-α-ethyl-metatyramine. Eur. J. Pharmacol. *5*, 357–366 (1969)

Carlton, P.L.: Potentiation of the behavioral effect of amphetamine by imipramine. Psychopharmacologia *2*, 364–376 (1961)

Christmas, A.J., Coulson, C.J., Maxwell, D.R., Riddell, D.: A comparison of the pharmacological and biochemical properties of substrate-selective monoamine oxidase inhibitors. Br. J. Pharmacol. *45*, 490–503 (1972)

Consolo, S., Dolfini, S., Garattini, S., Valzelli, L.: Desipramine and amphetamine metabolism. J. Pharm. Pharmacol. *19*, 253–256 (1967)

Coppen, A., Gupta, R., Montgomery, S., Ghose, K., Bailey, J., Burns, B., Deridden, J.J.: Mianserin hydrochloride: A new antidepressant. Br. J. Psychiatry *129*, 342–345 (1976)

Corrodi, H., Fuxe, K.: Decreased turnover in central 5-HT nerve terminals induced by antidepressant drugs of the imipramine type. Eur. J. Pharmacol. *7*, 56–59 (1969)

Davey, M.J., Farmer, J.B., Reinert, H.: The effects of nialamide on adrenergic functions. Br. J. Pharmacol. *20*, 121–134 (1963)

Dengler, H.J., Spiegel, H.E., Titus, E.O.: Uptake of tritium-labeled norepinephrine in brain and other tissues of cat in vitro. Science *133*, 1072–1073 (1961)

Domenjoz, T., Theobald, W.: Zur Pharmakologie des Tofranil. Arch. Int. Pharmacodyn. Ther. *120*, 450–489 (1959)

Edwards, D.J., Burns, M.O.: Effects of tricyclic antidepressants upon human platelet monoamine oxidase. Life Sci. *15*, 2045–2058 (1974)

Escobar, J.I., Schiele, B.C., Zimmerman, R.: The tranylcypromine isomers: A controlled clinical trial. Am. J. Psychiatry *131*, 1025–1026 (1974)

Evetts, K.D., Iversen, L.L.: Effects of protriptyline on the depletion of catecholamines induced by 6-hydroxydopamine in the brain of the rat. J. Pharm. Pharmacol. *22*, 540–543 (1970)

Fowler, C.J., Callingham, B.A., Mantle, T.J., Tipton, K.F.: Monoamine oxidase A and B: A useful concept? Biochem. Pharmacol. *27*, 97–101 (1978)

Frazer, A., Mendels, J.: Do tricyclic antidepressants enhance adrenergic transmission? Am. J. Psychiatry *134*, 1040–1042 (1977)

Freeman, J.J., Sulser, F.: Iprindole-amphetamine interactions in the rat: The role of aromatic hydroxylation of amphetamine in its mode of action. J. Pharmacol. Exp. Ther. *183*, 307–315 (1972)

Freeman, J.J., Sulser, F.: The role of parahydroxylation of amphetamine in its peripheral mode of action. J. Pharm. Pharmacol. *27*, 38–42 (1975)

Fuller, R.W.: Kinetic studies and effects in vivo of a new monoamine oxidase inhibitor, N-[2-(0-chlorophenoxy)-ethyl]-cyclopropylamine. Biochem. Pharmacol. *17*, 2097–2106 (1968)

Fuller, R.W.: Selective inhibition of monoamine oxidase. Adv. Biochem. Psychopharmacol. *5*, 339–354 (1972)

Fuller, R.W., Snoddy, H.D., Molley, B.B.: Blockade of amine depletion by nisoxetine in comparison to other uptake inhibitors. Psychopharmacol. Commun. *1*, 455–464 (1975)

Fuxe, K., Ungerstedt, U.: Histochemical studies on the effect of (+) amphetamine, drugs of the imipramine group and tryptamine on central intraventricular injection of catecholamines and 5-hydroxytryptamine. Eur. J. Pharmacol. *4*, 135–144 (1968)

Gabay, S., Valcourt, A.J.: Biochemical determinants in the evaluation of monoamineoxidase inhibitors. Rec. Adv. Biol. Psychiatr. *10*, 29–41 (1968)

Glowinski, J., Axelrod, J.: Effect of drugs on the uptake release and metabolism of norepinephrine in the rat brain. J. Pharmacol. Exp. Ther. *149*, 43–49 (1965)

Goodlet, I., Mireyless, S.E., Sugrue, M.F.: Effects of mianserin, a new antidepressant, on the in vitro and in vivo uptake of monoamines. Br. J. Pharmacol. *61*, 307–313 (1977)

Goodrich, C.A.: Effect of monoamineoxidase inhibitors on 5-hydroxytryptamine output from perfused cerebral ventricles of anesthetized cats. Br. J. Pharmacol. *37*, 87–93 (1969)

Goridis, C., Neff, N.H.: Monoamine oxidase in sympathetic nerves: A transmitter specific enzyme type. Br. J. Pharmacol. *43*, 814–818 (1971)

Green, J.P., Maayani, S.: Tricyclic antidepressant drugs block histamine H_2 receptor in brain. Nature *269*, 163–165 (1977)

Groppetti, A., Costa, E.: Tissue concentrations of p-hydroxynorephedrine in rats injected with d-amphetamine: Effect of pretreatment with desipramine. Life Sci. *8*, 653–665 (1969)

Hall, D.W.R., Logan, B.W., Parsons, G.H.: Further studies on the inhibition of monoamine oxidase by M & B 9320 (clorgyline) – I, substrate specificity in various mammalian species. Biochem. Pharmacol. *18*, 1447–1454 (1969)

Halliwell, G., Quinton, R.M., Williams, F.E.: A comparison of imipramine, chlorpromazine and related drugs in various tests involving autonomic functions and antagonism of reserpine. Br. J. Pharmacol. *23*, 330–350 (1964)

Hendley, E.D., Snyder, S.H.: Relationship between the action of monoamine oxidase inhibitors on the noradrenaline uptake system and their antidepressant efficacy. Nature *220*, 1330–1331 (1968)

Horn, A.S.: Conformational aspects of the inhibition of neuronal uptake of noradrenaline by tricyclic antidepressants. In: Frontiers in catecholamine research. Usdin, E., Snyder, S.H. (eds.), pp. 411–413. New York: Pergamon Press 1973

Horn, A.S., Snyder, S.H.: Steric requirements for catecholamine uptake by rat brain synaptosomes: Studies with rigid analogs of amphetamine. J. Pharmacol. Exp. Ther. *180*, 523–530 (1972)

Horn, A.S., Coyle, J.R., Snyder, S.H.: Catecholamine uptake by synaptosomes from rat brain: Structure-activity relationships of drugs with differential effects on dopamine and norepinephrine neurons. Mol. Pharmacol. *7*, 66–80 (1971)

Horvitz, D., Lovenberg, W., Engelman, K., Sjoerdsma, A.: Monoamine oxidase inhibitors, tyramine and cheese. J. Am. Med. Assoc. *188*, 1108–1110 (1964)

Houslay, M.D., Tipton, K.F.: The nature of the electrophoretically separable multiple forms of rat liver monoamine oxidase. Biochem. J. *135*, 173–186 (1973)

Houslay, M.D., Tipton, K.F., Youdim, M.B.H.: Multiple forms of monoamine oxidase: Fact or artefact. Life Sci. *19*, 467–478 (1976)

Hrdina, R.D., Ling, G.M.: Effects of desipramine and reserpine on "free" and "bound" acetylcholine in rat brain. J. Pharm. Pharmacol. *25*, 504–507 (1973)

Huang, M., Ho, A.K.S., Daly, J.W.: Accumulation of adenosine 3′,5′ monophosphate in rat cerebral cortical slices. Mol. Pharmacol. *9*, 711–717 (1973)

Hunt, P., Kannengiesser, M.H., Raynaud, J.P.: Nomifensine: A new potent inhibitor of dopamine uptake into synaptosomes from rat brain corpus striatum. J. Pharm. Pharmacol. *26*, 370–371 (1974)

Hyttel, J.: Neurochemical characterization of a new potent and selective serotonin uptake inhibitor: Lu 10-171. Psychopharmacology *51*, 225–233 (1977)

Iversen, L.L.: The inhibition of noradrenaline uptake by drugs. Adv. Drug Res. *2*, 1–46 (1965)

Iversen, L.L.: Neuronal and extraneuronal catecholamine uptake mechanisms. In: Frontiers of catecholamine Research. Usdin, E., Snyder, S.H. (eds.), pp. 403–408. New York: Pergamon Press 1973

Iversen, L.L.: Uptake mechanisms for neurotransmitter amines. Biochem. Pharmacol. *23*, 1927–1935 (1974)

Jain, M.: Monoamine oxidase: Examination of multiple forms. Life Sci. *20*, 1925–1934 (1977)

Johnston, J.P.: Some observations upon a new inhibitor of monoamine oxidase in brain tissue. Biochem. Pharmacol. *17*, 1285–1297 (1968)

Kalisker, A., Rutledge, C.H.O., Perkins, J.P.: Effect of nerve degeneration by 6-hydroxydopamine on catecholamine-stimulated adenosine 3′,5′ monophosphate formation in rat cerebral cortex. Mol. Pharmacol. *9*, 619–629 (1973)

Karobath, M.E.: Tricyclic anti-depressive drugs and dopamine-sensitive adenylate cyclase from rat brain striatum. Eur. J. Pharmacol. *30*, 159–163 (1975)

Kato, R., Chiesara, E., Vassanelli, P.: Mechanism of potentiation of barbiturates and meprobamate actions by imipramine. Biochem. Pharmacol. *12*, 357–364 (1963)

Knoll, J., Magyar, K.: Some puzzling pharmacological effects of monoamine oxidase inhibitors. Adv. Biochem. Psychopharmacol. *5*, 393–408 (1972)

Kim, H.C., D'Iorio, A.: Possible isoenzymes of monoamine oxidase in rat tissues. Can. J. Biochem. *46*, 295–297 (1968)

Koe, B.K.: Molecular geometry of inhibitors of the uptake of catecholamines and serotonin in synaptosomal preparations of the rat brain. J. Pharmacol. Exp. Ther. *199*, 649–661 (1976)

Lahti, R.A., Maickel, R.P.: The tricyclic antidepressants – inhibition of norepinephrine uptake as related to potentiation of norepinephrine and clinical efficacy. Biochem. Pharmacol. *20*, 482–486 (1971)

Leishman, A.W.D., Matthew, H.L., Smith, A.J.: Antagonism of guanethidine by imipramine. Lancet *1*, 112 (1963)

Leitz, F.H.: Mechanisms by which amphetamine and desipramine inhibit the metaraminol-induced release of norepinephrine from sympathetic nerve endings in rat heart. J. Pharmacol. Exp. Ther. *173*, 152–157 (1970)

Lewander, T.: Influence of various psychoactive drugs on the in vivo metabolism of d-amphetamine in the rat. Eur. J. Pharmacol. *6*, 38–44 (1969)

Lidbrink, P., Toussan, G., Fuxe, K.: The effect of imipramine-like drugs and antipsychotic drugs on uptake mechanisms in the central noradrenaline and 5-hydroxytryptamine neurons. Neuropharmacology *10*, 521–536 (1971)

Liu, S.J., Wang, R.I.H.: Increased analgesia and alterations in distribution and metabolism of methadone by desipramine in the rat. J. Pharmacol. Exp. Ther. *195*, 94–104 (1975)

Maître, L., Staehelin, M., Bein, H.J.: Blockade of noradrenaline uptake by 34276-Ba, a new antidepressant drug. Biochem. Pharmacol. *20*, 2169–2186 (1971)

Maître, L., Waldmeier, P.C., Baumann, P.A., Staehelin, M.: Effect of maproptiline, a new antidepressant drug on serotonin uptake. Adv. Biochem. Psychopharmacol. *10*, 297–304 (1974)

Mandell, A.J., Knapp, S.: Adaptive regulation in central biogenic amine neurons. In: Psychopharmacology: A generation of progress. Lipton, M.A., Dimascio, A., Killam, K.F. (eds.), pp. 205–216. New York: Raven Press 1978

Marley, E., Blackwell, B.: Interaction of monoamine oxidase inhibitors, amines and foodstuffs. Adv. Pharmacol. *8*, 185–239 (1970)

Maxwell, R.A., Keenan, P.D., Chaplin, E., Roth, B., Eckhardt, S.B.: Molecular features affecting the potency of tricyclic antidepressants and structurally related compounds as inhibitors of the uptake of tritiated norepinephrine by rabbit aortic strips. J. Pharmacol. Exp. Ther. *166*, 320–329 (1969)

Maxwell, R.A., Chaplin, E., Eckhardt, S.B., Soares, J.R., Hite, G.: Conformational similarities between molecular models of phenethylamine and of potent inhibitors of the uptake of tritiated norepinephrine by adrenergic nerves in rabbit aorta. J. Pharmacol. Exp. Ther. *173*, 158–165 (1970)

Meek, J., Werdinius, B.: 4-Hydroxytryptamine turnover decreased by the antidepressant drug chlorimipramine. J. Pharm. Pharmacol. *22*, 141–143 (1970)

Meek, J., Fuxe, K., Anden, N.E.: Effect of antidepressant drugs of the imipramine type on central 5-hydroxytryptamine neurotransmission. Eur. J. Pharmacol. *9*, 325–332 (1970)

Meek, J.L., Fuxe, K., Carlsson, A.: Blockade of p-chloromethamphetamine induced 5-hydroxy-tryptamine depletion by chlorimipramine, chlorpheniramine and meperidine. Biochem. Pharmacol. *20*, 707–709 (1971)

Mitchell, J.R., Cavanaugh, J.H., Arias, L., Pettinger, W.A., Oates, J.A.: Guanethidine and related agents: III. Antagonism by drugs which inhibit the norepinephrine pump in man. J. Clin. Invest. *49*, 1596–1604 (1970)

Mosnaim, A.D., Inwang, E.E., Sabelli, H.C.: The influence of psychotropic drugs on the levels of endogenous 2-phenylethylamine in rabbit brain. Biol. Psychiatry *8*, 227–233 (1974)

Muschek, L.D., McNeil, J.H.: The effect of tricyclic antidepressants and promethazine on 3′,5′ – cyclic AMP phosphodiesterase from rat brain. Fed. Proc. *30*, 330 (1971)

Neff, N.H., Costa, E.: The influence of monoamine oxidase inhibition on catecholamine synthesis. Life Sci. *5*, 951–959 (1966)

Neff, N.H., Yang, H.-Y.T.: Another look at the monoamine oxidases and the monoamine oxidase inhibitor drugs. Life Sci. *14*, 2061–2074 (1974)

Ngai, S.H., Neff, N.H., Costa, E.: Effect of pargyline treatment on the rate of conversion of tyrosine ^{14}C to norepinephrine ^{14}C. Life Sci. *7*, 847–855 (1968)

Nielsen, M., Braestrup, C.: Chronic treatment with desipramine caused a sustained decrease of 3,4,-dihydroxyphenylglycol-sulfate and total 3-methoxy-4-hydroxyphenylglycol in the rat brain. Naunyn-Schmiedeberg's Arch. Pharmacol. *300*, 87–92 (1977)

Nybäck, H.V., Walters, J.R., Aghajanian, G.K., Roth, R.H.: Tricyclic antidepressants: Effect on the firing rate of brain noradrenergic neurons. Eur. J. Pharmacol. *32*, 302–312 (1975)

Palmer, G.C.: Increased cyclic AMP response to norepinephrine in the rat brain following 6-hydroxydopamine. Neuropharmacology *11*, 145–149 (1972)

Palmer, G.C., Sulser, F., Robison, G.A.: Effect of neurohumoral and adrenergic agents on cyclic AMP levels in various areas of the rat brain in vitro. Neuropharmacology *12*, 327–338 (1973)

Pletscher, A., Gey, K.F.: Pharmakologische Beeinflussung des 5-hydroxytryptamin-Stoffwechsels im Gehirn und Monoaminoxydasehemmung in vitro. Helv. Physiol. Acta *17*, c35–c39 (1959)

Roberts, E., Simonsen, D.G.: Some properties of cyclic 3′5′-nucleotide phosphodiesterase of mouse brain: Effects of midazole 4-acetic acid, chlorpromazine, cyclic 3′5′-GMP, and other substances. Brain Res. *24*, 91–111 (1970)

Roffler-Tarlov, S., Schildkraut, J.J., Draskoczy, R.R.: Effects of acute and chronic administration of desmethylimipramine on the content of norepinephrine and other monoamines in the rat brain. Biochem. Pharmacol. *22*, 2923–2926 (1973)

Roffman, M., Kling, A., ; Cassens, G., Orsulak, P.J., Reigle, T.G., Schildkraut, J.J.: The effects of acute and chronic administration of tricyclic antidepressants on MHPG-SO$_4$ in rat brain. Commun. Psychopharmacol. *1*, 195–206 (1977)

Rosloff, B.N.: Studies on mechanism of action of tricyclic antidepressant drugs using iprindole as a tool. (Ph.D Thesis) Graduate School, Vanderbilt University 1975

Rosloff, B.N., Davis, J.M.: Effect of iprindole on norepinephrine turnover and transport. Psychopharmacologia *40*, 53–64 (1974)

Ross, S.B., Renyi, A.L.: Inhibition of the uptake of tritiated catecholamines by antidepressant and related agents. Eur. J. Pharmacol. *2*, 181–186 (1967)

Ross, S.B., Renyi, A.L.: Inhibition of the uptake of tritiated 5-hydroxytryptamine in brain tissue. Eur. J. Pharmacol. *7*, 270–277 (1969)

Ross, S.B., Renyi, A.L., Ogren, S.O.: A comparison of the inhibitory activities of iprindole and imipramine on the uptake of 5-hydroxytryptamine and noradrenaline in brain slices. Life Sci. *10*, 1267–1277 (1971)

Roth, J.A., Gillis, C.N.: Inhibition of rabbit mitochondrial monoamine oxidase by iprindole. Biochem. Pharmacol. *24*, 151–152 (1975a)

Roth, J.A., Gillis, C.N.: Some structural requirements for inhibition of type A and B forms of rabbit monoamine oxidase by tricyclic psychoactive drugs. Mol. Pharmacol. *11*, 28–35 (1975b)

Salama, A.I., Insalaco, J.R., Maxwell, R.A.: Concerning the molecular requirements for the inhibition of the uptake of racemic ^{3}H-norepinephrine into rat cerebral cortex slices by tricyclic antidepressants and related compounds. J. Pharmacol. Exp. Ther. *178*, 474–481 (1971)

Sandler, M., Youdim, M.B.H.: Multiple forms of monoamine oxidase: Functional significance. Pharmacol. Rev. *24*, 331–348 (1972)

Sanghvi, I., Gershon, S.: Effect of acute and chronic iprindole on serotonin turnover in mouse brain. Biochem. Pharmacol. *24*, 2103–2104 (1975)

Scheckel, C.L., Boff, E.: Behavioral effects of interacting imipramine and other drugs with d-amphetamine, cocaine and tetrabenazine. Psychopharmacologia *5*, 198–208 (1964)

Schildkraut, J.J.: The catecholamine hypothesis of affective disorders: A review of supporting evidence. Am. J. Psychiatry *122*, 509–522 (1965)

Schildkraut, J.J., Winokur, A., Applegate, C.W.: Norepinephrine turnover and metabolism in rat brain after long term administration of imipramine. Science *168*, 867–869 (1970)

Schildkraut, J.J., Winokur, A., Dreskoczy, P.R., Hensle, J.H.: Changes in norepinephrine turnover in rat brain during chronic administration of imipramine and protriptyline: A possible explanation for the delay in onset of clinical antidepressant effects. Am. J. Psychiatry *27*, 72–79 (1971)

Schmidt, M.J., Thornberry, J.F.: Norepinephrine stimulated cyclic AMP accumulation in brain slices in vitro after serotonin depletion or chronic administration of selective amine reuptake inhibitors. Arch. Int. Pharmacodyn. Ther. *229*, 42–51 (1977)

Schultz, J.: Psychoactive drug effects on a system which generates cyclic AMP in brain. Nature *261*, 417–418 (1976)

Segal, D.S., Kuczenski, R., Mandell, A.J.: Theoretical implications of drug induced adaptive regulations for a biogenic amine hypothesis of affective disorders. Biol. Psychiatry *9*, 147–159 (1974)

Shah, H.C., Lal, H.: The potentiation of barbiturates by desipramine in the mouse: Mechanism of action. J. Pharmacol. Exp. Ther. *179*, 404–409 (1971)

Shand, D.G., Oates, J.A.: Metabolism of propranolol by rat liver microsomes and its inhibition by phenothiazine and tricyclic antidepressant drugs. Biochem. Pharmacol. *20*, 1720–1723 (1971)

Sheard, M.H., Zolovick, A., Aghajanian, G.K.: Raphé neurons: Effect of tricyclic antidepressant drugs. Brain Res. *43*, 690–694 (1972)

Sigg, E.B.: Pharmacological studies with tofranil. Can. Psychiatr. Assoc. J. *4*, 575–585 (1959)

Sjöqvist, R., Hammer, W., Schumacher, H., Gillette, J.R.: The effect of desmethylimipramine and other "anti-tremorine" drugs on the metabolism of tremorine and oxotremorine in rats and mice. Biochem. Pharmacol. *17*, 915–934 (1968)

Spector, S., Gordon, R., Sjoerdsma, A., Udenfriend, S.: End-product inhibition of tyrosine hydroxylase as a possible mechanism for regulation of norepinephrine synthesis. Mol. Pharmacol. *3*, 549–555 (1967)

Squires, R.F.: Multiple forms of monoamine oxidase in intact mitochondria as characterized by selective inhibitors and thermal stability: A comparison of eight mammalian species. Adv. Biochem. Psychopharmacol. *5*, 355–370 (1972)

Stein, L., Seifter, J.: Possible mode of antidepressant action of imipramine. Science *134*, 286–287 (1961)

Steinberg, M.I., Smith, C.B.: Effects of desmethylimipramine and cocaine on the uptake, retention, and metabolism of H^3-tyramine in rat brain slices. J. Pharmacol. Exp. Ther. *173*, 176–192 (1970)

Stone, C., Porter, C., Stavorski, J., Ludden, C., Totaro, J.: Antagonism of certain effects of cat-echolamine depleting agents by antidepressants and related drugs. J. Pharmacol. Exp. Ther. *144*, 196–204 (1964)

Strada, S.J., Sulser, F.: Effect of monoamine oxidase inhibitors on metabolism and in vivo re-lease of H³ norepinephrine from the hypothalamus. Eur. J. Pharmacol. *18*, 303–308 (1972)

Sullivan, J.L., Dackis, C., Stanfield, C.: In vivo inhibition of platelet MAO activity by tricyclic antidepressants. Am. J. Psychiatry *134*, 188–190 (1977)

Sulser, F.: Functional aspects of the norepinephrine receptor coupled adenylate cyclase system in the limbic forebrain and its modification by drugs which precipitate or alleviate de-pression: Molecular approaches to an understanding of affective disorders. Pharmakopsy-chiatr. Neuropsychopharmacol. *11*, 43–52 (1978)

Sulser, F., Robinson, S.E.: Clinical implications of pharmacological differences among anti-psychotic drugs. In: Psychopharmacology: A generation of progress. Lipton, M.A., Di-Mascio, A., Killam, K.F. (eds.), pp. 943–954. New York: Raven Press 1977

Sulser, F., Vetulani, J.: The noradrenergic cyclic AMP generating system in the limbic fore-brain: A functional postsynaptic norepinephrine receptor system and its modification by drugs which either precipitate or alleviate depression. In: Animal models in psychiatry and neurology. Hanin, I., Usdin, E. (eds.), pp. 189–199. New York: Pergamon Press 1977

Sulser, F., Watts, J., Brodie, B.B.: On the mechanism of antidepressant action of imipramine-like drugs. Ann. N.Y. Acad. Sci. *96*, 279–286 (1962)

Sulser, F., Bickel, M.H., Brodie, B.B.: The action of desmethylimipramine in counteracting se-dation and cholinergic effects of reserpine-like drugs. J. Pharmacol. Exp. Ther. *144*, 321–330 (1964)

Sulser, F., Owens, M.L., Dingell, J.V.: On the mechanism of amphetamine potentiation by de-sipramine (DMI). Life Sci. *5*, 2005–2010 (1966)

Sulser, F., Owens, M.L., Strada, S.J., Dingell, J.V.: Modification by desipramine of the avail-ability of norepinephrine released by reserpine in the hypothalamus of the rat. J. Pharma-col. Exp. Ther. *168*, 272–282 (1969)

Todrick, A., Tait, A.C.: The inhibition of human platelets 5-hydroxytryptamine uptake by tri-cyclic antidepressive drugs. The relation between structure and potency. J. Pharm. Pharma-col. *21*, 751–762 (1969)

Tuomisto, J.: Nomifensine and its derivatives as possible tools for studying amine uptake. Eur. J. Pharmacol. *42*, 101–106 (1977)

U'Prichard, D.C., Greenberg, D.A., Sheehan, P.P., Snyder, S.H.: Tricyclic antidepressants: Therapeutic properties and affinity for α-noradrenergic receptor binding sites in the brain. Science *199*, 197–198 (1978)

Usdin, E., Usdin, V.R.: Effects of psychotropic compounds on enzyme systems, II. In vitro in-hibition of monoamine oxidase. Proc. Soc. Exp. Biol. Med. *108*, 461–463 (1961)

Valzelli, L., Consolo, S., Morpurgo, C.: Influence of imipramine-like drugs on the metabolism of amphetamine. In: Antidepressant drugs. Garattini, S., Dukes, M.N.G. (eds.), pp. 61–69. Amsterdam: Excerpta Medica Foundation 1967

Vetulani, J., Sulser, F.: Action of various antidepressant treatments reduces reactivity of nor-adrenergic cyclic AMP generating system in limbic forebrain. Nature *257*, 495–496 (1975)

Vetulani, J., Stawarz, R.J., Sulser, F.: Adaptive mechanisms of the noradrenergic cyclic AMP generating system in the limbic forebrain of the rat: Adaptation to persistent changes in the availability of norepinephrine (NE). J. Neurochem. *27*, 661–666 (1976a)

Vetulani, J., Stawarz, R.J., Dingell, J.V., Sulser, F.: A possible common mechanism of action of antidepressant treatments. Naunyn-Schmiedeberg's Arch. Pharmacol. *293*, 109–114 (1976b)

Voigtlander, P.F. von, Losey, E.G.: Inhibition of phenylethylamine metabolism in vivo – effect of antidepressants. Biochem. Pharmacol. *25*, 217–218 (1976)

Waldmeier, P.C., Delini-Stula, A., Maître, L.: Preferential deamination of dopamine by an A type monoamine oxidase in rat brain. Naunyn-Schmiedeberg's Arch. Pharmacol. *292*, 9–14 (1976)

Weiss, B., Strada, S.: Neuroendocrine control of the cyclic AMP system of brain and pineal gland. Adv. Cyclic Nucl. Res. *1*, 357–374 (1972)

Wong, D.T., Bymaster, F.P., Horng, F.S., Molloy, B.B.: A new selective inhibitor for uptake of serotonin into synaptosomes of rat brain: 3-(p-trifluoromethylphenoxy)-N-methyl-3-phenylpropylamine. J. Pharmacol. Exp. Ther. *193*, 804–811 (1975)

Yang, H.-Y.T., Neff, N.H.: β-Phenylethylamine: A specific substrate for type B monoamine oxidase of brain. J. Pharmacol. Exp. Ther. *187*, 365–371 (1973)

Yang, H.-Y.T., Neff, N.H.: The monoamine oxidases of brain: Selective inhibition with drugs and the consequences for the metabolism of the biogenic amines. J. Pharmacol. Exp. Ther. *189*, 733–740 (1974)

Youdim, M.B.H., Collins, G.G.S., Sandler, M.: Multiple forms of rat brain monoamine oxidase. Nature *223*, 626–628 (1969)

Zirkle, C.L., Kaiser, C., Tedeschi, D.H., Tedeschi, R.E., Burger, A.: 2-Substituted cyclopropylamines. II. Effect of structure upon monoamine oxidaseinhibitory activity as measured in vivo by potentiation of tryptamine convulsions. J. Med. Chem. *5*, 1265–1284 (1962)

Biochemical Effects of Antidepressants in Man

G. Langer and M. Karobath

A. General Introduction

Hypotheses of a relationship between functional abnormalities of CNS neurotransmitters such as norepinephrine (NE), dopamine (DA) or 5-hydroxytryptamine (5-HT, serotonin), and depressive disorders have been advanced by inductive reasoning based on pharmacologic studies in animals (Bunney and Davis, 1975; Schildkraut and Kety, 1967; Goodwin and Murphy, 1974). Within this conceptional framework antidepressant drugs such as the "tricyclics" and the monoamine oxidase (MAO) inhibitors have been extensively studied with regard to their effects on the neurotransmitter systems mentioned above. It has been shown that tricyclic antidepressants inhibit the uptake of NE and 5-HT into respective neurons (Carlsson, 1965). Further differentiation of the pharmacologic effects revealed that tricyclic antidepressants with terminal tertiary amines (e. g., imipramine, amitriptyline, chlorimipramine) affected reuptake of mainly 5-HT. Their desmethylated metabolites, the secondary amines desmethylimipramine, nortriptyline, and desmethylchlorimipramine, were found to inhibit predominantly NE uptake (for review, Maas, 1975). To what extent the clinical effects of tricyclics are indeed contingent on uptake inhibition of respective neurotransmitters, whether the concomitant MAO inhibitory effects might also play a role (Roth, 1976), or whether both biochemical properties are merely secondarily related to the therapeutic effect are still an unresolved question. The absence of a valid animal model of human depression renders the necessary test of the validity of any pharmacologic hypothesis in man extremely difficult. Another methodological problem is posed by the fact that the human brain is generally not amenable to direct biochemical investigation, with the exception of postmortem studies. Being aware of these methodological constraints, biochemical research of the effects of antidepressant drugs *in man* focused on measuring levels of biogenic amines (NE, DA, 5-HT) and their respective metabolites in the body fluids (urine, blood, CSF) of depressive patients before and during antidepressant drug treatment. Such studies will mainly be reviewed. We will exclude studies on biogenic amines and metabolites in postmortem human brain tissues (for review, Goodwin and Post, 1975); in these studies brain tissues of suicide victims were analyzed but the diagnoses of those patients and their history of antidepressant medication have been poorly established.

The biochemical effects of the tricyclic antidepressants imipramine and amitriptyline, their respective metabolites desmethylimipramine and nortriptyline (the latter are also used as antidepressants in their own right), and chlorimipramine were mainly studied in man. These studies will be reviewed together with biochemical studies in depressives treated with MAO inhibitors. Human studies with lithium will be reviewed elsewhere in this handbook (see Chap. 3.11); we shall only report a few studies at appropriate place for heuristic purposes. It is equivocal whether precursors of biogenic amines (e. g., levodopa, tryptophan, or 5-hydroxytryptophan (5-HTP) may be considered as antidepressants; nevertheless, we will review controlled studies which report biochemical effects along with therapeutic improvement.

B. Biochemical Effects of Antidepressants as Reflected in the Urine

I. Introduction

The biogenetic amines, NE, DA, 5-HT, cannot penetrate the blood brain barrier. Thus, their concentrations in the urine reflect peripheral neuro (-hormo)nal activity. 5-Hydroxyindoleacetic acid (5-HIAA) is the major metabolite of 5-HT, both centrally and peripherally (LOVENBERG and ENGELMAN, 1971). Since the peripheral contribution to urinary 5-HIAA is large and varying in amount, urinary 5-HIAA is not considered to be a suitable indicator of brain 5-HT metabolism. Similar reasoning applies to DA, which is metabolized principally to homovanillic acid (HVA) and, to a lesser extent, to dihydroxyphenylacetic acid (DOPAC), (GOODALL and ALTON, 1968). Urinary HVA does not reflect brain DA metabolism as exemplified by the fact that patients suffering from parkinsonism have been reported to excrete HVA in amounts not different from controls (RINNE and SONNINEN, 1968; WEIL-MALHERBE and VAN BUREN, 1969). Biochemical studies in depressive patients have, therefore, focused on the urinary excretion of 3-methoxy-4-hydrophenylglycol (MHPG), which is believed to be the major metabolite of NE in the brain (ERWIN, 1973). These studies have been advanced despite the ignorance as to what percentage of *human* urinary MHPG reflects CNS activity of NE and whether this unknown ratio of central to peripheral MHPG in urine is constant at least within an individual (GOODALL and ROSEN, 1963, MAAS and LANDIS, 1968; SCHANBERG et al., 1968; MAAS et al., 1973; EBERT and KOPIN, in press). In contrast to MHPG, urinary concentrations of the other metabolite of NE, vanillylmandelic acid (VMA), appear to reflect virtually exclusively peripheral NE metabolism (EBERT and KOPIN, in press).

II. Effects of Tricyclics and MAO Inhibitors

An early clinical study reported that the urinary excretion of normetanephrine, a NE metabolite, was significantly higher in patients during treatment with imipramine than before treatment (SCHILDKRAUT et al., 1965, 1966). This finding reflects the effects of imipramine on peripheral NE activity since the blood–brain barrier does not allow passage of NE or normetanephrine (GLOWINSKY et al., 1965; SCHANBERG et al., 1968).

Treatment of depressives with imipramine or amitriptyline (BECKMANN and GOODWIN, 1975), with the MAO inhibitor phenelzine (BECKMANN and MURPHY, 1977) or with d-amphetamine (BECKMANN et al., 1976) all reduced urinary MHPG excretion. Attempts have then been made to relate therapeutic response to an antidepressant drug with pretreatment MHPG levels. The therapeutic efficacy of imipramine and desmethylimipramine was reported to be greater when pretreatment concentrations of MHPG were low rather than normal or high (MAAS et al., 1973; BECKMANN and GOODWIN, 1975). Likewise, the short-term antidepressive effect of d-amphetamine was reported to be more pronounced in the "low MHPG excretors" (FAWCETT et al., 1972). The therapeutic improvement to amitriptyline, however, was found to be correlated with normal or high excretion of MHPG; patients who failed to respond to amitriptyline were retrospectively found to be "low MHPG excretors" (SCHILD-KRAUT, 1973; BECKMANN and GOODWIN, 1975). On the other hand, another longitudinal study of MHPG excretion did not support any relationship between pretreatment, MHPG excretion, and therapeutic response to amitriptyline (SACCHETTI et al., 1976). We would like to mention, for heuristic purposes, that the antidepressant response to lithium was reported to be best in patients with low MHPG levels whose MHPG excretion consequently increased on lithium, whereas the patients who had failed to improve on lithium showed no change in their MHPG excretion (BECKMANN et al., 1975).

In the attempt to clarify which pharmacologic properties of imipramine (the effects on NE or 5-HT systems) were involved in the therapeutic improvement, α-methylparatyrosine (α-MPT) or parachlorphenylalanine (PCPA) were given to patients in addition to imipramine. α-MPT, an inhibitor of NE synthesis, did not alter the therapeutic improvement due to imipramine, despite a significant reduction in MHPG excretion. PCPA, however, an inhibitor of serotonin synthesis, rapidly reversed the imipramine-induced improvement of the patient (SHOPSIN et al., 1975) and also reversed the improvement induced by the MAO inhibitor tranylcypromine (SHOPSIN et al., 1977).

The relationship between imipramine treatment and urinary excretion of cyclic AMP has also been studied; low pretreatment levels were reported to normalize with clinical improvement on imipramine (ABDULLAH and HAMADAH, 1970; PAUL et al., 1970).

III. Discussion

Most studies report a decrease of urinary excretion in depressive patients treated with various antidepressant drugs. A relationship between therapeutic improvement and change of MHPG excretion is not established. This may be exemplified by a study which particularly focused on investigating this relationship in depressives treated with the MAO inhibitor, phenelzine (BECKMANN and MURPHY, 1977). While pretreatment levels of urinary MHPG excretion were significantly correlated with platelet MAO activity, the phenelzine-induced reduction in both variables failed to correlate significantly. Likewise, no relationship was found between the amount of MHPG excretion and the clinical improvement to phenelzine.

While clinical studies at hand support the hypothesis that various antidepressant drugs in therapeutic dosages may indeed affect (CNS) NE neuronal activity (as partially reflected by MHPG in the urine) the significance of this pharmacologic effect for the antidepressant efficacy remains to be elucidated.

C. Biochemical Effects of Antidepressants as Reflected in the Blood

I. Introduction

Effects of antidepressants particularly on the activities of catechol-O-methyltransferase (COMT) and MAO and the relationship to clinical response have been studied in the blood. COMT is a major degradatory enzyme for NE, DA, epinephrine and their deaminated metabolites. COMT activity has been identified in human erythrozytes and leukozytes (BALDESSARINI and BELL, 1966; AXELROD and COHN, 1971).

Human platelet MAO is a mitochondrial enzyme that catalyzes the oxidative deamination of many biogenic amines. In tissue, several forms of MAO have been described based on different affinities to substrates or pharmacologic inhibitors (Murphy and Wyatt, 1975). MAO inhibitors such as tranylcypromine and phenelzine, in doses which yield to antidepressive effects, were found to markedly inhibit human platelet MAO (Robinson et al., 1968).

A higher activity of MAO was found in platelets and postmortem brains of normal women than in men and the activity was found to increase with age. Since epidemiologic studies revealed a higher incidence of unipolar depression in women of middle age, the hypothesis was advanced that increased MAO activity might be a pathogenetic factor of depression in elderly women (Robinson et al., 1972). If this were true, treatment with MAO inhibitors would indeed be the specific therapy for these women. Unfortunately, clinical studies with MAO inhibitors did not reveal unanimously beneficial therapeutic effects which should be expected if the hypothesis is valid in its narrow formulation. Furthermore, studies in depressive patients, postmortem, analyzing brain tissues for MAO activity did not find a significant difference compared to normal controls (Grote et al., 1974).

II. Effects of Tricyclics and MAO Inhibitors

An early clinical study, a combined biochemical-physiological approach, reported a correlation between the uptake inhibition of NE into peripheral neurons, the concentration of nortriptyline in plasma, and the elevation of a patients blood pressure to a certain degree by variable doses of tyramine (Engelman and Sjoerdsma, 1964; Freyschuss et al., 1970). In another study, imipramine, 25 mg, or dimetrazine, 32.5 mg, were injected intravenously into eight patients. In all patients a marked increase in plasma NE, accompanied by an elevation in blood pressure, was observed (Biamino et al., 1976).

Most investigations were interested in the study of the two major degradatory enzymes for biogenic amines, COMT and MAO. COMT activity was not found to fluctuate over a period of 6 months and was not affected by tricyclics, lithium, electrotherapy, α-MPT, PCPA, phenothiazines, or clinical improvement. When these data of depressed patients were stratified for sex, a reduced activity of COMT in erythrocytes of depressed women has been reported whereas depressed men were found not to differ from controls (Cohn et al., 1970). Two other studies investigated the relationship to clinical outcome. A significant linear negative correlation was found between COMT-activity in erythrocytes of unipolar depressed women and the therapeutic response of the patients to imipramine (Davidson et al., 1976).

MAO inhibitors are potent inhibitors of platelet MAO in clinical doses. However, change of platelet MAO activity in depressives treated with MAO inhibitors does not appear to correlate with therapeutic response (Murphy and Wyatt, 1975). It is interesting that treatment of depressives with the tricyclics imipramine or amitriptyline for 3 weeks also decreased platelet MAO activity by 40% (Sullivan et al., 1977); whether this pharmacologic "side effect" is of therapeutic relevance is unknown. Lithium, levodopa, tryptophan, or phenothiazines do not appear to affect MAO activity (Murphy and Wyatt, 1975).

The effects of amitriptyline treatment on various metabolic variables have been studied in 40 depressed patients. Upon clinical recovery a significant decrease of fasting levels of glucose and growth hormone were reported together with a normalization of glucose responses in the glucose tolerance test and the insulin tolerance test (HENINGER et al., 1976). In contrast to this study is a study in normal volunteers in which amitriptyline 100 mg, given for 28 days, failed to affect weight or glucose tolerance tests, i.e., glucose and insulin responses (NAKRA et al., 1977).

In studying the effects of tricyclics on various pituitary hormones it was found that thyroid activity was not significantly altered in depressed patients by 4 weeks of imipramine therapy; the latter yielded to clinical recovery (COPPEN et al., 1972). Liothyronine given with imipramine appears to accelerate and increase the antidepressive effect of imipramine, but only in women (PRANGE et al., 1969; COPPEN et al., 1972); likewise, thyroid-stimulating hormone plus imipramine also appears to potentiate imipramine's therapeutic efficacy (PRANGE et al., 1970, 1976). These findings are consistent with the clinical observation that MAO inhibitors and tricyclic antidepressants in usual doses are more toxic in hyper- than in hypothyroidism (BAILEY et al., 1959; CARRIER and BUDAY, 1961). Imipramine or amitriptyline, given acutely and chronically, did not affect baseline plasma prolactin levels in depressives (MELTZER et al., 1977). On the other hand, acute administrations of desmethylimipramine, either 75 mg intramuscularly or 100 mg orally, induced a prompt growth hormone peak in all normal subjects tested; chlorimipramine, given in the same manner, released growth hormone in only half the subjects (LAAKMANN et al., 1977).

The acute effects of amitriptyline, intravenously, on cyclic AMP and plasma renin activity (PRA) were measured in the renal vein of medically ill patients. Cyclic AMP increased by 50% whereas the PRA was found to be unaltered (ZEHNER et al., 1976).

Maprotiline, a tetracyclic and secondary amine, and chlorimipramine, a tricyclic and tertiary amine, were compared with regard to their effects on plasma tryptophan binding and inhibition of serotonin uptake in platelets. Either drug was given to healthy volunteers for 4 days. Neither drug affected tryptophan binding; only chlorimipramine was, as expected, found to be a strong inhibitor of serotonin uptake (GREENGRASS et al., 1976).

III. Discussion

Tricyclics and MAO inhibitors, given in therapeutic dosages, clearly affect peripheral noradrenergic activity as evidenced by influences on blood pressure and MAO activity. The impact of these pharmacologic properties, if any, for the therapeutic response is still obscure. This is also true for the effects of antidepressants on various metabolic variables which are only now being investigated in man. The benefical effects of hormone of the hypothalamic-pituitary-thyroid axis, administered in conjunction with tricyclics, appear to be established, at least for a portion of the depressive population. The pharmacologic and biochemical mechanism, however, of this potentiating effects of hormones with tricyclics is unknown.

D. Biochemical Effects of Antidepressants as Reflected in the CSF

I. Introduction

It is generally believed that the concentrations of 5-HIAA, HVA, and DOPAC, and MHPG in the human cerebrospinal fluid (CSF) reflect CNS neuronal activity of 5-HT, DA, and NE, respectively. Thus, the precursor tryptophan given peripherally raises 5-HIAA levels in human lumbar CSF whereby levels of CSF tryptophan and 5-HIAA appear to be significantly correlated (ASHCROFT et al., 1973). Conversely, parachlorophenylalanine, an inhibitor of tryptophan hydroxylase, significantly lowers 5-HIAA levels in CSF (CHASE, 1972). Factors which affect brain amine turnover also effect their metabolic concentrations in human CSF in the appropriate manner. Thus, in Parkinson's disease, which involves a decrease in brain dopamine (HORNYKIEWICZ, 1966), low concentrations of HVA are found in lumbar CSF (BERNHEIMER et al., 1966). α-Methylparatyrosine, an inhibitor of tyrosine hydroxylase, and fusaric acid, an inhibitor of dopamine-β-hydroxylase, both cause a decrease of MHPG in human lumbar CSF (CHASE et al., 1973). Peripherally administered MHPG, however, does not penetrate into the CSF (CHASE et al., 1973); likewise, no relationship between the concentrations of MHPG in urine and CSF were found (SHAW et al., 1973).

Several methodological considerations, nevertheless, have to be raised (for review, GOODWIN and POST, 1975). The relationship of the concentrations of these metabolites to the firing rate of respective neurons, one indicator of functional significance, is unknown (this is, certainly, a general methodological consideration of all amine and metabolite studies). The question as to the proportions of the brain metabolites which are removed via the CSF rather than directly by the blood is also unresolved. It has been suggested, e. g., that a substantial portion of brain 5-HIAA never enters the CSF but is directly removed into the blood (MEEK and NEFF, 1973). Another methodological point of particular significance for studies in man (samples for evaluating the CSF are, due to clinical reasons, mostly taken from the lumbar CSF) is the question as to what relationship exists between the concentrations of metabolites in lumbar CSF relative to the concentrations at "pertinent" brain sites. While this question appears to face paramount methodological problems in man, it is at least possible to evaluate to what degree the spinal cord contributes to the concentrations of amine metabolites found in the lumbar CSF. Human 5-HIAA in lumbar CSF most likely reflects both spinal cord and brain metabolism (GARELIS et al., 1974). This was also suggested by clinical observation of brain-stem lesions (GUILLEMINAULT et al., 1973) or spinal fluid blocks (CURZON et al., 1971). It is furthermore supported by studies investigating, in man, the timecourse of 5-HIAA increase in ventricular and lumbar CSF following tryptophan infusion (ECCLESTON et al., 1970; GOODWIN et al., 1973 a) and by studies in hydrocephalic children (ANDERSON and ROSS, 1969). Human HVA in lumbar CSF most likely originates in sites cranial to the spinal cord. This is suggested, in man, by timecourse studies with radioactive levodopa (PLETSCHER et al., 1967) and by clinical observations of spinal fluid block (CURZON et al., 1971; GARELIS et al., 1973; YOUNG et al., 1973) and cord transsection (POST et al., 1973). In addition, the proportion of human brain HVA which enters the CSF appears to be high (SOURKES, 1973). With regard to human MHPG in lumbar CSF, a considerable portion appears to reflect spinal cord metabolism. Thus, in man, no gradient between ventricular and lumbar CSF MHPG has been found (CHASE et al., 1973) unlike HVA, gradient 10:1, or 5-HIAA, gradient 10:3 (SOURKES, 1973). Furthermore, clinical observations revealed that spinal cord transsections show significantly decreased MHPG levels in lubar CSF whereas a mere block of spinal fluid flow rendered MHPG levels in lumbar CSF unaltered (POST et al., 1973). Since a gradient was found for HVA and 5-HIAA in human CSF, the amount of CSF fluid withdrawn and other factors (e. g., prior bed rest) are pertinent methodological variables and should be standardized (BERTILSSON et al., 1974; SIEVER et al., 1975).

A recent elaboration of the CSF technology has involved the development of the probenecid technique. Probenecid can inhibit the transport system responsible for the removal of 5-HIAA and HVA from the CSF (MOIR et al., 1970); thus, by measuring the accumulation of respective metabolites rather than the baseline levels, a more dynamic indicator of CNS amine function is thought to be assessed (GOODWIN and POST, 1975). It is clear that the degree of probenecid-induced uptake blockade of these acids is a crucial variable which has to be standardized. Furthermore the implicit assumption that probenecid itself and/or the artificial accumulation of amine metabolites has no bearing on the metabolism being investigated awaits to be substantiated.

II. Effects of Tricyclics, MAO Inhibitors, and Precursors of Biogenic Amines

Treatment of depressives with amitriptyline was found to reduce, relative to the pretreatment level, the accumulation of 5-HIAA induced by probenecid (BOWERS, 1972). In another study imipramine or amitriptyline were given in doses of 150–300 mg/day for 3–4 weeks; both drugs reduced probenecid-induced accumulations of 5-HIAA by about 35% (POST and GOODWIN, 1974). In both studies no effect on HVA was found. In studying a possible relationship between therapeutic improvement and the amount of decrease of 5-HIAA accumulation no significant correlation was found. It was reported, however, that MHPG had increased slightly in the patients who improved on imipramine or amitriptyline, in contrast to a significant decrease of MHPG in the therapeutic nonresponders (POST and GOODWIN, 1974). However, if the means of the MHPG levels were compared between the patients when depressed and after recovery, no difference in levels was found regardless of whether patients were treated with tricyclics, lithium, electrotherapy, or placebo (GOODWIN and POST, 1975). The authors then compared pretreatment levels of probenecid-induced 5-HIAA, HVA, and MHPG accumulations with subsequent therapeutic response to imipramine or amitriptyline; higher pretreatment levels of 5-HIAA and HVA were positively correlated with therapeutic response, whereas MHPG was not found to predict clinical improvement. It is interesting to note that the authors found the therapeutic response to lithium to be negatively correlated with pretreatment levels of 5-HIAA and HVA. Lithium, given for 2–4 weeks, reduced probenecid-induced accumulations of 5-HIAA and HVA without affecting MHPG (GOODWIN et al., 1973 b). For reasons of comparison, we would like to mention that in the latter study improvement with electrotherapy was reported to correlate with a decrease in probenecid-induced 5-HIAA levels, whereas HVA or MHPG levels were found to remain unaltered.

Chlorimipramine treatment of depressives significantly reduced 5-HIAA and MHPG levels; HVA levels were increased in some patients and decreased in others with the mean being unaltered. The decrease of 5-HIAA in CSF was correlated with the in vitro uptake inhibition of 5-HT by the patient's plasma; no analogous relationship was found between CSF MHPG reduction and NE plasma uptake (ASBERG et al., 1977). In studying the relationship between pretreatment levels of 5-HIAA and therapeutic response to nortriptyline the following relationship was found (ASBERG et al., 1973). Depressives with low pretreatment 5-HIAA levels did not significantly ameliorate during treatment with nortriptyline (nortriptyline has negligible effects on serotonin) in contrast to patients with higher 5-HIAA levels who improved significantly. The depressives with the low 5-HIAA levels showed increased 5-HIAA levels during nortriptyline treatment, whereas the same drug reduced 5-HIAA levels in the patients with high pretreatment levels of 5-HIAA.

Another study investigated the relationship between decrease of probenecid-induced 5-HIAA levels during chlorimipramine treatment and therapeutic response; a linear significant correlation was found in 30 patients (VAN PRAAG, 1977). Eight of these patients did not improve on chlorimipramine; they were consequently treated with nortriptyline, a NE-potentiating antidepressant; five patients then improved whereas no relationship of therapeutic response with pretreatment CSF MHPG was found (VAN PRAAG, 1977). Urinary MHPG had not been measured in this study which is unfortunate since urinary MHPG rather than CSF MHPG is expected to reflect cerebral NE metabolism (GARELIS et al., 1974); furthermore, only a poor correlation between MHPG in CSF and urine can be expected (SHAW et al., 1973). VAN PRAAG also studied these patients longitudinally when they were free of symptoms for 6 months and free of antidepressant medication for at least a month. Only half of these recovered patients showed a normalization of the probenecid-induced 5-HIAA accumulation in the CSF (VAN PRAAG, 1976).

The serotonin-uptake inhibitor chlorimipramine and nomifensine, a stimulator of postsynaptic DA receptors, were given to depressives with low and normal probenecid-induced HVA accumulation. Nomifensine was significantly more effective in the low HVA patients in contrast to chlorimipramine (VAN PRAAG, 1977).

In contrast to the report by POST and GOODWIN (1974), JORI and collaborators (1975) found no difference between probenecid-induced accumulations of 5-HIAA and HVA before and after treatment with imipramine or electrotherapy. They also reported that, without probenecid, imipramine increased rather than decreased 5-HIAA and HVA levels.

Patients who did not improve with amitriptyline alone were treated with triiodothyronine (T_3) additionally (BANKI, 1977). The T_3 combination yielded to a significant clinical improvement in contrast to a control group of amitriptyline nonresponders whose dose of amitriptyline had been increased. However, no difference in 5-HIAA or HVA levels was observed between the patients who responded to treatment and the ones who did not.

Various tricyclics, lithium, or electrotherapy were not found to affect CSF levels of cyclic AMP compared to unmedicated depressed controls (POST et al., 1977). There was also no correlation found between baseline or probenecid-induced levels of cyclic AMP and 5-HIAA, HVA, and MHPG levels. Likewise no correlation with severity of depression was found.

The serotonin precursors, tryptophan and 5-hydroxy-tryptophan (5-HTP), stimulate central serotonin synthesis as evidenced in man by the increased probenecid-induced accumulation of 5-HIAA in the CSF (DUNNER and GOODWIN, 1972; VAN PRAAG and KORF, 1975). The antidepressant effect of L-tryptophan in a biochemically undifferentiated group of depressives is controversial; some authors report a therapeutic efficacy (COPPEN et al., 1967; HERRINGTON et al., 1974), others do not (CARROL et al., 1970; MENDELS et al., 1975). It appears, however, that tryptophan in combination with a MAO inhibitor (COPPEN et al., 1963; GLASSMAN and PLATMAN, 1969) or with clomipramine (WALINDER et al., 1975) potentiates the therapeutic efficacy of respective drugs. 5-HTP alone might be therapeutically effective in a biochemically defined subgroup of depressives characterized by a relatively small probenecid-induced accumulation of 5-HIAA in CSF before treatment outset (VAN PRAAG et al., 1972).

The overall therapeutic effect of L-Dopa, studied in a biochemically undifferentiated group of depressives, was reported to be not significantly different from placebo (GOODWIN et al., 1970; MATUSSEK et al., 1970). The score of motor retardation, however, which was positively correlated with pretreatment levels of probenecid-induced HVA accumulation did improve in those patients who showed low levels of HVA accumulation in the CSF. The increase of probenecid-induced HVA accumulation on L-Dopa treatment was similar in the low and normal HVA patients (VAN PRAAG, 1974).

Treatment with the MAO inhibitor phenelzine decreased probenecid-induced accumulations of 5-HIAA and HVA (BOWERS and KUPFER, 1971). The invariable reduction of CSF HVA levels by phenelzine was suggested to be one biochemical discriminator between the MAO inhibitors and the tricyclics; the latter showed variable effects on HVA (BOWERS, 1974b). The relationship between 5-HIAA and HVA was further substantiated by a study aimed at comparing in depressed patients the amount of probenecid-induced accumulation of 5-HIAA, HVA, and MHPG. A significant correlation was found only between 5-HIAA and HVA levels (GOODWIN and POST, 1975). We like to mention for purpose of comparison that various neuroleptics or narcotics do not influence the probenecid-induced accumulation of 5-HIAA (GOODWIN and POST, 1975).

III. Discussion

The "paradoxical" reduction of amine-metabolite levels during antidepressant treatment is believed to reflect a decrease of transmitter synthesis (BOWERS, 1974a) due to negative feedback inhibition (SCHUBERT et al., 1970). The latter is possibly initiated by increased stimulation of the postsynaptic receptors (MODIGH, 1973) due to the tricyclics which are supposed to block neurotransmitter reuptake.

E. General Discussion

Studies on the effect of antidepressant drugs on biogenic amine metabolism in man have been stimulated by the formulation of several hypothesis linking changes in the functional activity of biogenic amines with the etiology and clinical pathophysiology of depression. Based on evidence alluded to in this review it appears rather unlikely that the reported biochemical effects of antidepressant drugs, reflected by the body fluids in man, reveal pharmacologic effects on the etiology of the depressive disorder or on the mechanism of action of these compounds. Clinical studies on the biochemical effects of antidepressant drugs in man have also not led to the discovery of new forms of pharmacotherapy of depression.

Clinically, successful treatment with various antidepressant agents does not normalize the biochemical parameters believed to reflect a respective neuronal dysfunction. Attempts to correlate pretreatment values of biogenic amine metabolism in patients with the therapeutic improvement induced by antidepressant drugs have not led to unequivocal conclusions. They have led to the tendency to formulate subdivisions of diagnostic categories in order to make predictions of therapeutic outcome possible. While there are certainly several subtypes of mania and depression it has not been possible to correlate biochemical changes in these patients with psychopathological syndroms. The fact that parameters of biogenic amine metabolism measurable in man exhibit severe intraindividual and interindividual variations and mainly reflect metabolism of peripheral tissues renders a demonstration of such correlations, if they exist at all, more difficult. Furthermore a postulated functional deficiency of a biogenic amine, even if it is not restricted to the central nervous system, but a general metabolic derangement, does not necessarily imply that the metabolism of this amine is decreased. Depending on the hypothetical site where such a functional deficiency is located within an aminergic synapse one could expect a decrease or an increase in the metabolism of the respective amine.

The data on the metabolism of NE, DA, and 5-HT do not support original hypotheses of a single functional deficiency of one of these amines in manic or depressive disorders. This bewildering situation has led to attempts to develop more extended hypotheses based on a variable involvement of the functional activity of catecholamines, serotonin and acetylcholine in order to find sufficient variables to fit diagnostic systems.

Thus, in reviewing the clinical literature on biochemical changes in depression and on biochemical changes introduced by antidepressant medication one is forced to conclude that "it is the attribute to the persuasiveness and attractiveness of current pharmacologic theories concerning the biogenic amines that they have persisted in spite of conflicting and inconsistant findings" (Baldessarini, 1975).

Acknowledgement. We thank J. Reisenhofer for her help during the preparation of this manuscript.

References

Abdullah, Y.H., Hamadah, K.: 3',5'Cyclic Adenosine monophosphate in depression and mania. Lancet *I*, 378 (1970)

Anderson, H., Ross, B.E.: 5-Hydroxyindoleacetic acid in cerebrospinal fluid of hydrocephalic children. Acta Paediatr. Scand., *58*, 601–608 (1969)

Asberg, M., Bertilsson, L., Tuck, D., Cronholm, B., Sjöqvist, F.: Indoleamine metabolites in the cerebrospinal fluid of depressed patients before and during treatment with nortriptyline. Clin. Pharmacol. Ther. *14*, 277–286 (1973)

Asberg, M., Ringberger, V.A., Sjöqvist, F., Thoren, P., Traeksman, L., Tuck, J.R.: Monoamine metabolites in cerebrospinal fluid and serotonin uptake inhibition during treatment with chlorimipramine. Clin. Pharmacol. Ther. *21*, 201–207 (1977)

Ashcroft, G.W., Crawford, T.B.B., Cundall, R.L., Davidson, D.L., Dobson, J., Dow, R.C., Eccleston, D., Loose, R.W., Pullar, I.A.: 5-Hydroxytryptamine metabolism in affective illness: the effect of tryptophan administration. Psychol. Med. *3*, 326–332 (1973)

Axelrod, J., Cohn, C.K.: Methyltransferase enzymes in red blood cells. J. Pharmacol. Exp. Ther. *176*, 650–654 (1971)

Bailey, S.d'a, Bucci, L., Gosline, E., Kline, N.S., Park, Q.H., Rochline, D., Sanders, J.C.: Comparison of iproniazid with other monoamine oxidase inhibitors. Ann. N. Y. Acad. Sci. *80*, 652 (1959)

Baldessarini, R.J., Bell, W.R.: Methionine-activating enzyme and catechol-O-methyl transferase activity in normal and leucemic white blood cells. Nature *209*, 78–79 (1966)

Baldessarini, R.J.: Biogenic amine hypotheses in affective disorders. In: The nature and treatment of depression. Flach, F.F., Draghi, S.C. (eds.), pp. 347–384. New York: Wiley & Sons 1975

Banki, C.M.: Cerebrospinal fluid amine metabolites after combined amitriptyline-triiodothyronine treatment of depressed women. Eur. J. Clin. Pharmacol. *11*, 311–315 (1977)

Beckmann, H., Goodwin, F.K.: Antidepressant response to tricyclics and urinary MHPG in unipolar patients. Arch. Gen. Psychiatry *32*, 17–23 (1975)

Beckmann, H., Murphy, D.L.: Phenelzine in depressed patients – effects on urinary MHPG excretion in relation to clinical response. Neuropsychobiology *3*, 49–55 (1977)

Beckmann, H., St. Laurent, J., Goodwin, F.: The effect of lithium on urinary MHPG in unipolar and bipolar depressed patients. Psychopharmacology 42, 277–282 (1975)

Beckmann, H., Van Kammen, D.P., Goodwin, F.K., Murphy, D.L.: Urinary excretion of MHPG: Modifications by amphetamine and lithium. Biol. Psychiatry 11, 377–387 (1976)

Bernheimer, H., Birkmayer, W., Hornykiewicz, O.: Homovanillinsäure im Liquor cerebrospinalis: Untersuchungen beim Parkinson-Syndrom und anderen Erkrankungen des ZNS. Wien. Klin. Wochenschr. 78, 417–419 (1966)

Bertilsson, L., Asberg, M., Thorén, P.: Differential effect of chlorimipramine and nortriptyline on cerebrospinal fluid metabolites of serotonin and noradrenaline in depression. Eur. J. Clin. Pharmacol. 7, 365–368 (1974)

Biamino, G., Schueren, K.P., Ramdohr, B., Lohmann, F.W.: Effect of tricyclic antidepressant agents on hemodynamics and plasma norepinephrine levels in man during rest and exertion. Z. Cardiol. 65, 319–327 (1976)

Bowers, M.B.: CSF 5HIAA and HVA following probenecid in unipolar depressives treated with amitriptyline. Psychopharmacologia 23, 26–30 (1972)

Bowers, M.B.: Amitriptyline in man: Decreased formation of central 5-hydroxyindolacetic acid. Clin. Pharmacol. Ther. 15, 167–170 (1974a)

Bowers, M.B.: Lumbar CSF 5-hydroxyindolacetic acid and homovanillic acid in affective syndromes. J. Nerv. Ment. Dis. 158, 325–330 (1974b)

Bowers, M.B., Kupfer, D.J.: Central monoamine oxidase inhibition and REM sleep. Brain Res. 35, 561–564 (1971)

Bunney, W.E., Jr., Davis, J.M.: Norepinephrine in depressive reactions. Arch. Gen. Psychiatry 13, 483–494 (1965)

Carlsson, A.: Drugs which block the storage of 5-hydroxytryptamine and related amines. In: Handbuch der experimentellen Pharmakologie, Vol. 19, Erspamer, U. (ed.), pp. 529–592. Berlin, Heidelberg, New York: Springer 1965

Carrol, B.J., Mowbray, R.M., Davies, B.M.: Sequential comparison of L-tryptophan with ECT in severe depression. Lancet I, 967–969 (1970)

Carrier, R.N., Buday, P.V.: Augmentation of toxicity of monoamine oxidase inhibitor by thyroid feeding. Nature 191, 1107 (1961)

Chase, T.N.: Serotonergic mechanisms in Parkinson's disease. Arch. Neurol. 27, 354–356 (1972)

Chase, T.N., Gordon, E.K., Ng, L.K.Y.: Norepinephrine metabolism in the central nervous system of man: studies using 3-methoxy-4-hydroxyphenylethylene glycol levels in cerebrospinal fluid. J. Neurochem. 21, 581–587 (1973)

Cohn, C.K., Dunner, D.L., Axelrod, J.: Reduced catechol-0-methyltransferase activity in red blood cells of women with primary affective disorder. Science 170, 1323–1324 (1970)

Coppen, A., Shaw, D.M., Farrell, J.P.: Potentation of the antidepressive effects of a monoamine oxidase inhibitor by tryptophan. Lancet I, 79–80 (1963)

Coppen, A., Shaw, D.M., Herzberg, B., Maggs, R.: Tryptophan in treatment of depression. Lancet II, 1178 (1967)

Coppen, A., Whybrow, P.C., Noguera, R., Maggs, R., Prange, A.J.: The comparative anti-depressant value of L-tryptophan and imipramine with and without attempted potentation by liothyronine. Arch. Gen. Psychiatry 26, 234 (1972)

Curzon, G., Gumpert, E.J.W., Sharpe, D.M.: Amine metabolites in the human cerebrospinal fluid of humans with restricted flow of cerebrospinal fluid. Nature 231, 189–191 (1971)

Davidson, J.R.T., McLeod, M.N., White, H.L., Raft, D.: Red blood cell catechol-0-methyltransferase and response to imipramine in unipolar depressive women. Am. J. Psychiatry 133, 952–955 (1976)

Dunner, D.L., Goodwin, F.K.: Effect of L-tryptophan on brain serotonin metabolism in depressed patients. Arch. Gen. Psychiatry 26, 364–370 (1972)

Ebert, M., Kopin, I.J.: Origins of urinary catecholamine metabolites: differential labeling by dopamine C^{14}. Abstract. Clin. Res. (in press)

Eccleston, D., Ashcroft, G.W., Crawford, T.B.B., Stanton, J.B., Wood, D., McTurk, P.H.: Effect of tryptophan administration on 5HIAA in cerebrospinal fluid in man. J. Neurol. Neurosurg. Psychiatry 33, 269–272 (1970)

Engelman, K., Sjoerdsma, A.: A new test for pheochromocytoma. J. Am. Med. Assoc. 2, 81–86 (1964)

Erwin, G.V.: Oxidative-reductive pathways for metabolism of biogenic aldehydes. In: Frontiers of catecholamine research. Usdin, E. (ed.), pp. 161–166. New York: Pergamon 1973

Fawcett, J., Maas, J.W., Dekirmenjian, H.: Depression and MHPG excretion: response to dextroamphetamine and tricyclic antidepressants. Arch. Gen. Psychiatry 26, 246–252 (1972)

Freyschuss, U., Sjöqvist, F., Tuck, D.: Tyramine pressor effects in man before and during treatment with nortriptyline or ECT: Correlation between plasma level and effect of nortriptyline. Pharmacol. Clin. 2, 72–78 (1970)

Garelis, E., Sourkes, T.L.: Sites of origin in the central nervous system of monoamine metabolites measured in human cerebrospinal fluid. J. Neurol. Neurosurg. Psychiat. 4, 625–629 (1973)

Garelis, E., Young, S.N., Lal, S., Sourkes, T.L.: Monoamine metabolites in lumbar CSF: The question of their origin in relation to clinical studies. Brain Res. 79, 1–8 (1973)

Glassman, A., Platman, S.R.: Potentation of a monoamine oxidase inhibitor by tryptophan. J. Psychiat. Res. 7, 83–90 (1969)

Glowinski, J., Kopin, I.J., Axelrod, J.: Metabolism of (H³)-norepinephrine in rat brain. J. Neurochem. 12, 25 (1965)

Goodall, Mc.C., Alton, H.: Metabolism of 3-hydroxytryptamine (dopamine) in human subjects. Biochem. Pharmacol. 17, 905–914 (1968)

Goodall, Mc.C., Rosen, L.: Urinary excretion of noradrenaline and its metabolites at ten-minute intervals after intravenous injection of dl-noradrenaline-2-C¹⁴. J. Clin. Invest. 42, 1578–1588 (1963)

Goodwin, F.K., Murphy, D.L.: Biological factors in the affective disorders and schizophrenia. In: Psychopharmacological agents. Gordon, E. (ed.), pp. 9–32. New York: Academic Press 1974

Goodwin, F.K., Post, R.M.: Studies of amine metabolites in affective illness and in schizophrenia: A comparative analysis. In: Biology of the major psychoses: A comparative analysis. Freedman, D.X. (ed.), pp. 299–322. New York: Raven Press 1975

Goodwin, F.K., Brodie, H.K.H., Murphy, D.L., Bunney, W.E., Jr.: L-Dopa, catecholamines, and behavior: a clinical and biochemical study in depressed patients. Biol. Psychiatry 2, 341–350 (1970)

Goodwin, F.K., Post, R.M., Dunner, D.L., Gordon, E.K.: Cerebrospinal fluid amine metabolites in affective illness: the probenecid technique. Am. J. Psychiatry 130, 73–79 (1973a)

Goodwin, F.K., Post, R.M., Murphy, D.L.: Cerebrospinal fluid amine metabolites and therapies for depression. Sci. Proc. Am. Psychiatr. Assoc. 126, 24–25 (1973b)

Greengrass, P.M., Waldmeier, P.C., Imhof, P.R., Maître, L.: Comparison of the effects of maprotiline and clomipramine on serotonin uptake and tryptophan-binding in plasma. Biol. Psychiatry 11, 91–100 (1976)

Grote, S.S., Moses, S.G., Robins, E., Hudgens, R.W., Croninger, A.B.: A study of selected catecholamine metabolizing enzymes: A comparison of depressive suicides and alcoholic suicides with controls. J. Neurochem. 23, 791–801 (1974)

Guilleminault, C., Cathola, J.P., Castaigne, P.: Effects of 5-hydroxytryptophan on sleep of a patient with a brain-stem lesion. Electroencephalogr. Clin. Neurophysiol. 34, 177–184 (1973)

Heninger, G.R., Mueller, P.S., Davis, L.S.: Responsiveness of endocrine-energy metabolism systems in depression and schizophrenia: Relationships to symptomatology. In: Hormones behavior and psychopathology. Sachar, E.J. (ed.), pp. 237–242. New York: Raven Press 1976

Herrington, R.N., Bruce, A., Johnstone, E.C., Lader, M.H.: Comparative trial of L-tryptophan and ECT in severe depressive illness. Lancet II, 731 (1974)

Hornykiewicz, O.: Dopamine (3-hydroxytyramine) and brain function. Pharmacol. Rev. 18, 925–964 (1966)

Jori, A., Dolfini, E., Casati, C., Argenta, G.: Effect of ECT and imipramine treatment on the concentration of 5HIAA and HVA in the CSF of depressed patients. Psychopharmacologia 44, 87–90 (1975)

Laakmann, G., Schumacher, G., Benkert, O.: Stimulations of growth hormone secretion by desimipramine and chlorimipramine in man. J. Clin. Endocrinol. Metab. 44, 1010–1013 (1977)

Lovenberg, W., Engelman, K.: Assay of serotonin, related metabolites and enzymes. Meth. Biochem. Anal. *19*, 1–34 (1971)

Maas, J.W.: Biogenic amines and depression. Biochemical and pharmacological separation of two types of depression. Arch. Gen. Psychiatry *32*, 1357 (1975)

Maas, J.W., *In vivo* studies of metabolism of norepinephrine in the central nervous system. J. Pharmacol. Exp. Ther. *163*, 147–162 (1968)

Maas, J.W., Dekirmenjian, H., Garver, D., Redmond, D.E., Landis, D.H.: Excretion of catecholamine metabolites following intraventricular injection of 6-hydroxydopamine in the macaca speciosa. Eur. J. Pharmacol. *23*, 121–130 (1973)

Matussek, N., Benkert, O., Schneider, K., Otten, H., Pohlmeier, H.: Wirkung eines Decarboxylasehemmers (Ro 4-4602) in Kombination mit L-Dopa auf gehemmte Depressionen. Arzneim. Forsch. *20*, 934–937 (1970)

Meek, J.L., Neff, N.H.: Is cerebrospinal fluid the major avenue for the removal of 5-hydroxyindoleacetic acid from the brain? Neuropharmacology *12*, 497–499 (1973)

Meltzer, H.Y., Piyakalmaza, S., Schyve, P., Fang, U.S.: Lack of the effect of tricyclic antidepressants on serum prolactin levels. Psychopharmacology *51*, 185–187 (1977)

Mendels, J., Stinnet, J.L., Burns, D., Frazer, A.: Amine precursors and depression. Arch. Gen. Psychiatry *32*, 22–28 (1975)

Modigh, K.: Effect of chlorimipramine on the rate of tryptophan hydroxylation in the intact and transected spinal cord. J. Pharm. Pharmacol. *25*, 926–928 (1973)

Moir, A.T.B., Ashcroft, G.W., Crawford, T.B.B., Eccleston, D., Guldberg, H.C.: Central metabolites in cerebrospinal fluid as a biochemical approach to the brain. Brain *93*, 357–368 (1970)

Murphy, D.L., Wyatt, R.J.: Neurotransmitter-related enzymes in the major psychiatric disorders: Catechol-0-methyl transferase, monoamine oxidase in the affective disorders, and factors affecting some behaviorally correlated enzyme activities. In: Biology of the Major Psychoses: A Comparative Analysis. Friedman, D.X. (ed.), pp. 227–228. New York: Raven Press 1975

Nakra, B.R., Rutland, P., Verma, S., Gaind, R.: Amitriptyline and weight gain: A biochemical and endocrinological study. Curr. Med. Res. Opin. *4*, 602–606 (1977)

Paul, M.I., Ditzion, R.R., Pauk, G.L., Janowski, D.S.: Urinary adenosine 3′,5′-monophosphate excretion in affective disorders. Am. J. Psychiatry *126*, 1493 (1970)

Pletscher, A., Bartholini, G., Tissot, R.: Metabolic fate of L-(^{14}C)Dopa in cerebrospinal fluid and blood plasma of humans. Brain Res. *4*, 106–109 (1967)

Post, R.M., Goodwin, F.K.: Effect of amitriptyline and imipramine on amine metabolites in the cerebrospinal fluid of depressed patients. Arch. Gen. Psychiatry *30*, 234–239 (1974)

Post, R.M., Goodwin, F.K., Gordon, E., Watkin, D.M.: Amine metabolites in human cerebrospinal fluid: effects of cord transection and spinal fluid block. Science *179*, 897–899 (1973)

Post, R.M., Goodwin, F.K., Cramer, H.: Cyclic adenosine monophosphate in cerebrospinal fluid of patients with affective illness: effects of probenecid, activity, and psychotropic medications. In: Neuroregulators and psychiatric disorders. Usdin, E., Hamburg, D.A., Barchas, J.D. (eds.), pp. 464–469. New York: Oxford Univ. Press 1977

Prange, A.J., Wilson, I.C., Rabon, A.M., Lipton, M.A.: Enhancement of imipramine antidepressant activity by thyroid hormone. Am. J. Psychiatry *126*, 457 (1969)

Prange, A.J., Wilson, I.C., Knox, A., McLane, T.K., Lipton, M.A.: Enhancement of imipramine by thyroid stimulating hormone. Am. J. Psychiatry *127*, 191 (1970)

Prange, A.J., Wilson, I.C., Breese, G.R., Lipton, M.A.: Hormonal alterations of imipramine response: A review. In: Hormones, Behavior, and Psychopathology. Sacher, E.J. (ed.), pp. 41–67. New York: Raven Press 1976

Rinne, U.K., Sonninen, U.: Dopamine and Parkinson's disease. Ann. Med. Intern. Fenn. *57*, 105–113 (1968)

Robinson, D.S., Lovenberg, W., Keiser, H., Sjoerdsma, J.: Effects of drugs on human blood platelet and plasma amine oxidase activity *in vitro* and *in vivo*. Biochem. Pharmacol. *17*, 109–119 (1968)

Robinson, D.S., Davis, J.M., Nies, A., Colburn, R.W., Davis, J.N., Bourne, H.R., Bunney, W.E., Shaw, S.M., Coppen, A.J.: Ageing monoamines, and monoamine-oxidase levels. Lancet *I*, 290–291 (1972)

Roth, J.E.: Multiple forms of monoamine oxidase and their interactions with tricyclic psy-
chomimetric drugs. Gen. Pharmacol. 7, 381–386 (1976)

Saccetti, E., Smeraldi, E., Cagnasso, B., Biondi, F.A., Bellodi, L.: MHPG, amitriptyline and
affective disorders. A longitudinal study. Int. Pharmacopsychiatry 11, 157–162 (1976)

Schanberg, S.M., Schildkraut, J.J., Breese, G.R., Kopin, I.J.: Metabolism of Normetanephrine-
H^3 in rat brain-Identification of conjugated 3-methoxy-4-hydrophenylglycol as the major
metabolite. Biochem. Pharmacology 17, 247–254 (1968)

Schildkraut, J.J.: Norepinephrine metabolites as biochemical criteria for classifying depressive
disorders and predicting responses to treatment: Preliminary findings. Am. J. Psychiatry
130, 695–698 (1973)

Schildkraut, J.J., Kety, S.S.: Biogenic amines and emotion. Science 156, 21–30 (1967)

Schildkraut, J.J., Gordon, E.K., Durell, J.: Catecholamine metabolism in affective disorders.
1. Normetanephrine and VMA excretion in depressed patients treated with imipramine. J.
Psychiatr. Res. 3, 213 (1965)

Schildkraut, J.J., Green, R., Gordon, E.K., Durell, J.: Normetanephrine excretion and affective
state in depressed patients treated with imipramine. Am. J. Psychiatry 123, 690 (1966)

Schubert, J., Nybäck, H., Sedvall, G.: Effect of antidepressant drugs on accumulation and disappearance of monoamines formed in vivo from labelled precursors in mouse brain. J.
Pharm. Pharmacol. 22, 136–139 (1970)

Shaw, D.M., O'Keeffe, R., Mac Sweeney, D.A., Brooksbank, B.W.L., Noguera, R., Coppen,
A.: 3-Methoxy-4-hydroxyphenylglycol in depression. Psychol. Med. 3, 333–336 (1973)

Shopsin, B., Gershon, S., Goldstein, M., Friedman, E., Wilk, S.: The use of synthesis inhibitors
in defining a role for biogenic amines during imi- pramine treatment in depressed patients.
Psychopharmacol. Commun. 1, 239–249 (1975)

Shopsin, B., Friedman, E., Gershon, S.: PCPA reversal of tranylcypramine effects in depressed
patients. Arch. Gen. Psychiatry 33, 811–819 (1977)

Siever, L., Kraemer, H., Sack, R., Angwin, P., Berger, P., Zarcone, V., Barchas, J., Brodie,
K.H.: Gradients of biogenic amine metabolites in cerebrospinal fluid. Dis. Nerv. Syst. 36,
13–16 (1975)

Sourkes, T.L.: Enzymology and sites of action of monoamines in the central nervous system.
Adv. Neurol. 2, 13–35 (1973)

Sullivan, J.L., Dackis, C., Stanfield, C.: In vivo inhibition of platelet MAO activity by tricyclic
antidepressants. Am. J. Psychiatry 134, 188–190 (1977)

Van Praag, H.M., Korf, J., Dols, L.C.W., Schut, T.: A pilot study of the predictive value of
the probenecid test in application of 5-hydroxytryptophan as an antidepressant. Psychopharmacologia 25, 14–17 (1972)

Van Praag, H.M.: Towards a biochemical typology of depression? Pharmacopsychiatry 7, 281–
285 (1974)

Van Praag, H.M., Korf, J.: Central monoamine deficiency in depressions: causative or secun-
dary phenomenon. Pharmacopsychiatr. Neuropsychopharmacol. 8, 322–325 (1975)

Van Praag, H.M.: Depression and schizophrenia. A contribution on their chemical pathology.
New York: Spectrum Publications 1976

Van Praag, H.M.: Significance of biochemical parameters in the diagnosis, treatment, and prevention of depressive disorders. Biol. Psychiatry 12, 101–131 (1977)

Walinder, J., Skott, A., Nagy, A., Carlsson, Á., Ross, B.-E.: Potentiation of antidepressant action of clomipramine by tryptophan. Lancet I, 984–985 (1975)

Weil-Malherbe, H., Van Buren, J.M.: The excretion of dopamine and dopamine metabolites
in Parkinson's disease and the effect of diet thereon. J. Lab. Clin. Med. 74, 305–318 (1969)

Young, S.N., Lal, S., Martin, J.B., Ford, R.M., Sourkes, T.L.: 5-Hydroxyindoleacetic acid,
homovanillic acid and tryptophan levels in CSF above and below a complete block of CSF
flow. Psychiatr. Neurol. Neurochir. 7 439–444 (1973)

Zehner, J., Klaus, D., Klumpp, F., Lemke, R.: Cyclic AMP and renin activity in renal vein
blood after amitriptyline, theophylline, furosemid, and beta adrenergic blocking substances. Klin. Wochenschr. 54, 1085–1093 (1976)

Drug-Induced Alterations in Animal Behavior as a Tool for the Evaluation of Antidepressants: Correlation with Biochemical Effects

A. DELINI-STULA

A. Introduction

Since the fortuitous discovery of the antidepressant activity of imipramine by KUHN (1957), psychopharmacologists have been striving to elaborate an animal model faithfully reproducing the clinical features of human depression. Such a model would not only make it possible to develop better and more specific drugs for the treatment of depression, but also to advance and facilitate the investigation of the aetiological and pathophysiological mechanisms underlying the disease. Many scientists and psychiatrists doubt, however, that a valid model of depression in animal will ever become available. This point of view arises partly from the assumption that depression is a uniquely human disease, inherent in which are the verbal communication and the expression of the state of the mind.

Nevertheless, within the framework of the current catecholamine hypothesis of depression (BUNNEY and DAVIS, 1965; SCHILDKRAUT, 1965) different animal models have been developed allowing more or less rational evaluation of the therapeutic antidepressant potential of new drugs.

According to the basic concept of the catecholamine hypothesis, the primary cause of depression is a relative deficiency in the functioning of the noradrenergic, probably also serotoninergic, and dopaminergic neural transmission systems. This deficiency is supposed to be due to a decreased availability of transmitters or, alternatively, changes in postsynaptic brain catecholamine receptor sensitivity (SULSER et al., 1978).

There is a prodigious amount of data in both the pharmacological and neurobiochemical literature relating to the influence of antidepressants on aminergic transmission systems. Strictly comparative data, however, are rather scarce. The relations that may exist between the functional manifestations and the neurobiochemical changes produced by drugs are, nevertheless, a matter of practical as well as theoretical importance. Some aspects of this problem as well as general considerations about pharmacological models are presented by reference to antidepressants that may be regarded as representative from both the clinical and the pharmacological standpoints.

B. Amine-Depleted Animals as a Model for the Study of Antidepressants, Correlations with Biochemical Effects

In the retrospective search for pharmacological correlates of antidepressant activity, the analogy between depressive states in man and psychomotor inhibition produced by reserpine in animals led pharmacologists to make use of reserpine and similar substances as tools in the determination of antidepressant properties of drugs. In the early 1960s, many reports appeared describing antagonistic action of imipramine against various autonomic and behavioral effects of reserpine (Domenjoz and Theobald, 1959; Garattini et al., 1960; Costa et al., 1960; Chen and Bohner, 1961; Sulser et al., 1961, 1962; Brodie et al., 1961).

The findings of Axelrod and his group, (Axelrod et al., 1961; Herting et al., 1961; Axelrod et al., 1962; Glowinski and Axelrod, 1964; Iversen et al., 1967) that these compounds block the principle pathway leading to the inactivation of noradrenaline (NA) released from the nerve terminals, i.e. its re-uptake into the peripheral and central adrenergic neurones offered at the same time a plausible explanation of the mode of action of antidepressants.

I. Parameters Used for the Determination of Antidepressant Effects in Amine-Depleted Animals

Among a variety of functional disturbances produced by amine-depleting agents in animals, hypothermia and the closure of the eyelids are among those which were most commonly used as parameters for quantitative and qualitative evaluation of drug activity (Garattini et al., 1962; Askew, 1963; Halliwell et al., 1964; Lapin, 1967b; Tedeschi, 1974). The specificity and selectivity of action of antidepressants in reversing these symptoms has been copiously discussed in the literature (Metyšova et al., 1964; Garattini and Jori, 1967; Lapin, 1967a, b; Maxwell, 1964; Barnett et al., 1969; Morpurgo and Theobald, 1965; Dhawan et al., 1970; Nimegeers, 1975; Simon and Boissier, 1975).

It is generally agreed that the reversal of hypothermia is not specific for antidepressants. The fall in body temperature that occurs in amine-depleted animals can be reversed by many other drugs with no proved clinical antidepressant activity such as antihistamines, analgesics, sympathomimetics and anticholinergics, although by the latter only under certain experimental conditions (Lapin, 1967 a, b). Nevertheless, the antagonizing effect of antidepressants seem to be selective for NA-mediated hypothermic responses. Doggett (Doggett et al., 1975a) for instance, found that hypothermia produced by blockade of dopamine (DA) receptors by pimozide is not counteracted by desipramine. The hypothermia induced by high doses of apomorphine, which is a direct DA-receptor stimulant drug, can be, however, counteracted by certain antidepressants such as imipramine, desipramine, maprotiline, amitriptyline and dibenzepin (Maj et al., 1974; Schelkunov, 1977), whereas some others like iprindole, clomipramine, doxepine, azaphen, and trimeprimine are ineffective. But as suggested by Schelkunov the effect also appears to correlate with adrenergic-stimulating properties of these compounds.

The tricyclic antidepressants prevent, but also reverse the already established hypothermia in animals pretreated with reserpine-like drugs. Figure 1 (a) illustrates the typical effect of antidepressants on the example of maprotiline. The time-course of action is quite characteristic and appears to be consistent among tricyclic as well as non-tricyclic drugs. In general maximal effects are seen 2 or 3 h after the drug administration. The failure of some authors to demonstrate antagonism of reserpine-induced hypothermia by some antidepressants could possibly be due to the rather short observation times that they have used (Nimegeers, 1975).

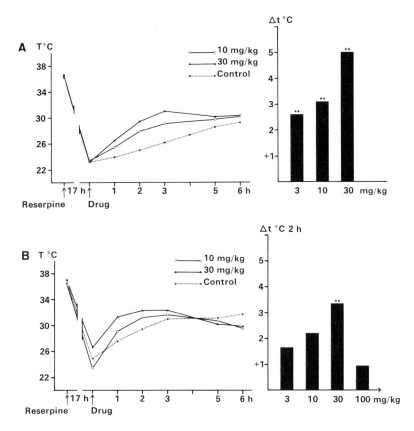

Fig. 1A and B. Reversal of reserpine-induced hypothermia by maprotiline in the mouse. Maprotiline **A** and mianserine **B** were administered orally to mice (*n*, six per group) 17 h after reserpine 2 mg/kg s.c. Each point on the curves represents the mean rectal temperature of six mice. The *black columns* (right) indicate the maximal differences in rectal temperature between drug-treated (T_D) and control (T_C) animals ($\Delta t = T_D - T_C$). Doses are indicated under the columns. For other details see Table 1. ** $P < 0.01$. (Student's *t*-test)

FELL et al. (1973) and FLEISCHHAUER et al. (1973) reported also that mianserine does not counteract the effects produced by either tetrabenazine or reserpine in mice. Neither of these reports, however, gave any methodological details.

Figure 1 (b) illustrates that in reserpine-pretreated mice this drug can also increase the rectal temperature. However, a clear-cut decrease in antagonism occurs when the dose is increased. Taking into account that the mechanisms involved in the control of body temperature are complex and that besides NA-activating (BRITTAIN and HANDLEY, 1967; GARATTINI and JORI, 1967; JORI and BERNARDI, 1970; LANKIER, 1969; SVENSSON, 1971; COX, 1975), other concomittant actions of antidepressants (e. g., postsynaptic α-receptor blockade, THEOBALD et al., 1965, CALLINGHAM, 1967) can interfere with magnitude of the antihypothermic effect, such bell-shaped dose-response curves are not surprising. The dose range in which the compounds are investigated is therefore of importance, as this is also stressed by PETERSEN (PETERSEN et al., 1966).

Table 1. Comparative potencies of antidepressants in inhibiting reserpine-induced hypothermia and NA-uptake in the heart[a]

Drug	Reversal of hypothermia ED$_{50}$ mg/kg p.o. (95% confidence limits) Mouse	No. of mice per group	NA-uptake inhibition heart[b]	
			ED$_{50}$ mg/kg i.p. Mouse	ED$_{50}$ mg/kg p.o. Rat
Imipramine	4.2 (1.10–16.0)	18	12	7
Desipramine	2.1 (0.65–6.8)	18	6	5
Clomipramine	2.2[c]	18	20	40
Amitryptiline	1.5 (0.45–5.03)	12	14	15
Nortryptiline	3.4 (1.6–10.88)	12	15	8.5
Maprotiline	2.2 (0.74–6.56)	12	—	20

[a] The reversal of reserpine-induced hypothermia was determined according to the method described by ASKEW (1963). Drugs were given orally 17 h after 2 mg/kg s.c. reserpine. The percentage of effect was calculated by using the formula:

$$\frac{T_D - T_R}{T_C - T_R} \times 100 \qquad (T_D \text{ drug-treated}; \; T_R \text{ reserpine-treated}; \; T_C \text{ saline-treated mice}).$$

ED$_{50}$ values were calculated according to LITCHFIELD and WILCOXON
[b] Data derived from CARLSSON et al. (1969a) and WALDMEIER et al. (1976)
[c] The dose response curve was rather flat and the effect decreased after high doses

The antihypothermic effect of antidepressants, with the exception of iprindole, coincides with NA-uptake inhibitory properties of these compounds. Direct comparisons of the potencies of these two actions are, however, impeded by the fact that in most cases biochemical assays have been carried out in rats, whereas the estimations of antihypothermic effects have been done in mice. In general, however, it does not appear that the potency of action determined in mice predicts the potency of the biochemical action in rats (Table 1).

As for hypothermia the same limitations are valid in respect to the specificity of the action of antidepressants in reversing the ptosis induced by reserpine or related drugs (GARATTINI et al., 1960; LAPIN, 1967b; SIGG et al., 1965; NIMEGEERS, 1975). In most cases, however, the effects of other types of drugs can be discriminated from those exerted by antidepressants. Directly acting sympathomimetic agents for instance, produce exophtalmos in untreated animals and in terms of doses this effect coincides with their antagonistic action against ptosis. This also applies for indirectly acting stimulating drugs like amphetamine (WILSON and TISLOW, 1962).

In Fig. 2 the relative potencies of ten antidepressants in preventing the ptosis induced by reserpine and tetrabenazine in rats are illustrated. With the exception of mianserine there was no difference in the magnitude of the effects observed in these two test systems, although the pretreatment times were different. The order of potency in the tetrabenazine tests: desipramine > imipramine > amitriptyline > nortriptyline > clomipramine, is identical with that determined in the reserpine-treated animals by SCHMITT and SCHMITT (1966).

It is recognized that antidepressants prevent the ptosis induced by amine-depleting agents by virtue of their ability to increase central adrenergic output (HALLIWELL et

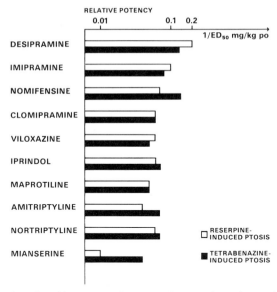

Fig. 2. Relative potencies of antidepressants in preventing tetrabenazine and reserpine-induced ptosis in the rat. Ptosis was rated according to the rating scale described by Rubin et al. (1957). Drugs were administered orally 1 h before either tetrabenazine (20 mg/kg i.p.) or reserpine (2 mg/kg s.c.). The closure of the eyes in the control and in drug-treated animals was evaluated 1 h after tetrabenazine and 4 h after reserpine injection. Individual scores were alloted to each rat (*n*=ten per group). Mean scores of the group were calculated and expressed in percentage change in comparison to the control. ED_{50} was calculated by graphical interpolation. Each column in the Fig. represents the reciprocal ED_{50} values in mg/kg p.o. on a logarithmic scale

al., 1964; TEDESCHI, 1974) through inhibition of NA uptake [a peripheral mode of action has also been indicated by some authors (FIELDEN and GREEN, 1965)]. The dose-response curves of reversal of tetrabenazine-induced ptosis and NA-uptake inhibition in the rat heart produced by desipramine and maprotiline, illustrated in Fig. 3, are examples of the parallelity of these two effects.

Linear regression of double-logarithmic plots of ED_{50} (in mg/kg p. o.) for NA uptake inhibition in the heart and reversal of reserpine-induced ptosis demonstrates that there is a highly significant correlation between these two effects (Fig. 4, $r = 0.931$, $P < 0.01$).

In contrast, no significant correlation was found if the effects of the same drugs on ptosis were compared to the inhibition of the NA-uptake in the brain. (Spearman coeff: $= 0.48$, $df = 8$, $r = 0.69$, $P > 0.05$).

If it can be assumed that drugs which inhibit NA-uptake in the heart will also produce functional effects manifested in prevention of reserpine symptoms, the example of iprindole, which is inactive in this respect (GLUCKMAN and BAUM, 1969; Ross et al., 1972; FANN et al., 1972), shows that the opposite is not the case.

Besides the antagonisms of hypothermia and ptosis already in the early stage of the development of antidepressants SULSER (SULSER et al., 1962, 1964) described the ability of these compounds to "reverse" sedation and produce hyperactive behavior in animals treated with amine-depletors [for the sake of clarity it should be mentioned

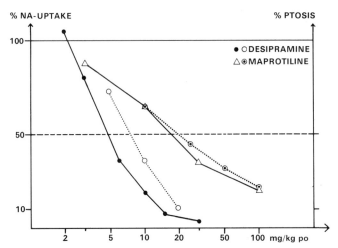

Fig. 3. Dose-response curves of desipramine and maprotiline relating to the NA-uptake inhibition in the heart and inhibition of ptosis in tetrabenazine-treated rats. Inhibition of the NA-uptake in the heart was determined as described by WALDMEIER et al. (1976) and inhibition of tetrabenazine-induced ptosis as described in Fig. 2. Each point on the curves is the mean of 5–10 observations. ●, △: NA-uptake inhibition; ○, ⊙: inhibition of tetrabenazine ptosis. In all experiments the drugs were given orally

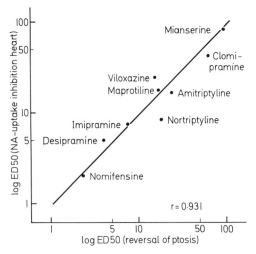

Fig. 4. Correlation between NA-uptake inhibition in the heart and inhibition of reserpine-induced ptosis by antidepressants in the rat. The ED_{50} values are in mg/kg p.o. Data are either unpublished results from this laboratory or derived from WALDMEIER et al. (1976)

that classical antidepressants do not produce a true reversal of symptoms which are already established because their activity depends on the presence of functionally active amines (SCHECKEL and BOFF, 1964)]. In many later studies such effects of various antidepressants related to imipramine were not fully confirmed. This was particularly true if attempts were made to quantify the increase in locomotion. GIURGEA (GIURGEA

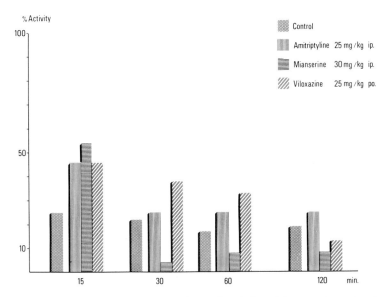

Fig. 5. Effect of antidepressants on motor depression induced by tetrabenazine in the rat. Drugs were administered either intraperitoneally 30 min or orally 1 h before tetrabenazine (10 mg/kg i.p.). The activity was evaluated by placing the animals on an open square surface (145 cm²) for 15 s and by rating their exploratory behavior from 0–4 (0–no exploration, 4–normal activity). Mean score of the group was expressed in percentage of activity of normal rats (score 4 = 100%). Normal untreated rats run away from the square surface in less than 10 s. Each column represents the average of six rats

et al., 1963) found, for instance, that fairly high doses of desipramine (60 mg/kg i. p.) were needed to restore normal activity in tetrabenazine-treated rats. The increase in activity produced by low doses (3–30 mg/kg) was weak and was seen in less than 50% of animals. Neither imipramine nor amitriptyline counteracted the depression more effectively.

SCHMITT and SCHMITT (1966) likewise found that various imipramine-like drugs did not reduce signs of motor depression to an appreciable extent. According to our own experiences antidepressants produce in general rather weak, inconsistent and mostly short-lived activating effects in amine-depleted animals. The example of the kinetic of this action is illustrated in Fig. 5.

Determination of the antagonism against motor depression produced by tetrabenazine by means of other criteria (THEOBALD et al., 1964, 1967) than the observation and rating scales (as in above mentioned studies), leads to the essentially same results (Fig. 6).

The alteration of cataleptic immobility (catalepsy, i. e. the failure of animals to correct the imposed body posture should be discriminated from symptoms of general depression and hypoactivity of animals) is another criterion often used for the determination of antidepressant potency in amine-depleted animals. SCHMITT and SCHMITT (1966), however, found that various tricyclic antidepressants were, in general less active in antagonizing catalepsy in the rat than ptosis or hypothermia produced by amine-depleting agents.

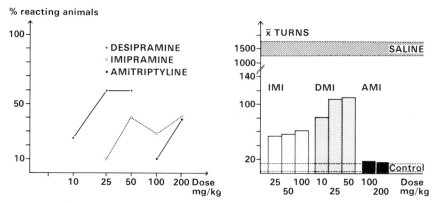

Fig. 6. Effect of antidepressants on locomotor activity in tetrabenazine treated rats. Drugs were given orally 1 h before 20 mg/kg i.p. tetrabenazine to groups of ten rats. Single animals were placed in rotating wheels (Theobald et al., 1967) and the number of turns produced by the movements of a rat was automatically recorded by a counter during an observation period of 30 min. **a** The percentage of animals completing ten or more turns of the wheel during a 30-min interval. **b** Average number of completed turns by ten rats during a 30-min interval. Control: average number of turns±SD of 30 rats treated with tetrabenazine. Saline: average number of turns±SD exerted by rats (*n*, 30) treated with physiological 0.9% NaCl solution. IMI, imipramine; DMI, desipramine; AMI, amitrityline

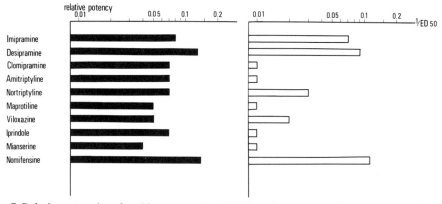

Fig. 7. Relative potencies of antidepressants in inhibiting the tetrabenazine-induced ptosis and catalepsy in the rat. Drugs were given orally 1 h before tetrabenazine 20 mg/kg i.p. to rats (*n*, ten per group). Ptosis was evaluated as described in Fig. 2. Cataleptic stance was evaluated 1 h after tetrabenazine injection according to the methods described by Wirth et al. (1958) and Delini-Stula and Morpurgo (1968). A dose producing 50% inhibition of either ptosis (black) or catalepsy (white) was determined by graphical interpolation. Each column represents reciprocal ED_{50} values in mg/kg p.o. on logarithmic scale

In the study on pharmacological properties of antidepressants, Stille (1968) also showed that, with the exception of desipramine, other related drugs only protected rats from tetrabenazine-induced catalepsy when administered in quite high doses. The rank order, estimated in terms of median effective doses was as follows: desipramine > imipramine > dibenzepine > nortriptyline > protriptyline > amitriptyline > clomipramine.

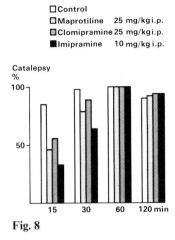

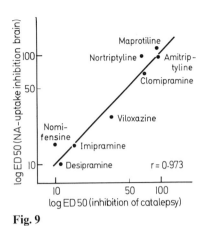

Fig. 8   **Fig. 9**

Fig. 8. Inhibition of tetrabenazine-induced catalepsy by antidepressants. Drugs were given intraperitoneally 30 min before tetrabenazine 10 mg/kg i.p. Catalepsy was evaluated using the method described by STANLEY and GLICK (1976). Each column represents the average catalepsy (in percentage) of six rats

Fig. 9. Correlation between the NA-uptake inhibition in the brain and inhibition of tetrabenazine-induced catalepsy by antidepressants in the rat. Data related to NA-uptake inhibition in the brain are derived either from WALDMEIER et al. (1976) or are unpublished results from this laboratory. Catalepsy was evaluated as stated in Fig. 7. The ED_{50} values are in mg/kg p.o.

Figure 7 illustrates the relative anticataleptic potencies of several antidepressants in comparison to their potencies to antagonize ptosis in tetrabenazine-treated animals determined in parallel experiments. In accordance with previously mentioned studies the anticataleptic effect of antidepressants was (with a few exceptions) weaker than their antiptotic effect. There is another particularity of this anticataleptic action. With the exception of nomifensine all these drugs did not produce a true attenuation of cataleptic rigidity. As illustrated in Fig. 8, by using a technique of repeated estimation of catalepsy in shortly spaced intervals (as described by STANLEY and GLICK, 1976), an appreciable extent of inhibition could be observed only during the first of several closely following trials (unpublished). This type of effect differentiates antidepressants from dopamine-stimulating drugs or monoamine oxidase inhibitors, which produce a long lasting and complete suppression of catalepsy. (MAÎTRE et al., 1976).

In general, however, the rank order of potency of antidepressants in reversing tetrabenazine-induced catalepsy (estimated by classic methods) appears to be similar to their potencies in inhibiting the NA-uptake in the brain (WALDMEIER et al., 1976; CARLSSON et al.,1969a; LIPPMANN and PUGSLEY, 1976; HUNT et al.,1974; SCHACHT and HEPTNER, 1974; KRUSE et al., 1977). Figure 9 shows that there is a highly significant correlation between these effects (Spearman coeff. 0.88, $df = 8$, $r = 0.971$, $P < 0.01$). It should also be mentioned that the ability of nomifensine to fully antagonize an already established catalepsy in amine-depleted animals, which is not shared by other antidepressants (HOFFMANN, 1973), relates to its additional dopamine-stimulating effects.

C. Drug-Induced Behaviors Implicating Aminergic Stimulation in the Evaluation of Antidepressants

In parallel with the development of models simulating depression state, models in which behavioral excitation induced by drugs believed to activate directly or indirectly central adrenergic functions have been introduced as tools for the evaluation of antidepressant qualities (CARLTON, 1961; QUINTON and HALLIWELL, 1963; HALLI-WELL et al., 1964; EVERETT, 1967; STEIN and SEIFTER, 1961; CORNE et al., 1963; MOR-PURGO and THEOBALD, 1967). But, in this respect most of these models have proved to be less valid than amine-depleted animal models and less apt to discriminate antidepressants from other types of drugs. The most widely used test-systems are listed in Table 2. However, in view of the recently postulated role of dopamine in affective diseases like mania and depression (for ref. see RANDRUP et al., 1975) interest has been regained in some of those models, because ultimately they can serve to indicate dopaminergic stimulating component in the spectrum of antidepressant activity.

Table 2. Animal models implicating monoaminergic stimulation used for the assessment of antidepressant properties of drugs

Agonists	Parameters	Authors
Amphetamine and amphetamine-like drugs	Hyperthermia Stereotyped behavior Self-stimulation	MORPURGO and THEOBALD (1967) HALLIWELL et al. (1964) CARLTON (1961) STEIN (1962)
Apomorphine	Hypothermia Stereotyped behavior	MAJ et al. (1974) SCHELKUNOV (1977) THER and SCHRAMM (1962)
L-Dopa	Behavioral excitation	EVERETT (1967) MOLANDER and RANDRUP (1976a)

I. Behavioral Responses Induced by Indirect Stimulation of Catecholaminergic Receptors

MORPURGO and THEOBALD (1965, 1967) have described the ability of various drugs related to imipramine to potentiate and prolong the hyperthermic response due to amphetamine.

However, effects similar to those produced by imipramine and its congeneers were also observed after administration of anticholinergics and some antihistamines. Furthermore, thioridazine and promazine, which can be characterized as weak neuroleptics, also prolonged the duration of amphetamine-induced temperature increase (MORPURGO and THEOBALD, 1967). In contrast to imipramine-like antidepressants, however, maprotiline has been shown to diminish the magnitude of, in doses comparable to that of imipramine, hyperthermia (DELINI-STULA, 1972).

Enhancement of amphetamine-induced behavioral stimulation by imipramine in the rat has been described by CARLTON (1961). Similar effects of other drugs structurally related to imipramine have been subsequently reported by several investigators

(QUINTON and HALLIWELL, 1963; HALLIWELL et al., 1964; SCHMITT and SCHMITT, 1966; MORPURGO and THEOBALD, 1967). In all these studies behavioral excitation was assessed globally (by means of rating scales) and no attempt has been made to differentiate between the effects of antidepressants on particular symptoms such as increase in locomotion, or intensification of only stereotyped behavioral patterns.

Imipramine and amitriptyline as well as monoamine oxidase inhibitors (MAOIs) such as iproniazide also increase the rate of self-stimulation in amphetamine-treated rats (STEIN, 1962; STEIN, 1964). Similar effects have been reported for iprindole (GLUCKMAN and BAUM, 1969).

It is not possible at present to draw a parallel between the biochemical events and functional manifestations of the interaction between amphetamines and antidepressant drugs. Imipramine, desipramine, and iprindole, which consistently potentiate and prolong the effects of amphetamine have been shown to inhibit its metabolic degradation and decrease the rate of its disappearance from the brain (SULSER et al., 1966; VALZELLI et al., 1967; CONSOLO et al., 1967; LEMBERGER et al., 1970; FREEMAN and SULSER, 1972). Therefore, the increase in brain concentration of amphetamine after treatment with these drugs can be very well correlated with increased behavioral responses. This is further supported by the observation of YOUNG and GORDON (1962) that the time-course of behavioral stimulation paralleled the levels of amphetamine in the brain. Almost nothing is known about the effects of other antidepressants on various parameters of amphetamine-induced stimulation and even less so whether or not they interfere with the metabolism of amphetamine.

The catecholamine precursor 3,4-dihydroxyphenlalanine (Dopa), or its active levorotatory form (L-Dopa), produces in animals autonomic and behavioral changes (piloerection, sweating, and salivation, acceleration of the respiratory rate, hyperactive and irritability) which have been attributed to the newly formed products of its catabolic degradation: NA, DA, and adrenaline.

In mice pretreated with MAOI, imipramine and related tricyclic antidepressants enhance signs of excitation induced by L-Dopa (EVERETT, 1967). They are, however, inactive if the enzymatic deamination of catecholamines formed from L-Dopa is not prevented by MAO inhibition. Recently MOLANDER and RANDRUP (1976a) have investigated the L-Dopa potentiating effects of a series of tricyclic antidepressants in mice pretreated with peripheral amino acid decarboxylase inhibitor Ro 4-4602 [N(DL-seryl)N-2,3,4-trihydroxybenzyl-hydrazine]. Under such experimental conditions they found that all investigated drugs potentiate L-Dopa induced stereotyped gnawing response, at least within a certain range of doses (Fig. 10). It should be noted that the differences in the shapes of the dose-response curves of various antidepressants were marked.

The ability to potentiate the stimulant effects of L-Dopa in mice pretreated with MAOI is not restricted to imipramine-like antidepressants. Similar effects were observed by antihistaminic drugs and anticholinergics. Among the latter, quaternery compound methyl-atropine, which does not pass the blood–brain barrier was also found to be highly active (SIGG and HILL, 1967).

Furthermore, it has been demonstrated that certain hormones, such as thyrotropin-releasing (TRH), or luteinizing hormone releasing (LH-RH) and growth hormone release inhibiting (somatostatin GHRIH) hormones markedly increase behavioral effects produced by L-Dopa (PLOTNIKOFF et al., 1971, 1972, 1975).

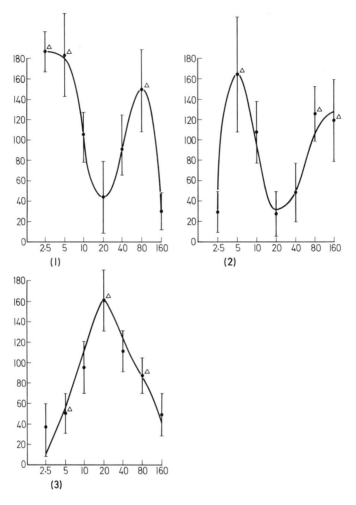

Fig. 10. Potentiation of L-Dopa response in mice pretreated with amino acid decarboxylase inhibitor Ro 4-4602. The gnawing behavior (estimated by means of a number of biting marks on the corrugate paper, Scheel-Krüger, 1970) was counted during a 1-h period after L-Dopa administration. All injections were made intraperitoneally (Molander and Randrup, 1976a with permission).

1. The effect of 40 mg/kg of imipramine on gnawing intensity (ordinate) induced by Ro 4-4602 (mg/kg, abscissa) and 400 mg/kg of L-Dopa. The deviations shown are standard errors of the means. Each point of the curve is based on experiments with 5–7 animals. $\triangle$ designates: significantly different from control. $P < 0.05$. Value for 2.5 mg/kg of Ro 4-4602 vs. value for 20 mg/kg of Ro 4-4602, $P < 0.008$; 20 mg/kg vs. 80 mg/kg, $P < 0.048$; 80 mg/kg vs. 160 mg/kg, $P < 0.008$ (Mann-Whitney U-test).

2. The effect of 40 mg/kg of desipramine on gnawing intensity (ordinate) induced by Ro 4-4602 (mg/kg, abscissa) and 400 mg/kg of L-Dopa. Value for 2.5 mg/kg og Ro 4-4602 vs. value for 5 mg/kg of Ro 4-4602, $P < 0.004$; 5 mg/kg vs. 20 mg/kg, $P < 0.015$; 20 mg/kg vs. 160 mg/kg, $P < 0.015$ (Mann-Whitney U-test).

3. The effect of 20 mg/kg of amitriptyline on gnawing intensity (ordinate) induced by Ro 4-4602 (mg/kg, abscissa) and 400 mg/kg of L-Dopa. Value for 2.5 mg/kg of Ro 4-4602 vs. value for 20 mg/kg of Ro 4-4602, $P < 0.026$; 20 mg/kg vs. 160 mg/kg, $P < 0.015$ (Mann-Whitney U-test)

Similar action was also described for some peptides and morphine (PLOTNIKOFF et al., 1976).

In the study on L-Dopa potentiation by antidepressants EVERETT (1967) showed that pretreatment with imipramine, norimipramine or amitriptyline did not increase the levels of catecholamines more than L-Dopa alone. He suggested therefore a relation between the ability of antidepressants to block the uptake mechanisms of the presynaptic nerve endings and their ability to increase pharmacological effects produced by L-Dopa. This relation was contested by MOLANDER and RANDRUP (1976a) who found that the potentiation of L-Dopa gnawing by antidepressants can not be considered as proportional to their biochemical NA-uptake inhibiting potencies. They suggested an association between the behavioral effects and biochemical effects of antidepressants on dopamine metabolism in the brain (MOLANDER and RANDRUP, 1976a; RANDRUP and BRAESTRUP, 1977).

At present it does not seem that a clear parallel between either of the biochemical effects of antidepressants and the potentiation of L-Dopa response can be drawn. However, although in the series of investigated antidepressants the potencies in inhibiting the NA-uptake in the brain (CARLSSON et al., 1969a) and variable effects on L-Dopa-induced gnawing in mice do not appear proportional, evidence favouring a facilitating effect of noradrenergic activation on behavioral items linked to DA has been presented by several authors (ANDÉN et al., 1973; STRÖMBOM, 1975; DOLPHIN et al., 1976; PYCOCK et al., 1977).

II. Behavioral Responses Induced by Direct Stimulation of Monoaminergic Receptors

Potentiation of stereotyped gnawing, licking or biting response induced by apomorphine, a direct DA-receptor stimulant, has been reported for a large number of antidepressant drugs including imipramine, desipramine, amitriptyline, clomipramine, nortriptyline, and protriptyline (THER and SCHRAMM, 1962; PEDERSEN, 1968; MENGE and BRAND, 1971; MOLANDER and RANDRUP, 1976b).

Most studies indicate that antidepressants augment the response to apomorphine only after rather large intraperitoneal or oral doses. In the study of MOLANDER and RANDRUP (1976b) imipramine was found to be among the most active tricyclics, producing a significant increase in the gnawing score (which was taken as a measure of the intensity of behavioral response) at intraperitoneal doses of 10 mg/kg and higher. Large variations of the response to apomorphine were observed after the treatment with desipramine, clomipramine, and amitriptyline. It is noteworthy, that amitriptyline also induced a suppression of gnawing, but at remarkably high dose of 50 mg/kg.

Intensification of certain stereotyped responses induced by apomorphine, such as licking and biting, has been also reported for iprindole, a non-tricyclic antidepressant (c. f. MOLANDER and RANDRUP, 1976b).

Potentiation of apomorphine effects is not a specific feature of antidepressants. Many drugs belonging to various pharmacological classes produce the same effects. In particular they have been described for anticholinergics (SCHEEL-KRÜGER, 1970), certain antihistamines and analgesics (THER and SCHRAMM, 1962; PEDERSEN, 1968). MOLANDER and RANDRUP (1976b) reported facilitation of apomorphine-induced stereotypies by clonidine, a drug considered to exert a direct NA-receptor stimulating effect (Andén et al., 1970).

The biochemical changes which underly to the functional effects manifested as potentiation of apomorphine-induced excitation by antidepressants, remain to be elucidated. On the basis of comparisons between the activities of several antidepressants and cholinergic and anticholinergic drugs, Molander and Randrup (1976 b) found no evidence that antidepressants produce their effects by a mechanism similar to that of anticholinergics. Facilitating effect of noradrenergic stimulation exerted upon behavioral responses induced by direct stimulation of DA-receptors which has been demonstrated by many authors would suggest such mode of action also for antidepressants. On the other hand, the interactions between the noradrenergic and dopaminergic nervous systems and the consequences of such interactions upon the behavior are neither simple (Molander and Randrup, 1974; Costall and Naylor, 1972; Mogilnicka and Braestrup, 1976) nor completely elucidated.

III. Behavioral Response Related to Serotoninergic Stimulation

The stimulation of functional responses related to NA and possibly DA as revealed in pharmacological models and biochemical assays is not the only property of antidepressants which has been related to their ability to relieve depressed mood and drive in mentally ill patients. Already in the early stage of the development of tricyclic drugs it has been recognized that they also facilitate functional effects of serotonin in the periphery (Gyermek and Possemato, 1960; Sabelli, 1960; Sigg et al., 1963) and it has been suggested that such effects may participate in the mechanism of the central action of these drugs.

Corne and colleagues (1963) have described a simple method for quantitative and qualitative assessment of effects of drugs on behavioral responses produced by administration of 5-hydroxytryptophan (5-HTP).

They showed that in parallel with the increase of the brain concentration of serotonin a particular head-twitch phenomenon occurs in mice and that the presence or frequency of this head-twitch can be taken as a sensitive measure of agonistic or antagonistic effect of drugs.

Among a large number of investigated compounds Corne found that imipramine, desipramine, and amitriptyline inhibit the head-twitch response, whereas MAOI consistently potentiate it. However, in mice pretreated with MAOI the antidepressants can increase the response to the 5-HTP (Ross et al., 1972). Likewise potentiation of 5-HTP can be observed in animals pretreated with MK-486 (L-α-hydrazine-α-methyl-β-(3,4,-dihydroxyphenyl propionic acid), a peripheral but not central amino acid decarboxylase inhibitor (Modigh, 1973, 1974).

The correlation between the ability of antidepressant drugs to potentiate the behavioral responses to 5-HTP in animals pretreated either with MAOI or inhibitors of aromatic amino acid decarboxylase and their 5-HTP uptake inhibiting properties has been suggested by Ross (Ross et al., 1972) and Modigh (1973, 1974). Modigh also found that under such conditions clomipramine but not protriptyline potentiated the behavioral effects of 5-HTP. According to biochemical studies protiptyline is comparable to desipramine in respect to its preferential and strong inhibitory action on the neuronal uptake of NA (Carlsson et al., 1969 a, b). In general there seems to be a

Table 3. Comparative potencies of antidepressants in potentiating 5-HTP-induced head-twitch and in inhibiting 5-HT uptake

Drug	Potentiation of 5-HTP MED[a] mg/kg p.o. Mouse	Inhibition of 5-HT uptake in the brain. ED_{50} mg/kg p.o.[b] Rat
Imipramine	100	50
Desipramine	> 300	200
Clomipramine	3	15
Amitriptyline	100	100
Nortriptyline	30	100
Maprotiline	300 (no effect)	300 (no effect)
Nomifensine	100	60
Viloxazine	> 100	150
Mianserine	> 100 s.c.	> 100 s.c.

[a] Minimal dose producing significant effect ($P<0.05$; Fourfold test: $n_1=n_2=20$). Methodological details have been previously reported (DELINI-STULA et al., 1978)
[b] From WALDMEIER et al. (1976) and WALDMEIER and BAUMANN (to be published). 5-HT uptake inhibition was determined indirectly (H 75/12 method) as described by CARLSSON et al. (1969b)

good agreement between the relative potencies of a number of antidepressants in potentiating the 5-HTP effects in mice and inhibiting the 5-HT-uptake in rats (Table 3).

The hyperactive behavior induced either by combination of L-tryptophan and MAOI (GRAHAME-SMITH, 1971 a, b; GREEN and GRAHAME-SMITH, 1974) or by L-tryptophan alone (JACOBS, 1976) has been also used for the evaluation of serotonin-stimulating properties of antidepressants (MODIGH and SVENSSON, 1972). Thus, the potentiation of L-tryptophan effects in MAOI pretreated rats by clomipramine and fluoxetine has been reported by FULLER (FULLER et al., 1974) and HOLMAN (HOLMAN et al., 1976). ORTMANN (ORTMANN et al., submitted) studiing a series of 5-HT uptake and MAOI found that there is a good correlation between the biochemically demonstrated selectivity of drugs for inhibition of uptake or deamination (MAO A inhibition) of serotonin and potentiation of L-5-HTP syndrome in rats. It seems therefore that these simple pharmacological models allow quite reliably the assessement of central 5-HT stimulating properties of antidepressants.

D. Final Conclusion and Remarks

The validity of the catecholamine hypothesis of depression has been frequently questioned in the past. Nevertheless, in view of the present state of knowledge it is still the most plausible theory which reconciles a great number of clinical and experimental findings. By reviewing the biochemical pathology of depressive disorders in his extensive monograph VAN PRAAG concluded that: "... the arguments in favour (of it) outweigh the arguments against" (VAN PRAAG, 1977).

The postulate that deficiency in the functioning of the catecholaminergic transmission system is one of the major contributing factors in the pathogenesis of depressive desease offers a rational basis for the use of animal models which can reveal amine-influencing properties of drugs. However, the limits of the usefulness of classic models, such as the amine-depleted animal, have been discussed in the past, the reasons for these limitations are summarized as follows:

1) The model of amine-depleted animal predicts the antidepressant action of such drugs which are chemically and pharmacologically tricyclic derivatives (KLERMAN, 1975).
2) Classical models do not specifically assess the activity of antidepressant drugs.
3) Antidepressants in generally prevent but do not reverse the fully established signs of depression in amine-depleted animals.
4) The effects of current antidepressants are immediate in animals, whereas under clinical conditions they appear only after a period of latency.

Undoubtedly, some of these objections are justified. But some of them can be reconsidered in the light of recent developments. Several antidepressant drugs which have been introduced into the clinics during the last years are chemically and pharmacologically distinctly different from classic tricyclics. They have, however, one property in common with tricyclics: the ability to increase to a greater or lesser extent, the responses mediated by catecholamines. With few exceptions, the effects observed in the behavioral studies correlated with the inhibition of the uptake of catecholamines found in the biochemical studies. But, drugs operating by other mechanisms were not completely inactive in these behavioral tests, which means that they could be discovered by careful analysis of behavioral responses and by astute observations. The fact that drugs not designed for psychiatric indications can demonstrate an activity in classic amine-depleted animal models does not necessarily argue against the predictive value of these models. In most cases such drugs have not been tested for their antidepressant properties clinically. Few of these drugs which have undergone clinical trials, however, have exerted some therapeutic activity. This is exemplified by cyclozacine (c.f. DOGGETT et al.,1975b). Naturally, their utility in the treatment of depression is largely limited by their predominant other properties.

The immediate onset of effects in animal experiments after single administration of antidepressants also does not negate the importance of the underlying mechanisms for the clinical action of these compounds (SCHILDKRAUT et al., 1971). Several lines of evidence demonstrate that by the virtue of their catecholamine potentiating effects, the antidepressants can produce adaptive changes in the functional state of the receptors in the brain, the mechanism which may ultimately be related to the desired therapeutic effect (SULSER et al., 1978).

Finally, except for MAOI which have established antidepressant action, drugs selectively influencing processes involved in the regulation of catecholaminergic transmission, other than membrane uptake, have not yet been developed. Such drugs could offer a challenging approach to the testing of the validity of experimental models on one hand and the theoretical concept of depression on the other hand.

The animal models which were outlined here appear to cover one aspect of depression: the consequences of catecholaminergic deficiency. In this respect they remain to be useful tools in the evaluation of drugs, which should compensate for this deficiency. However, neither the study of these models nor of the drugs which are used in the therapy of depression have helped to elucidate the most important question: what is the causative factor in the chain of events leading to the disease? In view of this both the drugs and the models used for their evaluation remain imperfect.

In this respect the advanced understanding of the mechanisms involved in the regulation of impulse-mediated release of noradrenaline (LANGER, 1974; STARKE, 1977; WESTFALL, 1977) and mechanisms leading to functional changes in receptor sensitivity (SULSER et al., 1978; DE MONTIGNY and AGHAJANIAN, 1978; CREWS and SMITH, 1978; TANG et al., 1978) may lead to new strategies and possibly to the development of new types of antidepressant drugs.

Acknowledgement. For the valuable help in the preparation of the manuscript the author wishes to thank Mrs. A. VASSOUT, Mrs. D. FIDALGO and Mr. J.-G. MEISBURGER. Technical assistance of Mrs. E. RADEKE is also greatfully acknowledged. For the generous permission to incorporate biochemical findings from their laboratories into the manuscript, the thanks are due to Drs. P. WALDMEIER, P. BAUMANN, and L. MAÎTRE.

References

Andén, N.E., Corrodi, H., Fuxe, K., Hökfelt, B., Hökfelt, T., Rydin, C., Svensson, T.: Evidence for a central noradrenaline receptor stimulation by clonidine. Life Sci. *9*, 513–523 (1970)

Andén, N.E., Strömbom, U., Svensson, T.: Dopamine and noradrenaline receptor stimulation: Reversal of reserpine-induced suppression of motor activity. Psychopharmacology *29*, 289–298 (1973)

Askew, B.M.: A simple screening procedure for imipramine-like antidepressant agents. Life Sci. *10*, 725–730 (1963)

Axelrod, J., Whitby, L.G., Herting, G.: Effect of psychotropic drugs on the uptake of ^{3}H-norepinephrine by tissues. Science *133*, 383–384 (1961)

Axelrod, J., Hertting, G., Polter, L.: Effect of drugs on the uptake and release of ^{3}H-norepinephrine in the rat heart. Nature *194*, 297 (1962)

Barnett, A., Taber, R.I., Roth, F.E.: Activity of antihistamines in laboratory antidepressant tests. Int. J. Neuropharmacol. *8*, 73–79 (1969)

Brittain, R.T., Handley, S.L.: Temperature changes produced by the injection of catecholamines and 5-hydroxytryptamine into the cerebral ventricles of the consious mouse. J. Physiol. (Lond.) *192*, 805–813 (1967)

Brodie, B.B., Bickel, M.H., Sulser, F.: Desmethylimipramine, a new type of antidepressant drug. Med. Exp. *5*, 454–458 (1961)

Bunney, W.E., Davis, J.M.: Norepinephrine in depressive reactions. Arch. Gen. Psychiatry *13*, 483–494 (1965)

Callingham, B.A.: The effects of imipramine and related compounds on the uptake of noradrenaline into sympathetic nerve endings. In: Anti-depressant drugs. Proc. 1 st Int. Symp., Milan, 1966. Garattini, S., Dukes, M.N.G. (eds.), pp. 35–43. Amsterdam: Excerpta Medica 1967

Carlsson, A., Corrodi, H., Fuxe, K., Hökfelt, T.: Effects of some antidepressant drugs on the depletion of intraneuronal brain catecholamine stores caused by 4,alpha-dimethylmeta-tyramine. Eur. J. Pharmacol. *5*, 357–366 (1969 a)

Carlsson, A., Corrodi, H., Fuxe, K., Hökfelt, T.: Effect of antidepressant drugs on the depletion of intraneuronal brain 5-hydroxytryptamine stores caused by 4-methyl-alpha-ethyl-meta-tyramine. Eur. J. Pharmacol. *5*, 367–366 (1969 b)

Carlton, P.L.: Potentiation of the behavioral effects of amphetamine by imipramine. Psychopharmacology *2*, 364–376 (1961)

Chen, G., Bohner, B.: The anti-reserpine effects of certain centrally – acting agents. J. Pharmacol. Exp. Ther. *131*, 179–184 (1961)

Consolo, S., Dolfini, E., Garattini, S., Valzelli, L.: Desipramine and amphetamine metabolism. J. Pharm. Pharmacol. *19*, 253–256 (1967)

Corne, S.J., Pickering, R.W., Warner, B.T.: A method for assessing the effects of drugs on the central actions of 5-hydroxytryptamine. Br. J. Pharmacol. *20*, 106–120 (1963)

Costa, E., Garattini, S., Valzelli, L.: Interactions between reserpine, chlorpromazine and imipramine. Experientia *16*, 461–463 (1960)

Costall, B., Naylor, R.J.: Possible involvement of noradrenergic area of the amygdala with stereotyped behavior. Life Sci. *11*, 1135–1146 (1972)

Cox, B.: The role of dopamine and noradrenaline in temperature control of normal and reserpine-pretreated mice. J. Pharm. Pharmacol. *27* (4), 242–247 (1975)

Crews, F.T., Smith, C.B.: Presynaptic alpha-receptor subsensitivity after longterm antidepressant treatment. Science *202*, 322–325 (1978)

Delini-Stula, A., Morpurgo, C.: Influence of amphetamine and scopolamine on the catalepsy induced by diencephalic lesions in rats. Int. J. Neuropharmacol. *7*, 391–394 (1968)

Delini-Stula, A.: The pharmacology of ludiomil: Depressive illness. Kielholz, P. (ed.), pp. 113–123. Int. Symp., St. Moritz, 1972. Bern: Huber

Delini-Stula, A., Radeke, E., Vassout, A.: Some aspects of the psychopharmacological activity of maprotiline (ludiomil): Effects of single and repeated treatments. J. Int. Med. Res. *6*, 421–429 (1978)

De Montigny, C., Aghajanian, G.K.: Tricyclic antidepressants: long term treatment increases responsivity of rat brain neurons to serotonin. Science *202*, 1303–1305 (1978)

Dhawan, K.N., Jaju, B.P., Gupta, G.P.: Validity of antagonism of different effects of reserpine as test for antidepressant activity. Psychopharmacologia *18*, 94–98 (1970)

Doggett, N.S., Reno, H., Spencer, P.S.J.: The effect of drugs with antidepressant activity upon the hypothermia and behavioral depression induced in mice by pimozide or centrally administered noradrenaline. Neuropharmacology *14*, 85–90 (1975a)

Doggett, N.S., Reno, H., Spencer, P.S.J.: Possible involvement of 5-hydroxytryptamine in the antidepressant activity of narcotic analgesics. Neuropharmacology *14*, 81–84 (1975b)

Dolphin, A.C., Jenner, P., Marsden, C.D.: The relative importance of dopamine and noradrenaline receptor stimulation for the restoration of motor activity in reserpine or alpha-methyl-p-tyrosine pretreated mice. Pharmacol. Biochem. Behav. *4*, 661–670 (1976)

Domenjoz, R., Theobald, W.: Zur Pharmakologie des Tofranil [N-(3-Dimethylaminopropyl)-iminodybenzylhydrochlorid]. Arch. Int. Pharmacodyn. Ther. *120*, 450–489 (1959)

Everett, G.M.: The dopa response potentiation test and its use in screening for antidepressant drugs. In: Antidepressant drugs. Proc. 1st Int. Symp., Milan, 1966. Garattini, S., Dukes, M.N.G. (eds.), pp. 164–167. Amsterdam: Excerpta Medica 1967

Fann, W.E., Davis, J.M., Janowsky, D.S., Kaufmann, J.S., Griffith, J.D., Oates, J.A.: Effect of iprindole on amine uptake in man. Arch. Gen. Psychiatry *26*, 158–162 (1972)

Fell, P.J., Quantock, D.C., Van der Burg, W.J.: The human pharmacology of GB 94 – a new psychotropic agent. Eur. J. Clin. Pharmacol. *5*, 166–173 (1973)

Fielden, R., Green, A.L.: Validity of ptosis as measure of the central depressant action of reserpine. J. Pharm. Pharmacol. *17*, 185–187 (1965)

Fleischhauer, J., Al-Shaltchi, B., Brändli, A.: Bericht über eine erste klinische Prüfung von Mianserin (GB 94), einem tetrazyklischen Antidepressivum im offenen Versuch. Arzneim. Forsch. *23* (12), 1808–1813 (1973)

Freeman, J.J., Sulser, F.: Iprindol-amphetamine interactions in the rat: the role of aromatic hydroxylation of amphetamine in its mode of action. J. Pharmacol. Exp. Ther. *183* (2), 307–315 (1972)

Fuller, R.W., Perry, K.W., Molloy, B.B.: Effect of an uptake inhibitor on serotonin metabolism in rat brain: studies with 3-(p-trifluoromethylphenoxy)-N-methyl-3-phenylpropylamine. (Lilly 110140) Life Sci. *15*, 1161–1171 (1974)

Garattini, S., Giachetti, A., Pieri, L., Re, R.: Antagonists of reserpine induced eyelid ptosis. Med. Exp. *3*, 315–320 (1960)

Garattini, S., Giachetti, A., Jori, A., Pieri, L., Valzelli, L.: Effect of imipramine, amitriptyline and their monomethyl derivatives (analogs) in reserpine activity. J. Pharm. Pharmacol. *14*, 509–514 (1962)

Garattini, S., Jori, A.: Interactions between imipramine-like drugs and reserpine on body temperature. In: Antidepressant drugs. Proc. 1st Int. Symp., Milan, 1966. Garattini, S., Dukes, M.N.G. (eds.), pp. 179–193. Amsterdam: Excerpta Medica 1967

Giurgea, M., Dauby, J., Levis, S., Giurgea, C.: Un test antitétrabénazine modifié, pour le screening des produits antidepressifs. Med. Exp. *9*, 249–262 (1963)

Glowinski, J., Axelrod, J.: Inhibition of uptake of tritiated-noradrenaline in the intact rat brain by imipramine and structurally related compounds. Nature *204*, 1318–1319 (1964)

Gluckman, M.I., Baum, T.: The pharmacology of iprindole, a new antidepressant. Psychopharmacologia *15*, 169–185 (1969)

Grahame-Smith, D.G.: Studies in vivo on the relationship between brain tryptophan, brain 5-HT synthesis and hyperactivity in rats treated with a monoamine oxidase inhibitor and L-tryptophan. J. Neurochem. *18*, 1053–1066 (1971 a)

Grahame-Smith, D.G.: Inhibitory effect of chlorpromazine on the syndrome of hyperactivity produced by L-tryptophan or 5-methoxy-N,N-dimethyltryptamine in rats, treated with amonoamine oxydase inhibitor. Br. J. Pharmacol. *43*, 856–864 (1971 b)

Green, A.R., Grahame-Smith, D.G.: The role of brain dopamine in the hyperactivity syndrome produced by increased 5-hydroxytryptamine synthesis in rats. Neuropharmacology *13*, 949–959 (1974)

Gyermek, L., Possemato, C.: Potentiation of 5-hydroxytryptamine by imipramine. Med. Exp. *3*, 225–229 (1960)

Halliwell, G., Quinton, R.M., Williams, F.E.: A comparison of imipramine, chlorpromazine and related drugs in various tests involving autonomic functions and antagonism of reserpine. Br. J. Pharmacol. *23*, 330–350 (1964)

Herting, G., Axelrod, J., Whitby, L.G., Patrick, R.: Effect of drugs on the uptake and metabolism of ³H-norepinephrine. J. Pharmacol. Exp. Ther. *134*, 146–153 (1961)

Hoffmann, I.: 8-Amino-2-methyl-4-phenyl-1,2,3,4-tetrahydroisoquinoline, a new antidepressant. Arzneim. Forsch. *23* (1), 45–50 (1973)

Holman, R.B., Seagraves, E., Elliot, G.R., Barchas, J.D.: Stereotyped hyperactivity in rats treated with tranylcypromine and specific inhibitors of 5-HT re-uptake. Behav. Biol. *16*, 507–514 (1976)

Hunt, P., Kannengiesser, M.-H., Raynaud, J.P.: Nomifensine a new potent inhibitor of dopamine uptake into synaptosomes from rat brain corpus striatum. J. Pharm. Pharmacol. *26*, 370–371 (1974)

Iversen, L.L., Axelrod, J., Glowinski, J.: The effect of antidepressant drugs on the uptake and metabolism of catecholamines in the brain. In: Neuropsychopharmacology. Proc. 5th Meeting CINP Washington, 1966. Brill, H., Cole, J.O., Deniker, P., Hippius, H., Bradley, P.B. (eds.), pp. 362–366. Amsterdam: Excerpta Medica 1967

Jacobs, B.L.: An animal behavior model for studying central serotonergic synapses. Life Sci. *19*, 777–786 (1976)

Jori, A., Bernardi, D.: Importance of catecholamines for the interaction between reserpine and desipramine on body temperature in rats. Pharmacology *4*, 235–241 (1970)

Klerman, G.L.: Relationship between preclinical testing and therapeutic evaluation of antidepressant drugs: The importance of new animal models for theory and practice. In: Predictability in psychopharmacology: Preclinical and clinical correlations. Sudilowsky, A., Gershon, S., Beer, B. (eds.), pp. 159–176. New York: Raven Press 1975

Kruse, H., Hoffmann, I., Gerhards, H.J., Leven, M., Schacht, U.: Pharmacological and biochemical studies with three metabolites of nomifensine. Psychopharmacology *51*, 117–123 (1977)

Kuhn, R.: Über die Behandlung depressiver Zustände mit einem Iminodibenzylderivat (G 22355). Schweiz. Med. Wochenschr. *87*, 1135–1140 (1957)

Lankier, S.I.: A calorigenic effect of imipramine in the mouse? Eur. J. Pharmacol. *7*, 224–226 (1969)

Langer, S.Z.: Presynaptic regulation of catecholamine release. Biochem. Pharmacol. *23*, 1793–1800 (1974)

Lapin, I.P.: Simple pharmacological procedures to differentiate antidepressants and cholinolytics in mice and rats. Psychopharmacologia *11*, 79–87 (1967 a)

Lapin, I.P.: Comparison of antireserpine and anticholinergic effects of antidepressants and of central and peripheral cholinolytics. In: Antidepressant drugs. Proc. 1st Int. Symp., Milan, 1966. Garattini, S., Dukes, M.N.G. (eds.), pp. 266–278. Amsterdam: Excerpta Medica 1967 b

Lemberger, L., Sernatinger, E., Kunzman, R.: Effect of desmethylimipramine, iprindole and DL-erithro-alpha-(3,4-dichlorophenyl)-beta-(t-butyl amino) propanol HCl on the metabolism of amphetamine. Biochem. Pharmacol. *19*, 3021–3028 (1970)

Lippmann, W., Pugsley, T.A.: Effects of viloxazine, an antidepressant agent, on biogenic amine uptake mechanisms and related activities. Can. J. Physiol. *54*, 494–509 (1976)

Maître, L., Delini-Stula, A., Waldmeier, P.C.: Relations between the degree of monoamine oxidase inhibition and some psychopharmacological responses to monoamine oxidase inhibitors in rats. In: Monoamine oxidase and its inhibition. Ciba Foundation Symp. 39, pp. 247–270. Amsterdam: Elsevier/Excerpta Medica 1976

Maj, J., Pawlowski, L., Wiscniowska, G.: The effect of tricyclic antidepressants on apomorphine-induced hypothermia in the mouse. Pol. J. Pharmacol. Pharm. *26*, 329–336 (1974)

Maxwell, D.R.: The relative potencies of various antidepressant drugs in some laboratory tests. In: Neuropharmacology. Proc. 3rd Meeting CINP, pp. 501–506. Munich, 1962. Amsterdam: Elsevier 1964

Menge, H.G., Brand, U.: Untersuchungen über die Stereotypen nach Amphetamin und Apomorphin sowie deren pharmakologische Beeinflussung. Psychopharmacologia *21*, 212–228 (1971)

Metyšova, J., Metys, J., Votava, Z.: Attempt to differentiate thymoleptics and neuroleptics by means of their influence on the effects of reserpine. Int. J. Neuropharmacol. *3*, 361–368 (1964)

Modigh, K., Svensson, T.H.: On the role of central nervous system catecholamines and 5-hydroxytryptamine in the nialamide-induced behavioral syndrome. Br. J. Pharmacol. *46*, 32–45 (1972)

Modigh, K.: Effect of clorimipramine and protriptyline on the hyperactivity induced by 5-hydroxytryptophan after peripheral decarboxylase inhibition in mice. J. Neural. Transm. *34*, 101–109 (1973)

Modigh, K.: Studies on DL-5-hydroxytryptophan-induced hyperactivity in mice. Adv. Biochem. Psychopharmacol. *10*, 213–217 (1974)

Mogilnicka, E., Braestrup, C.: Noradrenergic influence on the stereotyped behavior induced by amphetamine, phenethylamine and apomorphine. J. Pharm. Pharmacol. *28*, 253–255 (1976)

Molander, L., Randrup, A.: Investigation of the mechanism by which L-dopa induces gnawing in mice. Acta Pharmacol. Toxicol. (Kbh.) *34*, 312–324 (1974)

Molander, L., Randrup, A.: Effects of thymoleptics on behavior associated with changes in brain dopamine. Potentiation of dopa-induced gnawing of mice. Psychopharmacologia *45*, 261–265 (1976 a)

Molander, L., Randrup, A.: Effects of thymoleptics on behavior associated with changes in brain dopamine. Modification and potentiation of apomorphine-induced stimulation of mice. Psychopharmacology *49*, 139–144 (1976 b)

Morpurgo, C., Theobald, W.: Influence of imipramine-like compounds and chlorpromazine on the reserpine hypothermia in mice and the amphetamine-hyperthermia in rats. Med. Pharmacol. Exp. *12*, 226–232 (1965)

Morpurgo, C., Theobald, W.: Pharmacological modifications of the amphetamine-induced hyperthermia in rats. Eur. J. Pharmacol. *2*, 287–294 (1967)

Nimegeers, C.: Antagonism of reserpine-like activity. In: Industrial pharmacology 2. Antidepressants. Fielding, S., Lal, H. (eds.), pp. 73–98. New York: Futura 1975

Pedersen, V.: Role of catecholamines in compulsive gnawing behavior in mice. Br. J. Pharmacol. *34*, 219–220 (1968)

Petersen, P.V., Lassen, N., Hansen, V., Huld, T., Hjortkjaer, J., Holmbald, J., Møller-Nielsen, I., Nymark, M., Pedersen, V., Jørgensen, A., Hougs, W.: Pharmacological studies of a new series of bicyclic thymoleptics. Acta Pharmacol. Toxicol. (Kbh.) *24*, 121–133 (1966)

Plotnikoff, N.P., Kastin, A.J., Anderson, M.S., Schally, A.V.: Dopa potentiation by a hypothalamic factor, MSH release inhibiting hormone (MIF). Life Sci. *10* (1), 1279–1283 (1971)

Plotnikoff, N.P., Prange, A.J., Breese, G.R., Anderson, M.S., Wilson, I.C.: Thyrosine releasing hormone: enhancement of Dopa activity by a hypothalamic hormone. Science *178*, 417–418 (1972)

Plotnikoff, N.P., White, W.F., Kastin, A.J., Schally, A.V.: Gonadotropine releasing hormone (GnRH): Neuropharmacological studies. Life Sci. *17*, 1685–1692 (1975)

Plotnikoff, N.P., Kastin, A.J., Coy, D.H., Christensen, C.W., Schally, A.V., Spirtes, M.A.: Neuropharmacological actions of enkephalin after systemic administration. Life Sci. *19*, 1283–1288 (1976)

Pycock, C.J., Jenner, P.G., Marsden, C.D.: The interaction of clonidine with dopamine-dependent behavior in rodents. Naunyn Schmidebergs Arch. Pharmacol. *297*, 133–141 (1977)

Quinton, R.M., Halliwell, G.: Effects of alpha-methyl DOPA and DOPA on the amphetamine excitatory response in reserpinized rats. Nature *200*, 178–179 (1963)

Randrup, A., Munkvad, I., Fog, R., Gerlach, J., Molander, L., Kjellberg, B., Scheel-Krüger, J.: Mania, depression and brain dopamine. Current developments in psychopharmacology, Vol. 2. New York: Spectrum 1975

Randrup, A., Braestrup, C.: Uptake inhibition of biogenic amines by newer antidepressant drugs: Relevance to the dopamine hypothesis of depression. Psychopharmacology *53*, 309–314 (1977)

Ross, S.B., Renyi, A.L., Oegren, S.O.: Inhibition of the uptake of noradrenaline and 5-hydroxytryptamine by chlorphentermine and chlorimipramine. Eur. J. Pharmacol. *17*, 107–112 (1972)

Rubin, B., Malone, M.H., Waugh, M.H., Burke, J.C.: Bioassay of rauwolfia roots and alkaloids. J. Pharmacol. Exp. Ther. *120*, 125–135 (1957)

Sabelli, H.C.: Pressor effects on adrenergic agents and serotonin after administration of imipramine. Drug Res. *10*, 935–936 (1960)

Schacht, U., Heptner, W.: Effect of nomifensine (Hoe 984), a new antidepressant, on uptake of noradrenaline and serotonin and on release of noradrenaline in rat brain synaptosomes. Biochem. Pharmacol. *23*, 3413–3422 (1974)

Scheckel, C.L., Boff, E.: Behavioral stimulation in rats associated with a selective release of brain norepinephrine. Arch. Int. Pharmacodyn. Ther. *152* (3–4), 479–490 (1964)

Scheel-Krüger, J.: Central effect of anticholinergic drugs measured by the apomorphine gnawing test in mice. Acta Pharmacol. Toxicol. (Kbh.) *28*, 1–16 (1970)

Schelkunov, E.L.: Efficacy of neuroleptics and antidepressants in the test of apomorphine hypothermia and some data concerning neurochemical mechanisms of the test. Psychopharmacology *55*, 87–95 (1977)

Schildkraut, J.J.: The catecholamine hypothesis of affective disorders: a review of supporting evidence. Am. J. Psychiatry *122*, 509–522 (1965)

Schildkraut, J.J., Winokur, A., Draskóczy, P.R., Hensle, J.H.: Changes in norepinephrine turnover in rat brain during chronic administration of imipramine and protriptyline: a possible explanation for the delay in onset of clinical antidepressant effects. Am. J. Psychiatry *127*, 1032–1039 (1971)

Schmitt, H., Schmitt, H.: Valeur de pharmacologie prévisionelle dans le domaine des antidépresseurs dérivés de l'iminodibenzyle. Therapie *21*, 653–674 (1966)

Sigg, E.B., Soffer, L., Gyermek, L.: Influence of imipramine and related psychoactive agents on the effect of 5-hydroxytryptamine and catecholamines on the cat nictitating membrane. J. Pharmacol. Exp. Ther. *142*, 13–20 (1963)

Sigg, E.B., Gyermek, L., Hill, R.T.: Antagonism to reserpine induced depression by imipramine, related psychoactive drugs, and some autonomic agents. Psychopharmacologia *7*, 144–149 (1965)

Sigg, E.B., Hill, R.T.: The effect of imipramine on central adrenergic mechanisms. In: Neuropsychopharmacology. Proc. 5th CINP Congress, Washington, 1966. Brill, H. (ed.), pp. 367–372. Amsterdam, New York: Excerpta Medica 1967

Simon, P., Boissier, J.R.: Evaluating potential antidepressants in animals. J. Int. Med. Res. *3*,, Suppl. 3, 14–17 (1975)

Stanley, M.E., Glick, S.D.: Interaction of drug effects with testing procedures in the measurement of catalepsy. Neuropharmacology *15*, 393–394 (1976)

Starke, K.: Regulation of noradrenaline release by presynaptic receptor systems. Rev. Physiol. Biochem. Pharmacol. *77*, 1–124 (1977)

Stein, L., Seifter, J.: Possible mode of antidepressive action of imipramine. Science *134*, 286–287 (1961)

Stein, L.: New methods for evaluating stimulants and antidepressants. Psychosomatic medicine. 1st Hahnemann Symposium. Nodine, J.H., Moyer, J.H. (eds.), pp. 297–311. Philadelphia: Lea & Febiger 1962

Stein, L.: Self-stimulation of the brain and the central stimulant action of amphetamine. Fed. Proc. *23*, 836–850 (1964)

Stille, G.: Pharmacological investigations of antidepressant compounds. Neuropsychopharmacology *1*, 92–106 (1968)

Strömbom, U.: On the functional role of pre- and postsynaptic catecholamine receptors in brain. Acta Physiol. Scand. [Suppl.] *431*, 1–43 (1975)

Sulser, F., Watts, J.S., Brodie, B.B.: Blocking of reserpine action by imipramine, a drug devoid of stimulatory effects in normal animals. Fed. Pro c. *20*, 321 (1961)

Sulser, F., Watts, J.S., Brodie, B.B.: On the mechanism of antidepressant action of imipraminelike drugs. Ann. N.Y. Acad. Sci. *96*, 279–288 (1962)

Sulser, F., Bickel, M.H., Brodie, B.B.: The action of desmethylimipramine in counteracting sedation and cholinergic effects of reserpine-like drugs. J. Pharmacol. Exp. Ther. *144*, 321–330 (1964)

Sulser, F., Langlois Owens, M., Dingell, J.V.: On the mechanism of amphetamine potentiation by desipramine (DMI). Life Sci. *5*, 2005–2010 (1966)

Sulser, F., Vetulani, J., Mobley, P.L.: Commentary: Mode of action of antidepressant drugs. Biochem. Pharmacology *27*, 257–261 (1978)

Svensson, T.H.: On the role of central noradrenaline in the regulation of motor activity and body temperature in the mouse. Naunyn Schmiedebergs Arch. Pharmacol. *271*, 111–120 (1971)

Tang, S.W., Helmeste, D.M., Stancer, H.C.: The effect of acute and chronic desipramine and amitriptyline treatment on rat brain total 3-methoxy-4-hydroxyphenylglygol. Naunyn Schmiedebergs Arch. Pharmacol. *305*, 207–211 (1978)

Tedeschi, D.: Ptosis as a model of depression. J. Pharmacol. (Paris), Suppl. 2 (5), 98 (1974)

Theobald, W., Büch, O., Kunz, H.A., Morpurgo, C., Stenger, E.G., Wilhelmi, G.: Vergleichende pharmakologische Untersuchungen mit Tofranil, Pertofran und Insidon. Arch. Int. Pharmacodyn. Ther. *148*, (3–4), 560–596 (1964)

Theobald, W., Büch, O., Kunz, H.A.: Vergleichende Untersuchungen über die Beeinflussung vegetativer Funktion durch Psychopharmaka im akuten Tierversuch. Arzneim. Forsch. *15*, 117–125 (1965)

Theobald, W., Büch, O., Kunz, A., Morpurgo, C.: Zur Pharmakologie des Antidepressivums 3-chlor-5-(3-dimethylamino-propyl)-10, 11-dihydro-5H-dibenz(b,f) azepin. HCl. Arzneim. Forsch. *17*, 561–564 (1967)

Ther, L., Schramm, H.: Apomorphin-Synergismus (Zwangsnagen bei Mäusen) als Test zur Differenzierung psychotroper Substanzen. Arch. Int. Pharmacodyn. Ther. *138*, 302–310 (1962)

Valzelli, L., Consolo, S., Morpurgo, C.: Influence of imipramine-like drugs on the metabolism of amphetamine. In: Antidepressant drugs. Proc. 1st Int. Symp., Milan, 1966. Garattini, S., Dukes, M.N.G. (eds.), pp. 61–69. Amsterdam: Exerpta Medica 1967

Van Praag, H.M.: Depression and schizophrenia: A contribution to their chemical pathologies. New York: Spectrum 1977

Waldmeier, P.C., Baumann, P., Greengrass, P.M., Maître, L.: Effects of clomipramine and other tricyclic antidepressants on biogenic amine uptake and turnover. Postgrad. Med. J. *52*, Suppl. 3, 33–39 (1976)

Waldmeier, P.C., Baumann, P.A.: Effects of clomipramine, nomifensine, viloxazine and mianserine on the uptake and metabolism of biogenic amines. A review of the literature and some comparative studies. Br. J. Clin . Pract. to be published

Westfall, T.C.: Local regulation of adrenergic neurotransmission. Physiol. Rev. *57*, 659–728 (1977)

Wilson, S.P., Tislow, R.: Differential antagonism of reserpine eyelid closure by imipramine and amphetamine. Proc. Soc. Exp. Biol. Med. *109*, 847–848 (1962)

Wirth, W., Gösswald, R., Hörlein, U., Risse, K.H., Kreiskott, H.: Zur Pharmakologie acylierter Phenothiazin-Derivate. Arch. Int. Pharmacodyn. Ther. *115*, 1–31 (1958)

Young, R.L., Gordon, M.W.: The disposition of (^{14}C) amphetamine in rat brain. J. Neurochem. *9*, 161–167 (1962)

CHAPTER 22

Toxicology of Antidepressant Drugs

P. Thomann and R. Hess

A. Introduction

As many pharmacodynamic effects carry over from animals to man, many toxic effects may also be predicted from observations made in animals. However, some important toxic effects are not predictable from animal studies (WHO, 1966) and this limitation may apply particularly to drugs acting on the central nervous system, such as the antidepressants. Nevertheless, the recognition of species differences and similarities in responses is considered as an important means of predicting toxic effects in man. In the following, some degree of correlation is attempted by the comparison, whenever feasible, between toxicity in laboratory animals and adverse effects described in man, particularly in cases of acute intoxication. However, due to the differing amount of data that was available on various drugs and the widely varying experimental conditions employed, such a comparison may not always prove to be reliable.

The following review has been restricted to antidepressants in clinical use and, as far as evidence was available from the literature, concentrated on two main categories of antidepressants, the monoamine oxidase (MAO) inhibitors and the tricyclics. The lithium salts are considered in a separate chapter of this volume. Emphasis is placed on the systemic toxicity and on adverse effects on particular organs or tissues. Attention has also been directed to problems of possible adverse reactions arising from the concurrent application of several drugs and the attempt has been made to re-assess the sometimes controversial issue of effects on reproduction and embryonal-fetal development.

B. Monoamine Oxidase Inhibitor

I. Animal Toxicity

1. General Toxicology

The acute i.p. LD 50 of nialamide, phenelzine sulfate, and iproniazide in mice was reported to be 820, 640, and 135 mg/kg, respectively (Lapin and Samsonova, 1969). In the rat, i.p. administration of tranylcypromine was found to be associated with high mortality, multifocal cardiac necrosis with inflammatory reaction, and mononuclear cell infiltration. If the animals survived, myocardial fibrosis ensued. The injury was found to resemble that due to isoproterenol (Heggtveit, 1967). Panisset et al. (1965) reported species differences for intravenously administered tranylcypromine in dogs on the one hand and in cats and rabbits on the other hand. In dogs, the blood pressure increased while in cats and rabbits tranylcypromine caused an elevation followed by a fall in blood pressure.

The continuous lifetime administration of phenelzine sulfate (0.015 % in drinking water) to Swiss mice gave rise to an increased incidence of adenoma and adenocarcinoma of the lungs and to angioma and angiosarcoma of blood vessels in female mice. The treatment had no statistically significant effect on the development of tumors in males. The sex difference was explained by the increased mortality due to toxic effect in the males, before tumors had arisen (TOTH, 1976).

Some of the MAO inhibitors used as antidepressants were reported to cause embryotoxicity, but when given to pregnant animals, at high doses well exceeding the maximum recommended human dose, no congenital malformations were produced in the surviving offspring (SHARDEIN, 1976). Nialamide, at oral doses of 60–80 mg/kg, markedly diminished fertility in the rat and caused fetal resorptions. The treatment caused marked changes in the estrus cycle. This still prevailed at 10 mg/kg, a dose level that reduced fertility but had no fetotoxic action (TUCHMANN-DUPLESSIS and MERCIER-PAROT, 1961, 1962, 1963). Similar to nialamide, other amine oxidase inhibitors (including iproniazid, tranylcypromine, and phenelzine) have also been reported to prevent embryonic development in mice when administered in early pregnancy (POULSON and ROBSON, 1963). This effect was neither dependent on the amine oxidase inhibitory activity nor on the chemical structure. Hydrazines, for instance, claimed to interact with bacterial DNA (FREESE et al., 1968), appeared no more embryotoxic than other compounds. In the case of phenelzine it was suggested that the antifertility effect, brought about in mice at a daily subcutaneous dose of 25 mg/kg, was due to partial depression of pituitary gonadotropin activity (POULSON and ROBSON, 1964).

2. Interaction Experiments

The combined administration of ethanol and phenelzine to mice increased the duration of coma and loss of righting reflex due to alcohol (MILNER, 1968). The acute toxicity of isocarboxazid to mice increased when the mice were kept under crowded conditions (DOGGETT et al., 1977). Tranylcypromine caused fetal hyperpyrexia in rats pretreated with lithium chloride for 4 consecutive days (SHIMOMURA et al., 1977). In rabbits pretreated with MAO inhibitors, in contrast to nonpretreated rabbits, ethoheptazine consistently produced substantial hyperpyrexia, motor restlessness, hyperexcitability, tremors and tachypnea and, eventually, death (SINCLAIR, 1972). The acute toxicity of morphine, pethidine, and phenazocine in mice was increased by pretreatment with iproniazid or tranylcypromine. The reaction was related to an increased concentration of 5-hydroxytryptamine in the brain (ROGERS et al., 1968, 1969). Nialamide, iproniazid, and tranylcypromine potentiated the actions of histamine on cat blood pressure and on the tracheobronchial muscle of guinea pigs. It was concluded that side effects occurring with MAO inhibitors may be due to increased sensitivity to histamine (ALLEN et al., 1969). All MAO inhibitors, regardless of chemical type or biologic potency, increased the toxicity of amphetamine in mice (O'DEA et al., 1969). While parachlorphenylalanine had no protective effect on early mortality following tranylcypromine administration, it appeared to have protected the mice from late tranylcypromine toxicity (GESSNER et al., 1972). Anesthesia may protect mice against the potentiation of toxic effects resulting from MAO inhibition and concurrent L-Dopa administration by preventing an increase in central dopamine concentration and by reducing hyperthermia. Halothane had the most consistent beneficial effect (MÄNNISTÖ et al., 1971). In mice, the LD 50 of meperidine was markedly reduced by tranylcypromine pretreatment (FULLER and SNODDY, 1975). Chlorpromazine, parachlorphenylalanine, and cooling decreased the lethal effect of the combined treatment of tranylcypromine and meperidine in mice (GESSNER, 1973; GESSNER and SOBLE, 1973; GESSNER et al., 1974).

II. Intoxication in Man

1. Effects of Acute Overdose

In parallel to the more limited use of MAO inhibitors when compared to tricyclic antidepressants, new publications have become rare and relatively few cases of attempted suicide are reported. Fatalities after tranylcypromine overdosage have occurred at doses as low as 170 mg though most cases involve a dose range above 300 mg. With phenelzine, lethal outcome may be encountered in the range of 375–1500 mg. Doses up to 1,500 mg nialamide have been treated successfully but 5,000 mg have been fatal (DAVIS et al., 1968).

While a MAO inhibitor alone can result in death if taken at a high enough dose it should be mentioned here that a number of fatalities have occurred due to interaction of MAO inhibitors with other drugs or certain types of food. MAO inhibitors not only block the deamination of biogenic amines thus inducing pharmacodynamic changes, but also interfere with various other enzymes and are able to prolong and intensify the effects of other drugs and to interfere with the metabolism of naturally occurring substances. Interference occurs with central depressant agents such as barbiturates, alcohol, and potent analgesics; with anticholinergic agents and tricyclic antidepressants; with meperidine and with precursors of biogenic amines. The action of sympathomimetic amines are potentiated following treatment with MAO inhibitors and this is of considerable practical importance when food containing higher amounts of tyramine (cheese – especially aged cheese, beer, wine, pickled herring, chicken liver, yeast extracts such as Marmite or Bovril, cream, coffee, broad beans, etc.) are ingested by patients under treatment (DAVIS et al., 1968; GOODMAN and GILMAN, 1975).

Switching a patient from one MAO inhibitor to another or to a tricyclic antidepressant requires a rest period of 10–14 days (GOODMAN and GILMAN, 1975). A combined tricyclic-MAO inhibitor therapy for refractory depression, if carefully initiated, is, however, possible (GOLDBERG and THORNTON, 1978).

The clinical symptoms of acute overdosage appear after a lag period of several hours starting with motor uneasiness, agitation, violent motor activity with moaning and grimacing, profuse sweating and hallucinations. Temperature increases steadily well over 42 ° C within 24 h. The full clinical picture is characterized by coma with hyperthermia, tachypnea, tachycardia, dilated pupils, and hyperactive deep tendon reflexes. Convulsions and renal complications may also occur (DAVIS et al., 1968; GOODMAN and GILMAN, 1975).

2. Treatment of Acute MAO Inhibitor Overdose

Since various types of supra-additive effects from possible antidotes in clinical use may be expected, caution must be exercised in their use. In most reported cases, conservative treatment aimed at maintaining normal temperature and at supporting respiration, blood pressure, fluid and electrolyte balance has proven successful. The lag period between ingestion and the appearance of severe symptoms and hyperthermia should be used for therapeutic intervention. Osmotic diuresis, forced fluids, acidification of urine and in severe cases, hemodialysis, have been successful for elimination of the drug.

Chlorpromazine is a useful drug and in a hypertensive crisis phentolamine may be helpful, their actions being related to the α-adrenergic blocking properties.

Patients who took overdoses of MAO inhibitors should be observed in the hospital for at least a week after poisoning as late toxic effects may appear. Their diet should be controlled (DAVIS et al., 1968; GOODMAN and GILMAN, 1975).

3. Chronic Toxicity of MAO Inhibitors

MAO inhibitors possess a considerable potential for chronic toxic effects. Though the incidence of hepatotoxicity with currently used MAO inhibitors is low, hepatic effects are among the most dangerous. Liver involvement does not seem to be related to dosage or duration of therapy. Excessive central stimulation is observed covering the range from tremors and insomnia over agitation and, on rare occasions, hallucinations or confusion to convulsions. Finally, orthostatic hypotension occurs with all currently used MAO inhibitors (GOODMAN and GILMAN, 1975; HAMILTON and MAHAPATRA, 1972).

C. Tricyclic Antidepressants

I. Animal Toxicity

1. General Toxicology

The LD 50 values for a number of tricyclic antidepressants, when administered to mice and rats in single oral or parenteral doses, are listed in Table 1. Acute poisoning by tricyclic antidepressants usually leads to symptoms of central excitation followed at

Table 1. Acute LD_{50} values[a] of some tricyclic antidepressants

		Imipramine	Doxepine	Nortriptyline	Viloxazine	Maprotiline
Mouse	i.v.	35	15– 20	26	60	31
	p.o.	666	148–178	327	1000	660– 900
Rat	i.v.	22	13– 19	22	60–77	38– 52
	p.o.	625	346–460	502	2000	760–1050
		THOMANN (1970)	PDR (1973)	MEYERS et al. (1966a)	BROSNAN et al. (1976)	HESS et al. (1973)

[a] The values given are for LD_{50}, single administration, in mg/kg body weight

the higher and lethal dose levels by central inhibition. The symptomatology includes muscular weakness, twitching, stupor, respiratory disorders, ataxia, and tonic–clonic convulsions.

It is evident from Table 1 or from the reports of PLUVIAGE (1969) and of UEKI et al. (1974) that no major differences in the acute toxicity of tricyclic antidepressants are apparent. Information on animal studies relating to the tolerance of tricyclic antidepressants upon repetitive administration is relatively scarce. A large amount of animal data on individual compounds are contained in the documentation that is submitted to the Health Authorities. Published information on the results of long term tolerance in animals covering the whole range of toxicity assessment is, however, scarce and generally lacking in detail. Upon reviewing the data available in the literature the following conclusions may be drawn:

a) In response to comparatively small doses of imipramine in the range of 10 mg/kg, rats show a decrease in appetite and fail to gain weight at the normal rate.

b) In guinea-pigs treated with i.p. doses of 60–90 mg/kg imipramine daily, some renal tubular dilatation was observed after 30–60 days; there was no sign of cardiotoxicity however. Intramuscular injections of 30 and 40 mg/kg daily for 30 days resulted in cerebral, hepatic, and renal changes.

c) In rabbits, the striking feature of the response to repeated doses of imipramine is the discrepancy between the tolerance to the drug given by the oral and by the subcutaneous routes. Whereas oral treatment did not affect the animals' body weight until a dosage level of 100 mg/kg daily was reached, subcutaneous injections of 10 mg/kg daily were sufficient to cause a decrease in body weight gain (THOMANN, 1970).

d) Oral treatment with imipramine in daily doses of 20 mg/kg was relatively well tolerated by rats for 1 year, and by dogs for 6 months, the internal organs showing no histologic changes at autopsy. However, daily oral doses of 60 and 160 mg/kg administered for 360 days, resulted in some hepatotropic effects. In another group of rats treated with oral doses of 60 mg/kg daily the same histologic picture was observed after 168 days.

e) In dogs which had received imipramine in daily oral doses of 60 mg/kg for 6 months, examination at autopsy disclosed no treatment-related changes of organs or tissues (THOMANN, 1970).

f) Rats treated orally with 10 mg maprotiline/kg daily for up to 78 weeks showed minimal effects; 30 mg/kg was tolerated by about two-thirds of the animals and 60 mg/kg/day resulted in the death of more than half of the animals within a 1 year period. Apart from some fatty change in the liver of a number of rats at the higher dose levels that was reversible on withdrawal of medication, no pathology was produced by the treatment.

g) On repetitive oral administration of maprotiline to dogs, 20 mg/kg daily was tolerated by most animals over a 1 year period. A dose of 10 or 1 mg/kg daily given for the same amount of time did not give rise to any adverse effects. At all dose levels, no drug-related changes were seen in any organs or tissues (HESS et al., 1973).

h) Rats tolerated daily s.c. doses of 20 mg nortriptyline hydrochloride per kg body weight for 246 days with no drug-induced pathological changes except a local irritant effect at the site of injection. There was no significant alteration in food intake. Dogs given a daily dose of 40 mg/kg succumbed and prior to death showed emesis, mydriasis, ataxia, and occasional seizures. 20 mg/kg daily for 1 year was tolerated with no deleterious drug effects. Rats maintained for 1 year on a diet containing 1,500 ppm of nortriptyline showed no hematologic or histologic changes. A dose-dependent retardation in growth rate was seen in rats given 750 and 1,500 ppm in the diet (MEYERS et al., 1966a).

i) Dogs treated with doxepin at 25 and 50 mg/kg daily for up to 12 months exhibited slight emesis, ptosis, sedation, and twitching but showed no histopathological changes of their tissues attributable to the drug treatment.

k) When doxepin hydrochloride was fed to rats at dose levels of up to 100 mg/kg daily, fatty metamorphosis of the liver was observed primarily in the male rats at 100 mg/kg. At the same dose level there was an inhibition of body weight gain in the females. Doses of 50 mg/kg daily may be considered as a threshold level in that these dose levels produced no adverse effects in an 18 months study while in another study of 12 months duration, slight hepatic fatty metamorphosis was observed. Lower doses were tolerated without adverse effects (PDR, 1973).

2. Interaction Experiments

The toxicity of a number of tricyclic compounds has been shown to depend on a variety of conditioning factors such as stress, hormonal influences, and the effects of other pharmacologically active agents.

In mice, the acute LD 50 of imipramine depends on the number of animals per cage (LAL and BROWN, 1968). Crowding also increased the toxicity of desmethylimipramine in mice. The regression line from desmethylimipramine was steeper under crowded conditions than under uncrowded conditions (DOGGETT et al., 1977). In hyperthyroid animals, tricyclic antidepressants proved more toxic than in euthyroid condition (ASHFORD and ROSS, 1968; WINTER, 1966). In rats, orally administered activated charcoal was found to have only limited value as an antidotal adsorbent in imipramine or desipramine poisoning (RAUWS and OLLING, 1976).

Pretreatment with α- or β-receptor blockers had no measurable effect on the toxicity of imipramine, but the drug's toxicity was increased when it was injected simultaneously with ethanol. The combined administration of ethanol together with amitriptyline, trimipramine, imipramine, and nortriptyline to mice increased the duration of coma and loss of righting reflex due to alcohol, mostly two to fourfold, while desipramine protected the mice from ethanol-induced loss of righting reflexes (THOMANN, 1970; MILNER,, 1968).

A normal corticosteroid level is the most favourable prerequisite for survival during the first 6 h after an animal has received a toxic dose of imipramine. In the subsequent recovery phase, treatment with adrenocortical hormones improves the animal's chances of survival (THOMANN, 1970).

A higher death rate was observed when imipramine was given together with a MAO inhibitor than when it was administered alone (THOMANN, 1970). MAXWELL (1965) showed that the administration of imipramine and amitriptyline to rabbits premedicated with high doses of tranylcypromine, nialamide, or phenelzine was followed by hyperexcitement and fatal hyperpyrexia in a large proportion of animals. The author also found that imipramine, amitriptyline, and trimipramine differed in their ability to produce side effects in rabbits premedicated with MAO inhibitors and that the particular MAO inhibitors used also played a role. In a study on the effects of a number of drugs on the ECG changes induced by amitriptyline, NYMARK and RASMUSSEN (1966) reported that dichloroisoprenaline and propranolol slowed down heart rates but otherwise did not affect the electrocardiogram. ATTREE et al., (1972) reported on the effects of the administration of tricyclic antidepressants on the cardiotoxicity of digoxin in the rat. In some experiments, rats were stressed by repeated transfer from cage to cage. After acute administration only desmethylimipramine caused a significant increase in the toxicity of digoxin. While stress itself did not significantly increase the lethality of digoxin, stress in the presence of either amitriptyline or imipramine did increase digoxin lethality. When administered chronically, both imipramine and desmethylimipramine significantly increased the cardiotoxicity of digoxin.

A series of experiments was run on the effects of cholinesterase inhibitors, propranolol, and mecamylamine on the toxicity of amitriptyline or protriptyline. Amitriptyline induced tachycardia and neurological signs in all animals at subcutaneous doses of 50 or 70 mg/kg. The chronotropic actions were reversed by all drugs used and the neurological effects favorably influenced only by physostigmine. Protriptyline at 50 mg/kg produced less tachycardia, no neurological signs, and its effect on the heart were less sensitive to physostigmine antagonism. The results suggested that the toxicity of amitriptyline or protriptyline may be due to the anticholinergic activity of the drugs; the effects on the heart resulting from sympathetic activation (TORCHIANA et al., 1972).

The interaction of various tricyclic drugs with d-amphetamine toxicity has been studied under standard conditions in nonaggregated mice. Pre- or posttreatment with promazine protected the animals in all cases. The tertiary amines, imipramine and amitriptyline, had either no effect or exerted a protective action; the secondary amines, desmethylimipramine and nortriptyline, either potentiated or reduced the toxicity of d-amphetamine, depending on the dosage schedule with respect to time (SOKOL and MAIKEL, 1972).

In mice treated with lethal doses of amitriptyline, the number of fatalities was significantly reduced by physostigmine, pilocarpine and pyridostigmine (SCHAERER, 1965). In another study, NYMARK and RASMUSSEN (1966) reported that drugs which interfered with cholinergic transmission (e.g. prostigmine, pyridostigmine) markedly increased the survival of animals poisoned by amitriptyline and exercised a beneficial effect on the ECG changes.

VANCE et al. (1977) reported that subtoxic doses of physostigmine potentiated the convulsive toxicity and lethality of amitriptyline and imipramine in mice. The seeming discrepancy with the results reported by SCHAERER (1965) is explained by the 100- to 1,000-fold increased doses of physostigmine used in this study. SCHAERER (1965) reported that in his experiments higher doses of cholinergic agents increased the lethality since the gut peristalsis which is reduced in tricyclic intoxication is increased by the cholinergic drugs, suggesting the effect of increased resorption.

Based on their experiments, LEE and SPENCER (1977) showed that morphine would better be combined with maprotiline than with clomipramine. TOFANETTI et al. (1977) reported that doses of doxepin, in themselves lacking any analgesic effect, remarkably enhanced the analgesic activity of propoxyphene. On the other hand, the data proved that doxepin did not significantly alter the acute toxicity of propoxyphene.

In amitriptyline-treated mice, luminal and chlordiazepoxide halved fatalities (SCHAERER, 1965); imipramine convulsions could be prevented by diazepam (BEAUBIEN et al., 1976). In a study on the effects of prolonged treatment of rats with nortriptyline and amitriptyline on the acute toxicity of 26 neuropharmacologic agents, MEYERS et al. (1966a) showed that the toxicity of Na-pentobarbital, Na-secobarbital, methapyrilene-HCl, chlordiazepoxide and physostigmine was increased but the toxicity of isoproterenol, atropine sulfate, chlorpromazine, and ephedrine was reduced.

3. Cardiovascular Effects

Pharmacologic studies indicate that overdosage with tricyclic antidepressants has a complex action on the heart, affecting α- and β-adrenergic receptors, cholinergic receptors, catecholamine metabolism, and atrioventricular and intraventricular conduction (BACHMANN and ZBINDEN, 1978). In response to relatively high i.v. doses of tricyclic antidepressants, evidence of disturbances affecting cardiac conduction and repolarization was observed in the ECG (BOISSIER et al., 1965).

Experiments on anesthetized guinea pigs which were infused until death and additional in vitro studies on guinea pig atria revealed that i.v. infusion of imipramine, amitriptyline, nortriptyline, and doxepin produced sinus tachycardia, repolarization disturbances, prolongation of the corrected QT-interval and disturbances of atrioventricular and intraventricular conduction with atrioventricular and cardiac arrest in asystole. No significant difference between the tricyclic antidepressants was observed. The in vivo model was, therefore, considered to relate to the situation observed in humans suffering from acute intoxication of a tricyclic antidepressant. Guinea pigs infused with doxepin at a constant infusion rate survived significantly longer than those infused with amitriptyline, imipramine, or nortriptyline. In these experiments, sodium bicarbonate had no effects on the arrhythmias induced by tricyclic antidepressants; propranolol, apart from counteracting the tachycardia induced, was without further effect on the ECG.

In the isolated spontaneously beating guinea-pig atria, a slight but significant decrease in the rate and force of contraction was found with several tricyclic drugs at $10^{-2}mM$. It was concluded that an interference in impulse conduction could be responsible for the arrhythmogenic effect of tricyclic antidepressants (DUMOVIC et al., 1976, 1977). Further experiments performed on perfused isolated guinea-pig hearts and on intact guinea pigs, rats, and rabbits showed that amitriptyline had a negative inotropic effect but increased the coronary flow and influenced cardiac frequency, modified the electric axis of the heart, and caused disturbances of ventricular repolarization including block of right branch, supraventricular tachycardia and auricular –ventricular dissociation (LAMARCHE et al., 1966). When the effect of imipramine on the rat and guinea-pig isolated myocardial fiber was studied by means of intracellular electrodes, it was shown that imipramine decreased the membrane and action potentials, increased the conduction time and excitation threshold and slowed the depolarization velocity. The effect of imipramine on the action potentials of the isolated myocardial fiber was transiently abolished by sodium lactate, sodium bicarbonate, and calcium chloride. Whereas the calcium salt did not modify the increase in conduction time, the sodium salts almost completely abolished the action of imipramine (AUCLAIR et al., 1969). In rabbits, large doses of imipramine also gave rise to changes affecting cardiac activity (FOURNIER et al., 1966). In the rabbit isolated atrium and aortic strip, the cardiac effects of four tricyclic antidepressants correlated better to their "receptor blocking effect" than to their effect on the noradrenaline uptake (ELONEN and MATTILA, 1972).

Experiments on dogs showed that, depending on the dose, the force and rate of heart contractions as well as the aortic and coronary flow were increased. This was followed by a marked depression of contactility with decreased aortic flow and blood pressure followed by death in ventricular arrhythmia (DHUMMA-UPAKORN and COBBIN, 1975). In dogs with an artificial atrioventricular block, increasing doses of tricyclic antidepressants provoked changes in ventricular automaticity consisting of markedly lengthened ventricular intervals. In dogs treated with 200 mg amitriptyline/kg, administration of 25 mcg mestinon per kg, i.m., brought about rapid normalization of the severely raised heart rate and the altered ECG (SCHAERER, 1965). In studies in young anesthetized dogs, hyperventilation, sodium bicarbonate, or trishydroxya-minomethane abolished the arrhythmia produced by tricyclic antidepressants when the blood pH was over 7.4. The best treatment of the intoxication was either physostigmine or sodium bicarbonate (BROWN, 1974). In cats, cardiac changes involving ST-T wave and myocardial conduction were demonstrated during chronic amitriptyline treatment. Further investigations in the same experimental model led to the conclusion that stress increases the prominence of tricyclic-induced electrocardiographic abnormalities (GLISSON et al., 1978).

In rats given oral doses of tricyclic antidepressants twice daily, uncoupling of oxidative phosphorylation in heart mitochondria with concomitant changes in oxygen consumption was seen. With maprotiline, the effect appeared after 2 weeks while with amitriptyline, protriptyline, and imipramine it was seen after only two doses. It was concluded that the treatment had caused a mild to moderate impairment of the heart mitochondrial function suggesting that the effect is due to nonspecific binding of the drugs to lipid mitochondrial membranes (BACHMANN and ZBINDEN, 1978).

4. Induction of Myeloid Body Formation

A variety of drugs and other compounds may, upon single or repeated administration of high enough doses, induce the formation of lamellated cytoplasmic particles with distinct morphology resembling so-called myeloid bodies (HRUBAN et al., 1972) in cells of the parenchyma of the liver (Fig. 1) and in other tissues of laboratory animals. This morphological alteration, usually associated with intracellular accumulation of polar lipids, is elicited by compounds consisting of a hydrophobic ring system linked to a hydrophilic aliphatic side chain bearing a terminal cationic amine group (LUELL-MANN et al., 1973). Agents of that sort, also termed amphiphilic may interact with complex membranous structures forming complexes with phospholipids by virtue of electrostatic and hydrophobic forces (LUELLMANN et al., 1975). A number of psychotropic drugs, including tricyclic antidepressants, belong to this category and it may be speculated that distinct biologic effects (such as the interference with catecholamine uptake through the cell membrane of sympathetic neurons) may depend on the particular type of membrane interaction (STAEUBLI et al., 1974).

Based on ultrastructural studies, the antidepressants iprindole, imipramine, clomipramine, noxiptiline, maprotiline, amitryptiline and the experimental drug l-chloro-

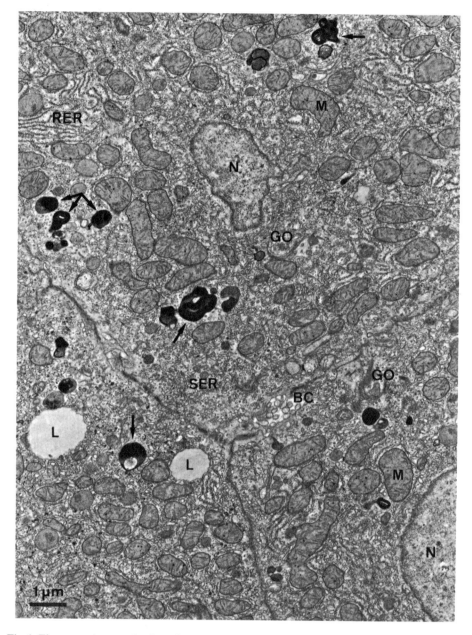

Fig. 1. Electron micrograph of rat liver following oral treatment with maprotiline (100 mg/kg per day for 4 days). L, lipid droplets; BC, bile canaliculus; M, mitochondria; N, nucleus; GO, Golgi complex; RER, rough surfaced, and SER, smooth surfaced endoplasmic reticulum. Arrows denote myeloid bodies. Magnification ×14,625. (Courtesy Dr. W. Stäubli)

amitryptiline have been reported to induce myeloid body-like changes in animals (LUELLMANN et al., 1975; STAEUBLI et al., 1974; TANAKA et al., 1975; THEISS et al., 1973). The latter compound, similar to chlorphentermine and to a number of tricyclic compounds (LUELLMANN et al., 1975), induced, apart from lamellated inclusion bodies, a remarkable increase in alveolar macrophages together with a change in their phospholipid pattern (KARABELNIK et al., 1974). Although induced formation of myeloid bodies is usually reported in the liver and, with certain compounds, in steroid-producing endocrine tissues, myeloid bodies may form in a variety of other cell types. The degree of formation of these particles appears to depend both on the amphiphilic compound used and on the local tissue response (HRUBAN et al., 1972); the latter being dependent, at least in part, on the pharmacokinetics and tissue distribution. Myeloid bodies have been produced in in vitro systems (LUELLMANN et al., 1975). They have been described in cells of normal animals (HRUBAN et al., 1972).

It has been conclusively demonstrated that myeloid bodies can be assigned to the lysosomal class of cytoplasmic organelles (ABRAHAM et al., 1968; LUELLMANN et al., 1975 STAEUBLI et al., 1974) and that their formation is a reversible process (HRUBAN et al., 1972). The reversibility of the alterations induced by amphiphilic drugs has been documented for a number of compounds. It is thought to depend on the dissociation rate constant of the complex formed between the amphiphilic compound and the phospholipoprotein, and on the actual concentration of drug present (LUELLMANN et al., 1975).

Among the antidepressants, maprotiline has been extensively studied with regard to the morphogenetic, cytochemical and biochemical aspects of myeloid bodies formed in rat liver (STAEUBLI et al., 1978). The behavior of subcellular fractions obtained from livers of rats receiving five consecutive daily doses of 200 mg/kg and subjected to velocity-centrifugation in shallow sucrose gradients supported the assumption, on cytochemical evidence, that the induced inclusion bodies are lysosomes. The appearance of these particles, morphologically distinct from normal lysosomes, did not substantially alter the distribution of constitutive enzymes (and hydrolases) which were, however, reversibly displaced to lower sucrose densities, possibly due to the accumulation of phospholipid-rich material within the myeloid bodies. Since the enzyme distribution among the various cell compartments and their fractional activity was virtually unaltered, there is every reason to assume that myeloid body formation per se does not indicate a toxic effect but is compatible with the normal physiology of the cell.

The observations made with maprotiline caution against the indiscriminate use of the term "drug-induced phospholipidosis" coined by SHIKATA et al., (1972) to describe the tissue changes induced in man and in rats by 4,4'-dimethylaminoethoxyhexoestrol, an amphiphilic coronary vasodilator. The rationale of this term, used in analogy with inborn lipid storage diseases, consists mainly of the structural resemblance of the phospholipid-rich myeloid bodies to the inclusion bodies found in some human gangliosidoses (VOLK et al., 1975). Biochemically however, the various inborn lysosomal storage diseases are characterized by a primary defect of a particular hydrolase or biosynthetic enzyme and the progressive accumulation of storage material in a hypertrophied lysosomal compartment, i.e., features that are quite different from the effects produced by maprotiline (STAEUBLI et al., 1978).

The available evidence on maprotiline is compatible with the conception that myeloid bodies induced in the animal by this drug, as well as presumably by other tricyclic antidepressants in common use, represent transient structures, reversible after discontinuation of treatment (Staeubli et al., 1974; Tanaka et al., 1975). The limited toxicologic relevance of this feature is borne out further by the fact that long-term treatment of rats with this drug did not produce any tissue changes of an irreversible nature (Hess et al., 1973).

II. Teratology

Antidepressants comprise only a small portion in the vast assortment of drugs that may be taken by pregnant women. In a sample of 3,072 subjects, the number of gravid women receiving antidepressant drugs was estimated to be in the order of 0.1 % (Peckham and King, 1963). Similar to other drugs that are used much more frequently during pregnancy (Forfar and Nelson, 1973), particularly during the first trimester (the most sensitive period of embryonal development), some antidepressants have been suspected to carry a teratogenic risk.

In a short note published 1972, McBride reported on one child with amelia and mentioned two others with a similar limb deformity he felt were caused by imipramine taken by the mothers in early pregnancy. Two further cases were subsequently reported (Freeman, 1972; Barson, 1972). Doubt was, however, cast upon the validity of the McBride's notion of a causal relation between imipramine or other tricyclic antidepressants such as amitriptyline and congenital abnormalities. The Australian Drug Evaluation Committee (1973) and the results of further clinical and epidemiologic studies failed to associate the ingestion of these drugs in early pregnancy with malformations (Crombie et al., 1972; Morrow et al., 1972; Rachelefsky et al., 1972; Banister et al., 1972; Sim, 1972; Bourke, 1974). Likewise, neither on account of the review presented by one manufacturer (Jacobs, 1972) nor on the basis of the survey of a series of 15,000 pregnancies in Scotland (Kuennsberg and Knox, 1972) and the review of 2,784 cases of birth defects in Finland (Idänpään-Heikkila and Saxen, 1973), was it inferred that imipramine or amitriptyline were causally related to congenital abnormalities. More recently, the results of an extensive surveillance program in the United Kingdom, relating to drug histories for the first trimester of pregnancy for mothers of congenitally malformed children and for an equal number of control mothers of normal babies, presented no evidence that antidepressants (tricyclics or MAO inhibitors) were teratogenic (Greenberg et al., 1977).

It is of interest to survey the experimental studies that were conducted to determine the effects of various antidepressants on the embryonal and foetal development of laboratory animals. A review of the literature pertaining to the various groups of antidepressant drugs is given by Tuchmann-Duplessis (1975) and by Schardein (1976). In the following, a survey is given of studies conducted in the laboratory animal with tricyclic antidepressants in therapeutic use.

The basic principles for testing for teratogenicity are similar to those underlying the detection of general toxicity except that two interdependent variables are involved, the pregnant female and the embryo. The reaction of each may be entirely different. According to present knowledge, rodents (rats or mice) and/or a lagomorph (the rabbit) can be expected to yield results that are of relevance to man. The predictive value of studies in these species appears to be at least as great as that of experiments in other species, including nonhuman primates. The rationale for testing and the present methods used in teratogenicity studies have been summarized by an expert committee of the Swiss Academy of Medical Sciences (1974).

Imipramine has been extensively studied in a variety of animal species. In the rat, a species in which the metabolism of imipramine has a certain resemblance to that of man (DINGELL et al., 1964), the drug was shown to be toxic to the mother animal and to the embryo or fetus at daily oral dose levels of 10 – 50 mg/kg body weight (STENGER et al., 1965; JELINEK et al., 1967; AEPPLI, 1969). Toxicity was increased about twofold by s.c. administration (AEPPLI, 1969) and by i.p. administration. Reduction in litter size was observed when 5 mg/kg was given continuously to rats prior to and during pregnancy (SINGER and COYLE, 1973). In none of these studies was teratogenicity produced and the effects were ascribed mainly to toxic effects on the mother animal (HARPER et al., 1965; AEPPLI, 1969). In contrast to the rat, pregnant mice proved resistant and doses up to 150 mg/kg were without effect (HARPER et al., 1965).

Whereas oral doses of imipramine (up to 50 mg/kg) given to pregnant rabbits were without effect on the foetus (HARPER et al., 1965; STENGER et al., 1965), the application of high parenteral doses (10–50 mg/kg) caused maternal toxicity and abnormalities in the fetuses, in a dose related fashion (HARPER et al., 1965; AEPPLI, 1969). Malformations of the CNS, the extremities, and of other parts of the skeleton being predominant. These findings corroborate to some extent earlier observations in this species by LARSEN (1963) and by ROBSON and SULLIVAN (1963). Their significance is doubtful, however, since in contrast to the human and the rat, the rabbit produces large amounts of 2-hydroxy-imipramine, which is the metabolite held responsible for the maternal and foetal toxicity and in consequence, for the teratogenic effects in this species (AEPPLI, 1969).

On the basis of these data, imipramine produces maternal toxicity when given in high enough doses to the pregnant animal. Only when this effect prevails, may embryotoxicity and abnormal development be induced. Nontoxic doses to the mother animal are without effect on the fetus. It is of interest to compare this secondary or nonspecific action in rats and rabbits to the results of experiments conducted in nonhuman primates. HENDRICKX (1975) administered imipramine hydrochloride to bonnet and Rhesus monkeys during the critical periods of organogenesis, including limb development and palatal closure, at daily oral doses ranging from 100 to 1000 mg, i.e., from 19 to 244 mg/kg per day. Signs of maternal toxicity (convulsions) occurred at the high dose level but no teratologic changes were produced. By and large, results similar to imipramine were also obtained with its desmethyl metabolite desipramine (AEPPLI, 1969).

Of other antidepressants in therapeutic use, the information available in the literature is less extensive. Amitriptyline was reported to induce malformations in rabbits, but it produced no such effects in mice (KHAN and AZAM, 1969) or rats (JELINEK et al., 1967). This drug and butriptyline were reported to cause an increasing degree of retardation of skeletal ossification in rats at doses of 5–25 mg/kg. Apart from this entirely nonspecific effect, no maternal or fetal toxicity was observed (DI CARLO and PAGNINI, 1971). Maprotiline, an antidepressant dibenzobicyclo-octadiene, likewise caused slight retardation of fetal growth when administered orally throughout the organogenetic phase at a dose level of 10 mg/kg (i.e., about five times the maximum therapeutic dose). No effects whatever were observed in pregnant mice. In rabbits, at a dose that produced maternal toxicity (6 mg/kg), the offspring were unaffected. The compound did not adversely effect fertility, general reproductive performance, perinatal behavior and lactation in rats (HESS et al., 1973).

III. Intoxication in Man

1. Effects of Acute Overdose

Most of the numerous publications on acute intoxication with tricyclic antidepressants deal with attempted suicide in adults or with accidental selfpoisoning in children. Taking into account the difficulty in establishing the dose ingested – particularly in the case of children and of successful suicides – it is not surprising that it is difficult to predict the severity of an acute intoxication from the dose apparently taken. In children, fatalities have occurred with doses below 500 mg and survival with doses as high as approximately 1,700 mg. In adults, doses below 1,000 mg may already prove fatal but survival has been reported with doses up to 4,000 mg or higher (MANOGUERRA and WEAVER, 1977; THOMANN, 1970). In children, the critical dose level for imipramine seems to lie around 500 mg. Of a survey comprising 34 cases, only two children who had ingested less died whereas only three with larger doses survived. (THOMANN, 1970). Adults, who have ingested 1,000 – 2,000 mg still have a good chance of recovery whereas the risk of a fatality becomes far greater at levels of over 2,000 mg (DAVIES et al., 1968; THOMANN, 1970). In relation to body weight, an LD 50 value for imipramine has been determined for children at 40 – 50 mg/kg and for adults at 30 – 50 mg/ kg (THOMANN, 1970).

The symptoms from poisoning with these tricyclic antidepressants may be characterized as follows: After a lag period of 1 – 12 h, patients may show motor disturbance, dryness of the mouth, sometimes mydriasis, then go through a phase of agitation with visual or auditory hallucination. While awake, they may complain of blurred vision photophobia, and difficulty with speech. After a few hours and depending on the dose ingested, coma usually sets in, the progress from a state of alertness to unconsciousness sometimes occurs over a short period of time. A striking feature in children is extreme agitation alternating with periods of drowsiness. At the height of the clinical picture, the patient is in coma with shock, respiratory depression, temporary agitation, and diminished or absent pupillary or corneal reflexes, hyperreflexive tendons, and positive Babinski's sign. Generalized twitching and clonic movements may progress to seizures, particularly following external stimuli such as examination of pain reflexes or endotracheal intubation. Mucous membranes may be dry, bowel and bladder function depressed or paralyzed. Hyperpyrexia is a common finding and disturbances of cardiac function such as tachycardia, atrial fibrillation, ventricular flutters, atrioventricular or intraventricular block have to be expected. Coma is usually not protracted over 24 h though prolonged coma has been reported and death from cardiac arrhythmias may occur even after several days. In the presence of an increased QRS-complex, normal vital signs and level of consciousness do not ensure that the patient is not a medical risk (BIGGS et al., 1977; DAVIES, 1968; FOURNIER, 1973; JUKES, 1975; MANOGUERRA and WEAVER, 1977; NOBLE and MATTHEW, 1969; PETIT and BIGGS, 1977; SEDAL et al., 1972; THOMANN, 1970; WOOD et al., 1976). Besides measuring plasma levels, the following symptoms appear to offer a guide to the dose ingested: onset and depth of coma, occurrence of grand mal seizures, abnormal deep tendon reflexes and, despite somewhat conflicting evidence (SPIKER et al., 1975), a positive Babinski sign, presence of respiratory and cardiovascular disorders especially prolongation of the QRS-duration (BIGGS et al., 1977; FOURNIER, 1973; GOEL and SHANKS, 1974; PETIT et al., 1976; THOMANN, 1970) – the duration over 100 ms having proven to be the most reliable clinical sign for evaluating the seriousness of tricyclic drug overdosage (BIGGS et al., 1977; PETIT and BIGGS, 1977; PETIT et al., 1976; SPIKER et al., 1975; THORSTRAND, 1975, 1976).

The main toxic effects of tricyclic antidepressants are related to the anticholinergic action of these drugs, which is apparent at relatively low concentrations. The symptoms of the toxic confusional state are not unlike those seen in poisoning with other anticholinergic drugs. The hyperreflexia, twitching, and seizure activity are also thought to result from the anticholinergic properties leading to competitive inhibition of acetylcholine in the central nervous system and an excess of dopamine influence (HOLLINGER and KLAWANS, 1976; MANOGUERRA and WEAVER, 1977).

Since the re-uptake of noradrenaline is blocked, the levels of circulating catecholamines rise. At high concentrations, these drugs depress myocardial contractility, heart rate and coronary flow. Further cardiovascular changes suggest that, in toxic doses, they may also exert a quinidine-like action (THORSTRAND, 1975; VOHRA, 1974; VOHRA et al., 1975; WOOD et al., 1976). Further cardiovascular effects may be produced by inducing metabolic or respiratory acidosis and by interference with intracellular sodium and potassium exchange. Acidosis has been shown to reduce plasma protein binding and, as it is the unbound fraction of the drug that is pharmacologically active, acidosis will worsen the toxicity. In addition, acidosis will directly increase the hazard of a depression of myocardial contractility (BURROWS et al., 1976; MANOGUERRA and WEAVER, 1977; VOHRA, 1974). These factors should be born in mind when taking supportive measurements in the treatment and may explain the rapid deterioration in the clinical picture which is frequently seen in patients.

One of the most dangerous consequences of tricyclic drug poisoning is circulatory collapse. Profound hypotension may occur with a variety of ECG changes, most of which are indicative of disturbances affecting impulse formation and proximal and distal cardiac conduction (DAVIES et al., 1968; FOURNIER, 1973; SEDAL et al., 1972; THOMANN, 1970; VOHRA, 1974; VOHRA et al., 1975; WOOD et al., 1976). While ECG changes invariably occurred in small children who had taken 200 mg of a tricyclic antidepressant or more, in the majority of adults 1000 mg were found to be necessary to provoke changes. Still higher doses are generally a prerequisite for the development of serious arrhythmias (THOMANN, 1970; THORSTRAND, 1976).

The usual sequential electrocardiographic findings in patients who die from overdosage of tricyclic drugs are sinus tachycardia, conduction defects, supraventricular tachycardia, ST and T-wave abnormalities, ventricular arrhythmias, profound bradycardia, and finally asystole (BURROWS et al., 1976). Cardiac arrest arose within the first 24 h after TCA ingestion (SERAFIMOVSKI et al., 1975). A QRS-prolongation (in the characteristic case over 100 ms) is always present in patients with a major overdose. Unlike the prolonged QT-time it is not correlated to heart rate (THORSTRAND, 1976).

A direct toxic effect of the drug in reducing the contractility of the myocardium, combined with an increased adrenergic strain possibly accounts for the serious arrhythmias. These often take the form of a nodal rhythm with aberrant intraventricular conduction. This effect may become enhanced by the acidosis and hypokalemia which may occur. The direct effect has been postulated to be an inhibition of the ATP phosphohydralase which is thought to be the enzyme involved in the maintenance of sodium and potassium balance across the myocardial cell membrane (Burrows et al., 1976; Manoguerra and Weaver, 1977; Thorstrand, 1975; Vohra, 1974; Wood et al., 1976).

Tricyclic drugs may have a direct toxic effect on the respiratory system in addition to the ability to centrally depress respiration. Amitriptyline has been reported to cause a respiratory distress syndrome, bronchiolitis and interstitial pneumonitis resulting in death (Wood et al., 1976).

In the electroencephalogram, the changes provoked by imipramine poisoning are atypical and relatively mild, i.e., they bear no relationship to the severity of the poisoning nor do they provide any guide to the prognosis (Thomann, 1970). Comparatively little has been published concerning findings obtained at autopsy, or the results of histological examinations. In cases of death due to imipramine poisoning, no specific changes were apparent in organs or tissues (Thomann, 1970).

In many cases of attempted suicide, several drugs are taken simultaneously. From the literature it would seem that, where a tricyclic drug is consumed together with other drugs in an attempt to commit suicide, these latter drugs usually consist of barbiturates or other psychopharmaceuticals. In the patients with mixed overdoses, it is as a rule the tricyclic drug which determines both the symptomatology of the poisoning and the clinical course which it assumes (Thomann, 1970). An increased rate of respiratory distress and a higher incidence of ventricular tachycardia has been reported under these circumstances (Biggs et al., 1977).

2. Treatment of Tricyclic Antidepressant Overdose

Treatment should always be performed in an intensive care unit. Vital signs and ECG should be monitored continuously for at least 72 h and preparation made for support of respiratory and cardio-vascular function. Plasma electrolytes should be examined as well as blood gas analysis performed to judge the degree of existing acidosis (Manoguerra and Weaver, 1977; Wood et al., 1976). Since the drug is rapidly absorbed, rapid removal from the stomach is important, either by inducing vomiting or by gastric lavage. To prevent re-absorption of the parent drug and active metabolites secreted via the bile, activated charcoal should be administered and the reduced bowel movements should be stimulated with a saline laxative (Bickel, 1975; Davies, 1968; Fournier, 1973; Jukes, 1975; Manoguerra and Weaver, 1977; Munoz, 1976; Wood et al., 1976). Forced diuresis and peritoneal dialysis are not effective owing to the firm protein binding of the drug (Davies et al., 1968; Manoguerra and Weaver, 1977; Moeschlin, 1972; Wood et al., 1976).

The further treatment depends on the particular signs exhibited:
a) For counteracting the central and peripheral anticholinergic effects, a vast amount of evidence speaks in favour of using physostigmine (Burks et al., 1974; Goodman and Gilman, 1975; Janson et al., 1977; Johnson, 1976b; Manoguerra and Weaver, 1977; Munoz, 1976; Petit and Biggs, 1975; Slovis et al., 1971; Tobis and Das, 1976; Wood et al., 1976) which has been said to approach a specific antidote (Johnson, 1976b) and to be the drug of choice when treating life-threatening symptoms

caused by tricyclic antidepressants (WOOD et al., 1976). Because it is a tertiary amine, physostigmine readily crosses the blood-brain barrier and thus is at present the only parasympathomimetic drug (neostigmine, for example, is a quaternary amine) capable of reversing both the central and peripheral manifestations of the anticholinergic syndrome. Physostigmine acts rapidly, dramatically reversing the toxic effects. Despite some controversy, the side effects are said to be minimal, provided a rapid i.v. injection is avoided. The drug is quickly degraded, allowing recurrence of symptoms of intoxication and may have to be readministered every 30 – 60 min (JOHNSON, 1976 b; MUNOZ, 1976; WOOD et al., 1976).

b) Seizures can be controlled with i.v. diazepam if they are not already counteracted by physostigmine. Barbiturates should be avoided even if they have previously been reported to be useful because their CNS depressant effect may be increased in the presence of a tricyclic drug overdosage. External stimulation should be minimized (GOOD-MAN and GILMAN, 1975; MANOGUERRA and WEAVER, 1977; MUNOZ, 1976; WOOD et al., 1976).

c) Ventricular tachycardia is best treated with procainamide or lignocaine and sodium lactate or bicarbonate. Physostigmine is also effective (BROWN, 1976 a, b; FOURNIER, 1973; GOODMAN and GILMAN, 1975; MANOGUERRA and WEAVER, 1977; WOOD et al., 1976). Propranolol may be helpful but should be used with care (FREE-MAN and LOUGHHEAD, 1973; GOODMAN and GILMAN, 1975; MANOGUERRA and WEAVER, 1977).

d) Hypotension is counteracted with i.v. fluids, if necessary with a vasopressor such as phenylephrine that does not increase the heart rate (MANOGUERRA and WEAVER, 1977; MUNOZ, 1976).

e) Hyperpyrexia is relieved by physical cooling, e.g., with ice packs (GOODMAN and GILMAN, 1975; MUNOZ, 1976).

The basic approach has been summarized by WOOD et al. (1976) and involved:

(1) Administering physostigmine to treat life threatening symptoms

(2) Removing the drug from the stomach by emesis or gastric lavage

(3) Administering activated charcoal for at least 24 h

(4) Taking general supportive measures

(5) Monitoring the patient's cardiovascular and respiratory system for an adequate time period

In view of the serious intoxication and the still-limited possibilities of treatment, BICKEL (1975) recommends preventive measures, e.g., that the products be stored safely out of the reach of children and that so-called child resistant containers are used. He relates that the use of these drug containers on a limited scale have reduced childhood poisoning by about 90%

D. Conclusions

Toxic reactions occurring in man with tricyclic antidepressants are most commonly associated with their pharmacodynamic properties, anticholinergic responses and neurological symptoms; the effects associated with their aminergic actions being prominent. Moreover, adverse effects on the cardiovascular system are observed. Toxic reactions of this type, although occasionally seen at therapeutic doses, usually form part of the toxicity due to acute overdosage. Since these effects are related to the action spectrum of this type of drug, there is a close correlation between animal and human studies.

MAO inhibitors may produce serious acute and chronic toxicity, involving the central nervous system, blood pressure, and hepatotoxicity. There is a considerable danger of potentiation of the actions of endogenous biogenic amines and of interaction with other drugs, in particular with tricyclic antidepressants. A number of these toxic effects including conditioning factors can also be studied in laboratory animals.

Less reliance can be placed upon animal reproduction data as a predictive method of assessing the teratogenicity of antidepressants. At present, there is no evidence of interference with human reproduction when these drugs are used at the recommended dosages.

References

Abraham, R., Hendy, R., Grasso, P.: Formation of myeloid bodies in rat liver lysosomes after chloroquine administration. Exp. Mol. Pathol. 9, 212–229 (1968)

Aeppli, L.: Teratologische Studien mit Imipramin an Ratte und Kaninchen. Ein Beitrag zur Planung und Interpretation teratologischer Untersuchungen unter Berücksichtigung von Biochemie und Toxikologie der Prüfsubstanz. Arzneim. Forsch. 19, 1617–1640 (1969)

Allen, G.S., Rand, M.J.: Interaction between histamine and monoamine oxidase inhibitors. J. Pharm. Pharmacol. 21, 317–322 (1969)

Ananth, J.: Side effects on fetus and infant of psychotropic drug use during pregnancy. Int. Pharmacopsychiatry 2, 246–260 (1976)

Ashford, A., Ross, J.W.: Toxicity of depressant and antidepressant drugs in hyperthyroid mice. Br. Med. J. 1968/II, 217–218

Attree, T., Sawyer, P., Turnbull, M.J.: Interaction between digoxin and tricyclic antidepressants in the rat. Eur. J. Pharmacol. 19, 294–296 (1972)

Auclair, M.C., Gulda, O., Lechat, P.: Analyse electrophysiologique des effects de l'imipramine sur la fibre myocardique ventriculaire. Arch. int. Pharmocodyn. 181, 218–231 (1969)

Australian Drug Evaluation Committee: Tricyclic antidepressants and limb reduction deformities. Med. J. Aust. 1, 768–769 (1973)

Bachmann, E., Zbinden, G.: Effect of antidepressant and neuroleptic drugs on mitochondrial function in rat heart and liver. 20th Congress of the European Society of Toxicology West Berlin, 25–28 June 1978

Banister, P., Dafoe, C., Smith, E.S.O., Miller, J.: Possible teratogenicity of tricyclic antidepressants. Lancet 1972/I, 838

Barson, A.J.: Malformed infant. Br. Med. J. 1972/II, 45

Baum, T., Peters, J.R., Butz, F., Much, D.R.: Tricyclic antidepressants and cardiac conduction: changes in ventricular automaticity. Eur. J. Pharmacol. 39, 323–329 (1976)

Beaubien, A.R., Carpentier, D.C., Mathieu, L.F., MacConaill, M., Hrdina, P.D.: Antagonism of imipramine poisoning by anticonvulsants in the rat. Toxicol. Appl. Pharmacol. 38, 1–6 (1976)

Bickel, M.H.: Poisoning by tricyclic antidepressant drugs. Int. J. Clin. Pharmacol. 11, 145–176 (1975)

Biggs, J.T., Spiker, D.G., Petit, J.M., Ziegler, V.E.: Tricyclic antidepressant overdose. JAMA 238, 135–138 (1977)

Boissier, J.R., Simon, P., Witchitz, S.: Etude chez le Cobaye de la toxicité cardiaque de l'imipramine, de l'amitriptyline et de leurs dérivés monoadesméthyles. Therapie 20, 67–75 (1965)

Bourke, G.M.: Antidepressant teratogenicity? Lancet 1974/I 98

Brosnan, R.D., Busby, A.M., Holland, R.P.C.: Cases of overdosage with viloxazine hydrochloride. J. Int. Med. Res. 4, 83–85 (1976)

Brown, T.C.K.: The use of sodium bicarbonate in the treatment of tricyclic antidepressant-induced arrhythmias. Anaesth. Intensive Care 1, 203–210 (1973)

Brown, T.C.K.: Treatment of tricyclic antidepressant overdosage arrhythmias. Pediatrics *54*, 386–387 (1974)

Brown, T.C.K.: Tricyclic antidepressant overdosage: experimental studies on the management of circulatory complications. Clin. Toxicol. *9*, 255–272 (1976a)

Brown, T.C.K.: Sodium bicarbonate treatment for tricyclic antidepressant arrhythmias in children. Med. J. Aust. *2*, 380–382 (1976b)

Burkhardt, D., Raeder, E., Mueller, V., Imhof, P., Neubauer, H.: Cardiovascular effects of tricyclic and tetracyclic antidepressants. JAMA *239*, 213–216 (1978)

Burks, J.S., Walker, J.E., Rumack, B.H., Ott, J.E.: Tricyclic antidepressant poisoning. Reversal of coma, choreoathetosis, and myoclonus by physostigmine. JAMA *230*, 1405–1407 (1974)

Burrows, G.D., Vohra, J., Hunt, D., Sloman, J.G., Scoggins, B.A., Davies, B.: Cardiac effects of different tricyclic antidepressant drugs. Br. J. Psychiatry *129*, 335–341 (1976)

Cocco, G., Strozzi, C.: Interazioni cliniche fra farmaci cardioattivi ed antidepressivi. Clin. Ter. *76*, 107–110 (1976)

Crombie, D.L., Pinsent, R.J., Fleming, G.: Imipramine in pregnancy. Br. Med. J. *1972/I*, 745

Davis, J.M., Bartlett, E., Termini, B.A.: Overdosage of psychotropic drugs: A review. Dis. Nerv. Syst. *29*, 246–256 (1968)

Dhumma Upakorn, P., Cobbin, L.B.: Cardiovascular toxicity of tricyclic antidepressant drugs. Clin. Exp. Pharmacol. Physiol. *2*, 429–430 (1975)

Di Carlo, R., Pagnini, G.: Comparative action of amitriptyline and butriptyline on skeletal development on the rat embryo. Teratology *4*, 486 (1971)

Dingell, J.V., Sulser, F., Gillette, J.R.: Species differences in the metabolism of imipramine and desmethylimipramine (DMI). J. Pharmacol. exp. Ther. *143*, 14–22 (1964)

Doggett, N.S., Reno, H., Spencer, P.S.J.: A comparison of the acute toxicity of some centrally acting drugs measured under crowded and uncrowded conditions. Toxicol. Appl. Pharmacol. *39*, 141–148 (1977)

Dumovic, P., Burrows, G.D., Vohra, J., Davies, B., Scoggins, B.A.: The effect of tricyclic antidepressant drugs on the heart. Arch. Toxicol. *35*, 255–262 (1976)

Dumovic, P., Burrows, G.D., Vohra, J., Davies, B., Scoggins, B.A.: Cardiac effects of tricyclic antidepressants. Clin. Exp. Pharmacol. Physiol. *4*, 207 (1977)

Eckmann, F., Schwalb, H., Hanika, R.: Psychopharmaka und Veränderungen im Elektrokardiogramm. Pharmakopsychiat. Neuropsychopharmakol. *8*, 57–58 (1975)

Elonen, E., Mattila, M.J.: Comparison of tricyclic antidepressants as to their cardiotoxic action in conscious rabbits. Acta Pharmacol. Toxicol. *31*, 64 (1972)

Escande, M., Gayral, L., Goldberger, E., Jarrige, A., Kulik, J.: Accidents convulsif et modifications E.E.G. au cours des traitements par les antidépresseurs tricycliques. Encéphale *2*, 133–151 (1976)

Forfar, J.O., Nelson, M.M.: Epidemiology of drugs taken by pregnant women: drugs that may affect the fetus adversely. Clin. Pharmacol. Ther. *14*, 632–642 (1973)

Forrest, W.A.: Maprotiline (Ludiomil) in depression: a report of a monitored release study of 10,000 patients in general practice. J. Int. Res. *5*, 42–47 (1977)

Fournier, E.: Intoxications par les antidepresseurs tricycliques. Therapie *28*, 307–320 (1973)

Fournier, P.E., Mellerio, F., Efthymion, M.L.: Etude expérimentale de l'intoxication aiguë par l'imipramine. Anesth. Analg. (Paris) *25*, 263–269 (1966)

Fowler, N.O., McCall, D., Chou, T., Homes, J.C., Hanenson, I.B.: Electrocardiographic changes and cardiac arrhythmias in patients receiving psychotropic drugs. Am. J. Cardiol. *37*, 223–230 (1976)

Freeman, R.: Limb deformities: possible association with drugs. Med. J. Aust. *1*, 606–607 (1972)

Freeman, J.W., Loughhead, M.G.: Beta blockade in the treatment of tricyclic antidepressant overdosage. Med. J. Aust. *1*, 1233–1235 (1973)

Freese, E., Sklarow, S., Freese, E.B.: DNA damage caused by antidepressant hydrazines and related drugs. Mutat. Res. *5*, 343–348 (1968)

Fuller, R.W., Snoddy, H.D.: Inhibition of serotonin uptake and the toxic interaction between meperidine and monoamine oxidase inhibitors. Toxicol. Appl. Pharmacol. *32*, 129–134 (1975)

Gessner, P.K.: Antagonism of the tranylcypromine-meperidine interaction by chlorpromazine in mice. Eur. J. Pharmacol. *22*, 187–190 (1973)

Gessner, P.K., Soble, A.G.: A study of the tranylcypromine-meperidine interaction: effects of p-chlorophenylalanine and 1-5-hydroxytryptophan. J. Pharmacol. Exp. Ther. *186*. 276–287 (1973)

Gessner, P.K., Soble, A.G., Buffalo, N.Y.: Antagonism by p-chlorophenylalanine of late tranylcypromine toxicity. J. Pharm. Pharmacol. *24*, 825–827 (1972)

Gessner, P.K., Clarke, C.C., Adler, M.: The effect of low environmental temperature on the tranylcypromine-meperidine interaction in mice. J. Pharmacol. Exp. Ther. *189*, 90–96 (1974)

Glisson, S.N., Fajardo, L., El-Etr, A.A.: Amitriptyline therapy increases electrocardiographic changes during reversal of neuromuscular blockade. Anesth. Analg. (Cleve) *57*, 77–83 (1978)

Goel, K.M., Shanks, R.A.: Amitriptyline and imipramine poisoning in children. Br. Med. J. *1974/I*, 261–263

Goldberg, R.S., Thornton, W.E.: Combined tricyclic-MAOI therapy for refractory depression: a review, with guidelines for appropriate usage. J. Clin. Pharmacol. *18*, 143–147 (1978)

Goodman, L.S., Gilman, A.: The pharmacological basis of therapeutics, New York: Macmillan 5th ed. 1975

Greenberg, G., Anman, W.H.W., Weatherall, J.A.C., Adelstein, A.M., Haskey, J.C.: Maternal drug histories and congenital abnormalities. Br. Med. J. *1977/II*, 853–856

Hallstrom, C., Gifford, L.: Antidepressant blood levels in acute overdose. Postgrad. Med. J. *52*, 687–688 (1976)

Hamilton, M., Mahapatra, S.B.: Antidepressive drugs: side effects of drugs. Amsterdam: Excerpta Medica, 1972

Harper, K.H., Palmer, A.K., Davies, R.E.: Effect of imipramine upon the pregnancy of laboratory animals. Arzneim. Forsch. *15*, 1218–1221 (1965)

Heggtveit, H.A., Grice, H.C., Wiberg, G.S.: Cardiac necrosis induced by a monoamine oxidase inhibitor (tranylcypromine). Am. J. Pathol. *50*, 2a–3a (1967)

Hendrickx, A.G.: Teratologic evaluation of imipramine hydrochloride in bonnet (Macaca radiata) and rhesus monkeys (Macaca mulatta). Teratology *11*, 219–222 (1975)

Hess, R., Diener, R.M., Fritz, H., Pericin, C., Heywood, R., Newman, A.J., Rivett, K.F.: Tossità ed effetti sulla riproduzioni nell'animale del nuovo farmaco antidepressivo maprotilina (Ludiomil). Boll. Chim. Farm. *112*, 782–791 (1973)

Hollinger, P.C., Klawans, H.L.: Reversal of tricyclic-overdosage-induced central anticholinergic syndrome by physostigmine. Am. J. Psychiatry *133*, 1018–1023 (1976)

Hollister, L.E.: Adverse reactions to psychotherapeutic drugs: drug treatment of mental disorders. Simpson, L. L. (ed.), pp. 267–288. New York: Raven 1976

Hruban, Z., Slesers, A., Hopkins, E.: Drug-induced and naturally occurring myeloid bodies. Lab. Invest. *27*, 62–70 (1972)

Hurwitz, A., Azarnoff, D.L.: Clinical principles of drug interactions in the adult patient. Ann. N.Y. Acad. Sci. *281*, 98–105 (1976)

Idänpään-Heikkila, J., Saxen, L.: Possible teratogenicity of imipramine/chloropyramine. Lancet *1973/II*, 282–284

Jacobs, D.: Imipramine (Tofranil). S. Afr. Med. J. *46*, 1023 (1972)

Janson, P.A., Brooks Watt, J., Hermos, J.A.: Doxepin overdose: success with physostigmine and failure with neostigmine in reversing toxicity. JAMA *237*, 2632–2633 (1977)

Jelinek, V., Zikmund, E., Reichlova, R.: L'influence de quelques médicaments psychotropes sur le développement du foetus chez le rat. Therapie *22*, 1429–1433 (1967)

Johnson, G.F.S.: Clinical use of anti depressant drugs. Curr. Ther. *17*, 33–34, 37, 40–41 (1976a)

Johnson, P.B.: Physostigmine in tricyclic antidepressant overdose. JACEP *5*, 443–445 (1976b)

Jukes, A.M.: Maprotiline (Ludiomil): side-effects and overdosage. J. Int. Res. *3*, 126 (1975)

Karabelnik, D., Zbinden, G., Baumgartner, E.: Drug-induced foam cell reactions in rats. I. Histopathologic and cytochemical observations after treatment with chlorphentermine, RMI 10 393 and Ro 4-4318. Toxicol. Appl. Pharmacol. *27*, 395–407 (1974)

Khan, I., Azam, A.: Teratogenic activity of trifluoperazine, amitriptyline, ethionamide, and thalidomide in pregnant rabbits and mice. Proc. Eur. Soc. Study Drug Toxic *10*, 235–242 (1969)

Kuennsberg, E.V., Knox, J.D.E.: Imipramine in pregnancy. Br. Med. J. *1972/II*, 292

Lal, H., Brown, R.M.: Enhanced toxicity of imipramine and desimipramine in aggregated mice. J. Pharm. Pharmacol. *20*, 581–582 (1968)

Lamarche, M., Royer, R., Weiller, M., Denis, P.: Etude pharmacodynamique de la toxicité cardiaque de l'amitriptyline. Therapie *21*, 59–71 (1966)

Lapin, I.P., Samsonova, M.L.: Comparison of pharmacological activity and toxicity of the antidepressants – nialamide, phenelzine and iproniazid. Farmacol. Toksikol. *32*, 526–530 (1969)

Larsen, V.: The teratogenic effects of thalidomide, imipramine HCl and imipramine-N-oxide HCl on white Danish rabbits. Acta Pharmacol. *20*, 186–200 (1963)

Lee, R.L., Spencer, P.S.J.: The effect of clomipramine and other amine-uptake inhibitors on morphine analgesia in laboratory animals. Postgrad. Med. J. *53*, 53–61 (1977)

Lippmann, S., Moskovitz, R., O'Tuama, L.: Tricyclic-induced myoclonus. Am. J. Psychiatry *134*, 90–91 (1977)

Luellmann, H., Luellmann-Rauch, R., Wassermann, O.: Arzneimittelinduzierte Phospholipidspeicherkrankheit. Dtsch. Med. Wochenschr. *98*, 1616–1625 (1973)

Luellmann, H., Luellmann-Rauch, R., Wassermann, O.: Drug-induced phospholipidosis. CRC Crit. Rev. Toxicol. *4*, 185–218 (1975)

Männistö, P., Nikki, P., Rissanen, A.: The toxicity of two MAO inhibitors combined with 5-HTP or L-DOPA in anaesthetized mice. Acta Pharmacol. Toxicol. *29*, 441–448 (1971)

Manoguerra, A.S., Weaver, L.C.: Poisoning with tricyclic antidepressant drugs. Clin. Toxicol. *2*, 149–158 (1977)

Maxwell, D.R.: Combining the antidepressant drugs. Lancet *1965/II*, 904–905

McBride, W.G.: Limb deformities associated with iminodibenzyl hydrochloride. Med. J. Aust. *1*, 492 (1972)

Meyers, D.B., Kanyuck, D.O., Anderson, R.C.: Effect of chronic nortriptyline pretreatment on the acute toxicity of various medicinal agents in rats. J. Pharm. Sci. *55*, 1317–1318 (1966a)

Meyers, D.B., Small, R.M., Anderson, R.C.: Toxicology of nortriptyline hydrochloride. Toxicol. Appl. Pharmacol. *9*, 152–159 (1966b)

Milner, G.: The effect of antidepressants and "tranquillizers" on the response of mice to ethanol. Br. J. Pharmacol. *34*, 370–376 (1968)

Moeschlin, S.: Klinik und Therapie der Vergiftungen. Stuttgart: Thieme 1972

Morrow, A.W., Pitt, D.B., Wilkins, G.D.: Limb deformities associated with iminodibenzyl hydrochloride. Med. J. Aust. *1*, 658–659 (1972)

Munoz, R.A.: Treatment of tricyclic intoxication. Am. J. Psychiatry *133*, 1085–1087 (1976)

Noble, J., Matthew, H.: Acute poisoning by tricyclic antidepressants: clinical features and management of 100 patients. Clin. Toxicol. *2*, 403–421 (1969)

Nymark, M., Rasmussen, J.: Effect of certain drugs upon amitriptyline induced electrocardiographic changes. Acta Pharmacol. Toxicol. *24*, 148–156 (1966)

O'Dea, K., Rand, J.: Interaction between amphetamine and monoamine oxidase inhibitors. Eur. Pharm. J. *6*, 115–120 (1969)

Panisset, J.C., Boivin, P., Napke, E., Murphy, J.B.: Effect of tranylcypromine on the blood pressure response of tyramine. Nature *206*, 311–312 (1965)

Paton, A.: Diseases of the alimentary system. Drug jaundice. Br. Med. J. *2*, 1126–1127 (1967a)

Paton, A.: Diseases of the alimentary system. Gastrointestinal reactions to drugs. Br. Med. J. *2*, 1179–1180 (1976b)

Peckham, C.H., King, R.W.: A study of intercurrent conditions observed during pregnancy. Am. J. Obstet. Gynecol. *87*, 609–624 (1963)

Petit, J.M., Biggs, J.T.: Tricyclic antidepressant overdoses in adolescent patients. Pediatrics *59*, 283–287 (1977)

Petit, J.M., Spiker, D.G., Biggs, J.T.: Psychiatric diagnosis and tricyclic plasma levels in 36 hospitalized overdose patients. J. Nerv. Ment. Dis. *163*, 289–293 (1976)

Petit, J.M., Spiker, D.G., Ruwitch, J.F., Ziegler, V.E., Weiss, A.N., Biggs, J.T.: Tricyclic antidepressant plasma levels and adverse effects after overdose. Clin. Pharmacol. Ther. *21*, 47–51 (1977)

Physicians Desk Reference (PDR): Oradell: Medical Economics 1973

Pluvinage, R.: La protriptyline, antidépresseur tricycline majeur. Etude clinique et thérapeutique. Therapie *24*, 273–282 (1969)

Poulson, E., Robson, J.M.: The effect of amine oxidase inhibitors on pregnancy. J. Endocrinol.
27, 147–152 (1963)

Poulson, E., Robson, J.M.: Effect of phenelzine and some related compounds on pregnancy
and on sexual development. J. Endocrinol. 30, 205–215 (1964)

Rachelefsky, G.S., Flynt, J.W., Ebbin, A.J., Wilson, M.G.: Possible teratogenicity of tricyclic
antidepressants. Lancet 1872/I, 838–839

Rauws, A.G., Olling, M.: Treatment of experimental imipramine and desipramine poisoning
in the rat. Arch. Toxicol. 35, 97–106 (1976)

Reid, W.H., Blouin, P., Schermer, M.: A review of psychotropic medications and the glau-
comas. Int. Pharmacopsychiatry 11, 163–174 (1974)

Report From Boston Collaborative Drug Surveillance Program: Adverse reactions to the tri-
cyclic-antidepressant drugs. Lancet 1972/I, 529–531

Robson, J.M., Sullivan, F.M.: The production of foetal abnormalities in rabbits by imipramine.
Lancet 1963/I, 638–639

Rogers, K.J., Thornton, J.A.: Pharmacological observations on the interaction between monoamine oxidase inhibitors and narcotic analgesics in animals. Br. J. Anaesth. 40, 146 (1968)

Rogers, K.J., Thornton, J.A.: The interaction between monoamine oxidase inhibitors and narcotic analgesics in mice. Br. J. Pharmacol. 36, 470–480 (1969)

Rossi, G.V.: Pharmacology of tricyclic antidepressants. A review. Am. J. Pharm. 148, 37–45
(1976)

Schaerer, K.: Toxizitätsstudien mit Amitriptylin. Therapeutische Richtlinien aus experimentellen Untersuchungen. Schweiz. Med. Wochenschr. 95, 173–176 (1965)

Schardein, J.L.: Drugs as teratogens. Cleveland (Ohio): CRC Press 1976

Sedal, L., Korman, M.G., Williams, P.O., Mushin, G.: Overdosage of tricyclic antidepressants.
A report of two deaths and a prospective study of 24 patients. Med. J. Aust. 2, 74–79 (1972)

Serafimovski, N., Thorball, N., Asmussen, I., Lunding, M.: Tricyclic antidepressive poisoning
with special reference to cardiac complications. Acta Anaesth. Scand. 57, 55–63 (1975)

Shikata, T., Kanetaka, T., Endo, Y., Nagashima, K.: Drug-induced generalized phospholipidosis. Acta Pathol. Jpn. 22, 517–531 (1972)

Shimomura, K., Hashimoto, M., Honda, F.: A fatal hyperpyrexia caused by tranylcypromine
in LiCl-pretreated rats. Jap. J. Pharmacol. 27, 124 P (1977)

Sim, M.: Imipramine and pregnancy. Br. Med. J. 1972/II, 45

Sinclair, J.G.: Ethoheptazine-monoamine oxidase inhibitor interaction in rabbits. Can. J.
Physiol. Pharmacol. 50, 923–926 (1972)

Singer, G., Coyle, I.R.: The effect of imipramine administered before and during pregnancy on
litter size in the rat. Psychopharmacologia 32, 337–342 (1973)

Slovis, T.L., Ott, J.E., Teitelbaum, D.T., Lipscomb, W.: Physostigmine therapy in acute tricyclic antidepressant poisoning. Clinical Toxicology, 4, 451–459 (1971)

Sokol, G.H., Maikel, R.P.: Toxic interactions of d-amphetamine and tricyclic antidepressants
in mice. Res. Commun. Chem. Pathol. Pharmacol. 3, 513–521 (1972)

Soulairac, A., Baron, J.B., Geier, S., Mijolla, A. de, Aymard, N.: Etude clinique et experimen-
tale de l'amitriptyline sur la vascularisation retinienne des sujets atheromateux. Ann. Med.
Psychol. 1, 208–216 (1965)

Spiker, D.G., Biggs, J.T.: Tricyclic antidepressants. Prolonged plasma levels after overdose. J.
Am. Med. Assoc. 236, 1711–1712 (1976)

Spiker, G.D., Weiss, N.A., Chang, S.S., Ruwitch, J.F., Biggs, J.T.: Tricyclic antidepressant
overdose: Clinical presentation and plasma levels. Clinical Pharm. Therap. 18, 539–546
(1975)

Staeubli, W., Schweizer, W., Suter, J., Hess, R.: Ultrastructure and biochemical study of the
actions of benzoctamine and maprotiline on the rat liver. Agents Actions 4, 391–403 (1974)

Staeubli, W., Schweizer, W., Suter.: Some properties of myeloid bodies induced in rat liver by
an antidepressant drug (maprotiline). Exp. Mol. Pathol. 28, 177–195 (1978)

Stenger, E.G., Aeppli, L., Fratta, I.: Zur Frage der keimschädigenden Wirkung von N-(α-Di-
methylaminopropyl)-iminodibenzyl-HCl am Tier. Arzneim. Forsch. 15, 1222–1224 (1965)

Stokes, G.S.: Drug-induced hypertension. Pathogenesis and management. Drugs 12, 222–230
(1976)

Swiss Academy of Medical Sciences: Evaluation of drugs and other chemical agents for teratogenicity. Joint report of the Expert Committee on Teratogenicity Testing and Evaluation. Bull. Schweiz. Akad. MED. Wiss. *30*, 1–62 (1974)

Tanaka, H., Furusato, M., Takasaki, S., Watanabe, M., Hattori, Y.: Morphological and biochemical alteration in the rat liver induced by maprotiline. Acta Pathol. Jpn. *25*, 413–437 (1975)

Tobis, J., Das, B.N.: Cardiac complications in amitriptyline poisoning. JAMA, *235*, 1474–1476 (1976)

Theiss, E., Hummler, H., Lengsfeld, H., Staiger, G.R., Tranzer, J.P.: Lipidspeicherung bei Versuchstieren nach Verabreichung trizyklischer Amine. Schweiz. Med. Wochenschr. *103*, 424 (1973)

Thomann, P.: Toxicology of Tofranil: Tofranil. pp. 145–159. Bern: Stämpfli 1970

Thorstrand, C.: Cardiovascular effects of poisoning by hypnotic and tricyclic antidepressant drugs. Acta Med. Scand. *583*, 1–34 (1975)

Thorstrand, C.: Clinical features in poisonings by tricyclic antidepressants with special reference to the ECG. Acta Med. Scand. *199*, 337–344 (1976)

Tofanetti, O., Albiero, L., Galatulas, I., Genovese, E.: Enhancement of propoxyphene-induced analgesia by doxepin. Psychopharmacology *51*, 213–215 (1977)

Torchiana, M.L., Wenger, H.C., Lagerquist, B., Morgan, G.M., Stone, C.A.: Pharmacological antagonism of the toxic manifestations of amitriptyline and protriptyline in dogs. Toxicol. Appl. Pharmacol. *21*, 383–389 (1972)

Toth, B.: Tumorigenicity of β-phenylethylhydrazine sulfate in mice. Cancer Res. *36*, 917–921 (1976)

Tuchmann-Duplessis, H.: Drug effects on the fetus. Monographs on drugs, Vol. 2. New York, London, Hongkong, Mexico, Sidney, Auckland: Adis Press 1975

Ueki, S., Fujiwara, M., Inoue, K.: Behavioral effects of maprotyline (Ciba 34 376-Ba). A new antidepressant. Jpn. J. Pharmacol. *24*, [Suppl. 55] (1974)

Vance, M.A., Ross, S.M., Millington, W.R., Blumberg, J.B.: Potentiation of tricyclic antidepressant toxicity by physostigmine in mice. Clin. Toxicol. *11*, 413–421 (1977)

Vohra, J.K.: Cardiovascular abnormalities following tricyclic antidepressant drug overdosage. Drugs *7*, 323–325 (1974)

Vohra, J., Burrows, G., Hunt, D., Sloman, G.: The effect of toxic and therapeutic doses of tricyclic antidepressant drugs on intracardiac conduction. Eur. J. Cardiol. Excerpta Medica *3*, 219–227 (1975)

Volk, B.W., Adachi, M., Schneck, L.: The gangliosidoses. Hum. Pathol. *6*, 555–569 (1975)

Winter, D.: Toxizitätsveränderung neurotroper Pharmaka bei Versuchstieren mit experimentell hervorgerufener Hyperthyreoidie. Med. Pharmacol. EXP. *14*, 391–394 (1966)

Wood, C.A., Brown, J.R., Coleman, J.H., Evans, W.E.: Management of tricyclic antidepressant toxicities. Dis. Nerv. Syst. *37*, 459–461 (1976)

WHO; Report of a WHO Scientific Group: Principles for pre-clinical testing of drug safety. WHO Technical Report Series No. 341 (1966)

Handbook of Experimental Pharmacology, Vol. 55/I
Edited by F. HOFFMEISTER/G. STILLE

Erratum

Page 551
Second paragraph should read:

Apart from the early and largely obsolete monoamine oxidase inhibitors, imipramine was the first antidepressant (thymoleptic). Surprisingly, during the 20 years of this drug's existence it has remained the prototype and the clinical standard among antidepressants. In addition, imipramine is increasingly used as a model drug in experimental and biochemical pharmacology. The following are some of the reasons for this: The drug is widely used and reaches millions of in- and out-patients each year; it has a wide spectrum of pharmacologic actions, including fascinating membrane effects; it is a highly lipophilic basic drug with a large apparent volume of distribution, thereby representing many of the modern, potent drugs. In particular, the metabolism of only a few drugs has been investigated as thoroughly as that of imipramine. This process started during the drug's introduction into therapy after which it was found to form active metabolites such as desmethylimipramine. Due to several points of metabolic attack, the drug molecule undergoes metabolism by multiple pathways leading to a variety of metabolites. These metabolites, differing in chemical structure, display a remarkable spectrum of both physicochemical and pharmacologic properties. Imipramine has, therefore, become a model drug for the study of complex drug metabolism situations and their pharmacokinetic and pharmacodynamic implications.

Springer-Verlag
Berlin Heidelberg New York 1980

CHAPTER 23

Metabolism of Antidepressants

M.H. BICKEL

A. Introduction

In the most general terms, the fate of a drug in the body can be summarized as follows: The drug undergoes absorption, i.e., transfer from the site of administration into the blood circulation. It is then further transferred to sites of metabolism, sites of excretion, sites of storage (nonspecific receptors), and sites of action (specific receptors). Within this complex interplay, drug metabolism is of particular importance because it influences both the pharmacokinetic as well as the pharmacodynamic situation. Thus, each of the metabolites formed may again be subject to the processes of transfer, distribution, excretion, and binding. Furthermore the action of the drug may be shortened, prolonged or qualitatively altered according to the activity of the metabolites.

Apart from the early and largely obsolete monoamine oxidase inhibitors, imipramine was the first antidepressant (thymoleptic). Surprisingly, during the 20 years of this: The drug is widely used and reaches millions of in- and out-patients each year; antidepressants. In addition, imipramine is increasingly used as a model drug in experimental and biochemical pharmocology. The following are some of the reasons for this: The drug is widely used and reaches millions of in- and out-patients each year; it has a wide spectrum of pharmacologic actions, including fascinating membrane effects; it is a highly lipophilic basic drug with a large apparent volume of distribution, thereby representing many of the modern, potent drugs. In particular, the metabolism of only a few drugs has been investigated as thoroughly as that of imipramine. This process started during the drug's introduction into therapy after which it was found to form active metabolites such as desmethylimipramine. Due to several points of metabolic attack, the drug molecule undergoes metabolism by multiple pathways leading to a variety of metabolites. These metabolites, differing in chemical structure, display a remarkable spectrum of both physicochemical and pharmacologic properties. Imipramine has, therefore, become a model drug for the study of complex drug metabolism situations and their pharmacokinetic and pharmacodynamic implications.

This chapter covers only metabolism, whereas the remaining pharmacokinetic processes of antidepressants are reviewed in the preceeding chapter. The subdivision follows the chemical structure types of the major antidepressants. A first section describes the metabolism of imipramine and other dibenzazepines (iminodibenzyls), the two following sections summarize the metabolic data of the major antidepressants belonging to other chemical groups. A few previous reviews have dealt with the metabolism of antidepressants (BICKEL, 1968; GRAM, 1974; JUDD and URSILLO, 1975).

B. Dibenzazepines

I. Imipramine and Its Therapeutically Used Metabolites

Imipramine and several other antidepressants are derivates of the tricyclic skeleton, dibenzazepine or iminodibenzyl (Table 1). Desipramine (desmethylimipramine) and imipramine-N-oxide, but not the other compounds of Table 1, are metabolites of imipramine. Their metabolism is therefore part of the metabolism of imipramine and need not be dealt with separately.

Table 2 shows the *metabolically vulnerable groups* or bonds of the imipramine molecule. It discloses that among some 20 atom groups or bonds only five or six are known as potential points of metabolic attack. All biotransformations of imipramine result in peripheral molecular changes only, leaving the tricyclic skeleton intact. Thus, all metabolites still belong to the one chemical family of dibenzazepine derivates.

Table 1. Imipramine and other dibenzoazepine antidepressants

	R_1	R_2	R_3
Imipramine	H	$CH_2-CH_2-CH_2-N(CH_3)_2$	H
Desipramine	H	$CH_2-CH_2-CH_2-N(H)(CH_3)$	H
Imipramine–N–oxide	H	$CH_2-CH_2-CH_2-N^+(\rightarrow O)(CH_3)_2$	H
Chlorimipramine	Cl	$CH_2-CH_2-CH_2-N(CH_3)_2$	H
Trimepramine	H	$CH_2-CH(CH_3)-CH_2-N(CH_3)_2$	H
Lofepramine	H	$CH_2-CH_2-CH_2-N(CH_3)(CH_2-CO-C_6H_4-Cl)$	H
Ketipramine	H	$CH_2-CH_2-CH_2-N(CH_3)_2$	O

Table 2. Metabolically vulnerable parts of the imipramine molecule and metabolic pathways

ALH = aliphatic hydroxylation, ARH = aromatic hydroxylation,
GAC = glucuronic acid conjugation, NOX = N–oxidation,
OND = oxidative N–demethylation, OSD = oxidative side chain dealkylation

Table 3. Metabolites of imipramine (IP)

Metabolite	References (first mentions)
2–Hydroxy–IP[a]	SCHINDLER (1960)
Desmethyl–IP (Desipramine)	HERRMANN and PULVER (1960)
2–Hydroxy–IP glucuronide[a]	HERRMANN and PULVER (1960)
2–Hydroxy–desmethyl–IP	HERRMANN et al. (1960)
2–Hydroxy–desmethyl–IP glucuronide	HERRMANN et al. (1960)
Desdimethyl–IP	HERRMANN et al. (1960)
IP–N–Oxide[a]	FISHMAN and GOLDENBERG (1962)
Iminodibenzyl	IM OBERSTEG and BÄUMLER (1962)
2–Hydroxy–iminodibenzyl	IM OBERSTEG and BÄUMLER (1962)
10–Hydroxy–IP[a]	CRAMMER and SCOTT (1966)
10–Hydroxy–desmethyl–IP	CRAMMER and SCOTT (1966)
10–Hydroxy–desdimethyl–IP	CRAMMER and SCOTT (1966)
10–Hydroxy–iminodibenzyl	CRAMMER and SCOTT (1966)
10–Hydroxy–IP glucuronide[a]	CRAMMER and SCOTT (1966)
10–Hydroxy–desmethyl–IP glucuronide	CRAMMER and SCOTT (1966)
10–Hydroxy–desdimethyl–IP glucuronide	CRAMMER and SCOTT (1966)
10–Hydroxy–iminodibenzyl glucuronide	CRAMMER and SCOTT (1966)
Unidentified glucuronides	CHRISTIANSEN et al. (1967)
	BICKEL and WEDER (1968a)
Unid. nonconjugated metabolites	CHRISTIANSEN et al. (1967)
	BICKEL and WEDER (1968a)
2–Hydroxy–desdimethyl–IP	BICKEL and WEDER (1968a)
2–Hydroxy–desdimethyl–IP glucuronide	BICKEL and WEDER (1968a)
2–Hydroxy–Iminodibenzyl glucuronide	BICKEL and WEDER (1968a)
Unid. nonglucuronide conjugates	CRAMMER et al. (1969)
Desmethyl–IP–N–glucuronide	BICKEL et al. (1973)
Desdimethyl–IP–N–glucuronide	BICKEL et al. (1973)
N–Hydroxy–desmethyl–IP	BECKETT and AL–SARRAJ (1973)
N–Hydroxy–desdimethyl–IP	BECKETT and AL–SARRAJ (1973)

[a] Metabolites of IP only; all others are also metabolites of desmethylimipramine (desipramine)

Table 3 is a list of all *imipramine metabolites* known to date. The order of the metabolites follows the chronology of their discoveries. It is important to notice that the number of metabolites far surpasses the number of metabolically vulnerable positions. This is because two or more positions can be attacked simultaneously or in sequence, leading to the formation of "combination metabolites", e.g., imipramine which is both demethylated and hydroxylated. As a matter of fact, some 24 metabolites have been identified so far, and about six have been detected without being chemically identified. It is likely that even more metabolites are formed which have escaped detection. The number of theoretically possible combinations considerably exceeds 30. On the other hand it is remarkable that certain combinations of metabolic attack seemingly exclude each other. Thus, hydroxylated N-oxides or metabolites hydroxylated both in 2- and 10-position have never been found.

Obviously, there are vast differences in the amounts of individual metabolites formed. The *major imipramine metabolites* in most species are desmethylimipramine, the 2-hydroxylated metabolites of the two compounds, and the 0-glucuronides of the hydroxylated metabolites. These five metabolites were identified soon after the introduction of imipramine by the first team of investigators dealing with the metabolism of this drug (SCHINDLER, 1960; HERRMANN and PULVER, 1960; HERRMANN et al., 1960). In certain species, imipramine-N-oxide, iminodibenzyl and possibly others may have quantitative importance. Most of the remaining compounds listed in Table 3 must usually be considered minor metabolites, trace metabolites, or absent at all in some species. It must be emphasized, however, that a so-called minor metabolite may well be qualitatively important, e.g., in terms of potential pharmacologic or toxic action.

Studies on the formation of the multitude of metabolites of imipramine and desipramine have been performed on various *biologic levels*. The most frequently used experimental systems are the following:

1) *Humans* under therapeutic conditions or volunteers, where urine was most frequently used as a source of metabolites (CHRISTIANSEN et al., 1967; CRAMMER et al., 1969; GRAM et al., 1971);

2) *Whole animals*, where metabolite analyses were also performed in feces and tissues (HERRMANN et al., 1960; BICKEL and Weder, 1968a; Minder et al., 1971; BICKEL et al., 1973);

3) *Perfused rat livers* (BICKEL and MINDER, 1970a; MINDER et al., 1971; VON BAHR and BORGA, 1971; BICKEL and BÖRNER, 1974; STEGMANN and BICKEL, 1977);

4) *Incubated liver slices* (CRAMMER and ROLFE, 1970; BICKEL and GIGON, 1971);

5) *Liver microsomes*, incubated in the presence of appropriate cofactors, such as NADPH for oxidative pathways and UDP-glucuronic acid for glucuronide conjugations (BICKEL and BAGGIOLINI, 1966; MINDER et al., 1971; VON BAHR and BERTILSSON, 1971). The use of the latter systems is based on the fact that the majority of drug metabolizing enzymes are localized in the hepatic endoplasmic reticulum.

Knowledge of individual metabolic pathways (Table 2) first emerged from metabolic analyses in urine and other biologic material. The suggested pathways were confirmed and others dicovered by using metabolites as substrates and studying the time course of metabolite formation (BICKEL and BAGGIOLINI, 1966; VON BAHR and BORGA, 1971; BICKEL andBOERNER, 1974). These investigations also shed light on the sequence of the metabolic process, i.e., on the formation of primary, secondary, and terminal metabolites (Table 4). The following 12 metabolic pathways are known to contribute to the metabolism of imipramine in various species and compartments (for references see also Table 3):

1) *Oxidative N-demethylation* may occur in two steps, transforming imipramine to its secondary (desmethyl) and primary (desdimethyl) amine along.

2) *Oxidative side-chain dealkylation*, leading to the formation of iminodibenzyl, is another N-dealkylation which now is directed towards the nonbasic nitrogen atom in the cyclic skeleton rather than towards the basic side-chain nitrogen. In contrast to chlorpromazine, a compound with an identical side chain, no evidence has been obtained for a consecutive deamination, β-oxidation, and ring nitrogen dealkylation. Formation of iminodibenzyl may also occur nonenzymatically.

3) *Aromatic hydroxylation* in position 2 is a major pathway.

4) *Aliphatic hydroxylation* in position 10 is of minor importance. The phenolic and alcoholic metabolites resulting from the latter pathways serve as substrates for the important pathway of O-glucuronidation.

5) *O-glucuronidation* is often so efficient that few unconjugated hydroxylated metabolites can de detected.

6) *N-glucuronidation* can apply to secondary and primary amine metabolites only.

7) *Hydrolysis or deconjugation of O-glucuronides* takes place, whereby the unconjugated hydroxylated metabolites (aglycons) are formed (BICKEL and WEDER, 1968a; CRAMMER et al., 1969).

8) *N-oxidation of the tertiary amine* leads to the formation of imipramine-N-oxide. This metabolite or drug undergoes both N-oxide reduction and demethylation.

9) *N-oxide reduction* leads back to imipramine (BICKEL, 1972; SUGIURA et al., 1977)

10) *N-oxide demethylation*, a nonoxidative process, results in the formation of desmethylimipramine (BICKEL, 1972)

11) *N-oxidation of the secondary and primary amine* analogs results in the formation of N-hydroxylated metabolites (hydroxylamines).

12) *N-methylation* of desmethylimipramine has also been reported in at least one species (DINGELL and SANDERS, 1966).

The predominant pathways leading to the major metabolites of imipramine are represented schematically in Table 4.

Table 4. Scheme of the major pathways and metabolites of imipramine

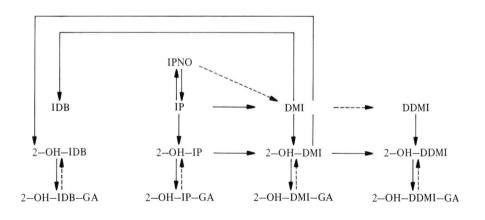

DMI = desmethylimipramine,DDMI = desdimethylimipramine, IDB = iminodibenzyl, GA = glucuronide, IP = imipramine

The metabolic reactions of imipramine are catalyzed by *enzymes or enzyme systems* localized in a variety of tissues and subcellular sites. A liver microsomal multienzyme system catalyzing the sequence of oxidations and subsequent glucuronide conjugation is the centerpiece of the metabolic machinery for this as well as for many other drugs. The oxidative system responsible for the initial pathways of demethylation and aromatic hydroxylation is known as the monooxygenase system which involves the flavoprotein, NADPH-cytochrome c reductase (= NADPH-cytochrome P-450 reductase), and cytochrome P-450. The reactions dependent on this electron transport chain can be simulated in vitro with liver microsomes, oxygen, and NADPH (BICKEL and BAGGIOLINI, 1966; VON BAHR and BERTILSSON, 1971; GIGON and BICKEL, 1971). Imipramine forms a complex with cytochrome P-450 which results in a "type I" spectral change (SCHENKMAN et al., 1967). The same has been observed with the major nonconjugated metabolites. Imipramine and desipramine exhibit particularly high binding affinities to P-450 when compared with other drugs (VON BAHR and ORRENIUS, 1971). The monooxygenase system is located predominantly in the smooth endoplasmic reticulum of hepatocytes (VON BAHR et al., 1972b). Minor activities have also been detected in extrahepatic tissues such as lung and kidney, but not adrenals, intestine, brain, blood, and others (MINDER et al., 1971). Controversial results have been reported with respect to lung and brain (CRAMMER and ROLFE, 1970; ROSENBLOOM and BASS, 1970; JUNOD, 1972; ROUBEIN and KEUP, 1975). N-demethylation of imipramine also occurs with intestinal contents, possibly as a nonoxidative process (MINDER et al., 1971). O-glucuronidation is catalyzed by UDP-glucuronyltransferase. It can be studied in vitro with liver microsomes and UDP-glucuronic acid (VON BAHR and BERTILSSON, 1971). This enzyme seems to be equally distributed between rough and smooth endoplasmic reticulum (VON BAHR et al., 1972b). Large amounts of glucuronides excreted with the bile are deconjugated by enterobacterial β-glucuronidase (BICKEL andWEDER, 1968a). Since this enzyme is also found in most tissues, including liver, the possibility exists that there are conjugation–deconjugation–reconjugation cycles. Finally, the discovery of N-oxide metabolites has introduced additional problems. Formation of N-oxides from tertiary amines has been shown to be independent of cytochrome P-450, but dependent on a flavoprotein, amine oxidase, which is also located in hepatic microsomes (ZIEGLER et al., 1969; BICKEL, 1971, 1972). Imipramine-N-oxide formed metabolically or given as substrate then undergoes both reduction (and demethylation) by liver microsomal cytochrome P-450 (SUGIURA et al., 1977) and/or an extramicrosomal enzyme system located in several tissues (BICKEL, 1972).

Considerable *species differences* in the metabolism of imipramine and its metabolites have been observed (DINGELL et al., 1964; GIGON and BICKEL, 1971; BICKEL, 1971; QUINN et al., 1976). Demethylation is the predominant initial pathway in rats and guinea pigs, while in pigs it is N-oxidation. Desmethylimipramine undergoes further metabolism rapidly in mice and rabbits but accumulates in rats and humans. In addition to these pronounced species differences, sex (PSCHEIDT, 1962) and strain differences (SULSER et al., 1962; JORI et al., 1970) have also been shown. All these qualitative and quantitative metabolic differences demonstrate the importance of the genetically determined biochemical background. In humans, a genetically heterogeneous species, similar interindividual differences have been detected, e.g., patients on a fixed dose regimen of desipramine attained steady state plasma levels varying between 8 and 280 ng/ml (HAMMER and SJÖQVIST, 1967; HAMMER et al., 1969; ALEXANDERSON, 1972).

The way imipramine is metabolized in an organism is obviously significant for the *pharmacologic and therapeutic action* of the drug. This is due to the formation of both inactive metabolites and desmethylimipramine which is an active metabolite and an antidepressant used in therapy. A pharmacologic screening of seven major metabolites of imipramine (THEOBALD et al., 1966) showed that all of them had peripheral activities, but that central actions were not elicited by the polar metabolites, particularly glucuronides. Similarly, the highly polar N-methylimipramine cation, which is not a metabolite, is peripherally active, but devoid of central actions (GYERMEK, 1966; LAPIN, 1969). These findings may reflect the exclusion of the polar metabolites by the blood brain barrier rather than intrinsic activities.

When desmethylimipramine was found to accumulate in the brains of imipramine-treated rats and to be responsible for the striking central antireserpine effects (GILLETTE et al.,1961; SULSER et al.,1962), it was believed to mediate the antidepressant action of imipramine. This extreme view had to be dismissed when more insight into the pharmacologic and therapeutic profiles of imipramine and desipramine was achieved. The therapeutic action of imipramine may be a function of the balance of the two compounds which is determined by metabolic factors. The pharmacologic differences between the tertiary and secondary amines are seen with many tricyclic drugs (BICKEL et al., 1963; BICKEL and BRODIE, 1964). Metabolism, and hence the balance of the active compounds, is also dependent on the species (DINGELL et al., 1964; BICKEL et al., 1967), the route of administration (BICKEL and WEDER, 1968b; NAGY and JOHANSSON, 1975), and other factors. Imipramine-N-oxide, a clinically active antidepressant is a special case in that this drug does not cross the blood–brain barrier but rather is rapidly metabolized into the active compounds, imipramine and desmethylimipramine. Imipramine-N-oxide must therefore be considered a prodrug or metabolic precursor. Finally, 2-hydroxy-imipramine has been reported to be the most active imipramine metabolite in terms of cardiac toxicity (BUCKLEY et al., 1975 JANDHYALA et al., 1977), which is of major importance in accidental or intentional overdosage (BICKEL, 1975)

In order to understand the pharmacokinetic behavior of individual or groups of metabolites, a knowledge of the *physicochemical properties* of imipramine and its major metabolites becomes imperative. Of particular importance are the polarity, usually estimated by determination of partition coefficients or buccal absorption, and the degree of ionization, which is dependent on the difference between the pK_a of the molecule and the pH of its surrounding biologic medium. Some of these key data are summarized in Table 5 which allows the following interpretations. Partition coefficients indicate low polarity (lipophility) of imipramine and desipramine, medium polarity of hydroxylated metabolites and imipramine-N-oxide, and high polarity (hydrophility) of the glucuronides. Lipophility is reflected in biologic transfer processes such as absorption by the mucosa of the human buccal cavity or the permeation across the blood–brain barrier which is known to sharply discriminate against polar foreign compounds. Characteristically, the mainstream of the metabolism of the lipophilic drug, imipramine, is the formation of increasingly polar metabolites, i.e., compounds increasingly restricted to the extracellular spaces and fitted to use the renal and hepatic excretory mechanisms.

One of the factors modifying drug metabolism is the *route of administration*. The rate of metabolism is slow when imipramine is absorbed into the systemic circulation as is the case after intramuscular or subcutaneous injection. On the other hand, metabolites are rapidly formed after oral or intraperitoneal administration, i.e., when the drug is absorbed into the portal system and hence is funneled through the liver in a first passage. In this case bioavailability is considerably reduced due to high hepatic extraction and first-pass elimination (GRAM and CHRISTIANSEN, 1975; NAGY and JO-HANSSON, 1975; NIAZI, 1976a; STEGMANN and BICKEL, 1977). Once absorption has oc-curred and metabolites have been formed, the *gross distribution* reflects the polarity-dependent diffusion processes discussed above. Thus, the lipophilic compounds, imip-ramine and desipramine, reach considerable concentrations in all tissues including brain (BICKEL and WEDER, 1968a,b, 1969; CHRISTIANSEN and GRAM, 1973; BICKEL, 1975). All polar metabolites, however, are restricted to extracellular compartments such as plasma, urine, bile, and lower intestinal lumen (BICKEL and WEDER, 1968a). Even in the liver, as the main site of metabolite formation, the concentration of polar metabolites is minute.

Renal excretion is the major route whereby imipramine metabolites are eliminated from the organism, even though a single dose takes several days to reach near-total excretion (CHRISTIANSEN et al., 1967; CRAMMER et al., 1968). Between 30% and 50% of the dose is excreted within the first 24 h. The urine, which may contain over 20 me-tabolites, characteristically contains only 10% or less unchanged imipramine and/or desipramine; the bulk of total urinary drug consists of polar metabolites, particularly glucuronides (CHRISTIANSEN et al., 1967; BICKEL and WEDER, 1968a; CRAMMER et al., 1969). This fact is explained by the fate of these compounds in the renal tubules. While polar metabolites are hardly reabsorbed and therefore efficiently excreted, unchanged drug or lipophilic metabolites undergo reabsorption by nonionic diffusion. Indeed, the excretion of the latter compounds is pH-dependent (BICKEL and WEDER, 1969; SJÖQVIST et al., 1970; GRAM et al., 1971) and therefore obeys the pH-partition law.

Table 5. Sequence of major metabolic pathways of imipramine and physicochemical properties of metabolites[a]

Metabolic scheme	BA %	P Hexane %	P DCE %	BBB	pK$_a$	Type
IP	57	99	99	+	8.0	LD
DMI	45	65	98	+	9.4	LM
2–OH–IP IPNO	36 18	25 10	71 71	(−)	8.0 4.7	MM
2–OH–DMI	2	6	50		9.3	
2–OH–IP–GA 2–OH–DMI–GA	<2	0	0	−	<4	HM

[a] BICKEL and WEDER (1969)
for abbreviations of metabolites and pathways see *Table 4*.
BA = % Buccal absorption under standardized conditions at pH 7.4.
P = Partition coefficient against buffer pH 7.4; % in organic phase. DCE dichloroethane.
BBB = Blood brain barrier permeation (+) or nonpermeation (−).
Type = LD low polarity drug; LM, MM, HM low, medium and high polarity metabolites.

Considerable amounts of nonconjugated hydroxylated metabolites are excreted with the feces (CRAMMER et al., 1968, 1969). The source of this material is *biliary excretion* which is a major excretory pathway for imipramine-like drugs (BICKEL and WEDER, 1968a VON BAHR and BORGA, 1971; RYRFELD and HANSSON, 1971). The major metabolites in the bile are glucuronides, while hydroxylated and lipophilic compounds comprise a minor fraction (BICKEL and MINDER, 1970a; VON BAHR and BORGA, 1971; BICKEL and BÖRNER, 1974). Glucuronides are known to use an active anion transport system in the canalicular membrane and for this reason attain bile/plasma concentration ratios up to 1,000. The lipophilic compounds, imipramine and desipramine, are in small absolute amounts in the bile, however, their bile/plasma ratios are still of the order of 50 which is indicative of a concentrative transfer. These compounds, but not their polar metabolites, have been shown to be incorporated into the bile salt/phospholipid micelles of the bile (BICKEL and MINDER, 1970b). Finally, the glucuronides excreted into the bile are deconjugated by enterobacterial β-glucuronidase to yield the hydroxylated aglycones which are largely excreted with the feces. The lipophilic compounds together with a fraction of the hydroxylated metabolites are reabsorbed from the intestine, thereby resulting in an enterohepatic circulation. Since both renal and fecal excretion of unchanged drug is almost negligible, the rate of elimination of imipramine is largely dependent on previous metabolism, particularly on the hydroxylation-glucuronidation pathway.

II. Derivatives of Imipramine

Chlorimipramine, trimepramine, lofepramine, and ketipramine are derivatives, but not metabolites of imipramine. Their structural formulae are given in Table 1, together with imipramine, desipramine and imipramine-N-oxide. Metabolic information on the four derivatives is scanty, however, it indicates considerable formal analogy with the metabolic pathways for imipramine (Table 2).

1. Chlorimipramine (Clomipramine, 3-Chloroimipramine)

This imipramine derivative which is widely used in several countries also resembles imipramine in terms of metabolism. Thus, the major metabolites are the mono-demethylated and several hydroxylated compounds, as well as the N-oxide and 3-chloro-iminodibenzyl (HERRMANN, 1967; FAIGLE and DIETERLE, 1973). The demethylated metabolite is likely to participate in the therapeutic action of chlorimipramine. In rabbit urine the nonconjugated fraction exceeds the glucuronides. More recently it has been shown that the urine of chronically-dosed patients contained the 8-hydroxylated metabolite in addition and in higher amounts than the 2-hydroxylated metabolite (PEREL and MANIAN, 1977). These authors also detected the isomeric pair of the demethylated 8- and 2-hydroxychlorimipramine. Unlike imipramin, there is no molecular symmetry in chlorimipramine and therefore the positions 2 and 8 are no longer identical.

2. Trimepramine (Trimeprimine)

According to a single study (POPULAIRE et al., 1970), this imipramine derivative with the branched side-chain also undergoes mono- and didemethylation, side-chain dealkylation (formation of iminodibenzyl), and hydroxylation. The hydroxylated metabolites are excreted as glucuronic and/or sulfuric acid conjugates which represent the major urinary metabolite fraction in dogs, rabbits, and humans. The authors obtained 26 chromatographic spots which may represent individual metabolites.

3. Lofepramine (Lopramine, Clofepramine, Leo 640)

This drug differs from imipramine in that one of its N-methyl groups is replaced by a p-chlorobenzoylmethyl moiety which increases the lipophility. Lofepramine also differs from other thymoleptics by its considerably lower lethal and cardiac toxicity. In rats and humans the large N-substituent is dealkylated so that desipramine is formed which is further metabolized to 2-hydroxydesipramine, 2-hydroxyiminodibenzyl and their glucuronides (Forshell, 1975). As a consequence of the first N-dealkylation, p-chlorobenzoic acid is formed which is likely to be excreted as p-chlorohippuric acid. Fecal desipramine may be due to deconjugation of its N-glucuronide. Finally, in microsomes in vitro, N-formyldesipramine has been detected as an unusual metabolite (Forshell, 1977).

4. Ketipramine (10-Ketoimipramine)

Ketipramine is an experimental compound although it has been claimed to be therapeutically active. Its metabolism is remarkably different from that of other imipramine derivatives which may be due to the presence of a keto group and the decreased lipophility of the compound. Extremely rapid biotransformation is indicated by a half-life of only 15 min in the rabbit. The major pathway with this drug is reduction of the keto groups resulting in the formation of 10-hydroxyimipramine (Herrmann, 1967) which is also a minor metabolite of imipramine. Large amounts of 10-hydroxyiminodibenzyl were also present in urine, together with demethylated and possibly phenolic compounds.

C. Dibenzocycloheptadienes (Amitriptyline, Nortriptyline)

Amitriptyline and nortriptyline are among the most frequently used antidepressants. Similar to imipramine, amitriptyline consists of a tricyclic skeleton connected to a dimethylaminopropyl side chain. Nortriptyline, similar to desipramine, is the N-demethylated, secondary amine analog. In contrast to imipramine and other dibenzazepines, amitriptyline contains a C-atom rather than a N-atom in position 5, hence its tricyclic skeleton is a dibenzocycloheptadiene. Due to the close chemical similarity, the physicochemical properties of the two classes of compounds are nearly identical and so are the general pharmacokinetic characteristics. On the other hand, the one structural difference in the tricyclic system creates a different electron distribution and thus a difference in chemical reactivity which influences its mode of reaction with drug-metabolizing enzymes. Indeed, the pattern of metabolic pathways of the dibenzocycloheptadienes is remarkably different from that of dibenzazepines. This is summarized in Table 6 (compare with Table 2).

Similar to imipramine, one of the major metabolic pathways is oxidative N-demethylation leading from amitriptyline to nortriptyline and on to desmethylnortriptyline. As with most tricyclic drugs the second demethylation step proceeds at a slower

Table 6. Metabolically vulnerable parts of amitriptyline (and nortriptyline[a]) and metabolic pathways

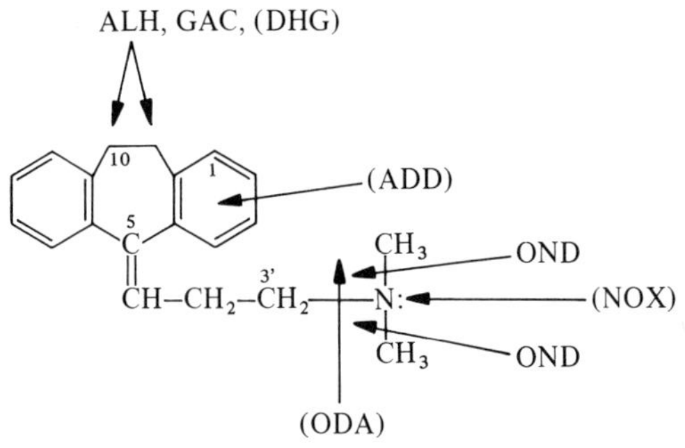

ALH, GAC, (DHG)

(ADD)

CH₃ ——OND

(NOX)

CH₃ ——OND

(ODA)

ADD = aromatic dihydrodiol formation
ALH = aliphatic hydroxylation
DHG = dehydrogenation
GAC = glucuronic acid conjugation
NOX = N—oxidation
ODA = oxidative deamination
OND = oxidative N—demethylation

[a] Nortrityline is desmethylamitriptyline. Minor pathways in brackets.

rate (BICKEL et al., 1967). In sharp contrast to dibenzazepines, no evidence has been obtained for aromatic hydroxylations. Rather, aliphatic hydroxylation in positions 10 or 10, 11 is a major pathway in the case of amitriptyline and its desmethyl analog. The alcoholic metabolites formed seem to be largely conjugated, mainly with glucuronic acid (BORGA and GARLE, 1972; HUCKER et al., 1977). Whereas aliphatic hydroxylation is a minor pathway with imipramine, two minor pathways seem to apply to dibenzo-cycloheptadienes only: dehydrogenation which introduces a double bond into the 10,11-bridge, and oxidative deamination giving rise to a propionic acid side chain after removal of the amine function. Finally, the recent identification of dihydro-diol derivatives of amitriptyline and nortriptyline (HUCKER et al., 1977) is suggestive of the formation of arene oxides and thus, possibly, of reactive intermediates. The me-tabolites of amitriptyline and nortriptyline detected so far in urine, bile, tissues and tissue preparations of various species are summarized in Table 7.

According to most authors the 10-hydroxylated derivatives are the major metab-olites of dibenzocycloheptadienes. In human urine, collected for one week after a single dose of amitriptyline, the following metabolites and percentages of the dose were determined: 10-hydroxy-nortriptyline 41%, 10-hydroxy-amitriptyline 28%, nor-triptyline 6%, unchanged drug 5%, amitriptyline-N-oxide 1% (SANTAGOSTINO et al., 1974). The amounts of N-oxide originally formed may considerably surpass the amount excreted since amitriptyline-N-oxide is reduced by various tissues (BICKEL, 1972; HAWKINS et al., 1977). 10-Hydroxy-nortriptyline was also detected as the major urinary metabolite in humans given the drug nortriptyline (DE LEENHEER and HEYN-DRICKX, 1971; HAMMAR et al., 1971). Due to the double bond connecting the tricyclic system and the side chain of dibenzocycloheptadienes, the monohydroxylated deriv-

Table 7. Metabolites of amitriptyline (AT) and nortriptyline
(NT, desmethylamitriptyline)

Metabolite	References (see also text)
10–Hydroxy–AT[a]	Hucker (1962): Corona and Facino (1968); Facino and Corona (1969); Eschenhof and Rieder (1969)
10–Hydroxy–AT glucuronide[a]	Cassano et al. (1965); Corona and Facino (1968); Eschenhof and Rieder (1969)
10, 11–Dihydroxy–AT[a]	Hucker (1962); Cassano et al. (1965); Corona and Facino (1968); Facino and Corona (1969); Corona et al. (1972)
10, 11–Dihydroxy–AT glucuronide[a]	Cassano et al. (1965)
NT (= desmethyl–AT)	Hucker and Porter (1961); Hucker (1962); Cassano et al. (1965); Corona and Facino (1968); Facino and Corona (1969); Eschenhof and Rieder (1969); Corona et al. (1972); Hucker et al. (1976; 1977)
Desmethyl–NT	Cassano et al. (1965); Eschenhof and Rieder (1969); McMahon et al. (1963); Hammar et al. (1971); Whitnack et al. (1972); Knapp et al. (1972)
10–Hydroxy–NT (cis and trans)	Hucker (1962); Corona and Facino (1968); Facino and Corona (1969); Eschenhof and Rieder (1969); Corona et al. (1972); Hucker et al. (1976); McMahon et al. (1963); Amundson and Manthey (1966); Hammar et al. (1971); De Leenheer and Heyndrickx (1971); Knapp et al. (1972)
10–Hydroxy–NT glucuronide	Eschenhof and Rieder (1969); Hucker et al. (1977); McMahon et al. (1963);
10, 11–Dihydroxy–NT	Corona and Facino (1968); Facino and Corona (1969); Corona et al. (1972)
10–Hydroxy–desmethyl–NT	Eschenhof and Rieder (1969); Hammar et al. (1971); Knapp et al. (1972)
10–Hydroxy–desmethyl–NT glucuronide	Eschenhof and Rieder (1969)
AT–N–Oxide[a]	Eschenhof and Rieder (1969); Hucker et al. (1976)
Deaminated 3'–acid (see *Table 6.*)	Facino et al. (1970)
N–Hydroxy–NT and –desmethyl–NT	Beckett and Al–Sarraj (1973)
10, 11–Dehydro–AT[a] or –NT	Caddy et al. (1976)
Aromatic dihydrodiol of AT[a] and NT	Hucker et al. (1976; 1977)

[a] Metabolites of AT only; all others are also metabolites of NT

atives can occur in two stereospecific forms. Indeed, nortriptyline has been found to undergo stereospecific hydroxylation giving rise to both cis- and trans-10-hydroxy-nortriptyline (Mc Mahon et al., 1963). The two isomers have been isolated and their ratio in the urine of healthy volunteers was 1:4–1:5 (Bertilsson and Alexanderson, 1972). In the serum of a patient on amitriptyline therapy the two trans-10-hydroxyl-ated metabolites of amitriptyline and nortriptyline were detected (Kraak and Bijster, 1977). Another investigation (von Bahr, 1972) showed that amitriptyline and nortrip-tyline bind to cytochrome P-450 with high affinity, whereas the binding of their hy-droxylated metabolites is much weaker. The compounds, therefore, are likely to influence each other's metabolism by competition for microsomal interaction. Furthermore, the demethylation rates of the two drugs and of 10-hydroxy-nortriptyline correlated with their binding to P-450, and finally, pretreatment of rats with phenobarbital increased the microsomal demethylation of amitriptyline, but decreased the 10-hydroxylation of nortriptyline.

Like many basic, lipophilic drugs, amitriptyline attains high tissue levels and low blood levels (CASSANO et al., 1965; ESCHENHOF and RIEDER, 1969). Plasma half-lives of 3 h have been reported for rats and of 44–76 h for humans (DIAMOND, 1965; ESCHENHOF and RIEDER, 1969). As with other tricyclic drugs, considerable interpatient variation in the steady-state plasma levels of nortriptyline have been reported (HAMMER and SJÖQVIST, 1967) and ascribed to individual variation in hydroxylation rates (ALEXANDERSON and BORGA, 1973). Again in accordance with other tricyclic drugs, nortriptyline is characterized by a high hepatic extraction and thus displays a first-pass effect (VON BAHR et al., 1972a; 1973) which reduces the bioavailability of the drug to values within the 41%–85% range according to the various authors (GRAM and OVERØ, 1975; GIBALDI, 1975; NIAZI, 1976b; ALVAN et al., 1977).

D. Other Antidepressants

1. Noxiptiline (Table 8)

This drug is structurally closely related to amitriptyline except for a modification within the side chain. According to an extensive study on the metabolism of noxiptiline in various species (DUHM et al., 1969), the same pathways as with amitriptyline are operative. However, there are striking quantitative and other differences. Thus, N-oxidation is a major pathway (23% of dose in rat urine, 12% dog), whereas N-demethylation is of minor importance. As with amitriptyline and nortriptyline, hydroxylation in position 10 and 10,11 is predominant, and a large proportion of these metabolites are further conjugated. In contrast to imipramine and amitriptyline, noxiptiline gives rise to the formation of metabolites which are both hydroxylated and N-oxidized, e.g., 10-hydroxy- and 10,11-dihydroxynoxiptiline-N-oxide. Thus, the total N-oxide metabolites excreted in rat urine amount to 32% of the dose, whereas total demethylation is only 4%, conjugation 43%, and excretion of unconjugated hydroxylated metabolites 16%. A total of 20 metabolites have been detected.

2. Opipramol (Table 8)

Little information is available on the metabolism of this iminostilbene antidepressant (HERRMANN, 1964). In the urine of rats and rabbits seven metabolites have been detected in addition to 1% of unchanged drug and a small glucuronide fraction. In a much later study (FRIGERIO and PANTAROTTO, 1976) the formation of a small percentage of the relatively stable 10,11-epoxide has been reported.

3. Protriptyline (Table 8)

Protriptyline differs from nortriptyline in having a double bond in the 10,11-bridge (making it a cycloheptatriene ring) and in having the side chain attached through a saturated C–C bond. An early study (CHARALAMPOUS and JOHNSON, 1967) concluded

Table 8. Various antidepressants I

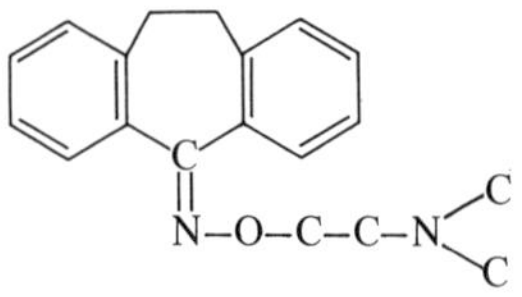

Noxiptiline

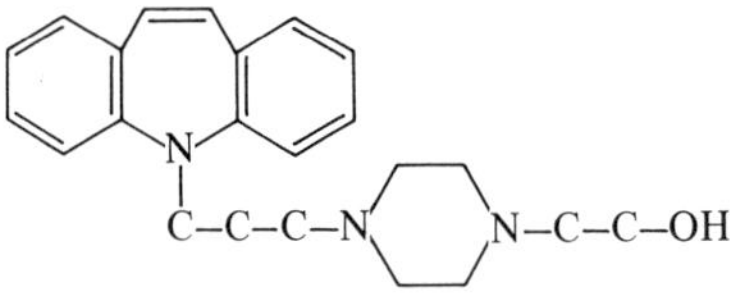

Opipramol

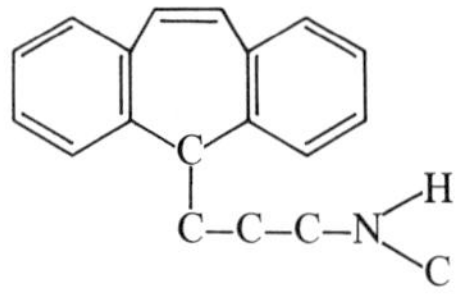

Protriptyline

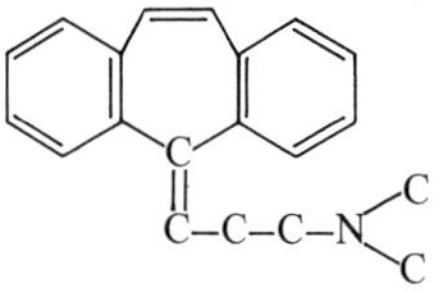

Proheptatriene
Cyclobenzaprine

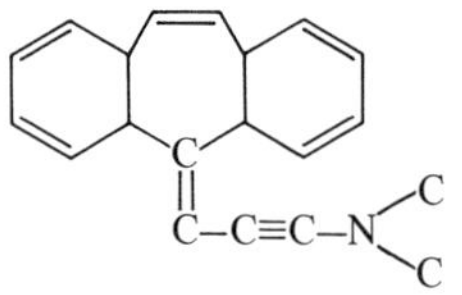

Intriptyline

from the drug's slow excretion that it was not rapidly converted to readily excreted metabolites. Later the following metabolites of protriptyline could be identified in urine of man, pig, and dog (SISENWINE et al., 1970): 10-hydroxy-, 10,11-dihydroxy- and their glucuronides, as well as a formylanthracene derivative, in which the 2-C bridge of the center ring has become a 1-C bridge with an attached aldehyde group. In dogs only, the primary amine metabolite, desmethylprotriptyline, is excreted. Chronic administration of the drug did not increase its rate of metabolism. Finally, rat urine revealed the presence of the 1o,11-epoxides of protriptyline and desmethylprotriptyline (HUCKER et al., 1975). In contrast to opipramol where epoxides were minor metabolites, the two epoxide metabolites of protriptyline amounted to no less than 40% of the total drug excreted in urine.

Since many epoxides (arene oxides and alkene oxides) are known as reactive and toxic intermediates their occurrence as metabolites of tricyclic antidepressants and anticonvulsive drugs might be regarded with concern. However, the following line of thoughts has been emphasized (FRIGERIO et al., 1976): The fact that these epoxides can be detected in urine is indirect evidence that they are not highly reactive and therefore are not available for covalent binding to intracellular macromolecules which is considered the basis of toxic effects. Indeed, some of these epoxides have been tested and were devoid of mutagenic activity under conditions where epoxides of known carcinogens proved active.

4. Proheptatriene (Table 8)

Proheptatriene (Cyclobenzaprine) has been reported to form the N-oxide, the des-methyl metabolite, and also the 10,11-epoxide upon incubation with rat liver micro-somes (BELVEDERE et al., 1975). Some characteristics of the mono-oxygenase-catalyzed epoxidation have been studied (PACHECKA et al., 1976).

5. Intriptyline (Table 8)

Intriptyline, a dibenzocyclotriene with a triple bond in the side chain, has also been found to form a stable 10,11-epoxide (FRIGERIO and PANTAROTTO, 1976).

6. Doxepine (Table 9)

Doxepine differs from amitriptyline only by the replacement of carbon by oxygen on one of the bridge positions. The following metabolites have been reported from stud-ies in dogs and rats (HOBBS, 1969): Mono- and didemethylated doxepine, hydroxyl-ated (in unknown position) and glucuronidated drug, doxepine-N-oxide, and de-methylated hydroxylated combination. In the metabolites the same ratio of cis- and

Table 9. Various antidepressants II

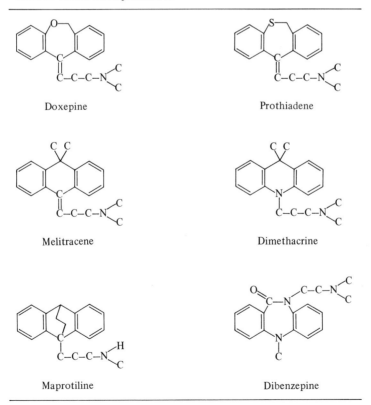

trans isomers as in the administered drug was present. It has been suggested that the clinical response is related to the desmethyl metabolite rather than to the unchanged drug (Kline et al., 1976).

7. Prothiadene (Table 9)

Metabolite formation of prothiadene, the thio analog of doxepine, has been studied in rat urine (Horesovsky et al., 1967). Seven metabolites were detected; the demethylation products, sulfoxide, and 3-hydroxy metabolite were identified.

8. Melitracene (Table 9)

The tricyclic skeleton of this antidepressant is a 10,10-dimethylated anthracene. Only the N-demethylated metabolite has become known so far (Eberholst and Huus, 1966).

9. Dimethacrine (Table 9)

This acridine analog of melitracene has been shown in various animal species to yield demethylated, 2-hydroxylated, combined and glucuronidated metabolites, and dimethacrine-N-oxide (Schatz et al., 1968). The finding of the tricyclic skeleton and the side chain fragment, $HO—CH_2—CH_2—N\overset{CH_3}{\underset{CH_3}{\diagdown}}$, suggested the existence of a less usual metabolic pathway.

10. Maprotiline (Table 9)

In the strict chemical sense this antidepressant is a tetracyclic compound since an ethylene bridge spans the center ring of the system. The metabolism of maprotiline, which has been studied in man and several animal species (Keberle et al., 1969; Riess et al., 1972), shows some complexities and unusual features. In addition to demethylation there is both aliphatic hydroxylation at the free position of the bridge head and aromatic mono-, di-, and tri-hydroxylation in unidentified positions. One phenolic group can undergo O-methylation by the action of a methyltransferase. In addition to combinations of demethylation and hydroxylation, oxidative deamination to metabolites with a propanol and propionic acid side chain occurs.

11. Dibenzepine (Table 9)

Dibenzepine differs from antidepressants dealt with so far in that its center ring is a diazepine which has the side chain attached to the amide nitrogen and a methyl group to the amine nitrogen (position 5). The metabolism of dibenzepine has been investigated in both animals and man (Hunziker and Schindler, 1965; Lehner et al., 1967; Michaelis, 1967). In man and dogs N-demethylation is the major pathway. There is mono- and didemethylation in the side chain as well as ring demethylation in position 5. Indeed, all five combinations have been identified. In rabbits, on the other hand, hydroxylation followed by conjugation predominates. The likely positions of hydroxylation are 4, 6, or 9. In autopsy material from suicide cases, unchanged dibenzepine dominated over the side-chain demethylated and other metabolites (BROCHON et al., 1969; CHRISTENSEN and FELBY, 1975). Desmethyldibenzepine was also the major metabolite in the plasma of patients (GAUCH and MODESTIN, 1973)

12. Miscellaneous Antidepressants

Some information is available on the metabolism of antidepressants which are not widely used or which have not yet been introduced on a large scale. *Thiazesim* has been found to form its sulfoxide as well as hydroxylated and other metabolites (DREYFUSS et al., 1968a,b). The metabolism of the bicyclic thymoleptics, *Lu 3-010* (FORSHELL et al., 1968), and its thio analog, *Lu 5-003* (OVERØ et al., 1970), is characterized by oxidative deamination and N-demethylation and, with the latter drug, sulfoxidation. *Nomifensine*, another bicyclic antidepressant, is biotransformed into an active monohydroxylated and two inactive methoxylated metabolites (KRUSE et al., 1977). *Iprindol*, which has become an important experimental antidepressant, appears to be extensively metabolized. Twenty metabolites have been detected but none accounted for more than a few percent of urinary radioactivity in various species tested (RUELIUS, 1977). *Mianserine*, a tricyclic compound with an additional "side chain cycle," has been reported to undergo the unusual metabolic reaction of N-(3-oxo-butyl) formation (VAN DER VEEN and DE JONG, 1977). Metabolic information on mianserin as well as the new antidepressants, *trazodone*, and *vivalen*, has been reviewed (MATUSSEK and GREIL, 1977).

References

Alexanderson, B., Borga, O.: Urinary excretion of nortriptyline and five of its metabolites in man after single and multiple oral doses. Eur. J. Clin. Pharmacol. 5, 174–180 (1973)

Alexanderson, B.: Pharmacokinetics of desmethylimipramine and nortriptyline in man after single and multiple oral doses – a cross-over study. Eur. J. Clin. Pharmacol. 5, 1–10 (1972)

Alvan, G., Borga, O., Lind, M., Palmer, L., Siwers, B.: First pass hydroxylation of nortriptyline: Concentrations of parent drug and major metabolites in plasma. Eur. J. Clin. Pharmacol. 11, 219–224 (1977)

Amundson, M.E., Manthey, J.A.: Excretion of nortriptyline HCl in man. I. Detection and determination of urinary nortriptyline. J. Pharm. Sci. 55, 277–280 (1966)

Beckett, A.H., Al-Sarraj, S.: Metabolism of amitriptyline, nortriptyline, imipramine and desipramine to yield hydroxylamines. J. Pharm. Pharmacol. 25, 335–336 (1973)

Belvedere, G., Rovei, V., Pantarotto, C., Frigerio, A.: Identification of cyclobenzaprine-10,11-epoxide and other metabolites after incubation of cyclobenzaprine with rat liver microsomes. Xenobiotica 5, 765–771 (1975)

Bertilsson, L., Alexanderson, B.: Stereospecific hydroxylation of nortriptyline in man in relation to interindividual differences in its steady-state plasma level. Eur. J. Clin. Pharmacol. 4, 201–205 (1972)

Bickel, M.H.: Untersuchungen zur Biochemie und Pharmakologie der Thymoleptica. Prog. Drug Res. 11, 121–225 (1968)

Bickel, M.H.: N-oxide formation and related reactions in drug metabolism. Xenobiotica 1, 313–319 (1971)

Bickel, M.H.: Liver metabolic reactions: Tertiary amine N-dealkylation, tertiary amine N-oxidation, N-oxide reduction, and N-oxide N-dealkylation. I. Tricyclic tertiary amine drugs. Arch. Biochem. Biophys. 148, 54–62 (1972)

Bickel, M.H.: Poisoning by tricyclic antidepressant drugs. General and pharmacokinetic considerations. Int. J. Clin. Pharmacol. Biopharm. 11, 145–176 (1975)

Bickel, M.H., Baggiolini, M.: The metabolism of imipramine and its metabolites by rat liver microsomes. Biochem. Pharmacol. *15*, 1155–1169 (1966)

Bickel, M.H., Börner, H.: Uptake, subcellular distribution, and transfer processes of imipramine and its metabolites formed in rat liver perfusion systems. Naunyn Schmiedeberg's Arch. Pharmac. *284*, 339–352 (1974)

Bickel, M.H., Brodie, B.B.: Structure and antidepressant activity of imipramine analogues. Int. J. Neuropharmacol. *3*, 611–621 (1964)

Bickel, M.H., Gigon, P.L.: Metabolic interconversions and binding of imipramine, imipramine-N-oxide, and desmethylimipramine in rat liver slices. Xenobiotica *1*, 631–641 (1971)

Bickel, M.H., Minder, R.: Metabolism and biliary excretion of the lipophilic drug molecules, imipramine and desmethylimipramine in the rat. I. Experiments in vivo and with isolated perfused livers. Biochem. Pharmacol. *19*, 2425–2435 (1970a)

Bickel, M.H., Minder, R.: Metabolism and biliary excretion of the lipophilic drug molecules, imipramine and desmethylimipramine in the rat. II. Uptake into bile micelles. Biochem. Pharmacol. *19*, 2437–2443 (1970b)

Bickel, M.H., Weder, H.J.: The total fate of a drug: Kinetics of distribution, excretion, and formation of 14 metabolites in rats treated with imipramine. Arch. Int. Pharmacodyn. Ther. *173*, 433–463 (1968a)

Bickel, M.H., Weder, H.J.: Demethylation of imipramine in the rat as influenced by SKF 525-A and by different routes of administration. Life Sci. *7*, 1223–1230 (1968b)

Bickel, M.H., Weder, H.J.: Buccal absorption and other properties of pharmacokinetic importance of imipramine and its metabolites. J. Pharm. Pharmacol. *21*, 160–168 (1969)

Bickel, M.H., Sulser, F., Brodie, B.B.: Conversion of tranquilizers to antidepressants by removal of one N-methyl group. Life Sci. *4*, 247–253 (1963)

Bickel, M.H., Flückiger, M., Baggiolini, M.: Vergleichende Demethylierung von tricyclischen Psychopharmaka durch Rattenleber-Mikrosomen. Arch. Pharmak. Exp. Path. *256*, 360–366 (1967)

Bickel, M.H., Minder, R., Di Francesco, C.: Formation of N-glucuronide of desmethylimipramine in the dog. Experientia *29*, 960–961 (1973)

Borga, O., Garle, M.: A gas chromatographic method for the quantitative determination of nortriptyline and some of its metabolites in human plasma and urine. J. Chromatogr. *68*, 77–88 (1972)

Brochon, R., Lehner, H., Gauch, R., Rudin, O.: The detection and determination of dibenzepine and its metabolites in autopsy material. Arch. Toxikol. (Berl.) *24*, 249–259 (1969)

Buckley, J.P., Steenberg, M.L., Jandhyala, B.S., Perel, J.M.: Effects of imipramine, desmethylimipramine and their 2-OH-metabolites on hemodynamics and myocardial contractility in dogs. Fed. Proc. *34*, 450 (1975)

Caddy, B., Fish, F., Tranter, J.: Studies on the oxidation of amitriptyline. Analyst *101*, 244–254 (1976)

Cassano, G.B., Sjöstrand, S.E., Hansson, E.: Distribution and fate of ^{14}C-amitriptyline in mice and rats. Psychopharmacologia *8*, 1–11 (1965)

Charalampous, K.D., Johnson, P.C.: Studies of ^{14}C-protriptyline in man: Plasma levels and excretion. J. Clin. Pharmacol. *7*, 93–96 (1967)

Christensen, H., Felby, S.: Dibenzepine and its metabolites in blood, muscle, liver, vitreous body and urine from fatal poisoning. Acta Pharmacol. Toxicol. *37*, 393–401 (1975)

Christiansen, J., Gram, L.F.: Imipramine and its metabolites in human brain. J. Pharm. Pharmacol. *25*, 604–608 (1973)

Christiansen, J., Gram., L.F., Kofod, B., Rafaelsen, O.J.: Imipramine metabolism in man. A study of urinary metabolites after administration of radioactive imipramine. Psychopharmacologia *11*, 255–264 (1967)

Corona, G.L., Facino, R.M.: Identification and evaluation of amitriptyline and its basic metabolites in rabbits urine. Biochem. Pharmacol. *17*, 2045–2050 (1968)

Corona, G.L., Zerbi, F., Facino, R.M., Santagostino, G., Pirillo, D.: Valutazione dell' amitriptilina e dei suoi metaboliti basici nelle urine di soggetti sani e depressi. Boll. Soc. Ital. Biol. Sper. *48*, 545–547 (1972)

Crammer, J.L., Rolfe, B.: Metabolism of ^{14}C-imipramine. III. Conversion by rat tissues. Psychopharmacologia *18*, 26–37 (1970)

Crammer, J.L., Scott, B.: New metabolites of imipramine. Psychopharmacol. *8*, 461–468 (1966)

Crammer, J.L., Scott, B., Woods, H., Rolfe, B.: Metabolism of ^{14}C-imipramine. I. Excretion in the rat and in man. Psychopharmacologia *12*, 263–277 (1968)

Crammer, J.L., Scott, B., Rolfe, B.: Metabolism of ^{14}C-imipramine: II. Urinary metabolites in man. Psychopharmacologia *15*, 207–225 (1969)

De Leenheer, A., Heyndrickx, A.: Identification of a major metabolite of nortriptyline in human urine. J. Pharm. Sci. *60*, 1403–1405 (1971)

Diamond, S.: Human metabolization of amitriptyline tagged with carbon 14. Curr. Ther. Res. *7*, 170–175 (1965)

Dingell, J.V., Sanders, E.: Methylation of desmethylimipramine by rabbit lung in vitro. Biochem. Pharmacol. *15*, 599–605 (1966)

Dingell, J.V., Sulser, F., Gillette, J.R.: Species differences in the metabolism of imipramine and desipramine. J. Pharmacol. Exp. Ther. *143*, 14–23 (1964)

Dreyfuss, J., Swoap, J.R., Chinn, C., Hess, S.M.: Excretion and distribution of thiazesim-^{14}C with its biotransformation in vivo and in vitro. J. Pharm. Sci. *57*, 1497–1505 (1968a)

Dreyfuss, J., Cohen, A.I., Hess, S.M.: Metabolism of thiazesim, 5-(2-dimethylaminoethyl)-2,3-dihydro-2-phenyl-1,5-benzothiazepin-4(5H)-one, in the rat in vivo and in vitro. J. Pharm. Sci. *57*, 1505–1511 (1968b)

Duhm, B., Maul, W., Medenwald, H., Patzschke, K., Wegner, L.: Untersuchungen mit ^{14}C-markiertem Noxiptilin. Stoffwechsel und Kinetik. Arzneim. Forsch. *19*, 858–870 (1969)

Eberholst, I., Huus, I.: Studies on the metabolism of melitracen (N 7001) in rats. Arzneim. Forsch. *16*, 876–878 (1966)

Eschenhof, E., Rieder, J.: Untersuchungen über das Schicksal des Antidepressivums Amitriptylin im Organismus der Ratte und des Menschen. Arzneim. Forsch. *19*, 957–966 (1969)

Facino, R.M., Corona, G.L.: Identification and evaluation of amitriptyline and its basic metabolites by thin-layer chromatography in rabbit organs. J. Pharm. Sci. *58*, 764–765 (1969)

Facino, R.M., Santagostino, G., Corona, G.L.: Presence of an acid metabolite of amitriptyline in rabbit urine. Biochem. Pharmacol. *19*, 1503–1505 (1970)

Faigle, J.W., Dieterle, W.: The metabolism and pharmacokinetics of clomipramine (anafranil). J. Int. Med. Res. *1*, 281–290 (1973)

Fishman, V., Goldenberg, H.: Identification of a new metabolite of imipramine. Proc. Soc. Exp. Biol. Med. *110*, 187–190 (1962)

Forshell, G.P.: The distribution and excretion of (^{3}H,^{14}C)lofepramine in the rat. Xenobiotica *5*, 73–82 (1975)

Forshell, G.P.: personal communication, 1977

Forshell, G.P., Schauman, P., Hansen, V., Larsen, U.D., Jørgensen, A., Overø, K.F.: Distribution and metabolism of 3,3-dimethyl-1-(3-methyl-aminopropyl)-1-phenylphthalane (Lu 3-010), a bicyclic compound with thymoleptic properties. Acta Pharmacol. Toxicol. *26*, 507–520 (1968)

Frigerio, A., Pantarotto, C.: Epoxide-diol pathway in the metabolism of tricyclic drugs. J. Pharm. Pharmacol. *28*, 665 (1976)

Frigerio, A., Cavo-Briones, M., Belvedere, G.: Formation of stable epoxides in the metabolism of tricyclic drugs. Drug Metab. Rev. *5*, 197–218 (1976)

Gauch, R., Modestin, J.: Zur Pharmakokinetik von Dibenzepin. Arzneim. Forsch. *23*, 687–690 (1973)

Gibaldi, M.: Comparison of observed and predicted bioavailability of nortriptyline in humans following oral administration. J. Pharm. Sci. *64*, 1036–1037 (1975)

Gigon, P.L., Bickel, M.H.: N-demethylation and N-oxidation of imipramine by rat and pig liver microsomes. Biochem. Pharmacol. *20*, 1921–1931 (1971)

Gillette, J.R., Dingell, J.V., Sulser, F., Kuntzman, R., Brodie, B.B.: Isolation from rat brain of a metabolic product, desmethylimipramine, that mediates the antidepressant activity of imipramine. Experientia *17*, 417–418 (1961)

Gram, L.F.: Metabolism of tricyclic antidepressants. Dan. Med. Bull. *21*, 218–231 (1974)

Gram, L.F., Christiansen, J.: First-pass metabolism of imipramine in man. Clin. Pharmacol. Ther. *17*, 555–563 (1975)

Gram, L.F., Overø, K.F.: First-pass metabolism of nortriptyline in man. Clin. Pharmacol. Ther. *18*, 305–314 (1975)

Gram, L.F. Kofod, B., Christiansen, J., Rafaelsen, J.: Imipramine metabolism: pH-dependent distribution and urinary excretion. Clin. Pharmacol. Ther. *12*, 239–244 (1971)

Gyermek, L.: The pharmacology of imipramine and related antidepressants. Int. Rev. Neurobiol. *9*, 95–143 (1966)

Hammer, W., Sjöqvist, F.: Plasma levels of monomethylated tricyclic antidepressants during treatment with imipramine-like compounds. Life Sci. *6*, 1895–1903 (1967)

Hammer, W., Martens, S., Sjöqvist, F.: A compartive study of the metabolism of desmethylimipramine, nortriptyline, and oxyphenylbutazone in man. Clin. Pharmacol. Ther. *10*, 44–49 (1969)

Hammar, C.G., Alexanderson, B., Holmstedt, B., Sjöqvist, F.: Gas chromatography-mass spectrometry of nortriptyline in body fluids of man. Clin. Pharmacol. Ther. *12*, 496–505 (1971)

Hawkins, D.R., Midgley, I., Chasseaud, L.F.: The metabolism of amitriptyline N-oxide in man. (abstr.) 2nd Int. Symp. Biol. Oxidation of Nitrogen in Organic Molecules, p. 64. London: 1977

Herrmann, B.: Untersuchungen über den Stoffwechsel von Insidon. Arzneim. Forsch. *14*, 219–222 (1964)

Herrmann, B.: Aspects of the metabolism of imipramine. In:Neuro-Psychopharmacology (Cole, J.O., Brill, H., eds.), p. 557. Washington: 1967

Herrmann, B., Pulver, R.: Der Stoffwechsel des Psychopharmakons Tofranil. Arch. Int. Pharmacodyn. Ther. *126*, 454–469 (1960)

Herrmann, B., Schindler, W., Pulver, R.: Papierchromatographischer Nachweis von Stoffwechselprodukten des Tofranil. Med. experimentalis *1*, 381–385 (1960)

Hobbs, D.C.: Distribution and metabolism of doxepin. Biochem. Pharmacol. *18*, 1941–1954 (1969)

Horesovsky, O., Franc, Z., Kraus, P.: Biochemistry of drugs. XI. The metabolic fate of a new psychotropic drug, 11-(3-dimethylaminopropylidene)-6,11-dihydrodibenz(b,e)-thiepine (prothiadene). Biochem. Pharmacol. *16*, 2421–2429 (1967)

Hucker, H.B.: Metabolism of amitriptyline. Pharmacologist *4*, 171 (1962)

Hucker, H.B., Porter, C.C.: Studies on the metabolism of amitriptyline. Fed. Proc. *20*, 172 (1961)

Hucker, H.B., Balletto, A.J., Demetriades, J., Arison, B.H., Zacchei, A.G.: Epoxide metabolites of protriptyline in rat urine. Drug Metab. Dispos. *3*, 80–84 (1975)

Hucker, H.B., Balletto, A.J., Demetriades, J., Arison, B.H., Zacchei, A.G.: Biotransformation of amitriptyline in the dog. Fed. Proc. *35*, 244 (1976)

Hucker, H.B., Balletto, A.J., Demetriades, J., Arison, B.H., Zacchei, A.G.: Urinary metabolites of amitriptyline in the dog. Drug Metab. Dispos. *5*, 132–142 (1977)

Hunziker, F., Schindler, O.: Zum Stoffwechsel von Noveril: ¹⁴C-Markierung und Synthese von Metaboliten. Helv. Chim. Acta *48*, 1590–1597 (1965)

Im. Obersteg, J., Bäumler, J.: Suicid mit dem Psychopharmakon Tofranil. Arch. Toxicol. (Berl.) *19*, 339–344 (1962)

Jandhyala, B.S., Steenberg, M.L., Perel, J.M., Manian, A.A., Buckley, J.P.: Effects of several tricyclic antidepressants on the hemodynamics and myocardial contractility of the anesthetized dogs. Eur. J. Pharmacol. *42*, 403–410 (1977)

Jori, A., Bernardi, D., Pugliatti, C., Garattini, S.: Strain differences in the metabolism of imipramine by rat. Biochem. Pharmacol. *19*, 1315–1321 (1970)

Judd, C.I., Ursillo, R.C.: Absorption, distribution, excretion, and metabolism of antidepressants. In: Antidepressants (Fielding, S., Lal, H., eds.), pp. 231–265. New York: Futura 1975

Junod, A.F.: Accumulation of ¹⁴C-imipramine in isolated perfused rat lungs. J. Pharmacol. Exp. Ther. *183*, 182–187 (1972)

Keberle, H., Riess, W., Meyer-Brunot, H.G., Schmid, K.: Species differences in absorption, metabolism, and excretion illustrated by reference to the psycho-active drugs from the dibenzo-bicyclo-octadiene series. In: Excerpta Medica Foundation (Cerletti, A., Bové, F.J., eds.), Int. Congr. Series *180*, pp. 123–127. Amsterdam: 1969

Kline, N.S., Cooper, T., Johnston, B.: Doxepin and desmethyldoxepin serum levels and clinical response. In: Pharmacokinetics of Psychoactive Drugs (Gottschalk, L.A., Merlis, S., eds.), pp. 221–228. New York: Spectrum 1976

Knapp, D.R., Gaffney, T.E., Mc Mahon, R.E., Kiplinger, G.: Studies of human urinary and biliary metabolites of nortriptyline with stable isotope labeling. J. Pharmacol. Exp. Ther. *180*, 784–790 (1972)

Kraak, J.C., Bijster, P.: Determination of amitriptyline and some of its metabolites in blood by high-pressure liquid chromatography. J. Chromatogr. *143*, 499–512 (1977)

Kruse, H., Hoffmann, I., Gerhards, H.J., Leven, M., Schacht, U.: Pharmacological and biochemical studies with three metabolites of nomifensine. Psychopharmacology *51*, 117–123 (1977)

Lapin, I.P.: Pharmacological activity of quaternary derivatives of imipramine and diethylaminopropionyl-iminodibenzyl. Pharmakopsychiatr. Neuropsychopharmakol. *2*, 14–27 (1969)

Lehner, H., Gauch, R., Michaelis, W.: Zum Stoffwechsel von 5-Methyl-10-β-dimethylaminoäthyl-10,11-dihydro-11-oxo-5H-dibenzo-(b,e)(1,4) diazepin HCl. III. Isolierung und Identifizierung von im Urin ausgeschiedenen Metaboliten der Substanz bei Mensch und Tier. Arzneim. Forsch. *17*, 185–189 (1967)

Matussek, N., Greil, W.: New antidepressants. In: Psychotherapeutic Drugs (Usdin, E., Forrest, I.S., eds.), pp. 1251–1266. New York: Marcel Dekker, 1977

Mc Mahon, R.E., Marshall, F.J., Culp, H.W., Miller, W.M.: The metabolism of nortriptyline-N-methyl-14C in rats. Biochem. Pharmacol. *12*, 1207–1217 (1963)

Michaelis, W.: Zum Stoffwechsel von 5-Methyl-10-β-dimethylaminoäthyl-10,11-dihydro-11-oxo-5H-dibenzo-(b,e)(1,4)-diazepin HCl. II. Resorption, Verteilung in den Organen und Ausscheidung der mit ^{14}C markierten Substanz beim Tier. Arzneim. Forsch. *17*, 181–185 (1967)

Minder, R., Schnetzer, F., Bickel, M.H.: Hepatic and extrahepatic metabolism of the psychotropic drugs chlorpromazine, imipramine, and imipramine-N-oxide. Naunyn Schmiedeberg's Arch. Pharmacol. *268*, 334–347 (1971)

Nagy, A., Johansson, R.: Plasma levels of imipramine and desipramine in man after different routes of administration. Naunyn Schmiedeberg's Arch. Pharmacol. *290*, 145–160 (1975)

Niazi, S.: Comparison of observed and predicted first-pass metabolism of imipramine in humans. J. Pharm. Sci. *65*, 1063–1064 (1976a)

Niazi, S.: Comparison of observed and predicted first-pass metabolism of nortriptyline in humans. J. Pharm. Sci. *65*, 1535 (1976b)

Overø, K.F., Jorgensen, A., Hansen, V.: Metabolism, distribution and excretion of the thiophthalane Lu 5-003, a bicyclic thymoleptic. Acta Pharmacol. Toxicol. *28*, 81–96 (1970)

Pachecka, J., Salmona, M., Cantoni, L., Mussini, E., Pantarotto, C., Frigerio, A., Belvedere, G.: Activity of liver microsomal mono-oxygenases on some epoxide-forming tricyclic drugs. I. Kinetics in vitro. Xenobiotica *6*, 593–598 (1976)

Perel, J.M., Manian, A.A.: Metabolism of 3-chloroimipramine in humans. Fed. Proc. *36*, 939 (1977)

Populaire, P., Terlain, B., Pascal, S., Lebreton, G., Decouvelaere, B.: Résorption, excrétion et biotransformation de la triméprimine (7162 R.P.) chez le chien et le lapin. Contribution à l'identification de plusieurs métabolites. Biotransformation chez l'homme. Produits et Problèmes Pharmaceutiques *25*, 632–645 (1970)

Pscheidt, G.R.: Demethylation of imipramine in male and female rats. Biochem. Pharmacol. *11*, 501–502 (1962)

Quinn, G.P., Hurwic, M.J., Perel, J.H.: Interspecies differences in drug metabolism. In: Psychotherapeutic Drugs (Usdin, E., Forrest, I.S., eds.),pp. 605–623. New York: Marcel Dekker, 1976

Riess, W., Rajagopalan, T.G., Keberle, H.: Metabolismus und Pharmakokinetik von Ludiomil (Maprotilin). In: Depressive Zustände. Erkennung, Bewertung, Behandlung (Kielholz, P., ed.), p. 140. Berne: Hans Huber, 1972

Rosenbloom, P.M., Bass, A.D.: A lung perfusion preparation for the study of drug metabolism. J. Appl. Physiol. *29*, 138–144 (1970)

Roubein, I.F., Keup, W.: On the origin of desmethylimipramine in rat brain. Res. Commun. Chem. Pathol. Pharmacol. *10*, 633–640 (1975)

Ruelius, H.W.: personal communication, 1977

Ryrfeld, A., Hansson, E.: Biliary excretion of quaternary ammonium compounds and tertiary amines in the rat. Acta Pharmacol. Toxicol. *30*, 59–68 (1971)

Santagostino, G., Facino, R.M., Pirillo, D.: Urinary excretion of amitriptyline N-oxide in humans. J. Pharm. Sci. *63*, 1690–1692 (1974)

Schatz, F., Jahn, U., Adrian, R.W., Molnar, I.: Untersuchungen über Resorption und Metabolismus des Antidepressivums 9,9-Dimethyl-10-(3-dimethylaminopropyl)acridan-hydrogentartrat. Arzneim. Forsch. *18*, 862–871 (1968)

Schenkman, J.B., Remmer, H., Estabrook, R.W.: Spectral studies of drug interaction with hepatic microsomal cytochrome. Mol. Pharmacol. *3*, 113–123 (1967)

Schindler, W.: Über die Konstitutionsermittlung und Synthese eines Metaboliten von N-(γ-dimethylaminopropyl)-iminodibenzyl-HCl (Tofranil). Helv. Chim. Acta *43*, 35–42 (1960)

Sisenwine, S.F., Tio, C.O., Shrader, S.R., Ruelius, H.W.: The biotransformation of protriptyline in man, pig and dog. J. Pharmacol. Exp. Ther. *175*, 51–59 (1970)

Sjöqvist, F., Berglund, F., Borga, O., Hammer, W., Andersson, S., Thorstrand, C.: The pH-dependent excretion of monomethylated tricyclic antidepressants. Clin. Pharmacol. Ther. *10*, 826–833 (1970)

Stegmann, R., Bickel, M.H.: Dominant role for tissue binding in the first-pass extraction of imipramine by the perfused rat liver. Xenobiotica *7*, 737–746 (1977)

Sugiura, M., Iwasaki, K., Kato, R.: Reduced nicotinamide adenine dinucleotide-dependent reduction of tertiary amine N-oxide by liver microsomal cytochrome P-450. Biochem. Pharmacol. *26*, 489–495 (1977)

Sulser, F., Watts, J., Brodie, B.B.: On the mechanism of antidepressant action of imipramine-like drugs. Ann. N.Y. Acad. Sci. *96*, 279–286 (1962)

Theobald, W., Büch, O., Kunz, H.A., Morpurgo, C.: Zur Pharmakologie von Metaboliten des Imipramins. Med. Pharmacol. experimentalis *15*, 187–197 (1966)

Van der Veen, F., De Jong, G.D.: N-(3-oxo-butyl) formation: A new metabolic transformation. Xenobiotica *7*, 99–100 (1977)

Von Bahr, C.: Binding and oxidation of amitriptyline and a series of its oxidized metabolites in liver microsomes from untreated and phenobarbital-treated rats. Xenobiotica *2*, 293–306 (1972)

Von Bahr, C., Bertilsson, L.: Hydroxylation and subsequent glucuronide conjugation of desmethylimipramine in rat liver microsomes. Xenobiotica *1*, 205–212 (1971)

Von Bahr, C., Borga, O.: Uptake, metabolism and excretion of desmethylimipramine and its metabolites in the isolated perfused rat liver. Acta Pharmacol. Toxicol. *29*, 359–374 (1971)

Von Bahr, C., Orrenius, S.: Spectral studies on the interaction of imipramine and some of its oxidized metabolites with rat liver microsomes. Xenobiotica *1*, 69–78 (1971)

Von Bahr, C., Fellenius, E., Fried, I.: On the "first-pass" effect in the liver of nortriptyline, lidocaine and propanolol. Acta Pharmacol. Toxicol. *31 Suppl.*, 92 (1972a)

Von Bahr, C., Hietanen, E., Glaumann, H.: Oxidation and glucuronidation of certain drugs in various subcellular fractions of rat liver: Binding of desmethylimipramine and hexobarbital to cytochrome P-450 and oxidation and glucuronidation of desmethylimipramine, aminopyrine, p-nitrophenol and l-naphthol. Acta Pharmacol. Toxicol. *31*, 107–120 (1972b)

Von Bahr, C., Borga, O., Fellenius, E., Rowland, M.: Kinetics of nortriptyline (NT) in rats in vivo and in the isolated perfused liver: Demonstration of a "first-pass disappearance" of NT in the liver. Pharmacology *9*, 177–186 (1973)

Whitnack, E., Knapp, D.R., Holmes, J.C., Fowler, N.O., Gaffney, T.E.: Demethylation of nortriptyline by the dog lung. J. Pharmacol. Exp. Ther. *181*, 288–291 (1972)

Ziegler, D.M., Mitchell, C.H., Jollow, D.: The properties of a purified hepatic microsomal mixed function amine oxidase. In: Microsomes and drug oxidations (Gillette, J.R., Conney, A.H., Cosmides, G.J., Estabrook, R.W., Fouts, J.R., Mannering, G.J., eds.), pp. 173–188. New York-London: Academic Press 1969

CHAPTER 24

Physiological and Psychological Effects of Antidepressants in Man

M. Lader and S. Bhanji

A. Introduction

The physiological and psychological effects in depressed patients of tricyclic or mono-amine oxidase inhibitor (MAOI) antidepressants have been investigated in order to explore: (1) the mode of action of these compounds, (2) to elucidate the physiological and psychological concomitants of depression by studying patients before and after recovery, and (3) to determine which objective measures predict or record the outcome of treatment. To correctly interpret the findings of such studies, changes deriving from alterations in depressive symptoms must be carefully distinguished from the direct effects of the drug under investigation. As a consequence, the effects of antidepressant drugs on nondepressed subjects merit systematic study.

Physiological measures can be conveniently divided into central (electroence-phalographic) and peripheral. Psychological measures, however, are less easily classified. Thus, reaction time estimates, in which the subject reacts in some prescribed way as quickly as possible to the presentation of a specified stimulus, are used as measures of psychomotor response speed but are also affected by changes in alertness, perception, and motor coordination. Furthermore, in depressed patients the results of such tests may be influenced by factors such as motivation, selfconfidence, and the patient's ability to understand and remember the instructions.

B. Central Physiological Effects

The MAOI antidepressants, phenelzine, isocarboxazid, iproniazid, and nialamide, have only minimal effects on spontaneous EEG activity (FINK and ITIL, 1968). In contrast, several changes occur during administration of imipramine or amitriptyline. BORENSTEIN and DABBAH (1959) treated a variety of patients with imipramine (about 100 mg/day) and discerned EEG changes in 15 of their 22 depressives; the commonest change being more marked α activity. FINK (1959) employed a dosage of 100–200 mg/day for over 4 weeks in treating 16 depressed patients. EEG changes were minor but included increased fast activity and, in four patients, the occurrence of theta activity. ZAPPOLI (1959) investigated a larger series of depressed patients who received up to 400 mg imipramine each day and described five, occasionally coexisting, EEG patterns. The two commonest were a diffusely hyperexcitable EEG and an increase in dysrhythmic activity. Other changes observed were a tendency to desynchronization with reduced α and increased β activity, an accentuation of pre-existing abnormalities, and an epileptiform dysrhythmia. The development of an irritable EEG pattern during the course of imipramine treatment was confirmed by DELAY et al. (1960) in a series of psychiatric patients, mainly endogenous or reactive depressives receiving 50–400 mg/day, and by Lecompte et al. (1963) in depressives receiving up to 200–400 mg each day. Both reports mentioned that these changes were most noticeable during photic stimulation; the former adding that they disappeared as clinical improvement commenced, the latter that the effect was dose-related. Imipramine tends to diminish EEG frequency in patients above the age of 50 but to increase or not alter that of younger subjects (Delay et al., 1960)

Fink and his co-workers have compared the effects of imipramine (maximum daily dosage 300 mg), chlorpromazine, and placebo on the EEGs of depressed and schizophrenic patients. Imipramine increased slow and fast wave activity but diminished α activity (Andermann and Fink, 1963; Fink, 1965; Fink et al., 1964). Fink and Itil (1968) suggested that these changes were typical of the tricyclic antidepressants. However, a recent investigation carried out by the authors at the Institute of Psychiatry (Bhanji, 1977; Bhanji and Lader, 1977) suggests that EEG changes occurring during the course of imipramine therapy are minor. Ten psychotic depressives received imipramine (150 mg/day) for 4 weeks; during this time the only significant EEG alteration was a transient increase in the percentage of the total (2.4–26.0 Hz) voltage lying within the 2.4–4.0 Hz waveband.

A number of authors have investigated the effects of a single intravenous dose of antidepressant on the EEG. Fink (1959) gave intravenous imipramine to 28 consecutive inpatients of mixed diagnoses at a dose-rate of 10 mg/40 s until EEG or behavioral changes were observed (a total of 40–125 mg). The tendency was for α activity to diminish and β activity to increase. After about 20 min, low voltage theta waves appeared. Similar changes were reported by Andermann and Fink (1963) who administered intravenous imipramine, chlorpromazine, or placebo to 56 psychiatric patients. α activity was reduced and slow activity moderately increased.

Kiloh et al. (1961), as part of an investigation into the possible analeptic effects of imipramine, administered single 75 mg intravenous doses to 24 nonepileptic patients, most of whom were depressed. α activity was diminished in most of the patients, but increased in those who became drowsy. Less common changes were the development of diffuse theta activity and a moderate increase in fast activity. A similar investigation into the effects of 20 mg amitriptyline showed the changes in nonepileptic depressives to be nonspecific (Davison, 1965)

There have been few studies of the effects of antidepressants on the EEGs of normal subjects. Itil et al. (1969) reported that intravenously administered imipramine (0.3–0.4 mg/kg) increased slow activity and decreased α and slow β activity. A more recent study (Bhanji, 1977) compared the effects on the EEG of two oral doses of imipramine (1.0 and 0.67 mg/kg) and placebo in 12 normal subjects. The total voltage of the EEG (2.4–26.0 Hz) was increased by the higher dose; both doses of imipramine increased the total within the 13.5–26.0 Hz waveband. The lower dose decreased the percentage of the total voltage within the 2.4–4.0 Hz and 4.0–7.5 Hz wavebands. The higher dose decreased the percentage within the 7.5–13.5 Hz band but had no effect compared with placebo on the other wavebands.

The EEG-evoked potential is a low voltage multiphasic wave recordable from the scalp following sensory stimulation. The first component of the evoked response occupies the 50 ms or so following stimulation and is generally thought to represent the arrival of thalamocortical impulses; the second component occurs during the next

300 ms and probably represents the arrival of sensory impulses via less direct pathways. The form of the evoked response depends on the sensory modality of the stimulus, the site of the electrodes, the level of attention of the subject, and the intensity, frequency, and significance of the stimulus. More stable influences are age, sex, personality, and intelligence. In addition, the evoked response is likely to be contaminated by muscle potentials and it has been suggested that the early component is in fact a myogenic artefact.

Both imipramine (SHAGASS et al., 1962) and amitriptyline (SHAGASS et al., 1973) reduce the amplitude of the early somatosensory-evoked scalp potential which comprises a negative wave occurring 20 ms, and a positive wave 25 ms, after stimulation of the ulnar nerve at the wrist. The later evoked potential following auditory stimulation consists of two peaks (P1 latency at 50–60 ms, P2 at 170–200 ms) and two troughs (N1 at 95–105 ms, N2 at 300 ms). BHANJI and LADER (1977) found that the P2 latency increased during the first 4 days of imipramine therapy and then declined. The P1–N1 and N1–P2 amplitudes showed a similar increase and remained elevated. The early onset of these changes suggested they were direct effects of the drug.

SALETU et al. (1973) investigated the effects of placebo and two dosages (0.45 mg/kg and 0.62 mg/kg) of imipramine and amitriptyline on the somatosensory-evoked response of normal subjects. The early latencies were shortened and the later increased. The effect on the later components was greater following amitriptyline, possibly because of its greater sedative effects.

Differences in drug dosage and administration, as well as in EEG technique and terminology, make it difficult to draw any clear conclusions from the above studies. Further problems arise from the loose usage of the term "depression" in studies on patients and the largely subjective manner in which EEG changes are discerned and interpreted. The use of objective computerized EEG evaluation techniques may clarify matters, particularly if any changes observed could be correlated with plasma drug concentrations.

C. Peripheral Physiological Effects

I. Skin Conductance

The electric conductance of the skin is one of the most widely used indices of the level of arousal. In states of heightened arousal, the basal conductance level is raised, the frequency of spontaneous skin conductance fluctuations is increased, and the rise in conductance following stimulation (the galvanic skin response or GSR) is increased and shows delayed habituation following repeated stimuli. It is now accepted that changes in skin conductance represent changes in sweat gland activity mediated by cholinergic sympathetic fibers. As GSR activity is reduced in retarded depression and increased in agitated depression, changes arising during treatment may reflect clinical change as well as the pharmacological effects of the drug used.

ALEXANDER (1961) investigated the effects of a number of drugs on the GSRs of a variety of psychiatric patients. Those who responded to iproniazid, isocarboxazid, nialamide, and imipramine showed a decrease in GSR activity. Patients who failed to improve with imipramine treatment showed increased GSR activity. In contrast, patients receiving amitriptyline had reduced GSR activity irrespective of clinical outcome. In a recent study of imipramine-treated depressives (BHANJI, 1977), the basal skin conductance decreased during the first week of treatment but 3 weeks later had returned to its pretreatment level. The skin conductance values did not correlate significantly with the depression rating scores nor with the plasma concentrations of imipramine and desmethylimipramine. In a companion study carried out on normal subjects receiving placebo or imipramine at 0.67 mg/kg and 1.0 mg/kg, the active drug decreased skin conductance and decreased spontaneous fluctuation rate in a dose-related fashion.

II. Finger Tremor

In primary depressive illness finger tremor can occur as a normal phenomenon, a manifestation of anxiety, or as a side-effect of treatment. Tremor occurring in the course of imipramine therapy has been described as fine, rapid, and persistent. A coarser, extra-pyramidal type of tremor may occur following high doses. BHANJI (1977) recorded finger tremor by means of a miniaturized accelerometer and used power spectral density analyses. Imipramine-treated depressives displayed an increase in power at 8 Hz during the first 15 days. The 8 Hz power correlated positively with imipramine and desmethylimipramine plasma concentrations and negatively with scores on depression rating scales. Single doses of imipramine administered to normal subjects increased tremor power within the physiological range (7–12 Hz) in a dose-related manner.

III. Pupil Diameter

Pupillary dilatation is a common clinical finding in patients receiving tricyclic antidepressants. Imipramine treatment was associated with an increase in the pupil diameter under bright illumination (BHANJI, 1977). This measure correlated significantly and positively with the plasma concentrations of imipramine and desmethylimipramine. Single oral doses of imipramine and desmethylimipramine (50, 100, and 200 mg) appear to have no effect on the pupil diameter of normal subjects (DIMASCIO et al., 1964). However, LAUBER et al. (1967) reported that single intravenous 25 mg doses of imipramine resulted in pupillary dilatation but that amitriptyline (10 mg) caused constriction.

Amplitude of accommodation and pupillary size were measured before and during therapy with nortriptyline, 25–50 mg three times a day, in 41 depressed in-patients ranging in age from 20 to 72 years (ASBERG and GERMANIS, 1972). Subjective complaints of blurred vision occurred in 7 patients but were not related to objective changes in accommodation. In younger patients amplitude of accommodation was somewhat decreased and this decrease correlated positively with plasma nortriptyline concentrations. Accommodation was unaffected in the older patients. Pupillary size showed no change in any patients.

IV. Cardiovascular Changes

Tachycardia and hypotension, which may be postural, are clinically well-recognized side-effects of the tricyclic antidepressants. As well as directly affecting the myocardium, the tricyclic antidepressants also inhibit the carotid and orthostatic vasopressor reflexes.

GERSHON et al. (1962) investigated the effects of imipramine (3 mg/kg/day) on a variety of psychiatric patients but did not include any depressives in their sample. Pulse rate was increased but no blood pressure changes were reported. FINK et al. (1964) administered imipramine (maximum dose 300 mg/day) or chlorpromazine to 144 psychiatric patients of whom a quarter were depressed and observed an increase in blood pressure during the course of treatment with imipramine. This finding, however, may have derived from the preponderance of schizophrenics in the sample. BLUMBERG et al. (1964) analyzed blood pressure changes in relation to age, initial levels, and diagnosis. Imipramine increased the mean systolic pressure of the schizophrenics, but, similar to placebo, was associated with a slight fall in that of the depressives. The effect on blood pressure was less marked in the elderly and in patients with high pretreatment levels. BHANJI (1977) recorded no significant changes in pulse rate amongst imipramine-treated depressives. However, the sitting and standing blood pressures fell during the first week, leveled out and then tended to rise during the fourth week of treatment. The standing systolic pressure correlated negatively but weakly with the plasma imipramine concentration. ZIEGLER et al. (1977) administered 50–150 mg nortriptyline at night to 17 depressives for at least 3 weeks. There was a highly significant increase in pulse rate and a weak positive correlation between change in heart rate and plasma nortriptyline concentration. This finding contrasts with that of FREYSCHUSS et al. (1970) who reported no significant relationship between plasma nortriptyline concentration and heart-rate changes in 40 depressed patients treated with 50 mg three times a day for 3 weeks.

HEIMANN et al. (1968) administered single doses of imipramine (75 mg), opipramol (75 mg), perphenazine (10 mg), and placebo to normal subjects. Apart from an increase in blood pressure one hour after imipramine, no cardiovascular changes were observed. IDESTROM and CADENIUS (1964) administered 25 mg and 50 mg doses of imipramine and desmethylimipramine to normal subjects: the former drug had no effect on pulse and blood pressure after 1 and 3 h, the latter was followed by a tachycardia. Normal subjects receiving imipramine 25 mg three times a day developed a tachycardia and moderate hypertension following a test dose of 50 mg after 1 and 2 weeks. On standing up, the tachycardia increased but the blood pressure fell. DIMASCIO et al. (1964), using higher doses of these drugs (50, 100, and 200 mg), also reported a tachycardia following single doses of desmethylimipramine.

In spite of the value of forearm blood flow as an objective correlate of anxiety and agitation, only one study has examined the effects of antidepressants on it. THORSTRAND and LINDBLAD (1976) infused amitriptyline into the left brachial arteries of normal subjects and detected an increase in forearm blood flow. Four dosage levels were employed: 0.05, 0.10, 0.15, and 0.20 mg/min for 5 min. At doses over 0.10 mg/min the effects on blood flow were dose-related. No changes in heart rate, blood pressure, and blood flow in the contralateral forearm were detected.

V. Salivation Rate

In spite of the difficulty in controlling for such factors as appetite, diet, smoking habits, facial mobility, and oral hygiene, it is generally accepted that saliva output is diminished in endogenous depression. It is well recognized also that patients receiving tricyclic antidepressants frequently complain of a dry mouth, and widely assumed that this effect derives from the anticholinergic actions of these drugs. However, PALMAI et al. (1967) have suggested that a direct effect on the salivation centres cannot be ruled out.

PALMAI et al. (1967) recorded saliva flow before and during treatment of depressive illness. Patients treated with ECT showed a steady return to normal salivation flow rates. In contrast, the salivation rates of imipramine-treated patients fell during the first week of treatment (200 mg/day) and then increased. LOEW and KOENIG (1967) administered imipramine, amitriptyline, and dibenzepine to depressed patients: all three inhibited salivation. After completion of treatment whole-mouth salivation rates and clinical improvement did not correlate but the former bore an inverse relationship to the pretreatment level of salivation. A more recent study compared the effects of ECT and antidepressant drugs on whole mouth and parotid gland secretion in depressed patients (BOLWIG and RAFAELSEN, 1972). The antidepressant drugs (unfortunately not specified) reduced whole-mouth saliva flow but not that from the parotid gland alone. The authors acknowledge, however, that parotid secretion may have been artificially enhanced by mechanical stimulation during measurement of whole-mouth salivation. Finally, BHANJI (1977) found that whole-mouth saliva flow was reduced during the first 4 days of imipramine treatment and remained low. The correlations between salivation rate and plasma imipramine and desmethylimipramine concentrations were negative and highly significant. In contrast, the correlations between saliva flow and depression scores were positive and barely significant.

BLACKWELL et al. (1972) investigated the effects of imipramine on salivation rates in normal subjects. Following single 100 mg doses, reduction in saliva flow was maximal after 3 h and persisted for 72 h. A multidose study using placebo, 25 mg, 50 mg, and 100 mg doses of imipramine established a logarithmic dose-response curve.

D. Psychological Effects

Many depressed patients perform poorly on tests of intellect, psychomotor ability, and memory. However, the existence of a psychological deficit specific to endogenous depression has not been established. The prevailing view is that such impairment derives from depressive symptoms such as low motivation, poor confidence, and lack of concentration. Hence the need for caution in assessing the cause of altered psychological performance during the course of treatment. Similarly, in assessing the effects of antidepressant drugs on the psychological abilities of normal subjects it must be borne in mind that a number of them include drowsiness, visual disturbances, and tremor amongst their side-effects.

PISHKIN (1962) treated 52 depressed chronic schizophrenics with imipramine or nialamide (maximum dosage of both drugs 400 mg) for 6 weeks. Nialamide was associated with improved performance on a continuous performance task (a measure of sustained attention) and shortened the visual choice reaction time (a measure of the rapidity with which subjects can respond in a specified fashion depending on which visual stimulus is presented). Imipramine did not affect the performance on either test. By contrast GERSHON et al. (1962) found a trend toward a general improvement in psychological performance amongst their sample of schizophrenics, nonschizophrenic psychotics (not including depressives), and neurotics who received imipramine 3 mg/

kg/day for 3 weeks. In two further studies concerning heterogeneous psychiatric populations, this time including depressives, 6 weeks of imipramine impaired hand coordination and arithmetic ability (FINK et al., 1964; POLLACK et al., 1964). In an early clinical trial, KENNING et al. (1960) compared the effects of imipramine and placebo on patients with neurotic and psychotic depression. Over half the patients studied completed the digit symbol substitution test (a measure of coding and associative ability as well as psychomotor speed), a word naming task, and two tests of motor speed and precision. After a month's treatment, the performance of the imipramine-treated group had improved more than that of patients receiving placebo, but this difference was not statistically significant. Unfortunately no information is given as to the diagnoses of the patients actually involved in the psychological tests nor as regards the relationship between therapeutic outcome and improved performance. WITTENBORN et al. (1962) reported that for a sample of depressed patients, imipramine (up to 200 mg/day) was the most effective antidepressant agent but had the same effect on various psychological tests as placebo and ECT. However, no psychological data were presented and the patients were reported as being in the main neurotically depressed. FRIEDMAN et al. (1966) investigated psychotic depressives and reported that imipramine (maximum dose 300 mg/day) had little effect on either clinical state or performance on a battery of 23 psychological tests. Nevertheless, those changes that were observed suggested that imipramine may improve psychomotor functioning. More recently, LEGG and STIFF (1976) investigated the effects of 3 weeks' treatment with chlorpromazine, imipramine (mean dose 275 mg/day), or placebo on patients with the symptom of depression but drawn from a variety of diagnostic categories. Imipramine impaired performance on the digit symbol substitution test and reduced the performance intelligence quotient (a composite measure of visuomotor, as opposed to verbal or numerical ability). Visual and auditory reaction times were unaffected as was tapping rate (a test of sustained psychomotor speed). BHANJI and LADER (1977) found that imipramine-treated depressives had improved visual choice reaction time, tapping speed, Gibson maze time (a measure of psychomotor speed and accuracy), digit symbol substitution score, symbol copying score (a means of recording copying speed and accuracy,) and digit cancellation time (which measures attention and psychomotor speed). No changes occurred with respect to simple auditory reaction times, nor in the number of errors made on the choice reaction time, Gibson maze, and digit cancellation tests. The improved psychological performance closely paralleled clinical improvement, but was also related to the plasma imipramine concentrations.

HENRY et al. (1973) specifically investigated the effect of imipramine (100–250 mg daily) on memory and learning, and LEGG and STIFF (1976) and BHANJI and LADER (1977) included a memory test amongst their psychological measures. HENRY et al. (1973) found learning ability and memory to be impaired in depressed patients and to fail to improve in spite of recovery from the illness. LEGG and STIFF (1976) found imipramine adversely affected verbal and logical memory, whereas BHANJI and LADER (1977) reported no effect on their test of memory storage.

The level of arousal is reflected in any test requiring attention and speed. A more direct measure of arousal is the flicker fusion threshold (FFT) – the minimum frequency at which separate flashes of light are perceived as continuous. In states of heightened arousal the FFT is increased. BLACK et al's (1975) finding that amitriptyline (25 mg i.v.) increased the FFT of four severely depressed patients was unexpected in view of amitriptyline's sedative effects and may have been due to pupillary dilatation increasing the area of retinal illumination (TURNER, 1975).

Single 200 mg doses of imipramine resulted in drowsiness and also impaired the performance of normal subjects on tests of arithmetic, coding, and psychomotor ability (DIMASCIO et al., 1964). However, desmethylimipramine and lower doses of imipramine had no such effect. IDESTROM and CADENIUS (1964) reported that 25 mg and 50 mg doses of these drugs did not alter the FFT, reaction time, and tests of psychomotor speed, attention, and coordination. Weekly 50 mg doses of imipramine were followed by a reduction in FFT when given to subjects taking imipramine 25 mg thrice daily. The view that single doses of antidepressant drugs have minimal effects on psychological test scores received further support from HEIMANN et al. (1968) who investigated the effects of 75 mg imipramine, 75 mg opipramol, and 10 mg perphenazine. In contrast to the above, 2 weeks of medication with imipramine 25 mg four times a day reduced visual reaction time (KEELER et al. 1966) and it was suggested that this might follow an increase in alertness. The possibility that imipramine might enhance psychomotor performance was raised also by BHANJI (1977) who reported that a dose of 0.67 mg/kg increased the score on the symbol copying test and reduced the time taken to complete a digit cancellation task. Higher (1.0 mg/kg) doses, however, impaired performance on these tests and also on a memory test.

Because of differences in the types of patients studied and the dosages administered to the normal subjects, it is difficult to draw any conclusions regarding the effects of antidepressants on psychological performance. Where effects have been demonstrated it is likely that these reflect either clinical changes or drug side-effects, especially drowsiness, rather than a direct effect of the drug in question.

E. Conclusions

Of the various goals set in the study of the physiological and psychological effects of antidepressant drugs, few are even in sight, let alone near attainment. Thus, the mode of action of these compounds, both tricyclic and MAOI, seems most likely to be elucidated in biochemical rather than physiological or behavioral terms. The concomitants of depression are not clearly established, as witnessed by the total lack of any diagnostic laboratory tests for this condition. Objective measures are not available for the prediction of therapeutic outcome and it is still very difficult to identify potential responders and nonresponders. Only in two areas is the outlook promising. Firstly, in evaluating the unwanted side-effects of antidepressant medication, objective measures of autonomic effects on glandular, ocular, and other functions add some worthwhile precision. Secondly, some psychological tests appear to be useful monitors of the patient's psychiatric progress.

Such limited progress is not unexpected. Depression is a complex topic – symptom, syndrome, and illness – and its biologic substrate remains largely unknown. The antidepressant drugs, both tricyclic and MAOI, were discovered and developed largely by accident and their pharmacologic effects were only established later. They are also complex drugs, with many actions in the body. It is not surprising that the physiological and behavioral effects of these drugs in depressed patients should be poorly documented and imperfectly elucidated.

References

Alexander, L.: Effects of psychotropic drugs on conditional responses in man. In: Neuropsychopharmacology, Vol 2, Rothlin, E. (ed.) pp. 93–123 Amsterdam: Elsevier Publ. Comp. 1961

Andermann, K., Fink, M.: EEG changes on acute and chronic administration of chlorpromazine and imipramine. Electroenceph. Clin. Neurophysiol. *15*, 133 (1963)

Asberg, M., Germanis, M.: Ophthalmological effects of nortriptyline: relationship to plasma level. Pharmacology *7*, 349–356 (1972)

Bhanji, S.: The clinical, physiological and psychological effects of imipramine in depressed inpatients and normal subjects. M.D. thesis, Univ. of London (1977)

Bhanji, S., Lader, M.: The electroencephalographic and psychological effects of imipramine in depressed patients. Eur. J. Clin. Pharmacol. *12*, 349–354 (1977)

Black, S., Franklin, L.M., De Silva, F.P.R., Wijewickrama, H.S.D.S.: The flicker-fusion threshold in schizophrenia and depression. N. Z. Med. J., *81*, 244–246 (1975)

Blackwell, B., Lipkin, J.O., Meyer, J.H., Kuzma, R., Boulter, W.V.: Dose responses and relationship between anticholinergic activity and mood with tricyclic antidepressants. Psychopharmacology *25*, 205–217 (1972)

Blumberg, A.G., Klein, D.F., Pollack, M.: Effects of chlorpromazine and imipramine on systolic blood pressure in psychiatric patients: relationship to age, diagnosis and initial blood pressure. J. Psychiatr. Res. *2*, 51–60 (1964)

Bolwig, T.G., Rafaelsen, O.J.: Salivation in affective disorders. Psychol. Med. *2*, 232–238 (1972)

Borenstein, P., Dabbah, M.: Action du Tofranil (G. 22. 355) sur l'electroencephalogramme. Ann. Med. Psychol. *117*, 1, 923–931 (1959)

Davison, K.: EEG activation after intravenous amitriptyline. Electroencephalogr. Clin. Neurophysiol. *19*, 298–300 (1965)

Delay, J., Verdeaux, G. and J., Mordret, M., Quetin, A.M.: Controle E.E.G. due traitment par le G 22355 (Tofranil). Rev. Neurol. *102*, 345–355 (1960).

Dimascio, A., Heninger, G., Klerman, G.L.: Psychopharmacology of imipramine and desipramine: a comparative study of their effects in normal males. Psychopharmacologia *5*, 361–371 (1964)

Fink, M.: Electroencephalographic and behavioral effects of Tofranil. Can. Psychiatr. Assoc. J. *4*, S166–S171 (1959)

Fink, M.: Quantitative EEG and human psychopharmacology. In: Applications of electroencephalography in psychiatry, pp. 226–240 N. Carolina: Duke University Press 1965

Fink, M., Itil, T.M.: EEG and human psychopharmacology: clinical antidepressants. In: Psychopharmacology, a review of progress 1957–1967. Efron, D.M. (ed.) pp 671–682 Washington, D.C.: U.S. Govt. Printing Office 1968

Fink, M., Pollack, M., Klein, D.F., Blumberg, A.G., Belmont, I., Karp, E., Kramer, J.C., Willner, A.: Comparative studies of chlorpromazine and imipramine. I. Drug discriminating patterns. In: Neuropsychopharmacology, Vol 3, Bradley, P.B., Flugel, F., Hoch, P., (eds.)., pp 370–372 Amsterdam. Excerpta Medica Foundation 1964

Freyschuss, U., Sjoqvist, F., Tuck, D.: Tyramine pressor effects in man before and during treatment with nortriptyline or ECT: correlations between plasma levels and effects of nortriptyline. Pharmacol. Clin. *2*, 72–78 (1970)

Friedman, A.S., Granick, S., Cohen, H.W., Cowitz, B.: Imipramine (Tofranil) vs. placebo in hospitalised psychotic depressives (a comparison of patient's self-ratings, psychiatrists' ratings and psychological test scores). J. Psychiatr. Res. *4*, 13–36 (1966)

Gershon, S., Holmberg, G., Mattsson, E., Mattsson, N., Marshall, A.: Imipramine hydrochloride, its effect on clinical, autonomic and psychological functions. Arch. Gen. Psychiat. *6*, 96–101 (1962)

Heimann, H., Reed, C.F., Witt, P.N.: Some observations suggesting preservation of skilled motor acts despite drug induced stress. Psychopharmacologia *13*, 287–298 (1968)

Henry, G.M., Weingartner, H., Murphy, D.L.: Influence of affective states and psychoactive drugs on verbal learning and memory. Am. J. Psychiatry *130*, 966–971 (1973)

Idestrom, C-M., Cadenius, B.: Imipramine – desmethylimipramine: pharmacological study on human beings. Psychopharmacology *5*, 431–439 (1964)

Itil, T.M., Shapiro, D.M., Fink, M., Kiremitci, N., Hickman, C.: Quantitative EEG studies of chlordiazepoxide, chlorpromazine and imipramine in volunteer and schizophrenic subjects. In: The psychopharmacology of the normal human. Evans, W.O., Kline, N.S., (eds.), pp. 231–241 Springfield: Charles C. Thomas 1969

Keeler, M.H., Prange, A.J., Reifler, C.R.: Efforts of imipramine and thioridazine on set and attention. Dis. Nerv. Syst. 27, 798–802 (1966)

Kenning, I.S., Richardson, N.L., Tucker, F.G.: The treatment of depressive states with imipramine hydrochloride. Can. Psychiatr. Assoc. J. 5, 60–64 (1960)

Kiloh, L.G., Davison, K., Osselton, J.W.: An electroencephalographic study of the analeptic effects of imipramine. Electroenceph. Clin. Neurophysiol. 13, 216–223 (1961)

Lauber, H., Hartmann, R., Herman, D.: The effects of tranquillisers and thymoleptic drugs on the human pupil. German Medical Monthly (Stuttgart) 12, 232–234 (1967)

Lecompte, G., Fadeville, A., Alcalay, R.: Paralelle clinique et electroencephalographique au cours du traitement de 14 syndromes melancholiques par l'imipramine. Ann. Med. Psychol. 121, 1, 246–251 (1963)

Legg, J.F., Stiff, M.P.: Drug-related test patterns of depressed patients. Psychopharmacology, 50, 205–210 (1976)

Loew, D., Koenig, U.: Salivation in depressed patients: a means to evaluate drug-patient evaluations. In: Neuropsychopharmacology. Brill, H., Cole, J.O., Deniker, P., Hippius, H., Bradley, P.B., (eds.), p. 1211 Amsterdam: Exerpta Medica Foundation 1967

Palmai, G., Blackwell, B., Maxwell, A.E., Morgenstern, F.: Patterns of salivary flow in depressive illness and during treatment. Br. J. Psychiatry 113, 1297–1308 (1967)

Pishkin, V.: CPT and VCRT performances as functions of imipramine and nialamide. J. Clin. Psychol. 18, 83–86 (1962)

Pollack, M., Karp, E., Belmont, I., Willner, A., Klein, D.F., Fink, M.: Comparative studies of chlorpromazine and imipramine II: psychological performance profiles. In: Neuropsychopharmacology. Bradley, P.B., Flugel, F., Hoch, P., (eds.), pp. 373–376. Amsterdam: Excerpta medica foundation 1964

Saletu, B., Saletu, M., Itil, M.: Effect of tricyclic antidepressants on the somatosensory evoked potential in man. Psychopharmacologia 29, 1–12 (1973)

Shagass, C., Schwarz, M., Amadeo, M.: Some drug effects on evoked cerebral potentials in man. J. Neuropsychiatry 3, S49–S58 (1962)

Shagass, C., Straumanis, J.J., Overton, D.A.: Effects of lithium and amitriptyline therapy on somatosensory evoked responses. Psychopharmacologia 29, 185–196 (1973)

Thorstrand, C., Lindblad, L.E.: The effect of amitriptyline on forearm blood flow. Scand. J. Clin. Lab. Invest. 36, 17–21 (1976)

Turner, P.: Flicker fusion threshold in mental illness. N. Z. Med. J. 82, 98 (1975)

Wittenborn, J.R., Plante, M., Burgess, F., Maurer, H.: A comparison of imipramine, electroconvulsive therapy and placebo in treatment of depressions. J. Nerv. Ment. Dis. 135, 131–137 (1962)

Zappoli, R.: Electroencephalographic study of patients affected by depressive states treated with imipramine hydrochloride (iminodibenzylderivative G 22355 - Tofranil). Electroenceph. Clin. Neurophysiol. 11, 849 (1959)

Ziegler, V.E., Bun, T.C., Biggs, J.T.: Plasma nortriptyline levels and ECG findings. Am. J. Psychiatry 134, 441–443 (1977)

Pharmacology and Toxicology of Lithium

M. Schou

Lithium is distinguished by its therapeutic action in mania and its prophylactic action in recurrent manic-depressive disorder of the bipolar and unipolar type. By prophylactic action is meant the ability to attenuate or prevent manic and depressive recurrences. Lithium has a relatively low therapeutic index, and knowledge of its pharmacology and toxicology is important for safe and effective usage.

A. Human Data, Animal Data, in Vitro Data

The clinical pharmacology and toxicology of lithium (lithium ions, lithium salts) can be studied only in man. Animal work and in vitro experiments may, however, provide useful information about mechanisms, provided the interpretation of such data takes into account the experimental conditions. It is, for example, unlikely that useful information can be obtained from studies in which lithium, substituted partly or completely for sodium in the medium, is present in a concentration of 50–150 mM when, during lithium treatment of patients, even in cases of poisoning, lithium concentrations in serum and tissues do not exceed 10 mM or mmol/kg wet weight.

The duration of the experiments is of importance. Acute and chronic lithium administration may produce entirely different effects as shown by brain amine concentration and turnover (CORRODI et al., 1967, 1969; GENEFKE, 1972), liver glycogen concentration (PLENGE et al., 1970; OLESEN and THOMSEN, 1974), thirst and urine flow (THOMSEN, 1970), and thyroid iodide transport and metabolism (BERENS and WOLFF, 1975). The way lithium is administered to the animals also plays a role. Intraperitoneal and subcutaneous injections lead to high concentration peaks but administration with food produces almost constant serum lithium levels and consequent differences in biologic effects (OLESEN et al., 1976). Further, the electrolyte composition of the food is important. It is possible to maintain rats for a long time at serum lithium levels as high as 1.0–1.5 mM, if they are given a free choice between water and a hypertonic (0.46 M) sodium chloride solution (THOMSEN, 1973; THOMSEN et al., 1974; THOMSEN and OLESEN, 1974). Addition of potassium to the food counteracts the development of polyuria, prevents poisoning, and serves to maintain health and normal growth of rats given high lithium doses (THOMSEN and OLESEN, 1974; OLESEN et al., 1975; OLESEN and THOMSEN, 1976).

B. Pharmacokinetics

Lithium is not metabolized. Its pharmacokinetics are determined solely by absorption, distribution, and excretion. Use of sustained-release tablets leads to slower absorption, attenuation of serum lithium variations, and reduction of side effects (AM-

Disen, 1975; Grof et al., 1976; Tyrer et al., 1976; Persson, 1977). The apparent distribution volume of lithium is about 70% of the body weight. Under steady-state conditions serum and tissue lithium levels are determined by intake and elimination. The latter takes place almost exclusively through the kidneys. Factors which influence renal lithium clearance are, therefore, of paramount importance for the safe use of lithium.

C. Renal Elimination and Mechanism of Poisoning

Lithium is filtered freely through the glomerular membrane. Eighty per cent of the filtered load is reabsorbed with sodium and water in the proximal tubules. Little or no lithium is reabsorbed distally, and the remaining 20% is therefore excreted. Under ordinary circumstances the excretion fraction is accordingly about 0.20 (Thomsen and Schou, 1968).

Lithium poisoning may be caused by (1) intake of a large single dose, e. g., with suicidal intent, or (2) reduction of the renal lithium clearance without corresponding reduction of the lithium dosage. The renal lithium clearance may be reduced as a result of kidney disease, sodium deficiency, or dehydration.

Manifest or threatening sodium deficiency is accompanied by a compensatory increase of the renal reabsorption of sodium and hence of the proximal reabsorption of lithium. This leads to a fall in the lithium clearance and a rise of the serum lithium concentration. When the kidneys are exposed to lithium concentrations above a critical level, the lithium clearance is reduced further, and a vicious circle is started, which may lead to grave intoxication, possibly death (Thomsen et al., 1974, 1976; Thomsen, 1976). The following circumstances may produce sodium deficiency with consequent lowering of the lithium clearance and risk of intoxication: (1) intake of a sodium-poor diet, (2) slimming diet without additional salt, (3) treatment with diuretics, (4) extrarenal sodium loss, (5) intercurrent disease, (6) rise of the serum lithium concentration above a certain critical level. This critical level varies with the sodium intake and with the factors that determine the minimum sodium requirement of the organism (Thomsen and Schou, 1973; Petersen et al., 1974; Thomsen et al., 1976; Thomsen and Olesen, 1978).

Whereas sodium deficiency affects primarily the lithium clearance, dehydration influences the glomerular filtration rate and leads to parallel decreases of the creatinine clearance and the lithium clearance. Many patients with impending lithium intoxication suffer from lithium-induced polyuria; in their slightly muddled state they fail to drink enough and become dehydrated with consequent impairment of kidney function, lowering of the lithium excretion, and aggravation of the poisoning (Hansen et al., 1976).

Lithium poisoning affects in the first line the central nervous system and the kidneys (Schou et al., 1968; Hansen and Amdisen, 1975). The patients are often comatose with increased muscle tone and hyperactive tendon reflexes. Epileptiform seizures may be seen. In a few cases cerebellar disturbances have been observed as lasting aftereffects (Hartitzsch et al., 1972; Juul-Jensen and Schou, 1973; Hansen and Amdisen, 1975). Lithium poisoning may lead to death in acute renal failure. Treatment is partly supportive and corrective (electrolyte and fluid balance, pulmonary function, infection prophylaxis, etc.) and partly aims at removing lithium from the body. In all but the mildest cases hemodialysis is advisable (HANSEN and AMDISEN, 1975; PEDERSEN and SVENDSEN, 1976).

D. Adverse Effects

I. Neuromuscular System

Lithium treatment may produce hand tremor (often relieved by β receptor blocking agents), EEG-changes, muscle hypertonicity or rigidity, and muscle fatigue. A few cases of myasthenia gravis have developed during lithium administration (NEIL et al., 1976; GRANACHER, 1977; VOETMANN, 1977).

II. Mind

Lithium effects on the normal mind are inconspicuous. Patients occasionally complain of tiredness, memory impairment, and lowered libido and potency. In some cases the disturbances may have been caused by depressive relapse or undiagnosed myxedema. Successful lithium prophylaxis may initially lead to problems of readjustment for patient and family and to a lowering, usually temporary, of creative power (SCHOU and BAASTRUP, 1973).

III. Heart

T-wave changes, ventricular arrhythmias, sinus node abnormality, atrioventricular block, and myocarditis have been reported during lithium treatment. The role played by lithium is not always clear, and cardiac complaints do not play any significant role in lithium treatment.

IV. Thyroid

Goiter and myxedema occasionally develop in lithium-treated patients, and cases of hyperthyroidism have recently been reported (BROWNLIE et al., 1976; BAFAQEEH and MYERS, 1976; CUBITT, 1976; CHAUDHRI and BEBBINGTON, 1977; SPAULDING et al., 1977). Among several effects of lithium on the thyroid, inhibition of hormone release seems the most important. Treatment with thyroxine concurrently with lithium invariably leads to disappearance of goiter and myxedema. One should note the risk that mild myxedema may be taken for a depressive relapse and treated accordingly with adverse results.

V. Kidneys

Polyuria and polydipsia are the most frequent renal side effects. Primary polydipsia may play a role, but lack of response to ADH seems to be the main factor; other mechanisms have been proposed. Refractoriness to ADH may be partial or complete. It is not known why some patients develop polyuria/polydipsia while others do not, but the lithium preparation and the administration pattern may play a role (OLESEN et al., 1976).

Lithium-induced polyuria/polydipsia occasionally respond to treatment with DDAVP, a vasopressin analog (Sørensen et al., 1973; Widerlöv et al., 1977). Treatment with diuretics seems more effective but is not without danger due to the lowering effect on the renal lithium clearance. Polyuria and polydipsia usually disappear after discontinuation of lithium, but cases are known in which the concentrating ability of the kidneys had not yet become normal 1–2 years after discontinuation of lithium (Simon et al., 1977).

Morphologic changes have recently been found in the kidneys of lithium-treated patients (Hestbech et al., 1977); they involve nephron atrophy and interstitial fibrosis. The 13 patients examined had all had previous lithium intoxications or suffered from lithium-induced impairment of renal concentrating ability or both. It is not clear whether patients not presenting these features may also show morphologic kidney changes. The functional and prognostic significance of the findings is at present under investigation.

VI. Skin

Lithium treatment may produce or aggravate various skin complaints, primarily acne and psoriasis. In the latter condition, lithium may act through inhibition of adenyl cyclase and further lowering of the already too low concentration of cyclic AMP in the psoriatic plaques (Voorhees et al., 1975).

VII. Body Weight

Weight gain during lithium treatment is fairly frequent and may have several causes. One is that polydipsic patients quench their thirst with drinks with a high content of calories (Vendsborg et al., 1976), but other mechanisms may be involved. Weight loss can be achieved under intake of slimming diets, but the patients should take extra salt to avoid lowering of the lithium clearance.

VIII. Edema

Transitory edema formation is not of great importance in itself, but it may lead to increased risk of lithium poisoning if treated incautiously with diuretic drugs.

E. Teratogenicity

The International Register of Lithium Babies at present contains records of 189 children (Schou and Weinstein, 1977). A "lithium baby" is a child born to a mother who was given lithium during the first trimester of the pregnancy. Among the lithium babies reported, 20 had malformations, 15 malformations involving the heart and the large vessels, 5 malformations involving other organ systems. The smallness of the material and the possibility that abnormal cases are overreported render definitive interpretation of the data difficult. However, the high relative frequency of cardiovascular malformations indicates that it is advisable for female patients to avoid lithium treatment during the first trimester of pregnancy. Lithium babies who are not malformed at birth do not seem to be at higher risk of somatic or mental anomalies than children in a control group consisting of their siblings (Schou, 1976e).

F. Lactation

Lithium passes from the blood into the milk, and the nursing infants' serum concentration is one-tenth to one-half of the mother's (SCHOU and AMDISEN, 1973; SYKES et al., 1976). The advisability of bottle-feeding rather than breast-feeding is the subject of debate.

G. Interaction with Other Drugs

The most important interaction clinically is that between diuretics and lithium, which was mentioned above. Combination of lithium with neuroleptics may slightly increase the incidence of side effects, particularly tremor (DEGKWITZ et al., 1976). Neurotoxicity resulting from the combined use of lithium and haloperidol has been reported in some cases (MARHOLD et al., 1974; COHEN and COHEN, 1974; THORNTON and PRAY, 1975; LOUDON and WARING, 1976), but usually drug doses were high, and examination of extensive series of patients treated with the combination has not revealed serious complications (BAASTRUP et al., 1976; JUHL et al., 1977).

Administration of antidepressant drugs together with lithium may offer therapeutic or prophylactic advantage. Adverse interaction seems limited to the appearance of extrapyramidal symptoms not seen with either drug given alone (MÜLLER and KRÜGER, 1975; GABRIEL et al., 1976).

Lithium may prolong the effect of neuromuscular blocking agents (BORDEN et al., 1974; HILL et al., 1976, 1977; REIMHERR et al., 1977), but the clinical significance of this is unclear. Experiments on humans and animals have shown interaction between lithium and a number of centrally acting drugs: morphine, codeine, dextropropoxyphene, reserpine, amphetamine, and alcohol. Interactions have not led to clinical side effects.

H. Literature

Reviews of the pharmacology, toxicology, and side effects of lithium, and bibliographies on its biology and pharmacology have been published by SCHOU (1969, 1972, 1976 a, b, c, d, 1977), GERSHON and SHOPSIN (1973), JOHNSON (1975), JEFFERSON and GREIST (1977), and AMDISEN and SCHOU (1978).

Manuscript completed December 1977.

References

Amdisen, A.: Sustained release preparations of lithium. In: Lithium Research and Therapy. Johnson, F.N. (ed). London, New York, San Francisco: Academic Press 1975

Amdisen, A., Schou, M.: Lithium. Side effects of Drugs Annual 2, 17–29 (1978)

Baastrup, P.C., Hollnagel, P., Sørensen, R., Schou, M.: Adverse reactions in treatment with lithium carbonate and haloperidol. J. Am. Med. Assoc. 236, 2645–2646 (1976)

Bafaqeeh, H.H., Myers, D.H.: Lithium and thyrotoxicosis. Lancet I, 1409 (1976)

Berens, S.C., Wolff, J.: The endocrine effects of lithium. In: Lithium Research and Therapy. Johnson, F.N. (ed.). London, New York, San Francisco: Academic Press 1975

Borden, H., Clarke, M.T., Katz, M.: The use of pancuronium bromide in patients receiving lithium carbonate. Can. Anaesth. Soc. J. 21, 79–82 (1974)

Brownlie, B.E.W., Chambers, S.T., Sadler, W.A., Donald, R.A.: Lithium associated thyroid disease – a report of 14 cases of hypothyroidism and 4 cases of thyrotoxicosis. Aust. N.Z.J. Med. *6*, 223–229 (1976)

Chaudhri, M.A., Bebbington, P.E.: Lithium therapy and ophthalmic Graves' disease. Br. J. Psychiatr. *130*, 420 (1977)

Cohen, W.J., Cohen, N.H.: Lithium carbonate, haloperidol, and irreversible brain damage. J. Am. Med. Assoc. *230*, 1283–1297 (1974)

Corrodi, H., Fuxe, K., Hökfelt, T., Schou, M.: The effect of lithium on cerebral monoamine neurons. Psychopharmacology *11*, 345–353 (1967)

Corrodi, H., Fuxe, K., Hökfelt, T., Schou, M.: The effect of prolonged lithium administration on cerebral monoamine neurons in the rat. Life Sci. *8*, 643–652 (1969)

Cubitt, T.: Lithium and thyrotoxicosis. Lancet *I*, 1247–1248 (1976)

Degkwitz, R., Consbruch, U., Haddenbrock, S., Neusch, B., Oehlert, W., Unsöld, T.: Therapeutische Risiken bei der Langzeitbehandlung mit Neuroleptika und Lithium. Klinische, histol ogische und biochemische Befunde. Nervenarzt *47*, 81–87 (1976)

Gabriel, E., Karobath, M., Lenz, G.: Extrapyramidale Symptomatik bei Kombination der Lithiumlangzeittherapie mit Nortriptylin. Ein kasuistischer Beitrag zur Pathogenese-Hypothesenbildung. Nervenarzt *47*, 46–48 (1976)

Genefke, I.K.: The concentration of 5-hydroxytryptamine (5-HT) in hypothalamus, grey and white brain substance in the rat after prolonged oral lithium administration. Acta Psychiatr. Scand. *48*, 400–404 (1972)

Gershon, S., Shopsin, B.: Lithium. Its Role in Psychiatric Research and Treatment. New York, London: Plenum 1973

Granacher, R.P.: Neuromuscular problems associated with lithium. Am. J. Psychiatr. *134*, 702 (1977)

Grof, P., MacCrimmon, D., Saxena, B., Daigle, L., Prior, M.: Bioavailability and side effects of different lithium carbonate products. Neuropsychobiol. *2*, 313–323 (1976)

Hansen, H.E., Amdisen, A.: Acute renal insufficiency in lithium intoxication. Abs. 12th Congr. Eur. Dialysis Transplant Assoc. 223 (1975)

Hansen, H.E., Hestbech, J., Amdisen, A., Olsen, S.: Lithium induced nephrogenic diabetes insipidus associated with chronic renal disease. Abs. 13th Congr. Eur. Dialysis Transplant Assoc. 304 (1976)

Hartitzsch, B. von, Hoenich, N.A., Leigh, R.J., Wilkinson, R., Frost, T.H., Weddel, A., Posen, G.A.: Permanent neurological sequelae despite haemodialysis for lithium intoxication. Br. Med. J. *4*, 757–759 (1972)

Hestbech, J., Hansen, H.E., Amdisen, A., Olsen, S.: Renal lesions following long-term treatment with lithium salts. Kidney Int. *12*, 205–213 (1977)

Hill, G.E., Wong, K.C., Hodges, M.R.: Potentiation of succinylcholine neuromuscular blockade by lithium carbonate. Anesthesiology *44*, 439–442 (1976)

Hill, G.E., Wong, K.C., Hodges, M.R.: Lithium carbonate and neuromuscular blocking agents. Anesthesiology *46*, 122–126 (1977)

Jefferson, J.W., Greist, J.H.: Primer of Lithium Therapy. Baltimore: Williams & Wilkins 1977

Johnson, F.N. (ed.): Lithium Research and Therapy, London, New York, San Francisco: Academic Press 1975

Juhl, R.P., Tsuang, M.T., Perry, P.J.: Concomitant administration of haloperidol and lithium carbonate in acute mania. Dis. Nerv. Syst. *38*, 675–680 (1977)

Juul-Jensen, P., Schou, M.: Permanent brain damage after lithium intoxication. Br. Med. J. *4*, 673 (1973)

Loudon, J.B., Waring, H.: Toxic reactions to lithium and haloperidol. Lancet *II*, 1088 (1976)

Marhold, J., Zimanová, J., Lachman, M., Král, J., Vojtechovský, M.: To the incompatibility of haloperidol with lithium salts. Act. Nerv. Sup. (Praha) *16*, 199–200 (1974)

Müller, D., Krüger, E.: Nebenwirkungen der Lithiumtherapie. Psychiatr. Neurol. Med. Psychol. *27*, 172–180 (1975)

Neil, J.F., Himmelhoch, J.M., Licata, S.L.: Emergence of myasthenia gravis during treatment with lithium carbonate. Arch. Gen. Psychiatr. *33*, 1090–1092 (1976)

Olesen, O.V., Thomsen, K.: Effect of prolonged lithium ingestion on glucagon and parathyroid hormone responses in rats. Acta Pharmacol. Toxicol. (Kbh.) *34*, 225–231 (1974)

Olesen, O.V., Thomsen, K.: A preventive effect of potassium against fatal lithium intoxication in rats. Neuropsychobiol. *2*, 112–117 (1976)

Olesen, O.V., Jensen, J., Thomsen, K.: Effect of potassium on lithium-induced growth retardation and polyuria in rats. Acta Pharmacol. Toxicol. (Kbh.) *36*, 161–171 (1975)

Olesen, O.V., Schou, M., Thomsen, K.: Administration of lithium to rats by different routes. Neuropsychobiol. *2*, 134–138 (1976)

Pedersen, R.S., Svendsen, O.: Lithiumforgiftning behandlet med hæmodialyse. Ugeskr. Læg. *138*, 3325–3327 (1976)

Persson, G.: Lithium side effects in relation to dose and to levels and gradients of lithium in plasma. Acta Psychiatr. Scand. *55*, 208–213 (1977)

Petersen, V., Hvidt, S., Thomsen, K., Schou, M.: The effect of prolonged thiazide treatment on the renal lithium clearance of humans. Br. Med. J. *3*, 143–145 (1974)

Plenge, P., Mellerup, E.T., Rafaelsen, O.J.: Lithium action on glycogen synthesis in rat brain, liver and diaphragm. J. Psychiatr. Res. *8*, 29–36 (1970)

Reimherr, F.W., Hodges, M.R., Hill, G.E., Wong, K.C.: Prolongation of muscle relaxant effects by lithium carbonate. Am. J. Psychiatr. *134*, 205–206 (1977)

Schou, M.: The biology and pharmacology of lithium: A bibliography. Psychopharmacol. Bull. *5*, No. 4, 33–62 (1969)

Schou, M.: A bibliography on the biology and pharmacology of lithium – Appendix I. Psychopharmacol. Bull. *8*, No. 4, 36–62 (1972)

Schou, M.: A bibliography on the biology and pharmacology of lithium – Appendix II. Psychopharmacol. Bull. *12*, No. 1, 49–74, No. 2, 69–83, No. 3, 86–89 (1976a)

Schou, M.: Bibliography on the biology and pharmacology of lithium. 4. Neuropsychobiol. *2*, 161–191 (1976b)

Schou, M.: Advances in lithium therapy. Curr. Psychiatr. Ther. *16*, 139–162 (1976c)

Schou, M.: Pharmacology and toxicology of lithium. Ann. Rev. Pharmacol. *16*, 231–243 (1976d)

Schou, M.: What happened later to the lithium babies? A follow-up study of children born without malformations. Acta Psychiatr. Scand. *54*, 193–197 (1976e)

Schou, M.: Bibliography on the biology and pharmacology of lithium. 5. Neuropsychobiol. *4*, 40–64 (1977)

Schou, M., Amdisen, A.: Lithium and pregnancy – III, Lithium ingestion by children breast-fed by women in lithium treatment. Br. Med. J. *2*, 138 (1973)

Schou, M., Amdisen, A., Trap-Jensen, J.: Lithium poisoning. Am. J. Psychiatr. *125*, 520–527 (1968)

Schou, M., Baastrup, P.C.: Personal and social implications of lithium maintenance treatment. In: Psychopharmacology, Sexual Disorders and Drug Abuse, Ban, T.A., Boissier, I.R., Gessa, G.J., Heimann, H., Hollister, L., Lehmann, H.E., Munkvad, I., Steinberg, H., Sulser, F., Sundwall, A., Vinař, O. (eds.), pp. 65–68. Amsterdam, London: North-Holland 1973 Prague: Avicenum 1973

Schou, M., Weinstein, M.R.: Problems of lithium maintenance treatment during pregnancy, delivery and lactation. Agressologie (in press).

Simon, N.M., Garber, E., Arieff, A.J.: Persistent nephrogenic diabetes insipidus after lithium carbonate. Ann. Intern. Med. *86*, 446–447 (1977)

Sørensen, R., Jensen, J., Mulder, J., Schou, M.: Lithium side effects and their treatment. Polyuria/polydipsia. Acta Psychiatr. Scand., Suppl. *243*, 39 (1973)

Spaulding, S.W., Burrow, G.N., Ramey, J.N., Donabedian, R.K.: Effect of increased iodide intake on thyroid function in subjects on chronic lithium therapy. Acta Endocrinol. *84*, 290–296 (1977)

Sykes, P.A., Quarrie, J., Alexander, F.W.: Lithium carbonate and breast-feeding. Br. Med. J. *4*, 1299 (1976)

Thomsen, K.: Lithium-induced polyuria in rats. Int. Pharmacopsychiatr. *5*, 233–241 (1970)

Thomsen, K.: The effect of sodium chloride on kidney function in rats with lithium intoxication. Acta Pharmacol. Toxicol. (Kbh.) *33*, 92–102 (1973)

Thomsen, K.: Renal elimination of lithium in rats with lithium intoxication. J. Pharmacol. Exp. Ther. *199*, 483–489 (1976)

Thomsen, K., Olesen, O.V.: Long-term lithium administration to rats. Lithium and sodium dosage and administration, avoidance of intoxication, polyuric control rats. Int. Pharmacopsychiatr. *9*, 118–124 (1974)

Thomsen, K., Olesen, O.V.: Precipitating factors and renal mechanisms in lithium intoxication. Gen. Pharmacol. *9*, 85–89 (1978)

Thomsen, K., Schou, M.: Renal lithium excretion in man. Am. J. Physiol. *215*, 823–827 (1968)

Thomsen, K., Schou, M.: The effect of prolonged administration of hydrochlorothiazide on the renal lithium clearance and the urine flow of ordinary rats and rats with diabetes insipidus. Pharmakopsychiatr. *6*, 264–269 (1973)

Thomsen, K., Jensen, J., Olesen, O.V.: Lithium-induced loss of body sodium and the development of severe intoxication in rats. Acta Pharmacol. Toxicol. (Kbh.) *35*, 337–346 (1974)

Thomsen, K., Jensen, J., Olesen, O.V.: Effect of prolonged lithium ingestion on the response to mineralocorticoids in rats. J. Pharmacol. Exp. Ther. *196*, 463–468 (1976)

Thornton, W.E., Pray, B.J.: Lithium intoxication: A report of two cases. Can. Psychiatr. Assoc. J. *20*, 281–282 (1975)

Tyrer, S., Hullin, R.P., Birch, N.J., Goodwin, J.C.: Absorption of lithium following administration of slow-release and conventional preparations. Psychol. Med. *6*, 51–58 (1976)

Vendsborg, P.B., Bech, P., Rafaelsen, O.J.: Lithium treatment and weight gain. Acta Psychiatr. Scand. *53*, 139–147 (1976)

Voetmann, C.: Myastenisk reaktion fremkaldt af lithiumkarbonatbehandling. Ugeskr. Læg. *140*, 2375–2376 (1978)

Voorhees, J.J., Marcelo, C.L., Duell, E.A.: Cyclic AMP, cyclic GMP, and glucocorticoids as potential metabolic regulators of epidermal proliferation and differentiation. J. Invest. Dermatol. *65*, 179–190 (1975)

Widerlöv, E., Sjöström, R., Söderberg, U.: D.D.A.V.P. and lithium-induced polyuria/polydipsia. Lancet *II*, 1080 (1977)

CHAPTER 26

Antipsychotics and Experimental Seizure Models

R. KRETZSCHMAR and H.J. TESCHENDORF

A. Introduction

Shortly after the introduction of chlorpromazine into the therapy of schizophrenic psychosis the occurrence of epileptic fits was observed under that therapy. Since then these side effects were also found with numerous other neuroleptics of the phenothiazine type and with reserpine (BEIN, 1956; SCHENKER and HERBST, 1963). Synoptic papers on the literature compiled by LOGOTHETIS (1967), ITIL (1970), and ITIL and MYERS (1973) mention the incidence of seizures as a clinical side effect of various neuroleptic drug therapies. ITIL also considers the changes of the human EEG induced by neuroleptic drugs. In his papers ITIL hardly deals with findings obtained in animal experiments on the behavior of neuroleptic drugs in seizure models.

The question of a convulsive action of neuroleptics is, however, of interest with regard to potential side effects particularly when administering high doses for the treatment of psychosis. This question is of decisive importance in the treatment of diseases in which there is a combination of psychotic and epileptic symptoms (see SLATER and BEARD, 1963, and DAVISON and BAGLEY, 1968).

Besides the predisposition of the patient and dosage, the chemical structure of the neuroleptic drug is said to play a particular role in the possible incidence of seizures. Clinical experience has shown that there is a greater risk of seizures after administration of phenothiazines with aliphatic side chain than after phenothiazines with piperazinyl side chain (ITIL, 1970; ITIL and MYERS, 1973).

A summary on the influence of neuroleptics upon experimentally induced seizures is so far not available. The survey below deals with the different tricyclic neuroleptic drugs, butyrophenones, and diphenylbutylpiperidines (as well as reserpine, although this substance is probably no longer of significance in antipsychotic therapy).

B. Neuroleptics

The data found in the literature on the effects of neuroleptics on seizures in animal experiments are shown in the Tables. Table 1 gives the findings on electrically induced seizures (minimal and maximal electroshock), Table 2 the findings on pentetrazole (PTZ)-induced seizures, Table 3 the findings on other chemically induced seizures (e. g., nikethamide, picrotoxin, strychnine, nicotine). Table 4 gives the findings on seizures induced by other methods (e. g., audiogenic seizures).

Within each table the neuroleptics are arranged as follows:
Tricyclic compounds
Chlorpromazine
Other phenothiazines with aliphatic side chain

Phenothiazines with piperidyl side chain
Phenothiazines with piperazinyl side chain
Azaphenothiazines and thioxanthenes
Clozapine
Butyrophenones and diphenylbutylpiperidines
Chlorpromazine is the substance most often tested; therefore, it will be discussed in detail in
a separate section.

I. Tricyclic Compounds

1. Chlorpromazine

a) Electroshock (see Table 1)

Chlorpromazine at low dose levels has no effects on tonic extensor seizures in mice
due to maximal electroshock. ED_{50} values can be found only at very high dose levels
[150 mg/kg p. o. according to SCHALLEK et al. (1956), 261 mg/kg p. o. according to
FINK and SWINYARD (1959)]. In the minimal electroshock test TESCHENDORF et al.
(1978) found an ED_{50} of 57 mg/kg. These findings are in compliance with investigations by CHEN and BOHNER (1960) who determined the seizure thresholds. The seizure threshold is elevated only after high doses of chlorpromazine (40 mg/kg i. p. or
more).

In low doses it has a threshold lowering effect on clonic (SWINYARD et al., 1959)
and tonic seizures (TEDESCHI et al., 1958). After oral administration of chlorpromazine
to rats GUJRAL et al. (1956) found an ED_{50} of 23 mg/kg (inhibition of tonic extensor
seizure). Chlorpromazine doses of up to 25 mg/kg s. c. are ineffective according to
other authors (e. g., BERTRAND et al., 1954; MERCIER, 1955).

The threshold for the after-discharge induced by electrical stimulation of the thalamus is decreased by chlorpromazine, the duration is prolonged (DELGADO and MI-
HAILOVIC, 1956; GANGLOFF and MONNIER, 1957; SAYERS, 1979). High doses of chlorpromazine increase the spontaneous seizure discharge in the amygdala (PRESTON,
1956; TAKAGI et al., 1958). In conscious rabbits chlorpromazine (5 mg/kg i. v.) lowers
the threshold for the after-discharge in the hippocampus dors. and in the N. amyg-
dalae; the duration of after-discharge is prolonged and generalization facilitated
(SCHALLEK et al., 1964; KOBAYASHI and ISHIKAWA, 1965; SAYERS, 1979). According to
SAYERS these findings suggest seizure facilitating properties of chlorpromazine.

b) Chemically Induced Seizures

α) Pentetrazole (see Table 2)

As reported by most authors chlorpromazine has no effect on pentetrazole-induced seizures (tonic or clonic) in mice. CHRISTENSEN et al. (1965) and SCHALLEK et
al. (1956) indicate ED_{50} values for a protective effect (50 mg/kg s. c. and 400 mg/kg
p. o.). These values are found at very high dose levels as was also seen in the electroshock test. NIESCHULZ et al. (1955) describe an anticonvulsant effect after intravenous administration of 0.5–10 mg/kg of chlorpromazine, 25 mg/kg having no effect.
In contrast to the electroshock, chlorpromazine in doses of up to 40 mg/kg i. p. elevates the threshold doses of pentetrazole for clonic seizures, higher doses (up to
140 mg/kg) lower the seizure threshold according to CHEN and BOHNER (1960).

In rats chlorpromazine has no effect or intensifies the EEG changes observed after
low pentetrazole doses (ARUSHANIAN and AVAKIAN, 1978).

Table 1. Effects of neuroleptics on electrically induced seizures

Substance	Species	Route of administration (dose mg/kg)	Pretreatment time	Induction of seizures	Parameter measured	Effect	Reference
Chlor-promazine	Mice	p. o.	60 min	Electroshock	Tonic extension	ED_{50}: 150 mg/kg	SCHALLEK et al. (1956)
		p. o. (2–27)	Peak time		Threshold for minimum seizures	Decrease in doses from 9–18 mg/kg	TEDESCHI et al. (1958)
		p. o.	Peak time		Tonic extension	$ED_{50} > 100$ mg/kg	TEDESCHI et al. (1959)
		p. o. (7.5–15)	90 min		Threshold for clonic seizures	Significant decrease	SWINYARD et al. (1959)
		p. o. (up to 60)	90 min		Tonic extension	No effect	SWINYARD et al. (1959)
		p. o.	60–120 min		Tonic extension	Up to ataxic doses no effect	PIALA et al. (1959)
		p. o.	90 min		Tonic extension	ED_{50}: 261 mg/kg	FINK and SWINYARD (1959)
		p. o. (2.15–100)	60 min		Tonic extension	Max. 20% protection	TESCHENDORF et al. (1980)
		p. o.	60 min		Clonic convulsions (minimum electroshock)	ED_{50}: 57 mg/kg	TESCHENDORF et al. (1980)
		i. p. (10–80)	30 min		Threshold for tonic seizures CD_{50} (mA)	10–40 mg/kg: no effect; 60–80 mg/kg: increase of the CD_{50}	CHEN and BOHNER (1960)
		i. p. (1–100)	120 min		Threshold for tonic extension (CD_{50})	3–60 mg/kg: decrease; 100 mg/kg: increase of the CD_{50}	MEYER and MEYER-BURG (1964)

Table 1. (Continued)

Substance	Species	Route of administration (dose mg/kg)	Pretreatment time	Induction of seizures	Parameter measured	Effect	Reference
Chlor-promazine	Mice	i. p. (2–60)	15–30 min	Electroshock	Threshold for tonic seizures CD_{50} (mA)	40–60 mg/kg: increase of the CD_{50}; 2–20 mg/kg: decrease; (pretreatment: diphenylhydantoin or methazolamide)	CHEN et al. (1968)
		i. v. (1–10) s. c.	30 min		Tonic extension Tonic seizures	No effect $ED_{50} \sim 90$ mg/kg	MANIAN et al. (1965) COURVOISIER et al. (1958)
		s. c.			Tonic seizures	$ED_{50} > 50$ mg/kg	CHRISTENSEN et al. (1965)
	Rats	p. o. s. c. (20)	90 min 3 h		Tonic convulsions Tonic seizures	ED_{50}: 23.7 mg/kg No effect	GUJRAL et al. (1956) BERTRAND et al. (1954, 1955)
		s. c. (25)			Threshold for tonic extension	No effect	MERCIER (1955)
		s. c. (10/die)			Threshold	Decrease of the threshold	HEMING et al. (1956)
		s. c. (15)			Tonic extension	No effect	ARRIGONI-MARTELLI and KRAMER (1959)
	Rabbits	i. v. (10)	30–40 min		Clonic seizures	20% protection	BALESTRIERI (1955a, b)
Promazine	Mice	p. o. (6–53)	Peak time		Threshold for minimum seizures	Decrease of the threshold (22–50 mg/kg)	TEDESCHI et al. (1958)
		p. o. (2–20)	60 min		Tonic extension	ED_{50}: 175 mg/kg	FINK and SWINYARD (1959)

Drug	Species			Electroshock			Reference
Promazine	Mice	i. p. (2–20)	30 min		Threshold for tonic extension	2 mg/kg: decrease; 20 mg/kg: increase (pretreatment: diphenylhydantoin 8 mg/kg)	CHEN et al. (1968)
Triflupromazine		p. o. (2–40)	90 min		Tonic extension	ED_{50}: 280 mg/kg	FINK and SWINYARD (1959)
		p. o.	60–120 min		Tonic extension	Up to ataxic doses no effect	PIALA et al. (1959)
		i. p. (2–40)	30 min		Threshold for tonic extension	2 mg/kg: decrease; 40 mg/kg: increase of the threshold (pretreatment: diphenylhydantoin 8 mg/kg)	CHEN et al. (1968)
Thioridazine		p. o. (up to 120)	90 min		Tonic extension	No effect	SWINYARD et al. (1959)
		p. o. (15–30)	90 min		Threshold for clonic seizures	15 mg/kg: decrease of the threshold; 30 mg/kg: no effect	
		p. o. (4.64–147)	60 min		a) Tonic extension b) Clonic convulsions	a) Max. 30% protection b) Max. 30% protection	TESCHENDORF et al. (1980)
Mepazine		i. p. (2.5–10)	60 min		Seizures	No effect	MAJ et al. (1974)
		p. o. (45–224)	Peak time		Threshold for minimum seizures	Decrease of the threshold (112–224 mg/kg)	TEDESCHI et al. (1958)
Perphenazine		i. p. (10, 40)	30 min		Threshold for tonic extension	10 mg/kg: decrease; 40 mg/kg: increase of the threshold (pretreatment: diphenylhydantoin 8 mg/kg)	CHEN et al. (1968)

Table 1. (Continued)

Substance	Species	Route of administration (dose mg/kg)	Pretreatment time	Induction of seizures	Parameter measured	Effect	Reference
Perphenazine	Rats	s. c. (2, 15)		Electroshock	Tonic extension	No effect	ARRIGONI-MARTELLI and KRAMER (1959)
Trifluo-perazine	Mice	p. o. (0.4–33)	Peak time		Threshold for minimum seizures	0.4–17 mg/kg: no effect; 33 mg/kg: decrease (−21%)	TEDESCHI et al. (1958, 1959)
		p. o. (20, 60)	Peak time		Tonic extension	ED$_{50}$: 100 mg/kg	TEDESCHI et al. (1959)
		s. c. (20, 60)	30 min		Threshold for tonic extension	20 mg/kg: decrease; 60 mg/kg: increase of the threshold (pretreatment: diphenylhydan-toin 8 mg/kg)	CHEN et al. (1968)
Prochlor-perazine		p. o. (1.5–18)	Peak time		Threshold for minimum seizures	1.5–6.5 mg/kg: increase of the threshold	TEDESCHI et al. (1958)
Chlorpro-thixen		i. p.			Tonic extension	ED$_{50}$: 11.5 mg/kg	PETERSEN and MØLLER NIELSEN (1964)
		i. p. (0.1–1.6)			Threshold	Decrease of the threshold	PETERSEN and MØLLER NIELSEN (1964)
Clopen-thixol		i. p.			Tonic extension	ED$_{50}$: 32.5 mg/kg	PETERSEN and MØLLER NIELSEN (1964)

Drug	Species	Route (dose)	Time		Parameter	Result	Reference
Clozapine Haloperidol	Mice	i. p. (2–8) p. o. (0.464–10)	60 min 3 h	Electroshock	Seizures a) Tonic extension b) Minimum seizures	No effect a) No effect b) Max. 20% protection	MAJ et al. (1974) TESCHENDORF et al. (1980)
		i. p. (0.1, 15)	30 min		Threshold for tonic extension	0.1 mg/kg: decrease of the threshold (pretreatment: diphenylhydantoin)	CHEN et al. (1968)
		i. p. (0.1)	2–6 h		Threshold for tonic extension	No effect	KILIAN and FREY (1973)
		s. c.			Tonic extension	ED_{50}: 6.0 mg/kg	CHRISTENSEN et al. (1965)
Melperone		p. o.			a) Tonic extension b) Minimum seizures	a) ED_{50}: 83.6 mg/kg b) ED_{50}: 50.3 mg/kg	TESCHENDORF et al. (1978)
		s. c.			Tonic extension	ED_{50}: 11 mg/kg	CHRISTENSEN et al. (1965)

β) Other Chemically Induced Seizures (see Table 3)

In nikethamide seizures chlorpromazine prolongs the time up to the occurrence of seizures, reduces the duration and intensity of seizures and protects the animals (mice and rats) against death.

However, acetaldehyde-induced seizures are potentiated. Low doses of chlorpromazine inhibit procaine or cocaine seizures but have no effect on picrotoxin seizures. Chlorpromazine is very potent in nicotine seizures. All components of the nicotine seizure (clonic, tonic seizures, death) are inhibited at low doses, the tonic seizures being most readily inhibited. The data given concerning strychnine seizures are ambiguous. No effects, potentiation of seizures (NIESCHULZ et al., 1955), and protection against strychnine-induced death (SACRA and McCOLL, 1958) are reported for the low chlorpromazine doses tested. Low doses of chlorpromazine inhibit bicuculline seizures, higher doses potentiate tonic seizures (WORMS and LLOYD, 1978; dose range tested 0.1–10 mg/kg i. p.).

c) Seizures Induced by Other Methods (see Table 4)

Seizures which occur spontaneously in connection with withdrawal syndromes in barbiturate or ethanol dependent animals or which are provoked by additional stimuli, are not influenced or potentiated by chlorpromazine.

Chlorpromazine has an anticonvulsant effect on audiogenic seizures whereby the tonic component of the seizure pattern can be more easily influenced than the symptoms running or jumping.

2. Other Tricyclic Neuroleptics

a) Electroshock (see Table 1)

As was the case with chlorpromazine, these substances are ineffective at the dose levels used to establish the pharmacologic findings typical of neuroleptics. The ED_{50} values, if indicated at all, are very high. Studies of the seizure threshold mostly bring about the same result as with chlorpromazine: small doses lower the seizure threshold, high doses increase it. Trifluoperazine and prochlorperazine are exceptions; TEDESCHI et al. (1958) did not find the seizure threshold lowered but found it increased by these substances.

As with chlorpromazine SAYERS (1979), reports of changes of the after-discharge (such as lowering of the stimulus threshold or prolongation of the duration) following administration of promazine, chlorprothixene, and clozapine, which suggest a possible potentiation of seizures by these substances.

b) Chemically Induced Seizures

α) Pentetrazole (see Table 2)

In general the substances do not influence pentetrazole-induced clonic or tonic seizures. Threshold doses of pentetrazole are not changed either. CHEN and BOHNER (1960) report of a promazine-induced inhibition of tonic pentetrazole seizures in the mouse, the clonic seizures, however, remain uninfluenced. With trifluoperazine WARDELL and STAPLES (1969) observed an up to 50% inhibition of clonic pentetrazole seizures in the rat which was not dose-dependent.

Table 2. Effects of neuroleptics on pentetrazole-induced seizures

Substance	Species	Route of administration (dose mg/kg)	Pretreatment time	Induction of seizures	Parameter measured	Effect	Reference
Chlorpro-mazine	Mice	p. o. (5)	60 min	Pentetrazole (PTZ) s. c. 100 mg/kg	Clonic convulsions	ED_{50}: 400 mg/kg	Schallek et al. (1956)
		p.o.	60 min	PTZ s. c. 150 mg/kg	Convulsions	Up to ataxic doses no effect	Piala et al. (1959)
		p.o. (up to 60)	Peak time	PTZ i.v.	Seizure threshold	No effect	Swinyard et al. (1959)
		p.o. (10)	60 min	PTZ i.v. infusion 2 mg/min	Time up to persistent convulsions	Shortened	Bastian et al. (1959)
		p.o. (2–80)	60 min	PTZ i.p.	Threshold for convulsions (CD_{50})	No effect	Coscia et al. (1966)
		i. p. (10)	15 min	PTZ i.p.	Threshold for clonic convulsions	No effect	Sacra and McColl (1958)
		i. p. (10–140)	30 min	PTZ i.m.	Threshold for clonic seizures (CD_{50})	5–40 mg/kg: increase; 60–140 mg/kg: decrease	Chen and Bohner (1960)
		i. p. (5–40)	30 min	PTZ i.v. 50 mg/kg	Clonic and tonic seizures	No effect	Chen and Bohner (1960)
		i. p. (5)	60 min	PTZ i.p. 75 mg/kg	Convulsions	No effect	Sanders (1967)
		i. v. (0.5–25)	Immediately after the PTZ injection	PTZ i.p. 60 mg/kg	Convulsions	Inhibition (40–50%) in doses of 0.5–10 mg/kg; 25 mg/kg: no effect	Nieschulz et al. (1955)
		s. c. (5)	45 min	PTZ i.v.	Threshold for clonic and tonic seizures	No effect	Kobinger (1959)

Table 2. (Continued)

Substance	Species	Route of administration (dose mg/kg)	Pretreatment time	Induction of seizures	Parameter measured	Effect	Reference
Chlorpromazine	Mice	s.c. (5–40)	30 min	PTZ s.c. 150 mg/kg	Clonic and tonic seizures	ED_{50}: 50 mg/kg	Christensen et al. (1965)
	Rats	i.p. (10)	30 min	PTZ i.p. cumulative up to 40 mg/kg	a) Myoclonic jerks; spike and wave complexes in EEG	a) Increased	Arushanian and Avakian (1978)
					b) Duration of the cortical response to electric striatal stimuli	b) Prolonged	
		s.c. (20)	30 min	PTZ i.p. 45 mg/kg	Convulsions and death	No effect	Koch (1957)
		s.c. (4, 15)		PTZ s.c. 80 mg/kg	Clonic seizures time up to convulsions	No effect	Arrigoni-Martelli and Kramer (1959)
	Rabbits	i.v. (1–10)	30–40 min	PTZ i.v. 25 mg/kg	Clonic – tonic seizures	No effect	Balestrieri (1955a, b)
		i.m. (1.5)	20 min	PTZ i.m. 50 mg/kg	Clonic seizures EEG	Decrease of number of convulsions	Suarez et al. (1957)
	Frogs	Lymph sac (25–100)	20 min	PTZ 10 mg/kg	Convulsions with and without external stimuli	Potentiation of the pentetrazole effects	Deshpande et al. (1963)
Promazine	Mice	i.p. (5–40)	30 min	PTZ i.v. 50 mg/kg	a) Clonic b) Tonic seizures	a) No effect b) 20–80% inhibition	Chen and Bohner (1960)
Triflupromazine		p.o.	60 min	PTZ s.c. 150 mg/kg	Convulsions	Up to ataxic doses no effect	Piala et al. (1959)
Thioridazine		p.o. (up to 120)	Peak time	PTZ i.v.	Seizure threshold	No effect	Swinyard et al. (1959)

Drug	Species	Route (mg/kg)	Time	PTZ	Parameter	Effect	Reference
Thioridazine	Mice	p.o. (1.5–60)	60 min	PTZ i.p.	Threshold for convulsions CD_{50} (mg/kg)	No effect	Coscia et al. (1966)
		i.p. (2.5–10)	60 min	PTZ s.c. 80 mg/kg	Number of mice seizures	Slight, insignificant decrease	Maj et al. (1974)
Perphenazine		p.o. (0.1–4)	60 min	PTZ i.p.	Threshold for convulsions; CD_{50} (mg/kg)	No effect	Arrigoni-Martelli and Kramer (1959)
	Rats	s.c. (4, 15)		PTZ s.c. 80 mg/kg	Clonic seizures, time up to seizures	No effect	
Prochlor-perazine	Frogs	Lymph sac	20 min	PTZ i.p.	Convulsions with and without external stimulation	Potentiation of the pentetrazole action	Deshpande et al. (1963)
Trifluoperazine	Rats	p.o. (0.25–40)	45 min	PTZ i.v. 22.5 mg/kg	Clonic seizures	40–50% protection	Wardell and Staples (1969)
Clozapine	Mice	i.p. (2–8)	60 min	PTZ s.c. 80 mg/kg	Seizures	Slight, insignificant decrease	Maj et al. (1974)
Haloperidol		i.p. (0.1)	2–6 h	PTZ i.v. infusion	Threshold for clonic and tonic seizures	No effect	Kilian and Frey (1973)
		s.c.	30 min	PTZ s.c. 150 mg/kg	a) Clonic seizures b) Tonic seizures	a) No effect b) ED_{50}: 15 mg/kg	Christensen et al. (1965)
	Rats	i.p. (3)	30 min	PTZ i.p. cumulative up to 20–40 mg/kg	a) Myoclonic jerks; spike and wave complexes in EEG b) Duration of cortical responses to striatal electric stimuli	a) Increased b) Prolonged	Arushanian and Avakian (1978)
Melperone	Mice	p.o.	60 min	PTZ s.c. 121 mg/kg	Tonic seizures	ED_{50}: 107 mg/kg	Teschendorf et al. (1980)
Pimozide		i.p. (1)	30 min	PTZ i.p. 50 mg/kg	Clonic-tonic seizures	40% protection	Chimote and Moghe (1977)

β) Other Chemically Induced Seizures (see Table 3)

Trifluopromazine protects mice against strychnine-induced death (Piala et al., 1959). In nikethamide seizures mepazine has effects similar to chlorpromazine. The latency phase up to the occurrence of seizures is prolonged, the incidence of death is reduced. Thioridazine and clozapine potentiate tonic seizures following bicuculline. All substances administered at low dose levels antagonize nicotine seizures (clonic, tonic seizures or death).

c) Seizures Induced by Other Methods (see Table 4)

Promazine and trifluopromazine inhibit audiogenic seizures whereby the tonic seizure component is inhibited at low dose levels, as is observed with chlorpromazine. Very high doses are necessary to inhibit the initial symptom "running".

II. Butyrophenones and Diphenylbutylpiperidines

a) Electroshock (see Table 1)

According to Christensen et al. (1965) haloperidol in a s. c. dose of 6 mg/kg inhibits the electroshock in mice; an oral dose of 10 mg/kg is ineffective (Teschendorf et al., 1980). In after-discharge experiments haloperidol induced a generalization of seizures, the threshold for after-discharges or their duration was not influenced (Sayers, 1979). Melperone, which is chemically closely related to haloperidol but has substantially less pronounced neuroleptic effects, is active in electroshocks (Christensen et al., 1965). According to Teschendorf et al. (1980) relatively high doses are required with oral administration to inhibit clonic and tonic seizures. As compared to other neuroleptics, the dose interval between neuroleptic effects and anticonvulsant effects is smaller with this compound.

b) Chemically Induced Seizures (see Tables 2 and 3)

According to Christensen et al. (1965) haloperidol inhibits tonic pentetrazole seizures, it does not, however, inhibit clonic seizures. In the rat 3 mg/kg of haloperidol increase the seizure equivalents visible in the EEG after pentetrazole. Haloperidol at low doses ($ED_{50} = 0.14$ mg/kg) inhibits bicuculline-induced convulsions. Melperone is effective in protecting against pentetrazole (tonic seizures) (Teschendorf et al., 1978).

In a dose of 1 mg/kg pimozide has a partly protective effect on tonic–clonic seizures induced by pentetrazole, but is ineffective against strychnine; it inhibits mortality but not the seizures after procaine, and antagonizes bicuculline seizures.

C. Reserpine

Reserpine induces a facilitation of experimental seizures. This finding first established by Jenney (1954) and Chen et al. (1954) could be confirmed by numerous authors in many seizure models. The individual findings are summarized in Table 5. Reserpine administered to mice, rats, or rabbits in the electroshock in parenteral doses of 0.25 mg/kg or more has an effect on the various parameters measured in terms of a facilitation or potentiation of seizures. The threshold values for the induction of clonic or tonic seizures are reduced, subthreshold stimuli cause seizures, latency phases up to the occurrence of seizures are shortened.

The finding established by KOSLOW and ROTH (1971) in the electroshock on rats is an exception. Besides a facilitation of seizures (increased incidence of tonic extensor seizures) at reserpine doses of up to 0.5 mg/kg, the authors also report of an anticonvulsant effect at doses of 2.5–10 mg/kg becoming manifest in a decrease in the duration of the tonic extensor seizure.

The seizure facilitating effect of reserpine can also be demonstrated by chemically induced seizures. After the administration of different substances (pentetrazole, bemegride, nikethamide, hydralazine, acridone, caffeine, camphor, cocaine, procaine) seizures occur more often or are more pronounced after pretreatment with low doses of reserpine. Seizures induced by picrotoxin, strychnine, or nicotine are not influenced. The results established with regard to the effect on audiogenic seizures vary. TRIPOD et al. (1954), PLOTNIKOFF (1958, 1960), and PLOTNIKOFF and GREEN (1957) describe a protective effect of reserpine against audiogenic seizures while other authors do not note any influence (FINK and SWINYARD, 1959) or potentiation of seizures (BEVAN and CHINN, 1957; BIELEC, 1959; SCHLESINGER et al., 1968, 1970; BOGGAN and SEIDEN, 1971, 1973).

The threshold lowering or seizure facilitating effect of reserpine is attributed to biogenic amine depletion. Monoaminoxydase inhibitors, capable of preventing amine depletion, suppress the seizure facilitating effect of reserpine (PROCKOP et al., 1959 a, b; CHEN et al., 1967, 1968).

Other substances inducing amine depletion, such as tetrabenazine or RO 4-1284 (a benzoquinolizine derivative), are like reserpine also able to induce an increased susceptibility to seizures. Tetrabenazine lowers the maximal electroshock threshold (CHEN et al., 1967, 1968), increases the incidence of minimal electroshock seizures (AZZARO et al., 1972), reduces the survival time following pentetrazole infusions (LESSIN and PARKES, 1959) and enhances the intensity of audiogenic seizures (LEHMANN, 1967; SCHLESINGER et al., 1968). RO 4-1284 increases the intensity of electroshock seizures (STULL et al., 1973) and of audiogenic seizures (JOBE et al., 1973).

A detailed literature survey concerning the influence of neurotransmitters upon epileptic fits is given by MAYNERT et al. (1975). The tests, which were to demonstrate that the seizure facilitating action of reserpine or tetrabenazine is due to the depletion of a certain neurotransmitter did not yield uniform results. According to PFEIFER and GALAMBOS (1967), JONES and ROBERTS (1968) a noradrenaline deficiency is primarily responsible for the seizure facilitating action of reserpine in the pentetrazole shock of the mouse. As indicated by RUDZIK and JOHNSON (1970) the seizure thresholds for the electroshock and chemoshock induced by caffeine or bemegride are dependent on noradrenaline, but the seizure threshold for pentetrazole is dependent on serotonin. The presence of noradrenaline is more important than that of dopamine in the audiogenic seizure of the rat (JOBE et al., 1973).

The investigations by DE SCHAEPDRYVER et al. (1962) revealed that the threshold lowering effect of reserpine to electroshock in rabbits is primarily conditioned by the dopamine deficiency, noradrenaline or serotonin are negligible in this respect. Dopamine is of significance in audiogenic seizures in mice since a reduction of both noradrenaline and dopamine provokes an increased susceptibility of the animals and only an increased dopamine level leads to reduced susceptibility (BOGGAN and SEIDEN, 1971). According to BOGGAN and SEIDEN (1973) serotonin is also an important factor for the susceptibility to audiogenic seizures and LESSIN and PARKES (1959) report of a relationship between serotonin level and susceptibility to pentetrazole.

Table 3. Effects of neuroleptics on chemically induced seizures

Substance	Species	Route of administration (dose mg/kg)	Pretreatment time	Induction of seizures	Parameter measured	Effect	Reference
Chlorpro-mazine	Mice	i. v. (1–20)	10 min	Nikethamide 300 mg/kg i. p.	a) Time up to convulsions b) Convulsions c) Death	a) Time prolonged (not dose-dependent) b) Convulsions diminished c) 20 mg: 100% protection against death	NIESCHULZ et al. (1955)
		s. c. (80–100)		Nikethamide 500 mg/kg s. c.	Convulsions and death	Convulsions diminished no lethality	COURVOISIER et al. (1953)
	Rats	s. c. (10)	30–35 min	Nikethamide 300 mg/kg i. p.	Duration and intensity diminished	Convulsions diminished	KOCH (1957)
		s. c. (10)	3–35 min	Aminophena-zone i.p. 200 mg/kg	Convulsions	No effect	KOCH (1957)
	Mice	i. p. (10)	15 min	Acetaldehyde i.p. 200 mg/kg	Score (handling convulsions)	Slight increase	ORTIZ et al. (1973)
		i. p. (5)	60 min	Procaine 200 mg/kg	Convulsions	100% protection	SANDERS (1967)
		i. p. (5)	60 min	Cocaine 80 mg/kg	Convulsions and death	90–100% protection	SANDERS (1967)
		p. o.	120 min	Nicotine LD 95% i. v.	Tonic extension and death	ED_{50}: 3.0 mg/kg	ACETO (1974)
		i. p. (10)	15 min	Nicotine i.p.	Threshold for clonic con-vulsions (CD_{50})	77% increase of threshold	SACRA and McCOLL (1958)
		i. p. (5–40)	30 min	Nicotine 200 mg/kg i. v.	Clonic and tonic seizures	No effect	CHEN and BOHNER (1960)

Drug	Species	Route (dose)	Time	Agent/dose	Parameter	Effect	Reference
Chlorpromazine	Mice	i.p.	30 min	Nicotine 8.4 mg/kg i.p.	Clonic seizures	ED$_{50}$: 30 mg/kg	YAMAMOTO et al. (1966)
		i.p.	30 min	Nicotine 17 mg/kg i.p.	Tonic extension and death	ED$_{50}$: 4.0 mg/kg	YAMAMOTO et al. (1966)
		i.v. (5–20)	10 min	Nicotine 0.7 mg/kg i.v.	Convulsions	13–27% protection	NIESCHULZ et al. (1955)
	Rats	i.v. (2–20)	10 min	Nicotine 20 mg/kg i.v.	Death	30–70% protection	NIESCHULZ et al. (1955)
	Rabbits	i.v. (1.25–5)	5 min	Nicotine 0.5 mg/kg i.v.	Intensity of convulsions	Diminished	COURVOISIER et al. (1953)
	Mice	i.p. (10)	15 min	Picrotoxin i.p.	Threshold for clonic convulsions	No effect	SACRA and McCOLL (1958)
		p.o.	120 min	Strychnine 0.75 mg/kg i.v.	Protection against death	ED$_{50}$: 6.4 mg/kg	PIALA et al. (1959)
		i.p. (10)	15 min	Strychnine i.p.	Clonic seizures	No effect	SACRA and McCOLL (1958)
	Rats	p.o. (3)	120 min	Strychnine infusion i.v.	Threshold for clonic and tonic seizures	Increase	DE SALVA and EVANS (1960)
		i.v. (2–10)	10 min	Strychnine 2.5 mg/kg i.p.	Seizures and death	Potentiation of the strychnine effects	NIESCHULZ et al. (1955)
		s.c.	20 min	Strychnine 10 mg/kg s.c.	Time up to convulsions, convulsions and death	No effect	COURVOISIER et al. (1953)
	Rabbits	s.c. (20)	30–35 min	Strychnine 3 mg/kg i.p.	Clonic – tonic seizures, death	No effect	BALESTRIERI (1955a, b)
		i.v. (10)		Strychnine 0.3 mg/kg i.v.	Clonic – tonic seizures	No effect	

Table 3. (Continued)

Substance	Species	Route of administration (dose mg/kg)	Pretreatment time	Induction of seizures	Parameter measured	Effect	Reference
Chlorpro-mazine	Mice	i.p. (0.1–10)	30 min	Bicuculline 0.45 mg/kg	Convulsions	Protection (−50%) in low doses, in higher doses enhancement of tonic seizures	WORMS and LLOYD (1978)
Promazine		i.p. (5–40)	30 min	Nicotine 200 mg/kg i.v.	Clonic and tonic seizures	10–40 mg/kg: 50–90% protection against clonic, 20–40 mg/kg: 10–30% protection against tonic seizures	CHEN and BOHNER (1960)
Triflupro-mazine		p.o.	60–120 min	Strychnine 0.75 mg/kg (0.12 mg/min) i.v.	Protection against death	ED_{50}: 6.4 mg/kg	PTALA et al. (1959)
Levomepro-mazine		i.p.		Nicotine LD_{90} i.v. (−17 mg/kg)	Death	ED_{50}: 4.2 mg/kg	YAMAMOTO et al. (1967)
Thioridazine		p.o.	120 min	Nicotine LD_{95} i.v.	Tonic seizures and death	ED_{50}: about 3.0 mg/kg	ACETO (1974)
		i.p. (0.3–10)	30 min	Bicuculline 0.45 mg/kg	Convulsions	Up to 3 mg/kg about 50% protection, higher doses enhancement of tonic seizures	WORMS and LLOYD (1978)

Drug	Animal	Route (mg/kg)	Time	Convulsant	Endpoint	Result	Reference
Mepazine	Mice	i.v. (1–20)	10 min	Nikethamide 300 mg/kg i.p.	a) Time up to convulsions b) Convulsions c) Deaths	a) Prolonged b) No effect c) Diminished	Nieschulz et al. (1955)
		i.v. (5–20)	10 min	Nicotine bitartrate 0.7 mg/kg i.v.	Convulsions	8–93% protected	Nieschulz et al. (1955)
	Rats	i.v. (2–20)	10 min	Nicotine 20 mg/kg i.v.	Death	10 mg/kg: max. protection (70%) 2, 5, 20 mg/kg: 20–30% protected	Nieschulz et al. (1955)
Perphenazine	Mice	i.p.	30 min	Nicotine 8.4 mg/kg i.p.	Clonic seizures	ED_{50}: 1.75 mg/kg	Yamamoto et al. (1966)
		i.p.	30 min	Nicotine 17 mg/kg i.p.	Tonic seizures and death	ED_{50}: 3.0 mg/kg	Yamamoto et al. (1967)
Trifluoperazine		p.o.	120 min	Nicotine LD_{95}	Tonic extension and death	ED_{50}: 19 mg/kg	Aceto (1974)
Prochlorperazine		i.p.	30 min	Nicotine 17 mg/kg i.p.	Tonic seizures and death	ED_{50}: 40 mg/kg	Yamamoto et al. (1967)
Chlorprotixene		i.p.	30 min	Nicotine 17 mg/kg i.p.	Tonic seizures and death	ED_{50}: 1.9 mg/kg	Yamamoto et al. (1967)
Clozapine		i.p. (0.3–10)	30 min	Bicuculline 0.45 mg/kg	Convulsions	No effect against clonic convulsions, enhancement of tonic seizures	Worms and Lloyd (1978)
Haloperidol		p.o.	120 min	Nicotine LD_{95}	Tonic extension and death	ED_{50}: 10 mg/kg	Aceto (1974)
		i.p.	30 min	Bicuculline 0.45 mg/kg	Convulsions	ED_{50}: 0.14 mg/kg	Worms and Lloyd (1978)
Pimozide		i.p. (1.0)	30 min	Procaine-HCl 180 mg/kg i.p.	a) Convulsions b) Death	a) No effect b) 100% protection	Chimote and Moghe (1977)
		i.p. (1.0)	30 min	Strychnine 0.4 mg/kg i.p.	Convulsions and death	No effect	Chimote and Moghe (1977)
		i.p.	30 min	Bicuculline 0.45 mg/kg	Convulsions	ED_{50}: 0.55 mg/kg	Worms and Lloyd (1978)

Table 4. Effects of neuroleptics on other experimentally induced seizures

Substance	Species	Route of administration (dose mg/kg)	Pretreatment time	Induction of seizures	Parameter measured	Effect	Reference
Chlorproma-zine	Mice	i.p. (40)	15 min	Oxygen at raised pressure (65 p.s.i.g.) (1b/sq in)	Time up to convulsions	Prolonged	PATON (1967)
		i.p. (10, 20)	5 h after withdrawal	Withdrawal of ethanol dependent mice	Scoring system clonic – tonic seizure	Intensification of withdrawal syndrome	GOLDSTEIN (1972)
	Rats	s.c. (10/die)		Withdrawal of barbiturate dependent rats	Clonic–tonic convulsions	No effect	NORTON (1970)
	Mice	p.o.	60 min	Audiogenic	Score: (running jumping circling convulsing)	50% protection 11 mg/kg	PLOTNIKOFF and GREEN (1957) PLOTNIKOFF (1958)
		p.o. (15.7)	Peak time		Tonic seizures	50% protected	SWINYARD et al. (1959)
		p.o.	90 min		a) Running b) Tonic extension	a) ED_{50} >157 mg/kg b) ED_{50}: 21 mg/kg	FINK and SWINYARD (1959)
		p.o.	60 min		Clonic–tonic seizures	ED_{50}: 4.8 mg/kg or no effect (dependent on the strain of mice used)	PLOTNIKOFF (1960)
		i.p. (5–20)	30 min	Audiogenic	a) Time up to clonic seizures b) Tonic seizures	a) No effect b) ED_{50}: 6.2 mg/kg	MANIAN et al. (1965)

Substance	Species	Route of administration (dose mg/kg)	Pretreatment time	Induction of seizures	Parameter measured	Effect	Reference
Promazine	Mice	p.o.	60 min		a) Running b) Tonic extension	a) ED_{50}: 235 mg/kg b) ED_{50}: 24 mg/kg	Fink and Swinyard (1959)
Triflupro-mazine	Mice	p.o.	90 min		a) Running b) Tonic extension	a) ED_{50}: > 100 mg/kg b) ED_{50}: 18 mg/kg	Fink and Swinyard (1959)
Thioridazine	Mice	p.o. (30)	Peak time		a) Tonic seizures b) Death	a) 25% protection b) Increased incidence	Swinyard et al. (1959)

Table 5. Effects of reserpine on experimental seizures

Substance	Species	Route of administration (dose mg/kg)	Pretreatment time	Induction of seizures	Parameter measured	Effect	Reference
Reserpine	Mice	p.o. (10–100)	8–24 h	Electroshock	a) Seizure latency b) Threshold for tonic seizures	a) Shortened b) Decreased	Everett et al. (1955)
		p.o.	4 h		a) Tonic extension b) Time up to tonic extension	a) ED_{50}: 165 mg/kg b) Shortened	Fink and Swinyard (1959)
		i.p. (8)	$4^{1}/_{2}$ h		Low frequency stimulation: stunning response or convulsion	Potentiation (tonic extension)	Chen et al. (1954)
		i.p. (5)	6 h		Threshold for tonic extension	Decreased	Chen et al. (1954) Chen and Bohner (1957)
		i.p. (0.0125–8)	24 h		Threshold for tonic seizure (CD_{50})	As of 0.25 mg/kg decrease	Chen et al. (1954, 1968) Chen and Bohner (1957)

Table 5. (Continued)

Substance	Species	Route of administration (dose mg/kg)	Pretreatment time	Induction of seizures	Parameter measured	Effect	Reference
Reserpine	Mice	i.p. (4)	5 h	Electroshock	Threshold for max. seizure (CD_{50})	Decreased	GRAY et al. (1963)
		i.p. (2)	2 h		Clonic or tonic seizures	Incidence of seizures increased	SCHLESINGER et al. (1968)
		i.p. (2.5)	4 h		Threshold for tonic extension	Decreased	RUDZIK and JOHNSON (1970)
		i.p. (0.1–5.0)	6 h		Number of animals convulsing at subthreshold stimuli	Convulsions in 20–50% of the animals	AZZARO et al. (1972)
		i.p. (1)	2–24 h		Clonic convulsions	Increased susceptibility (max. 6 h after reserpine)	WENGER et al. (1973)
	Rats	i.p. (5)	2 h		a) No. of full seizure pattern b) Latency up to tonic extension	a) Increased b) Shortened	PROCKOP et al. (1959 a, b)
		i.p. (2.5)	4 h		Threshold for tonic extension	Decreased	RUDZIK and JOHNSON (1970)
		i.p. (0.25–10)	2 h		a) Incidence of extension phase b) Incidence of flexion-phase c) Duration of extension phase	a) 0.25–0.5 mg/kg increased b) 2.5–10 mg/kg decreased c) 2.5–10 mg/kg decreased	KOSLOW and ROTH (1971)
	Rabbits	i.v. (10)	1 h		Threshold for tonic flexion	Decreased	JURNA and REGÉLHY (1968)
		i.v.	16 h		Threshold for clonic–tonic seizures	Decreased	DE SCHAEPDRYVER et al. (1962)

Drug	Species	Dose (route)	Time	Stimulus	Test	Effect	Reference
Rauwolfia alkaloids Reserpine	Mice	p.o. (50/die for 10 days)	3 h	Electroshock	CD$_{50}$ for tonic seizures	Decreased	JENNEY (1954)
		p.o. (up to 300)	4 h	Pentetrazole (PTZ) 40 mg/kg i.v.	Convulsions	No effect	TRIPOD et al. (1954)
		p.o. (10)	720 min	PTZ i.v. 100 mg/kg/min	Time up to persistent convulsions	Reduced to 60% of the controls	BASTIAN et al. (1959)
		i.p. (1–8)	1–4 h	PTZ i.v. infusion	Threshold for a) clonic seizure b) tonic seizure c) death	a) No change b) Decreased c) Decreased	CHEN et al. (1954); CHEN and BOHNER (1956, 1957, 1958, 1961)
		i.p. (10)	4 h	PTZ i.p.	Threshold for clonic convulsions	Decreased (−36%)	SACRA and McCOLL (1958)
		i.p. (5)	3 h	PTZ i.v. infusion (0.05 ml/10 s, 0.5%)	Threshold for a) clonic seizures b) tonic seizures	a) No effect b) Decreased	KOBINGER (1959)
		i.p. (2.0)	1–72 h	PTZ i.v. infusion (0.05 ml/10 s, 0.5%)	Survival time	Decreased	LESSIN and PARKES (1959)
		i.p. (0.1–8)	4 h	PTZ i.p.	Threshold for tonic seizures	Decreased	WEISS et al. (1960)
		i.p. (2)	240 min	PTZ i.p. 75 mg/kg	a) Convulsions b) Death	a) No effect b) Increased	SANDERS (1967)
		i.p. (2.5)	2 h	PTZ i.v. (0.05 ml/10 s, 0.5%)	Threshold for tonic seizures	Decreased	PFEIFER and GALAMBOS (1967)
		i.p. (2)	2 h	PTZ i.p. 32 mg/kg	Incidence of seizures	Increased	SCHLESINGER et al. (1968)
		i.p. (2.5)	4 h	PTZ i.v. 0.5%	Threshold for tonic seizures	Decreased	RUDZIK and JOHNSON (1970)
		i.p. (2.5)	6 h	PTZ i.p.	Convulsions	Decreased	NAIK RATAN et al. (1974)
		i.p. (2.0)	1/2 h	PTZ i.p. 20 mg/kg	Incidence of seizures	Increased (control 0%, reserpine 100%)	CHIMOTE and MOGHE (1977)

Table 5. (Continued)

Substance	Species	Route of administration (dose mg/kg)	Pretreatment time	Induction of seizures	Parameter measured	Effect	Reference
Reserpine	Mice	i.p. (2.0)	1/2 h	PTZ i.p. 50 mg/kg	Incidence of death	Increased (0 to 60%)	CHIMOTE and MOGHE (1977)
		s.c. (30.0)	3 h	PTZ i.p. 49 or 81 mg/kg (CD$_5$)	Clonic–tonic seizures	Increased	BIANCHI (1956)
Rauwolfia alkaloids Reserpine		p.o. (50/die for 10 days)	3 h	PTZ	Threshold for convulsions	Decreased	JENNEY (1954)
Reserpine		i.p. (8)	5 h	Bemegride 0.05 ml/10 s, 0.25%	Threshold for a) clonic seizures b) tonic c) death	a) No effect b) Decreased c) Decreased	CHEN and BOHNER (1958)
		i.p. (2.5)	4 h	Bemegride 0.25% i.v.	Threshold for tonic seizures	Decreased	RUDZIK and JOHNSON (1970)
		i.p. (2.0)	1/2 h	Bemegride 5 mg/kg i.p.	Incidence of seizures	Increased (0–70%)	CHIMOTE and MOGHE (1977)
		i.p. (2.0)	1/2 h	Bemegride 20 mg/kg i.p.	Incidence of death	Increased (30–60%)	CHIMOTE and MOGHE (1977)
		i.p. (8)	5 h	Nikethamide 1.5%; 0.05 ml/10 s	Threshold for a) clonic seizures b) tonic c) death	a) No effect b) Decreased c) Decreased	CHEN and BOHNER (1956)
		i.p. (8)	5 h	Hydralazine 1.0%; 0.05 ml/10 s	Threshold for a) clonic seizures b) tonic c) death	a) No effect b) Decreased c) Decreased	CHEN and BOHNER (1958)
		i.p. (8)	5 h	Acridone 0.05%; 0.05 ml/10 s	Threshold for a) clonic seizures b) tonic c) death	a) No effect b) Decreased c) Decreased	CHEN and BOHNER (1958)
		i.p. (8)	5 h	Ammonium-acetate 5% 0.05 ml/10 s	Threshold for a) tonic seizures b) death	a) Increased b) Increased	CHEN and BOHNER (1956)

Reserpine	Mice	i.p. (4)	3 h	Caffeine 1% i.v.	Threshold for tonic seizures	Decreased	Chen et al. (1954) Chen and Bohner (1961)
		i.p. (8)	5 h	Caffeine 1%; 0.05 ml/10 s	a) Clonic b) Tonic seizures c) Death	a) Decreased b) Decreased c) Decreased	Chen and Bohner (1956)
		i.p. (2.5)	4 h	Caffeine 1% i.v.	Threshold for tonic seizures	Decreased	Rudzik and Johnson (1970)
		s.c. (30.0)	3 h	Camphor i.p. CD_5 (66 mg/kg)	Clonic–tonic seizures	Increased	Bianchi (1956)
		i.p. (2)	4 h	Cocaine 80 mg/kg i.p.	Clonic–tonic seizures	Significant decrease	Sanders (1967)
		i.p. (2)	4 h	Procaine 200 mg/kg i.p.	Clonic–tonic seizures	Decreased	Sanders (1967)
		i.p. (2)	1/2 h	Procaine 180 mg/kg i.p.	Convulsions and death	Incidence of death	Chimote and Moghe (1977)
		i.p. (2)	1/2, 18 h	Procaine 90 mg/kg i.p.	Convulsions and death	No effect	Chimote and Moghe (1977)
		i.p. (10)	4 h	Nicotine i.p.	Clonic seizures	No effect	Sacra and McColl (1958)
		i.p. (8)	5 h	Nicotine 200 mg/kg i.v.	Clonic and tonic seizures	No effect	Chen and Bohner (1960)
		i.p. (8)	5–6 h	Picrotoxin 0.05 ml/10 s; 0.15% i.v.	Clonic–tonic seizures and death	No effect	Chen and Bohner (1956, 1958)
		i.p. (10)	4 h	Picrotoxin i.p.	Clonic convulsions (CD_{50})	Decrease (−50%)	Sacra and McColl (1958)
		i.p. (2)	1/2 h	Picrotoxin i.p. 7 mg/kg	Convulsions and death	No effect	Chimote and Moghe (1977)
		i.p. (8)	5 h	Strychnine i.v. 0.05 ml/10 s, 0.005%	Tonic seizures and death	No effect	Chen et al. (1954) Chen and Bohner (1956)
		i.p. (10)	4 h	Strychnine i.p. CD_{50}	Clonic con-vulsions	No effect	Sacra and McColl (1958)

Table 5. (Continued)

Substance	Species	Route of administration (dose mg/kg)	Pretreatment time	Induction of seizures	Parameter measured	Effect	Reference
Reserpine	Mice	i.p. (2)	2 h	Strychnine 0.4 mg/kg i.p.	Convulsions and death	No effect	CHIMOTE and MOGHE (1977)
		s.c. (30)	3 h	Strychnine i.p. 0.66 mg/kg (LD₅)	Death	Increased	BIANCHI (1956)
	Rats	p.o. (1)	4 h	Strychnine i.v. infusion	Threshold for clonic and tonic seizures	Increased	DE SALVA and EVANS (1960)
	Mice	i.p. (2)	1 h	Audiogenic	a) Wild running b) Clonic seizures c) Tonic seizures d) Death	a) No change b) Increased c) Increased d) Increased	BOGGAN and SEIDEN (1971, 1973)
		p.o.	1 h		Score: (running jumping circling convulsing immobility)	Protective dose 100 mg/kg 300–400 mg/kg increase of convulsing	PLOTNIKOFF and GREEN (1957), PLOTNIKOFF (1958)
		p.o.	4 h		a) Running b) Tonic extension	ED₅₀: 165 mg/kg	FINK and SWINYARD (1959)
		i.p. (5–100)	24 h		Score: (running jumping circling convulsing immobility)	30–100% protection	PLOTNIKOFF (1958)
	Mice (different strains)	i.p.	24 h		Score: (running jumping circling convulsing immobility)	Protective ED₅₀ 5.0–9.0 mg/kg	PLOTNIKOFF (1960)

Reserpine	Mice	i.p. (1, 2)	1–168	Susceptibility for seizures	Increased	Schlesinger et al. (1968, 1970)
		i.p. (5.0)	3–72 h	Seizures	Increased	Bielec (1959)
	Rats	p.o.	4 h	Seizures	ED$_{50}$: 100 mg/kg	Tripod et al. (1954)
		i.m. (0.037–0.9)	5 h	Running clonic seizures tonic	Increase of frequency and intensity	Bevan and Chinn (1957)
	Mice	i.p. (0.625–5.0)	4 h	Hyperbaric oxygen		
				a) Incidence of clonic convulsions	a) No effect	Oliver et al. (1970)
				b) Incidence of tonic convulsions	b) Increased	
				c) Time up to convulsions	c) Decreased	

According to Azzaro (1970) and Azzaro et al. (1972) the change of the seizure threshold is not due to the changed content of only one transmitter. Both catecholamines and serotonin are responsible for a normal susceptibility to seizures. According to Wenger et al. (1973) the seizure threshold is better correlated with the ability of the brain tissue to store transmitters than with the total content of transmitters in the brain.

D. Influence of Neuroleptics and Reserpine on the Effects of Anticonvulsant Drugs

Animal experiments on the effects of neuroleptic and anticonvulsant drugs following combined administration are rarely described in the literature and their results are partly contradictory.

Bertrand et al. (1954) observed a potentiation of the anticonvulsant effect of diphenylhydantoin by chlorpromazine. Simultaneous administration of 20 mg/kg of subcutaneous chlorpromazine shifts to the left the dose-effect curve of diphenylhydantoin in the maximal electroshock of the rat and reduces the ED_{50} of diphenylhydantoin from 35 to 22 mg/kg. Administration of a dose of 20 mg/kg of chlorpromazine alone has no effect.

As mentioned above neuroleptics administered at low dose levels lower the seizure threshold in electroshock, high doses cause an elevation (Chen et al., 1968). The threshold lowering effect of neuroleptics becomes particularly evident, according to Chen et al., if the seizure threshold has been raised by pretreatment with an anticonvulsant substance. Chen et al. describe such an antagonistic effect on the threshold elevating, i. e., anticonvulsant effect of diphenylhydantoin for small doses of chlorpromazine, promazine, trifluopromazine, perphenazine, trifluoperazine, and haloperidol. Similarly, low doses of chlorpromazine provoke a lowering of the seizure thresholds increased by methazolamide, and low doses of haloperidol reduce those increased by phencyclidine. On the other hand, with this experimental design, somewhat higher doses of chlorpromazine and haloperidol – which, when being administered alone, do not influence the seizure threshold – increase the seizure threshold in the presence of anticonvulsant pretreatment and thus potentiate the anticonvulsant effect.

Hauschild (1955) indicates an antagonistic behavior of the combination chlorpromazine and phenacemide without giving detailed information on the dosage.

The findings of Gujral et al. (1956) are completely contrary to the findings of Bertrand et al. (1954) and Chen et al. (1968). In the maximal electroshock on rats the authors found a potentiation of the diphenylhydantoin effect following low doses of chlorpromazine (1–5 mg/kg); after higher doses (20–40 mg/kg) there was, however, an antagonistic effect.

According to more recent studies of Teschendorf et al. (1978, 1980) various neuroleptics (chlorpromazine, thioridazine, haloperidol, melperone) show – particularly at low dose levels – an antagonistic behavior towards diphenylhydantoin in the maximal electroshock on mice. A study of the behavior of the neuroleptics mentioned, when being combined with diazepam, revealed, however, a potentiating effect in all cases. The results were not uniform as compared to valproic acid and trimethadione, potentiating, additive, and antagonistic behavior could be observed. According to these studies the effects of an interaction between neuroleptic and anticonvulsant drugs do not depend on the neuroleptic but rather on the anticonvulsant drug.

The influence upon the effect of anticonvulsant drugs following concomitant administration of reserpine was primarily investigated by CHEN and BOHNER (1956, 1957, 1958). On the one hand the interactions observed are dependent on the anticonvulsant drug used and on the other hand on the seizure model.

Reserpine suppresses or diminishes the effect of diphenylhydantoin on tonic seizures induced either by electroshock (RUDZIK and MENNEAR, 1965; RUDZIK and JOHNSON, 1970; GRAY et al., 1963; GRAY and RAUH, 1967) or chemically by pentetrazole, bemegride or picrotoxin (BIANCHI, 1956; CHEN and BOHNER, 1956, 1957, 1958). In the maximal electroshock the anticonvulsant effect of methazolamide and acetazolamide is suppressed by reserpine, that of phenobarbital is attenuated (GRAY et al., 1963; GRAY and RAUH, 1967, 1971; RUDZIK and JOHNSON, 1970). The inhibition of pentetrazole-induced tonic extensor seizures by anticonvulsant drugs (phenobarbital, succinimide, phensuximide, trimethadione, phenacemide) or anticonvulsant sedatives-hypnotics (cabromal, barbital, NaBr) as well as by mephenesin is abolished by reserpine (8 mg/kg i. p., 5 h pretreatment) (CHEN and BOHNER, 1956). The lethal doses of pentetrazole increased by anticonvulsant treatment are again reduced by reserpine (except for barbital).

The doses of pentetrazole required to induce clonic seizures are increased by the anticonvulsant drugs mentioned (exceptions: diphenylhydantoin and phenacemide), but are not influenced or even further increased by pretreatment with reserpine. The effects of phenobarbital, phensuximide, trimethadione, cabromal, barbital, and sodium bromide on tonic and even clonic seizures induced by caffeine are lessened by reserpine. The antitonic effect on strychnine of the anticonvulsant drugs mentioned is potentiated by reserpine.

E. Conclusions

The discussed animal experimental findings on the effects of neuroleptics and of reserpine on seizures are hardly uniform so that a summarizing assessment can be made only with difficulty.

In general, neuroleptics are ineffective in relation to electroshocks if administered in doses which normally provoke effects typical of these substances. Protective effects can be observed only at very high dose levels. An appropriate experimental design (e. g., determination of the threshold for clonic and tonic seizures or after-discharge) allows evidence to be given of an intensification of seizures after small doses. In the electroshock reserpine has seizure intensifying effects.

There are no uniform results within the group of chemically induced seizures either. Potentiation and attenuation of seizures are observed. Neuroleptics are ineffective or have only minor effects in the pentetrazole shock, a commonly used and appropriate model for testing anticonvulsant actions. Determination of the threshold shows, e. g., for chlorpromazine, an effect opposite to that in the electroshock; low doses elevate the threshold, high doses lower it. Again reserpine is seizure facilitating. Exceptions are nicotine-induced seizures which are inhibited by low doses of all neuroleptics tested. However, reserpine has no anticonvulsant effect on nicotine seizures. Moreover, neuroleptic drugs are highly effective in inhibiting the tonic component of audiogenic seizures. In this respect reserpine is described as having seizure inhibiting and seizure facilitating effects.

The seizure potentiating effect of neuroleptics may be demonstrated after combined administration with anticonvulsant drugs by eliminating the anticonvulsant effect. This is, however, dependent on the anticonvulsant drug used. The effect of diphenylhydantoin is antagonized whereas that of diazepam is potentiated. Reserpine, too, attenuates or suppresses the action of anticonvulsant drugs, with the exception of the antitonic effect of the anticonvulsant drugs in the strychnine seizure which is potentiated by reserpine. The seizure potentiating effect of reserpine is attributed to its amine depleting effect, the potentiation of seizures not being due to the depletion of a certain neurotransmitter.

References

Aceto, M.D.: Effects of CNS agents on nicotine extensor convulsions and lethality in mice and their sedative-antianxiety effects in man. Pharmacologist *16*, 205 (1974)

Arrigoni-Martelli, E., Kramer, M.: Studio farmacologico di un nuovo derivato fenotiazinico: La perfenazina. Arch. Int. Pharmacodyn. Ther. *119*, 311–333 (1959)

Arushanian, E.B., Avakian, R.M.: Metrazol-induced petit mal: the role played by monoaminergic mechanisms and striatum. Pharmacol. Biochem. Behavior *8*, 113–117 (1978)

Azzaro, A.J.: The role of biogenic amines in drug induced alterations of the minimal electroshock seizure threshold in the mouse. Dissertation Abstr. Int. *31*, 2863-B-64-B (1970)

Azzaro, A.J., Wenger, G.R., Craig, C.R., Stitzel, R.E.: Reserpine-induced alterations in brain amines and their relationship to changes in the incidence of minimal electroshock seizures in mice. J. Pharmacol. Exp. Ther. *180*, 558–568 (1972)

Balestrieri, A.: Le azioni di alcuni derivati della fenotiazina nei confronti di agenti convulsivanti. Arch. Int. Pharmacodyn. Ther. *100*, 361–372 (1955a)

Balestrieri, A.: Azione anticonvulsivante e struttura molecolare di derivati fenotiazinici. Arch. Int. Pharmacodyn. Ther. *103*, 1–12 (1955b)

Bastian, J.W., Krause, W.E., Ridlon, S.A., Ercoli, N.: CNS drug specificity as determined by the mouse intravenous pentylenetetrazol technique. J. Pharmacol. Exp. Ther. *127*, 75–80 (1959)

Bein, H.J.: The pharmacology of Rauwolfia. Pharmacol. Rev. *8*, 435–483 (1956)

Bertrand, I., Quivy, D., Gayet-Hallion, Th.: Sur la potentialisation, par la chlorpromazine, de l'effet anticonvulsivant de la diphényl-hydantoine. Compt. Rend. Soc. Biol. *148*, 1170–1172 (1954)

Bertrand, I., Gayet-Hallion, Th., Quivy, D.: Influence exercée par certains ganglioplégiques et neuroplégiques sur l'effet anticonvulsivant de la diphényl-hydantoine. Arch. Int. Pharmacodyn. Ther. *100*, 283–297 (1955)

Bevan, W., Chinn, R.McC.: Sound-induced convulsions in rats treated with reserpine. J. Comp. Physiol. Psychol. *50*, 311–314 (1957)

Bianchi, C.: Anticonvulsant action of some anti-epileptic drugs in mice pre-treated with Rauwolfia alkaloids. Br. J. Pharmacol. *11*, 141–146 (1956)

Bielec, S.: Influence of reserpine on the behavior of mice susceptible to audiogenic seizures. Arch. Int. Pharmacodyn. Ther. *119*, 352–357 (1959)

Boggan, W.O., Seiden, L.S.: Dopa reversal of reserpine enhancement of audiogenic seizure susceptibility in mice. Physiol. Behav. *6*, 215–217 (1971)

Boggan, W.O., Seiden, L.S.: 5-Hydroxytryptophan reversal of reserpine enhancement of audiogenic seizure susceptibility in mice. Physiol. Behav. *10*, 9–12 (1973)

Chen, G., Bohner, B.: A study of the neuropharmacologic properties of certain convulsants, anticonvulsants and reserpine. J. Pharmacol. *117*, 142–148 (1956)

Chen, G., Bohner, B.: A method for the biological assay of reserpine and reserpine-like activity. J. Pharmacol. *119*, 559–565 (1957)

Chen, G., Bohner, B.: A study of central nervous system stimulants. J. Pharmacol. Exp. Ther. *123*, 212–215 (1958)

Chen, G., Bohner, B.: A study of certain CNS depressants. Arch. Int. Pharmacodyn. Ther. *125*, 1–20 (1960)

Chen, G., Bohner, B.: The anti-reserpine effects of certain centrally-acting agents. J. Pharmacol. Exp. Ther. *131*, 179–184 (1961)

Chen, G., Ensor, C.R., Bohner, B.: A facilitation action of reserpine on the central nervous system. Proc. Soc. Exp. Biol. Med. *86*, 507–510 (1954)

Chen, G., Ensor, C.R., Bohner, B.: The participation of biogenic amines in electrically induced extensor-seizures to certain drugs. Pharmacologist *9*, 189 (1967)

Chen, G., Ensor, C.R., Bohner, B.: Studies of drug effects on electrically induced extensor seizures and clinical implications. Arch. Int. Pharmacodyn. Ther. *172*, 183–218 (1968)

Chimote, K.V., Moghe, P.J.: Putative neurotransmitters in CNS and chemoconvulsions. Arch. Int. Pharmacodyn. Ther. *228*, 304–313 (1977)

Christensen, J.A., Hernestam, S., Lassen, J.B., Sterner, N.: Pharmacological and toxicological studies on γ-(4-methylpiperidino)-p-fluorobutyrophenone (FG 5111) – A new neuroleptic agent. Acta Pharmacol. Toxicol. (Kbh.) *23*, 109–132 (1965)

Coscia, L., Sansone, M., Causa, P.: Fenotiazinici e convulsioni da metrazolo nel topo. Arch. Int. Pharmacodyn. Ther. *159*, 48–52 (1966)

Courvoisier, S., Fournel, J., Ducrot, R., Kolsky, M., Koetschet, P.: Propriétés pharmacodynamiques du chlorhydrate de chloro-3 (diméthylamino-3'propyl)-10 phénothiazine (4.560 R. P.). Arch. Int. Pharmacodyn. Ther. *92*, 359 (1953)

Courvoisier, S., Ducrot, R., Fournel, J., Julou, L.: Propriétés pharmacologiques générales d'un nouveau dérivé de la phénothiazine, neuroleptique puissant a action neurovégétative discrete, le chlorhydrate de (méthyl-2' diméthylamino-3' propyl-1')-10 phénothiazine (6.549 R. P.). Arch. Int. Pharmacodyn. Ther. *115*, 90–113 (1958)

Davison, K., Bagley, C.R.: Schizophrenia-like psychoses associated with organic disorders of the central nervous system: A review of the literature. Br. J. Psychiatry *114*, 113–184 (1968)

Delgado, J.M.R., Mihailovic, L.: Use of intracerebral electrodes to evaluate drugs that act on the central nervous system. Ann. N.Y. Acad. Sci. *64*, 644–666 (1956)

De Salva, S., Evans, R.: Continuous intravenous infusion of strychnine in rats: II. Antagonism by various drugs. Arch. Int. Pharmacodyn. Ther. *125*, 348–354 (1960)

De Schaepdryver, A.F., Piette, Y., Delaunois, A.L.: Brain amines and electroshock threshold. Arch. Int. Pharmacodyn. Ther. *140*, 358–367 (1962)

Deshpande, V.R., Sharma, M.L., Dashputra, P.G., Kherdikar, P.R., Grewal, R.S.: Effect of chlorpromazine and prochlorperazine on metrazol induced convulsions in frogs. Arch. Int. Pharmacodyn. Ther. *141*, 525–531 (1963)

Everett, G.M., Toman, J.E.P., Smith, Jr., A.H.: Reduction of electroshock seizure latency and other central actions of reserpine. Fed. Proc. *14*, 337 (1955)

Fink, G.B., Swinyard, E.A.: Modification of maximal audiogenic and electroshock seizures in mice by psychopharmacologic drugs. J. Pharmacol. Exp. Ther. *127*, 318–324 (1959)

Gangloff, H., Monnier, M.: Topic action of reserpine, serotonin, and chlorpromazine on the unanesthetized rabbit's brain. Helv. Physiol. Acta *15*, 83–104 (1957)

Goldstein, D.B.: An animal model for testing effects of drugs on alcohol withdrawal reactions. J. Pharmacol. Exp. Ther. *183*, 14–22 (1972)

Gray, W.D., Rauh, C.E.: The anticonvulsant action of inhibitors of carbonic anhydrase: Relation to endogenous amines in brain. J. Pharmacol. Exp. Ther. *155*, 127–155 (1967)

Gray, W.D., Rauh, C.E.: The relation between monoamines in brain and the anticonvulsant action of inhibitors of carbonic anhydrase. J. Pharmacol. Exp. Ther. *177*, 206–218 (1971)

Gray, W.D., Rauh, C.E., Shanahan, R.W.: The mechanism of the antagonistic action of reserpine on the anticonvulsant effect of inhibitors of carbonic anhydrase. J. Pharmacol. Exp. Ther. *139*, 350–360 (1963)

Gujral, M.L., Saxena, P.N., Kulsreshtha, J.K.: Effect of chlorpromazine on dilantin-protection against electroshock convulsions. J. Indian Med. Prof. *3*, 1141–1142 (1956)

Hauschild, F. ct. by Feller, K.: Gasstoffwechselversuche mit einigen Phenothiazinkörpern. Arch. Exp. Pathol. Pharmacol. *225*, 90–91 (1955)

Heming, A.E., Holtkamp, D.E., Huntsman, D.B., Doggett, M.C., Mansor, L.F.: The effect of chlorpromazine on electroshock seizure threshold, eosinopenia, and inflammation. J. Pharmacol. Exp. Ther. *116*, 28 (1956)

Itil, T.M.: Convulsive and anticonvulsive properties of neuro-psycho-pharmaca. In: Epilepsy. Mod. Probl. Pharmacopsychiat., Vol. 4, pp. 270–305. Basel, New York: Karger 1970

Itil, T.M., Myers, J.P.: Epileptic and anti-epileptic properties of psychotropic drugs. In: Anticonvulsant drugs. Mercier, J. (ed.), Vol. II, pp. 599–622. International encyclopedia of pharmacology and therapeutics, Section 19. Oxford, New York: Pergamon Press 1973

Jenney, E.H.: Changes in convulsant thresholds after Rauwolfia serpentina, reserpine and veriloid. Fed. Proc. *13*, 370–371 (1954)

Jobe, P.C., Picchioni, A.L., Chin, L.: Role of brain norepinephrine in audiogenic seizure in the rat. J. Pharmacol. Exp. Ther. *184*, 1–9 (1973)

Jones, B.J., Roberts, D.J.: The effects of intracerebroventricularly administered noradnamine and other sympathomimetic amines upon leptazol convulsions in mice. Br. J. Pharmacol. *34*, 27–31 (1968)

Jurna, I., Regélhy, B.: The antagonism between reserpine and some antiparkinson drugs in electroseizure. Naunyn-Schmiedebergs Arch. Pharmakol. Exp. Pathol. *259*, 442 (1968)

Kilian, M., Frey, H.-H.: Central monoamines and convulsive thresholds in mice and rats. Neuropharmacology *12*, 681–692 (1973)

Kobayashi, T., Ishikawa, T.: Effects of psychotropic drugs on hippocampal after-discharges in the rabbit. Neuropsychopharmacology *4*, 320–326 (1965)

Kobinger, W.: Zusammenhang zwischen experimenteller Katatonie und Förderung von tonischen Streckkrämpfen. Naunyn-Schmiedebergs Arch. Exp. Pathol. Pharmakol. *235*, 87–95 (1959)

Koch, R.: Das Verhalten antikonvulsiver Substanzen gegen Aminophenazon- und Strychnin-Krämpfe. Arzneim. Forsch. *7*, 461 (1957)

Koslow, S.H., Roth, L.J.: Reserpine and acetazolamide in maximum electroshock seizures in the rat. J. Pharmacol. Exp. Ther. *176*, 711–717 (1971)

Lehmann, A.: Audiogenic seizures data in mice supporting new theories of biogenic amines mechanisms in the central nervous system. Life Sci. *6*, 1423–1431 (1967)

Lessin, A.W., Parkes, M.W.: The effects of reserpine and other agents upon leptazol convulsions in mice. Br. J. Pharmacol. *14*, 108–111 (1959)

Logothetis, J.: Spontaneous epileptic seizures and electroencephalographic changes in the course of phenothiazine therapy. Neurology *17*, 869–877 (1967)

Maj, J., Sowinska, H., Baran, L., Palider, W.: The central action of clozapine. Pol. J. Pharmacol. Pharm. *26*, 425–435 (1974)

Manian, A.A., Efron, D.H., Goldberg, M.E.: A comparative pharmacological study of a series of monohydroxylated and methoxylated chlorpromazine derivatives. Life Sci. *4*, 2425–2438 (1965)

Maynert, E.W., Marczynski, T.J., Browning, R.A.; The role of the neurotransmitters in the epilepsies. In: Advances in Neurology, Friedlander, W.J. (ed.), Vol. 13, pp. 79–147. New York: Raven Press 1975

Mercier, J.: Sur l'action anticonvulsivante expérimentale de la chlorpromazine. Comp. Rend. Soc. Biol. *149*, 370–382 (1955)

Meyer, H.J., Meyer-Burg, J.: Hemmung des Elektrokrampfes durch die Kawa-Pyrone Dihydromethysticin und Dihydrokawain. Arch. Int. Pharmacodyn. Ther. *148*, 97–110 (1964)

Naik Ratan, S.R., Naik Rucha, S., Sheth, A., Sheth, U.K.: Role of mono-amines in pentylenetetrazol induced seizures in mice. Indian J. Med. Res. *62*, 1562–1570 (1974)

Nieschulz, O., Popendiker, K., Hoffmann, I.: Weitere pharmakologische Untersuchungen über N-Methyl-piperidyl-(3)-methyl-phenothiazin. Arzneim. Forsch. *5*, 680 (1955)

Norton, P.R.E.: The effects of drugs on barbiturate withdrawal convulsions in the rat. J. Pharm. Pharmacol. *22*, 763–766 (1970)

Oliver, J.H., Little, J.M., Pirch, J.H.: Effect of reserpine and other drugs on the CNS and lethal effects of hyperbaric oxygen in mice. Arch. Int. Pharmacodyn. Ther. *183*, 215–223 (1970)

Ortiz, A., Littleton, J.M., Griffiths, P.J.: A simple screening test for drugs of potential use in ethanol withdrawal. J. Pharm. Pharmacol. *25*, 1020–1021 (1973)

Paton, W.D.M.: Experiments on the convulsant and anaesthetic effects of oxygen. Br. J. Pharmacol. Chemother. *29*, 350–366 (1967)

Petersen, P.V., Møller Nielsen, I.: Thioxanthene derivatives. In: Medicinal Chemistry. Gordon, M. (ed.), Vol. 4, pp. 301–324. New York, London: Academic Press 1964

Pfeifer, A.K., Galambos, E.: The effect of reserpine α-methyl-m-tyrosine, prenylamine, and guanethidine on metrazol-convulsions and the brain monoamine level in mice. Arch. Int. Pharmacodyn. Ther. *165*, 201–211 (1967)

Piala, J.J., High, J.P., Hassert, Jr., G.L., Burke, J.C., Craver, B.N.: Pharmacological and acute toxicological comparisons of triflupromazine and chlorpromazine. J. Pharmacol. Exp. Ther. *127*, 55–65 (1959)

Plotnikoff, N.P.: Bioassay of potential tranquilizers and sedatives against audiogenic seizures in mice. Arch. Int. Pharmacodyn. Ther. *116*, 130–135 (1958)

Plotnikoff, N.: Ataractics and strain differences in audiogenic seizures in mice. Psychopharmacologia *1*, 429–432 (1960)

Plotnikoff, N., Green, D.M.: Bioassay of potential ataraxic agents against audiogenic seizures in mice. J. Pharmacol. Exp. Ther. *119*, 294–298 (1957)

Preston, J.B.: Effects of chlorpromazine on the central nervous system of the cat: A possible neural basis for action. J. Pharmacol. *118*, 100–115 (1956)

Prockop, D.J., Shore, P.A., Brodie, B.B.: Anticonvulsant properties of monoamine oxidase inhibitors. Ann. N.Y. Acad. Sci. *86*, 643–651 (1959 a)

Prockop, D.J., Shore, P.A., Brodie, B.B.: An anticonvulsant effect of monoamine oxidase inhibitors. Experientia *15*, 145–147 (1959 b)

Rudzik, A.D., Johnson, G.A.: Effect of amphetamine and amphetamine analogs on convulsive thresholds. In: Amphetamines and related compounds. Costa, E., Garattini, S. (eds.), pp. 715–728. New York: Raven Press 1970

Rudzik, A.D., Mennear, J.H.: The mechanism of action of anticonvulsants. I. Diphenylhydantoin. Life Sci. *4*, 2373–2382 (1965)

Sacra, P., McColl, J.D.: Effects of ataractics on some convulsant and depressant agents in mice. Arch. Int. Pharmacodyn. Ther. *117*, 1–8 (1958)

Sanders, H.D.: A comparison of the convulsant activity of procaine and pentylenetetrazol. Arch. Int. Pharmacodyn. Ther. *170*, 165–177 (1967)

Sayers, A.C.: Prediction of possible convulsive activity in man. Pharmacol. Ther. *5*, 563–570 (1979)

Schallek, W., Kuehn, A., Seppelin, D.K.: Central depressant effects of methylprylon. J. Pharmacol. Exp. Ther. *118*, 139–147 (1956)

Schallek, W., Zabransky, F., Kuehn, A.: Effects of benzodiazepines on central nervous system of the cat. Arch. Int. Pharmacodyn. Ther. *149*, 467–483 (1964)

Schenker, E., Herbst, H.: Phenothiazine und Azaphenothiazine als Heilmittel. Fortschritte der Arzneimittelforschung. Jucker, E. (ed.), Vol. 5, pp. 268–627. Basel, Stuttgart: Birkhäuser 1963

Schlesinger, K., Boggan, W.O., Freedman, D.X.: Genetics of audiogenic seizures: II. Effects of pharmacological manipulation of brain serotonin, norepinephrine, and gamma-aminobutyric acid. Life Sci. *7*, 437–447 (1968)

Schlesinger, K., Boggan, W.O., Freedman, D.X.: Genetics of audiogenic seizures: III. Time response relationship between drug administration and seizure susceptibility. Life Sci. *9*, 721–729 (1970)

Slater, E., Beard, A.W.: The schizophrenia-like psychoses of epilepsy i. psychiatric aspects. Br. J. Psychiatry *109*, 95–150 (1963)

Stull, R.E., Jobe, P.C., Geiger, P.F., Ferguson, G.G.: Effects of dopamine receptor stimulation and blockade on Ro 4-1284-induced enhancement of electroshock seizures. J. Pharm. Pharmacol. *25*, 842–844 (1973)

Suarez, M., Teijeira, J., Dominguez, J., Sierra, G.: Estudio experimental sobre clorpromazina y convulsiones. Rev. Esp. Pediatr. *13*, 165–170 (1957)

Swinyard, E.A., Wolf, H.H., Fink, G.B., Goodman, L.S.: Some neuropharmacological properties of thioridazine hydrochloride (Mellaril). J. Pharmacol. Exp. Ther. *126*, 312–317 (1959)

Takagi, H., Yamamoto, S., Takaori, S., Ogiu, K.: The effect of LSD and reserpine on the central nervous system of the cat. The antagonism between LSD and chlorpromazine or reserpine. Jpn. J. Pharmacol. *7*, 119–134 (1958)

Tedeschi, D.H., Benigni, J.P., Elder, C.J., Yaeger, J.C., Flanigan, J.V.: Effects of various phenothiazines on minimal electroshock seizure threshold and spontaneous motor activity of mice. J. Pharmacol. Exp. Ther. *123*, 35–38 (1958)

Tedeschi, D.H., Tedeschi, R.E., Cook, L., Mattis, P.A., Fellows, E.J.: The neuropharmacology of trifluoperazine: A potent psychotherapeutic agent. Arch. Int. Pharmacodyn. Ther. *122*, 129 (1959)

Teschendorf, H.J., Worstmann, W., Kretzschmar, R.: Interactions of anticonvulsants in experimental seizures. Naunyn Schmiedebergs Arch. Pharmacol. *302*, R56 (1978)

Teschendorf, H.J., Safer, A., Worstmann, W., Kretzschmar, R.: Untersuchungen zur Wirkung von Antikonvulsiva-Neuroleptika-Kombinationen auf experimentelle Krämpfe. Arzneim. Forsch. (in preparation) (1980)

Tripod, J., Bein, H.J., Meier, R.: Characterization of central effects of serpasil (reserpine, a new alkaloid of Rauwolfia serpentina B.) and of their antagonistic reactions. Arch. Int. Pharmacodyn. Ther. *96*, 406–425 (1954)

Wardell, J.R., Jr., Staples, R.G., III: Animal studies comparing the neuropharmacological profile of a trifluoperazine HCl-Amobarbital combination with that of the individual components. Arch. Int. Pharmacodyn. Ther. *179*, 106–120 (1969)

Weiss, L.R., Nelson, J.W., Tye, A.: The facilitative action of reserpine on metrazol convulsions when modified by iproniazid. J. Am. Pharmacol. Assoc. *49*, 514–517 (1960)

Wenger, G.R., Stitzel, R.E., Craig, C.R.: The role of biogenic amines in the reserpine-induced alteration of minimal electroshock seizure thresholds in the mouse. Neuropharmacology *12*, 693–703 (1973)

Worms, P, Lloyd, K.G.: Differential blockade of bicuculline convulsions by neuroleptics. Eur. J. Pharmacol. *51*, 85–88 (1978)

Yamamoto, I., Otori, K., Inoki, R.: Pharmacological studies on antagonists against nicotine-induced convulsions and death. Jpn. J. Pharmacol. *16*, 402–415 (1966)

Yamamoto, I., Inoki, R., Iwatsubo, K.: Antagoniststic effects of phenothiazine derivatives on nicotine-induced death in mice. Jpn. J. Pharmacol. *17*, 133–134 (1967)

Author Index

Page numbers *in italics* refer to bibliography

Subject Index

Handbook of Experimental Pharmacology

Continuation of "Handbuch der experimentellen Pharmakologie"

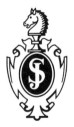

Springer-Verlag
Berlin
Heidelberg
New York

Handbook of Experimental Pharmacology

Continuation of "Handbuch der experimentellen Pharmakologie"

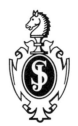

Springer-Verlag
Berlin
Heidelberg
New York

PAGES DEMAGED
232, 233, 271, 333, 335, 583, 587